Contents

UNIT 1
Introduction to Nursing 1

CHAPTER 1   The Vista of Nursing 3
CHAPTER 2   Health Care Delivery and Economics 15
CHAPTER 3   Nursing Ethics and Law 29
CHAPTER 4   The Nursing Process and Decision Making 47
CHAPTER 5   Documentation 79

UNIT 2
Communicating and Understanding 113

CHAPTER 6   Communication and Relationships 115
CHAPTER 7   Promoting Health and Wellness 133
CHAPTER 8   Ethnic, Cultural, and Spiritual Aspects of Care 147
CHAPTER 9   Growth and Development Throughout the Life Span 167
CHAPTER 10   Loss, Grief, and Dying 187
CHAPTER 11   Complementary and Alternative Medicine 209
CHAPTER 12   Patient Teaching 221

UNIT 3
Nursing Basics 231

CHAPTER 13   Safety 233
CHAPTER 14   Medical Asepsis and Infection Control 255
CHAPTER 15   Personal Care 279
CHAPTER 16   Moving and Positioning Patients 311
CHAPTER 17   Vital Signs 343
CHAPTER 18   Applying Heat and Cold 377
CHAPTER 19   Pain Management, Rest, and Restorative Sleep 391
CHAPTER 20   Admission, Transfer, and Discharge 407
CHAPTER 21   Physical Assessment 421
CHAPTER 22   Surgical Asepsis 455

UNIT 4
Clinical Skills and Care 473

CHAPTER 23   Nutrition 475
CHAPTER 24   Nutritional Care and Support 497
CHAPTER 25   Diagnostic Tests 539
CHAPTER 26   Wound Care 557
CHAPTER 27   Musculoskeletal Care 591
CHAPTER 28   Respiratory Care 611
CHAPTER 29   Fluids, Electrolytes, and Acid-Base Balance 645
CHAPTER 30   Bowel Elimination and Care 675
CHAPTER 31   Urinary Elimination and Care 709
CHAPTER 32   Care of Elderly Patients 745
CHAPTER 33   Care of the Surgical Patient 769
CHAPTER 34   Phlebotomy and Blood Specimens 805

UNIT 5
Medication Administration 825

CHAPTER 35   Researching and Preparing Medications 827
CHAPTER 36   Administering Oral, Topical, and Mucosal Medications 851
CHAPTER 37   Administering Intradermal, Subcutaneous, and Intramuscular Injections 879
CHAPTER 38   Peripheral Intravenous Therapy 913
APPENDIX A: Answers to Review Questions 967
APPENDIX B: Photo and Illustration Credits 981

Fundamentals of Nursing Care
Concepts, Connections & Skills

**Marti A. Burton,
RN, BS**
Curriculum Developer
Instructor, Link to Nursing Program
Canadian Valley Technology Center
Yukon, Oklahoma

**Linda J. May Ludwig,
RN, BS, MEd**
Nursing Instructor
Canadian Valley Technology Center
El Reno, Oklahoma

F.A. Davis Company • Philadelphia

Make The

FUNDAMENTALS OF
NURSING
CARE
Concepts, Connections & Skills

Clinical Connection

Your Assignment: You have been assigned to care for a patient in the hospital with multiple health problems. He is a 68-year-old male with congestive heart failure, diabetes, and emphysema. He has had two significant heart attacks (myocardial infarctions) in the past 6 years. You are also assigned to write your first student plan of care concerning this patient. You are supposed to arrive for your first day of clinical with a list of probable and a possible nursing diagnoses, appropriate nursing interventions for each, and a patient goal for each.

Your Actions: You have no idea where to even start finding this information. In addition to that, you do not see how you even see how any instructor can expect you to f... nursing diagnoses before you even see the patient... you are being asked to work o... evening prior to your clinical e... don't know what you are supp...

Clinical Connections
guide you through the chapter and identify the information you'll need to consider and the actions you'll need to take when caring for a patient.

Knowledge Connection

What is the difference between the role of the RN and the role of the LPN/LVN in the nursing process? What does ADPIE stand for?

Real-World Connection

Critical Thinking in Patient Care

An elderly woman who was visiting the area was admitted to the hospital with shortness of breath. Eventually she required mechanical ventilation because she could not breathe well on her own. A tracheostomy was performed to prevent problems of a long-term ventilator run. After time and treatment, she was being weaned from the ventilator. The weaning process was rocky, however, because she kept having severe respiratory distress and having to go back onto the ventilator. Some of the nurses thought she was just anxious, but others felt there was something more going on.

This went on for over a week. She would be weaned off the ventilator and be doing fine. Then, in a few hours, she would go into respiratory distress and have to go back on the ventilator. Some of the staff thought she was just dependent on the ventilator and would never be able to breathe on her own. Yet, she did breathe on her own and would do well for hours, then suddenly relapse.

A nurse and a respiratory therapist decided to think critically about this case. They shared the observation that within...

Knowledge Connections
are brief questions to jog your memory and improve retention.

People and Places Connection

Communicating Across Developmental Stages

Language is part of a person's psychosocial and intellectual development, which occurs in varying stages over a lifetime. Knowledge of a patient's stage of development allows the nurse to tailor communication appropriately. Nurses care for patients in many stages of development from childhood to elderly patients, as well as mentally challenged patients, and you cannot take a cookie-cutter approach to communication. Adapt your communication strategies to coincide with the patient's stage of development. As a nurse, you will need to be aware of developmental stages and work within them to establish effective, patient-centered communication, including patient teaching.

People and Places Connection
are tips to help you care for patients of all ages in all settings, and include concepts and skills for home care and long-term care.

Real-World Connections
feature stories that illustrate positive and negative experiences in clinical situations.

Connections!

Supervision/Delegation Connection
provide specific examples of appropriate delegation, as well as examples of critical tasks that should not be delegated.

Laboratory and Diagnostic Connection
How Laboratory and Diagnostic Results Affect Patient Care
Sometimes nurses think that analyzing laboratory and diagnostic test results is strictly in the realm of the physician. Although the physician and other health care providers will review the results of laboratory and diagnostic tests, it is important for nurses to examine them as well. As you learn more about abnormal results of such tests, you will understand how they affect the patient's nursing care. For example, if you have a patient whose white blood cell count is very low, you know he or she is at high risk for developing an infection, as white blood cells are responsible for fighting invading pathogens. That information is important when you think about how to care for your patient and how to protect him or her from potential infections.

Supervision/Delegation Connection
There Are Times When You Should Not Delegate Vital Signs
Vital sign assessment is commonly delegated, but because the skill of measuring vital signs is simple to perform and is performed many times a day, day after day, it is possible to take the process and the delegation of vital sign assessment for granted and to become totally dependent upon unlicensed personnel for their measurement. Though it is appropriate in most cases to delegate this task to CNAs or UAPs, keep in mind that vital sign assessment is ultimately your responsibility. You are responsible for analyzing the vital sign findings and for determining when further action is necessary, whether you take the vital signs yourself or not.

Laboratory and Diagnostic Connection
explain laboratory results and how specific tests are used to help determine diagnoses.

Anatomy and Physiology Connection
The Nervous System's Role in Communication
The brain and nervous system directly affect our ability to communicate. Activities that precede, initiate, or support communication are controlled by the brain and nervous system. A variety of communication problems occur when there is a brain or nervous system malfunction. P... disease, CVA (also known as "brain attack" or stroke) trauma cause damage to the brain and nervous ... often affect a person's ability to engage in the c... process.
    The cerebral cortex of the brain has several ... control voluntary muscle movement, sensory ... and sensory interpretation—all of which are ne... communication process. The left frontal lobe ... motor speech area, which co...

Patient Teaching Connection
Teaching About Child Safety
Young adults starting families may need instruction on child safety. Teach parents of toddlers the importance of safety to prevent accidental deaths. You can do this in two ways: teach parents about the developmental stage of the toddler and about the causes of accidents so they can work to maintain their child's safety.
    Motor vehicle accidents are one cause of injury and death among toddlers. Encourage parents to use car seats correctly. Teach them about the importance of vigilance when driving in areas where toddlers may be playing. It is very difficult to see a small child when you are backing out or pulling into a driveway. In addition, a child this age may ... front of a car without realizing it is dangerous...

Patient Teaching Connection
demonstrate how to communicate effectively with patients and families, and improve and support patient wellness.

Post Conference
You provided care for your patient who, according to the automatic vital sign machine, had abnormal vital signs. In evaluation of your nursing care, you review the actions you took:
• You further assessed the patient and found him to be awake, alert, oriented, and smiling; skin pink, warm, and dry; oral mucosa and nailbeds pink; respirations normal depth, regular, and effortless at 19 breaths per minute; and radial pulse regular at strong at 69 bpm.
• You reviewed the 8 a.m. vital signs: BP – 126/74, T – 98°F, P – 64, SpO₂ – 98% on room air.
• You compared the 8 a.m. vital signs to those obtained at noon, which were BP – 94/46, T – 96.6°F, P – 51, and SpO₂ – 70% on room air, indicated dramatic differences from those obtained at 8 a.m.
• You performed manual reassessment of vital signs with an aneroid blood pressure cuff and portable pulse oximeter, with the following results: BP – 122/78, AP – 69, R – 10, SpO₂ – 96%.
• You determined that the automatic vital sign machine was inaccurate and removed it from use until repairs and calibration could be completed. This event reinforced in your mind the importance of looking at all of the

Anatomy and Physiology Connection
provide more in-depth content on A & P and the effects of disease on the body.

Post Conference Boxes
review the concepts and skills you've learned in each chapter so you can evaluate your performance and identify areas for additional study.

Clear, step-by-step presentation makes every skill and concept easy to grasp.

Over **120 Skills** with appropriate rationales reflect real world nursing procedures.

Skills Safety Guidelines outline the important information you need to know to ensure patient safety and avoid harmful situations.

Nursing Care Plans are a clear, comprehensive presentation of interventions and evaluations that are easy to understand.

shoulders to his or her knees. *This keeps the patient centered on the draw sheet for turning and moving.*

8. Fanfold the fitted sheet and draw sheet toward the patient. Tuck them beneath the tightly folded soiled linens. *Safety: If there is a danger that the soiled linens are wet or could contaminate the clean ones, place a towel or waterproof pad between the clean and dirty linens.*

12. Assist the patient to turn onto his or her back in the center of the bed.
13. Unfold the clean top sheet so it is centered on the bed. Be sure the seams are away from the patient.
14. Remove the bath blanket by pulling it from beneath the clean top sheet. Put it in the laundry bag or hamper and avoid touching it to your scrubs.
15. Replace the blanket or spread so it is centered on the bed and the top edge is approximately 4 inches lower than the top edge of the sheet.
16. Tuck the sheet and blanket together at the foot of the bed. Make a mitered corner (see Skill 15-10).

other side of the bed and tuck the sheet
et together at the foot of the bed. Make a
orner.

10. Go to the other side of the bed and lower the side rail. Pull the soiled linen off of the bed and put it in the laundry bag or hamper. *Safety: Do not allow the soiled linens to touch your scrubs to prevent contamination.* NEVER put soiled linen on the floor *because this spreads microorganisms.*

Table 4-1   Nursing Care Plan Interventions and Evaluation

Nursing Diagnosis: Acute pain r/t decreased oxygenation of the myocardium
Outcome: Patient will rate chest pain 0–1 by discharge.

Interventions	Evaluation
Monitor for chest pain episodes. If chest pain occurs, report to nurse immediately and take vital signs. Evaluate effectiveness of nitroglycerin spray in relieving chest pain. Monitor vital signs after use of nitro spray.	Pt had no chest pain during morning prior to arteriography. BP stable at 146/80, P – 92 and irreg, R – 20, T – 98.
Maintain telemetry monitoring by ensuring that electrodes and wires are in place.	Telemetry maintained until pt left floor for cath lab.
Assist pt to dangle first and evaluate response before getting up to BR. If pt c/o chest pain, return to bed.	Pt dangles and tol without c/o chest pain.
Ambulate pt to BR slowly, stay close and be prepared to lower to floor if pt becomes weak or loses consciousness.	VS remained stable when dangling at 140/82, P – 94, R – 24. Assisted to BR ×2 without problem. Stopped to rest ×1 when returning to bed. No loss of consciousness.
Consider asking for order for BSC if pt unable to make to the bathroom.	Unneccesary—able to amb to BR.

contamination. NEVER put soiled linen on the floor *because this spreads microorganisms.*

11. Spread the fitted sheet and draw sheet across the bed. Slip the corners over the mattress corners. Smooth the draw sheet by grasping the middle and pulling tightly across and down. Tuck it between the mattress and springs. Repeat with the top and bottom edges of the draw sheet. *This helps make a tight bed with fewer wrinkles, which is more comfortable for the patient.*

12. Assist the patient to turn onto his or her back in the center of the bed.
Unfold the clean   rit is   d on the

Full Color Photographs and Illustrations showcase important concepts and skills.

Midsternal line — Midclavicular line

Anterior axillary line

Apical pulse before age 4

Apical pulse in adult

Body of sternum

his toddler is mastering sphincter control
become toilet trained.

Figure 17-7   Location of apical pulse for adults and
children.

A complete multi-media learning experience!

Study Guide*

- **Exercises** and **activities** develop your critical-thinking and problem-solving skills.
- **Each chapter** emphasizes **real-world nursing connections.**
- **Perforated pages** make it easy for you to submit your assignments for evaluation.

Learning Connection CD-ROM
(Mac and PC compatible.)

- **IQ Question Bank** features over 300 NCLEX-style questions that cover the topics found in the book and on the NCLEX-PN® exam.
- **Auscultation Sounds** offer examples of the heart, lung, and bowel, followed by quizzes for review.
- **Over 1,000 Audio Pronunciations** from **Taber's Cyclopedic Medical Dictionary, 21st Edition** teach the language of nursing.
- **Dosage Calculator** lets you find answers to the most common dosage problems.
- **Abbreviation tables** and **documentation forms** prepare you for administrative tasks.

LPN Skills Videos*
(On two DVDs.)

- **70 real skills performed by real nurses** prepare you for class and clinical and help you evaluate your progress.
- **Visual and Auditory versions** let you choose the approach that works best for your learning style.

Online at Davis*Plus*

(No fee. No password. No registration.)

http://davisplus.fadavis.com. Keyword: Durton.

- **Animations** and **videos** offer a visual learning experience.
- **Flash cards, care-planning templates,** and a **wound care tutorial** make handy learning and reference tools.

*Sold separately or as part of a package.

Instructor's Resources available upon adoption on Davis*Plus* and on CD-ROM

- **Instructor's Guide**—Helpful teaching tips and classroom activities.
- **ExamView Pro Testbank**—Almost 1,000 NCLEX-style questions with rationales.
- **PowerPoint Presentation**—Slides for each chapter compatible with iClicker technology.
- **Image Bank**—Over 500 photographs and illustrations from the text.
- **Web Resource Kits**—For web classes and activities, available online only at Davis*Plus*.

F. A. Davis Company
1915 Arch Street
Philadelphia, PA 19103
www.fadavis.com

Printed in the United States of America

Last digit indicates print number: 10 9 8 7 6 5 4 3 2 1

Acquisitions Editor: Jonathan D. Joyce
Senior Developmental Editor: William F. Welsh
Director of Content Development: Darlene D. Pedersen
Senior Project Editor: Christina C. Burns
Illustration & Design Manager: Carolyn O'Brien

Interior design art and cover art (c) 2009 Jose Ortega c/o the ipsot.com.
Additional cover images courtesy istock.com.

As new scientific information becomes available through basic and clinical research, recommended treatments and drug therapies undergo changes. The author(s) and publisher have done everything possible to make this book accurate, up to date, and in accord with accepted standards at the time of publication. The author(s), editors, and publisher are not responsible for errors or omissions or for consequences from application of the book, and make no warranty, expressed or implied, in regard to the contents of the book. Any practice described in this book should be applied by the reader in accordance with professional standards of care used in regard to the unique circumstances that may apply in each situation. The reader is advised always to check product information (package inserts) for changes and new information regarding dose and contraindications before administering any drug. Caution is especially urged when using new or infrequently ordered drugs.

Library of Congress Cataloging-in-Publication Data

Burton, Marti.
  Fundamentals of nursing care : concepts, connections & skills / Marti A. Burton, Linda J. May Ludwig.
    p. ; cm.
  Includes bibliographical references and index.
  ISBN-13: 978-0-8036-1970-8 (alk. paper)
  ISBN-10: 0-8036-1970-7 (alk. paper)
  1. Nursing—Textbooks. I. Ludwig, Linda J. May. II. Title.
  [DNLM: 1. Nursing Care. 2. Ethics, Nursing. 3. Nurse's Role. 4. Nurse-Patient Relations.
5. Nursing Process. WY 100.1]
  RT41.B92 2011
  610.73—dc22   2010027925

Special Features

Skills

10-1	Postmortem Care	205
13-1	Using a Bed/Chair or Leg Monitor	247
13-2	Applying Restraints	248
13-3	Using Body Mechanics	250
14-1	Performing Hand Hygiene	271
14-2	Donning Personal Protective Equipment	272
14-3	Removing Personal Protective Equipment	274
15-1	Administering a Complete Bed Bath	294
15-2	Administering Perineal Care	296
15-3	Administering a Back Massage	298
15-4	Administering Oral Care for an Unconscious Patient	298
15-5	Administering Oral Care for a Conscious Patient	299
15-6	Providing Denture Care	300
15-7	Shaving a Male Patient	301
15-8	Providing Nail Care	302
15-9	Shampooing Hair With the Patient in Bed	303
15-10	Making an Unoccupied Bed	304
15-11	Making an Occupied Bed	306
16-1	Performing Passive Range-of-Motion Exercises	327
16-2	Positioning Patients	331
16-3	Moving a Patient Up in Bed	332
16-4	Turning a Patient in Bed	333
16-5	Transferring a Patient from Bed to a Stretcher, Chair, or Wheelchair	335
16-6	Transferring a Patient With a Mechanical Lift	336
16-7	Assisting a Patient to Dangle	337
16-8	Assisting With Ambulation	338
17-1	Assessment of Blood Pressure	364
17-2	Assessment for Orthostatic Hypotension	366
17-3	Assessing Body Temperature by Various Routes	367
17-4	Assessing the Radial and Apical Pulses	369
17-5	Assessing Peripheral Pulses	370
17-6	Using Doppler Ultrasound to Assess Nonpalpable Pulses	372
17-7	Assessing Respirations	372
17-8	Assessing Oxygen Saturation	373
18-1	Application of Dry or Moist Heat	385
18-2	Application of Aquathermia Pad (K-pad)	386
18-3	Administering a Sitz Bath	386
18-4	Application of Cold Packs	387
19-1	Application of TENS Unit	403
21-1	Measuring a Patient's Height	447
21-2	Measuring a Patient's Weight	448
21-3	Measuring an Infant's Weight and Length	448
21-4	Performing an Initial Head-to-Toe Shift Assessment	449
21-5	Performing a Basic Neurological Examination	450
21-6	Auscultating Breath Sounds	451
21-7	Auscultating Heart Sounds	452
22-1	Setting up a Sterile Field, Opening Sterile Packs, and Pouring Sterile Liquids	461
22-2	Donning Sterile Gloves—Open Method	463
22-3	Performing a Surgical Hand Scrub	466
22-4	Donning a Sterile Gown and Sterile Gloves—Closed Method	467
24-1	Assisting a Patient with Feeding	527
24-2	Recording Intake and Output	528
24-3	Inserting a Nasogastric Tube	530
24-4	Irrigating a Nasogastric Tube	532
24-5	Removing a Nasogastric Tube	532
24-6	Administering Intermittent Bolus Enteral Feedings	533
24-7	Using a Feeding Pump	534
25-1	Assisting with Aspiration Procedures: Bone Marrow, Lumbar Puncture, and Paracentesis	551
25-2	Performing a 12-Lead Electrocardiogram (EKG)	552
26-1	Removing Sutures and Staples	578
26-2	Caring for Drainage Devices	579
26-3	Irrigating a Wound	580
26-4	Obtaining a Wound Culture	582
26-5	Changing Sterile Dressings and Wet-to-Damp Dressings	582
26-6	Applying Transparent and Hydrocolloid Dressings	585
27-1	Performing Neurovascular Checks	605
27-2	Setting Up a Continuous Passive Motion Machine	605
27-3	Applying Elastic Bandages	606
28-1	Obtaining a Sputum Specimen	631
28-2	Obtaining a Throat Culture Specimen	632
28-3	Assisting With Incentive Spirometry	632
28-4	Administering a Nebulizer Treatment	633
28-5	Administering Supplemental Oxygen	634
28-6	Performing Nasopharyngeal and Oropharyngeal Suctioning	635
28-7	Performing Endotracheal and Tracheostomy Suctioning	637
28-8	Performing Tracheostomy Care	639
28-9	Maintaining Chest Tubes	640
30-1	Administering an Enema	698
30-2	Obtaining a Stool Specimen for Culture, and Ova and Parasites	700
30-3	Performing Guaiac Testing: Testing Stool Specimen for Occult Blood	701
30-4	Removing a Fecal Impaction	702
30-5	Applying/Changing an Ostomy Appliance	703
30-6	Irrigating a Colostomy	705
31-1	Assisting the Male Patient With a Urinal	731
31-2	Assisting With a Bedpan	731
31-3	Obtaining a Clean-catch Midstream Urine Specimen	732

31-4   Inserting an Indwelling Urinary Catheter   733
31-5   Obtaining a Urine Specimen From an   736
        Indwelling Catheter
31-6   Inserting a Straight Catheter   737
31-7   Performing Continuous Bladder Irrigation   739
31-8   Applying a Condom Catheter   740
31-9   Irrigating a Closed Urinary Drainage System   741
31-10   Discontinuing an Indwelling Urinary Catheter   742
33-1   Applying Antiembolism Hose   799
33-2   Applying Sequential Compression Devices   801
34-1   Applying a Tourniquet   818
34-2   Performing Venipuncture   819
34-3   Collecting a Blood Culture Specimen   821
34-4   Performing Skin Puncture for a Finger Stick   822
        Blood Sugar
36-1   Administering Oral Medications   865
36-2   Administering Medications Through an   866
        Enteral Tube
36-3   Administering Topical and Transdermal   868
        Medications
36-4   Administering Eye and Ear Medications   869
36-5   Irrigating the Eye and Ear   870
36-6   Administering Vaginal Medications   871
36-7   Administering Rectal Suppositories   872
36-8   Administering Inhaled Medications   873
37-1   Reconstituting and Withdrawing Medication   902
        From a Vial
37-2   Withdrawing Medication From an Ampule   903
37-3   Administering an Intradermal Injection   903
37-4   Combining and Administering Insulin   904
        Subcutaneously
37-5   Administering an Intramuscular Injection   906
37-6   Administering a Z-track Injection   907
38-1   Administering IV Push Medication   946
        via PRN Lock or IV Line
38-2   Administering IV Piggyback Medication   948
38-3   Converting an IV Infusion to a PRN Lock   951
38-4   Calculating IV Infusion Rate   953
38-5   Adding Medications to Primary IV   953
        Solution
38-6   Initiating Peripheral Venipuncture   955
38-7   Adding a New Bag of IV Solution to   959
        Existing IV Line
38-8   Discontinuing an IV Infusion or PRN Lock   960
38-9   Preparing, Initiating, and Monitoring   961
        Infusion of Blood and Blood Products

Nursing Care Plans

Nursing Care Plan for Patients at Risk for Falls   245
Nursing Care Plan for a Patient with a MRSA   267
Infection
Nursing Care Plan for a Patient Post-CVA With   520
a PEG Tube
Nursing Care Plan for a Patient With an Infected   575
Stage II Pressure Ulcer
Nursing Care Plan for a Patient With Total   600
Left Knee Replacement
Nursing Care Plan for a Patient With COPD and   627
Pneumonia
Nursing Care Plan for a Patient With a Fluid   669
Imbalance
Nursing Care Plan for a Patient With a   692
New Colostomy of the Descending Colon
Nursing Care Plan for a Patient With a Urinary   727
Tract Infection
Nursing Care Plan for an Elderly Patient   763
Nursing Care Plan for a Patient Who Is   795
Postoperative Following Colectomy

Concept Maps

Sample of a Concept Map Care Plan   76
Concept Map Care Plan for a Patient with Total   602
Left Knee Replacement
Concept Map Care Plan for a Patient with COPD   629
and Pneumonia
Concept Map Care Plan for a Patient with a UTI   728
Concept Map Care Plan for a 78-year-old Female   764
Patient with Bradycardia, Nausea, Congestive Heart
Failure, and Hypokalemia
Concept Map Care Plan for a Patient having   795
Abdominal Surgery

Anatomy and Physiology Connection

Differentiating Abnormal From Normal Anatomy and   38
Physiology
The Nervous System's Role in Communication   129
The Fight-or-Flight Response   140
The Spine, the Nerves, and Correcting Interference   212
Hair, Nails, and Glands   282
What Makes the Heart Beat?   357
The Lungs   435
Digestion   478
Gastrointestinal Tract   508
Blood   541
The Inflammatory Process   564
The Hip Joint   596
The Pleura   613
The Brain and Acid-Base Balance   667
Gastrointestinal Tract   676
Urinary System   711
Metabolization and Elimination of Medications   754
Veins and Arteries   807
Anatomy of the Tissues You Inject   890
Maintaining Compartmental Fluid Balance   918

Laboratory and Diagnostic Connection

Feature Overview   9
Confidentiality of HIV and AIDS Test Results   35
How Laboratory and Diagnostic Results Affect   55
Patient Care
Your Laboratory and Diagnostic Documentation   100
Responsibilities

Approaches to Procedures for Different Developmental Stages — 177
Hypercalcemia — 203
Identifying Bacteria in the Laboratory — 256
Hematocrit Impacts Blood Pressure — 346
Diabetes — 504
Testing to Determine if a Wound Is Infected — 567
Testing for Musculoskeletal Conditions — 593
Arterial Blood Gases — 616
Diarrhea — 681
Assessing Kidney Function and Failure — 719
Standard Preoperative Laboratory Tests — 774
Drawing Blood Culture Specimens — 815
Determining Digoxin Toxicity — 831
Coordinating Medication Administration With Blood Specimens — 862
Prothrombin Time and Activated Partial Thromboplastin Time — 896

Patient Teaching Connection

Teaching About HMO Regulations — 25
Meeting Patient Needs First — 56
Documenting Patient Teaching — 102
Patient Teaching to Decrease Stress — 144
Teaching About Child Safety — 181
Teaching Family Members How to Comfort the Patient — 201
Teaching About CAM and Medical Conditions — 216
Teaching Safe Oxygen Use in the Home — 241
Incorporating Hand Hygiene in Patient Teaching — 263
Teaching About Antibacterial Soaps — 285
Explaining to Promote Cooperation — 320
Children With Viruses: No Aspirin! — 356
Heating Pad Use Carries Risk — 382
We Need to Educate Parents About Sleep — 401
Discharge Teaching — 415
Pregnancy: Weight Gain and Diet — 491
Diabetes — 505
Diagnostic Tests — 541
Wound Care — 568
Incentive Spirometry — 618
Furosemide — 655
Preventing Recurrent Constipation — 684
Teaching Patients About Medications for Multiple Conditions — 763
Preoperative Teaching for Outpatient Laparoscopic Cholecystectomy — 776
Using a Metered-Dose Inhaler — 861
Insulin Self-administration — 894

People and Places Connection

Feature Overview — 8
Communicating Across Developmental Stages — 130
Communicating With Older Adults — 130
Respect the Beliefs of Others — 159
Patient Populations in Home Health and Long-Term Care — 184

Patient Teaching for Different Age Groups in Different Locations — 226
Teaching Children — 226
Teaching Elderly Patients — 226
Home Health Care Considerations — 226
Personal Care Considerations for Children, for the Elderly, and in Special Settings — 283
Newborns Cannot Shiver — 350
The Skin of Seniors and Children Is Fragile — 382
Separation Anxiety Is Real — 410
Cultural Beliefs in Assessment — 425
Sterile Technique and Different Practice Settings — 461
Home Health and Nutritional Support — 520
Wound Care of Elderly Patients — 574
Wound Care in Home Health Care — 574
Promoting Mobility in Home Health Care and Long-Term Care — 600
Promoting Mobility in Long-Term Care — 600
Fluid Intake in Elders — 652
Bowel Elimination and Aging — 680
Home Health Care and Catheterizations — 726
Long-term Care and Catheterizations — 726
Pediatric Considerations for Urinary Care — 726
Working in Home Health Care and Long-term Care — 758
Skin Puncture Sites — 817
Age-Related Concerns of Medication Administration — 847
Medication Organizers — 857
Punch Card Systems — 857
Injection Variations for Infants, Toddlers, Children, and the Older Adult — 901
Performing Venipuncture in Elders — 937

Real-World Connection

Becoming a "Good Nurse" — 12
How Easy Is It to Accidently Breach HIPAA Laws? — 35
Critical Thinking in Patient Care — 49
How Many Can There Be? — 108
Communicating With a Smile — 117
Meeting Rachael's Spiritual Needs — 150
A School Nurse Supervisor's Experience — 184
To Give the Medication or Not? — 189
Being a Medical and CAM Practitioner — 213
The Focus of Patient Teaching — 224
Participating in a Disaster During Clinical Experience — 242
Who Is Responsible for Maintaining a Clean Patient Environment? — 262
Safety Tips for Stretchers — 326
How Much Good Can Application of Heat Really Accomplish? — 381
Over-the-Counter Pain Relief Carries Risks — 398
The Importance of Sterile Supplies — 460
If a Little Is Good, Is More Better? — 490
Inserting an NG Tube — 512
EKG Imperfection — 549
How Deep Can a Pressure Ulcer Be? — 561
Researching the Right Condition — 596
Effects of Hypoxia on Thinking — 614
The Dangers of Potassium Chloride — 661
Monitoring Urinary Output — 716

Alzheimer's Disease	752
Postoperative Complications	789
Drug Abuse in Nursing	829
Consequences of Medications Not Administered	864
Ventrogluteal Injection Site	899
Reduced-strength Heparin Versus Regular-strength Heparin	925

Supervision/Delegation Connection

Feature Overview	11
The Secret to Good Supervision	23
Responsibility of Patient Advocacy	39
Collaboration, Not Delegation in Care Planning	51
Must "You" Document Everything?	108
Delegating the Care of Infants and Children	180
Patient Teaching and Delegation	227
Delegation of Restraint Checks and Releases	238
Supervising the Use of Medical Asepsis, Standard Precautions, and Transmission-based Precautions	266

Determining Delegation of a Bed Bath	283
Safety in Numbers	326
There Are Times When You Should Not Delegate Vital Signs	344
Delegation of Tasks Does Not Relieve You of Your Responsibilities	402
Admission Assessments	414
Sterile Technique and Assistive Personnel	458
Tube Feedings	518
Wound Care and Unlicensed Assistive Personnel	574
Delegating Administration of an Enema	688
Monitoring Intake and Output	716
Caring for Confused Elderly Patients	748
Postoperative Assessment	792
Phlebotomy	817
Medication Administration	845
Unlicensed Personnel and Medication Administration	856
You Must Administer Injections Yourself	881
IV Push and IVPB Medications	938

Dedications

To our past, present, and future nursing students: You are the inspiration for this book. May you each be not just a nurse, but a *good* nurse with passion.... passion to always strive to reach your individual potential, never settling for just being an average nurse. May you each be a patient advocate in every sense of the word.

To our fellow nursing instructors: You, too, inspired us to write this book. We wanted this book to explain concepts the way you explain them to your students, to provide you with *real world connections* to illustrate what can and does happen and to emphasize what is truly important in nursing.

To my wonderful husband, Barry: You went above and beyond anything I could have asked of as you supported my efforts to write this book. I cannot thank you enough for all you have done. Without you and your loving encouragement, I would have given up long ago. You are my rock, and I love you.

To my precious daughter, Kelsea: You have done without so many things while I wrote this book. Thank you for understanding when there was no time for me to bake cookies or prepare special dinners to celebrate your achievements. I love you so much, and I am so proud of you.

To my "Chattanooga Sisters," whose caring, prayers, and friendship have been a great source of strength to me. You have been with me through this entire journey and I don't think I could have done it without you. I love you guys.

And, to all my friends and family who understood when I responded to every invitation with the words, "I can't. I have to write."

Marti A. Burton

To my husband, Allen, whose ability to problem-solve and always create *something that works better* has, for 37 years, amazed, excited, and challenged me to push myself to become a better person. You allow and encourage me to do whatever I want and become whomever I need to become in order to accomplish my goals. You knew when to encourage me and when to simply listen. I love you. You are my hero. Thank you for being my support.

To my doting parents, Winona and Bill, who always had unwavering faith in me and taught me that I could do anything I chose to do.

To my three younger sisters, Sheryl, Marla, and Kelly, of whom the four of us are simply referred to as "The Girls," and to my younger brother, Brent, the talented musician: The four of you have always supported me and respectfully valued my nursing opinions as if I knew everything there was to know about nursing. You gave me heart, strength, and bond.

To my best friend, almost a sister, Rhonda, who always supported me and tried to understand when I said, "I am sorry. I can't go. I have to write." You validate me.

To Sister Sandy, who trusted my opinion and told everyone that I had literally "written the book on nursing."

To Sister Karen, with whom I shared the extraordinary and priceless experience of caring for Our Margaret. Even though you had not one iota, not one inkling of nursing ability, you still excelled at making each moment meaningful as you were totally competent at wearing the wedding dress, dancing on the bed, and retrieving messages on new phones. Thank you for helping me to "see the need" for writing this book.

Linda J. May Ludwig

Acknowledgments

We want to express our thanks to the following people, without whom this book would have never been completed:

To Jonathan Joyce, Acquisitions Editor, for your encouragement and helpfulness throughout this project. You always were able to look at our concerns and offer us sage advice. You have come through for us so many times, especially towards the end when deadlines were looming. Thank you for believing that two nursing instructors from Oklahoma had what it took to write this book.

To Patti Cleary, Editor in Chief of Nursing, who believed in our proposal from the beginning and provided rich approval for meeting the schedule for release to production.

To William Welsh, Senior Development Editor, for all of your expertise and guidance during the writing and revisions of every chapter. We appreciate your dedication and your insights, and all that you did to make this an excellent book. You always managed to make us feel like our book was *one of the best*, and as first-time authors, we frequently needed that lift. Thank you for being so supportive.

To Christina Burns, Senior Project Editor, for prioritizing our tasks and keeping us organized through the writing of the book and workbook. We appreciate all of your encouragement as well as your hard work getting the details in order, even when we could no longer remember which details were missing. We really appreciated your assistance with last-minute figure changes. You were a life-saver.

To Kris Piersall, our photographer, for your kindness and patience during our multiple-day photo shoot. We appreciated so much your willingness to re-shoot from different angles until the shot was perfect. We also thank your wife, Janis, for all of her help coordinating the photo shoot and providing refreshments for the models. It really helped to make it a smooth process.

To Berta Steiner, for all your patience with our edits and re-edits, as well as your hard work throughout the production of this book.

To Marilee LeBon, for your wonderful work on the Instructor's Guide and PowerPoint presentations, as well as your willingness to help us out of some tight spots.

To Rhonda Reherman, Marcella Williams, Tracey Hopkins, and Patricia Delmoe, for their dedicated work on the ancillary package.

To our Family, Friends, Students, and Peers, who served as models for text photographs, you were such good sports. Thank you for your contribution to our book.

To Canadian Valley Technology Center, Cowan Campus, for the use of their new nursing laboratory and equipment for our photo shoot. We also want to thank Sharon Mitchell and Rhonda Reherman, our supervisors, for their support and understanding during this project. Rhonda, thank you for allowing us to use your program's care plan, the caliber of which is rare.

To Kingfisher Regional Hospital, Kingfisher, Oklahoma, for the generous use of your facility chart forms. For Linda, who worked at the facility from ages 15 to 37, it was especially meaningful.

Marti Burton, RN, BS

Marti has been an RN for 33 years. She worked in the areas of medical intensive care and coronary care for several years, and worked as a pulmonary nurse specialist. She also has worked in home health, as a field nurse, supervisor, and quality assurance specialist. She has taught in entry level health care education to adults and high school students for 27 years. She has been an instructor in several Practical Nursing programs. She currently teaches in the Link to Nursing program and designs and develops curriculum for new health care education programs.

Linda J. May Ludwig, RN, BS, MEd

Linda entered nursing as a nursing assistant at age 15, and graduated from St. Anthony Hospital School of Nursing, OKC, Oklahoma and has been an RN for 36 years. She has worked for over 20 years in medical-surgical nursing, coronary care, labor and delivery, newborn nursery, and emergency nursing. She also worked as a legal nurse consultant and expert witness for seven of those years. She is currently a nursing educator at Canadian Valley Technology Center where she has worked for 16 years. She develops curriculum, teaches in the classroom, provides skills training in the lab, and serves as clinical instructor. Linda resides in Kingfisher, Oklahoma with her husband of 37 years, Allen.

When we decided to write a nursing textbook, we wanted it to be written to the entry-level student, not about the student. We designed it so that students could truly understand what they are reading, without the need for prior nursing experience or knowledge. To that end, we ensured that its readability level is comfortably accessible. We wrote it to guide the student in developing simple problem-solving skills, then progressing to critical thinking in real-world nursing. We teach students to understand and connect the what, why, and how of safe, effective care.

Themes

We believe it is important to help the student understand that, just because a book lists certain nursing diagnoses as *common* to a particular medical diagnosis, this does not mean that every patient with that medical diagnosis will have those *common* nursing diagnoses or need the same nursing interventions. We wrote this book to help students assess patients for their individual problems and formulate personalized care plans that will be specific to each individual patient. We take the students through the steps of the nursing process as it applies to each selected patient and situation. The book's organization and content enable students to make their own connections without requiring an instructor's lecture to do so. Our book incorporates these themes:

1. **Making the Connection:** In this text, we assist students to see that each feature connects to something the student can relate to or something important the student will need to take into consideration. Students often memorize information to only retain it in their short-term memory. The knowledge obtained with this lower level of learning is limited and difficult—sometimes impossible—to retrieve when needed. The more a student can relate information to previous learning, anatomy or physiology, certain patients, specific scenarios, clinical experiences, or "war stories" of actual nurses, the more "mind connections" are made. These associations will provide easier and improved recall. This book uses multiple areas of focus to help make these connections.

2. **Thinking Like a Nurse:** Our book teaches students to identify patient problems and then relate those problems to the appropriate nursing diagnosis. We help students identify what problems a patient is experiencing or may be expected to experience and relate the problems, nursing diagnoses, and interventions to changes in normal body function. Our book provides students with a solid understanding of how to problem-solve in the clinical arena, holistically view their patients' needs, and apply a working knowledge of nursing fundamentals.

3. **Personalizing Care:** While listing NANDA-I diagnoses alone teaches students to categorize care, we teach students how to individualize care. We include situations that require students to think about the individual and his or her needs as opposed to a generic one-size-fits-all care plan guide. We want students to take individual patients' preferences and requirements into consideration as they plan and deliver care, rather than caring for all patients with the same diagnosis in the same manner.

4. **Utilizing Real-World Nursing:** Quite often there are gaps in how to take what is in a textbook and apply it to what the student sees during clinical experience. Often, as instructors, we have found ourselves saying, "I know what your book says, but in the real world...." This book is designed to help students learn to prioritize care and manage patients who have more than one illness. We also help students think through ways care might need to be adapted or could be more easily implemented. We emphasize the need for thorough care delivered by a thinking nurse, so that students are not tempted to take shortcuts.

Features

This book contains the following special features, each appearing as a different colored block. The 122 step-by-step skill presentations will be found at the end of the chapters to prevent interruption of the flow as the student reads.

- **Clinical Connection:** These clinical situations that nursing students commonly face are featured at the beginning of each chapter. They are designed to put the student in a realistic situation that could occur during clinical experiences. Each demonstrates the need to prepare for caring for patients in clinical. This feature helps students connect what is in the book to what they will be doing when they care for real patients.

- **Knowledge Connection:** These questions occur after sections of text so students can make certain they have understood the main ideas of the section. This feature is in addition to workbook questions and review questions at the end of each chapter.

- **Anatomy and Physiology Connection:** This feature provides students with the connection between anatomy and physiology and their nursing diagnoses and interventions. It is not designed as a system review, but rather intended to connect the concepts of anatomy and physiology with the critical aspects of nursing fundamentals.

- **Patient Teaching Connection:** This feature outlines the important points to emphasize when talking with patients or explaining their care; its emphasis is on helping students capture teachable moments during patient care.

- **Real-World Connection:** This feature shares stories to explain how errors have led to patient harm, how to improve patient compliance or care, and how situations could play out in the real world. We asked our contributing writers to share stories from their own experiences to illustrate a major concept of the chapter. We also drew from our experiences as staff nurses, instructors, and students to share illustrations that students will remember far beyond the course for which they use this book.

- **People and Places Connection:** This feature offers special considerations for pediatric and elderly populations, as well as different considerations for concepts and skills in home care and long-term care settings.

- **Laboratory and Diagnostic Connection:** These features relate elevated or decreased results for one laboratory test or a group of tests to effects in the body or explain the use of specific laboratory or diagnostic tests to help determine diagnoses. The laboratory tests chosen coordinate with the topic of the chapter.

- **Supervision/Delegation Connection:** These features point out aspects of appropriate delegation to nurse assistants and unlicensed assistive personnel, as well as the critical elements that should not be delegated to unlicensed personnel. Additional information included will help students learn to supervise care given by nursing assistants and unlicensed assistive personnel.

- **Skills:** We designed our book to be very comprehensive regarding the skills we present. We wanted this book to be the go-to book for skills for the entry-level nurse, with nothing important omitted. Our book includes step-by-step procedures with appropriate rationales for 122 skills. In addition, we are passionate about making the book about real-life nursing, so the steps in the skills are reasonable, rational, and understandable to the student.

End-of-Chapter Highlights

At the end of each chapter, the student will find questions reviewing key points, references to additional resources, and a "Post Conference" reflective of the student in the "Clinical Connection" feature, as he or she evaluates the effectiveness of his or her interventions. Some of the features to be included are:

- Bulleted summary of the key points
- Post Conference
- Review questions
- Critical thinking exercises

Ancillaries

Student Workbook

Accompanying our book is a student workbook, designed to assist the student to develop critical thinking skills. The workbook includes application-style questions, matching and multiple-choice questions, true-or-false questions, examples of "blank forms" such as incident reports, head-to-toe assessment flow sheets, graphic sheets, activity flow sheets, intake/output sheets, and progress notes. To assist the student with documentation, there will be assignments within the specific workbook chapters that will refer the student to the blank form on which the documentation is to be completed. Some of the sections in the workbook include:

- Key Terms Review
- Connection Questions
- General Review Questions
- Application and Critical Thinking Questions
- Scenarios for Documenting Patient Care
- Sample Chart Forms
- Documentation Practice

Electronic Study Guide

Additional resources on the student CD-ROM include:

- NCLEX review questions for each chapter
- Audio library of heart, lung, and bowel sounds
- Medical terminology pronunciations
- Documentation forms
- Abbreviation tables
- Dosage calculator

Web Site

DavisPlus.fadavis.com

DavisPlus, located at http://davisplus.fadavis.com, will carry many of the materials from the electronic study guide as well as additional instructional materials, including:

- Medication administration video clips
- Wound care tutorial
- Medication errors tutorial
- Skills check-off forms
- Animations
- Medical record activities
- Audio podcasts
- Flash cards
- Care planning templates

Instructor's Resource Disk

Accompanying the text will be a CD-ROM of teaching aids for the instructor. Included on this disk are:

- NCLEX-Style Question Test Bank
- PowerPoint Presentations with integrated iClicker questions
- Electronic Image Bank
- Instructor's Guide

Contributors

Sherry Baker, RN, BS/BM, CPHQ
Senior Supervisor Appeals/Grievances
Blue Cross Blue Shield of Oklahoma
Tulsa, Oklahoma
Chapter 2

Bertha Amy Barker, RN, BSN, MSN
Assistant Nurse Manager
St. Anthony's Medical Center
St. Louis, Missouri
Chapter 16

Stacy McDaniel Boruff, RN, PhD, MSN
Associate Professor of Nursing
Walters State Community College
Morristown, Tennessee
Chapter 23

Barry Burton, DC
Owner
Burton Chiropractic
Bethany, Oklahoma
Chapter 11

Patricia Fennessy, MSN
Educational Consultant
Connecticut Technical School System
Middletown, Connecticut
Chapter 9

Elizabeth J. Huntley, RN, CHPN
City Hospice
Oklahoma City, Oklahoma
Chapter 10

Linda Kimble, RN, MSN, CNP
Sole Proprietor
Linda Kimble Health Educator/Consultant
Director of Nursing
Ohio Valley College of Technology
East Canton, Ohio
Chapter 8 and Chapter 30

Kim Litwack, PhD, APNP, FAAN
Associate Professor of Nursing
University of Wisconsin
Milwaukee, Wisconsin
Chapter 33

Diane M. Mayo, RN, BA, MS
Nurse Educator
Healthcare Ventures Alliance
Erie, Pennsylvania
Chapter 6

Nancy McGowan, RN, PhD, CEN
Assistant Professor
The University of Texas Health Science Center at San
    Antonio School of Nursing
San Antonio, Texas
Chapter 7

Lila Self Moersch, RN, BSN, MSN
Clinical Nurse Educator
St. Anthony's Medical Center
St. Louis, Missouri
Chapter 16

Cindy Parsons, DNP, ARNP, BC, FAANP
Assistant Professor of Nursing
University of Tampa
Tampa, Florida
Chapter 24

Cherie R. Rebar, RN, PhD, MBA, FNP
Associate Professor
Kettering College of Medical Arts
Kettering, Ohio
Chapter 32

Beth E. Schultz, RN, MSN
Nursing Faculty
TriCounty Technical College
Pendleton, South Carolina
Chapter 31

Elizabethe Westgard, RN, MSN
Critical Care Nurse
Albert Einstein Medical Center
Elkins Park, Pennsylvania
Chapter 29

Ancillary & Workbook Contributors

Patricia Delmoe, RN, MN
Maricopa Community College
District Nursing Program
Boswell-Mesa Community College
Sun City, Arizona

Tracey B. Hopkins, RN, BSN
Ardmore, Pennsylvania

Marilee LeBon, BA
Developmental Editor
Brigantine, New Jersey

Rhonda Reherman, RN, BS, MEd
Practical Nursing Program Director
Canadian Valley Technology Center
El Reno and Chickasha, Oklahoma

Marcella Williams, RN, MS, AOCN®
Lansing Community Hospital and Sparrow Health System
Lansing, Michigan

Reviewers

Karin Allen, RN, BSN
Coordinator
Hutchinson Community College
McPherson, Kansas

Jocelyn Amberg, RN, MSN
Practical Nursing Program Director
Albuquerque Public Schools Career Enrichment Center
Albuquerque, New Mexico

Patrice Balkcom, RN, MSN
Director of Nursing Program
Central Georgia Technical College
Milledgeville, Georgia

LaVon Barrett, RN, MSN
Assistant Professor
Amarillo College
Amarillo, Texas

Wendy L. Batch-Wilson, RN, MSN
Director
Cuyahoga Community College
Cleveland, Ohio

Eileen Beck, ADN, BSN
Instructor of Nursing
Bates Technical College
Tacoma, Washington

Dianne R. Beedle, RN, MSN, FNP-BC
Nursing Instructor/Educator
Metropolitan Community Colleges
Kansas City, Missouri

Holli Benge, RN, BSN, LVN
Instructor
Tyler Junior College
Tyler, Texas

Korbi Berryhill, RN, MSN, CRRN
Vocational Nursing Program Director
South Plains College
Lubbock, Texas

Susan F. Bond, RN, MSN
Nursing Instructor
Pima Community College Center for Training and
    Development
Tucson, Arizona

Anne L. Brown, RN, BSN
Instructor
Broome-Tioga BOCES
Binghamton, New York

Kathy Burlingame, MS
Associate Dean of Nursing
Minnesota State Community and Technical College
Detroit Lakes, Minnesota

Michele Cislo, RN, MA
Associate Professor
Union County College
Plainfield, New Jersey

Jeanne M. Colia, RN, MSN, CNOR
Director of Nursing
Keiser Career College Greenacres
Greenacres, Florida

Leslie Z. Collier, RN, MSN
Lead Instructor
Brunswick Community College
Supply, North Carolina

Kim Cooper, RN, MSN
Nursing Department Chair
Ivy Technical Community College
Terre Haute, Indiana

Heather Cox, RN, MSN
Assistant Professor
Alfred State College
Alfred, New York

Timothy D. Curl, RN, BSN, MSN
Dean of Nursing
Beckfield College
Florence, Kentucky

Sally J. Flesch, RN, BSN, MA, EdS, PhD
Professor
Black Hawk College
Moline, Illinois

Katherine Fukuyama, RN, BSN, MEd
Department Head
Vancouver Community College
Vancouver, British Columbia, Canada

Jennifer Gambal, RN, MSN, CHPN
Adjunct Faculty
Pennsylvania State University
Bethlehem, Pennsylvania
DeSales University
Center Valley, Pennsylvania

Mary Moser Gautreaux,
 EdD, MSN, CEN, CNS
Director of Nursing
Apollo College
Albuquerque, New Mexico

Edith Gerdes, RN, BSHCA, MSN
Associate Professor of Nursing
Ivy Technical Community College
South Bend, Indiana

Tammy L. Giltner, RN, BSN
Director, Nursing Education Program
Academy of Medical & Health Science Incorporated
Pueblo, Colorado

Jillian Glouscher, RPN
Lab Technologist for Nursing Studies
Algonquin College
Ottawa, Ontario, Canada

Shari Gould, RN
Instructor
Victoria College
Gonzales, Texas

Evelyn F. Grigsby, RN, MSN
Practical Nursing Program Coordinator
Bluegrass Community and Technical College
Danville, Kentucky

Lisa Gutierrez, RN, BSN
Director of VOCN Program
Blinn College
Bryan, Texas

Elizabeth Gwyn
Instructor
Surry Community College
Dobson, North Carolina

Debby Hadley, RN, MSN, CNOR
Instructor
Alcorn State University
Natchez, Mississippi

Karen R. Hazzard, RN, BSN, MSN
Professor of Nursing
Horry Georgetown Technical College
Georgetown, South Carolina

Phyllis S. Howard, RN, BSN
Practical Nursing Program Coordinator
Ashland Community and Technical College
Ashland, Kentucky

Melodie Hull, RPN
Nursing Faculty
College of the Rockies
Cranbrook, British Columbia, Canada

Michael W. Hutton, RN, MSN
Instructor
Blinn College
Bryan, Texas

Patricia B. Lisk, RN, BSN
Instructor
Augusta Technical College
Augusta, Georgia

Gayla Love, RN, MSN, BSN, CCM
Practical Nurse Program Coordinator
Griffin Technical College
Griffin, Georgia

Deborrah K. Maita, RN
Adjunct Instructor
North Metro Technical College
Clinical Coordinator
WellStar Health System
Atlanta, Georgia

Cynthia Manning, RN, MSN, CCRN
Instructor
Blinn College
Bryan, Texas

Julie M. Marzano, RN, BSN, MSed
LPN Instructor
WF Kaynor Technical High School
Waterbury, Connecticut

Aimee W. McDonald, RN, MSN, ENP, CNE
Instructor of Practical Nursing
MCC-Penn Valley Pioneer
Kansas City, Missouri

Mickey McGinty, BSN
Vocational Nursing Instructor
Victoria County Junior College
Gonzales, Texas

Carrie E. McGuire, RN, BSN
Associate Professor
Ashland Community and Technical College
Ashland, Kentucky

Laura Smith McKenna, RN, MSN, DNSc
College Director
American College of Nursing
Concord, California

Hazel Mead, RN, MSN
Professor of Nursing
Dodge City Community College
Dodge City, Kansas

Sandra Melton, PhD, APRN, BC
Professor and Assistant Director
Ventura College
Ventura, California

Lori Moore, BSN, CIC
Nursing Faculty
Apollo College
Damascus, Oregon

Patricia H. Murphy, RN, EdD
Associate Professor
Daytona State College
Daytona Beach, Florida

Sallie Noto, RN, MS, MSN
Director, School of Practical Nursing
Career Technology Center
Scranton, Pennsylvania

Joann Oliver, RN, BSN, MNEd
Assistant Professor
Anne Arundel Community College
Arnold, Maryland

Pamela Owen, BSN
Theory Instructor
Canadian Health Care Academy
White Rock, British Columbia, Canada

Carmen M. Panai, RN, BSCN
Instructor
Palm Beach Community College
Lakeworth, Florida

Tina Peer, RN, MS
Associate Professor of Nursing
College of Southern Idaho
Twin Falls, Idaho

Patrice Pierce, RN, MSN
Director of Nursing Program
Central Georgia Technical College
Milledgeville, Georgia

Dianna Pledger, California Teaching Credential
Vocational Nursing Instructor
Boston Reed College
Napa, California

Judith Polaski-Brown, RN, BSN
Nursing Instructor
Mercyhurst College North East
North East, Pennsylvania

Mary Russo, MSN
LLCC LPN Program Director
Lincoln Land Community College
Jacksonville, Illinois

Crystal Schauerte, RN, MscN
Professor
Algonquin College
Ottawa, Ontario, Canada

Patricia L. Schrull, RN, MSN, MBA, MEd
Associate Professor
Lorain County Community College
Elyria, Ohio

Rebecca A. Shuttlesworth, RN, BSN
Skills Lab Coordinator and Nursing Instructor
San Jacinto College
Houston, Texas

Rosemary Thuet, RN, BSN, MSN
Nursing Program Director
Apollo College
Las Vegas, Nevada

Shawn Marie White, RN, BSN
Nursing Instructor
Griffin Technical College
Griffin, Georgia

Lynda Whitfield, RN, BSN, MS
Instructor
Windham Technical School
Willimantic, Connecticut

Ann Wiesen, BSN, MRA
Director of Practical Nursing
Erwin Technical Center
Tampa, Florida

Kelly Williams, RN, MSN
Department Chair, Nursing
Ivy Technical Community College
Kokomo, Indiana

Christina Wilson, RN, BAN, PHN
Faculty
Anoka Technical College
Anoka, Minnesota

Contents

UNIT 1
Introduction to Nursing 1

CHAPTER 1 The Vista of Nursing 3

History of Nursing —A Look at Where We Have Been 4

Options for Entering Nursing 6
Licensed Practical or Vocational Nurse 6
Associate Degree Nurse 6
Diploma Program Nurse 6
Baccalaureate Degree Nurse 6

Advancing Your Career 7

Specialization in Nursing 7
Scope of Practice 7

Being a Lifelong Learner 7

Characteristics of Nurses 8
Being Responsible 8
Being Honest 8
Being Caring 8
Being Organized 9

Professionalism in Nursing 9
Professional Appearance and Behavior 9
Professional Organizations 10

Nursing Theories and Theorists 11

The Impact of Nursing 11

CHAPTER 2 Health Care Delivery and Economics 15

The Health Care Team 16

Health Care Delivery 16
Medical Necessity 16
Appropriate Level of Care 16

Delivery of Nursing Care 22
Team Nursing 22
Client-Centered Care 22
Primary Care Nursing 23
Case Management 23

Health Care Economics 23
Public Health Insurance 24
Private Health Insurance 24
Health Insurance Plans for Specific Populations 25
Charitable Organizations 25
Self-Pay 25

CHAPTER 3 Nursing Ethics and Law 29

Ethics 30
Patients' Ethical Rights 31
Ethics Committees 33
Do-Not-Resuscitate Orders 33

Law 33
Types of Laws 34

Professional Accountability 38
Professional Liability Insurance 39
Professional Role Boundaries 39
Competency 39
Standards of Care 39
Continuing Education 39

Legal Documents 40
Patient Chart 40
Informed Consent 41
Advance Directives 42
Incident Reports 42

CHAPTER 4 The Nursing Process and Decision Making 47

Decision Making in Nursing 48
Critical Thinking Skills 48

The Nursing Process 49
Steps of the Nursing Process 49
Roles of RNs and LPN/LVNs in the Nursing Process 49
Performing the Steps of the Nursing Process 51

Nursing Care Plans 64
Types of Care Plans 64

Concept Maps 76
Steps for Concept Mapping of a Care Plan 76

CHAPTER 5 Documentation 79

Purposes of Documentation 80
Continuity of Care 80
Permanent Record of Care 81
Accountability 81
Legal Record 82

Confidentiality of Documentation 82

Forms of Documentation 83
Report Form 83
Kardex 85
Incident Reports 85

Care Plans 87
Patient Chart or Medical Record 87

Guidelines for Documentation 87
Use Black or Blue Ink 87
Write Neatly and Legibly 87
Sign Each Entry 87
Include the Date and Time With Each Entry 87
Follow Chronological Order 87
Make Entries in a Timely Manner 88
Be Succinct 88
Use Punctuation 88
Use Only Approved Abbreviations 88
Be Accurate 89
Do Not Leave Blank Lines 92
Use Continued Notes 92
Correct Mistaken Entries 92
Keep the Medical Record Intact 92

Documentation Systems 93
Source-Oriented Records 93
Problem-Oriented Records 95

Data to Document 96

Methods of Charting 96
SOAPIER Charting 96
PIE Charting 98
Focus Charting 99
Charting by Exception 100
Narrative Charting 100

Computerized Charting 102

Long-term Care and Home Health Care Documentation 103
Long-term Care 103
Home Health Care 104

Five Documentation Mistakes That Carry Increased Risks 104
Failure to Document Assessment Findings 104
Failure to Document Medications Administered 104
Failure to Document Pertinent Health History 104
Documenting on Wrong Chart or MAR 105
Failure to Accurately Document Physician's Orders 108

UNIT 2
Communicating and Understanding 113

CHAPTER 6 Communication and Relationships 115

The Communication Process 116

Types of Communication 116

Factors That Affect Communication 117
Personal Space 117
Body Position 117
Language 117
Culture 118
Attitude 118
Emotion 118

Active Listening 118

Styles of Communication 119
Learning a New Communication Style 119

Therapeutic Communication 119
Barriers to Therapeutic Communication 120

Communication in a Crisis 120
Anger or Hostility in Communication 120

Humor in Communication 121

Communication With the Health Care Team 121
Upward Communication 121
Downward Communication 123
Shift-to-Shift Reporting 123
Written Communication 125

The Nurse-Patient Relationship 126
Establishing Trust 126
Patient-Centered Communication 126
Communication During a Patient Interview 126

Special Communication Needs 127
People Who Are Deaf or Hard of Hearing 127
People Who Have Speech and Language Impairments 128
Patients on Mechanical Ventilation 129
Patients Who Are Unresponsive 129

CHAPTER 7 Promoting Health and Wellness 133

Theories of Wellness and Illness 134
The Wellness-Illness Continuum 134
Dunn's Theory of High-Level Wellness 135
Fitzpatrick's Rhythm Model 135

Promoting Wellness 135
Healthy People 2010 135

Illness 138
Types of Illness 138
Phases of Illness 139
Risk Factors for Illness 139

Stress and Adaptation 139
Effects of Stress on Illness 141
Recognizing the Symptoms of Stress 141
Stress Management 141

CHAPTER 8 Ethnic, Cultural, and Spiritual Aspects of Care 147

Ethnicity and Culture 148
Ethnicity and Culture in America 148

Transcultural Nursing and Cultural Competence 149
Cultural Diversity 149
Cultural Awareness 149
Cultural Competence 149

How Culture Affects Health Care 150

Death and Dying 156

Delivering Culturally Sensitive Care 157

Barriers to Health Care 157
Economics 157
Education 157
Geography 157
Language 157
Stereotyping 158
Prejudice and Discrimination 158
Misunderstanding 159
Religion, Spirituality, and Creativity 159
Spiritual Care 161

CHAPTER 9 Growth and Development Throughout the Life Span 167

Concepts of Growth and Development 168
Principles of Growth and Development 168
Factors That Influence Growth and Development 168
Theories of Development 169
Stages of Child Development 172
Infant 172
Toddlers 173
Preschoolers 175
School-Age Child 175
Adolescence 176
Health Concerns for Infants, Children, and Adolescents 177
Infants and Toddlers 177
Preschoolers and School-age Children 178
Adolescents 179
Stages of Adult Development 180
Young Adult 180
Middle Adult 181
Older Adult 181
Health Concerns for Young, Middle, and Older Adults 182

CHAPTER 10 Loss, Grief, and Dying 187

Dealing With the Terminal Patient 188
Medicating the Dying Patient 188
Palliative Care and Hospice Care 189
Living Until They Die 190
End-of-Life Documentation 190
Facing Loss 194
Five Traditional Stages of Grief 194
The Dying Process 198
Psychological and Emotional Changes 199
Physical Changes 199
Nursing Care 200
Listening 200
Teaching 201
Observation and Provision of Comfort 202
Symptom Management 203
Just Be There 204
Postmortem Care 204

CHAPTER 11 Complementary and Alternative Medicine 209

Alternative Therapy Versus Complementary Therapy 210
The Choice of Complementary and Alternative Therapies 210
Western Medicine 211
Eastern and Alternative Health Care 211
Mind-Body Connections 211
Types of Complementary and Alternative Medicine 212
Chiropractic 212
Massage Therapy 213
Acupuncture and Acupressure 214
Herbal Supplements 214
Yoga 214
Additional Forms of Complementary and Alternative Medicine 215
Lifestyle Changes That Reverse Disease 215
Nursing Care and CAM 216

CHAPTER 12 Patient Teaching 221

Learning 222
Learning Styles 222
Factors That Affect Learning 222
Repetition 223
Teaching About Health and Illness 223
Purposes of Patient Teaching 223
Teaching Plans 224
Documentation of Teaching 226
Teaching Patients About Internet Resources 226

**UNIT 3
Nursing Basics 231**

CHAPTER 13 Safety 233

Safe Environment for Patients 234
National Patient Safety Goals 234
Factors Contributing to an Unsafe Patient Environment 234
Promoting Patient Safety 235
Safe Environment for Nursing Staff 243
Minimizing Physical Hazards 243
Radiation Hazards 244
Chemical Hazards 244
Biological Hazards 245

CHAPTER 14 Medical Asepsis and Infection Control 255

Causes of Infection 256
Types of Pathogens 256
Common Illnesses Caused by Microbes 257
Chain of Infection 257

Types of Infection 260

Defenses Against Infection 260
Primary Defenses 260
Secondary Defenses 261
Tertiary Defenses 261
Factors That Decrease Defenses 261

Preventing Infection 261
Precautions for Preventing the Transmission of
Pathogens 262
Medical Asepsis 262
Psychological Aspects of Transmission-based
Precautions 266

CHAPTER 15 Personal Care 279

Routinely Scheduled Care 280

Bathing 281
Benefits of Bathing Patients 281
Patient Preferences and Abilities 282
Types of Baths 284
Nursing Responsibilities During Bathing 285

Grooming 286
Back Massage 286
Oral Care 286
Shaving 287
Nail Care 287
Hair Care 287
Caring for Piercings 288
Eye and Ear Care 289

Managing the Environment 291
The Patient Room 291
Furniture 291
Environment 291

**CHAPTER 16 Moving and Positioning
Patients 311**

Effects of Immobility 312
Physiological Effects 312
Psychological Effects of Immobility 319

Positioning Patients 320
Assisting Patients With Position Changes 320

Moving and Lifting Patients 322
Devices for Lifting and Moving Patients 323
Manual Transfers 326
Assisting With Ambulation 326
Lifting and Moving Obese Patients 327
Protecting Yourself and Your Patients 327

CHAPTER 17 Vital Signs 343

The Six Vital Signs 344

Blood Pressure 345
Factors Affecting Blood Pressure 346
Components of a Blood Pressure Reading 346
Blood Pressure Equipment 346
Assessment Sites 348
Korotkoff's Sounds 348
Hypertension 349
Hypotension 349

Body Temperature 350
Scales of Temperature Measurement 350
Thermogenesis 350
Thermoregulation 351
Factors Affecting Body Temperature 352
Types of Thermometers 352
Routes of Temperature Assessment 353
Normal Body Temperatures by Selected Routes 355
Elevated Temperature 355
Hypothermia 356

Pulse 356
Peripheral Pulse Sites 357
Pulse Assessment 358

Respiration 360
Inspiration 360
Expiration 360
Assessing Respiration 360

Oxygen Saturation 362

Pain Assessment 363
Site or Location 363
Characteristics 363
Pain Scale 363

Documenting Vital Signs 363

CHAPTER 18 Applying Heat and Cold 377

Heat Therapy 378
Indications for Heat Therapy 379
Contraindications for Heat Therapy 379
Methods of Heat Application 379
Nursing Care During Heat Therapy 382

Cold Therapy 383
Indications for Cold Therapy 383
Methods of Cold Application 384
Nursing Care During Cold Therapy 384

**CHAPTER 19 Pain Management, Rest,
and Restorative Sleep 391**

Pain 392
Nature and Physiology of Pain and Its Transmission 392
Classifications of Pain 393
Factors Affecting Pain 394
Responses to Pain 395
Management and Treatment of Pain 395

Rest and Restorative Sleep 399
What Happens During Restorative Sleep? 399
Amount of Sleep Required 400
Factors Affecting Rest and Restorative Sleep 401
Interventions to Promote Restorative Sleep 401

**CHAPTER 20 Admission, Transfer,
and Discharge 407**

Admission 408
Reactions to Admission 409
Cultural Considerations 411

Admitting Procedure 411

Authority to Treat 412
Identification Bands 412
Nursing Responsibilities During Patient
Admission 412

Discharge 414

Discharge Planning 414
Physician's Discharge Order 415
Reconcile Medications 415
Discharge Instructions 415
Notification of Business Office 417
Gathering of Belongings and Valuables 417

Patient Transfer 417

Transfer Within the Facility 417
Transfer to Another Facility 417

CHAPTER 21 Physical Assessment 421

What Is Physical Assessment? 422

Purpose of Physical Assessment 422
Three Levels of Physical Assessment 422
When Is Physical Assessment Performed? 423
Assessment Techniques 423

**Assessment Components Related to
Each Body System 427**

**Performing an Initial Head-to-Toe Shift
Assessment 428**

General Appearance 428
Vital Signs 429
Neurological Examination 429
Head and Neck 429
Chest and Abdomen 433
Extremities 442
Needs and Comfort 444

Documentation of Assessment Findings 445

CHAPTER 22 Surgical Asepsis 455

Disinfection and Sterilization 456

Types of Sterilization 456
Indications of Sterility 456
Sterile Settings 457
Using Sterile Technique in Other Settings 457

Principles of Sterile Technique 457

Sterile Conscience 458
Guidelines for Using Sterile Technique 458
When to Use Sterile Technique 460

UNIT 4
Clinical Skills and Care 473

CHAPTER 23 Nutrition 475

Nutrition 476

FDA Guidelines and Food Labels 476
Dietary Guidelines for Americans 477

**Essential Nutrients and Their General
Function 480**

Water 480
Protein 480

Fats 481
Carbohydrates 482
Vitamins 483
Minerals 484

Nutritional Deficiencies and Excesses 484

Protein 485
Fats 485
Carbohydrates 487
Vitamins 487
Minerals 487

**Differing Nutritional Needs Over the
Life Span 490**

Pregnancy 490
Toddlers and Preschool Children 490
School-age Children 491
Adolescents 491
Adulthood 491
Older Adults 492

Cultural Influences on Nutrition 492

Acculturation 493

**CHAPTER 24 Nutritional Care
and Support 497**

Supporting Nutritional Intake 498

Assessment 498
Mealtime Preparation 499
Assistance With Eating 500
Monitoring Intake and Output 500
Supporting Patients With Special Nutritional Needs 501

Therapeutic Diets 502

NPO 502
Regular Diet 502
Diets Modified by Consistency 502
Diets Modified for Disease 503
Nursing Responsibilities 504

Eating Disorders 505

Anorexia Nervosa 505
Bulimia Nervosa 505

Food-Drug Interactions 506

Drug Effects on Food Intake 506
Drug Effects on Absorption 506
Drug Effects on Metabolism 507
Drug Effects on Excretion 507

Enteral Tubes 508

Nasogastric and Nasointestinal Tubes 508

Gastric Decompression 509

Insertion of NG Tube for Gastric Decompression 510
Removing an NG Tube 513

Enteral Nutrition 513

Feeding Tubes 513
Tube Feeding Formulas 513
Enteral Feeding Methods 514

**Complications Associated With Tube
Feedings 517**

Parenteral Nutrition 518

Partial Parenteral Nutrition 518
Total Parenteral Nutrition 519
Monitoring Nutritional Status 520

CHAPTER 25 Diagnostic Tests 539

Nursing's Role in Diagnostic Testing 540

Categories of Diagnostic Tests 541
Laboratory Tests 541
Radiology and Imaging Tests 547
Ultrasonography 548
Endoscopic Examinations 548
Graphic Recording Tests 549

CHAPTER 26 Wound Care 557

Types of Wounds 558
Contusions 558
Abrasions 558
Puncture Wounds 558
Penetrating Wounds 558
Lacerations 558
Pressure Ulcers 558

Contamination of Wounds 558

Pressure Ulcers 559
Risk Factors for Pressure Ulcers 560
Staging Pressure Ulcers 560
Prevention of Pressure Ulcers 561

Other Wounds Found in Hospitalized Patients 563
Stasis Ulcers 563
Draining Sinus Tracts 563
Surgical Incisions 563

Wound Healing 563
Phases of the Healing Process 563
Types of Wound Closures for Healing 564
Factors Affecting Wound Healing 564
Complications of Wound Healing 565

Wound Treatment 569
Closure 569
Drains and Drainage 570

Measurement of Wounds and Observation of Drainage 571

Cleaning Wounds 571
Nursing Responsibilities for Cleaning Wounds 572
Obtaining a Wound Culture 572

Dressings 572
Wet-to-Damp and Wet-to-Dry Dressings 572
Securing Dressings 572
Nursing Responsibilities for Applying Dressings 574

Documenting Wound Care 574

CHAPTER 27 Musculoskeletal Care 591

Musculoskeletal Conditions Resulting in Limited Mobility 592
Common Musculoskeletal Conditions 592

Types of Immobilization 593

Caring for Patients With Musculoskeletal Immobilization 594
Caring for a Patient in a Cast 594
Caring for a Patient in Traction 595
Caring for a Patient After Joint Replacement 595
Caring for a Patient After Amputation 597

Assistive Devices for Ambulation 598
Crutches 598
Canes 598
Walkers 599

CHAPTER 28 Respiratory Care 611

Normal Oxygenation 612
The Mechanics of Breathing 612

Impaired Oxygenation 613
Causes of Impaired Oxygenation 614
Caring for Patients With Impaired Oxygenation 614
Nursing Interventions for Patients With Impaired Oxygenation 617
Nursing Interventions for Patients Needing Airway Assistance 623
Chest Tubes 625

CHAPTER 29 Fluids, Electrolytes, and Acid-Base Balance 645

Water 646
Distribution and Movement of Body Fluids 646
Functions of Water in the Body 649
Regulation of Body Fluids 650

Fluid Volume Disturbances 651
Fluid Volume Deficit 651
Fluid Volume Excess 653

Electrolytes 655
Sodium 655
Chloride 660
Potassium 661
Calcium 662
Magnesium 663
Phosphorus 664
Bicarbonate 664

Acid-Base Balance 664
pH Scale 665
Regulation of Acid-Base Balance 666
Acid-Base Imbalance 667

CHAPTER 30 Bowel Elimination and Care 675

Bowel Elimination 676
Frequency of Elimination 677
Timing of Elimination 677
Characteristics of Feces 677

Alterations in Bowel Elimination 678
Constipation 678
Diarrhea 679
Fecal Impaction 681
Fecal Incontinence 681

Promotion of Bowel Elimination 681
Subjective Assessment 681
Objective Assessment 682
Increased Activity 682
Adequate Fluid and Fiber Intake 683
Privacy 683
Positioning 683

Management of Alterations in Elimination 684
Dietary Considerations 684
Medications 684
Enemas 685
Perineal Care 688
Obtaining a Stool Specimen 688
Digital Removal of Impaction 688
Treatment of Fecal Incontinence 689

Alternative Bowel Elimination 689
Colostomy 690
Ileostomy 690
Nursing Care of Ostomies 691

CHAPTER 31 Urinary Elimination and Care 709

Normal Urinary Elimination 710
Characteristics of Urine 710
Normal Voiding Patterns 712

Assessing Urine and Urinary Output 713
Physical Assessment 713
Collecting Specimens and Testing Urine 713
Measuring Intake and Output 715

Alterations in Urinary Function 717
Altered Bladder Function 717

Caring for Patients With Altered Urinary Function 719
Urinary Catheters 719
Urinary Diversions 725
Urinary Tract Infections 725

CHAPTER 32 Care of Elderly Patients 745

A Description of Aging 746
Classifications of Age Groups 746
The Aging Population and Nursing 747
Myths About Aging 747

Physical Effects of Aging 747
Changes in Neurological Functioning 748
Changes in Sensory Functioning 753
Changes in Cardiovascular Functioning 753
Changes in Respiratory Functioning 753
Changes in Gastrointestinal Functioning 754
Changes in Endocrine and Genitourinary Functioning 754
Changes in Reproductive Functioning 755
Changes in Musculoskeletal and Integumentary Functioning 755
Assessment Considerations for Older Adults 755

Psychosocial Problems of Aging 756
Loss, Grief, and Dying 756
Safety From Scams and Crime 757
Elder Abuse 757
Financial Concerns 757

Positive Aspects of Aging 758

Long-term Care 758
Patient or Resident? 758
Residents' Needs 759
Assessment 762
Documentation 762

The Problem of Polypharmacy in Elders 762

CHAPTER 33 Care of the Surgical Patient 769

Purposes of Surgery 770

Degrees of Urgency 770

Various Surgical Settings 771
Outpatient Surgery 771
Inpatient Surgery 771

Preoperative Care of the Surgical Patient 772
Presurgical Assessment 772
Preoperative Diagnostic Testing 774
Preoperative Patient Teaching 774
Preoperative Medications 779
Informed Consent 779
Preoperative Checklist 781
The Holding Area 781

Intraoperative Care of the Surgical Patient 781
Surgical Team Members 781
Preparation of Surgical Suite 784
Types of Anesthesia 784
Intraoperative Interventions 786

Postoperative Care of the Surgical Patient 788
Postanesthesia Assessment and Care 788
Return to the Patient's Room 790
Postsurgical Complications 793

CHAPTER 34 Phlebotomy and Blood Specimens 805

Phlebotomy 806
Why We Draw Blood 806
Preparation of the Patient 806
Selecting an Appropriate Vein for Venipuncture 807
Cleansing the Site 809
Equipment and Supplies 809

Performing Venipuncture 814

Complications of Phlebotomy 815

Skin Punctures 816
Performing Skin Puncture 817

UNIT 5
Medication Administration 825

CHAPTER 35 Researching and Preparing Medications 827

Fundamentals of Medications 828
Names, Categories, and Routes of Medications 828
Legal Regulation of Medications 829
Effects and Interactions of Medications 829
Researching Medications 832
Classifications and Effects of Medications 833

Preparing to Administer Medications 840
Reading Medication Orders 840
Calculating Drug Dosages 841
Obtaining Medications 843
Rights Involving Medications 844

Safety Checks 845
Guidelines for Preparing Medications 845

Medication Errors 846

Handling a Medication Error 846

CHAPTER 36 Administering Oral, Topical, and Mucosal Medications 851

Routes of Administration 852

Oral Route 852
Enteral Tube Route 855
Topical Route 857
Transdermal Route 858
Mucosal Route 858

Nursing Responsibilities for Administering Oral, Topical, and Mucosal Medications 861

Documentation of Medication Administration 862

Documentation on a Paper MAR 862
Documentation on an Electronic MAR 863
Documentation on MARs in Long-term Care 863
Documenting Withheld or Refused Medications 864

Preventing Administration and Documentation Errors 864

If a Medication Error Occurs 864

CHAPTER 37 Administering Intradermal, Subcutaneous, and Intramuscular Injections 879

Injections 880

Supplies and Equipment 881
Handling Syringes and Needles 884

Medications 886

Reconstitution and Drawing up Medications 886
Mixing Medications 888

Comparison of Routes of Administration 890

Intradermal Injections 891
Subcutaneous Injections 892
Intramuscular Injections 896

CHAPTER 38 Peripheral Intravenous Therapy 913

Purposes of IV Therapy 914

Maintaining Fluids and Electrolytes 914
Replacing Fluid and Electrolyte Losses 914
Infusion of Intravenous Medications 915

Safe Administration of IV Drugs 917

IV Solutions 917

Isotonic Solution 917
Hypotonic Solution 918
Hypertonic Solution 918

IV Equipment 920

IV Needle Cannula 920
Winged Butterfly 922
IV Tubing 923
IV Infusion Pumps and Controllers 927
IV Start Kit 927

Asepsis and IV Therapy 928

Handwashing 928
Gloves 928
Supplies 928
Patient's Skin 929

Calculation of Infusion Rate 929

Practice 930

Initiating Peripheral Venipuncture 930

Medical Record Review 930
Preparing the Equipment 931
Selecting a Vein 932
Performing Final Preparation of Supplies 933
Cleaning the Site 934
Performing Venipuncture and Cannulation 934
Determining Proper Cannulation 935
Securing the IV Site 935
Starting the IV Pump 936
Setting Gravity Infusion Rate 936
Monitoring IV Infusions 936
Documenting the Venipuncture 937
Problem-Solving 937
Discontinuing an IV Infusion 938

Complications of Peripheral IV Therapy 938

Infiltration 939
Extravasation 939
Phlebitis and Thrombophlebitis 940
Localized Infection 940
Septicemia 941
Severed Cannula 941
Air Embolism 941
Circulatory Fluid Overload and Pulmonary Edema 942
Speed Shock 942

Blood and Blood Products 943

Transfusion 943

APPENDIX A: Answers to Review Questions 967

APPENDIX B: Photo and Illustration Credits 981

INDEX 987

Introduction to Nursing

The Vista of Nursing

Key Terms

Associate degree nurse

Baccalaureate degree nurse

Diploma program nurse

Health Occupations Students
 of America (HOSA)

Licensed practical/vocational nurse
 (LPN/LVN)

National Federation of Licensed
 Practical Nurses (NFLPN)

NCLEX-PN

NCLEX-RN

Nurse Practice Act

Scope of practice

Objectives

1. Define key terms associated with nursing practice.
2. Trace the providers of nursing care from ancient history until the mid-1800s.
3. Summarize the development of modern nursing.
4. Describe the history of nursing, both at the LPN/LVN level and at the RN level.
5. Differentiate four pathways for entering nursing education.
6. Discuss career ladders and specialization in nursing.
7. Define scope of practice.
8. Describe four characteristics of nurses.
9. Evaluate professional appearance and behavior.
10. Discuss the purposes of professional organizations you can join as a nursing student.
11. Discuss consequences of unprofessional conduct.
12. Explain the impact of nurses on patients' lives.

When you stand at the top of a mountain and look out, you see a vista—an open, unblocked view. If you look closely, you can see where you have been: the winding ribbon of road that you followed from the foot of the mountain to the top. As you move your eyes to change your view, you start to see where you can go. A trail begins to your left and leads along the crest of the mountain. Several miles away you can see an interesting ski lodge nestled on a second mountain. To your right is a scenic overlook ideal for taking pictures. Behind you stands a ski lift that you can ride to an even higher peak.

When you begin nursing school, it is like standing at the top of that mountain. You may have followed quite a winding path to get where you are now, and you bring many life experiences with you. After suffering through entrance examinations, waiting lists, and preference points, you are finally here—you have started nursing school. But "here" is only the beginning. This is just the first step in your nursing career.

Look out across the vista of nursing and see the possibilities. From here, you can go many places and work in a variety of settings. You may work in a hospital, outpatient surgery center, physician's office, or specialty clinic. Your path might take you to a career in home health care, long-term care, or assisted living. You may choose to continue your education. Some people work while they go on with college to obtain higher degrees in nursing. You may even decide to climb another mountain and become an advanced practice nurse. Sometimes students start out in nursing and then decide to go into other areas of health care, such as physical or occupational therapy, legal nurse consulting, or even medical school. Many possibilities are available in the vista of nursing.

History of Nursing—A Look at Where We Have Been

Through ancient history, nursing care was provided by family members and male priests. Around 1,000 AD, after the end of the Dark Ages, the Italian town of Salerno allowed women to attend school to study midwifery. As Christianity spread, care for the sick and poor was considered a valuable endeavor. Convents were then established for training

caregivers and providing care for the sick. Deaconesses, religious women who served by helping the poor and sick, administered care similar to today's public health nursing.

In the 1700s to 1800s, very little was known about antisepsis. Hospitals were not clean, nor were they places of hope. Educated women did not pursue nursing because it was considered beneath them. It was left to the poor, the low class, the "Sairy Gamps" to care for sick people. (Sairy Gamp was a fictional character, a drunken midwife, created by Charles Dickens. Her name became synonymous with low-class, poorly qualified health care workers.) Wealthier people cared for sick family members at home because it was considered a disgrace to send one's family away to a hospital.

Modern nursing began in the mid-1800s. In 1836, the first school of nursing was established in Kaiserworth, Germany, by pastor Theodore Fliedner. Many women were educated here, who then were assigned to various places in the world to teach other women to be nurses. They were referred to as *Kaiserworth deaconesses,* and the most famous of them was Florence Nightingale (Fig. 1-1). For information on women who helped mold modern nursing, see Table 1-1.

In 1897, in Baltimore, Maryland, the Nurses Associated Alumnae of the United States was formed in an effort to oversee training to protect patients from incompetent nurses.

Figure 1-1 Florence Nightingale during the Crimean War.

Table 1-1 **Women Who Molded Nursing History**

Person or People	Role in History
Clara Barton	Known as the "Angel of the Battlefield" during the U.S. Civil War, she cared for soldiers both from the North and the South. She was the first president of the Red Cross Association, now the American Red Cross.
Dorthea Dix	An activist for better mental health care and the establishment of psychiatric hospitals. She was appointed as the Superintendent of Female Nurses in the Army in 1861, where she organized staff and equipment for Army hospitals. She was not a nurse or a military officer, but a retired teacher.
Florence Nightingale	Seen as the person who established modern nursing, she attended the Kaiserworth School in Germany in 1851 and also studied in Paris under the Sisters of Charity. She is famous for her work giving nursing care during the Crimean War. She also kept records during that time, shared them with the Secretary of War, and influenced war strategy. She was instrumental in the establishment of the Nightingale School in London, England, which became a model for other nursing schools.
Mary Mahoney	The first African American nurse in the United States. She worked tirelessly to improve acceptance for African Americans in nursing. She established an association for this purpose, the National Association for Colored Graduate Nurses, and served as its first president.
Linda Richards	Recognized as the first "trained nurse" in the United States, she graduated from Boston's New England Hospital for Women and Children in 1872. Her system of noting information about her patients at Bellevue Hospital in New York became the foundation for modern nurse's notes. She later went to Japan on a medical mission and established the first school of nursing there.
Isabel Hampton Robb	An activist for nursing labor reform in the late 1800s. She helped usher in 12-hour shifts with meal breaks for nurses, when 24 hours had been standard. She also was instrumental in establishing a 3-year training program for nurses and worked for licensure examinations and nursing registration.
Mary Adelaid Nutting, Lillian Wald, and Annie Goodrich (the "Great Trio")	These three nurses made great strides in nursing education and community health nursing. Nutting graduated in the first nursing class from Johns Hopkins University and established the Nursing and Teachers College at Columbia University, where she was the first professor of nursing. Wald, known as the first visiting nurse, opening the Henry Street Settlement to provide health care to the poor. Goodrich was devoted to establishing nursing as a profession. She received the Distinguished Service Award for developing the Army School of Nursing. She also served as the director of the Visiting Nursing Service at the Henry Street Settlement. In addition, she served as the dean of Nursing at Yale University and President of the American Nurses Association.

Soon afterward, the American Society of Superintendents of Training Schools for Nurses was also established. This group later became the National League for Nursing Education. It was established to set standards and rules in nursing education and continues in that function today.

In the early 1900s, some states began to pass laws requiring the licensure of nurses. Requirements for entering nursing school also were established. The *American Journal of Nursing* was published for the first time during this era to help keep nurses aware of the newest medical information and newest information about nursing education.

In 1892, the first training program for practical nurses was established in New York City at the Young Women's Christian Association (YWCA). The next year, the first official school for practical nurses, called the Ballard School, was opened, also through the YWCA. This school was established to help meet the need for educated bedside nurses, recruiting those who "had a special way with the sick." Because many people were cared for at home during this era, these first practical nurses were essentially home health nurses. The training program was 3 months long and focused on homemaking skills as well as caring for the sick.

It was not until 1955 that all states required practical nurses to be licensed. The title Licensed Practical Nurse, or LPN, is used in all states except California and Texas. Those states use the title Licensed Vocational Nurse, or LVN.

Knowledge Connection
When did modern nursing begin, and who is recognized as its founder? When did states start requiring RN licensure? What type of training did the first practical nurses receive?

Options for Entering Nursing

When you decide to pursue a nursing career, many pathways are open to you (Box 1-1). It is unusual for so many choices to exist for entering a field of study, and often students find it confusing. Remember, too, that these options do not have to be selected in any certain order.

Licensed Practical or Vocational Nurse

The **licensed practical or vocational nurse (LPN/LVN)** is the most basic of all the entry-level options for nurses. The educational programs are from 9 months to 1 year for full-time programs, and generally 18 months to 2 years for part-time programs. Some college courses may be required before

Box 1-1
Nursing Education Levels

A number of entry-level and advanced practice education options are available to those entering the nursing field.

Entry-Level Education
- **Licensed Practical or Vocational Nurse:** 9 to 12 months of education at a technical college or career technology center
- **Registered Nurse, Associate Degree:** 2 to 3 years at a community college or state college
- **Registered Nurse, Diploma Program:** 3 years in a hospital-based program affiliated with a college or university
- **Registered Nurse, Baccalaureate Degree:** 4 years at a college or university

Advanced Practice Education
- **Masters of Science in Nursing (MSN):** 2 or more years in the graduate school of a university; may teach in BSN, ADN, and LPN/LVN programs; may also choose to specialize further in one of these areas:
  - Clinical Nurse Specialist
  - Nurse Practitioner
  - Certified Registered Nurse Anesthetist
  - Nurse Midwife
- **Doctorate in Nursing (PhD, DNP):** 2 or more years in a doctoral program at a university; may serve as the Dean of Nursing in university programs or Director of Nursing in large hospitals, may teach in MSN and doctorate programs; may direct and design formal research programs

entering LPN/LVN school, but in many states there are no requirements for previous education except a high school diploma or the equivalent.

When students finish their educational program, they will take the **NCLEX-PN** test to become licensed. Those letters stand for the National Council Licensure Examination for practical nursing. This examination is standardized in all 50 states and is taken by computer at a specified location. Results are mailed to graduates within a short period of time (5 to 7 days, usually), and the newly licensed LPN/LVN can quickly begin to work in health care.

Associate Degree Nurse

The **associate degree nurse** is an entry educational level for registered nurses. Students in these programs attend a private or community college for a minimum of 2 years to obtain their associate degree in nursing (ADN). An associate degree includes some basic general education courses, such as science, math, history, English, and social sciences, at the college level. In addition, these students take three to four semesters of nursing courses. If a student has not attended college previously, it is not uncommon for this educational preparation to take up to 3 years to complete.

When students complete all course work and graduate, they are eligible to take the **NCLEX-RN** or National Council Licensure Examination for registered nursing. Upon successfully passing the examination, the graduate becomes a Registered Nurse and uses the title "RN" after his or her name.

Diploma Program Nurse

Diploma program nurses are educated in hospital-based nursing education programs, of which few remain. Before universities and community colleges were numerous and easily accessed, nursing education was delivered through a hospital. Students worked on the patient units and gained experience while attending classes. Eventually, hospitals offering such programs affiliated with a college or university. The college or university faculty, either at the hospital or at a convenient location, provides general education courses such as the sciences, history, English, and math. The hospital oversees and employs the faculty who teach nursing courses. Diploma programs last about 3 years, often with required summer sessions. Graduates of these programs also take the NCLEX-RN for licensure to become Registered Nurses.

Baccalaureate Degree Nurse

The **baccalaureate degree nurse** program can also be an entry into nursing. Students who choose this option enter a university to pursue their nursing education. They take all required courses for a 4-year college degree: general education courses as well as four to five semesters of nursing courses. It is not uncommon for students to complete their first 2 years of college before they make application and are admitted to the university's school of nursing to obtain their bachelor of science in nursing (BSN) degree.

Upon completion of all course work, these students also take the NCLEX-RN. The focus of their nursing education puts more emphasis on management and leadership than do the ADN and diploma programs. Therefore, these nurses are more in demand for management positions.

Advancing Your Career

Career ladder options are available to every nurse (Box 1-2). The LPN/LVN may wish to obtain an ADN and become a registered nurse, but still focus mostly on direct care. The same nurse may later wish to go to a university for a BSN, then move into management or leadership opportunities. An associate degree nurse may return to school quickly and obtain a BSN, or may work several years before doing so. Some nurses choose not to obtain higher degrees and find working as LPN/LVNs, associate degree nurses, or diploma nurses very rewarding. You are the best judge of what level of education is best for you.

Knowledge Connection
How many ways can a person become a registered nurse? Which preparation for RN takes the longest? What is the advantage of a "One Plus One" Program?

Specialization in Nursing

Nursing students often ask about specializing in different areas, such as critical care or pediatrics. In nursing school, you will rotate through many areas of nursing care: medical-surgical floors, surgery and recovery, emergency, mental health, obstetrics, and pediatrics, just to list a few. As a newly graduated entry-level nurse, you may be encouraged to work in a medical-surgical unit for a year to gain experience in nursing and to develop good nursing judgment before obtaining a position in a specialty area. Many metropolitan hospitals limit specialty areas only to registered nurses. However, in more rural areas, LPN/LVNs may work in a greater variety of settings. Once you have completed school and passed the NCLEX, you may find one area of work that you prefer above all others.

Scope of Practice

All nurses are responsible for knowing their own **scope of practice**, that is, the limitations and allowances of what they can do as a nurse. In every state, a **Nurse Practice Act**, or the law governing nurses' actions, exists. This law is written to specifically address each level of nursing. In every state, licensed practical or vocational nurses are required by law to practice under the supervision of a registered nurse or physician, and registered nurses are required to practice under the supervision of a physician. The Nurse Practice Act in each state establishes the scope of practice for each level of nurse, based on educational preparation. The Board of Nursing in each state determines and enforces the contents of the Nurse Practice Act. Other specific allowances or limitations vary from state to state. For example, in some states, LPN/LVNs are prohibited by the Nurse Practice Act from initiating intravenous (IV) therapy. In other states, LPN/LVNs are allowed under the law to perform this skill. *It is your responsibility to know the content of the Nurse Practice Act in your state regarding your scope of practice and to follow it faithfully.*

Being a Lifelong Learner

Whatever choice you make for your basic nursing education, you will work hard to achieve your nursing license. You will be expected to learn an enormous amount of information in a relatively short period of time. You will be expected to remember what you have learned in previous courses and apply that knowledge to new situations in patient care. Nurses must constantly connect known information while absorbing new information. All nurses, whether LPN/LVN, RN, BSN, or advanced practice, should strive to deliver good nursing care. Although we may have different scopes of practice based on our initial time in school, we all share skills and knowledge, working together to provide excellent patient care. All nurses must continue to learn after they complete their basic nursing education. Whether you choose to do that through formal degree programs or through continuing education, seminars, and short courses, you will need to continue to learn to stay current in the ever-changing field of nursing.

Box 1-2
Career Ladder in Nursing

Once you become a nurse, you can continue your education in a variety of ways.

- **One Plus One Programs:** Offered at community and state colleges. In the first year, the curriculum prepares the student to take the NCLEX-PN. After passing the examination, the student can work as an LPN/LVN while completing the second-year curriculum. The student then takes the NCLEX-RN to be licensed as a Registered Nurse.
- **PN to ADN Programs:** Offered at community and state colleges. The student is given credit for LPN/LVN education that counts toward requirements for RN education, making the time spent in school shorter to complete coursework to become a registered nurse.
- **PN to BSN, ADN to BSN, and Diploma to BSN Programs:** All previous entry-level nursing education programs are credited toward the course requirements for a baccalaureate degree in nursing, making the time in school shorter.

As a nurse, you will work with a variety of people in a variety of places. For example, much of your educational program will focus on adults and adult health problems. However, the elderly population has additional health issues, such as multiple chronic illnesses, sensory deficits, and multiple prescription medications. Very young patients also have additional issues, including difficulty understanding what is happening and expressing their feelings during medical procedures. They have no previous experience to prepare them for illness or treatment, so they are often frightened.

Your educational program will focus mainly on hospital care. When you care for patients in the home care setting, there are differences in how care is delivered, with fewer available supplies and less equipment than in a hospital. You have to adapt and sometimes be creative. You are generally alone in the patient's home, with no other health professionals to help you make decisions about care. You must have good nursing judgment to make quick decisions in the home.

In the long-term setting, care is delivered in a more homelike environment that is less institutional than a hospital. Residents are surrounded by familiar items from home, and they may participate in activities together. When you work in this setting, you will encourage residents to participate in their care and decision making when possible. Because confusion and agitation can be a problem for some residents, it is essential to use an easy, calming approach when providing care. To help detect health problems in elderly individuals, it is as important to recognize changes in residents' behavior as it is to recognize changes in vital signs. This feature will provide tips to help you care for patients of all ages and in all settings.

Characteristics of Nurses

If you asked people on the street to choose one word to describe nurses, chances are great that the word you would hear most often is "caring." Other descriptions might include "compassionate," "comforting," and "helpful." According to several Gallup polls, nurses are considered to be honest, ethical, and trustworthy. Though you might not hear this from interviewing random strangers, words like "technologically savvy," "troubleshooter," "problem-solver," "intelligent," and "multi-talented" are equally appropriate for describing nurses. In this section, we will discuss four important characteristics—being responsible, honest, caring, and organized.

Being Responsible

The job of nursing requires that you be able to think critically about each patient, while carrying out all physicians' orders and handling unexpected admissions and emergencies that may arise. Nursing is a unique field in which to work, due to the amount of responsibility involved. You are responsible for:

- Caring for several patients, including their medications and comfort, and seeing that their physical, emotional, and spiritual needs are met
- Helping families understand what is happening to the patient and preparing them for his or her care after discharge
- Noticing changes in the patient's condition and notifying the appropriate health care professional if negative changes occur

Contrast this with the job of a bank teller, who is responsible for greeting customers, performing requested transactions such as deposits and withdrawals, cashing checks, and, at the end of the day, balancing his or her drawer with the transaction record. While handling money is certainly a big responsibility, the responsibilities of a nurse far outweigh those of most any other job.

Being Honest

Nurses have to be honest—far more honest than the average person. You can put patients at risk for developing infection, illness, or complications when you make an error in medication dosage, sterile technique, or assessment. It is extremely difficult for most of us to admit that we made a mistake. It is even harder to tell your supervising nurse or doctor about an error. And if you make an error while caring for patients, it is possible that no one would ever know unless you admit to it. However, for the sake of protecting patients from possible complications, you must be responsible and honest enough to admit your mistake. In other words, you must be willing and able to put your patients' well-being first, before your pride. Patients place their trust in you and depend on you, so you must be completely honest about anything that could potentially harm them.

Being Caring

Much has been written about nurses and caring. Dr. Jean Watson, a nurse, educator, and theorist, advocates stressing the art of nursing with an emphasis on caring. In this way, nurses respond to patients in a way that confirms their individuality, emotions, and needs. A caring nurse does not treat patients in a "one approach fits all" manner, but individualizes care for that particular patient. A caring nurse does not see a patient in terms of a cellular disorder or an illness to be cured. Instead, the caring nurse sees patients as people who have needs for touch and understanding as much as they have needs for IV fluids and antibiotics. In fact, "high-touch" nursing is just as important as "high-tech" nursing, as Figure 1-2 illustrates.

Figure 1-2 Caring and listening are some of the skills needed for the art of nursing.

Being Organized

There is also another side to nursing—the side that integrates information from laboratory values, normal structure and function, nursing diagnoses, patient needs and problems, supervision and delegation issues, vital sign readings, and medication orders to determine what nursing care to perform for each patient. In addition, the nurse is using highly technical equipment and troubleshooting for problems when alarms sound. It is extremely important that you be able to keep track of all this information about your patients. You also must deal with changing orders from the physician and meet the changing needs of your patient.

The only way to accomplish all of this for several patients during one shift is to be very organized. You will learn to make notes on a shift report or other form rather than to trust your memory with important information. You will also learn how to prioritize the care you give your patients so that nothing gets missed. In some ways, when you are striving to be organized and on time with treatments and medications, it is easy to lose sight of the fact that your patients are people who need a human touch, rather than a list of tasks to be completed.

Nursing is both an art and a science. The art of nursing describes the caring, creativity, communication, and compassion necessary to connect with patients in a meaningful way. The science of nursing describes the analysis and integration of data, the decision-making process, and the technical monitoring of patients. Figure 1-3 shows a nursing instructor teaching with a computerized manikin, one of many high-tech tools for learning about clinical patient care. Good nurses blend both the art and the science into their daily nursing practice.

Laboratory and Diagnostic Connection

Feature Overview
Most hospitalized patients have frequent laboratory and diagnostic tests performed to identify illnesses and to evaluate

the treatment of disease. Some medications affect balances in the body, so frequent laboratory tests are done to detect any potential imbalance. It is your responsibility as a nursing student to check laboratory and diagnostic tests often, to note any abnormal findings, and to notify the appropriate health care professionals of significant abnormal findings. In future chapters, this Laboratory and Diagnostic Connection feature will provide information to help you learn about different laboratory values and their significance in your patients' care.

Knowledge Connection
How is nursing different from other jobs? Why is it so important that nurses be honest? Explain how nursing can be both an art and a science.

Professionalism in Nursing

Sometimes beginning nursing students talk about past experiences with nurses that were both positive and negative. The students' motivation to become a nurse may be due to a desire to emulate a positive nurse role model or the aspiration to be a better nurse than one who was a negative example. As students learn more about nursing, they often discover that a "negative example nurse" simply failed to communicate what was about to happen and why. When you do not communicate well with your patients and their families, you will leave a negative impression about your abilities as a nurse.

Professional Appearance and Behavior

You can be a nurse, or you can be a good nurse. There is a difference. Good nurses communicate well. They tell patients what will happen and why before they begin a procedure. Good nurses take responsibility for their own behavior, including mistakes they may have made. Good nurses also see themselves as professionals and act in a corresponding manner. Not everyone views appearance as important, but you are judged as a nurse by how you look and present

Figure 1-3 A nursing instructor using a computerized manikin to teach students about the science of nursing, including managing monitors and equipment.

yourself. If you are not neat and clean, patients may feel that you will not provide meticulous nursing care. If you do not act like a professional, patients may feel that you are not competent to care for them (Box 1-3).

Unprofessional Conduct

Professional behavior is so important that the Nurse Practice Acts in many states define unprofessional conduct as a reason to revoke or suspend a nurse's license. Some examples of unprofessional conduct that could result in the loss of your nursing license include:

- Use of drugs or alcohol in a way that could endanger patients
- Diversion of drugs from prescribed patient use to personal use

- Failure to supervise certified nursing assistants and unlicensed assistive personnel adequately
- Failure to adequately care for patients or conform to minimum standards of nursing practice
- Criminal conduct

Professionalism is extremely important in nursing. You represent all nurses each time you care for a patient in any setting, so it is essential that you appear and conduct yourself in a manner that says you are not only a nurse, but you are a good nurse.

Professional Organizations

Another aspect of professional behavior is participation in professional organizations, both as a student and as a nurse. Professional organizations give you a collective voice that will be heard by those who enact laws and establish policy for health care. In addition, professional organizations provide opportunities for leadership in nursing.

RN Student Organizations

The National Student Nurse Association (NSNA) is an organization that RN students can join while they are in nursing school. One of the main benefits of joining this organization is developing leadership skills that future employers often see as a benefit. There is a national conference at different locations each spring where topics of interest to future nurses are discussed. This organization also gives students a chance to network with one another and with future employers at functions designed to bring both together.

The official publication of the NSNA is *Insight,* and is available to all members. To learn more about this organization, go to their website, www.nsna.org. Upon graduation, RNs can join their professional organization, the American Nurses Association (ANA).

LPN/LVN Student Organizations

While in nursing school, you can belong to the **Health Occupations Students of America (HOSA)** and the **National Federation of Licensed Practical Nurses (NFLPN)** as a student affiliate.

HOSA is a national organization specifically for students in health occupations educational programs. Membership is open to both high school and adult students, with separate chapters for each group. HOSA holds two state or regional events per school year. In the summer, a national conference is held in a different major city each year. The state or regional events include a fall leadership conference to provide training for chapter officers and the election of state officers. In the spring, a skills competition is held, allowing qualifying students to compete in a variety of contests. Some examples are job-seeking skills, outstanding chapter, CPR/First Aid, and practical nursing skills. For more information about HOSA, look on the website *www.hosa.org.*

Box 1-3

Professional Appearance and Behavior

You will be expected to appear and behave in a professional manner during your nursing education and in your nursing career.

Professional Appearance

- Shower or bathe and apply deodorant daily.
- Keep hair clean and styled appropriately.
- Wear clean undergarments.
- Wear a clean scrub suit or uniform that fits well, without tears or wrinkles.
- Wear shoes that are clean and in good condition with clean shoelaces.
- Cover any visible tattoos.
- Remove studs, barbells, and gauges from piercings as required by facility policy.
- Keep fingernails short and clean; this helps prevent scratching patients or injury to self.

Professional Behavior

- Arrive on time, prepared to work.
- Complete assigned care during your shift. If you are unable to do so, ask for help. If you are caught up on your assignment, offer to help someone who is behind.
- Give thorough care with no shortcuts that compromise patient safety or comfort.
- Take breaks on time and return on time so that others can go at their assigned times.
- Leave the unit only after you have ensured that another nurse is aware that you are gone and will be responsible for your patients while you are gone.
- Assume responsibility for other nurses' patients when they leave the unit.
- Be kind and supportive of other nurses and health care professionals.
- Avoid criticizing the mistakes of others, since you will undoubtedly make mistakes too.
- Look for the positives in people—patients, family members, coworkers, and supervisors.

NFLPN is the professional organization for licensed practical/vocational nurses. It was established in 1949 by Lillian Custer, and only those with an LPN or LVN license can join. Student affiliation is allowed. NFLPN offers updates on legislation affecting LPN/LVNs, recognition of practical nursing students with a B average or above who are recommended by their instructor in the NFLPN Student Honor Society, and participation in state events and the national convention. State affiliates often sponsor a Student Day at their annual convention, with topics of interest to students and new LPN/LVNs. The official publication of NFLPN is the journal *Advance* for LPNs. They also publish *NFLPN Extra!* for members. For more information about NFLPN, look on the website *www.nflpn.org*.

Supervision/Delegation Connection

Feature Overview

It will be your responsibility to know the scope of practice not only for yourself, but also for the unlicensed assistive personnel (UAPs) and certified nursing assistants (CNAs) that you supervise. If you delegate a task to a CNA or UAP that is not within his or her scope of practice, you put the assistant and yourself in legal jeopardy. In this book, we will include information about appropriate delegation and supervision to help you learn what you can and cannot delegate. We will also include tips for successfully supervising assistants.

Knowledge Connection

What professional organizations you can join as a nursing student? What can result when a nurse exhibits unprofessional conduct?

Nursing Theories and Theorists

Nursing theories are ideas that a particular nurse or nurse educator has developed to explain how he or she looks at the purpose and focus of nursing. Each theory addresses the theorist's views regarding the person, environment, health, and nursing itself. A variety of nursing theories have been developed over the past 160 years. Table 1-2 presents a brief outline of some of the best-known nurse theorists and the basic premise for their theories. As you might imagine, no one theorist is "right" and the others "wrong." Rather, each theory approaches the overall idea of nursing with a different view. The more you learn about nursing theories, the better you will understand every aspect of being a nurse.

The Impact of Nursing

Nurses have an amazing opportunity to impact patients' lives every day. People who are ill or recovering from illness or surgery have many needs. They are often unable to perform normal activities and rely on the nursing staff for help with the most basic needs.

Table 1-2   Selected Nurse Theorists

Theorist	Date	Theory
Peplau, Hildegard E.	1952	Interpersonal relationships model: interpersonal communication can improve mental health.
Henderson, Virginia	1955	14 basic needs addressed by nursing care; definition of nursing; do for the patient what he or she cannot do for himself or herself.
Abdellah, Faye G.	1960	21 nursing problems; deliver care to the whole person.
Orlando, Ida Jean	1961	Interpersonal process; nursing process theory
Wiedenbach, Ernestine	1964	The purpose of nursing is to support and meet patients' needs for help. Nursing is a helping art.
Levine, Myra	1967	Conservation model, published in 1973; designed to promote adaptation of the person while maintaining wholeness, or health.
Johnson, Dorothy	1968, 1980	The behavioral system model: incorporates five principles of systems thinking to establish a balance or equilibrium (adaptation) in the person. The patient is a behavioral system consisting of subsystems.

(table continues on page 12)

Table 1-2 **Selected Nurse Theorists** (continued)

Theorist	Date	Theory
Rogers, Martha	1970	The science of unitary human beings focuses on the betterment of humankind through new and innovative modalities. Maintaining an environment free of negative energy is important.
Orem, Dorothea	1971	The self-care deficit nursing theory explains what nursing care is required when people are not able to care for themselves. Goal is to help client attain total self-care.
King, Imogene	1971	First of two theories was the interacting systems framework, designed to explain the organized wholes within which nurses are expected to function: society, groups, and individuals. The first theory led to the theory of goal attainment, which focuses on mutual goal setting between a nurse and patient and the process for meeting the goals.
Neuman, Betty	1972	Neuman systems model is based on general systems theory (a non-nursing theory) and reflects the nature of living organisms as open systems.
Roy, Sr. Callista	1974	Adaptation model was inspired by the strength and resiliency of children. The model relates to the choices people make as they adapt to illness and wellness.
Leininger, Madeleine M.	1978, 1984	Cultural care diversity and universality theory; caring theory
Newman, Margaret	1979	Theory of health as expanding consciousness describes nursing intervention as nonintervention, where the nurse's presence helps patients recognize their own pattern of interacting with the environment.
Watson, Jean	1979	Caring theory. Nursing is an interpersonal process.
Parse, Rosemarie Rizzo	1981	Theory of human becoming focuses on the human-universe-health process and knowledge related to human becoming (or reaching one's potential)
Benner, Patricia and Wrubel, J.	1989	Primacy of caring model. Caring is central to the model and helps the client cope with stressors of illness.

While other health care professionals come in and out of patients' lives with short-term contact, nurses are the 24/7 caregivers. This gives nurses a number of opportunities to develop relationships with patients. In establishing such relationships, nurses can influence patients in many positive ways. For example, nurses teach healthier lifestyles, when and how to take medications, which side effects or complications to watch for, and when to notify the physician.

You will have opportunities to help patients and their families in countless ways throughout your nursing career. Often patients never know what could have happened were it not for a thinking nurse. And while not everyone will always say, "thank you," you will have the satisfaction of a job well done.

Real-World Connection

Becoming a "Good Nurse"

As one nursing instructor reflects over her 25 years of teaching LPN/LVN students, she says, "I have seen all kinds of students who came from all walks of life be successful in nursing school. The one thing they had in common was the desire to learn and to care for people. My desire was that they not just become nurses, but that they become good nurses, the kind of nurse I would want caring for my family members or me." Her advice to you is, "Do not settle for just being a nurse. Settle for nothing less than being a good nurse, a thinking nurse, one whose presence makes a difference."

🌐 **Post Conference**

The Post Conference at the end of each chapter will help you see how to evaluate the clinical experience of caring for the assigned patient in the Clinical Connection. You will participate in Post Conferences after you care for real patients in the long-term or acute care setting. You will find that you can learn something new from each experience of caring for people. What new things have you learned from reading and studying this chapter?

KEY POINTS

- Many educational opportunities and a variety of practice settings are available to nursing students after graduation.

- For much of history, nursing was provided by religious orders, then by the poor, lower classes.

- Modern nursing originated in the mid-1800s with Florence Nightingale as its founder.

- The standardization of nursing education came into being through the American Society of Superintendents of Training Schools for Nurses (now the National League for Nursing).

- Education for LPNs began in 1892 in New York City through the YWCA.

- The title LPN is used in all states except California and Texas, where the title LVN is used.

- Four entry-level options for nursing education are LPN/LVN, ADN (RN), diploma (RN), and BSN.

- It is your responsibility to know the content of your state's Nurse Practice Act and to follow it faithfully.

- Nurses must be responsible, honest, caring, and organized.

- You represent all nurses to your patients and their families, so it is extremely important to be professional in appearance and behavior.

- There is a difference between being a nurse and being a good nurse.

- RN students can join the NSNA while they are in school. After graduation, the professional organization for them is the American Nurses Association (ANA).

- Two organizations LPN/LVN students can join while in school are HOSA and NFLPN. After graduation, NFLPN is the professional organization.

- Unprofessional conduct is described in the Nurse Practice Acts of most states. If you are found guilty of certain conduct, you could lose your license and the legal right to practice as a nurse.

- Think about the kind of nurse you would want to take care of your family or to care for you. Be that kind of nurse.

REVIEW QUESTIONS

Select the answer that is most appropriate for each of the following questions. Some questions may have more than one correct answer. Check all that apply.

1. The first role for a woman in health care was that of a:

    a. nun.

    b. midwife.

    c. deaconess.

    d. teacher.

2. The most famous Kaiserworth deaconess was:

    a. Sairy Gamp.

    b. Clara Barton.

    c. Florence Nightingale.

    d. Mary Mahoney.

3. Which is true of a "One Plus One" program?

    a. One year after a student becomes an ADN, he or she can finish college with a BSN.

    b. One year after working as an RN, the nurse can achieve advanced practice status with 1 more year of college.

    c. One RN and one LPN/LVN work together for 1 year in a hospital setting; then the LPN/LVN can become an RN after passing the NCLEX.

    d. The first year of a 2-year program prepares the student to take the NCLEX-PN. The student can work as an LPN/LVN while completing the second year of nursing school to become an ADN.

4. The NCLEX is:

 a. an examination to determine entry into a practical/vocational nursing school.

 b. an examination taken to become licensed as a nurse.

 c. a review course to help students do well on their licensure examination.

 d. a national survey of all nurses to determine average age and work settings.

5. An RN student asks a friend who is an LPN/LVN student, "Will you be able to start IVs when you get out of school?" Which is the best response?

 a. "It will depend on the Nurse Practice Act of the state where I work."

 b. "Sure. I'm sure I will learn how to do that in school."

 c. "Maybe. If the hospital where I work allows it."

 d. "No. Licensed practical/vocational nurses are never allowed to do that."

6. Which is a description of professional behavior by a nurse?

 a. Taking several breaks when you need to make personal phone calls.

 b. Criticizing another nurse in the break room because of an error made when administering medications.

 c. Requesting assistance if you realize you will not be able to finish your assigned duties on time.

 d. Leaving the patient unit without notifying anyone to run to the gift shop for a few minutes.

FILL IN THE BLANK QUESTION

7. Write the type of entry-level nursing program next to its description.

 a. Minimum of 2 years at a private or community college: _____

 b. Two or more years in graduate school at a university: _____

 c. Nine months to 1 year at a technical college or career technology center: _____

 d. Four-year college degree at a university: _____

 e. Three years in a hospital-based program affiliated with a college or university: _____

CRITICAL THINKING EXERCISES

8. What would you do if you, a nursing student, made an error that could harm a patient?

9. How would you respond to this statement: "Nursing is more science than art in today's world. 'Caring' nurses are equated with subservient handmaidens."

ADDITIONAL RESOURCES

For additional Resources, Questions, and Activities, please see:

 Student Resource Disk

 http://davisplus.fadavis.com

 Student Study Guide

REFERENCES

Anderson MA. *Nursing Leadership, Management, and Professional Practice for the LPN/LVN.* 3rd ed. Philadelphia: FA Davis; 2005.
Cooper PG. A call for a return to patient-centered care. *Nurs Forum.* 2005;40(3):73-74.
Idczak SE. I am a nurse: nursing students learn the art and science of nursing. *Nurs Educ Perspect.* 2007;28:66-71.
Kleiman S. Revitalizing the humanistic imperative in nursing education. *Nurs Educ Perspect.* 2007;28:209-213.
Manojlovich M. Power and empowerment in nursing: looking backward to inform the future. *OJIN Online J Issues Nurs.* 2007;12(1):2.
McCabe S. What does it take to make a nurse? *Perspect Psychiatr Care.* 2006;42:252-255.
Metules T. Who cares about caring? *RN Magazine,* 2007;August 1.
Nursing Degree Guide. History of Nursing in the United States. Available at: www.nursingdegreeguide.org/articles/general/history_of_nursing_in_the_united_states/. Accessed June 26, 2009.
U.S. Department of Labor, Bureau of Labor Statistics. (2008). *Occupational Outlook Handbook.* Available at: www.stats.bls.gov/oco. Accessed June 26, 2009.

Health Care Delivery and Economics

Key Terms

Capitation

Case management

Client-centered care

Diagnosis-related groups (DRGs)

Health maintenance organization (HMO)

Home health care

Hospice

Inpatient

Managed care

Medicaid

Medicare

Outpatient

Point-of-service (POS) plan

Preferred provider organization (PPO)

Primary care nursing

Primary care physician

Referral

Rehabilitation

Team nursing

Third-party payer

Objectives

1. Identify the two most important factors in health care delivery and economics.
2. Describe members of the health care team and their functions.
3. Describe inpatient health care settings and their services.
4. Describe outpatient health care settings and their services.
5. Distinguish between types of nursing care delivery systems.
6. Contrast Medicare and Medicaid.
7. Describe various types of private health insurance.
8. Explain two types of rehabilitation services.

Clinical Connection

Your Assignment: You have been assigned to care for a 60-year-old female patient diagnosed with colon cancer. She has had abdominal surgery to remove the tumor, and now has an infected abdominal wound. Her care plan calls for dressing changes on the wound twice a day and IV antibiotics. She does not have any health insurance and is very concerned about the cost of her hospital stay.

Your Actions: As you care for your patient, you are concerned about the cost of every item you use. You do not want her to have to pay for supplies that are not needed. In addition, you wonder if there are ways to help her with her concerns about payment. She tells you that she thinks she might be eligible for Medicaid or Medicare, but she does not know the difference or how to enroll in either of them. You want to help her, but you do not really know about them either. What can you do to help this patient?

The Health Care Team

A patient in a health care facility sees an amazing number of different workers, all members of the health care team. These team members provide medical and mental health services to patients in various settings. They have a common goal of providing quality, cost-efficient care to all patients in order to restore their patients to their optimal level of functioning and wellness. You will work with a variety of team members with different types of training and focus (Table 2-1). It is important that you realize the valuable input of each health care team member. It takes all of us working together to deliver quality health care to our patients. Communication between members of the health care team is also extremely important. This is discussed further in Chapter 6. One way that all team members communicate with one another is during a patient care conference. Such conferences allow discussion of patient needs and involve input from all team members.

Health Care Delivery

While caring for patients on a busy day, the last thing on the minds of many nurses is who is paying for each patient's care. Yet, some entity is responsible for payment. When the economics of care is a foremost consideration, two factors help guide decisions about patient care: medical necessity and appropriate level of care. These factors are important for patients with health care insurance as well as those without it. Payment for medical care is most often through one of two major entities: Medicare and private insurance.

Medicare is the federal government's health insurance program for people older than 65 years of age or those with certain disabilities or conditions. Private insurance is provided by a number of companies and purchased by the individual or his or her employer. Often private insurers

adopt the requirements and payment policies determined by Medicare.

Today, most patients with health care insurance are automatically enrolled in some form of managed care. Mullahy and Jensen define **managed care** as "a system of health care delivery aimed at managing the cost and quality of access to health care." Patients without health care insurance will automatically be "managed" for the simple reason that they have no funding for their medical care and require health care services for which they cannot pay.

Medical Necessity

Insurers determine medical necessity by comparing the patient's clinical/medical information against accepted medical review criteria. According to government funding sources, *medical necessity* is defined as services or items reasonable and necessary for the diagnosis or treatment of illness or injury or to improve the functioning of a malformed body member. This means that the services must seem reasonable and necessary to the entity paying for them. For example, if a person had health insurance and submitted a claim for a face lift, the insurance company would not pay it because a face lift is not needed to diagnose or treat an illness or injury, nor does it improve the functioning of a malformed body member. However, another person could submit a claim for facial reconstruction surgery after a car accident, and that claim would be paid, because it was reasonable and necessary to repair the person's facial structures after an injury.

Appropriate Level of Care

Another aspect of paying for health care requires determining an appropriate level of care to meet the patient's needs. In today's health care environment, there is a continuum of care that the patient may travel in his or her efforts to reach an optimal level of health, function, and wellness. It

Table 2-1 **The Health Care Team**

Staff Member	Description
Medical Staff	
Medical Doctor (MD)	Responsible for diagnosing and treating disease, illness, and injury;
Doctor of Osteopathy (DO)	ordering diets, tests, medications, treatments, therapies, and procedures; and directing overall care of patients
Physician's Assistant (PA)	Employed by physician or hospital to work closely with physician and assist in directing patient care
Nursing Staff	
Nurse Practitioner (NP)	Masters-prepared registered nurse certified in a specific area of practice and identified with advanced practice license who diagnoses illnesses and prescribes medications and treatments for them
Registered Nurse (RN)	Practices nursing within a defined scope under the direction of a physician; provides direct patient care, manages departments, and supervises other nurses and assistive personnel
Licensed Practical/Vocational Nurse (LPN or LVN)	Practices within a defined scope under the supervision of a physician, dentist, or RN; provides direct patient care and supervises assistive personnel
Unlicensed Assistive Personnel (UAP)	Perform patient care duties and assist nursing staff
Certified Nursing Assistant (CNA)	UAPs perform more complicated tasks, including sterile procedures, in some states
Therapy Staff	
Respiratory Therapist (RT)	Evaluate, treat, and care for patients with breathing problems due to heart and lung disease
Respiratory Therapy Technician (RTT)	RTTs generally work under the supervision of an RT
Physical Therapist (PT)	Provide services to help improve or restore function and mobility, relieve pain, and prevent or limit permanent physical disabilities for patients suffering from injuries and disease
Physical Therapy Assistant (PTA)	PTAs generally work under the supervision of PTs and carry out their orders
Speech and Language Therapist (ST)	Assesses, diagnoses, treats, and helps to prevent disorders related to speech, language, voice, swallowing, and fluency
Occupational Therapist (OT)	Assist patients with disabilities to develop, recover, or maintain their skills for daily activities and work
Certified Occupation Therapy Assistant (COTA)	
Laboratory Staff	
Pathologist (MD)	Medical doctor who examines tissue and blood samples to determine the origin or existence of disease
Medical Laboratory Technologist (MLT)	Examine and analyze body fluids and tissues, match blood for
Medical Technician (MT)	transfusions, and test for blood levels of medications
Phlebotomist	Draws blood specimens from patients for testing
Radiology Staff	
Radiologist (MD)	Medical doctor who specializes in procedures involving x-rays and radiation therapy; reads radiographs and other radiologic films
Radiologic Technologist (Rad Tech)	Operates x-ray machines and other radiologic equipment, such as computed tomography (CT) scanners, as well as magnetic resonance imaging (MRI) and ultrasound equipment; assists the radiologist by performing ordered tests to determine diagnoses and treat certain diseases
Ancillary Staff	
Pharmacists	Pharmacists distribute prescription medications; advise patients and
Pharmacy Technicians	prescribers on the selection, dosages, interactions, and side effects of medications

(table continues on page 18)

Table 2-1 **The Health Care Team** (continued)

Staff Member	Description
	Pharmacy technicians assist pharmacists by helping to prepare prescribed medications, answering phones, stocking shelves
Registered Dietitian (RD)	RDs plan regular menus and develop special menus to meet the dietary needs of patients; work with physicians to meet special dietary needs; instruct patients on special diets
Dietary Technician	Dietary Technicians assist the RD by distributing and picking up selective menus and monitoring patient food intake
Medical Social Worker	Provide psychosocial support to patients, families, or vulnerable populations; advise caregivers, counsel patients, plan for patients' needs after discharge, and arrange for needed care such as home health care
Public Health Social Worker	
Chaplains	Provide spiritual care for patients in hospitals and hospice settings; meet spiritual needs of families and patients when diagnosis is terminal or when deaths occur; provide spiritual care for hospital staff as well

is important that the patient is cared for at the most cost-effective, yet safe and effective level. This may be either an inpatient or outpatient level.

Inpatient Settings

Inpatients stay overnight or longer in a health care facility. Inpatient care may be provided in an acute medical or mental health care hospital, a skilled nursing facility in a nursing home or hospital, a long-term acute care hospital, a long-term chronic care facility such as a nursing home or assisted living facility, or a rehabilitation facility.

The term *residential care* is used to describe care given in settings where the patients, or residents, stay for long periods of time. Box 2-1 lists examples of residential care facilities.

Acute Care Hospital or Medical Center

An acute care hospital may be the only hospital for many miles or one of several hospitals in a medical center complex, where a number of different specialty hospitals are grouped together and share resources. Acute care hospitals provide emergency care, surgeries, inpatient care, diagnostic testing, and usually some types of outpatient care. Staff is composed of a variety of doctors, nurses, assistants, therapists, laboratory workers, and other medical personnel. Rural hospitals may be smaller, with fewer departments and less staff than their larger city counterparts. Regardless of size or location, when a person is ill or injured, he or she generally seeks care at the closest hospital.

Long-term Acute Care Hospital

A long-term acute care hospital (LTACH) provides a level of care similar to that of an acute care hospital. However, an LTACH focuses on patients with serious medical problems that require intense, special treatment for a long period of time, usually about 20 to 30 days. These patients often trans-fer from intensive care units in traditional hospitals. It would not be unusual for a patient in an LTACH to need ventilator or other life support medical assistance.

The health care team in an LTACH is composed of members similar to those in the acute care hospital. A physician visit is required daily.

An example of the effective use of this level of care would be a situation in which a patient is in intensive care on a ventilator after lung surgery and develops an infection in the chest cavity. The patient is stable on the ventilator and will have to remain on it until the infection is completely cleared, which could be up to a month. It would be extremely expensive

Box 2-1

Examples of Residential Care Facilities

A client may live in a variety of residential care settings. Each provides a different level of assistance.

- **Long-term care facilities:** Also called nursing homes or convalescent homes, these facilities are where residents often live for many years. Nursing care is provided around the clock for the residents in these facilities.
- **Assisted living facilities:** These facilities provide less nursing care than that found in long-term care facilities. Residents are assisted with medications and personal care such as bathing and dressing. Meals are provided, and a choice of activities may be available.
- **Independent living facilities:** These facilities do not provide nursing care. They generally have staff available around the clock to respond to urgent situations by contacting emergency medical services for the residents. Meals are usually available, as well as transportation and activities.

for the patient to remain in an acute care hospital during that time. The patient is transferred to an LTACH for continued treatment of the lung infection and ventilator support.

Skilled Nursing Facility

A skilled nursing facility (SNF) may be associated with a hospital or long-term care facility. The SNF provides a less intense level of care than that found in a traditional or long-term acute care hospital. It is usually a transitional care setting. Patients may stay in an SNF for a few days or as long as 100 days, but they eventually move to a rehabilitation, nursing home, or home care setting.

SNF care consists of skilled nursing care and physical, occupational, and speech therapy as needed. Physicians usually do not visit daily and are more likely to see patients on a weekly basis. Laboratory, radiology, or surgical services are not usually available at an SNF. An SNF level of care is usually covered by Medicare and most private insurers, but there are certain requirements:

- The patient must have been hospitalized for at least 3 days prior to admission.
- The patient must enter the nursing home within 30 days of a hospitalization.
- There is a 100-day stay maximum per year related to any one hospitalization and diagnosis.
- The patient must be making regular progress as documented by the medical professionals.

An example of the effective use of this level of care would be a situation in which an elderly man falls at home and suffers a fractured hip. While in the acute care hospital, he has surgery to repair the fracture but does not want to eat after surgery. Eventually a feeding tube is placed and the patient is fed through the tube. He begins to eat a bit, but not enough to take out the tube. The surgery was successful, but the patient is not strong enough to return home. He is placed in an SNF unit for skilled nursing care. He continues to increase his oral intake and is discharged to his home in 40 days.

Rehabilitation Facility

Rehabilitation, often shortened to rehab, is a level of care in which the patient can receive intense physical, occupational, and speech therapy services. The rehabilitation facility may be part of a hospital or it may be a freestanding facility. A physician specialist in physical medicine and rehabilitation oversees the patient's care during his or her stay. Other health care team members who may participate in patient care include nurses, therapists, therapist assistants, nursing assistants, and technicians. As a rule of thumb, the patient must be capable of participating in at least 3 hours of therapy a day to be admitted to a rehabilitation facility. If the patient becomes ill or has other medical problems while in rehabilitation, he or she may be transferred back to an acute care hospital.

An example of this level of care would be a situation in which a female patient suffers a stroke and has weakness on the left side of her body. She is discharged from the hospital to a rehabilitation facility for 2 months of intensive therapy to regain as much strength and use as possible in her affected side. The therapy sessions are held every morning and afternoon. She is also expected to perform activities such as bathing and grooming with assistance. As her stay lengthens, she is expected to need less assistance.

Another type of rehabilitation facility focuses on treating patients with chemical dependency and mental health issues. Some of these facilities provide medical care in the form of *detoxification,* or the removal of drugs and alcohol from the person's body, which generally takes several days.

If the rehabilitation facility does not provide this type of care, the patients have to be admitted to an acute care hospital for the detoxification process, as it can lead to a medical emergency. After going through the detoxification process, the patient can then be admitted to a rehabilitation facility designed to treat chemical dependency and mental health issues. Most generally, the physician who oversees the patient's care is a psychiatrist who specializes in treating mental or behavioral disorders. The health care team in this type of rehabilitation setting consists of nurses; nursing assistants; clinical social workers, usually functioning as therapists or counselors; and psychologists.

An example of the effective use of this level of care would be the treatment of a young male patient who is addicted to the pain medication OxyContin. He cannot really begin treatment for addiction until the drug is completely out of his body and the withdrawal symptoms are past. He goes through detoxification the first few days after stopping the drug. He is monitored closely by the health care staff for physical problems related to withdrawal, such as seizures, sweating, hallucinations, muscle pain, and nausea and vomiting. He then begins individual and group counseling sessions and group activities to deal with issues that led to his addiction.

Assisted Living Facilities

Assisted living facilities provide relatively independent seniors with assistance and limited health care services in a homelike atmosphere, but there is no common definition for assisted living facilities. Assisted living services include 24-hour protective oversight, food, shelter, and a range of services that promote the quality of life of the individual. The health care team in an assisted living facility may consist of one or more RNs, several LPN/LVNs, and numerous nursing assistants and certified medication aides. In some assisted living facilities, a nurse is not on the premises 24 hours per day, but one is available by telephone. Therapies such as physical, occupational, or speech therapies may be available but are not part of the facilities' regular services. These are generally provided by contracted home health care agencies.

Long-term Care Facilities

Long-term care (LTC) facilities provide 24-hour custodial care and some medical services for patients with chronic illness or disability, particularly older people who have mobility and eating problems who cannot be cared for at home. Some LTC facilities are also affiliated with skilled nursing units.

Staffing in LTC facilities depend on the level of care provided. If the residents are stable and need little nursing care, there may be one RN and several LPN/LVNs, certified medication aides, and nursing assistants providing care. If the residents require more skilled care, more RNs are generally on staff. Therapies such as physical, occupational, or speech therapies may be available through the facility or through home health care.

Knowledge Connection

Give an example of a procedure that would be considered medically necessary. List three settings for residential care. List four criteria that a patient must meet to be admitted to an SNF. What is the difference between an acute care hospital and a long-term acute care hospital?

Outpatient Care

Outpatient care is provided in many settings and is designed to meet the needs of the patient in 1 day and then allow him or her to return home. Care and services provided on an outpatient basis are usually less expensive than care provided on an inpatient basis. Outpatient care is preferred when possible to decrease costs while still providing quality care. A patient may require surgery that can be provided at an outpatient facility, but the appropriate level of care for this patient may be for the surgery to occur in an inpatient setting because the patient has other health conditions that could influence his or her recovery.

Hospital Outpatient Department

Hospitals offer a wide range of outpatient services. Most larger hospitals or medical centers provide outpatient surgery; cardiac, pulmonary, physical, occupational, and speech therapy/rehabilitation; laboratory, radiation, and diagnostic testing; and mental health services such as intensive outpatient or partial day treatment. Most hospitals also have a 23-hour observation setting in which patients can receive care and diagnostic testing to determine whether it is necessary for them to be admitted.

Outpatient surgery is performed in a hospital setting, but the patient is allowed to return home on the same day that the surgical procedure is performed. Outpatient surgery is also referred to as *ambulatory surgery* or *same-day surgery*. It is suited best for healthy people undergoing minor or intermediate procedures. Some outpatient surgeries may require a 23-hour observation stay to make sure the patient does not have any immediate complications after surgery. More than 60% of elective surgical procedures in the United States are currently performed as outpatient surgeries. Health experts expect this percentage will increase to nearly 75% over the next decade.

Ambulatory surgery centers (ASCs) are freestanding health care facilities providing outpatient surgery only. The type of surgeries performed at ASCs may be directed by certain state regulations.

An example of the appropriate use of this level of care would be a situation in which a patient has her gallbladder removed via a small abdominal incision, called *laparoscopic surgery*. The patient is monitored after waking from the anesthetic. The nurse assesses the patient to ensure that she can tolerate liquids and can urinate after surgery. Then she is discharged to home with follow-up instructions.

Outpatient Mental Health Services

Some hospital mental health outpatient services include intensive outpatient and partial day treatment programs. The intensive outpatient programs generally provide group counseling and therapy sessions for mental health and chemical dependency illnesses, lasting approximately 2 to 3 hours per day, two to five times per week. Partial day treatment programs provide group and individual counseling and therapy sessions for mental health and chemical dependency illnesses, lasting approximately 7 to 8 hours per day during the week.

An example of this level of care would be a continuation of the client we discussed earlier who was addicted to OxyContin. After detoxification and inpatient treatment, the patient would then be changed to partial day treatment, coming to the mental health facility daily for 8 hours. As the client improves, he begins a job during the day. He then comes back to the facility 2 nights per week for group therapy sessions.

Cardiac Rehabilitation

The American Heart Association describes cardiac rehabilitation as a medically supervised program to help patients with cardiac disorders recover quickly and improve their overall physical, mental, and social functioning. The goal is to stabilize, slow, or even reverse the progression of cardiovascular disease, thereby reducing the risk of worsening heart disease, another cardiac event, or death. Cardiac rehabilitation programs include:

- Counseling so the patient can understand and manage the disease process
- Exercise programs
- Nutritional counseling
- Risk factor modification
- Vocational guidance
- Instruction on physical limitations
- Emotional support
- Counseling on appropriate use of prescribed medications

The cardiac rehabilitation health care team consists of cardiologists (physicians who specialize in the diseases and treatments of the heart), nurses, physical/exercise therapists and assistants, and dietitians. Cardiac rehabilitation is provided through an outpatient setting of a hospital or at a freestanding facility.

Pulmonary Rehabilitation

Pulmonary rehabilitation is a program of education and exercise classes that teach patients about their lungs, how to exercise and perform activities with less shortness of breath, and how to live better with a lung condition. The health care team for pulmonary rehabilitation includes a pulmonologist (physician who specializes in diseases and treatments of the lungs), nurses, respiratory therapists, and respiratory assistants. Pulmonary rehabilitation is provided through an outpatient setting of a hospital or at a freestanding facility.

Ambulatory Care Clinics

Ambulatory care clinics operate much like a physician's office and provide the same type of services. Some may specialize in one type of care, such as urgent care or occupational health care. Ambulatory care clinics may provide a variety of health care services under one roof. These services may include medical, dental, laboratory, x-ray, psychological, and/or pharmaceutical care.

Health Departments

Health departments are public facilities that provide health care services. These facilities are funded by county, city, state, and federal governments. Therefore, the cost of care at these facilities is lower than the cost of care at private clinics. In some cases care is provided at no cost. The services provided are determined by the governing entity but may include immunizations, family planning, maternity education, well-baby clinics, adolescent health clinics, hearing and speech services, child developmental services, environmental health, and physical and occupational therapy.

Health departments are also responsible for the tracking and treatment of certain *communicable diseases,* which are diseases that are transmitted through direct contact with an infected individual or indirect contact through a carrier. Some examples of communicable diseases that health departments treat and track include tuberculosis, sexually transmitted diseases, measles, mumps, rubella, hepatitis, flu, and certain viruses.

An example of the use of this level of care might be a teenage mother who is pregnant with her second child. She does not work due to pregnancy and caring for her 18-month-old son. Her husband has been laid off from his construction job. She is seen at the health department for assistance with food and health care for herself and her child, through the Women, Infants, and Children (WIC) health program. She is provided with vouchers to buy healthy food, and her pregnancy is monitored for problems. Her son is provided with the appropriate immunizations and is monitored for normal growth and development.

Physician's Office

The physician's office setting provides evaluation, assessment, treatment, simple diagnostic testing, and simple surgical treatment. The physician may specialize in one particular area of health care, seeing only patients with specific health conditions. The health care team in a physician's office usually consists of the physician, a nurse or medical assistant, and medical office personnel. The administrative medical assistants are responsible for appointments, phone calls, collaboration with health insurance companies, billing, and other duties assigned by the physician.

Most physicians participate in some type of group practice. The group may consist of physicians in the same specialty or may be a group of different types of specialists in order to allow the patient to have a "one-stop shopping" type of opportunity. Physicians have developed group practices in order to cut administrative costs and receive assistance with health insurance contracting with the various insurance companies.

Home Health Care

Home health care can be one or many types of health or medical services provided to patients in their homes because they are confined to their homes by an illness or disability. Home health companies can be independent agencies or are sometimes part of a hospital-based health care system. They provide care in the form of skilled nursing visits with or without home health aide visits; physical, occupational, and speech therapy; medical social worker visits; infusion therapy; durable medical equipment; and hospice. The patient's primary care physician usually orders the home care services, but a specialist may also oversee and order home care. Home health services must be medically necessary in order to be covered by Medicare and private insurance plans.

Skilled services are those services that require a license to perform, and Medicare requires that a patient need skilled services to qualify for home health care. These skilled services may be a need for nursing, therapy, or social work. Skilled nursing visits include performing nursing assessment and evaluation, complicated dressing changes, and the administration of IV medications. Specially trained nursing assistants, or home health aides, provide nonskilled services. Examples of such services are assistance with bathing and grooming, housekeeping, transportation, and food preparation and delivery.

Physical, occupational, and speech therapy services can be provided in the home by therapists who make home visits through a home health agency. The patient must be homebound to receive these services, because otherwise the patient could go to an outpatient therapy center for this type of care.

Medical social worker visits can be ordered to assist patients and families with psychosocial support to help them deal with chronic, acute, or terminal illnesses. They also advise family caregivers, counsel patients, and help plan for patients' needs. They may arrange for community services such as Meals on Wheels, public transportation, medication assistance, and legal assistance.

Home health care allows people to stay in their homes rather than being forced by medical needs to live in a health care facility. Home visits for skilled care are a cost-effective way to provide limited care.

An example of a patient needing this level of care would be an elderly man whose wife died last year. He recently underwent abdominal surgery to repair a bowel perforation. His abdominal wound has not healed and he requires dressing changes twice each day. A home health nurse comes each morning and evening to change the dressing, and a home health aide comes 4 days per week to help him take a sponge bath, change his sheets weekly, and prepare a light lunch for him. The social worker has arranged for meals to be delivered through a neighborhood Meals on Wheels program. His wound gradually heals and he gains strength. He no longer needs home health assistance and goes to the senior center for his noon meal most days.

Hospice

The National Hospice and Palliative Care Organization defines **hospice** as "a medically-directed nurse-coordinated program providing a continuum of home and inpatient care for the terminally ill patient and family." The appropriate time for hospice care is when the patient is no longer seeking treatment to arrest or cure the disease and is expected to live 6 months or less. The patient is treated with medications and other measures to relieve pain and remain comfortable. Hospice services include management of the patient's pain and symptoms, emotional support to the patient and family, medications, medical supplies and equipment, caregiver instructions and support, coordination of all health care services, and grief support for surviving loved ones and friends.

The hospice team usually consists of home health aides, a hospice physician, nurses, social workers, a chaplain or clergy, and trained volunteers, and may include the patient's personal physician. For more information about hospice, see Chapter 10.

Knowledge Connection

How are inpatient and outpatient settings different? What types of diseases are treated and tracked by health departments? How are home health care and hospice care similar? How are they different?

Whatever the setting or level of care, nurses provide quality care to patients. This requires organization, in-depth knowledge of patient care, and application of that knowledge in a variety of situations.

Delivery of Nursing Care

When you care for patients, you deliver nursing care. This may be accomplished in several different ways. It is important for you to be familiar with these delivery systems to understand your role in each of them. Some systems are well suited to specific settings, but would not work as well in others. The most commonly used types of delivery for nursing care include team nursing, client-centered care, primary care nursing, and case management.

Team Nursing

Team nursing uses a team consisting of nurses and certified nursing assistants (CNAs) or unlicensed assistive personnel (UAPs) to provide care for a group of patients. This type of delivery system for nursing care is often used in the acute care hospital, rehabilitation setting, and long-term care setting. In team nursing, each member of the team provides nursing care depending on his or her skills, education, and licensure.

For example, a nursing care team in the acute care hospital might consist of an RN, an LPN, and a UAP or CNA, all of whom are responsible for the care of 10 patients. The RN might be responsible for assessing patients, administering some or all of the IV medications, maintaining the IV sites, communicating with physicians and obtaining orders, and ensuring that other team members have performed and documented care appropriately. The LPN/LVN might be responsible for administering medications to all of the patients as well as performing any treatments (for example, dressing changes), assessing the patient for any changes from baseline, evaluating pain levels and medicating appropriately, and providing patient teaching. The UAP or CNA might be responsible for helping each patient bathe and dress in a clean gown, changing sheets on the beds, assisting patients to the bathroom, and taking routine vital signs. The job duties are divided by the nursing team's level of knowledge and education. That is not to say that only nursing assistants should help a patient to the bathroom. The needs of the patients must be the first priority with everyone on the team.

A disadvantage of team nursing is that, without excellent communication between team members, care may become fragmented.

Client-Centered Care

Client-centered care empowers the patient to take control of and manage his or her care. This type of system is often seen in a rehabilitation setting. It allows patients to achieve independence within the limits of their disability by permitting them to have a voice in their rehabilitation, schedule, goals, and method of attaining those goals.

Client-centered care in the acute care hospital setting varies. In that setting, the goal is to decrease the number of people who give care to the patient so that there is less chance of miscommunication or error, and to provide care as soon as it is needed instead of having to wait for people from different departments to arrive. Health care workers are cross-trained to perform as many tasks as possible for each patient. For example, in some client-centered care settings, the nurse not only performs the usual nursing care, but also obtains needed blood specimens, runs an *electrocardiogram* or EKG (a tracing of electrical heart activity) when indicated, and may even administer respiratory therapy treatments. In this situation, no phlebotomist comes in to draw blood, no EKG technician is requested if the patient is having chest pain, and no respiratory therapy technician is needed to give a breathing treatment. One disadvantage of this type of care in the acute care hospital is the time and education needed for each staff member to cross-train in all of these areas.

Primary Care Nursing

In **primary care nursing**, one nurse is responsible for all aspects of nursing care for his or her assigned patients. This means that there is no UAP or CNA who takes vital signs, no other nurse to call the physician or take orders, no one else who bathes the patient or changes the bed. In this type of nursing, the nurse carries a great deal of responsibility. A secondary nurse is assigned care for the patient when the primary nurse is off duty.

The primary care nursing model is often used in intensive care units. An RN or LPN/LVN provides all aspects of nursing care to one or two critically ill patients. These nurses must be able to work quickly and efficiently in a crisis or under stress. In addition, they must be able to assess the patient carefully, making sure to note any small change in the patient's condition and correctly interpreting its significance. A disadvantage of this type of nursing delivery is that it works best when the number of patients assigned to the nurse is very limited, so it does not work well outside critical care areas.

Case Management

The delivery of nursing care via a **case management** system is associated with a managed care strategy. The nurses providing case management services act simultaneously as coordinators, facilitators, impartial advocates, and educators. These case managers can be found in hospitals, rehabilitation facilities, and home health agencies, and handling workers' compensation claims resulting from severe injury or disability. The process of case management involves seeing each patient as an individual and each situation as unique. The goal of case management is to assist patients who are vulnerable, at-risk, or cost intensive so that their care is coordinated, meets their specific needs, and is cost-effective while still bringing them to optimum health.

An example of case management would be a nurse employed by an insurance company who is managing the care of a patient who was injured in a bridge collapse, resulting in numerous broken bones. The hospital nearest the bridge is a small rural hospital without specialty care for orthopedics or bone specialists. The patient was taken there because it was the closest facility. The case manager arranges for the stable patient to be transferred to an appropriate specialty unit in a nearby city via helicopter. At that facility, the patient's injuries are quickly evaluated and treated. In a short time, the case manager arranges for the patient to transfer to a rehabilitation facility that specializes in multiple trauma. The patient gets the best possible care for his injuries and quickly moves into rehabilitation because the case manager was able to locate the most appropriate facilities for him and arrange to have him treated there.

Case managers may also supervise the care of a group of patients within one facility, such as an acute care hospital or home health agency. In that situation, the case manager ensures that each assigned patient is receiving cost-effective care while reaching goals of a return to optimal health and function.

A disadvantage of this type of nursing delivery is that case managers' options may be limited, depending on the availability of adequate facilities and funding to move the patient to the optimum facility.

Knowledge Connection
Give one advantage and one disadvantage for each type of nursing care delivery system. Which system seems the best for providing optimum patient care? Which system seems the most cost-effective?

Supervision/Delegation Connection
The Secret to Good Supervision
RNs and LPNs may function as managers or supervisors. It is important to remember that, when you supervise other nurses, you are supervising health care professionals. Avoid allowing a position of supervision to "go to your head." Put yourself in the place of the people you supervise. Always treat them with respect and avoid being overly critical. Everyone responds well to positive comments about their work. Find positives to praise, and if you must correct another nurse or nursing assistant, be as kind as possible.

Health Care Economics

Whose responsibility is it to pay the cost of health insurance? Is it an individual's responsibility or the government's? In the United States, there is a great deal of debate on this issue. Eighteen percent of the population younger than age 65 were without health insurance in 2007, according to the National Coalition on Health Care. The numbers have no doubt increased since then. Also in 2007, 62% of the population had employer-based health care, a number that is projected to fall due to job losses and health care costs. Because of the increasing number of uninsured, the cost of private and public health insurance is steadily increasing to help hospitals and doctors defray those health care costs. How does an uninsured person pay for insurance if he or she is unemployed or too ill to work? What are the most important factors in determining the need and payment for health care?

Health care and health care costs are two of the most important issues in the United States economy. According to the National Coalition on Health Care, total spending was $2.3 trillion in 2007, or $7,600 for each United States citizen. Health care costs are paid for in one of five ways:

• Public health insurance
• Private health insurance

- Insurance for special populations
- Charitable organizations
- Self-pay (those without health insurance)

Public Health Insurance

Public health insurance is funded by the government, either state or federal, or a combination of both. Medicare and Medicaid are forms of public health insurance, as is the Indian Health Service.

Medicare

As discussed at the beginning of this chapter, Medicare is the federal government's acute care health insurance program for people older than 65 years of age. It is also available to disabled individuals younger than 65 years of age, individuals with end-stage renal disease, or those with certain debilitating illnesses. Medicare includes four programs, which are described in Box 2-2.

Medicare employs a payment schedule based on **diagnosis-related groups (DRGs)**. These classifications of illnesses and diseases are used to determine the amount of money paid by Medicare to the hospital for the care of a patient with that particular illness or disease. For example, a patient might be admitted to the hospital with diabetes. According to the DRGs, Medicare will pay the hospital a certain amount for the care of this diabetic patient, which includes all nursing care, tests, treatments, and teaching. If the patient stays in the hospital longer than the allowed time or it costs the hospital more than the set amount for the patient's care, the payment will still be the set amount of the DRG. If the patient has complicating factors that affect the hospital stay, such as if the patient gets an infection or develops a new problem in addition to diabetes, the hospital can submit bills for the additional problems under a different DRG.

Box 2.2

Medicare Programs

Medicare includes several types of programs. Parts A through D each provide a different aspect of care for eligible patients.
- **Part A:** insurance for hospitalization, hospice, home health, and skilled nursing facility services.
- **Part B:** supplementary health insurance to help pay participating providers, such as physicians, laboratories, x-ray technicians, and home health nurses, and for durable medical equipment.
- **Part C:** also called Medicare Advantage Plans, which are health insurance plans administered by private insurance companies in place of traditional Medicare.
- **Part D:** also known as Medicare Prescription Drug Coverage, provides payment for prescribed medications and is run by insurance companies or other private companies approved by Medicare.

Medicaid

Medicaid is a federal-state government matching funding program. Because the state is required to set coverage policies and administer the program, the benefits are slightly different in each state. This program offers assistance for poor and medically indigent individuals, pregnant women with an income below the poverty level, children meeting certain income-level requirements, and certain disabled individuals meeting income-level requirements.

Indian Health Service

The Indian Health Service (IHS) provides government funding for health care for qualified Native American individuals. The IHS may fund hospitals, ambulatory medical and mental health care clinics, and dental care facilities. It may contract with one or more of the federally recognized tribes to fund health care services in that tribe's reservation territory. Individuals utilizing these health care services must meet criteria for a "certificate of degree of Indian blood (CDIB)" in order to be eligible to receive care. A CDIB card is issued when an individual meets the criteria set by the tribe. This card enables the individual to receive health care services at tribal and IHS facilities.

Private Health Insurance

When a person uses private health insurance, he or she, known as the beneficiary, pays premiums to the insurance company. When the beneficiary is cared for by a physician or hospital and the bill is sent to the insurance company, the insurance company is referred to as a third party or a **third-party payer**. Blue Cross Blue Shield, Aetna, United Health, and Prudential are a few of the largest private health insurance companies currently operating in the United States.

Private health insurance companies offer several types of health insurance plans and services. Box 2-3 provides a brief explanation of the most common types. The development of these plans came about as a strategy to help contain the cost of health care by restricting patients' access to only those groups of health care providers who have contracted to provide specific services at a negotiated price.

Capitation refers to the payment system employed by health maintenance organizations (HMOs). In this system, **primary care physicians** (PCPs) are paid a set amount per member per month to manage the health care of those members. This PCP is considered the gatekeeper to health services for the individual enrolled in the HMO. For example, a PCP may have 200 patients assigned to him or her. Perhaps the set amount per member is $40. The PCP is paid $8,000 per month to see all the patients who make appointments and perhaps to make hospital rounds as well. If the PCP is unable to successfully treat the patient's condition, he or she makes a **referral** to a specialist. The patient cannot self-refer, and the specialist cannot accept the patient without a referral. In this way, access to more costly care and potentially redundant testing is controlled.

Common Types of Health Insurance Programs

Health insurance programs fall under several main categories.

- **Health Maintenance Organization (HMO):** A cost containment program featuring a primary care physician (PCP) as the gatekeeper to eliminate unnecessary testing and procedures; this is a capitated system requiring the insured person to remain within the network.
- **Preferred Provider Organization (PPO):** A group of health care providers who contract with a health insurance company to provide services to a specific group of patients on a discounted basis.
- **Point-of-Service (POS) Plan:** This is similar to the HMO in that a primary care physician still serves as a gatekeeper, but it is not capitated. Insured people can seek care from physicians who are both in and out of the network. The patient pays a part of the bill (usually 20% to 30%) and the insurance company pays the remainder.

Patient Teaching Connection

Teaching About HMO Regulations

Teach patients enrolled in HMOs the importance of going through their PCPs before accessing care to ensure that the care will be covered. If it is not ordered by their PCP, the insurance company may deny the claim. It is extremely important that patients understand the requirements of their insurance plan. Teach patients that, before any procedures, surgeries, and tests are performed, the patient or physician's staff must obtain prior authorization by contacting the insurance company and acquiring approval for the treatment.

Private health insurance is available in different venues. Individuals may participate in group health insurance plans provided by employers. With this type of health insurance, the employer pays a portion or all of the cost of the premium. The company may offer one type of health plan or may offer a variety of plans, and the individual can choose from several types of coverage for different prices. The employer decides what types of policies are available to the employee. The options available to the employer may include HMO, preferred provider organization (PPO), or point-of-service (POS) plans.

The company may also define and fund its own benefits, and have a health insurance company administer the benefits according to the employer's defined requirements. The employer generally negotiates with the health insurance company to utilize their HMO, PPO, or POS networks to provide health care services to their members.

Individual policies may also be purchased directly from a health insurance company. This type of policy generally does not have the extent of benefits that the group policies offer. This policy is priced so that an individual can afford the full price of the premium, whereas with the group policy the employer and employee both pay a portion of the premium. Individual policies generally utilize PPO or POS networks.

Health Insurance Plans for Specific Populations

Some health insurance plans are designed to serve only a specific group of people. TRICARE is an insurance plan for active and retired military service members and their families, and CHAMPVA provides free health benefits for veterans of military service. Workers' compensation insurance provides for people who are injured on the job. It pays for medical costs and some living costs while the person is unable to work. Disability insurance is designed specifically for those who cannot work due to some type of temporary or permanent disability.

Charitable Organizations

There are also local, state, and national charitable organizations that provide free health care services to individuals. These organizations may be funded by religious denominations, private individuals, or national or community organizations such as the Catholic and Jewish health systems, the Shriners, the Kaiser family, and Robert Wood Johnson foundation, just to name a few.

Self-Pay

Many people in the United States do not fall into any of the above categories for obtaining health insurance. For example, those who are self-employed often make too much money to qualify for Medicaid, are too young to qualify for Medicare, and do not have enough employees to qualify for a group health policy. They must pay the full amount for any insurance they obtain, which can be cost-prohibitive for a small business owner. Some programs are available through certain small business associations, but they tend to be expensive because they require membership dues for the association as well as payment of insurance premiums.

Some small businesses are unable to provide health insurance as a benefit to their employees, especially as costs for health insurance continue to increase. The employer cannot pay a portion of the cost, and the employee is unable to pay the full cost, so he or she may not have health insurance.

Another example of those without insurance includes people who are between jobs. They may have been laid off from one position and been unable to find another position quickly. While they have the option of continuing the health care coverage provided during their earlier employment, they must pay the full premium, which may be more than they can afford when they are surviving on a reduced income.

Some people, while employed full time or part time, are classified as temporary employees and are not eligible for benefits such as employer-paid health insurance. Again, these individuals may not be able to afford the full cost of the insurance premiums for themselves and their families.

Another example of people who cannot afford to pay for insurance is those who have divorced from a husband or wife who carried insurance through his or her employer.

The uninsured spouse may not have skills to work for an employer who provides or offers insurance benefits.

 Post Conference

During Post Conference with your clinical group, a discussion about insurance and the lack of insurance ensues. Some people seem rather judgmental, saying, "The uninsured cost everyone else money." You explain that your patient had worked full time and did have insurance. She was laid off 8 weeks after being diagnosed with cancer and could not get another job because she was too ill. She could not afford to continue paying the insurance premiums from her previous job and had to let her insurance lapse. She cannot get a new insurance policy because she is considered uninsurable due to the cancer. It is also considered a pre-existing condition, so no new insurance company will cover it. You had no idea how to help her, but you learned a great deal from the RN in charge of her care. He brought in the hospital social worker to help the patient apply for Medicaid if she qualifies. He talked to her doctor about home health care to do the dressing changes, IV antibiotics, and assessments. The physician agreed and the RN got everything scheduled. The patient will be discharged today with the home health nurse to see her this evening.

KEY POINTS

- The two most important factors in payment for health care delivery are medical necessity and appropriate level of care.

- The health care team is made up of a number of professionals and assistants who include medical, nursing, therapeutic, laboratory, radiology, and ancillary staff. It is impossible to provide thorough health care without the help of everyone on the team.

- A variety of inpatient and outpatient settings exist to provide health care. It is important for patients to obtain needed care in the most appropriate setting to deliver cost-effective health care.

- Nursing care is delivered in a variety of ways. Some commonly used delivery systems are team nursing, client-centered care, primary care nursing, and case management.

- Health care is costly, and there are a number of ways the costs may be paid. These include public and private health insurance, insurance for special populations, charitable organizations, and self-pay.

- Public health insurance is funded by the federal government or state governments, or a combination of both. It includes Medicare, Medicaid, and the Indian Health Service.

- Private health insurance companies, also known as "third-party payers," include health maintenance organizations (HMOs), preferred provider organizations (PPOs), and point-of-service (POS) plans and variations of these services.

- HMOs pay primary care providers (PCPs) by a capitation system. The PCP is the gatekeeper for referrals to other health care professionals such as specialists and therapists.

- PPOs and POS plans rely on previously negotiated discount agreements between the insurance companies and the health care providers, including specialists.

- Many situations exist that prevent Americans from being able to afford health care insurance, and this is of great concern to those both inside and outside the health care system.

REVIEW QUESTIONS

Select the answer that is most appropriate for each of the following questions. Some questions may have more than one correct answer. Check all that apply.

1. Which of the following would NOT be considered medically necessary by an insurance company?

   a. Surgery to remove an infected gallbladder

   b. Breast implants to increase breast size

   c. Breast implants after breast cancer surgery

   d. Botox injections to decrease facial wrinkles

   e. Skin grafts to repair a spider bite injury

2. If an elderly person needed help with meals, medications, and personal care, but did not need continuous nursing care, which inpatient setting would be the most appropriate level of care?

   a. A skilled nursing facility

   b. A long-term acute care hospital

   c. An assisted living facility

   d. A long-term care facility

3. Which member of the therapy staff would be consulted if a patient had difficulty swallowing?

   a. Speech therapist

   b. Physical therapist

   c. Occupational therapist

   d. Respiratory therapist

4. A cost-efficient way to provide care to people who are confined to their homes due to illness or disability is the use of:

   a. the hospital outpatient department.

   b. a skilled nursing facility.

   c. the health department.

   d. home health care.

5. A patient who is terminally ill with cancer is no longer being treated with radiation or *chemotherapy* (cancer-attacking medication). The most appropriate level of care for this patient would be:

   a. home health care.

   b. hospice.

   c. a skilled nursing facility.

   d. a long-term care acute hospital.

6. You are working on a large medical unit with 30 patients requiring medications, therapies, dressing changes, and pain management. Nursing staff for the day shift consists of two RNs, three LPNs, and three CNAs. Which type of nursing care delivery would you expect to work best on this unit?

   a. Team nursing

   b. Client-centered care

   c. Primary care nursing

   d. Case management

7. Payment to hospitals for the care of Medicare patients is based on:

   a. a specified amount per member per month.

   b. the actual costs of all supplies, equipment, tests, and nursing care.

   c. diagnosis-related groups (DRGs).

   d. a previously negotiated discount rate.

8. Eligibility for Indian Health Service is:

   a. based on having a certificate of degree of Indian blood.

   b. available to all people with at least 25% Indian blood.

   c. set by each tribe.

   d. determined by presenting a family genealogy.

   e. determined by blood type.

CRITICAL THINKING EXERCISES

9. If a patient with HMO coverage wanted to see a specialist for a skin condition, what must the patient do *first*?

10. How would you respond to the following statement by a fellow nursing student? "People who do not have health insurance just make excuses. If they got a job and worked like the rest of us, they would have insurance."

ADDITIONAL RESOURCES

For additional Resources, Questions, and Activities, please see:

 Student Resource Disk

DavisPlus **http://davisplus.fadavis.com**

 Student Study Guide

REFERENCES

American Heart Association. What is cardiac rehabilitation? 2007. Available at: http://www.americanheart.org/downloadable/heart/119620120447745%20WhatIsCardiacRehab%209_07.pdf. Accessed July 29, 2009.

American Thoracic Society. Pulmonary rehabilitation. 2008. Available at: http://www.thoracic.org/sections/clinical-information/pulmonary-rehabilitation/index.html. Accessed July 29, 2009.

Beyers M, Phillips C. *Nursing Management for Patient Care.* Boston: Little, Brown; 1971.

eMedicineHealth. Outpatient surgery. 2008. Available at: http://www.emedicinehealth.com/outpatient_surgery/article_em.htm. Accessed July 29, 2009.

Medicare Information Source. Medicare Part A—Coverage for Skilled Nursing Facility Care. 2008. Available at: http://www.medicare.org. Accessed July 29, 2009.

Mullahy CM, Jensen DK. *The Case Manager's Handbook.* Boston: Jones and Bartlett; 2004.

National Center for Assisted Living. NCAL's guiding principles for quality in assisted living. 2008. Available at: http://www.ahcancal.org/ncal/about/Documents/GPAssistedLiving.pdf. Accessed July 29, 2009.

National Coalition on Health Care. Health insurance costs. July 31, 2008. Available at: http://www.nchc.org/issue-areas/cost.

National Hospice and Palliative Care Organization. Definition of hospice. May 25, 2008. Available at: http://www.caringinfo.org/CaringForSomeone/Hospice/TheHospiceTeam.htm.

The Princeton Review. Career profiles—hospital administrator. April 30, 2008. Available at: http://www.princetonreview.com.

U.S. Department of Labor, Bureau of Labor Statistics. Occupational Outlook Handbook, 2008. Available at: http://www.bls.gov/oco/. Accessed July 29, 2009.

Williams L, Hopper P. *Understanding Medical Surgical Nursing.* 3rd ed. Philadephia: FA Davis; 2007.

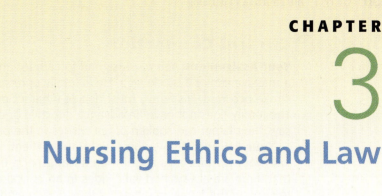

Nursing Ethics and Law

Key Terms

Abandonment

Advance directive

Advocate

Assault

Battery

Centers for Disease Control
and Prevention (CDC)

Emancipated minor

Empathy

Ethics

Good Samaritan Law

Health Insurance Portability
and Accountability Act (HIPAA)

Incident report

Informed consent

Malpractice

Negligence

Nurse Practice Act

Precedent

Scope of practice

Standards of care

Value

Objectives

1. Define key terms relating to nursing ethics and law.
2. Explain what it means to advocate for a patient.
3. Identify at least six types of unethical behavior that as a nurse you must report.
4. Describe ways in which you could violate HIPAA regulations within a hospital or clinic setting.
5. Locate your state's Nurse Practice Act using the Internet.
6. Read your state's Nurse Practice Act in its entirety.
7. Specify two areas of mandatory reporting for nurses.
8. Name five areas of tort law that apply to the nurse.
9. Identify at least five ways to keep your nursing practice up to date after graduating.
10. Explain ways to make your nursing entries in the patient's chart so that the chart would serve you well in a court of law.
11. Compare a proxy directive to an instructional directive.
12. Apply nursing ethics and laws to specific scenarios.

Clinical Connection

Your Assignment: You are assigned to care for an 86-year-old patient who had a massive stroke 2 weeks ago. He is totally unresponsive and has been since the stroke occurred. His family must decide whether or not to put in a feeding tube. The family does not have an advance directive or durable power of attorney, but says their father has spoken of his wishes in the past.

Your Actions: Before you care for this patient, you must first come to terms with your own feelings about the ethical aspects of this situation. Keep in mind that there are always two valid sides in an ethical dilemma. You must also plan to support the family in whatever they decide, and not judge them if they make a different decision than you would make. Although you are definitely a patient advocate, in this situation a case could be made for placing a feeding tube or for leaving it out. You may even be allowed to attend an ethics committee meeting in the hospital regarding this situation. You will plan to give complete care for this patient.

The goal of your nursing care should be to improve the quality of the patient's living and dying. As you strive to determine how to best accomplish this goal, there are many laws and regulatory guidelines that will be instrumental in determining what you can, cannot, should, and should not do. Once the legal and regulatory boundaries have been designated, you must then consider the codes of professional ethics and personal ethics. *Professional ethics* are published formal statements indicating the profession's expectations for its members. An example is the American Nurses Association (ANA) *Code of Ethics for Nurses* (Box 3-1).

One principle that can provide overall guidance during your career is the following: *Never do anything that you know is not in the patient's best interest.* This requires you to evaluate your own moral and ethical codes so you can more effectively deal with those of the patient. This self-evaluation does not happen overnight. It requires inquiry, thought, analysis, and time to identify the moral and ethical codes that dictate who you are and how you relate to others. We encourage you to initiate this process now as you begin your nursing education. Many nurses in practice today have never evaluated their own codes of ethics and morality.

Ethics

As a nurse, you will face many ethical dilemmas regarding honesty, organ transplantation issues, informed consent, child and elder abuse, surrogate mother issues, honoring advance directives, and other life-and-death decisions such

Box 3-1

American Nurses Association Code of Ethics for Nurses

1. The nurse, in all professional relationships, practices with compassion and respect for the inherent dignity, worth and uniqueness of every individual, unrestricted by considerations of social or economic status, personal attributes, or the nature of health problems.
2. The nurse's primary commitment is to the patient, whether an individual, family, group, or community.
3. The nurse promotes, advocates for, and strives to protect the health, safety, and rights of the patient.
4. The nurse is responsible and accountable for individual nursing practice and determines the appropriate delegation of tasks consistent with the nurse's obligation to provide optimum patient care.
5. The nurse owes the same duties to self as to others, including the responsibility to preserve integrity and safety, to maintain competence, and to continue personal and professional growth.
6. The nurse participates in establishing, maintaining, and improving healthcare environments and conditions of employment conducive to the provision of quality health care and consistent with the values of the profession through individual and collective action.
7. The nurse participates in the advancement of the profession through contributions to practice, education, administration, and knowledge development.
8. The nurse collaborates with other health professionals and the public in promoting community, national, and international efforts to meet health needs.
9. The profession of nursing, as represented by associations and their members, is responsible for articulating nursing values, for maintaining the integrity of the profession and its practice, and for shaping social policy.

Source: American Nurses Association, *Code of Ethics for Nurses with Interpretive Statements,* © 2001 Nursesbooks.org, Silver Spring, MD.

as abortion, assisted suicide, euthanasia, "do-not-resuscitate" (DNR) orders, and withdrawal of artificial nutrition or ventilators. The more technology provides for artificial ways to preserve life, the more those situations develop in which you will have to make ethical decisions.

Before you can comfortably make these decisions affecting your nursing practice, you must determine your own values and ethics. A **value** is related to your belief of something's worth and may differ from the values of others around you. Your values are learned from your life experiences and determine who you are. Your **ethics** are made up of the values that influence your decisions and behavior. They are partially determined by what you believe is morally right and wrong and further structured by numerous other principles, such as:

• The patient's welfare is our primary concern.
• Individuals have the right to make choices even if the choices are not in their best interest.

An *ethical dilemma* is a situation in which a decision must be made between two opposing alternatives when there is not an exact right or wrong answer. Ethical decisions are not made with one's emotions or feelings, but are based on principles and logical reasoning. Open communication with those involved in these decisions is vital. In preparation to entering nursing, a profession rich with ethical dilemmas, examine your feelings about life, death, health, disease, spirituality, and religion. Familiarize yourself with the profession's codes of ethics (refer to Box 3-1). Reflect on patient expectations in the American Hospital Association's *The Patient Care Partnership,* which can be found in Box 3-2.

Once you clarify your beliefs and study these principles, you will be better equipped to deal with ethical situations as they arise.

Patients' Ethical Rights

Patients have the right to be treated ethically with advocacy, respect, dignity, honesty, and compassion. To **advocate** for a patient means to stand up for that which is in the patient's best interest, as opposed to that which is in the best interest of the physician, hospital, or coworker. The nurse serves as the primary patient advocate. Respect includes honoring the patient's feelings, beliefs, opinions, and decisions

---

Box 3-2

American Hospital Association's The Patient Care Partnership

The Patient Care Partnership: Understanding Expectations, Rights and Responsibilities

Our goal is for you and your family to have the same care and attention we would want for our families and ourselves. The sections explain some of the basics about how you can expect to be treated during your hospital stay. They also cover what we will need from you to care for you better. If you have questions at any time, please ask them. Unasked or unanswered questions can add to the stress of being in the hospital.

What to Expect During Your Hospital Stay

• **High quality hospital care.** Our first priority is to provide you the care you need, when you need it, with skill, compassion, and respect. Tell your caregivers if you have concerns about your care or if you have pain. You have the right to know the identity of doctors, nurses and others involved in your care.

• **A clean and safe environment.** We use special policies and procedures to avoid mistakes in your care and keep you free from abuse or neglect. If anything unexpected and significant happens during your hospital stay, you will be told what happened, and any resulting changes in your care will be discussed with you.

• **Involvement in your care.** Please tell your caregivers if you need more information about treatment choices. When decision-making takes place, it should include:

• *Discussing your medical condition and information about medically appropriate treatment choices.* To make informed decisions with your doctor, you need to understand:

• The benefits and risks of each treatment, and whether the treatment is experimental or part of a research study.

• What you can reasonably expect from your treatment and any long-term effects it might have on your quality of life.

• What you and your family will need to do after you leave the hospital.

• The financial consequences of using uncovered services or out-of-network providers.

• *Discussing your treatment plan.* When you enter the hospital, you sign a general consent to treatment. In some cases, such as surgery or experimental treatment, you may be asked to confirm in writing that you understand what is planned and agree to it.

• *Getting information from you.* Your caregivers need complete and correct information about your health and coverage so that they can make good decisions about your care. That includes:

• Past illnesses, surgeries or hospital stays, past allergic reactions; any medicines or dietary supplements (such as vitamins and herbs) that you are taking; and any network or admission requirements under your health plan.

• *Understanding your health care goals and values.* Make sure your doctor, your family and your care team know your wishes.

• *Understanding who should make decisions when you cannot.* If you have signed a health care power of attorney stating who should speak for you if you become unable to make health care decisions for yourself, or a "living will" or "advance directive" that states your wishes about end-of-life care, give copies to your doctor, your family and your care team.

• **Protection of your privacy.** State and federal laws and hospital operating policies protect the privacy of your medical information. You will receive a Notice of Privacy Practices that describes the ways that we use, disclose and safeguard patient information and that explains how you can obtain a copy of information from our records about your care.

(box continues on page 32)

whether you agree with them or not. Maintaining a patient's dignity means allowing and honoring the patient's possession of self-respect. Every patient is considered worthy of dignity and self-respect. To maintain one's dignity may even mean allowing the patient the freedom of refusing an aspect of care that he or she does not want, such as a particular medication or procedure. Honesty means being completely truthful about the patient's condition, test results, treatment options, and potential for recovery. Occasionally, family members will request that a patient not be told his or her diagnosis, but every patient deserves to know the truth about his or her own body, health, and ensuing death. Honesty also means acknowledging when you make a mistake, rather than hiding the fact. It requires you to report any type of illegal, incompetent, or impaired medical or nursing practices that you may come across. Compassion involves delivering nursing care with a gentle and caring attitude.

The golden rule that allows you to provide all these ethical rights is to treat every patient as you would want to be treated yourself or as you would want the most important person in your life to be treated.

Knowledge Connection
Explain what it means to serve as the patient's advocate.

Advocating for the Patient
It is paramount to remember your number-one role: you are to serve as the patient's advocate. In the acute care setting, nurses care for the patient 24 hours a day, 7 days per week. In other longer term care settings, nurses may care for the patient over a period of months or years. Therefore, as the nurse, you will have the opportunity to learn things about a patient that he or she may never share with another individual. What an awesome honor and responsibility! You will have opportunities to validate patients' feelings, to provide physical care and comfort, and to assist patients to live and die with dignity. *You must stand with the patient, you must stand for the patient, and you must stand by the patient, always asserting yourself in the patient's best interest.*

Serving as the patient's advocate requires you to assist and provide care to the patient without imposing your own values upon the patient. Because your values change over time as you grow and experience life events, you should examine your values at this stage of your education and continue to re-evaluate them at intervals during your career.

To be a good nurse, you will need to develop empathy for patients and families as well as coworkers. **Empathy** is the ability to intellectually or emotionally understand the feelings of another person without actually experiencing or even agreeing with their situation, thoughts, feelings, distress, or pain. It is different from *sympathy,* which is sharing the feelings and distress of the other individual.

Reporting Unethical Behavior
Nurses are responsible for reporting unethical behavior and misconduct by other nurses. Not to do so is considered negligence. **Negligence** is defined as a patient injury that occurs because the nurse fails to meet his or her responsibility to the patient. If it seems like tattling, remember that you are the patient's advocate, not the nurse's advocate. *If you do not advocate for the patient...who will?*

The authority to which you report unethical behavior differs from state to state, requiring you to be familiar with your own state laws. Most unethical behaviors would be reported to your immediate supervisor and the Board of Nursing. Behaviors to be reported include but are not limited to:

- Impairment of a nurse by alcohol, prescription or illegal drugs, or severe fatigue
- Diverting drugs by taking a patient's medications, such as narcotics, for personal use but charting them as administered to the patient
- Abuse or mistreatment of patients, both known and suspected
- Fraudulent documentation
- Practicing without a license
- Incompetence
- Failure to follow physician's orders
- Failure to perform a necessary action
- Practice outside the individual's scope of practice

Ethics Committees

Most hospitals have an ethics committee responsible for reviewing ethical issues related to patient care. The committee members may serve the hospital by developing its policies and procedures for handling ethical issues such as DNRs and organ transplantation. When there is a decision to be made concerning cessation of life support or artificial nutrition, it may be reviewed by the ethics committee. The committee generally serves the patient and his or her rights as its focal point of concern. Family members may request that the ethics committee be consulted regarding differing opinions related to medical or nursing care issues.

Do-Not-Resuscitate Orders

You must initiate cardiopulmonary resuscitation if a patient stops breathing unless there is a written DNR order. In certain situations when a patient is in the terminal stages of a disease and not expected to live much longer, the physician may write a DNR order in the patient's chart. This order may be the result of a living will, a verbal request made by the patient to the physician, or, in the absence of a patient's ability to request it, a family's request made to the physician. This generally indicates that the care for the patient should be limited to that which allows for comfort and dignity, while withholding life-extending steps such as cardiopulmonary resuscitation, tube feeding, or use of a ventilator to breathe for the patient.

Law

As you are probably aware, we live in a world of increasing litigation, some justifiable and some not so justifiable. Individuals sue wealthy corporations for injuries resulting from the individual's own ineptness. Criminals, hurt in the act of breaking the law, sometimes sue their intended victim. Sometimes they even win monetary settlements. The world of nursing that you are entering is not exempt from the increasing frequency of lawsuits. While working as a nurse, you will constantly hold the lives of others in your hands. It is of the utmost importance that you understand the state and federal laws, rules, and regulations, as well as personal and professional ethics, that regulate your nursing practice. These laws and ethics define the boundaries in which nurses may work and still be protected. Without this knowledge, you will find yourself ill-prepared to protect your license and career, patients, and coworkers. Table 3-1 provides a list of commonly used legal terms and their definitions.

Table 3-1   Common Legal Terminology

Term	Definition
Abandonment of patient	To desert or forsake a patient in your charge; to leave a patient in your charge without appropriate nursing replacement; wrongful termination of care.
Advance directive	A written statement indicating a patient's wishes regarding future medical care in the event the patient becomes unable to voice his or her decisions. It may give consent for certain aspects of care as well as refusal of specific care.
Appeal	To challenge the decision of a court to a higher court, where the decision will either be confirmed or reversed.
Assault	To purposely threaten physical harm to an individual.
Battery	To touch an individual without consent.
Civil law	The individual or personal rights guaranteed by federal law, such as the Constitution and the Bill of Rights.
Competency	The legal qualification to make one's own decisions.
Consent	To give permission for, to agree to; the consent generally must be written.
Controlled substances	Drugs regulated by laws; drugs that have potential for abuse, such as narcotics.
Criminal law	Laws that protect the public or society.
Damages	Money awarded to a plaintiff upon proving injury by the defendant.

(table continues on page 34)

Table 3-1 **Common Legal Terminology** (continued)

Term	Definition
Defendant	The one accused of breaking criminal or civil law.
Durable medical power of attorney	Legal written designation making another person responsible for one's medical decisions.
Emancipated minor	Legal consideration of one younger than the age of 18 as an adult, due to living alone and supporting oneself, joining the military, marriage, or parenthood.
Liability	One's responsibility for his or her own actions, such as acts of negligence.
Libel	False written statements about another that are made publicly known, with intent to harm.
Malpractice	Injury, loss, or damage to a patient due to failure to provide a reasonable standard of care or demonstrate a reasonable level of skill.
Negligence	Failure to provide certain care that another person of the same education and locale would generally provide under the same circumstances.
Plaintiff	The one accusing another of criminal or civil law violation.
Statute	A written law.
Tort	A violation of a civil law; involves a wrong against an individual or his or her property.

One of the most important things you can do is to treat all patients with respect and dignity and to develop a trusting relationship with each patient. If your patient trusts you, feels secure that you have given your best effort, and believes that you have delivered your nursing care in a respectful manner and have consistently treated him or her with dignity, the patient is not likely to sue you, even if you do make a mistake. By assuming this active, rather than passive, role in establishing good nurse-patient rapport, you become proactive rather than being reactive. You will find it beneficial to become knowledgeable and proactive, as taking these steps can decrease your risk of being sued.

Knowledge Connection

Explain what it means to be proactive. Why is it better to be proactive rather than reactive? How do trust, respect, and dignity affect your likelihood of being sued?

Types of Laws

There are different types of laws that affect you as a nurse. The federal government provides two sources of laws that govern nurses: constitutional law and statutory law. An example of *constitutional law* is the U.S. Bill of Rights, which provides U.S. citizens with 10 rights, one of which, the right to privacy, directly affects your nursing practice. Patients have legal rights to privacy and confidentiality.

Federal, state, and local governments pass laws that are known as *statutory laws.* The most common statute governing licensed nurses is passed by the state legislature and known as the **Nurse Practice Act** (NPA), which provides the scope of nursing as designated by each state. The state legislature also creates agencies to supervise hospitals; health care professionals, including nurses; and licensure. These agencies write and enforce rules and regulations dictating the boundaries within which nurses must practice, termed *administrative laws.* These laws are designated to enforce statutes. One such agency created by the state legislature is the state Board of Nursing, which writes the rules and regulations for enforcement of each state's NPA.

Case or *judicial laws* are written in response to specific legal questions brought before the courts. Once these courts decide these questions, **precedents** are set by which similar future cases will be judged. All laws are designated as either criminal law or civil law. *Criminal laws* protect the public or society as a whole. *Civil laws* protect an individual's personal rights, such as life, liberty, thinking, speaking, privacy, and most health care issues.

Statutory Law

The layperson probably does not equate regulation of nursing with federal and state statutes or laws. However, as you begin your journey as a nurse, it is important that you recognize that your nursing practice and license are subject to federal laws such as the **Health Insurance Portability and Accountability Act (HIPAA)** of 1996 and state statutes, specifically your state's NPA. Even though you are not yet licensed, as a nursing student you are held to the same standards as a licensed nurse. You are responsible to meet all federal and state requirements while *competently* performing *only* those skills for which you have been trained.

Health Insurance Portability and Accountability Act of 1996

Better known as the privacy protector, HIPAA was implemented by regulations of the U.S. Department of Health and Human Services in 1996. It provides for confidential maintenance of protected health information.

HIPAA mandates that hospitals, clinics, and other health care providers handle patients' records in a manner that will protect record confidentiality. The presence of an individual as a patient may not be acknowledged to others without expressed patient permission, and patient records and charts may not be left open and visible to the public at the nurse's station. Facilities using computerized charting must institute measures to prevent patient records from being viewed or accessed by inappropriate individuals. Discussion of patients must be carefully guarded and held only in areas where privacy is ensured, ruling out conversations regarding patients in hallways, dining rooms, and elevators. HIPAA also ensures patients the right to view and amend their own health record, as well as obtain a copy of the entire medical record upon request. This is discussed further in Chapter 5.

The only health care providers who have a right to access the patient chart are those workers directly involved in the care of that patient. As a student, you are held to the same confidentiality rules and regulations as licensed health care providers.

Laboratory and Diagnostic Connection

Confidentiality of HIV and AIDS Test Results

When a patient's test results for HIV and AIDS are positive, this information must be handled confidentially. You must have patient permission to discuss these test results with a spouse or other family members. Discussing the results without obtaining permission is a violation of HIPAA.

Real-World Connection

How Easy Is It to Accidently Breach HIPAA Laws?

A licensed nurse was finishing up a long and difficult shift. The weather was icy, and the forecast was for even more ice. As the nurse was giving report to the oncoming shift, her husband called her on her cell phone. Due to the weather, cell connections had been difficult to maintain. She asked her husband to hold and laid down her cell phone, then continued to give the rest of her report. She was later called in by the facility's privacy officer and disciplined for violating HIPAA and patient confidentiality.

As you can see, you can violate confidentiality without intending to do so. A breach of confidentiality such as this could easily have resulted in a civil lawsuit, monetary fine, and termination from employment. A written disciplinary action was placed in the nurse's personnel file. Luckily, there were no lawsuits or fines and the nurse was not fired from her job...this time.

Nurse Practice Acts

Each state has in place an NPA that defines the scope of nursing within its state. States differ in the groups of people who are governed by their NPA. For example, California has two separate practice acts, one for LVNs (the equivalent of LPNs in other states) and another for RNs. Oklahoma's NPA covers LPNs, RNs, advanced practice RNs, and authorized UAPs. Ohio's NPA includes RNs, LPNs, dialysis technicians, certified medication assistants, and community health workers. In each state, the state agency designated to administer and enforce the NPAs is the state Board of Nursing. This board has the authority to:

- License nurses
- Take disciplinary measures against nurses who fail to follow the NPA
- Regulate the practice of nursing as well as nursing education

The primary purpose of NPAs is to protect the public's health, safety, and welfare from harm related to nursing care. The **scope of practice** sets legal boundaries for nursing care. For example, LPN/LVNs must work under the supervision of an RN, physician, or dentist. All NPAs require the nurse to be knowledgeable about his or her own state NPA, to perform within its constraints, and to maintain professional demeanor. NPAs stipulate that nurses will provide for patient confidentiality and safety, as well as demonstrate competency providing nursing care and administering medications. They generally provide a lengthy list of actions that will result in disciplinary judgment, probation, or licensure revocation. If these actions occur while the individual is still a student, it may prevent the student from being allowed to take the National Council Licensure Examination licensing examination.

Student nurses are held to the same legal standards as licensed nurses. Every student nurse and licensed nurse has a moral, ethical, professional, and legal responsibility to be familiar with his or her own state's NPA. To locate your state Board of Nursing, see the student resources for this textbook found at www.davisplus.com. It provides a complete listing of state boards of nursing, along with their corresponding address, phone, and other pertinent information. It is highly recommended that you locate the website of your state Board of Nursing at this time. Then access the NPA and read the entire document. If you do not read it and begin to absorb its content during the early stages of your education, it makes it more difficult to practice within its boundaries once you begin your clinical experiences.

Licensure

Each state requires nurses, both practical nurses and registered nurses, to become licensed in order to practice nursing. To obtain your nursing license, you will be required to demonstrate preparedness by passing the National Council Licensure Examination (NCLEX), a computerized test developed to determine nursing competence. There are separate examinations for practical nursing and registered nursing, dependent upon your level of education.

A fee is paid along with application to the National Council of the State Boards of Nursing to sit for the examination. Once you have successfully passed the NCLEX, you are eligible to apply for licensure in any of the 50 states. You must have a license for the specific state in which you work. Each state has its own procedures to follow for initial licensure application. Most states require payment of an application fee and demonstration that the individual can read, write, and understand English. An increasing number of states are making reciprocity agreements, which means they recognize licenses from other states and will grant you permission to practice in their state without repeating the entire process of applying for licensure.

Mandatory Reporting Laws

Most states have laws requiring certain conditions to be reported to the proper authorities. One of the most common is related to communicable diseases and immunizations. This reporting helps to protect the public, track outbreaks or occurrences of disease, and aid health authorities such as the **Centers for Disease Control and Prevention (CDC)** in determining steps to take regarding treatment and containment of illness, immunizations, and future research.

Another area of mandatory reporting is the abuse of children. All 50 states require that you report to authorities even suspected child abuse, including physical, verbal, sexual, and emotional abuse, and abuse by neglect. Reports can be made to local law officials or directly to specific group services such as the state Child Protective Services. Also required in some states, but not mandated by all, is reporting of abuse of disabled individuals and those older than 60 years of age. Most states have statutes that mandate reporting situations such as gunshot or stab wounds, rapes, and sexual assaults.

Knowledge Connection

List three categories of individuals for whom you must report suspected abuse.

Civil Law

Civil law is applicable when two or more private parties seek resolution to a dispute. The most common area of civil law that affects the health care provider is *tort law*, which usually involves a claim such as negligence or malpractice. **Malpractice** is when the nurse's action fails to meet professional standards of care and injures a patient. These two areas of tort law cover nearly any aspect of nursing care that can be provided. Three additional areas of tort law that apply to nurses are false imprisonment, assault and battery, and sexual harassment.

False Imprisonment

A competent patient has the right to leave a health care facility even if it may prove harmful to his or her health and his or her physician feels the patient should remain for medical treatment. Intentionally preventing a patient from leaving a facility or restricting his or her movement within the facility is considered false imprisonment.

The only time a patient may be forced to remain in a health care facility against his or her own will is under an involuntary admission for a psychiatric disorder. The criteria for involuntary admissions include a physician's belief that the person is a threat to self or others. The physician may petition the court for an order of involuntary admission for a limited length of time, most commonly 72 hours.

When the patient is not under a court order and expresses the desire to leave, your responsibility in this situation is to explain to the patient why it is important for him or her to remain under the physician's care. If the patient still refuses, have him or her sign the facility's Leaving Against Medical Advice (AMA) form, according to the facility policy (Fig. 3-1). Never attempt to physically prevent the patient from leaving.

Protective Restraint Devices

Inappropriate use of restraint devices, including bed rails, chemical restraints such as sedatives and tranquilizers, belts, tied sheets, wrist or ankle restraints, and vest or halter restraints can also be considered false imprisonment.

Before restraint devices can be used, the patient must present a clear danger to either self or others and other methods of protecting the patient from injury must have been attempted. When other methods fail to provide adequate safety, the physician must write an order for the restraint device to be used. You will learn more about safe use of restraints in Chapter 13.

Assault and Battery

To threaten a patient with harm or to show intent to touch him or her without permission is considered **assault**. An example would be threatening a resident of a long-term care facility that you will leave him or her lying in the wet bed if another "accident" occurs that messes the bed.

To intentionally cause a patient harm is termed **battery**. However there does not actually have to be a harmful result. Just touching a patient without permission, such as performing a procedure without informed consent, can be considered battery. Some other areas of potential liability for the nurse may be found in Box 3-3.

Sexual Harassment

Sexual harassment is a form of discrimination that violates the Civil Rights Act of 1964. It is sad to say this, but sexual harassment has become a real threat to male and female nurses alike. Sexual harassment is harassment that is based on sex

Leaving Before Medical Evaluation – Treatment Completed: ◆ LWBS ◆ Elopement ◆ AMA

Complete applicable section (1 or 2) only

Left Without Notification to Staff (LWBS or ELOPEMENT)

The patient has: ☐ LWBS ☐ Eloped

No answer when called: 1. Time: _____ Signature: _____

2. Time: _____ Signature: _____

3. Time: _____ Signature: _____

Searched ☐ Emergency Room ☐ Hospital Room ☐ Patient waiting areas ☐ Cafeteria ☐ Parking area

☐ Additional actions taken: _____ ☐ MD Notified:(as needed)

X_____

Nurse or EDT Signature

LWBS—Left Without Being Seen by a physician or nurse.

Elopement - An ER Patient who leaves after a physician or nurse initiates triage / initial Medical Screening Exam. Or an inpatient or outpatient leaving without authorization and/or notification of their departure.

Leaving Against Medical Advice (AMA) *To be completed by physician or nurse*

☐ This patient is leaving AMA despite being encouraged to stay for further examination and treatment

☐   The patient has been advised of the risks of leaving and benefits of remaining at Kingfisher Regional Hospital for further examination and treatment. The risks and benefits include:

☐ Potential threat to life, limb, and/or safety; including death or permanent disability.

☐ Other: (specific to presenting complaint) _____

☐ MD Notified: _____ Time:_____

• Reason(s) for leaving: _____

_____

Patient Acknowledgement

You have been advised to stay for further examination and treatment. Please follow up with your provider. Return to an Emergency Department if your symptoms persist or worsen.

I am voluntarily leaving or I am voluntarily taking _____ from the facility without a written discharge order from Dr. _____. I have been advised of the risk(s) involved, and against the advice and consent of the patient's doctor and/or healthcare providers.

I hereby release the physicians, hospital, and it's employees and agents from all responsibility for any ill effects that may result from my refusal of further medical examination and/or treatment for myself or the person I am taking from the facility.

X_____   X_____

Physician or Nurse Signature   Patients Signature or authorized representative

☐ *Patient refused to sign*

Figure 3-1 Leaving Against Medical Advice form. This form includes a section to be used when the patient leaves without the staff's knowledge; there is also a section for leaving against medical advice.

Box 3-3
Areas of Potential Liability

There are numerous areas of potential liability for you as a licensed nurse: the list is probably inexhaustible. These are the more common areas that you will want to be acutely aware of:

- Failure to carry out physician's orders
- Failure to clarify ambiguous physician's orders prior to performance
- Failure to maintain confidentiality
- Failure to perform adequate assessment of the patient's condition
- Failure to provide appropriate safety measures
- Failure to report pertinent changes in the patient's condition
- Falsification of patient records
- Inaccurate or incomplete documentation
- Medication errors
- Performing actions for which you are not trained
- Taking patient photographs without express permission
- Unprofessional conduct
- Untimely delivery of appropriate nursing care

and is unwelcome, causing what is termed a hostile or offensive work environment. It can be verbal, visual, or physical in presentation. Whenever a supervisor offers the nurse tangible job benefits in exchange for some type of sexual interaction, it is termed quid pro quo sexual harassment.

Because nurses often feel comfortable with the human body and its functions due to the nature of their work, they may not give a second thought to making comments that might be perceived by others as sexual and unwelcome. As a nurse, you will have to be even more careful than those in other professions. It is important that you understand the types of behavior and conversations that may be considered sexual harassment. A sampling of types of behaviors that might be so interpreted includes:

- Touching or rubbing against another person
- Physically standing within another's "personal space"
- Telling or playing jokes on another that are sexual in nature or carry a sexual innuendo
- Engaging in personal conversations regarding reproductive organs or sexual activity that can be overheard by one who is offended by the context
- Having leering or wandering eyes, or facial expressions that make the recipient uncomfortable
- Stalking
- Treating an individual of the opposite sex like he or she is just "one of the gang"

This is another situation in which being proactive is superior to just reacting. It is better to prevent situations that may be misconstrued as sexual harassment, rather than trying to defend yourself after you have offended someone.

Knowledge Connection
Name five areas of tort law that apply to the nurse. Explain the differences in them.

Good Samaritan Law

Most states have a law called the **Good Samaritan Law** that provides protection to the voluntary caregiver at sites of accidents and emergencies. It serves to provide protection to a citizen, nurse, or other health care provider who chooses to stop and render aid to someone in an emergency situation, such as an automobile accident. It is not for use in health care facilities and does not extend to individuals who are employed as emergency response workers.

Professional Accountability

As a nurse, you are held to a certain level of professional accountability: being responsible for your own actions. You are the patient advocate and must maintain professional boundaries, as well as meet certain standards of care and safety. Some of these standards include:

- Assuring that, when you accept a patient assignment, the assignment is within your level of education, training, experience, and ability.
- Refusing to take extra assignments if you are so fatigued that you are not a safe practitioner.
- Never walking away from patients without providing for continuity of care. If you leave or walk away from patient assignments without replacement by another nurse, you are guilty of **abandonment**. This term is defined as the premature cessation of the professional care nurse-patient relationship without adequate notice or the patient's permission.

You will be responsible for establishing and maintaining a nurse-patient relationship, one that is based on honesty, trust, and respect. This rapport develops as a direct result of safely meeting your patients' individual needs with caring, compassion, and competency.

Even though you are a student nurse, this does not relieve you of your accountability. You are expected to:

- Know your state's specific scope of practice.
- Know your school's policies and procedures that guide your clinical performance.
- Perform only those skills for which you have been prepared, trained, or guided by your instructor.
- Report changes in your patient's condition to your instructor or staff nurse in a timely manner.
- Make certain that you adequately prepare for each and every clinical experience. If you are in doubt as to what constitutes "adequate preparation," you are responsible for obtaining that information from your instructor.

Anatomy and Physiology Connection

Differentiating Abnormal From Normal Anatomy and Physiology

As a student, you must be prepared to care for patients assigned to you. This includes understanding the normal anatomy and physiology of the major body systems. Without this foundation of knowledge, you will be unable to accurately assess the patient's physical condition and apply it to the disease process, which is the abnormal anatomy and physiology.

Professional Liability Insurance

No one likes to think about being sued, but as litigation increases, it is pertinent that you give the matter of professional liability insurance serious thought and research. This is necessary to make an educated decision about whether or not to purchase this insurance. While most hospitals and other nursing employers may tell you that you are covered on their group liability policy, this should always be verified. Ask for a written verification, such as a certificate of insurance, which shows you are personally covered under their policy and specifies the limits of the coverage.

Even though your employer may tell you that the hospital's liability insurance protects you personally, make note that the insurance company's interest may lie with the hospital. It is argued that hospital insurance companies may not have the nurse's best interest at heart. There are documented cases in which the hospital's insurance carrier refused to pay a claim against the nurse. As a result, many nurses feel safer carrying their own individual liability policy as a supplement to their employer's insurance. The cost varies from state to state, but 1 million dollars of coverage can generally be purchased for $200 or less per year.

Supervision/Delegation Connection

Responsibility of Patient Advocacy

Patient advocacy is something that you may NEVER delegate to another individual. It is your primary responsibility to fill this role for your patient.

Professional Role Boundaries

It is important to make a distinction between advocacy and becoming personally involved with a patient. Caring about your patient and providing intimate nursing care are sometimes taken out of context and misinterpreted by vulnerable patients. A good nurse must make certain that the professional nurse-patient relationship boundaries are never crossed. Relationships with your patients must be kept on a professional level. Never allow personal feelings to affect your actions as a nurse. Take care to avoid:

• Emotional involvement with a patient
• Physical or sexual relationships with a patient
• Financial involvement with a patient
• Accepting gifts or tips from a patient

Competency

You must be able to competently apply the principles learned in nursing school in different scenarios. This requires you to individualize your nursing care to meet the specific needs of each patient. You are also accountable for wise delegation of nursing care: make certain the one to whom you are delegating is competent and legally qualified to perform the nursing action. This means the one to whom you delegate must be trained and that training must be documented.

You must always know when you need further guidance. The LPN must know when to solicit advice or assistance from the RN or physician. The RN must know when to solicit guidance or assistance from a supervisor or physician. A good nurse never performs a skill or procedure for which he or she has not been trained. Nor does a good nurse perform any assignment, task, or nursing action that raises doubt in the nurse's mind about whether it should be done or not.

Standards of Care

Standards of care, which may also be known as *standards of performance* or *clinical guidelines,* can come in many forms. They can be:

• Established within nursing textbooks
• Published in nursing journals
• Published by nursing accreditation and regulatory agencies
• Written by professional nursing associations
• Written in policy and procedure manuals

Regardless of their origin, standards of care represent the level of skill and nursing care that another nurse in the same area of the country, with the same educational level, would perform in the same situation. These standards of care serve as the nursing care templates by which you are measured. So it behooves you to familiarize yourself with the standards of care relevant to your licensure. An example is the *Standards of Practice and Educational Competencies of Graduates of Practical/Vocational Nursing Programs,* published by the National Association for Practical Nurse Education and Service, Inc. (NAPNES), which can be found in Box 3-4.

Continuing Education

Continuing education is postlicensure study done to maintain, improve, expand, and enhance your nursing knowledge. Because nursing is dynamic or ever-changing, continuing education is necessary for ensuring competence. Many states require a specified number of hours of continuing education each year as a licensure requirement; other states do not. However, even if your state does not have a mandatory continuing education requirement, you must ensure that your skills, training, and knowledge remain current. This can be difficult, especially considering how often scientific and medical discoveries are made and how quickly new drugs and technological advancements become available. Between the time you began your education and the day you graduate, there will be many significant discoveries that will

Box 3-4

NAPNES Standards of Practice and Educational Competencies of Graduates of Practical/Vocational Nursing Programs

Professional Behaviors

Professional behaviors, within the scope of nursing practice for a practical/vocational nurse, are characterized by adherence to standards of care, accountability for one's own actions and behaviors, and use of legal and ethical principles in nursing practice. Professionalism includes a commitment to nursing and a concern for others demonstrated by an attitude of caring. Professionalism also involves participation in life long self-development activities to enhance and maintain current knowledge and skills for continuing competency in the practice of nursing for the LP/VN, as well as individual, group, community and societal endeavors to improve health care.

Upon completion of the practical/vocational nursing program the graduate will display the following program outcome: Demonstrate professional behaviors of accountability and professionalism according to the legal and ethical standards for a competent licensed practical/vocational nurse.

The following competencies demonstrate that this outcome has been attained:

1. Comply with the ethical, legal, and regulatory frameworks of nursing and the scope of practice as outlined in the LP/VN nurse practice act of the specific state in which licensed.
2. Utilize educational opportunities for life long learning and maintenance of competence.
3. Identify personal capabilities and consider career mobility options.
4. Identify own LP/VN strengths and limitations for the purpose of improving nursing performance.
5. Demonstrate accountability for nursing care provided by self and/or directed to others.
6. Function as an advocate for the health care consumer, maintaining confidentiality as required.
7. Identify the impact of economic, political, social, cultural, spiritual, and demographic forces in the role of the LP/VN in the delivery of health care.
8. Serve as a positive role model within healthcare settings and the community.
9. Participate as a member of a practical/vocational nursing organization.

Source: Excerpted from *Standards of Practice and Educational Competencies of Graduates of Practical/ Vocational Nursing Programs.* © 2007 National Association for Practical Nurse Education and Service, Inc. To view the full document, refer to *www.napnes.org.*

affect your practice. The only way to be a good nurse is to continue your education as a nurse.

This does not necessarily mean you must go on to earn additional degrees, though we highly recommend this. However, it does mean that you must continue to learn and stay current so you are competent to practice safe nursing. Some ideas to assist you include:

- Subscribing to and reading nursing journals regularly
- Attending educational seminars and workshops
- Attending employer training opportunities
- Researching nursing topics and health-related issues in both current textbooks and professional websites
- Taking individual courses and workshops at a college or university
- Taking correspondence courses
- Taking continuing education for credit—found in professional journals and online, often requiring only 30 to 60 minutes to complete
- Staying up to date with the published Board of Nursing meeting reports
- Joining and participating in your professional organizations

We are passionate about this, live it ourselves, and encourage you to do the same. The day a nurse stops looking up unfamiliar medications, reviewing policies and procedures of his or her employer, researching new nursing trends and issues, seeking a way to improve nursing care, and reading and staying abreast of current changes in nursing is the

day that individual should *get out of nursing.* This is for the benefit of future patients as well as the nurse.

Make your career a challenging, problem-solving, and rewarding growth-filled journey by continually seeking new knowledge.

Knowledge Connection

What are five things you can do to maintain current knowledge and practice? When should a nurse *get out of nursing?*

Legal Documents

The entire patient chart is considered a legal document and must be handled accordingly. Though this is the primary document the nurse utilizes on a daily basis, there are numerous other documents with which you must be familiar and for which you must know your responsibilities.

Patient Chart

A patient chart or medical record is kept on each patient who enters into any aspect of the health care system. It provides data regarding the patient's health status and problems as well as the medical and nursing care provided to that patient. The patient chart is utilized as the health care providers' principle site for communication regarding a specific patient. It serves as a source of information about the patient's condition, test results, care provided, and effectiveness of care among other things.

The chart does not belong to the patient, but is the property of the hospital or of the physician in a clinic setting. The patient has the right to access the chart and to request copies of the chart as guaranteed by HIPAA. The chart is considered confidential and may only be accessed by health care workers providing care to the patient. With signed permission of the patient, copies of the chart may be made available to the patient's insurance company or other health care agencies or physicians. Charts may not be copied for students to use in their care planning or written assignments. Any data that you, the student, collect from the chart must be written in a way that it maintains confidentiality for the patient. In other words, the patient's name and identifying numbers should never be written on any of your paperwork that will be taken outside the facility.

In the United States, government hospitals forbid that any copy of any document in the patient chart be taken outside the hospital walls, even if the name is cut off the page. Notes that are written while caring for the patient, as well as copies of care plans or physician orders, should be transcribed to the patient chart as necessary and shredded before you leave the facility. Most agencies provide a shredder for this purpose.

When you make entries in the patient chart, keep in mind that it is a legal document and can be used as evidence in a court of law. Make your entries in a timely manner, being accurate and pertinent. Never use correction fluid or erase an entry. If you must correct an entry, make a single straight line through the incorrect information and write "incorrect entry" and your initials just above it. Then write the correct entry to follow. Record all pertinent data, including such things as assessment findings, a patient's refusal to allow certain care or tests, nursing care provided, results of care, a patient's verbal comments or complaints regarding any aspect of his or her problems or care, and any unusual occurrences. Keep entries factual, without your opinions or assumptions. Avoid editorializing. The standard accepted in a court of law is "if it's not charted, it wasn't done." Never document something that you did not actually do, do not document anything before it is actually done, and never document anything less than the full truth. To document under any of these circumstances constitutes fraud.

Charts should never be left open at the nurse's station or computer stations positioned close to patient rooms, and not even in the patient rooms. Charts and such things as laboratory reports must be secured in a manner that will not be conducive to the public casually glancing over or reading them. All patient information is considered confidential. Failure to handle charts appropriately breaches HIPAA.

Knowledge Connection

Who may legally access a patient's chart? To whom does the chart belong?

Informed Consent

Informed consent is written permission to allow medical treatment or surgical procedures. It indicates that the patient has voiced understanding of and agreement to participate in his or her medical care. Informed consent requires the patient (or a legal representative if the patient is a minor or is unconscious) to have knowledge and understanding of the procedure or process to be performed, along with its accompanying risks and possible outcomes. It is the responsibility of the person performing the procedure to make certain that the procedure or surgery and its risks and benefits have been explained using layperson's terminology to the patient or legal representative in such a way as to ensure understanding. While the physician may delegate the responsibility of obtaining the patient's signature on the consent form to the nurse, it is still the legal responsibility of the physician to explain the procedure and risks, making certain the patient understands. The patient must voluntarily give consent without any pressure to do so. Failure to obtain informed consent for a procedure or surgery may be construed as assault and battery in a court. Consent forms should never be signed after the patient has received mind-altering medications, or has consumed alcohol.

All persons signing the consent form must be at least 18 years old and *competent,* both mentally and legally fit. The only legal way for an individual younger than 18 to sign his or her own consent forms is if the individual is an emancipated minor. An **emancipated minor** is one who has established his or her independence from parental control by one of the following methods:

• Court order
• Marriage
• History of living independently and being self-supporting
• Service in the military

Signatures required on an informed consent form include those of the care provider, the patient or a parent or legal guardian, and a witness. Nurses should only sign as a witness to the patient's signature. If the patient is younger than 18 years of age and his or her parents are divorced, the consent must be signed by the custodial parent. In most states, stepparents do not have the legal authority to sign consent.

Your primary role is to make certain that informed consent has been obtained. If the patient tells you that he or she does not understand what is to be done or changes his or her mind about having a procedure after signing the consent form, it is your duty to inform the physician.

The only time that medical treatment may be provided without written consent is when a life-threatening emergency exists. The law then allows for what is termed *implied consent.* The emergency may also allow parental permission to be given via the telephone, but this must be witnessed by two individuals who heard the permission granted over the phone.

Knowledge Connection
What are the components of informed consent? Whose responsibility is it to inform the patient of the procedures for which consent is sought and its risks?

Advance Directives

Advance directives are written documents that provide guidelines for making medical decisions in the event a person becomes incapacitated and is unable to make his or her wishes known. All states recognize two types of advance directives: proxy directive, such as power of attorney, and instructional, such as a living will. However, from state to state, there are considerable differences in restrictions, interpretation, and the scope of decision making that may be included.

A proxy directive designates the individual legally responsible for making medical decisions once the person is unable to make decisions. Once a proxy has been appointed, an instructional directive such as a living will is required to specify aspects of care the person does or does not desire, as well as the circumstances in which to apply these wishes. Federal law requires hospitals, nursing homes, and home health agencies to ask each patient upon admission if he or she has a living will or other advance directive. This must be documented in the patient's chart. The patient should provide the facility with a copy of the directive so that it may be kept with the chart for use if needed.

Incident Reports

Incident reports may also be known as *unusual occurrence reports* or *variance reports*. They are to be completed in the event of an unusual occurrence or an accident. The incident report should include what happened, who was involved, witnesses to the event, and treatment provided. Most agencies have their own incident report form to use for patient or visitor occurrences and one to use for employee occurrences (Fig. 3-2).

When accidents or unusual occurrences happen, injuries, physical assessments, and care provided are documented in the chart, generally in the nurse's notes. Entries are kept factual and objective, without impressions, assumptions, or conclusions. Then an incident report is completed according to agency policy, including notification of the supervisor and designated personnel. The completion of an incident report is not mentioned in the patient's chart. Nor will the report be filed as part of the chart; it will be filed separately. Designated committees within agencies, such as quality assurance committees or risk management committees, review all incident or occurrence reports for the purpose of improving quality of care and risk reduction. Some states only require that the chart be made available during litigation unless the incident report is mentioned in the chart. Other states require the report to be made available in the case of a lawsuit. However, if the incident report is mentioned in the chart, it too may be subpoenaed.

Post Conference

After you began caring for the patient described in the Clinical Connection, you were notified that the decision was made not to insert a feeding tube. The family finally agreed that this decision was what their father would have wanted.
- Did you deliver the best possible care to the patient?
- Did you show support and kindness to the family, regardless of their decision?
- Did you allow the family to make the decision without trying to influence them?
- Did you show understanding of the family's difficult, almost unbearable, situation?

KEY POINTS

- The goal of all nursing care should be to improve the quality of the patient's living and dying processes.
- You must never do anything that you know is not in the patient's best interest.
- The nurse is the patient's primary advocate who stands up for that which is in the patient's best interest.
- Nurses are responsible for reporting unethical behavior and misconduct by other nurses. Behaviors to report include, but are not limited to, impairment of the nurse, diverting drugs, mistreatment of patients, fraudulent documentation, practice outside the scope of practice, practice without a license, incompetence, failure to follow physician's orders, and failure to perform a necessary action.
- The state Board of Nursing writes the rules and regulations for enforcement of each state's Nurse Practice Act.
- HIPAA provides for confidential maintenance of protected health information.
- The scope of practice sets legal boundaries within which each nurse must keep his or her practice.

| Report #_____ |
| Date Received:_____ |
| Initials:_____ |

Kingfisher Regional Hospital
Unusual Occurrence Report

Date of Event:_____   Time of Event:_____   Department:_____

Patient Last Name:	First Name:	MI
Patient #	Attending Physician:	
Visitor Last Name:	First Name	Phone:
Employee Name:	Dept:	
Physician Name:	Specialty:	

Occurrence Category: (Circle most appropriate)

Fall	Treatment/Procedure	Equipment/Supplies	AMA	Diet Related
HIPAA Compliance	Medication Related	Narcotic Related	Delay in Treatment	Security
Loss of Personal Property	Patient Injury	Order Not Executed	Peer Review Related	Agency Nurse Related
Employee Injury	Visitor Injury	Restraint Related	Other:	

Provide a Brief Description of the Event:

What are the Contributing Factors? (Circle all that apply)

Individual:	System:
Knowledge, Skills, Experience: Unclear or Incomplete	Policies/Procedures Not In Place: Unclear, Outdated
Standard of Care or Practice: Non-Adherence to	Environmental: Staffing, Patient Acuity, Congestion
Documentation: Incomplete or Not Adequate	Communications and Work Flow: Intra & Inter Departmental
	Equipment Failure

Other: (Please Explain)

Submitted by:	Dept.	Date:

This form is for the confidential use of the Quality and Risk Management Programs. Do Not Copy. Revised 3/09

Figure 3-2 This Unusual Occurrence Report form can be used for patients, visitors, and employee incidents. It includes sections to list factors that contributed to the occurrence, steps that would prevent a recurrence, and specific actions taken along with the follow-up plan.

Report #_____
Date Received:_____
Initials:_____

Page 2: To Be Completed By the Supervisor/Director—

What Steps Would Be Appropriate To Prevent A Recurrence? (Circle All That Apply)

Education:	Personnel/Credentials:
New Equipment/Supplies	Revise Job Description
Distribute Relevant Information	Modify Staffing
Focused Continuing Education	Informal Counseling
Modify Staff Orientation	Formal Counseling
Other:	Other:
Policies & Procedures:	**Equipment/Supplies:**
Circulate Policy/Procedure	Change Equipment/Supplies
Revise Policy/Procedure	Notification: MSDA, FDA, Vendor
Modify Communication	Repair Equipment
Other:	Other:

Specific Action & Follow-Up Plan:

☐ Met with Employee on (Date): _____ (See Above)
☐ Provided In-service Education at Dept. Meeting (See Meeting Minutes)
☐ Notified Department Leader of Action Needed (Name):
☐ Referred to Nursing Leadership Council
☐ Referred to Nursing Practice Council
☐ Referred to Medical Staff Quality Committee
☐ Referred to Patient Safety Team
☐ Referred to Safety/Fire/Disaster Preparedness Committee
☐ Referred to Senior Leadership Council
☐ Other:

Summary of Discussion with Initiator of Occurrence Report/Physician if indicated:

Supervisor/Director:	Date:

Please Forward *Within 7 Days of Report* to Chief Quality Officer

Level Key:

Level 0	No Patient Impact
Level 1	Minor Error/Mistake, Low Potential for Harm, No Harm Done/No Injury
Level 2	Moderate to High Potential for Harm, No Harm Done, No Injury
Level 3	Moderate to High Potential for Harm, Injury/Harm Occurred
Root Cause Analysis	Great Potential for Prevention of Same Occurrence in the Future
Near Miss	Error/Injury Intercepted Before it Causes Problems or Harm

Reviewed by CQO	Date:

This form is for the confidential use of the Quality and Risk Management Programs. Do Not Copy. Revised 3/09

Figure 3-2 cont'd

- All Nurse Practice Acts require the nurse to be knowledgeable about his or her own state Act, to perform within its constraints, and to maintain professional demeanor.
- It is mandatory to report suspected abuse of children, mentally disabled individuals, and individuals older than 60 years of age.
- Nurses are held accountable for their own actions.
- As a student nurse, you are held to the same accountability as a licensed nurse.
- You must stand with the patient, for the patient, and by the patient, always asserting yourself in the patient's best interest.
- It is vital to maintain professional boundaries with all patients.
- You must be competent in anything you do as a nurse...or else do not do it.
- The patient chart belongs to the hospital or to the physician in a clinic setting.
- The patient has a right to know what is in the chart and to have a copy of it if requested.
- Entries in the patient chart should be timely, accurate, and pertinent. Never use correction fluid or erase an entry. Make corrections by drawing a single line through the incorrect entry and writing "incorrect entry" and your initials above it. Keep entries factual and objective. Avoid editorializing. Never document anything before it is actually done.
- Charts should never be left open where they can be read by others who do not have a right to the information.
- Informed consent is required before performing medical treatment or surgical procedures.
- Incident reports are filed separately from the patient's chart.

REVIEW QUESTIONS

Select the answer that is most appropriate for each of the following questions. Some questions may have more than one correct answer. Check all that apply.

1. You are suspicious that a coworker might be diverting drugs from patients for her own personal use. Which of the following are *inappropriate* actions to take?

   a. Accuse her of being a drug addict.

   b. Tell your best friend with whom you work to see what she thinks about it.

   c. Report your suspicions to your supervisor.

   d. Ignore the situation because it is none of your business.

   e. Wait until you can catch her yourself before reporting it.

2. Which of the following can be construed as protective restraint devices?

   a. Bed rails

   b. Belts

   c. Tied sheets

   d. Sedatives

   e. Wrist restraints

   f. Vest restraints

3. Who is responsible for serving as the primary advocate for the patient?

   a. The nurse

   b. The physician

   c. The nurse supervisor

   d. The hospital

   e. The laboratory technician

4. Violation(s) of HIPAA would include:

   a. failure to comply with mandatory reporting of suspected abuse of children.

   b. documenting inaccurate information in your nurse's notes.

   c. discussing the patient's condition in the hospital dining room.

   d. filling out an incident report.

   e. leaving a chart lying open on top of the medication cart in the hallway outside the patient's room.

   f. telling your neighbor about a mutual friend hospitalized for treatment of a sexually transmitted disease.

SHORT ANSWER QUESTIONS

5. The primary purpose of Nurse Practice Acts is to ____
_____.

6. The standard is: If it is not charted, _____
_____.

FILL IN THE BLANK QUESTIONS

7. Failure to report unethical behavior or misconduct of another nurse is known as _____.

8. To legally sign his or her own consent forms, an individual younger than 18 years of age must be an emancipated minor. This required independence can be established by one of four methods, including _____
_____, _____, _____
_____, or _____.

CRITICAL THINKING EXERCISES

9. Your patient, who has already signed the informed consent for a surgical procedure, indicates to you that he does not understand the risks of the procedure nor exactly what will occur during the procedure. What should you do as the patient's advocate?

10. During the night, Jim Jones, a 46-year-old male, was admitted with alcohol intoxication and cirrhosis of the liver. His liver enzymes and bilirubin tests are elevated. He is severely distended and has multiple bruises covering much of his extremities and lower abdomen. The physician has ordered Mr. Jones to have nothing by mouth (NPO) and IV fluids to infuse at 100 mL/hr. Mr. Jones repeatedly asks for breakfast, stating he is going to "starve to death" if not fed. After explaining to the patient why he is NPO, Mr. Jones tells you to get his clothes for him and that he is going home. What are your responsibilities as his nurse?

ADDITIONAL RESOURCES

For additional Resources, Questions, and Activities, please see:

 Student Resource Disk

 http://davisplus.fadavis.com

 Student Study Guide

REFERENCES

American Nurses Association. *Code of Ethics for Nurses With Interpretive Statements.* Silver Spring, MD: Nursesbooks.org; 2001.

Brous EA. HIPAA vs. law enforcement. *Am J Nurs.* 2007;107(8):60-63.

Eden R. Criminal prosecution of human error: dangerous consequences. *StuNurse.com Magazine* [serial online]. 2007;Edition 5:20-21. Available at: http://www.stunurse.com.

Edmunds MW, Scudder L. The nurse's obligation to illegal immigrants seeking emergency care. March 2009. *Medscape Nurses* [serial online]. Available at: http://www.medscape.com/viewarticle/590328. Accessed July 18, 2009.

Fremgen BF. *Medical Law and Ethics.* Upper Saddle River, NJ: Pearson Prentice Hall; 2006.

Gibbs RR. Your patient wants to see his medical record. *LPN2007.* 2007;3(5):4-5.

Haddad A. The final word? RN Web. August 1, 2007. Available at: http://rn.modernmedicine.com/rnweb/Ethics+in+Action/The-final-word/ArticleStandard/Article/detail/447257. Accessed September 22, 2007.

Haddad, A. Ethics in Action: What the family needs to know. *RN.* 2007;70(11):23.

Kumekawa, J. HIPAA: how our health care world has changed. *OJIN Online J Issues Nurs.* 2005;10(2):1. Available at: http://www.medscape.com/viewarticle/506839. Accessed July 19, 2009.

Lewis MA, Tamparo CD. *Medical Law Ethics & Bioethics.* 6th ed. Philadelphia: FA Davis; 2007.

Macciocchi SN. Doing good: the pitfalls of beneficence. *J Head Trauma Rehabil.* 2009;24(1):72-74.

Medi-Smart Nursing Education Resources. Nursing legal issues—types of law. Available at: http://www.medi-smart.com/lawtypes.htm. Accessed September 17, 2007.

Mikos-Schild S. Educational ethics: a basis for guiding practice. *J Nurses Staff Dev.* 2008;24(6):300-301.

National Association for Practical Nurse Education and Service, Inc. (NAPNES). *Standards of Practice and Educational Competencies of Graduates of Practical/Vocational Nursing Programs.* Alexandria, VA: NAPNES; 2007.

Nelson R. The personal health record. *Am J Nurs.* 2007;107(9):27-28.

Nursing Service Organization. April 2009 legal case study. Available at: http://www.nso.com/case-studies/casestudy-article/249.jsp. Accessed July 19, 2009.

Nursing Service Organization. January 2009 legal case study. Available at: http://www.nso.com/case-studies/casestudy-article/245.jsp. Accessed July 19, 2009.

Nursing Service Organization. June 2009 legal case study. Available at: http://www.nso.com/case-studies/casestudy-article/252.jsp. Accessed July 19, 2009.

Nursing Service Organization. July 2009 legal case study. Available at: http://www.nso.com/case-studies/casestudy-article/253.jsp. Accessed July 19, 2009.

Sabatino CP. 10 legal myths about the advance medical directives. American Bar Association Commission on Legal Problems of the Elderly. Available at: http://www.abanet.org/aging/publications/docs/10legalmythsarticle.pdf. Accessed November 19, 2007.

Stokowski LA. Ethical dilemmas for healthcare professionals: can we avoid influenza? May 2009. *Medscape Nurses* [serial online]. Available at: http://www.medscape.com/viewarticle/702371. Accessed July 19, 2009.

Treas LS. *Fundamentals for Nursing Review Module Edition 5.0.* Overland Park, KS: Assessment Technologies Institute, LLC; 2005.

University of Buffalo Center for Clinical Ethics and Humanities in Health Care. Advance directives. Available at: http://wings.buffalo.edu/faculty/research/bioethics/adv-dir.html. Accessed September 17, 2007.

Oklahoma Board of Nursing. Violations of the Oklahoma nursing practice act and rules. Available at: http://www.ok.gov/nursing/violation.html. Accessed September 23, 2007.

Vivaldelli J. Ethical issues: therapeutic reciprocity. *Am J Nurs.* 2007;107(7):74-76.

Wilkinson JM, Van Leuven K. *Fundamentals of Nursing: Theory, Concepts & Applications.* Philadelphia: FA Davis; 2007.

The Nursing Process and Decision Making

Key Terms

Care plan

Collaborative interventions

Critical thinking

Defining characteristics

Dependent interventions

Direct patient care

Expected outcomes

Independent interventions

Indirect patient care

Nursing diagnosis

Nursing goal

Nursing process

Objective data

Primary data

Rapport

Secondary data

Subjective data

Validate

Objectives

1. Define key terms associated with the nursing process and decision making.
2. Discuss ways in which critical thinking is used in nursing.
3. Enumerate the steps of the nursing process.
4. Contrast subjective and objective data.
5. Explain how to conduct a nursing interview.
6. List techniques used to gather data during a physical assessment.
7. Describe how Maslow's hierarchy of human needs is used to prioritize nursing diagnoses.
8. Explain how NANDA-I nursing diagnoses are listed.
9. Compare one-part, two-part, and three-part nursing diagnoses.
10. Differentiate between long-term and short-term goals.
11. Explain how to write correct outcomes statements.
12. Compare types of nursing interventions.
13. Explain the importance of individualized nursing interventions.
14. Enumerate initial intervention steps.
15. List types of nursing care plans.
16. Explain the process for writing a student care plan.
17. Discuss the use of concept maps to plan care.

⊕ **Clinical Connection**

Your Assignment: You have been assigned to care for a patient in the hospital with multiple health problems. He is a 68-year-old male with congestive heart failure, diabetes, and emphysema. He has had two significant heart attacks (myocardial infarctions) in the past 6 years. You are also assigned to write your first student plan of care concerning this patient. You are supposed to arrive for your first day of clinical with a list of probable and possible nursing diagnoses, appropriate nursing interventions for each, and a patient goal for each.

Your Actions: You have no idea where to even start finding this information. In addition to that, you do not see how any instructor can expect you to figure out nursing diagnoses before you even see the patient or talk with him. You feel like you are being asked to work completely in the dark. You go to the hospital the evening prior to your clinical experience to research the patient's chart, but you don't know what you are supposed to find when you read it.

It can feel confusing to be asked to come prepared to care for a patient whom you know nothing about, and yet nurses care for patients every day who are newly admitted to the nursing unit. The nurse knows nothing about the patient, other than perhaps a working medical diagnosis, yet he or she must find out the pertinent information about the patient and develop an appropriate plan of care in an hour or less. In this chapter, you will learn about the steps of the **nursing process**, a decision-making framework used by all nurses to determine the needs of their patients and to decide how to care for them. You will also learn how to obtain pertinent information from various sources so that you make correct decisions about your patients' care. And, you will learn how to organize the information in a care plan that other nurses can follow, so patient care is both consistent and appropriate during the hospital stay. A **care plan** is a documented plan for giving patient care and includes physician's orders, nursing diagnoses, and nursing orders.

Decision Making in Nursing

How do nurses know what to do for patients, particularly patients with multiple problems who are very ill? Do they just perform the orders left by the physicians, nurse practitioners, and physician assistants? How do they know when or if it is necessary to call the health care provider?

Critical Thinking Skills

One way nurses make such decisions is by the use of critical thinking. Many definitions exist for this term, but to keep it simple and clear, **critical thinking** is using skillful reasoning and logical thought to determine the merits of a belief or action. To think critically, you must think about *how* you think so that you can improve your ability to make sound decisions about patients and their care.

Nurses who use critical thinking avoid jumping to conclusions about patients or patient care, and they also avoid making decisions based on assumptions. They **validate**, or ensure the correctness of, the information they obtain. It is sometimes tempting to simply "do what you are told" or to "just follow orders" rather than to think critically about your nursing practice. However, you must learn to think purposefully, using reasoning and logical thought, to determine whether your actions are appropriate for the optimal care of your patient. The following example depicts a nurse who uses critical thinking when caring for patients:

A nurse receives an order from the physician for an antibiotic to be administered IV to a patient who has developed pneumonia. The nurse remembers that the patient has an allergy to another medication in the same family of antibiotics and validates that memory by checking the patient's allergies in the chart. The nurse further validates the information by asking the patient to relate again the name of the medication and the type of reaction that occurred in a previous hospitalization, ensuring that it is entered in the chart. The nurse then notifies the physician of the potential for the patient to have a reaction to the ordered antibiotic.

This thinking nurse is not working on "automatic pilot" and simply carrying out the physician's orders. The nurse has promoted the patient's health and well-being, and prevented a potentially severe medication reaction.

You will use critical thinking skills many, many times during a shift when you work as a nurse. Your job now is to learn to think in a way that is perhaps different than you are accustomed to, and to practice that thinking at every opportunity. In addition to learning to think critically, you must learn to make nursing decisions using a framework for decision making known as the *nursing process*.

An elderly woman who was visiting the area was admitted to the hospital with shortness of breath. Eventually she required mechanical ventilation because she could not breathe well on her own. A tracheostomy was performed to prevent problems of a long-term ventilator run. After time and treatment, she was being weaned from the ventilator. The weaning process was rocky, however, because she kept having severe respiratory distress and having to go back onto the ventilator. Some of the nurses thought she was just anxious, but others felt there was something more going on.

This went on for over a week. She would be weaned off the ventilator and be doing fine. Then, in a few hours, she would go into respiratory distress and have to go back on the ventilator. Some of the staff thought she was just dependent on the ventilator and would never be able to breathe on her own. Yet, she did breathe on her own and would do well for hours, then suddenly relapse.

A nurse and a respiratory therapist decided to think critically about this case. They shared the observation that, within 30 minutes of getting a breathing treatment with medication to open her airways, the patient would be in distress and have to go back on the ventilator. One of them wondered aloud, "Could she be allergic to the medication, causing it to have the opposite effect?"

It was not easy, but the nurse approached the pulmonologist about discontinuing the medication in the breathing treatments. He was quite skeptical, but agreed to discontinue it. The patient never had to go back on the ventilator again...until the medication was reordered a week and a half later. The pulmonologist then discontinued the medication again and the patient's chart was marked with a red allergy tag.

If these two staff members were not willing to think outside the box and think critically, that patient may have remained on the ventilator when it was not necessary.

The Nursing Process

As early as the 1950s, nurses were attempting to define and explain the function of the nurse. We were not simply the handmaidens of the physicians, nor were we nonthinking and task-oriented assistants. Nurses see the whole patient and all of the patient's problems and needs, and we work to meet those needs. One way nursing function is defined is by the use of the five steps of the nursing process: assessment, diagnosis, planning, implementation, and evaluation.

Steps of the Nursing Process

Remember that the nursing process is a framework for decision making. By following these five steps, nurses determine actions to take and the effectiveness of those actions. An easy way to remember the first letter of each step is to use the mnemonic ADPIE:

- *Assessment* is the gathering of information through signs and symptoms, patient history, and objective findings. Just as a physician gathers information by performing a physical examination and a patient history, the nurse gathers information about the patient through asking questions (interviewing), performing a head-to-toe assessment, and reviewing laboratory and diagnostic tests.
- *Diagnosis* is the formulation of nursing diagnoses through analysis of the assessment information that you have gathered. The **nursing diagnoses** are related to the needs or problems the patient is experiencing. These are completely different than medical diagnoses and are selected based on definitions and defining characteristics.
- *Planning* is the process of determining priorities and what nursing actions should be performed to help resolve or manage each patient problem. In addition, the nurse determines expected outcomes for the patient to meet for the nursing diagnosis to be resolved, as well as a realistic time frame for that to occur. The nurse then decides on appropriate interventions to resolve each patient problem or nursing diagnosis.
- *Implementation* is the process of taking actions to resolve the patient's problems, the nursing diagnoses. These actions are also called *interventions*. When the nurse performs these interventions, it is called *implementation*. So the nurse implements the plan to help resolve the patient's problems.
- *Evaluation* is performed when the nurse reflects on the interventions he or she has performed and decides if they have brought the patient closer to achieving the goals and outcomes set in the planning step. If not, the nurse then revises and changes the interventions and perhaps the goals to better fit the needs of the patient.

While it looks like the steps are performed in a step-by-step sequence, that is often not the case. The steps may overlap, and the nurse may move among the steps as he or she makes decisions about patient care. Figure 4-1 presents an example of the overlapping aspects of the nursing process. Box 4-1 looks at the steps of the nursing process from a non-nursing perspective.

Roles of RNs and LPN/LVNs in the Nursing Process

According to the American Nurses Association (ANA) Standards of Practice for RNs, all the steps of the nursing process, from assessment through evaluation, are the responsibility of the RN. This also includes outcome identification in addition to planning. The National Federation of Licensed Practical Nurses (NFLPN) Nursing Practice Standards for the LPN/LVN identify assessment and nursing diagnosis as an RN function, and the LPN/LVN participates directly in

Figure 4-1 This diagram illustrates the interconnected steps of the nursing process, and how the nurse continuously uses this decision-making process.

Box 4-1

The Nursing Process From a Non-Nursing Perspective

As you look at the steps of the nursing process, you may realize that you use a similar method for making many decisions in your life. You gather information, analyze the information, develop a plan, execute the plan, and then decide how well it worked. Based on your evaluation, you may modify or change your plan. This way of making decisions is not really new to you, but using it to make nursing decisions will be different for you.

Let's look at a non-nursing example of this decision-making process: You are at a family gathering when you hear your son, Charlie, crying in the backyard. You can tell that he is hurt, so you rush out to see what has happened.

Assessment

You see Charlie standing at the side of the slide with blood coming from his left knee. As you look closer, you see a "goose egg" forming above his left eye, and you notice that his lower lip is swollen and bleeding. You ask your niece, "What happened?" She tells you that, as Charlie was going down the slide, he flew over the side and hit his head and face on the pole of the swing set. You ask Charlie, "How did you fall off of the slide?" He replies through his tears that his tennis shoe caught against the side of the slide, stopping him and causing him to fall over the side. Then you notice that he is holding onto his left wrist, so you ask him if it hurts. He nods, still crying, and says that it hurts a whole lot.

All of the above was the assessment phase of the nursing process. You gathered information by asking questions, observed Charlie's injuries, and asked about additional injuries that you might not be able to see at first glance.

Diagnosis

You began the diagnosis portion of the nursing process when, after assessment, you began to analyze the information you gathered and determined the problems that Charlie is experiencing. In this case, you wonder if his wrist could be broken. You must decide if you need to take him to the urgent care center for x-rays.

Planning

Now you have to decide what you will do to resolve the problems. This is the planning phase. Can you clean and bandage all the injuries yourself, or do you need to take him to the doctor or hospital? You know that you need to clean his knee and lip so they do not get infected. You also think that you had better check his teeth to be sure that he has not broken or loosened a permanent tooth. You plan to put some ice on the goose egg to keep it from getting any bigger.

Implementation

Next, you put your plan into action. You gently wash his knee and lip. You inspect his lower teeth for damage, but find none. You apply antibiotic ointment to his knee and cover it with a bandage to keep out dirt that could cause infection. You make an ice pack and place it on the goose egg over his left eye to help prevent further swelling.

While doing that, you check his eye for bruising or damage, but it seems uninjured. You notice that Charlie is not moving his left wrist during the time you are working on him. He keeps it close to his body with his elbow bent. You ask Charlie if he can move his hand without pain. He replies that it feels better not to move it. When you look closer, you can see a lump just above his wrist. Now you decide that you need to take him to the urgent care center for x-rays and help him into the car.

Evaluation

After performing your care (the planned interventions), you had thought this would resolve all of his problems. Now it is time to re-evaluate because you have now gathered more information about Charlie's wrist injury. The additional information helped you determine that Charlie needed to see a health care provider for further testing.

After his wrist was x-rayed, the health care provider determined that Charlie had fractured his wrist, and she applied a cast. She also checked his other injuries, validating your findings that nothing else was serious. You did the right things to get Charlie the help he needed, and now he will heal with time.

As you can see, you make similar decisions all the time. The nursing process is simply a way to help you make good, sound nursing decisions while caring for patients.

the remaining steps of planning, intervention, and evaluation. This does not mean that the LPN/LVN cannot perform assessment skills, but that the LPN/LVN's findings are shared with and sometimes confirmed by the RN. The same is true of formulating the nursing diagnosis. The LPN/LVN contributes greatly to the development of the nursing diagnosis. All data and information gathered by all nurses are considered when the nursing diagnoses are identified and prioritized.

All members of the health care team contribute to providing quality patient care for patients (Fig. 4-2). No one, from the housekeeping staff to the director of nursing, is less valuable than anyone else when it comes to providing care for our patients.

Supervision/Delegation Connection

Collaboration, Not Delegation in Care Planning

You cannot delegate nursing decisions or care planning. Those activities are strictly the role of the licensed nurse. However, it is absolutely necessary that all members of the health care team share observations and information about patients so that the best possible care can be provided. Everyone must work together in collaboration to develop a thorough care plan.

Knowledge Connection

What is the difference between the role of the RN and the role of the LPN/LVN in the nursing process? What does ADPIE stand for?

Performing the Steps of the Nursing Process

While you may now realize that you do use decision-making processes in your daily life, and that you also use critical thinking to decide what is important even in non-nursing settings, you may be confused about how to actually use the nursing process to make nursing decisions.

We will discuss each step in detail so that you can see how you, as a nursing student now and later as a licensed nurse, will gather information to determine patient needs, then decide what actions to take to meet those needs, and finally, evaluate the effectiveness of each action.

Assessment

As discussed earlier, there are three components to the assessment of patients when gathering information about their problems and needs. These are:

• Interviewing, which involves asking questions, listening, and using both verbal and nonverbal communication skills.
• Performing a focused body system assessment to determine deviations from normal in the patient's physical condition. (Chapter 21 gives you a complete guide to performing a physical assessment.)
• Reviewing the results of laboratory and diagnostic tests to determine problems and needs caused by abnormal findings.

Subjective and Objective Findings

When you gather information regarding a patient, your data will fall into one of two categories: objective or subjective. **Objective data** are those things that you can observe through your senses of hearing, sight, smell, and touch. Examples of objective data include "pale, cool, moist skin" and "dark brown, formed bowel movement." Box 4-2 shows how senses are used to gather objective data. Information that is known only to the patient and family members is **subjective data**. While some clues to these symptoms may be observable, only the patient knows exactly what he or she is feeling. Examples of subjective data include nausea, pain, anxiety, fear, depression, and discouragement. It is very important that you report and document objective data. If you are relaying subjective data, they must be attributed to the patient; for example, you would say that *the patient states* that she has a headache. The objective data that support this might include the fact that she is pale and holding her head in her hands. More information about documenting and reporting subjective and objective data can be found in Chapter 5.

Notice that objective data provide a description of what you see, hear, smell, and touch, but they do not involve drawing conclusions or inferences. If a patient is crying, your objective data are that the patient's eyes are red and that she is wiping away tears. If you draw a conclusion or an inference, you might assume that the patient is sad, depressed, or discouraged. However, you must validate your assumptions before acting on them. The patient may be crying due to happiness or relief about the results of a diagnostic test.

Interviewing

When you enter a patient's room or area to perform a nursing interview, it is important to first establish **rapport**, creating a relationship of mutual trust and understanding. You can do this by introducing yourself and explaining your role in the patient's care. For example, you would say, "I am John Smith and I will be your nurse until 7 p.m." To avoid

Figure 4-2 These nursing team members are collaborating on the care plan for a patient.

Box 4-2

Use of Senses to Obtain Objective Data

Objective data are limited to that which you can detect with your five senses. Because we no longer need to rely on our sense of taste, we only document that which we can see, hear, smell, or feel.

Use of Vision
- Make direct observation of patient's physical characteristics, facial expressions, actions, or behavior.
- Make direct observation of characteristics of eliminated bodily fluids, such as blood, urine, emesis, feces, or drainage.
- Read results of laboratory, x-ray, or diagnostic reports.
- Read reports and documentation within the patient's current or past medical records.
- Read results and detect function of equipment, such as sphygmomanometer, thermometer, pulse oximeter, various monitors, oxygen or suction flowmeters, or finger stick blood sugar equipment.
- Observe measured volume of urine or drainage in a graduated container, volume of fluid remaining in IV bag, or amount of liquid drunk from a cup with graduated markings.
- Read textbooks, medical journals, and multimedia devices used to research medical diagnoses or treatments.

Use of Hearing
- Note patient-made sounds heard with the naked ear, such as belching, passing flatus, crying, moaning, snoring, spoken words of patient or family, or laughter.
- Note sounds heard during auscultation.

Use of Smell
- Detect patient body- or bodily fluid–related odors, such as foul, fetid, sweet, fruity, acidic, ammonia-like, sulfurous, fresh, or musty.

Use of Touch
- Assess pulse rate.
- Palpate for edema, firmness or softness, nodules, papules, taut skin, masses, or mushy tissue.
- Detect temperature of patient's skin.
- Detect moisture of patient's skin.
- Detect texture of skin, hair, or nails.
- Measure strength of muscular contractions.

---

asking the patient the same questions he or she has already answered, review all the available information about the patient first. Then you can ask the patient to validate that information. Another way to establish rapport is to tell the patient the purpose of the interview and the approximate length of time it will take. Sometimes nurses take a few moments to ask some general questions and make small talk before beginning the interview, allowing the patient to relax with them. For example, the nurse might ask if the woman with the patient is his wife, then ask if they have children. Another nurse might comment about the weather or ask whether the patient is from the immediate area or an outlying one.

Once rapport is starting to be established, you will begin the nursing interview. While you begin your interactions with patients based on an admitting medical diagnosis, you are gathering evidence about patient problems that will be the foundation of your nursing care. The medical diagnosis is the disease or illness diagnosed by the physician. For example, the patient may be admitted with a diagnosis of appendicitis, pneumonia, or thrombophlebitis, all of which describe physical conditions. Nurses are concerned with how medical diagnoses affect patients' abilities to care for themselves and their families, as well as how the diagnoses affect their patients' lives.

During the interview, you will often obtain information from more than one source. When the patient provides information, it is considered **primary data**. When you obtain information from family members, friends, and the patient's chart, it is considered **secondary data**.

When interviewing your patients, avoid simply asking questions on a form and obtaining minimal answers. Rather, listen carefully to the answers and ask for additional information as it is appropriate. This requires you to think of and ask questions that may not appear on your nursing interview form. In many situations, patients do not volunteer important information simply because they do not realize it is important. If this happens, you may find out valuable facts that are crucial to providing appropriate nursing care much later than you needed to know about them. When questioned at that time, the patient will tell you, "No one asked me about that before."

Most facilities use an admission form that requires a nursing history to be performed as well as a head-to-toe assessment. Figure 4-3 shows an example of a hospital admission form. Such a form cues you to questioning the patient and completing a full assessment. However, it is appropriate to ask for additional information that is not specifically on the form if you identify additional problems as you talk with the patient. For example, if the admission form asks about previous hospitalizations and the patient responds by listing two recent surgeries, it is appropriate to say, "What about when you were a child, or a young adult? Were you ever hospitalized then?"

In addition to asking for further information, be alert to how the patient responds to questions. Notice the words the patient uses, or if he or she hesitates before answering. Box 4-3 shows ways to respond to different nuances of patient responses in order to obtain the most complete information from the patient.

Sometimes patients want to give more detail than is necessary for you to obtain pertinent information. For example, a patient may spend a great deal of time describing what was happening before he fell and injured his back. You

CODE   NA - NOT APPLICABLE   UTA - UNABLE TO ACQUIRE   0 - OTHER (SPECIFY IN NOTES)

COGNITIVE - PERCEPTUAL PATTERN

MENTAL STATUS

☐ ALERT   ☐ RECEPTIVE APHASIA   ☐ UNRESPONSIVE   ☐ COMBATIVE

☐ POOR HISTORIAN   ☐ ORIENTED ┬ ☐ PERSON   ☐ CONFUSED ┬ ☐ TOTAL
                                      ├ ☐ PLACE   ├ ☐ INTERMITTENT
                                      └ ☐ TIME   └ ☐ NIGHTTIME

CHANGE IN MEMORY   ☐ NO   ☐ YES SPECIFY _____

HEARING

☐ WNL   ☐ IMPAIRED

☐ RIGHT	☐ MILD	☐ MODERATE	☐ SEVERE	☐ PROFOUND
☐ LEFT	☐ MILD	☐ MODERATE	☐ SEVERE	☐ PROFOUND

☐ HEARING AID ┬ ☐ RIGHT   ☐ TINNITUS
              └ ☐ LEFT

VISION

☐ WNL   ☐ CORRECTIVE LENSES   ☐ BLIND ┬ ☐ RIGHT   ☐ CATARACT ┬ ☐ RIGHT
                                                └ ☐ LEFT   └ ☐ LEFT
          ☐ BLURRED

          ☐ DOUBLE   ☐ ARTIFICIAL EYE ┬ ☐ RIGHT   ☐ OTHER _____
                                             └ ☐ LEFT
          ☐ GLAUCOMA

SPEECH

☐ WNL   ☐ SLURRED   ☐ GARBLED   ☐ EXPRESSIVE APHASIA   ☐ LANGUAGE BARRIER (EXPLAIN)

SPOKEN LANGUAGE _____   INTERPRETER ☐ NO ☐ YES _____
                                                                              (NAME)

EYES

	R	L
CLEAR	☐	☐
DRAINING	☐	☐
REDDENED	☐	☐
OTHER _____	☐	☐

PUPILS

	R	L
REACTIVE	☐	☐
NONREACTIVE	☐	☐

☐ EQUAL   ☐ UNEQUAL

(CIRCLE NUMBER)

RIGHT SIZE (mm)   1 . 2 ● 3 ● 4 ● 5 ● 6 ● 7 ● 8 ●

LEFT SIZE (mm)   1 . 2 ● 3 ● 4 ● 5 ● 6 ● 7 ● 8 ●

MOUTH

GUMS/MUCOUS MEMBRANES   ☐ WNL   ☐ MOIST   ☐ DRY   ☐ LESIONS   ☐ OTHER _____

TEETH   ☐ WNL   ☐ CAPPED   ☐ ORTHODONTIA ☐ DENTURES   ☐ EDENTULOUS   ☐ OTHER _____

RESPIRATORY

☐ WNL   ☐ SHALLOW   ☐ RAPID   COUGH   ☐ NO   ☐ YES   ☐ DRY   ☐ MOIST

☐ LABORED   ☐ OTHER   ☐ PRODUCTIVE (DESCRIBE): _____

AUSCULTATION

COMMENTS

LEFT LUNG   ☐ CL   ☐ ABNORMAL   _____

RIGHT LUNG   ☐ CL   ☐ ABNORMAL   _____

CIRCULATORY

APICAL HEART RATE	☐ REG. ☐ IRREG. ☐ PACEMAKER		EDEMA	☐ NO ☐ YES	WHERE _____
NUMBNESS	☐ NO ☐ YES	WHERE _____	PAIN / ANGINA	☐ NO ☐ YES	WHERE _____
SYNCOPE	☐ NO ☐ YES	WHEN _____	LEG CRAMPS	☐ NO ☐ YES	WHEN _____
ANEMIA	☐ NO ☐ YES	_____	H / A	☐ NO ☐ YES	WHERE _____

COMMENTS:

ABDOMEN

☐ SOFT   ☐ FIRM   ☐ FLAT   ☐ DISTENDED   BOWEL SOUNDS   ☐ PRESENT   ☐ ABSENT

COMMENTS:

SKIN EXTREMITIES

COLOR ☐ WNL ☐ PALE ☐ CYANOTIC ☐ GRAY ☐ JAUNDICED ☐ FLUSHED

TEMP.   ☐ WARM   ☐ COOL   MOISTURE   ☐ DRY   ☐ DIAPHORETIC

TURGOR   ☐ WNL   ☐ POOR   AMPUTATION (SPECIFY)

INTEGRITY   ☐ INTACT   ☐ NO   SPECIFY AND LOCATE ON DIAGRAM ON RIGHT

LESIONS	☐ NO	☐ YES	_____
BRUISES	☐ NO	☐ YES	_____
REDDENED	☐ NO	☐ YES	_____
PRURITIS	☐ NO	☐ YES	_____
EDEMA	☐ NO	☐ YES	_____
OTHER	☐ NO	☐ YES	_____

RIGHT PEDAL PULSE   ☐ STRONG   ☐ WEAK   ☐ NON-PALPABLE

LEFT PEDAL PULSE   ☐ STRONG   ☐ WEAK   ☐ NON-PALPABLE

RN SIGNATURE _____   DATE _____   TIME _____

Figure 4-3   Sample assessment portion of an admission form.

DISCOMFORT/PAIN	☐ NONE ☐ ACUTE ☐ CHRONIC
	DESCRIPTION/LOCATION _____

RATING CODE
CIRCLE ONE NUMBER ▸

0	1	2	3	4	5	6	7	8	9	10

NONE   MINIMAL ————————————————➤ MODERATE ————————————————➤ SEVERE

PAIN MANAGEMENT AT HOME:

MUSCULOSKELETAL	RANGE OF MOTION ☐ FULL ☐ LIMITED SPECIFY: _____

HAND GRASPS   ☐ EQUAL   │ ☐ LEFT ☐ STRONG ☐ WEAK ☐ PARALYSIS │ ☐ RIGHT ☐ STRONG ☐ WEAK ☐ PARALYSIS

LEG MUSCLES   ☐ EQUAL   │ ☐ LEFT ☐ STRONG ☐ WEAK ☐ PARALYSIS │ ☐ RIGHT ☐ STRONG ☐ WEAK ☐ PARALYSIS

BALANCE AND GAIT   ☐ STEADY   ☐ UNSTEADY   ☐ BEDFAST

                         ☐ CONTRACTURES

COMMENTS:

NUTRITION   TYPE OF DIET: _____

APPETITE: ☐ GOOD ☐ FAIR   ☐ POOR   AVERAGE FLUID INTAKE: _____

TYPICAL DAILY FOOD INTAKE: NUMBER OF MEALS: _____   SUPPLEMENTS _____AMOUNT OF WEIGHT LOSS/GAIN: _____

NAUSEA / VOMITING   ☐ NO   ☐ YES   HEARTBURN   ☐ NO   ☐ YES

DYSPHAGIA   ☐ NO   ☐ YES   ☐ SOLIDS   ☐ LIQUIDS   ABD. PAIN / CRAMPING   ☐ NO   ☐ YES

COMMENTS:

ELIMINATION   BOWEL PROBLEM: ☐ NO   ☐ YES   DATE OF LAST BM: _____   LAXATIVE / DIETARY CONTROL: ☐ NO   ☐ YES

DIARRHEA: ☐ NO   ☐ YES   CONSTIPATION: ☐ NO   ☐ YES   BOWEL INCONTINENCE: ☐ NO   ☐ YES

URINARY FREQUENCY: ☐ NO   ☐ YES   URINARY PAIN, BURNING, HESITANCY: ☐ NO   ☐ YES   URINARY RETENTION: ☐ NO   ☐ YES

CATHETER / OSTOMY: ☐ NO   ☐ YES   LAST CHANGED _____   URINARY INCONTINENCE: ☐ NO   ☐ YES

COMMENTS:

REPRODUCTIVE   ☐ N/A   DATE OF LAST MENSTRUAL PERIOD: _____   LAST PAP SMEAR: _____   MENOPAUSE: ☐ NO   ☐ YES

BREAST: SELF EXAM ☐ NO ☐ YES ☐ NA   MENSES: ☐ NO ☐ YES

PROSTATE PROBLEMS: ☐ NO ☐ YES ☐ NA _____

COMMENTS:

ACTIVITY/EXERCISE PATTERN

1. MOBILITY STATUS: ☐ AMBULATORY   ☐ AMBULATORY WITH ASSIST   ☐ BEDREST   ☐ TRANSFER WITH ASSISTANCE

2. ASSISTIVE DEVICES: ☐ NONE ☐ CANE ☐ WHEELCHAIR ☐ WALKER ☐ CRUTCHES ☐ PROSTHESIS

        ☐ NO PROBLEM   ☐ CONTRACTURES   ☐ JOINT STIFFNESS   ☐ MUSCLE STIFFNESS ☐ FRACTURES   ☐ PARALYSIS   ☐ ARTHRITIS

        ☐ PROSTHESIS   ☐ PAIN   ☐ WEAKNESS   ☐ OTHER

COMMENTS: _____

COPING - STRESS TOLERANCE/SELF-PERCEPTION/SELF-CONCEPT PATTERN

DO YOU OR YOUR FAMILY HAVE ANY CONCERNS ABOUT YOUR HOSPITALIZATION OR ILLNESS?

☐ NO   ☐ YES   COMMENTS:

DO YOU FEEL: ☐ CALM   ☐ ANXIOUS   ☐ FEARFUL   ☐ HOPELESS   ☐ POWERLESS   ☐ OTHER

COMMENTS:

HAVE YOU HAD A MAJOR LOSS OR CHANGE IN YOUR LIFE IN THE PAST YEAR?   ☐ NO   ☐ YES

COMMENTS:

SUPPORT PERSON(S): ☐ MOTHER   ☐ FATHER   ☐ SISTER   ☐ BROTHER   ☐ GUARDIAN   ☐ OTHER

NAME(S):

SAFETY EVALUATION: SCORE 1 FOR EACH CRITERIA MARKED

☐ CONFUSION/DISORIENTATION   ☐ BOWEL/BLADDER INCONTINENCE/NOCTURIA   │ ☐ MINIMAL RISK FALL PRECAUTIONS - 1 OR 2 SELECTED

☐ HX OF FALLS   ☐ VERTIGO   │ ☐ HIGH RISK FALL PRECAUTIONS - 3 OR MORE SELECTED

☐ REQUIRES ASSIST TO AMBULATE

ADDITIONAL COMMENTS _____

RN SIGNATURE _____   DATE _____   TIME _____

KRH DISK #3

Figure 4-3 cont'd

Responses to Nuances in Patient Interviews

During the patient interview, the patient may respond to your questioning in a number of ways. The patient may be open, honest, and talkative, or quiet, evasive, or vague. It is up to you to get the appropriate response from your patient. Below are some possible tips to utilize when interviewing your patient.

Patient Response: Patient hesitates before answering a question.
Nurse's Response: Give the patient time, as he or she may be thinking through an answer. If the patient continues to hesitate, you may need to reword the question.
Patient Response: Patient responds with a vague answer, using phrases such as "not exactly," "sort of," "maybe," or "you could call it that" in reply.
Nurse's Response: Ask the patient for more detail or to be more specific. Ask him or her to be precise and accurate so that you can get a clear picture of what it is he or she is describing.
Patient Response: Patient looks away or acts uncomfortable when you ask a question.
Nurse's Response: Apologize if question seems intrusive and explain that the information is necessary for you to completely comprehend how the illness is affecting his or her life and relationships.

must listen carefully to extract what is important, but if the interview is taking an extended amount of time, it is appropriate to find a polite way to redirect the patient to the subject at hand. Some ways to do this include saying,

- "Can you tell me more about the pain you have been experiencing?"
- "Now, let's get back to what happened after you fell."
- "After that happened, what did you do to relieve the pain?"

You will use many techniques for interviewing and extracting pertinent information from your patients. Chapter 6 explains how to use open-ended questions when talking with patients and also includes phrases to avoid because they can shut down communication.

Physical Assessment

Physicians and nurse practitioners often perform extremely in-depth physical assessments to detect signs and symptoms that contribute to formulating medical diagnoses. Nurses in the acute care setting, both RNs and LPN/LVNs, perform thorough physical assessments to collect additional data used in formulating nursing diagnoses according to facility policy and the state Nurse Practice Act.

In general, the RN is responsible for performing a complete assessment when the patient is admitted to a nursing unit in the hospital. The RN will also establish the nursing diagnoses and goals for the patient during the

hospital stay. However, in many settings, the LPN/LVN may do all or part of the assessment, which is then confirmed by the RN. *Safety: Always follow facility policy and practice within the scope established by your state's Nurse Practice Act.* Nurses gather data about how the patient's body is functioning using the following techniques:

- *Inspection,* which is the visual examination of the patient's body for rashes, breaks in the skin, and normal appearance of eyes, ears, nose, mouth, limbs, and genitals
- *Palpation,* which is touching or feeling the torso and limbs for pulses, abnormal lumps, temperature, moisture, and vibrations
- *Auscultation,* or listening for abnormal sounds in the lungs, heart, or bowels
- *Percussion,* or using tapping movements to detect abnormalities of the internal organs

Physical assessment is usually performed in a head-to-toe pattern to avoid omitting any important data. Many hospital admission forms include a head-to-toe assessment guide for the nurse to follow. However, you are responsible for obtaining thorough data whether or not it is found on an assessment form. Performing a physical assessment is discussed in detail in Chapter 21.

Laboratory and Diagnostic Connection

How Laboratory and Diagnostic Results Affect Patient Care

Sometimes nurses think that analyzing laboratory and diagnostic test results is strictly in the realm of the physician. Although the physician and other health care providers will review the results of laboratory and diagnostic tests, it is important for nurses to examine them as well. As you learn more about abnormal results of such tests, you will understand how they affect the patient's nursing care. For example, if you have a patient whose white blood cell count is very low, you know he or she is at high risk for developing an infection, as white blood cells are responsible for fighting invading pathogens. That information is important when you think about how to care for your patient and how to protect him or her from potential infections.

Nursing Diagnosis

The formulation of nursing diagnoses is a uniquely nursing function. Physicians, physician assistants, and nurse practitioners all focus on medical diagnoses based on signs, symptoms, laboratory findings, and test results, but nurses focus on the needs of patients. As was discussed in the previous section, a medical diagnosis is a label for a disease, illness, or injury, such as coronary artery disease, pneumonia, or hematoma. A nursing diagnosis, however, is a label or statement for a problem that a patient is experiencing as a result of his or her medical diagnoses. This type of diagnosis is treated by the nurse using interventions to improve the patient's ability to function as normally as possible.

Prioritizing Diagnoses

Nursing diagnoses address physical, psychosocial, and environmental needs of patients, with some of them being a higher priority than others. For example, the nursing diagnosis "Ineffective airway clearance" would be considered a higher nursing priority than "Chronic low self-esteem." Both diagnoses are important, but the first is critical to the patient's ability to breathe. How will you decide which diagnoses are the most important?

Maslow's Heirarchy of Human Needs

One helpful tool for determining priority is Maslow's hierarchy of human needs. This pyramid identifies human needs in ascending order of importance. The first level is composed of physiological needs, those things a human being needs to survive. The next level addresses safety and security needs, those things a human being needs to remain alive and protected. The third level includes the need for love and belonging, such as meaningful relationships. The next level is the need for self-esteem and feelings of self-worth. This is followed by the level that addresses cognitive needs for learning and exploring. The sixth level is composed of aesthetic needs for beauty and order. The seventh level addresses the need for self-actualization, which is the need for reaching one's own growth potential, and the highest level is that of transcendence, or the need to help others reach their highest potential. Figure 4-4 shows Maslow's hierarchy of human needs depicted as ascending steps.

According to Abraham Maslow, who was an American psychologist, humans must meet their physiological needs first, before needs higher on the steps are of any concern. For example, a homeless person is focused on finding food and shelter in a safe area and would not be interested in joining a self-help group until his or her basic needs have been met. Nurses, therefore, must address the physiological needs of survival first with their patients, then the needs related to relationship issues in the love and belonging tier.

An example of this in the hospital setting would be a patient who has recently had an abdominal surgery, causing him or her to be in pain and not sleep well. This patient would not be ready or able to learn how to perform a dressing change on his or her abdominal wound until the basic physiological needs of pain relief and rest have been met.

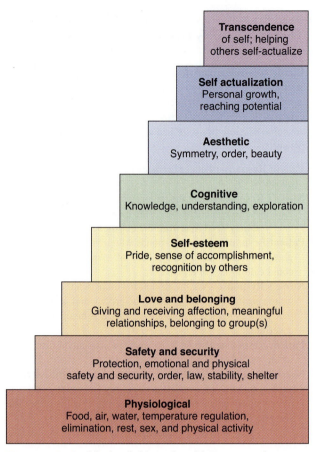

Figure 4-4 Maslow's hierarchy of human needs moves upward from survival needs to transcendence.

Selecting Nursing Diagnoses

Although formulation of nursing diagnoses is identified by the ANA and NFLPN as an RN function, all nurses, both LPN/LVNs and RNs, must be knowledgeable about the North American Nursing Diagnosis Association–International (NANDA-I) diagnoses list and the selection of appropriate nursing diagnoses, as all nurses contribute to the development of the care plan. NANDA-I, which was formerly known as the North American Nursing Diagnosis Association and has now added "International" to the title, is responsible for creating and maintaining an approved list of nursing diagnoses to be used throughout most countries, including the United States and Canada. By establishing and revising this list, nursing diagnoses are standardized for use by nurses everywhere and lend themselves more easily to computerized documentation than individually developed diagnoses.

NANDA-I Lists

Most lists are written to make the diagnoses easy to find. The main topic is listed first, then modifiers such as "risk for," "readiness for enhanced," "acute," "chronic," "family," "impaired," "disturbed," and "deficient" follow. When you write a nursing diagnosis on a care plan, you will write it as it would logically be read, not the way it appears on the

---

Patient Teaching Connection

Meeting Patient Needs First

It is important to remember what you have learned about Maslow's hierarchy when you prepare to teach patients. If a patient is uncomfortable, is in pain, needs to go to the bathroom, is too cold, too hot, nauseated, or hungry, or feels feverish, he or she will not be able to learn. You need to be alert to cues that the patient is not ready or able to learn due to lower level needs that have not been met. Do your best to determine what the problem is and take care of the physiological and safety needs first, then begin your patient teaching.

list. For example, on the list, one nursing diagnosis reads "Infection, risk for." This makes it easy to find within the list when infection is a potential problem. However, on the care plan, you would write it in the logical form of "risk for infection."

There are approximately 199 NANDA-I diagnoses on the 2009–2011 list. Authors and others have developed a variety of ways to group the diagnoses into clusters, or subdivisions. For the purposes of this book, we developed functional divisions that allow you to find and prioritize the nursing diagnoses based on body system, physiological or psychosocial functioning, or environmental influences (Box 4-4). We attempted to organize the list in such a way that a beginning student in nursing would be familiar with the subdivisions. Other ways to divide or organize the nursing diagnoses list exist, and you will want to find one that is easy for you to use. When you do, keep it close at hand when you are developing your care plans.

Determining Nursing Diagnoses

All data collected in the assessment step of the nursing process are analyzed to determine the correct nursing diagnoses. It is not simply a matter of choosing a diagnostic label from the list. Rather, the nurse must understand the definition of the nursing diagnosis as well as the **defining characteristics**, or signs and symptoms, exhibited by the patient.

Box 4-4

Simplified Divisions of Nursing Diagnoses

This list of nursing diagnoses is grouped by types of needs. First, the physiological needs are listed by body system, safety, activities of daily living, and growth and development. Then the diagnoses that pertain to psychosocial needs are listed by those that affect the individual, the family, and the community. Lastly, the diagnoses that pertain to environmental problems and needs are listed.

Diagnoses for Physiological Needs and Problems

Body System

Neurological System
Acute confusion
Acute confusion, risk for
Autonomic dysreflexia
Autonomic dysreflexia, risk for
Chronic confusion
Decreased intracranial adaptive capacity
Impaired environmental interpretation syndrome
Impaired memory
Ineffective cerebral tissue perfusion, risk for
Peripheral neurovascular dysfunction, risk for
Thermal regulation, ineffective
Unilateral neglect
Verbal communication, impaired
Wandering

Cardiovascular System
Bleeding, risk for
Decreased cardiac output
Decreased cardiac tissue perfusion, risk for
Ineffective gastric perfusion, risk for
Ineffective renal perfusion, risk for
Peripheral tissue perfusion, ineffective
Shock, risk for
Vascular trauma, risk for

Respiratory System
Airway clearance, ineffective
Aspiration, risk for
Breathing pattern, ineffective
Impaired gas exchange

Impaired spontaneous ventilation
Ventilator weaning response, dysfunctional

Integumentary System
Impaired skin integrity
Impaired skin integrity, risk for
Impaired tissue integrity

Urinary System
Functional urinary incontinence
Impaired urinary elimination
Overflow urinary incontinence
Reflex urinary incontinence
Stress urinary incontinence
Urge urinary incontinence
Urge urinary incontinence, risk for
Urinary elimination, readiness for enhanced
Urinary retention

Musculoskeletal System
Disuse syndrome, risk for
Impaired bed mobility
Impaired physical mobility
Impaired transfer ability
Impaired walking
Impaired wheelchair mobility

Sensory System
Disturbed sensory perception (Specify: visual, auditory, kinesthetic, gustatory, tactile, olfactory)

Endocrine System
Unstable glucose level, risk for

Digestive System
Bowel incontinence
Constipation
Constipation, perceived
Constipation, risk for
Diarrhea
Dysfunctional gastric mobility
Dysfunctional gastric mobility, risk for
Impaired liver function, risk for

(box continues on page 58)

Box 4-4

Simplified Divisions of Nursing Diagnoses (continued)

Impaired oral mucous membranes
Impaired swallowing
Nausea

Reproductive System/Childbirth
Childbearing process, readiness for enhanced
Disturbed maternal/fetal dyad, risk for
Sexual dysfunction
Sexuality pattern, ineffective

Fluid and Electrolyte Balance
Deficient fluid volume
Deficient fluid volume, risk for
Electrolyte imbalance, risk for
Excess fluid volume
Fluid balance, readiness for enhanced
Imbalanced fluid volume, risk for

Comfort and Rest
Comfort, readiness for enhanced
Disturbed sleep pattern
Fatigue
Impaired comfort
Insomnia
Pain, acute
Pain, chronic
Sleep, readiness for enhanced

Nutrition
Imbalanced nutrition: less than body requirements
Imbalanced nutrition: more than body requirements
Imbalanced nutrition, risk for more than body requirements
Impaired dentition
Infant feeding pattern, ineffective
Nutrition, readiness for enhanced

Safety
Falls, risk for
Hyperthermia
Hypothermia
Imbalanced body temperature, risk for
Infection, risk for
Injury, risk for
Latex allergy response
Latex allergy response, risk for
Perioperative positioning injury, risk for
Poisoning, risk for
Protection, ineffective
Self-mutilation
Self-mutilation, risk for
Sudden infant death syndrome, risk for
Suffocation, risk for
Suicide, risk for
Thermoregulation, ineffective
Trauma, risk for

Activities of Daily Living
Activity intolerance
Activity intolerance, risk for
Delayed surgical recovery

Self-care deficit, bathing
Self-care deficit, dressing
Self-care deficit, feeding
Self-care deficit, toileting
Self-care, readiness for enhanced

Growth and Development
Adult failure to thrive
Attachment, risk for impaired
Breastfeeding, effective
Breastfeeding, ineffective
Breastfeeding, interrupted
Delayed development, risk for
Delayed growth and development
Disorganized infant behavior
Disorganized infant behavior, risk for
Disproportionate development, risk for
Immunization status, readiness for enhanced
Neonatal jaundice
Organized infant behavior, readiness for enhanced
Parenting, impaired
Parenting, risk for impaired

Diagnoses for Psychosocial Problems and Needs

Affecting the Individual
Health Concerns
Activity planning, ineffective
Compromised human dignity, risk for
Decision making, readiness for enhanced
Deficient knowledge
Disturbed energy field
Diversional activity, deficient
Health maintenance, ineffective
Knowledge, readiness for enhanced
Noncompliance
Risk-prone health behavior
Sedentary lifestyle
Self–health maintenance, ineffective
Self–health maintenance, readiness for enhanced
Self-neglect

Emotional Concerns
Anxiety
Chronic low self-esteem
Chronic sorrow
Communication, readiness for enhanced
Compromised resilience, risk for
Coping, ineffective
Death anxiety
Decisional conflict
Defensive coping
Denial, ineffective
Disturbed body image
Disturbed personal identity
Fear
Grieving
Grieving, complicated

Box 4-4

Simplified Divisions of Nursing Diagnoses (continued)

Grieving, complicated, risk for
Hope, readiness for enhanced
Hopelessness
Impaired individual resilience
Loneliness, risk for
Other-directed violence, risk for
Post-trauma syndrome
Post-trauma syndrome, risk for
Power, readiness for enhanced
Powerlessness
Powerlessness, risk for
Rape-trauma syndrome
Relocation stress syndrome
Relocation stress syndrome, risk for
Self-concept, readiness for enhanced
Situational low self-esteem
Situational low self-esteem, risk for
Social isolation
Stress overload

Spiritual/Moral Concerns
Impaired religiosity
Moral distress
Religiosity, readiness for enhanced
Spiritual distress
Spiritual distress, risk for
Spiritual well-being, readiness for enhanced

Affecting the Family
Caregiver role strain
Caregiver role strain, risk for
Family coping, compromised
Family coping, disabled
Family coping, readiness for enhanced
Family processes, dysfunctional
Family processes, interrupted
Family processes, readiness for enhanced
Family therapeutic regimen management, ineffective
Impaired parenting
Impaired parenting, risk for
Parental role conflict
Parenting, readiness for enhanced

Affecting the Community and Society
Community coping, ineffective
Community coping, readiness for enhanced
Impaired social interaction
Ineffective role performance
Relationships, readiness for enhanced

Diagnoses for Environmental Problems and Needs
Contamination
Contamination, risk for
Impaired home maintenance

The following example will help you understand selection of a nursing diagnosis:

A male patient has been admitted with the medical diagnosis of pneumonia. The nursing assessment reveals that he is short of breath at rest, has a weak cough, and is unable to bring up mucus that can be heard in his lungs and throat. He complains of chest discomfort and has a temperature of 101.8°F (38.8°C), pulse of 112 beats per minute, respirations at 22 per minute, and blood pressure of 128/84 mm Hg. When the nurse listens to his lungs, the nurse hears crackles and wheezes. The patient breathes easiest when he is sitting upright in bed. He is very weak and unable to get out of bed without assistance; when he attempts to walk to the bathroom, he becomes short of breath and his pulse increases to 128. His laboratory results show normal oxygen levels in the blood when he is resting.

As you look at the NANDA-I list in Box 4-4, refer to the physiological section under the respiratory system because this patient is having problems with breathing. There you will see several nursing diagnoses, some about breathing and others about ventilation, and some about gas exchange. Several look like they might apply to this patient, so how does the RN determine which is appropriate? The nurse must use the definition of the diagnosis and the defining characteristics found in nursing diagnoses manuals. In this situation, the nurse narrows the possible diagnoses about the patient's respiratory problems down to two possibilities: "Impaired gas exchange" or "Ineffective airway clearance."

The nurse rules out "Impaired gas exchange" because that diagnosis is used when the patient's oxygen level is low or the carbon dioxide level is high. While this may be the case in a patient with a similar diagnosis, from the information the nurse has collected, the patient's oxygen level is now within normal limits. When the nurse looks at the definition and defining characteristics for "Ineffective airway clearance," the patient's symptoms match several of the defining characteristics as well as the definition. This diagnosis fits because it is used when the patient is unable to cough mucus up and out of the airway to keep the airway clear. Looking further, this patient matches several of the defining characteristics for this diagnosis, including crackles and wheezes in the lungs, needing to sit upright to breathe easily, and the inability to bring up mucus from his throat and airways.

As the nurse continues to review the assessment data, other clusters of data become evident, such as the patient's weakness and inability to tolerate getting out of bed. The nurse knows this is a physiological problem and affects the patient's ability to perform normal activities, or activities of daily living. Under those subheadings, the nurse finds the diagnosis, "Activity intolerance." After reading further, the nurse confirms that the patient fits this diagnosis due to his weakness and inability to ambulate to the bathroom due to shortness of breath and increased pulse rate.

Writing Nursing Diagnoses

Up to this point, we have discussed only one part of the nursing diagnosis: the first part, also referred to as the diagnostic label or diagnostic concept. This is the portion of the nursing diagnosis that is identified through definitions and defining characteristics, and it is the core of the diagnosis.

A complete nursing diagnosis may be a one-part, two-part, or three-part statement. The three-part statements are often called PES statements. This stands for problem, etiology, and signs and symptoms:

- The *problem* is the diagnostic concept or label based on the patients needs.
- The *etiology* refers to the causative factor(s) and is connected to the diagnostic label by the words "related to."
- The *signs and symptoms* include the data collected and evidence used to support the diagnostic label, and they are linked to the statement with the words "as evidenced by."

Using the diagnostic concepts selected for our patient in the previous section, the complete three-part nursing diagnosis statements are shown in Figure 4-5:

Ineffective airway clearance related to secretions in the airways as evidenced by abnormal lung sounds, orthopnea, and dyspnea
Problem · Etiology (cause) · Signs and symptoms (evidence)

Activity intolerance related to generalized weakness as evidenced by dyspnea on exertion, and elevated heart rate with activity
Problem · Etiology (cause) · Signs and symptoms (evidence)

Figure 4-5 Three-part nursing diagnosis statement samples.

In some circumstances, all three parts of the statement will not apply. In that case, a two-part statement may be a better fit. When the nursing diagnosis is one that expresses the risk for a problem, a possible problem, or certain actual problems, the two-part statement is used. This is referred to as a PE statement, or problem and etiology only. An example of a PE statement is shown in Figure 4-6:

Risk for poisoning related to risk factor of confusion
Problem · Etiology

Figure 4-6 Sample of a PE statement.

When the NANDA-I diagnosis falls into the category of "wellness," "syndrome," or "specified," a one-part statement is used. In this situation, the diagnostic label clearly states the patient's need without requiring further elaboration:

- A *wellness* diagnosis usually includes the phrase, "readiness for enhanced...," which means that the patient is willing to improve his or her lack of hope, knowledge, coping, or other needs.
- A syndrome is a label for a group of signs and symptoms, so *syndrome* diagnoses already refer to defining characteristics and do not need further elaboration. Examples of syndrome diagnoses include "Post-trauma syndrome," "Rape-trauma syndrome," and "Impaired environmental interpretation syndrome."
- *Specified* diagnoses are those that clearly apply to one defined patient need, so that any more description would only be redundant. An example of a specified diagnosis is "Latex allergy response." There is no need to say "related to allergy to latex" because it is the only cause of that response.

Another unique situation occurs when the nursing diagnosis from the list requires that you specify additional information. In that case, the word "specify" appears in parentheses after the nursing diagnosis. For example, one nursing diagnosis reads "Deficient knowledge (specify)." You might write it as "Deficient knowledge of diabetic foot care."

Sometimes the available nursing diagnoses do not really fit the situation with a patient. Rather than using a diagnosis that is not completely accurate, it is better to use your own words to describe the patient's problem. It is more important that you communicate effectively with the nursing staff regarding the patient's problems than that you use official NANDA-I language.

Once you have determined the patient's problems and needs, and you have selected the appropriate nursing diagnoses for the patient, you are ready for the next step of the process: planning.

Knowledge Connection

List three ways to obtain assessment data. How do nurses decide which nursing diagnoses have the highest priority? Write a three-part nursing diagnosis for a patient with constipation.

Planning

The planning step of the nursing process involves several areas: setting long-term and short-term goals, planning outcomes for each nursing diagnosis, and planning the interventions you will use in the implementation step.

Long-term and Short-term Goals

A **nursing goal** is the overall direction in which one must progress to improve a problem. Long-term goals are not expected to be met before the patient is discharged from the hospital. It may be an ongoing process of improvement or a gradual change in circumstances. Short-term goals are expected to be met by the time of discharge or transfer to another level of care. They may be met in a brief teaching session. Some facilities and schools do not include these broad long- and short-term goals. They use expected outcomes only.

Expected Outcomes

While goal statements are general, outcomes are specific. **Expected outcomes** are statements of measurable action for the patient within a specific time frame, in response to nursing interventions. According to the ANA Standards of Practice, expected outcomes are to be developed by the RN. Again, the LPN/LVN contributes information and provides input in the development of expected outcomes.

Just as NANDA-I creates and revises standardized nursing diagnoses, a similar classification and standardization process is underway for nursing expected outcomes. The Nursing Outcomes Classification (NOC), originally developed at the University of Iowa College of Nursing, currently contains a list of 330 nursing expected outcomes designed to coordinate with established NANDA-I diagnoses. For example, an expected outcomes label to go with the nursing diagnosis "Activity intolerance" could be *Endurance* or *Mobility*. Standardization of the terminology of expected outcomes is helpful for computer documentation and electronic medical records.

Expected outcomes statements are often the exact opposite of the problem or diagnostic label. For example, if the nursing diagnosis for a patient was "Self-care deficit related to weakness and pain after surgery," the outcome statement might be *Patient will shower with standby assistance by the second postoperative day.* However, once you are clear on the difference between nursing diagnoses and outcome statements, you will realize that these two components of the nursing process work hand-in-hand to help deliver only the best in patient care.

Outcomes statements should include the following information:

- **A realistic, specific action to be taken by the patient (not the nurse):** To be specific, the expected outcome must state precisely what is to be accomplished. To be realistic, the expected outcome must be something the patient is capable of doing. For example, *Patient will ambulate 30 feet in the hallway with walker* tells where and with what assistance the patient will perform the activity.
- **An action that the patient is willing and able to perform:** To be an action that the patient is willing and able to perform, the expected outcome must be something the patient wants to do and will cooperate in achieving. For example, the nurse may think that a good action for the patient is to ambulate in the hallway, but if the patient is too short of breath or in pain, he or she will be unable to meet the expected outcome.
- **An action is that measurable:** To be measurable, it is necessary to use verbs that can be evaluated. In the previous example, we can evaluate whether or not the patient was able to ambulate 30 feet.
- **A definite time frame for the action to have been accomplished:** To include a definite time frame, the expected outcome could be *Patient will ambulate 30 feet in the hallway with walker before discharge from hospital.*

Because expected outcomes are often required before a patient can be discharged from the hospital, they are sometimes referred to as *discharge criteria.* Long-term goals may require follow-up by health care providers such as physicians, nurse practitioners, physician assistants, home health care staff, and physical and occupational therapists.

As you plan expected outcomes and goals, you will also plan the nursing interventions you will use to improve the patient's health status and meet his or her health care needs. We will discuss the selection of interventions in the next step of the nursing process, implementation.

Implementation

Nursing actions, or interventions, are sometimes referred to as *nursing orders.* Just as the physician makes a medical diagnosis and writes physician's orders to improve the patient's condition, nurses formulate nursing diagnoses and write nursing orders to resolve the patient's problems. To a beginning nursing student, this may seem totally overwhelming. However, learning which nursing actions to take and the reasons behind each action will help you become a better nurse. Just as every skill prepares you to give needed care to patients, understanding how nursing diagnoses work helps you know when such care is indicated. You will become so familiar with nursing actions that, when you hear a nursing diagnosis, you will automatically begin thinking of nursing interventions for it.

In the same University of Iowa College of Nursing project that is standardizing and classifying nursing outcomes (NOC), a group is also working to do the same for nursing interventions. The standardized language for nursing interventions is found in the Nursing Interventions Classification (NIC).

Types of Nursing Interventions

Nurses must work together, as well as with other health care professionals, to accomplish established goals and outcomes. Nursing interventions may involve direct or indirect patient care. **Direct patient care** is performed when the nurse interacts directly with the patient, and includes such activities as bathing, teaching, listening, and administering medications. **Indirect patient care** is performed when the nurse provides assistance in a setting other than with the patient. Examples of indirect care would include documenting care, participating in care conferences, talking with the health care provider, and receiving new orders.

Nursing interventions can also be classified as independent, dependent, or collaborative. When nurses determine that interventions are needed, they may be able to provide the intervention without consulting anyone else. These are **independent interventions**, because a physician's order is not required to perform them. An example of this type of intervention would occur when the nurse assesses a patient's urine and notices that it is dark yellow and concentrated, and the amount is lower than normal. The nurse decides to put the patient on intake and output measurement because the patient has a risk for imbalanced fluid volume. This nursing action does not require a physician's order, but instead is a nursing order, and is a way to obtain more data about the patient's possible problems.

Some nursing interventions do require a health care provider's order before they can be performed, and these are referred to as **dependent interventions**. For example, if a patient was complaining of constipation, the nurse would assess the date of the last bowel movement and assess the abdomen. The nurse would use independent interventions to help promote peristalsis, such as increasing fluid intake, encouraging high-fiber foods, and assisting with ambulation if allowed. The nurse would also administer laxatives or stool softeners as ordered by the physician. If the patient still was unable to have a bowel movement and further orders were needed, the nurse would call the physician to obtain an order to administer an enema to the patient. *Nurses always need an order from a health care provider for diet, activity level, medications, IV therapy, treatments, diagnostic tests,*

and discharge. **Collaborative interventions** are those that involve working with other health care professionals in the hospital setting, such as therapists, social services workers, and dietitians. An example of this would be when the nurse caring for a resident in a long-term care facility learns that hospice has been called in to see the resident. The hospice nurse provides certain types of care to the resident related to his or her terminal diagnosis. The nurse employed by the long-term care facility also provides care to the resident, including medications and treatments. The two nurses work together to provide the best possible care to this terminally ill resident.

Individualized Nursing Interventions

In the world of computer lists and preprinted actions for nursing diagnoses, it is tempting to simply select nursing orders from a list of possible interventions without taking into account what is most appropriate for your particular patient and without considering the patient's likes or needs. However, such "cookie-cutter care" is dangerous because you can miss cues about a patient's unique problems that can lead to a life-threatening situation.

Individualized care for patients ensures better nursing care. Your patient is not just a diagnosis or the person in room 537, but a person with individual responses to being ill and in the hospital. It is important to remember that no two patients are the same; even though some patients share the same diagnoses, their care should reflect their individual needs. Box 4-5 provides an example of how to provide individualized nursing care.

Sometimes a nursing order is to carry out the physician's order. For example, a patient complains of a moderate

---

Box 4-5

Providing Individualized Nursing Care

You are caring for a female patient who has a nursing diagnosis of "Deficient fluid volume." The short-term goal is for the patient to increase her oral fluid intake to 1,500 mL/day. What will your nursing interventions be? You want the patient to drink, so you offered her iced tea between meals. However, she says she does not like it. How do you ensure that you and the other nursing staff know what fluids to provide to this patient and how often to do so?

First, ask the patient which fluids she likes. She responds that she likes fruit juices, and prefers grape, orange, and lemonade, as well as coffee with cream.

Next, you divide the 1,500 mL of fluid up so that she consumes it throughout the day and not all at once. You determine that the day shift fluid goal is 750 mL, the evening shift fluid goal is 500 mL, and the goal for the night shift is 250 mL.

You now write the following nursing orders:
• Offer 8 ounces of fruit juice every 2 hours, especially grape, orange, and lemonade.
• Record intake and output every shift to detect improvements in fluid balance.

• Offer coffee with cream with meals and between meals. Inform dietary department of dislike for tea.
• Encourage water intake from the bedside water pitcher for additional fluid intake.
• Assess mucous membranes, tongue, and skin turgor every shift to evaluate signs of dehydration.

If you looked at a standard care plan without individualization, it might list nursing interventions such as these:
• Encourage fluid intake.
• Record intake and output.
• Assess for signs and symptoms of dehydration.

You can see the difference in the detail of nursing care for this patient. In addition, other nursing staff will know specifically how to improve this patient's fluid status, and no one will bring fluids that the patient does not like to drink. As a bonus, the patient does not have to tell each nursing staff member which fluids she prefers.

headache, which he attributes to not sleeping well. The nursing orders include administering a back and neck rub, keeping the patient's room quiet, and dimming the lights. The nurse also administers 400 mg of ibuprofen, which was ordered by the physician for relief of mild to moderate pain. The nursing orders and the medical orders combine to improve the patient's health status. We are all working in collaboration toward the same goal.

Initial Intervention Steps

Nursing students learning to perform interventions soon discover that the initial steps for each intervention are very similar. Before you begin any intervention, you must be sure that you know how to perform it. *Safety: Never perform any skill or intervention that you have not been taught how to do.* In some situations, you will have the opportunity to observe a skill being performed before you learn how to do it yourself as you have not yet reached that area of your curriculum. In that case, you must be an observer only; you cannot try to perform a skill or intervention with a staff nurse attempting to "talk you through it." It is dangerous for the patient, and you put yourself in a position of liability in such a situation.

The initial steps of most nursing interventions include:

- Checking the chart to be certain of a physician's or other health care provider's order. *Safety: Always review the order before executing it, rather than simply going by what someone tells you is ordered. Misunderstandings can lead to serious consequences for patients.*
- Thinking critically about the order. Has the patient's condition changed in such a way that the order might no longer be appropriate?
- Gathering needed equipment and supplies.
- Introducing yourself to the patient if you have not previously done so. Include your name and title, such as "I'm Jane Johnson, a student nurse."
- Explaining the procedure to the patient. Use words the patient understands, avoiding nursing lingo. For example, you might say, "I must insert this tube into your nose and pass it down into your stomach," rather than "I am going to insert an NG tube."
- Identifying your patient using two methods of identification according to facility policy. In the hospital, patients will be wearing an armband for identification purposes. In addition, you will ask the patient his or her name. Avoid asking, "Are you Mr. Smith?" since some confused or hard-of-hearing patients may answer inappropriately. *Safety: Always ensure that you are providing ordered care to the correct patient. Patients may have similar names or the same name, so always check the armband and, if necessary, also compare the hospital number to the chart.*
- Re-evaluating the appropriateness of this intervention. Is this the correct time to proceed? For example, you enter a male patient's room to teach him how to correctly use a glucometer to check blood sugar levels. As you arrive, you hear the patient vomiting and find him pale and sweaty. You determine that this intervention can wait until a later time when the patient feels better.
- Providing privacy for the patient by closing the door to the room or drawing the privacy curtain around the bed. It may be necessary to ask family or friends to step out of the room briefly while you complete the intervention. Close window blinds if necessary also.
- Washing your hands or using hand sanitizer according to facility policy (see Chapter 14).
- Putting on gloves and other necessary protective equipment to protect yourself from blood and body fluids (see Chapter 14). *Safety: Raising the bed to a comfortable working height to prevent injury to your back.*

These "Initial Implementation Steps" are also listed inside the front cover of this book for quick reference when you are performing nursing interventions.

You will be caring for more than one patient at a time as a nurse, so you must learn to plan your shift in such a way that you implement all nursing and medical orders for all of your patients in a timely manner. In addition, you must document all the nursing interventions that you perform. Chapter 5 offers more information about organizing and documenting your nursing care.

During the implementation stage, it can feel like you are running around all day checking tasks off of a list. Sometimes you can lose your focus and forget why you are performing these interventions, and you can forget to add the human touch to the technology. Never lose sight of the individual patients that you care for. Step back to evaluate what is and what is not working, and whether or not goals are being accomplished. This is the next and last step in the nursing process—evaluation.

Evaluation

As you look at your patient's nursing diagnoses and desired outcomes, you will evaluate whether your nursing interventions brought about the desired outcomes. Evaluate the following factors:

- Are the nursing diagnoses correct?
- Have you established realistic, reachable goals?
- Have you determined the correct priorities for your nursing diagnoses?
- Have you selected and implemented the correct interventions?
- Has the patient's condition changed?

Box 4-6 illustrates the process of evaluating nursing care.

Knowledge Connection

What is the difference between short-term goals and expected outcomes? Give an example of an independent nursing intervention. Give an example of a dependent nursing intervention.

Box 4-6

Evaluating Your Nursing Care

You are caring for a patient whose nursing diagnosis was "Activity intolerance related to generalized weakness as evidenced by shortness of breath and increased heart rate when ambulating to the bathroom." The expected outcome was *Patient will ambulate to the bathroom with minimal assistance by the third hospital day.* Your interventions included gradually increasing activity to increase strength. Your nursing orders were:

• Get the patient up in the chair for 30 minutes three times per day, increasing the time by 30 minutes each day.
• Encourage protein-rich foods to help promote healing and strength.
• Assist the patient to ambulate from the bed to the chair and back two times before sitting up, starting on the second day.

Now it is time to evaluate this approach. On the third hospital day the patient is stronger, but now complains of left calf pain when taking steps. You must go back to the assessment step of the nursing process. When you assess the leg, you find that the calf is warm, red, and swollen. You notify the physician, who orders tests that confirm the presence of thrombophlebitis in the saphenous vein of the left leg. The physician orders bedrest for the patient to prevent a pulmonary embolus.

Now your nursing diagnosis changes to "Impaired physical mobility, level 4, related to impaired leg circulation as evidenced by redness, pain, and swelling of the left calf." Your nursing interventions change to:

• Maintaining bedrest
• Elevating the leg to reduce swelling
• Maintaining moist heat on the leg as ordered by the physician
• Assessing for changes in the leg, such as decreased swelling, decreased redness and warmth, and decreased pain
• Assessing for symptoms of a pulmonary embolus, such as chest pain and dyspnea
• Administering anticoagulants as ordered by the physician

The expected outcome changes to *Restored physical mobility when blood clot has resolved.* As you go through the evaluation process, you realize that everything has changed and nothing from your original plan applies now.

Your nursing day will be filled with similar scenarios when you care for patients. One hallmark of a good nurse is that he or she is ready to make changes and use a fresh approach when necessary.

Nursing Care Plans

Care plans are documented on various forms, depending on the type of facility and the policies of that facility. In hospitals, a detailed care plan of some type generally is included in the patient's chart. In addition, a short summary of specific care may be written on the Kardex. (See Chapter 5 for more information about the Kardex.)

Types of Care Plans

A care plan is often used as a basis for documentation, as in the problem-oriented medical record. (See Chapter 5 for more information about documentation.) A detailed care plan may be documented in a variety of ways.

Computerized Care Plans

In some hospitals, computerized care plans are the standard. The RN highlights or checks appropriate nursing diagnoses on the computer screen, then selects corresponding goals and nursing interventions listed for that diagnosis. The care plan is saved in the computer and may not be printed out at all. It is available to all nursing staff with computer passwords. Use of standardized language for nursing diagnoses (NANDA-I), outcomes (NOC), and interventions (NIC) is essential for the computerized care plan to be consistent from facility to facility. It is also necessary as electronic medical records become more of a reality. *Safety: Always turn off or shut down the computer monitor screen so that other people cannot see the patient's private information.*

Standardized Care Plans

Standardized care plans are preprinted documents with typical nursing diagnoses and corresponding nursing intervention choices to coordinate with a particular medical diagnosis. For example, a standardized care plan for a patient with pneumonia might include choices of the following nursing diagnoses:

• Ineffective airway clearance
• Impaired gas exchange
• Activity intolerance

The nurse checks the nursing diagnoses that match the assessment data, then selects from the listed interventions those that are appropriate for this patient. Many standardized care plans provide the opportunity to individualize further by writing details or dates in blank spaces. An advantage to these standardized care plans is that they help you remember most of the interventions for a specific diagnosis, preventing oversight.

Multidisciplinary Care Plans

Another type of care plan frequently used in hospitals is a collaborative or multidisciplinary plan of care. This type of care plan includes choices of different nursing diagnoses with options the nurse may select in order to individualize the patient's care (Fig. 4-7). It also contains blanks for the nurse to write in further detail or dates. In addition, the multidisciplinary care plan contains similar areas for respiratory therapists, social services workers, physical therapists, and dietitians to document their plans and the patient's response. One major advantage of this type of care plan is that all

MULTIDISCIPLINARY PLAN OF CARE

KINGFISHER REGIONAL HOSPITAL
500 S. 9th Street 375-3141
"Your Home Team Advantage"

PHYSICAL MEDICINE AND REHABILITATION

INITIAL EVAL.		PATIENT PROBLEMS	EXPECTED OUTCOMES / GOALS	INTERVENTIONS / APPROACHES	RESOLVED	
DATE	INITIALS				DATE	INITIALS
		☐ Activity Intolerance ☐ Pain 2° _____ ☐ Decreased Strength ☐ Decreased Endurance ☐ Decreased ROM _____	☐ Increased Activity Tolerance ☐ Decreases Pain ☐ Increase Strength ☐ Increase Endurance ☐ Increase ROM _____	☐ Therapy: ☐ Hot Packs ☐ Ultrasound ☐ Massage ☐ Tens ☐ Therapeutic Exercise ☐ Progressive Gait Training ☐ Other _____		
		☐ Impaired Physical Mobility ☐ Bed mobility _____ ☐ Transfers _____ ☐ Ambulation _____ ☐ Balance _____ ☐ Decreased Safety Awareness	☐ Bed mobility _____ ☐ Transfers _____ ☐ Ambulation _____ ☐ Balance _____ ☐ Improve Safety Awareness	☐ Bed mobility Training ☐ Transfers Training ☐ Progressive Gait Training ☐ Balance Training ☐ Safety Awareness ☐ Precautions ☐ Written Instructions - Precautions		
		☐ Wound	☐ Wound Cleansed ☐ Increased Circulation ☐ Healing Promoted ☐ Reduced Potential for Infection	☐ Whirlpool ☐ With Additive _____ ☐ Without Additive ☐ With Debridement ☐ Sterile Dressing ☐ Dry ☐ Dry with Topical Ointment ☐ Wet/Dry with Saline With Packing _____ Other _____		

Therapy, Evaluation. Treatment Flow Sheets and Progress Notes can be found in the Physical Therapy section of the patient's current medical record.

Additional Comments: _____

INIT.	SIGNATURE	INIT.	SIGNATURE	INIT.	SIGNATURE

FOOD & NUTRITION

INITIAL EVAL.		PATIENT PROBLEMS	EXPECTED OUTCOMES / GOALS	INTERVENTIONS / APPROACHES	RESOLVED	
DATE	INITIALS				DATE	INITIALS
		Actual / potential nutrition risk factors identified: ☐ Patient requires enteral and/or parenteral support _____ ☐ Knowledge deficit related to _____ _____ ☐ Dental status ☐ Protein/Energy Depletion ☐ Cultural Influence ☐ Other:	Maintain / improve nutritional status as evidenced by ☐ Weight maintenance or gain ☐ Improved PO intake > 75% meals ☐ Lab Values: _____ ☐ Improved: _____ ☐ Patient/Significant Other able to demonstrate comprehension of diet modification. ☐ Other:	☐ Provide supplement and/or snack _____ ☐ Provide consultation/recommendation _____ ☐ Provide education/counseling _____ ☐ Monitor tolerance/response to: Meals _____ Supplements _____ Snacks _____ Enteral feedings _____ Parenteral nutrition _____ ☐ Calorie counts _____ ☐ Monitor weight/lab values _____ ☐ Other _____ ☐ Refer to Pt. Nutrition Evaluation found in patient's Medical Record		

Additional Comments: _____

INIT.	SIGNATURE	INIT.	SIGNATURE	INIT.	SIGNATURE

Figure 4-7 Sample of a multidisciplinary care plan that combines a standardized nursing care plan with those of other disciplines.

RESPIRATORY MULTIDISCIPLINARY PLAN OF CARE (Continued)

RESPIRATORY

INITIAL EVAL.		PATIENT PROBLEMS	EXPECTED OUTCOMES / GOALS	INTERVENTIONS / APPROACHES	RESOLVED	
DATE	INITIALS				DATE	INITIALS
		□ Impaired Gas Exchange □ Dyspnea related to: _____ □ Ineffective airway clearance related to: _____ □ Secretions: _____ □ Knowledge deficit related to: _____ _____ _____ □ Other:	□ Improved Oxygenation □ Establish effective respiratory pattern □ Reduce potential for atelectasis □ Diminished or absence of rales □ Mobilize secretions □ Patient / significant other able to demonstrate: □ ABG's within normal limit _____ □ Respiratory rate normal _____ □ Other:	□ Assess respiratory function _____ □ Monitor: Breath Sounds _____ ABG _____ Oximeter _____ CXR _____ Other _____ □ Oxygen _____ □ HHN / MDI _____ □ IPPB _____ □ Incentive Spirometry _____ □ Aerosol Therapy _____ □ CP&PD _____ □ Bronchodilator _____ □ Suction _____ □ Other:		

Additional Comments: _____

_____

_____

_____

_____

_____

INIT.	SIGNATURE	INIT.	SIGNATURE	INIT.	SIGNATURE

DISCHARGE PLANNING / SOCIAL SERVICES

INITIAL EVAL.		PATIENT PROBLEMS	EXPECTED OUTCOMES / GOALS	INTERVENTIONS / APPROACHES	RESOLVED	
DATE	INITIALS				DATE	INITIALS
		□ Concern: patient's ability to return to premorbid living arrangements related to: □ Living alone □ Has disabling illness □ Not alert / disoriented □ Has no identified family / significant other □ Depressed / anxious □ Suspected abuse / neglect □ Conservatorship □ Other _____ □ Cultural Influences □ Agitated / Combative / Suicidal □ Hallucinations / Delusions	□ Patient / significant other will be aware of appropriate D/C arrangements as evidenced by verbalizing what services are being arranged □ Increased awareness of adjustments needed to cope with disabling illness □ Financial assessment will result in referral to eligible programs □ Other:	Arrange for: □ Home Health _____ □ Attendant care _____ □ Rehab _____ □ SNF / Sub-acute _____ □ Board & care _____ □ Durable medical equipment _____ □ Counseling / support group referrals ____ _____ □ Transportation _____ □ Nutrition program _____ □ SSI _____ □ IHSS _____ □ Medicaid □ Educ. re: Advanced Directive _____ □ Initiated short-term counseling _____ □ Other:		

Additional Comments: _____

_____

INIT.	SIGNATURE	INIT.	SIGNATURE	INIT.	SIGNATURE

Figure 4-7 cont'd

MULTIDISCIPLINARY PLAN OF CARE (Continued)

Page 3

NURSING CARE PLAN

INITIAL EVAL.		PATIENT PROBLEMS	EXPECTED OUTCOMES / GOALS	INTERVENTIONS / APPROACHES	RESOLVED	
DATE	INITIALS				DATE	INITIALS
		1 Knowledge deficit related to: _____ _____ _____	☐ Patient / family will verbalize and/or demonstrate understanding of education during hospitalization: _____ _____	☐ Initiate Education Profile ☐ Other: _____ _____ _____		
		2 Anxiety ☐ Potential ☐ Actual related to: ☐ Hospitalization ☐ Perceived threat to self concept or health status ☐ Perceived threat to significant other ☐ Other:	☐ Patient / family will verbalize decreased feeling of anxiety during hospitalization ☐ Other:	☐ Assess level of anxiety _____ ☐ Encourage patient / family to verbalize feelings _____ ☐ Give information regarding: test, disease process / surgery as patient is ready to learn _____ ☐ Answer questions appropriately and concisely _____ ☐ Encourage patient input into plan of care _____ ☐ Offer appropriate reassurance and support _____ ☐ Pastoral care referral _____ ☐ Social services referral _____ ☐ Other:		
		3 Alteration in Respiratory Status related to: ☐ Infection ☐ Loss of functioning lung tissue ☐ Post-op status ☐ Other:	☐ Patient will obtain adequate ventilation during hospitalization ☐ Other:	Monitor: ☐ CXR's _____ ☐ Respiratory status _____ ☐ Character of sputum _____ ☐ ABG's / Labs _____ ☐ O2 as ordered: _____ ☐ Respiratory therapy: _____ ☐ Assess Home Health needs _____ ☐ Other:		
		4 Alteration in Cardiac Status related to: ☐ Hemodynamic instability ☐ Potential ☐ Actual ☐ Dysrhythmia ☐ Hypo / hypertension ☐ Pulmonary congestion ☐ Edema ☐ Cardiac output, diminished ☐ Other:	Patient will exhibit, within potential: ☐ Hemodynamic stability _____ ☐ Rhythm stability ☐ Blood pressure stability ☐ Fluid and electrolyte balance _____ _____ ☐ Other:	Monitor: ☐ Cardiac rhythms _____ ☐ Vital signs per protocols _____ ☐ Invasive lines _____ ☐ Medications _____ ☐ Fluid balance / I&O _____ ☐ Daily weight - type of scale _____ ☐ Lab values per protocols _____ ☐ Test results (EKG, CXR, ECHO) _____ ☐ Cardiac teaching (diet, meds, activity, etc.) ☐ Other:		

		5 Alteration in Comfort related to:
		☐ Illness / surgery
		☐ Nausea / vomiting
		☐ Pain
		☐ Itching
		☐ Other:
			☐ Patient will verbalize and/or demonstrate relief of discomfort 30-60 minutes p intervention using pain scale 1-10 _____
			☐ Other:
				☐ Assess for discomfort and relief pos: intervention _____
				☐ PRN meds as ordered _____
				☐ Provide comfort measures _____
				☐ Position changes _____
				  Teach pain relief options _____
				  ☐ Breathing ☐ Relaxation exercises
				  ☐ Other:
				  ☐ Other:		

		6 Alteration in Bowel Elimination related to: ☐ Diarrhea ☐ Constipation ☐ Ileus ☐ Neurogenic bowel ☐ Other:	☐ Patient will _____ pattern of bowel elimination ☐ Patient demonstrate management ☐ Other:	☐ Assess and monitor causative factors _____ ☐ Increase fluids / bulk ☐ PRN meds as ordered _____ ☐ Monitor bowel sounds q _____ ☐ Bowel program _____ ☐ Other:		
		7 Alteration in Urinary Elimination related to: ☐ Incontinence ☐ Retention ☐ Neurogenic bladder ☐ Other:	☐ Patient will _____ pattern of urinary elimination ☐ Patient / family will demonstrate management _____ ☐ Other:	☐ Assess and monitor causative factors _____ ☐ Assess and monitor signs and symptions _____ ☐ Offer bedpan / urinal q _____ ☐ Comfort measures _____ ☐ Catheter _____ ☐ Teach patient / family _____ ☐ Other:		

Figure 4-7 cont'd

MULTIDISCIPLINARY PLAN OF CARE (Continued)

Page 4

NURSING CARE PLAN (Continue)

INITIAL EVAL.		PATIENT PROBLEMS	EXPECTED OUTCOMES / GOALS	INTERVENTIONS / APPROACHES	RESOLVED	
DATE	INITIALS				DATE	INITIALS
		8 Potential for physical injury related to: ☐ Unsteady gait ☐ Weakness ☐ Age ☐ Altered mental status ☐ Seizures ☐ Other ☐ Handicap	☐ Reduced potential from injury during hospitalization ☐ To ensure safety in event of fire / disaster ☐ Other:	☐ Assess for orientation to time & place & comprehension ability _____ ☐ Institute fall precautions _____ ☐ Soft restraints with order q 24 hours ☐ Identification sticker on chart & Kardax ☐ Pad side rails as needed _____ ☐ Other:		
		9 Self care deficit related to: ☐ Decreased strength and endurance ☐ Altered mental status ☐ Pain ☐ Restrictive devices ☐ Other:	☐ Patient will assist within potential with care during hospitalization _____ _____ ☐ Patient care needs will be met during hospitalization _____ _____ ☐ Other:	☐ Assess strengths and limitations _____ ☐ Encourage family involvement in care _____ ☐ Teach patient / family on importance of progression of self care activities _____ _____ ☐ Pain management _____ ☐ Other:		
		10 ☐ Potential ☐ Actual Impaired skin integrity related to: ☐ Decreased mobility ☐ Altered nutritional status ☐ Decreased tissue perfusion ☐ Chronic disease process ☐ Other:	☐ Patient's skin integrity will be maintained or improved during hospitalization _____ _____ ☐ Other:	☐ Assess and document skin condition _____ ☐ Reposition Q2h & pad pressure points _____ ☐ Instruct patient / family on importance of nutrition and mobility ☐ Pressure therapy device: _____ ☐ Nursing consultation _____ ☐ Pressure area protocol _____ ☐ Other:		
		11 ☐ Potential ☐ Actual Infection related to: ☐ Incision / wound ☐ Invasive lines: _____ _____ ☐ Other:	☐ Reduced potential for infection _____ _____ ☐ Patients will show improvement in Clinical signs of infection by time of discharge ☐ Other:	☐ Assess for signs and symptoms of infection ☐ Monitor vital signs _____ ☐ Monitor lab values _____ ☐ Isolation: _____ ☐ Other:		
		12 ☐ Potential ☐ Actual Spiritual distress related to: ☐ Grieving, Anticipatory ☐ Grieving, dysfunctional ☐ Coping, ineffective ☐ Decisional conflict _____ _____ ☐ Family coping altered ☐ Level of care decisions ☐ Cultural Influence	☐ Patient ☐ Family ☐ Spiritual distress is acknowledged ☐ able to describe coping strategies ☐ to achieve: ☐ comfort with decisions ☐ Spiritual calm ☐ _____ _____ _____	☐ Assess spiritual identity ☐ Assess reliance on spiritual activities ☐ Provide / arrange for ☐ Spiritual leader ☐ Meditation / quiet time, space ☐ Non-judgmental listening • Clergy • Social worker • Psychologist • Other _____ ☐ Reading materials _____ _____ ☐ Other:		
		13 ☐ Potential ☐ Actual ☐ ☐	☐ ☐ ☐	☐ ☐ ☐		

Additional Comments: _____

INIT.	SIGNATURE	INIT.	SIGNATURE	INIT.	SIGNATURE

DOCUMENT 24 HOUR CARE PLAN REVIEW

DATE	NAME	INIT.	DATE	NAME	INIT.

Figure 4-7 cont'd

health care professionals involved in the patient's care are working together and communicating with one another.

Critical Pathway

Critical pathways, also called clinical pathways, are similar to standardized care plans except that they are based on the progression expected for each day the patient is in the hospital.

Certain nursing interventions are provided each day, changing as the patient improves and less comprehensive nursing care is needed. The critical pathway uses the average length of stay for a particular medical diagnosis as the basis for the progression of care. When a patient has more than one major medical diagnosis, it becomes more difficult to use critical pathways. Figure 4-8 shows an example of a critical pathway.

Estimated Length of Stay: 7 Days – Variations from Designated Pathway Should Be Documented in Progress Notes						
Nursing Diagnoses and Categories of Care	Time Dimension	Goals and/or Actions	Time Dimension	Goals and/or Actions	Time Dimension	Discharge Outcome
Risk for injury related to CNS agitation					Day 7	Client shows no evidence of injury obtained during ETOH withdrawal
Referrals	Day 1	Psychiatrist Assess need for: Neurologist Cardiologist Internist			Day 7	Discharge with follow-up appointments as required.
Diagnostic studies	Day 1	Blood alcohol level Drug screen (urine and blood) Chemistry Profile Urinalysis Chest x-ray ECG	Day 4	Repeat of selected diagnostic studies as necessary.		
Additional assessments	Day 1 Day 1–5 Ongoing Ongoing	VS q4h I&O Restraints p.r.n. Assess withdrawal symptoms: tremors, nausea/ vomiting; tachycardia, sweating, high blood pressure, seizures, insomnia, hallucinations	Day 2–3 Day 6 Day 4	VS q8h if stable SC I&O Marked decrease in objective withdrawal symptoms	Day 4–7 Day 7	VS b.i.d.; remain stable Discharge; absence of objective withdrawal symptoms
Medications	Day 1 Day 2 Day 1–6 Day 1–6	*Librium 200 mg in divided doses Librium 160 mg in divided doses Librium p.r.n. Maalox ac & hs *NOTE: some physicians may elect to use Serax or Tegretol in the detoxification process	Day 3 Day 4	Librium 120 mg in divided doses Librium 80 mg in divided doses	Day 5 Day 6 Day 7	Librium 40 mg DC Librium Discharge; no withdrawal symptoms
Client education			Day 5	Discuss goals of AA and need for outpatient therapy	Day 7	Discharge with information regarding AA attendance or outpatient treatment

Figure 4-8 Sample of a critical pathway showing the progression of nursing care for a patient with alcohol withdrawal.

Student Care Plans

For many years in nursing education, student care plans have been used to help students make connections between the patient's medical diagnoses, medications, laboratory and diagnostic tests, assessment data, nursing diagnoses, nursing orders or interventions, and evaluations. It is true that, once you are out of school, you will no longer complete these detailed care plans due to time constraints. However, while you are a student, these care plans are excellent tools for sharpening your critical thinking skills and your nursing decision making. In fact, it is one major way that you learn to think like a nurse. Figure 4-9 shows an example of a student care plan.

Preparing to Care for Patients Prior to Clinical Experience

As a student, you may be required to prepare for your clinical experiences by completing a portion of your care plan form before you actually care for your patients. This gives you background and sparks ideas about types of problems and assessment data that you may find when you care for the patient. For example, suppose your instructor gives you the following information from the patient's Kardex:

- George Marquez, a 54-year-old male patient with medical diagnosis of coronary artery disease
- Admitted after experiencing radiating chest pain to left arm and jaw while bicycling with his son
- Scheduled for arteriogram at 1 p.m. tomorrow
- Nothing by mouth (NPO) after midnight
- Healthy heart diet
- Vital signs every 4 hours
- Bedrest with bathroom privileges
- IV line in left arm
- Intake and output
- *Telemetry* (a remote heart monitoring device)

Your instructor tells you that he has arranged for you to accompany Mr. Marquez to the catheterization laboratory and to observe the arteriogram procedure tomorrow. He also tells you that the patient is very anxious about the procedure and about what the doctors might find. He mentions that, as Mr. Marquez had chest pain ambulating to the bathroom on two different occasions, it looks like he probably has significant blockage in his coronary arteries.

Step 1—Research

With this information, you are ready to do some further research. Before you care for Mr. Marquez the next day, you need to know more about his likely problems and potential problems. What are the signs and symptoms of this condition? Which diagnostic tests do you expect? What is the usual treatment? You will learn more about diseases, diagnosis, and treatment in the medical-surgical portion of your nursing education. Early in school, you will need to research medical diagnoses in your medical-surgical textbook.

You learn that the common signs and symptoms of coronary artery disease are chest pain with or without radiation to other areas, chest pressure or discomfort, elevated blood pressure, dyspnea with exertion, and possibly an irregular heartbeat. Tests include *coronary arteriography,* which is taking x-rays after the injection of contrast media into the coronary arteries to detect blockages or narrowing that could lead to a myocardial infarction, or heart attack. The treatment is diet and lifestyle modifications, medications to dilate the coronary arteries (for example, nitroglycerin), medications to lower blood pressure, and possible stent placement or coronary artery bypass grafts if the blockages are severe. A *stent* is a device inserted into a blood vessel to keep it open, allowing blood to flow evenly through it.

Because you will be accompanying the patient when the arteriogram is obtained, you research what will be done during the procedure and what the patient can expect after the procedure. You learn that, if stents are necessary, they will be placed during the procedure. If the blockages cannot be treated with stents due to their location, the patient may have to undergo open heart surgery for coronary artery bypass grafts.

Now you know more about what to expect in the care of this patient. But how do you turn all of that medical information into nursing care? You must use the nursing process.

Step 2—Possible Nursing Diagnoses

Even though you cannot perform an assessment on your patient now, you are beginning to have ideas about the possible problems that your patient might have. For student care plans, it is often suggested that only three or four nursing diagnoses be required so the student can concentrate on learning specifics of those diagnoses. In this case, you can narrow down the possibilities to these diagnoses:

- Acute pain related to decreased oxygen to the heart muscle
- Activity intolerance related to decreased ability of the heart to respond to increased demand as evidenced by pain and dyspnea when ambulating
- Deficient knowledge about pending coronary arteriography

Step 3—Expected Outcomes

Expected outcomes for each nursing diagnosis could be similar to the following:

- Patient will rate chest pain at a 0–2 before discharge.
- Patient will ambulate 30 feet in the hallway without chest pain before discharge.
- Patient will verbalize what to expect during and after the coronary arteriography by noon tomorrow.

Step 4—Develop Your Interventions

You now need to determine what you will do for this patient. How will you help relieve his chest pain if it occurs? What do you need to monitor about his chest pain? You can find out more about managing pain in Chapter 19.

What, if anything, do you need to know about his telemetry unit? Are you supposed to do anything with it while you are caring for Mr. Marquez? What will you do with it

Level IV Master Clinical Written Assignment (100 pts)					
Admitting Diagnosis:	Admission Date:	Age:	M/F	Admitting Dr.	Student:
	Surgical Procedure (if applicable) & Date		Diet:		Instructor:
			Secondary Diagnosis:		
	History of Presenting Illness: (Get from patient interview & reading the History & Physical in the chart.)		Social History:		
			Past Medical History:		
Allergies:					

Nursing Care to be Provided	
Activity:	Fluid Balance: (I & O, Encourage Fluids, Fluid Restriction, etc.)
Safety:	
Vital Sign Frequency:	Treatments (dressings changes, irrigations, FSBS, etc.):
Hygiene & Type Bath:	
Respiratory Therapy:	
Physical Therapy:	

(Worth 5 pts.)					
Drug/Dose/ Route	Frequency/ Time	Classification	Why is Patient on This Drug? BE SPECIFIC	What assessment or lab result must be monitored prior to administering this drug?	Was Patient on this drug at home?

(Disease Research worth 5 pts.)
Diagnosis: _____
Disease Research of Admitting Diagnosis: *(Describe the processes/changes within the body that result in the signs and symptoms of the disease.)* **5 pts.**

(20 pts.)
Textbook Signs & Symptoms. Underline the signs and symptoms your patient had. **5 pts.**
Textbook Medical Care Typically Ordered to Diagnose & Treat the Disease: **3 pts.**
Dx.
Tx.
Textbook Nursing Care: **5 pts.**
Etiology: **2 pts.**   What lab or diagnostic test confirmed your pt's. Dx.? **5 pts.**

Figure 4-9   A student care plan for a student near graduation from an LPN/LVN program.

Secondary Admitting Diagnosis is: _____

Disease Research of Admitting Diagnosis: *(Describe the processes/changes within the body that result in the signs and symptoms of the disease.)*

Textbook Signs & Symptoms. Underline the signs and symptoms your patient had.

Textbook Medical Care Typically Ordered to Diagnose & Treat the Disease:

Dx.

Tx.

Textbook Nursing Care:

Diagnostic Studies: Level IV Master					
List routine lab tests/procedures for your patient, the results and possible significance of each. Worth 15 pts.					
Lab Test/X-ray/ Procedure	Normal Value	Admit Results & Date	Day 1 Results & Date	Day 2 Results & Date	Significance
WBC					
RBC					
HGB					
HCT					
PLT					
Glucose					
BUN					
Creatinine					
Sodium					
Potassium					
Chloride					

Lab Test/X-ray/ Procedure	Normal Values	Admit Results & Date	Day 1 Results & Date	Day 2 Results & Date	Significance
Urinalysis:					
Color/ Appearance					
Specific Gravity					
Urine PH					
Protein					
Glucose					
Ketone					
Bilirubin					
Blood					
Nitrate					
Bacteria					
UA WBC					

Figure 4-9 cont'd

Lab/X-rays/ Procedure:	Normal Values	Admit Results & Date	Day 1 Results & Date	Day 2 Results & Date	Significance
Cultures:					
Wound					
Blood					
Urine					
X-Rays: CXR, MRIs, CT scans, Ultrasounds, General x-rays					

Priority Of Problems	Problem/Nursing Diagnosis *(List #1 & #2 most important problems or potential problems according to Maslow's Hierarchy, that have been identified on the existing patient care plan. Some institutions write the patient problems/nursing diagnosis in the nurse's notes rather than a separate care plan. If **unable to locate** these patient problems/nursing diagnosis, **ask the nursing instructor to identify** two problems for you.*	Nursing Interventions **(10 pts.)** *(Identify the 3–4 most important interventions that **student can perform** to resolve, improve or prevent each problem. Number them.)*	Rationale **(10 pts.)** *(Write a rationale for each intervention. Number them.)*	Evaluation/Therapeutic Effectiveness **(15 pts.)** *(Evaluate the patient's response to each intervention. Number them.)*

Patient Teaching: (10 pts.)

a) Identify 1 or 2 of your most important interventions that you either taught or reinforced to your patient. Use an established teaching plan as the basis for your teaching.

b) Explain how you know your patient understood these things. (How did you chart their understanding?)

Discharging Planning: (5 pts.)

Answer both parts on question 1 **OR** answer question 2.

1.
a) What changes or adaptations will your patient and/or family have to make as a result of your patient's illness/condition and/or treatment?

b) Will your patient and/or family require a referral to a community agency to assist with those changes or adaptations?

OR

2. What additional teaching would be beneficial to your patient? (This is in reference to health maintenance or prevention.) Use an established teaching plan.

Figure 4-9 cont'd

while the arteriogram is being obtained? Chapter 25 has information about caring for patients on telemetry.

What will you do about his activity problems? How will you get him to the bathroom? What could you do instead? How can you help keep him from getting weak even though he is on bedrest with bathroom privileges? Chapter 16 contains information about moving and positioning patients.

What about his lack of knowledge leading to anxiety about the coronary arteriography? You need to teach him what to expect during the procedure and afterward. You have looked up the information, but how do you teach it to him? Chapter 12 contains information on patient teaching.

As you go through this book and learn to care for patients, you will use information from different chapters for different situations, because every patient is a unique individual. That is why it is so important for you to learn what is in this book, allowing you to think on your feet as you provide nursing care for a variety of patients.

Caring for the Patient During Clinical Experience

Step 5—Meet and Assess the Patient

Now it is the morning of your clinical experience, and you have met Mr. Marquez. He is pale and a bit shaky, and you wonder if he is nervous. He was glad to hear that you will be with him for the arteriogram procedure. As you perform your assessment, you obtain the following data:

• His father died suddenly at 60 with what was presumed to be a heart attack.
• He verbalizes concern that he "might end up like my dad."
• He verbalizes concern over "what they will find when they look at my heart. I don't want to have open heart surgery."
• His blood pressure is 160/90, temperature 99°F (38.2°C), pulse 94 and irregular, respirations 20.
• His skin is pale and moist.
• He has had no more chest pain since the nitroglycerin patch was put on last night; he is able to walk to the bathroom without pain, but does still have dyspnea with exertion.

• He owns his own business and is frequently on the telephone with his employees while in the hospital.
• He states that he does not want to know what they are going to do today, just wants them "to do it and get it over with."
• He has a history of smoking a pack of cigarettes per day since he was 16.

Step 6—Evaluate Your Nursing Diagnoses

Now that you have assessed your patient, do you need to make any changes to the nursing diagnoses that you developed last night? Or are they still the priorities in his care? Does another diagnosis need to take priority over these?

As you look at the diagnoses you formulated last night, they still seem to be appropriate. Although Mr. Marquez is no longer having chest pain when he ambulates to the bathroom, he has the potential for chest pain at any time, so it is appropriate to leave it as a priority diagnosis.

Step 7—Implement Your Interventions

Now you will implement the interventions that you developed last night as you asked yourself all those questions about taking care of Mr. Marquez. Table 4-1 shows the nursing diagnoses with related interventions.

Step 8—Evaluate Your Care Plan

Now you are finishing up your clinical day. You have completed everything that you had planned to accomplish. Mr. Marquez made it through the coronary arteriography and had two stents placed. He knew what to expect afterward because you had prepared him, so he was able to cooperate fully. He is scheduled for discharge tomorrow and already feels better than he did before the stents were placed.

Before he is discharged, he will need additional teaching about health promotion—diet and lifestyle choices, including smoking cessation. Although you will not be taking care of him again, you know the plans for this teaching are already underway. Table 4-1 shows the evaluations of your nursing interventions for Mr. Marquez.

Table 4-1 Nursing Care Plan Interventions and Evaluation

Nursing Diagnosis: Acute pain r/t decreased oxygenation of the myocardium
Outcome: Patient will rate chest pain 0–1 by discharge.

Interventions	Evaluation
Monitor for chest pain episodes. If chest pain occurs, report to nurse immediately and take vital signs. Evaluate effectiveness of nitroglycerin spray in relieving chest pain. Monitor vital signs after use of nitro spray.	Pt had no chest pain during morning prior to arteriography. BP stable at 146/80, P – 92 and irreg, R – 20, T – 98°.
Maintain telemetry monitoring by ensuring that electrodes and wires are in place.	Telemetry maintained until pt left floor for cath lab.

Table 4-1 **Nursing Care Plan Interventions and Evaluation** (continued)

Interventions	Evaluation
Notify monitor station before removing telemetry for any reason.	Monitor station notified and telemetry monitor removed.

Nursing Diagnosis: Activity intolerance r/t decreased ability of heart to respond to demands AEB pain and dyspnea when ambulating
Outcome: Pt will ambulate 30 feet in hallway without chest pain before discharge.

Interventions	Evaluation
Assist pt to dangle first and evaluate response before getting up to BR. If pt c/o chest pain, return to bed.	Pt dangles and tol without c/o chest pain.
Ambulate pt to BR slowly, stay close and be prepared to lower to floor if pt becomes weak or loses consciousness.	VS remained stable when dangling at 140/82, P – 94, R – 24. Assisted to BR ×2 without problem. Stopped to rest ×1 when returning to bed. No loss of consciousness.
Consider asking for order for BSC if pt unable to make to the bathroom.	Unneccesary—able to amb to BR.
Monitor VS when pt returns from BR.	VS remain fairly stable. BP – 160/86, P – 98, R – 26 on return from BR.
Provide active ROM exercises for pt to prevent muscle weakness while on bedrest.	Performed active ROM ×2 prior to going to cath lab.

Nursing Diagnosis: Deficient knowledge about coronary arteriography
Outcome: Pt will verbalize what to expect during and after scheduled arteriogram.

Interventions	Evaluation
Allow pt to talk about what he knows about procedure, and concerns and fears he may have.	Pt talked about his father's death and his fears that it could happen to him. Acknowledged that his father had ignored health problems, but he was not ignoring his.
Instruct pt on what to expect during arteriogram procedure: • Pt will be awake. • Staff will be dressed in gowns, gloves, masks, goggles. • Puncture will be made into femoral artery and cath will be inserted and passed through to heart. • Pt may feel a warm sensation when contrast medium is injected. • If necessary, stents will be placed in arteries to keep them open.	At first, pt was not interested in hearing this. Said it would make him more nervous, but as time drew closer, he started asking questions, leading to pt teaching. Able to verbalize to me what stents were and what they were for.
Instruct patient on what to expect after arteriogram is performed: • Must lie flat 6 hr afterward. • Cannot bend rt leg at groin for 24 hr. • Staff will check groin frequently for bleeding. • Pt will be attached to heart and BP monitor for 2 hr after procedure.	Pt verbalized what to expect after procedure; very cooperative afterward; kept leg straight and knew what would happen when the staff checked his leg.
	Pt to be d/c'd in a.m.

You can see that you definitely used the nursing process while developing your care plan. You also realize that you did not follow the exact order in which you learned it. When you are preparing for clinicals the evening before, you must adapt the process to fit your circumstances. It is very important for you to be prepared to care for your patients when you arrive for clinicals each day, and now you have a guide for how to prepare.

Concept Maps

Concept maps, also known as "mind maps," can be used to diagram and connect data about any subject. They can also be used to organize and plan nursing care, in effect making them a care plan as well. When you use a concept map to plan care, you still use the nursing process as your basis for decision making.

Concept maps can help you see relationships between nursing diagnoses and assessment data. They can also help you make connections between interventions and diagnoses, even though those are on a separate piece of paper. Sometimes you are not sure what to do with information. Should it be a nursing diagnosis or not? Where might it fit? You can put it on your concept map with a question mark, then see where it fits later. Visual learners often enjoy using concept maps.

Steps for Concept Mapping of a Care Plan

You will follow the steps of the nursing process as you plan care for your patient, but you will also follow steps for concept mapping:

Step 1: In the middle of a blank sheet of paper, write the reason the patient is hospitalized or seeking medical care. (Figure 4-10 presents an example of a concept map.) This is usually the medical diagnosis, but not always.

Step 2: Using rectangles, write the nursing diagnoses/patient problems around the reason for hospitalization, leaving room to write in additional information. Connect the nursing diagnoses to the patient with a solid line.

Step 3: List supporting information, or evidence, from your assessment and nursing history below each nursing diagnosis (see Fig. 4-10). Write nursing actions or additional information in a triangle beneath the nursing diagnosis or patient problem.

Step 4: Connect nursing diagnoses to other nursing diagnoses with a broken line if there is a relationship. Be prepared to explain your reasons for connecting them.

Step 5: On a separate sheet of paper, make a chart showing the first priority nursing diagnosis at the top, then list the desired outcome beneath the diagnosis. Make two columns beneath the headings (see Table 4-1).

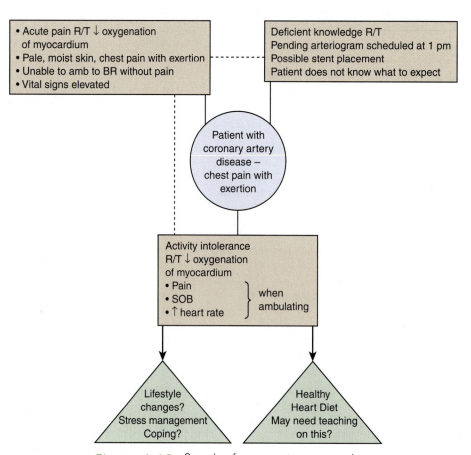

Figure 4-10 Sample of a concept map care plan.

Step 6: Write the nursing interventions in the left-hand column of the paper beneath the nursing diagnosis. Repeat this for each nursing diagnosis (see Table 4-1).

Step 7: Write your evaluation information in the right-hand column of the paper beneath the appropriate nursing diagnosis. Evaluate each intervention, nursing diagnosis, and goal and outcome (see Table 4-1).

This is just one way to create a concept map. You can make them look however you would like. Some students like to use different colors for different things, such as red for medications and green for nursing diagnoses. You can use different shapes to represent different aspects of your map, such as a square for diagnostic tests and a circle for medications. Be sure to follow any guidelines established by your school when you do concept mapping. Some people use very large sheets of paper and also include nursing interventions, outcomes, and evaluations in the concept map itself.

Whether you use a traditional care plan, a concept map, or a combination of the two, your main focus is integrating your knowledge and skills to provide the very best, individualized care for your particular patient.

Knowledge Connection

What types of care plans are available? Why do students write care plans? Which parts of a care plan can be done before your clinical experience and which parts must be done after you have met the patient?

Post Conference

After being frustrated and upset, you read your chapter and looked up your patient's major diagnoses. It was confusing to read about all of those signs and symptoms, tests, and treatments, so you decided to focus on his congestive heart failure. You were actually able to come up with about six nursing diagnoses, and some overlapped with his other diagnoses. Your instructor was impressed with your list. You still did not know how to select many interventions, but as the day went on, you began to understand better that nearly everything you did for your patient was a nursing intervention.

KEY POINTS

- Nurses make decisions using critical thinking and the nursing process.

- The steps of the nursing process are assessment, diagnosis, planning, intervention, and evaluation. RNs participate in all aspects of the nursing process. LPN/LVNs contribute to assessment and diagnosis, and participate in planning, intervention, and evaluation.

- Assessment includes collecting objective and subjective data through interviewing, physical assessment, and review of laboratory and diagnostic tests.

- Nursing diagnoses are prioritized using Maslow's hierarchy of human needs. Physiological or survival needs must be met before other needs are of concern to the patient.

- Nursing diagnoses are statements describing problems that patients are experiencing as a result of illness or health issues.

- The NANDA-I list contains nursing diagnoses developed and approved by the North American Nursing Diagnoses Association–International. The list is arranged with the primary topic first, then modifiers follow.

- Nursing diagnoses may be one-, two-, or three-part statements. All contain a diagnostic label.

Two-part statements also contain an etiology, and three-part statements contain both of these plus defining characteristics exhibited by the patient.

- Expected outcomes are specific measurable actions by the patient within a specific time frame. In care plans, there is an expected outcome for every nursing diagnosis. They are determined by the RN.

- Interventions are nursing actions taken to resolve the nursing diagnosis. When the nurse performs these interventions, it is called implementation.

- Nursing interventions may be direct or indirect, and independent, dependent, or collaborative.

- All aspects of the nursing process need to be evaluated to determine if changes in the plan are necessary. In addition, each step may be evaluated, depending on the patient's response and problems.

- Nursing care plans provide a communication tool for all nursing staff regarding the care of patients. They may be standardized, computerized, multidisciplinary, or critical pathways.

- Concept maps are alternate ways of making connections between the steps of the nursing process and determining interventions to be performed for each patient.

REVIEW QUESTIONS

Select the answer that is most appropriate for each of the following questions. Some questions may have more than one correct answer. Check all that apply.

1. Which of the following are examples of activities in which a nurse would need to use critical thinking?

   a. Prioritizing patient care

   b. Administering medications

   c. Writing nursing orders

   d. Questioning the appropriateness of an order

   e. Starting an IV infusion

2. Which of these is considered subjective data?

   a. The patient is resting on his side.

   b. The patient complains of a headache.

   c. The patient ambulated to the bathroom with assistance.

   d. The patient's mother states that he does not eat well.

3. Given that all of the following are appropriate nursing diagnoses for your patient, which would be the priority?

   a. Ineffective coping

   b. Sedentary lifestyle

   c. Risk for loneliness

   d. Self-care deficit: bathing

4. Which of these nursing diagnoses is correctly written?

   a. Readiness for enhanced knowledge related to problems with diabetes

   b. Risk for injury related to poor balance when walking

   c. Risk for falls as manifested by frequent falls in the past

   d. Anxiety and fear

SHORT ANSWER QUESTIONS

5. Give an example of the following types of nursing interventions:

   a. dependent.

   b. independent.

   c. collaborative.

6. List in correct order the steps of the nursing process.

7. Which steps of the nursing process does the LPN/LVN directly participate in? Which steps of the nursing process does the LPN/LVN contribute to?

CRITICAL THINKING EXERCISES

8. A patient is admitted with nausea and vomiting. She has lost a great deal of fluid and is dehydrated. The physician orders IV fluids and nothing by mouth. The patient is already very thin. Give two possible nursing diagnoses for this patient, using diagnostic labels only, and etiology if possible.

9. Draw a concept map of the information in and nursing diagnoses for the patient in Question 8.

ADDITIONAL RESOURCES

For additional Resources, Questions, and Activities, please see:

    Student Resource Disk

 DavisPlus **http://davisplus.fadavis.com**

   Student Study Guide

REFERENCES

American Nurses Association. *The Nursing Process: A Common Thread Amongst All Nurses.* Washington, DC: American Nurses Association; 2009.

Carlson S. A practical approach to the nursing process. *Am J Nurs.* 1972;72(9):1589-1591.

Castner J. Emergency nursing decisions: a proposed system of nursing diagnosis. *J Emerg Nurs.* 2008;34:33-36.

Doenges M, Moorhouse MF. *Application of Nursing Process and Nursing Diagnosis.* 5th ed. Philadelphia: FA Davis; 2008.

Doenges M, Moorhouse MF, Murr A. *Nursing Diagnosis Manual: Planning, Individualizing, and Documenting Client Care.* 2nd ed. Philadelphia: FA Davis; 2008.

Heaslip P. Critical thinking: to think like a nurse. 2008. Foundation for Critical Thinking Web site. Available at: http://www.criticalthinking.org/page.cfm?PageID=834&CategoryID=64. Accessed June 13, 2009.

Lown M. Editorial: content. *Teaching Learning Nurs.* 2007;2:1.

McNeill A, Porter-O'Grady T. Engaging transformation: constructing a new model for nursing education and practice. *Nurse Leader.* 2007;5(3):30-34.

Mundy K, Denham SA. Nurse educators—still challenged by critical thinking. *Teaching Learning Nurs.* 2008;3:94-99.

Quan K. The nursing process. 2007. Available at: http://www.thenursingsite.com/Articles/the%20nursing%20process.htm. Accessed June 3, 2009.

Senita J. The use of concept maps to evaluate critical thinking in the clinical setting. *Teaching Learning Nurs.* 2008;3:6-10.

Schuster P. *Concept Mapping: A Critical-Thinking Approach to Care Planning.* Philadelphia: FA Davis; 2002.

Venes D, ed. *Taber's Cyclopedic Medical Dictionary.* 20th ed. Philadelphia: FA Davis; 2005.

Wilkinson JM, Van Leuven K. *Fundamentals of Nursing: Theory, Concepts & Applications.* Philadelphia: FA Davis; 2007.

Williams LS, Hopper PD. *Understanding Medical-Surgical Nursing.* 3rd ed. Philadelphia: FA Davis; 2007.

Documentation

Key Terms

Charting by exception

Documentation

Focus charting

Kardex

Narrative charting

PIE charting

SOAPIER charting

Objectives

1. Define key terms associated with documentation.
2. Explain four purposes of written documentation.
3. Discuss confidentiality of patient records.
4. Summarize 12 guidelines for documentation.
5. Compare source-oriented and problem-oriented documentation systems.
6. List the common sections of a source-oriented documentation system.
7. Compare PIE charting and SOAPIER charting formats.
8. Contrast charting by exception and focus charting.
9. Explain how narrative charting is different from all other formats.
10. Enumerate the advantages and disadvantages of computerized charting.

Clinical Connection

Your Assignment: You are assigned to take care of a Native American Indian female who is 87 years old. She was admitted with congestive heart failure and to rule out myocardial infarction (a heart attack). You have already sailed through several clinical days and made pretty good grades, but you feel anxious about today because this is the first time that you will be expected to document your nursing care.

Your Actions: You have been mentally reviewing what all has to be charted and your mind has not come up with very many details. Plus, you are wondering which method of documentation is used at this clinical site. What if it is narrative documentation? That is one of the most detailed types of charting there is. You are afraid you will not know when to chart, let alone what to chart and how to do it correctly. While you are receiving the shift report before assuming care of the patient, a CNA on staff opens the report room door, sticks her head in, and says, "There is someone waiting at the nurse's station who is asking to view Minnie Whitefeather's chart. I did not know what to tell her. I do not know if she is a daughter or a neighbor or what, but she is insistent that she be allowed to read the chart. So hurry and come take care of her please." The nurse giving you the shift report says that she will let you take care of it because she needs to get home. Now what will you do?

Prior to entering nursing school, when you thought of nursing, you probably thought of the physical aspects of providing care to patients, such as administering injections, performing cardiopulmonary resuscitation, or holding the hand of a dying patient: the heroics of nursing. Those are all part of nursing, but nursing also encompasses the routine, daily tasks that every nurse must perform in order to ensure that every patient he or she cares for receives the utmost in care. **Documentation**, which is the act of charting or making written notation of all the things that are pertinent to each patient for whom you provide care, is one of the most important tasks you will perform on a daily basis. This written account of patient care will be maintained in a chart to serve as a permanent medical record; it is evidence of what transpired while treating a specific condition or during an event requiring medical care.

Because the patient's chart is a record of patient care you have delivered, it is imperative that you are as skilled in documentation as you are in assessing vital signs or drawing a blood sample. In this chapter, we will cover the purposes of and guidelines for documentation, explain the various documentation formats that you may see, and explain related legal concerns.

Purposes of Documentation

The process of providing ongoing medical and nursing care that meets patients' needs requires that an abundance of data be shared among all the health care providers involved with an individual patient's care. Pertinent data regarding the patient's condition, physician's orders, diagnostic results, procedures, treatment, and medications, as well as the effectiveness of each, is recorded within written, typed, or computer-generated documentation. This documentation constitutes the patient's *chart,* otherwise known as the *medical record.* Written documentation serves at least four purposes:

1. To communicate pertinent data that all health care team members need in order to provide continuity of care.
2. To provide a permanent record of medical diagnoses, nursing diagnoses, the plan of care, the care provided, and the patient's response to that care.
3. To serve as a record of accountability for quality assurance, accreditation, and reimbursement purposes.
4. To serve as a legal record for both the patient and the health care provider.

Knowledge Connection

Explain what documentation is. Relate the four purposes of documentation.

Continuity of Care

In the hospital setting, nurses are the only health care members who provide care for a patient 24 hours a day. Physicians, physical therapists, respiratory therapists, dietitians, laboratory personnel, and others provide care at intervals and sometimes on a daily basis, but not continually as does the nurse. It is nursing's responsibility to document an ongoing account of all pertinent patient data 24 hours a day. This documentation helps to provide physicians and other members of the health care team with a more complete picture of each patient's individual problems, treatments, and responses to treatment.

For patient care to be effective, it must be delivered and evaluated continuously, systematically, and smoothly from one hour to the next, including through the staffing changes between shifts. This cannot be done without communication of the patient's current condition, changes that have transpired, care that has been delivered and its effectiveness, and medications that have been administered and their effectiveness, as well as the care that is to be delivered in the oncoming hours. While some of these data can be provided through a verbal shift report, it is impossible to tell the next nurse everything that is contained within the patient's chart. The written documentation serves as a source of information that can be utilized to make decisions regarding care to be given (Fig. 5-1). You will learn more about the verbal shift report in Chapter 6.

Knowledge Connection

What is meant by *continuity of care*? Why is it so important?

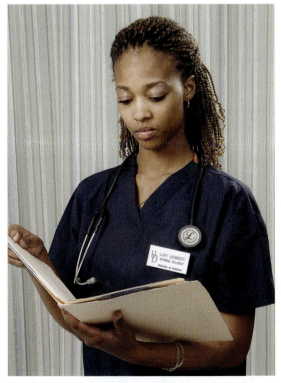

Figure 5-1 A nurse gathers data from the patient's medical record.

Permanent Record of Care

Another purpose of documentation is to produce a permanent record of the patient's condition, diagnoses, results of diagnostic tests and procedures that were performed, and all medical and interdisciplinary care that was provided, as well as the patient outcome. This record supplies a permanent source of medical history that can be used for reference when the patient requires additional health care in the future. It allows for future comparison of physical assessments, illnesses, injuries, or diagnostic test results with those previously recorded, as well as allowing for detection of any changes that may have occurred in the interval. It is not uncommon for medical records from decades past to shed light on present-day medical problems.

Accountability

Medical records, or charts, are utilized by facility quality assurance committees as they monitor the quality of care being delivered in their institution. Records help facilities to detect problems, less-than-desirable outcomes, or areas of weakness in their delivery systems so that improvements can be made. Statistics such as rates of hospital-acquired infections, mortality rates, success rates of specific procedures, and number of incidents and accidents serve as defining factors of a medical facility's reputation. This motivates continual internal assessment and evaluation of the care that is delivered.

Government and other accrediting agencies, such as The Joint Commission, also audit medical records to verify facility compliance in meeting established health care standards. The Joint Commission sets the standards by which the quality of health care is measured both nationally and internationally. It seeks to improve the safety and quality of the care that health care organizations provide to the public. Standards are written for different types of facilities, such as critical access hospitals, long-term care facilities, home health care, and outpatient surgery offices. To be accredited by The Joint Commission, a facility must practice in a manner that meets The Joint Commission's standards. This is determined by a team of reviewers who visit the facility to assess its policies, procedures, and actual performance and ensure that the standards are met.

Reimbursement by insurance companies and other third-party payers is generally dependent upon documentation of specific data in the medical record, making correct documentation an issue of financial survival for medical institutions. Researchers also utilize data from medical records in their experimental work and development.

Knowledge Connection

Explain what The Joint Commission has to do with documentation. How do quality assurance committees utilize documentation? Describe why insurance companies would have need of documentation.

Legal Record

The documentation in the permanent record serves as a legal record for both the patient and the health care providers. It can be used in a court of law by the patient to prove that malpractice or negligence occurred, but it can also be used by health care providers to defend or disprove claims of malpractice or negligence—that is, *if* adequate documentation was performed. From a legal standpoint, it is best to assume that, if it wasn't charted, it wasn't done. While that may not always be the case, in many courts that will be the standard, which is why it is so imperative to document thoroughly all patient care and pertinent data.

Not Charted, Not Done

The phrase *"Not charted, not done"* is interpreted to mean that, if something is not documented, then it was not done or did not occur. This can apply to an assessment finding, a change in a patient's condition or situation, or a nursing intervention that you performed, as well as many other things. The concept of "not charted, not done" has been treated as a literal truth in medical negligence and malpractice cases for many years. Quality assurance committees, accrediting agency examiners, attorneys, and nurses continue to function according to this idea, believing that, if something is not charted, then it was not done...period. However, this is inherently false if the documentation method is charting by exception (explained in more detail later in this chapter), which limits charting to only *abnormal* findings, situations, conditions, or results. Anything falling within the realm of normal would not be charted, making it difficult to prove that you did something.

The phrase "not charted, not done" is not limited to just this particular method of documentation; it may be applied to all documentation methods. It may also be used against you when you simply forget to chart something that is, or later turns out to be, pertinent. This requires you to always chart with a clear understanding of the following: Documentation that is lacking in full detail serves to support even false claims of negligence or malpractice.

Lawsuits often are not filed until years after the precipitating event, possibly long after the patient or event has been forgotten by the medical personnel who delivered care at that time. In some states, events occurring during labor and delivery can be called into evidence for a very long time—until the baby that was delivered is 21 years of age. The longer the interval is between occurrence and legal involvement, the more important the things you documented will be, because they will serve as the record of what actually happened. This record is considered much more credible than any one individual's memory.

If you should ever find yourself involved in a malpractice suit brought by one of your patients, especially one whom you do not remember, you will find it comforting to discover that you were careful to document objectively, accurately, and thoroughly. However, if you discovered charting omissions, misspellings, phrases that do not make sense, unapproved abbreviations, illegible handwriting, or any number of unwise shortcuts within your documentation, you would likely find it distressing and worrisome.

Knowledge Connection

Explain how documentation is pertinent during a lawsuit. What types of errors could possibly make you, the nurse, "look bad"?

Whose Medical Record Is It?

As you learned in Chapter 3, the original written or computerized medical record, even though it is about the patient, is the property of the hospital or facility. In a physician-owned medical office, the record is the property of the physician. *However, all the information within the chart belongs to the patient.* The patient is guaranteed by the Health Insurance Portability and Accountability Act (HIPAA) the right to view and obtain a copy of the medical record, but the patient does not have the right to take the original chart copy itself. HIPAA ensures the patient's right not only to view and copy his or her own medical record, but also to amend his or her own health information. HIPAA also requires hospitals and medical sites to disclose to each patient, in writing, the way the patient's health data will be used and to ask the patient to specify who can obtain the patient's personal health data. As a result, hospitals have become more careful regarding who may view the chart, and most require that the patient sign a document indicating who may view the medical record or obtain verbal reports about his or her condition or tests and surgery reports. You are responsible to know your facility's policy regarding this issue. Never allow anyone to access the chart until you have verified the facility's policy and ensured that the patient has granted consent in writing.

Confidentiality of Documentation

As you learned in Chapter 3, federal and state laws govern confidentiality of patients' medical data. HIPAA requires that medical data be maintained in a confidential manner at all times. This applies to the patient's chart, results of diagnostic procedures and consultations, and any notes you might write regarding the patient's health status. Remember that you cannot even confirm that an individual is a patient in your facility without specific permission from the patient. Therefore, all medical records must be protected and maintained in such a manner that no unauthorized individuals have access to them, only the health care providers that are directly involved in the patient's care. Take care to avoid leaving patient care notes, laboratory results, medication administration records (MARs), and patient charts lying open and accessible by other facility employees and the public. Before you are allowed to send medical records to even another physician to whom the patient is being referred, the patient must sign a written consent. Any handwritten notes or copies of confidential patient information should be shredded once their purpose has been fulfilled. Most nurses' stations have a paper shredder to aid you in keeping records private.

Faxing of medical information has become a common occurrence and brings with it another opportunity to breach confidentiality laws. Just before you fax the medical record, telephone the intended recipient to inform him or her of the impending confidential fax. This helps to ensure that the intended recipient is present to receive the fax in an effort to prevent it from lying unattended when it is received.

Knowledge Connection

To whom does the original patient medical record belong? Explain the rights of the patient regarding his or her medical record. What should you do prior to faxing a medical record?

Forms of Documentation

You will need to be familiar with various forms of documentation. In some facilities, a form of documentation is the **Kardex**, which is a type of flip chart with a page for each patient on the unit or floor that contains a summary of care required by the patient and requires continual updating and maintenance by nursing staff. Another type of documentation you will use is known as an *incident report* or *variance report*. When accidents, incidents, mistakes, or anything out of the ordinary occurs, you will be required to file a written report. There are also various forms in the patient's chart that you must complete every shift. If you work in a hospital or long-term care facility, at the beginning of your shift you will receive a report from the off-going nurse about each of your assigned patients. The shift report will be discussed more thoroughly in Chapter 6, but the written notes that you should make during the shift report will be included in this chapter as a form of written documentation.

Report Form

As your work shift will begin with an initial patient report, we will begin with the form on which you will document report information. Most facilities have a standard report form on which to document the report you receive at the beginning of your shift. An example may be seen in Figure 5-2. The notes that you take during the shift report should be detailed and all-inclusive so they can serve as your template for scheduled duties for the coming shift. This form will need specific areas to document the following:

- Room number; patient name, age, and gender; and attending physician
- Date of admission and diagnoses
- Frequency of vital signs and activity orders
- Type of diet ordered, nothing-by-mouth (NPO) status, fluid restrictions, IV, or intake and output totals
- Any diagnostics to be done and pertinent results of recent tests
- Personal care that may be needed
- All nursing care to be delivered

You will also need room to make additional notes throughout the shift as things occur. Nurses commonly refer to these notes as their "pocket-brains." Few nurses are able to accurately remember all the necessary details that should be documented and reported to the oncoming shift, without some form of pocket-brains. Some nurses prefer to create a self-designed format that works best for them. Figure 5-3 presents a sample of one nurse's pocket-brains. It was designed so that only a glance was required to identify the blank lines and the times of the tasks that were to be performed. One could be made for each patient during a shift; this one, which was handwritten, could be modified when additional nursing care was in order. If you make your own, figure out what works best for you and be certain to use the same order or format for each set of patient data and draw blank lines for marking each task completed. You will probably want to save time and use computer technology to create your pocket-brains.

The ideal method to ensure documentation accuracy is to consistently chart immediately after care is provided, after assessment data are obtained, and after any event or occurrence that has the potential to affect the patient. However, the reality of documentation is that it is not always possible to chart immediately. The very patient about whom you need to document something may require numerous other aspects of care before you can get to the chart. Other patients may have needs that are higher priority than charting. You simply get busy. However, no matter how busy you get, there are certain things that you can do to increase the accuracy of your documentation.

One thing you can do is to write a quick note on your pocket-brains right at the bedside or just outside the patient's room door, providing yourself with specific times and data that can be transcribed onto the chart as soon as possible. One might argue that to write something down and then be forced to copy or rewrite it on the chart provides another chance for error. This is true; but it is also true that, for most of us, it is safer to write notes as things happen, along with the exact time of occurrence, rather than to assume that we will remember everything we need to chart at some point later in the shift. We may remember what happened and think that we know the correct time it occurred. However, there are nurses who can testify to the hard lessons learned because of poor memory. It should be understood that our memories are fallible when we are trying to keep track of dozens of facts about multiple patients; especially when you throw in one or two episodes of adrenaline rush due to emergent situations. Excessive stimuli decrease the average individual's ability to recall details. A patient's improvement, even the patient's life, may be dependent upon the accuracy of your documentation.

Nursing Report

Room	Name	Dr	Diag.	Age/Sex	V. Signs	IV/Rate	FSBS	Diet	Guaiac	Tele	Tests/Notes
101		A G K M S			4 8 12		Da Bid Qid		Emesis 1 2 3 Stool 1 2 3		
102		A G K M S			4 8 12		Da Bid Qid		Emesis 1 2 3 Stool 1 2 3		
103		A G K M S			4 8 12		Da Bid Qid		Emesis 1 2 3 Stool 1 2 3		
104		A G K M S			4 8 12		Da Bid Qid		Emesis 1 2 3 Stool 1 2 3		
105		A G K M S			4 8 12		Da Bid Qid		Emesis 1 2 3 Stool 1 2 3		
107		A G K M S			4 8 12		Da Bid Qid		Emesis 1 2 3 Stool 1 2 3		
108		A G K M S			4 8 12		Da Bid Qid		Emesis 1 2 3 Stool 1 2 3		
109		A G K M S			4 8 12		Da Bid Qid		Emesis 1 2 3 Stool 1 2 3		
110		A G K M S			4 8 12		Da Bid Qid		Emesis 1 2 3 Stool 1 2 3		
111		A G K M S			4 8 12		Da Bid Qid		Emesis 1 2 3 Stool 1 2 3		
112		A G K M S			4 8 12		Da Bid Qid		Emesis 1 2 3 Stool 1 2 3		
114		A G K M S			4 8 12		Da Bid Qid		Emesis 1 2 3 Stool 1 2 3		
115		A G K M S			4 8 12		Da Bid Qid		Emesis 1 2 3 Stool 1 2 3		
116		A G K M S			4 8 12		Da Bid Qid		Emesis 1 2 3 Stool 1 2 3		
117		A G K M S			4 8 12		Da Bid Qid		Emesis 1 2 3 Stool 1 2 3		

Figure 5-2 A sample of a facility report form.

Rm 201	Matt Hau 54 y/o/m Dr. Evans Adm. 6/2/11 Dx: MI Allergic: PCN
	Ordered Tests: EKG today Meds @ ~~7:30, 9~~, 11:30, 2:00.
	IV Rt wrist. 18g. ¹/₂ NS @ 60 mL/hr per pump: new bag @_____
	Bedrest w/ BRP__✓__ Turn q 2 hrs: 8__✓__ 10__✓__ 12____ 2____
	VS @ 8___146/88__98-88irr-18_____12_____.
	O² @ 4 L/M per NC con't__✓__ SpO₂ @ 8___96%__ 12_____
	Reg diet: B__75 %__ L____% Foley__✓__
	Bedbath @__10:30_____ mouth & skin care q4hr 9__✓__ 1____
	I-____mL O-____mL BMs X__1 lg soft brown_____

Figure 5-3 An example of handwritten "pocket-brains."

Accuracy of the time at which things occur and tasks are performed can be momentous in regard to legal action as well. It would be difficult, if not impossible, to explain from the witness chair how Patient X could have been "Lying quietly with eyes closed. Respirations even and regular at 19/min" at 1930, when Patient X was actually in the imaging department having magnetic resonance imaging performed from 1910 until 1955. It is vital that you vigilantly document things at the correct time they were done and as soon as possible after the event or task.

Knowledge Connection
What is a report form? Explain the various types of data that you will document on the report form.

Kardex

Many facilities use a Kardex, which contains written data and is used for quick reference regarding each patient's care. A Kardex has a page for each patient on that floor or unit. Each page folds in half to fit into the Kardex chart holder. The Kardex page lists all the care that should be provided for that specific patient. It places the physician's orders and the nursing orders for each patient in one location, on a single page where it can be retrieved or referred to quickly, without having to go through an entire patient chart or medical record. Some facilities prefer not to use the Kardex chart holder, keeping each patient's Kardex page flat and placing it in the front of the patient's medical record. In facilities where medical records are in a computerized format rather than a hard-copy chart, the Kardex is really a necessity to use for shift reports and to quickly look up such things as diet, type of bath to be given, or frequency of vital signs assessment during the shift.

Kardex pages are usually made of card stock rather than regular paper so that they can withstand the many erasures that occur as orders change over days, weeks, or even months. Basic patient data and all physician's and nursing orders are noted along with the date ordered (Fig. 5-4). Each time a new order is written and an order is noted or processed by the nurse or unit clerk, it is added to the Kardex. Orders to discontinue specific care are recorded in the Kardex either by erasing the order that has been discontinued or by highlighting the discontinued order with yellow marker to indicate that it is no longer in effect. Each facility will have specific policies and procedures to follow regarding Kardex systems. Some facilities will file the Kardex page with the patient's medical record, while others shred it at the patient's discharge from the facility.

Incident Reports

Another type of documentation that is not part of the patient's medical record is the incident report, also known as the variance report. These reports are used to document out-of-the-ordinary things that happen in a facility. The incident or occurrence may or may not actually involve a patient. Occurrences that should be documented on an incident or variance report form include the following:

- Medication error
- Patient injury
- Visitor injury
- Employee injury
- Condition constituting a safety hazard, such as unsafe staffing situation or failure to repair reported broken or damaged equipment
- Failure of appropriate health care provider response to an emergency
- Failure to perform ordered care
- Loss of patient's personal belongings, prosthetic or assistive devices, home medications, or secured valuables
- Lack of availability of vital patient care supplies or equipment

Some nurses feel that completion of an incident report is punitive, but that is far from the truth. In fact, the report is designed to better protect the facility, you, and the patient when something unusual occurs, by providing accurate facts regarding the incident or occurrence. When completing an incident or variance report, be objective, documenting only what you were able to detect with your senses: what you saw, heard, smelled, or were able to feel with your hands. Avoid interpreting what you saw or heard, such as "Heard the patient fall from the chair to the floor." Keep it completely objective: "Heard loud crashing sound." Rather than write that the "patient fell out of bed," document only objective data such as "found patient lying face down on the floor beside the bed" and "patient reports he fell out of bed while trying to reach his telephone." Never document assumptions or drawn conclusions.

DOCTOR'S ORDERS

Activity _8/9 increase activity_
_____ _daily_

☐ Bedrest		☐ Up in Chair	
☒ BRP		☐ Up ad lib	
☐ Dangle		☒ TCDpBr q2°	
☒ Ambulate _T/D_		☐ BSC only	

DATE	ORDER
8/9	TED
8/9	Chg. abd drsg daily
8/8	DC foley in AM

IV #	SOLUTION	SIZE	ADDITIVE	RATE
2	D5¹/₂ NS	1000 mL	20 mEg KCL	125 mL/hr
3	D5¹/₂ NS	1000 mL	Ø	80 mL/hr

IV - Lt forearm 8-8-11 10pm

Restarted Rt hand 8-9 4pm

ALLERGIES | _PCN, Compazine_

Patient Classification Number _____
Room # _1126_ Name _Ruth Weaver_

PROSTHESIS
X Dentures
X Hearing Aide
___ Contact Lens
X Glasses
___ Limb _____
___ Eye _____ Rt. _____ Lt.

HOME MEDICATIONS
X None with Pt/(Home)
___ In Room With Pt.
___ In Pharmacy
___ In Drug Cart

BATH/HYGIENE
X Bed   X Complete
___ Tub   ___ Assist
___ Shower   ___ Self
___ Sizt   X Mouth Care
_____   X Skin Care

BLADDER/BOWEL
___ Independent
X Foley
___ Straight Cath.
___ Incontinent
___ BSC
___ Ostomy _____

ORDERED LAB & X-RAYS

Date	Test
8/8	CBC, UA, CXR.
	EKG, Chem 21,
	PT, PTT
8/9	CBC today
	Lytes in AM

ADM. DX. _8/8 abd pain & N/V_
unknown etiology
8/9 appendicitis

SMOKER
☐ Yes   ☒ No

DIET

Date	Type
8/8	NPO
8/10	Full liq

☒ Assist   ☒ Set up
☐ Self   ☐ Feed

FLUIDS
X I/O
___ Force Fluids
___ Restrict Fluids
   7–3 _____
   3–11 _____
   11–7 _____

SAFETY PRECAUTIONS
X Siderails _x2_
   ___ Night Only
   X Constant
___ Restraints
   ___ PRN
   ___ Constant
___ Smoking Precautions

ATTENTION
8/8 Exp lap in AM

Pre-op teaching

tonight

ADM. TIME _9:15 pm_
ADM. DATE _8-8-11_
DOCTOR _Keast_
AGE _73_

Figure 5-4 A sample Kardex page.

Incident forms will include not only the incident, but also the action taken and any care provided after the occurrence. They will have a section in which you will list any witnesses that observed the occurrence, the physician who was notified and any orders received, the signature of the employee involved or who discovered the variance, and the supervisor's signature. (Refer to the sample incident report form in Chapter 3, Figure 3-2.) These reports are kept separate from patient records, and are reviewed and analyzed by facility committees according to policy and procedure. The incident or variance report provides an accurate record of what happened for use if legal action results. Most importantly, however, it helps to identify unsafe conditions or situations for which a change in facility policy and procedure may prevent or at least reduce the risk for repeated occurrences.

Knowledge Connection

Describe what is meant by a Kardex form. What happens to the Kardex upon the patient's discharge from the hospital? Explain why incident or variance reports are not filed with the patient's medical record. List at least five types of occurrences for which an incident or variance report should be completed.

Care Plans

Another form of written documentation is the plan of care developed for each patient, which was covered in depth in Chapter 4. The care plan serves to communicate the patient's problems, what interventions are to be performed for each problem, and the effectiveness of each intervention. Revisions and modifications to the plan of care are made and documented within the plan as the patient's changing condition warrants, providing a current plan of action for health care providers to follow each day.

Patient Chart or Medical Record

The most lengthy and encompassing form of written documentation is the patient's chart or medical record. While some facilities still maintain only hard-copy, or paper, charts, most facilities have changed or are in the process of changing to computerized, also known as electronic, medical records. The format of both the paper medical record and the computerized medical record depends on the type of documentation system that is utilized within the medical facility. We will cover the two documentation system types later in this chapter.

Guidelines for Documentation

There are various guidelines that should direct your documentation in an effort to produce a more accurate, objective, complete, and reliable record of the patient's changing condition, the nursing care you provided, and the effectiveness of that care.

Use Black or Blue Ink

Dependent upon facility policy, write all entries in permanent black or blue ink. Avoid using pencil, erasable ink, or colored inks such as purple, red, or green. Black or blue ink will copy better than other colors.

Write Neatly and Legibly

If other health care providers are unable to read your handwritten notes, the risk of errors increases and continuity of care is inhibited. Avoid using swirls, curly-cues, large loops, or little circles or hearts to dot your "i" or "j." Keep handwriting neat and legible. If your cursive writing is not legible, print your notes. If you always remember that the chart is a *legal* document, it may help motivate you to keep it readable.

Sign Each Entry

Always sign each entry with your first initial, last name, and credentials according to facility policy. Your credentials are the formal initials of the specific nursing license and certifications that you hold. For example, a registered nurse signs RN and a licensed practical or vocational nurse signs LPN or LVN. Your signature must be legible.

Knowledge Connection

Explain why it is important that all entries are legible and why you must sign each entry. If your cursive handwriting is not clear and legible, what should you do when charting?

Include the Date and Time With Each Entry

Each entry generally requires the date and time in front of the entry. However, some facilities require the date to be written only once on each page. Many facilities now use military time in an effort to decrease confusion between a.m. and p.m. (Fig. 5-5). Military time is not difficult to learn. After 12:00 noon, for the p.m. hours, you simply add 12 to the hour. The colon is no longer used and the minutes remain the same. For example, to obtain the military equivalent for 3:00 p.m., add 12 to the hour. The time would be 1500. The equivalent for 3:50 p.m. would be 1550.

Follow Chronological Order

Documentation should begin at the start of your shift and continue in the order in which it occurs. Use specific times for each entry. Avoid documenting in blocks of time, such as from "8:30 to 12:30." Most acute care hospitals require that you make an entry at least every 2 hours. If an entry is inadvertently omitted, make a late entry by documenting the time you are writing the entry; then write "late entry for...,"

Figure 5-5 Many health care facilities use the 24-hour clock.

including the time of the actual occurrence. Make the entry and sign it as usual. For example:

07-10-12 0945 Late entry for 0830. Restlessly tossing and turning. Moaning. Ativan 1 mg administered IO push over 2 minutes.———— Nurse's signature and credentials

Make Entries in a Timely Manner

Document all assessment findings and provided care as soon as possible after the occurrence. If unable to document on the chart immediately, write a note on your pocket-brains, including time and pertinent details. Then transcribe the information to the patient's chart as soon as you are able. Otherwise, another staff member may make an entry before yours, making your out-of-sequence entry a late entry. Never chart something before it is done, as this is fraudulent.

> **Knowledge Connection**
> Why are date, time, chronological order, and documenting in a timely manner such a high priority? What is the military or 24-hour clock time for 10:15 p.m.? For 4:30 a.m.? For 3:45 p.m.?

Be Succinct

Make entries brief, concise, and to the point. It is not necessary to use complete and grammatically correct sentences when documenting. The accepted standard is to omit unnecessary words that are not pertinent to the clarity of the entry, such as "the" or "a." Because the chart is written about the patient, it is not necessary to use the word "patient." This applies equally to the other patient designations such as "client" or "resident." It is understood that you are documenting about the patient, client, or resident. Table 5-1 presents examples of succinct documentation.

Use Punctuation

Begin the first word of each phrase with an uppercase letter and use punctuation, usually a period, at the end of each phrase. Avoid using exclamation marks or question marks as they tend to imply emotion or doubt, which can make the entry appear subjective.

> **Knowledge Connection**
> Why do you think it is important to start each phrase with an uppercase letter and place a period at the end of the phrase?

Use Only Approved Abbreviations

It is your responsibility to know which abbreviations and symbols may be used in your documentation and which ones may not be used. Most facilities have their own list of approved abbreviations and symbols that may be used in documentation. The Joint Commission's 2009 National Patient Safety Goals also require that each facility has a documented standardized list of abbreviations, symbols, dose designations, and acronyms that are *not* to be used anywhere in the facility. The facility's list must include each of the items on The Joint Commission's official "Do Not Use" list (Table 5-2). Box 5-1 provides a list of commonly used health care abbreviations.

Table 5-1 Examples of Succinct Charting

When charting, remember that it is not necessary to use complete sentences as long as the correct meaning is imparted.

Lengthy Entry	Succinct Entry
"The patient got up to the bathroom to urinate and was able to go on her own without any help. She voided into the specimen pan. I measured 450 mL of real light yellow urine that does not have any sediment or particles in it. Then she walked from the bathroom back to bed."	"Ambulated unassisted to bathroom. Voided 450 mL clear, pale yellow urine. Back to bed."
"Upon entering the room, I found the patient just laying there. I spoke to him, but he did not answer me and did not open his eyes. He was pale and did not have as much color as he did this morning. His skin felt real moist and also cooler than it did at the beginning of the shift. He did not respond to me touching him either. Then I used pressure on one of his nailbeds on each hand, and he moaned softly. But he did not open his eyes at all. I took his blood pressure and got 84/46. I took his apical pulse and got 116. It was also irregular and quite hard to hear both the S_1 and the S_2...."	"Lying supine. Eyes closed. Responds only to pain stimuli: moans when pressure applied to nailbed. Pale, cool, & clammy. BP – 84/46. AP – 116 muffled & irregular. R – 9 shallow & irregular...."

Table 5-2 **List of The Joint Commission's "Do Not Use" Abbreviations**

Official "Do Not Use" List[1]

Do Not Use	Potential Problem	Use Instead
U (unit)	Mistaken for "0" (zero), the number "4" (four) or "cc"	Write "unit"
IU (International Unit)	Mistaken for IV (intravenous) or the number 10 (ten)	Write "International Unit"
Q.D., QD, q.d., qd (daily) Q.O.D., QOD, q.o.d., qod (every other day)	Mistaken for each other Period after the Q mistaken for "I" and the "O" mistaken for "I"	Write "daily" Write "every other day"
Trailing zero (X.0 mg)* Lack of leading zero (.X mg)	Decimal point is missed	Write X mg Write 0.X mg
MS MSO$_4$ and MgSO$_4$	Can mean morphine sulfate or magnesium sulfate Confused for one another	Write "morphine sulfate" Write "magnesium sulfate"

Additional Abbreviations, Acronyms, and Symbols[2]

> (greater than) < (less than)	Misinterpreted as the number "7" (seven) or the letter "L" Confused for one another	Write "greater than" Write "less than"
Abbreviations for drug names	Misinterpreted due to similar abbreviations for multiple drugs	Write drug names in full
Apothecary units	Unfamiliar to many practitioners Confused with metric units	Use metric units
@	Mistaken for the number "2" (two)	Write "at"
cc	Mistaken for U (units) when poorly written	Write "ml" or "milliliters"
μg	Mistaken for mg (milligrams) resulting in one thousand-fold overdose	Write "mcg" or "micrograms"

[1]Applies to all orders and all medication-related documentation that is handwritten (including free-text computer entry) or on pre-printed forms.

*Exception: A "trailing zero" may be used only where required to demonstrate the level of precision of the value being reported, such as for laboratory results, imaging studies that report size of lesions, or catheter/tube sizes. It may not be used in medication orders or other medication-related documentation.

[2]For possible future inclusion in the Official "Do Not Use" List.

Be Accurate

Make certain that all pertinent data are recorded. Be factual. Be specific. Chart the correct time for each entry. Make certain to use correct terminology and watch your spelling. Keep descriptions of behaviors and events objective. Avoid putting labels on them. Avoid using judgmental language. Do not document your opinions, assumptions, interpretations, or self-drawn conclusions. Refrain from using subjective terms such as *strange, well, average, normal, bad, poor,* *odd,* or *good* because they are vague and mean different things to different people. If you want to chart that you think the patient is acting "strangely," describe only what you see or hear that makes you think the behavior is "strange." Is the patient avoiding making eye contact with you? Is the patient picking at the air with his fingers, as if he were picking something out of the air? Is she talking aloud when no one else is present in the room? Specify what is happening to lead you to think the behavior is "strange," rather than

Box 5-1

Commonly Used Health Care **Abbreviations**

Abbreviations	Meaning	Abbreviations	Meaning
½NS	0.45% sodium chloride	ER	emergency room
¼NS	0.22% sodium chloride	ETOH	alcohol
⅓NS	0.33% sodium chloride	F	female
3%NS	3% sodium chloride	Fr	French (diameter size measurement)
ā	before		
AAO×4	awake, alert, and oriented times four spheres	FSB	fasting blood sugar
		FSBS	finger stick blood sugar
abd	abdomen	ft	foot or feet
ac	before meals	fx	fracture
ADL	activities of daily living	g	gram
ad lib	as patient desires	GI	gastrointestinal
AEB	as evidenced by	gr	grain
AKA	above-the-knee amputation	gtt(s)	drop/drops
amb	ambulate, ambulatory	GU	genitourinary
amp	ampule	GYN	gynecology
amt	amount	HA	headache
ASAP	as soon as possible	Hct	hematocrit
ax	axillary	Hgb	hemoglobin
BE	barium enema	h/o	history of
bid	twice per day	hob	head of bed
BKA	below-the-knee amputation	HOH	hard of hearing
BM	bowel movement	H&P	history and physical
BMR	basal metabolic rate	hr	hour
BP	blood pressure	HS	hour of sleep
bpm	beats per minute	ht	height
BR	bedrest	HTN	hypertension
BRP	bathroom privileges	hyper	above or high
BSC	bedside commode	hypo	below or low
c̄	with	ICU	intensive care unit
ca	cancer	ID	intradermal
cal	calories	IDDM	insulin-dependent diabetes mellitus
cath	catheter		
CBC	complete blood count	IM	intramuscular
CCU	coronary care unit; critical care unit	Inj	injection
		I/O	intake and output
chem.	chemistry	IV	intravenous
CHF	congestive heart failure	IVP	intravenous push
cm	centimeter	IVPB	intravenous piggyback
C/O, c/o	complained of	L	liter
CO₂	carbon dioxide	lb	pound
CPR	cardiopulmonary resuscitation	liq	liquids
CVA	cerebrovascular accident; stroke	LLE	left lower extremity
CXR	chest x-ray	LLL	left lower lobe
D5 ½NS	dextrose 5% in 0.45% sodium chloride	LLQ	left lower quadrant
		LMP	last menstrual period
D5RL	dextrose 5% in lactated Ringers' solution	LOC	level of consciousness
		LUE	left upper extremity
D5W	dextrose 5% in water	LUL	left upper lobe
D&C	dilation and curettage	LUQ	left upper quadrant
DM	diabetes mellitus	med	medication
Dp Br	deep breathe	mg	milligram
dsg or drsg	dressing	mL	milliliter
Dx	diagnosis	MN	midnight
ECG or EKG	electrocardiogram	NAS	no added salt
EEG	electroencephalogram	NG	nasogastric
EENT	eyes, ears, nose, throat	NGT	nasogastric tube

Box 5-1

Commonly Used Health Care Abbreviations (continued)

Abbreviations	Meaning	Abbreviations	Meaning
NKA	no known allergies	Ⓡ	rectal
NKDA	no known drug allergies	R	respirations
noc	night	RLE	right lower extremity
NPO	nothing by mouth	RLL	right lower lobe
NS	0.9% sodium chloride	RLQ	right lower quadrant
N/V/D	nausea, vomiting, diarrhea	RML	right middle lobe
O	oral	R/O	rule out
O_2	oxygen	Rt	right
OB	obstetrics	RUE	right upper extremity
OOB	out of bed	RUL	right upper lobe
OR	operating room	RUQ	right upper quadrant
ortho	orthopedics	Rx	prescription
os	mouth or opening	$\bar{s}$	without
OT	occupational therapy	SCD	sequential compression device
OTC	over the counter	SOB	shortness of breath
oz	ounce	SpO_2	percentage of hemoglobin saturated with oxygen
P	pulse		
$\bar{p}$	after	SSE	soapsuds enema
pc	after meals	stat	immediately
PCA	patient-controlled analgesia	STD	sexually transmitted disease
PEARL	pupils equal and reactive to light	T	temperature
		TB	tuberculosis
PEARLA	pupils equal and reactive to light and accommodation	tid	three times per day
		TO	telephone order
PERLA	pupils equally reactive to light and accommodation	TPR	temperature, pulse, respirations
		Tx	treatment
PERRLA	pupils equally round and reactive to light and accommodation	UA	urinalysis
		VO	verbal order
PO	by mouth	VS	vital signs
PPP	peripheral pulses palpated	WBC	white blood cell count
prn	as needed	W/C	wheelchair
PT	physical therapy	WDI	warm, dry intact
q	every	WNL	within normal limits
qid	four times per day	wt	weight

describing it as strange. If you think a patient tolerated the clear liquid diet "well," think of the reasons why you think the patient tolerated it well. Was it because the patient did not experience nausea or vomiting after consumption of the first liquids allowed following being NPO? Or was it because the patient with *dysphagia,* or difficulty swallowing, did not choke or aspirate the liquids? Whatever caused you to think the patient tolerated it "well" is what you should chart.

Do not allow *your* perspective or your personal feelings and emotions to be expressed in your documentation. Chart only those objective data that you can detect with your senses:

- What you can see, read, or observe with your eyes
- What you can smell with your olfactory sense
- What you can feel using your sense of touch

- What you can hear with your ears with or without a stethoscope, which also includes subjective data that the patient, family, or significant other may tell you

Refer back to Chapter 4, Table 4-1, for a description of different types of objective data. Table 5-3 shows the differences between subjective and objective entries. The only subjective data that you will chart will be things that the patient, family, or significant other tells you. When you chart direct quotations of the patient, you should use his or her *exact* words and place them in quotation marks. Correct examples of charting what the patient told you might include:

- States *"I have vomited everything I have eaten and drunk since yesterday."*
- Supine, holding lower abdomen with both hands. Moaning. States *"The pain is getting worse. I don't know if I can stand it or not."*

It would be incorrect to chart what the patient said in the following manner:

- States *"he vomited everything he ate and drank since yesterday."* (The bold underlined words are not the patient's exact words.)
- Supine, holding lower abdomen with both hands. Moaning. States *"his pain is getting worse and he doesn't know if he can stand it or not."*

Do Not Leave Blank Lines

Avoid leaving a blank line, or even a blank portion of a line. Blank lines serve as an invitation for another individual to write something in the middle of your charting that could be attributed to you. If you do not fill the line completely, draw a single straight line through the middle of the space, extending from the last word to your signature. Then sign your name and credentials (Fig. 5-6). If your charting completely fills the line, leaving no room for your signature, avoid crowding your signature at the end or in the margin. Simply draw a single straight line through the middle of the space on the next line, leaving room for your signature and credentials.

Use Continued Notes

When there is not enough room to complete your entry on a page, it must be continued on the next page. Stop writing on the last line at a point that leaves room for you to write *"(continued)—Nurse's signature and credentials"* (Fig. 5-7).

Correct Mistaken Entries

Upon making an incorrect entry, mark a single horizontal line through the incorrect word or phrase. Write "mistaken entry" and your initials just above the incorrect words (Fig. 5-8). Then proceed with the correct entry. *Never* use correction fluid or correction tape to totally blank out the mistaken entry. Avoid using markers or making multiple ink marks in an effort to blacken the incorrect entry so that it cannot be read, as this may raise suspicion regarding the entry. Also avoid trying to "write over" incorrect letters. This only serves to make documentation sloppy and difficult to read.

Keep the Medical Record Intact

The medical record must be kept intact. Never discard any part of the chart. Even if a page of your nurse's notes

Table 5-3 Subjective Versus Objective Entries

Subjective Entry*	Objective Entry
Ate *well* and tolerated it well.	Ate 80% full liquid diet unassisted. Tolerated without nausea or vomiting.
Ate *most* of lunch. Tolerated *well.*	Fed 90% clear liquid diet by wife, who stated he swallowed easily without choking or strangling.
Worried & nervous about impending surgery. Instructed about procedure.	Sitting in chair at bedside. Tapping fingertips on arm of chair. Bouncing left leg repeatedly. Inquired if he had any questions or concerns about his surgery tomorrow. Responded by asking several questions about surgery. Sat beside him for 15–20 minutes: answered questions, marked surgical sites on RUQ abdomen, & explained what to expect preop & postop. Laparoscopic Cholecystectomy Patient Teaching Brochure reviewed verbally with patient & left at bedside. Encouraged to read it and ask any questions that come to mind. States he already understands better and does not feel as nervous as he did, but will call if he has more questions. Posture more relaxed. No longer tapping fingers or bouncing left leg.
Wound *worse* today.	Wound measures larger than on 6-1-12. Now 2 cm × 2.5 cm. Wound bed bright red. Now draining green purulent drainage.
Had a *good* night.	1200 Left lateral position. Eyes closed. Resp reg & even. 0115 Supine. Eyes closed. Resp reg & even. 0320 Snoring softly. 0530 Assisted to bedside commode. Voided 350 mL clear, yellow urine. Assisted back to bed. 0615 Supine. Eyes closed. Resp reg & even.

*Note: words in *italics* are subjective terms.

William, Mayson #91208 Rm. # 804 BD 6-4-61 Admit 2-12-12		Mission Regional Hospital
Date	Time	Nurse's Notes
6-4-12	1330	C/O indigestion & mild nausea after eating pizza brought by
		wife. Requests antacid. Mylanta 30 mL given p.o. Instructed
		to call if no relief within 30 min. -------------J. Hammond, LPN
	1420	States nausea completely relieved & indigestion improving.
		-- J. Hammond, LPN

Figure 5-6   Sample documentation: leave no blank lines.

First Page:

6-3-12	1720	Dyspneic. Coughing decreasing. Skin cool, dry, pale. No
		cyanosis. BP-136/88 P-102 Irr. R-29 Shallow & regular.
		SpO² 90%. Breath sounds---(continued)-------J. Hammond, LPN

Second Page:

William, Mayson #91208 Rm. # 804 BD 6-4-61 Admit 2-12-12		Mission Regional Hospital
Date	Time	Nurse's Notes
6-3-12	1720	(continued) – auscultated: rales in LUL, LLL, RUL, rhonchi
		RML & RLL. HOB elevated to 45°. O² at 4 L/min applied
		via NC. Dr. Holsted notified of condition per phone. New
		orders received. -----------------------------------J. Hammond, LPN

Figure 5-7   Sample documentation: continued note.

Mistaken entry-LL
"Phenergan 50 mg IM Z-track method administered Lt. ~~dorsogluteal~~ ventral gluteal."
L. Ludwig, RN

Figure 5-8   Sample documentation: mistaken entry.

becomes saturated with the soda you were drinking, do not discard the page after you recopy it. If a portion of page 2 or the page in its entirety is so damaged that it is not legible, requiring that you rewrite the data, keep the damaged page in the chart. Make a notation on the damaged page indicating the portion of the page that will be rewritten and make reference to the recopied page ("Recopied to page 3"). Then, on the new blank page, write "Recopied from page 2" and include the current date and time, and your signature. Recopy the notes word-for-word from the damaged sheet and sign it. Leave both pages in the record to prevent doubt or suspicion regarding the recopied page.

Knowledge Connection

Give examples of subjective data and objective data. Explain how one knows the difference between the two types of data. Is cc an approved abbreviation? How about: >, U, mL, O₂, UA, @, and MS (for morphine sulfate)?

Documentation Systems

Each facility designates the type of system that is used to organize patient medical records. There are two basic formats: source-oriented records and problem-oriented records. Both systems may be utilized for handwritten medical records, known as hard copies, or for computerized records, which will be discussed later in this chapter.

Source-Oriented Records

Source-oriented medical records are organized according to the source or type of data, using specific forms for each, with each section designated by a labeled tab. The various health care providers and staff members will enter their data under the corresponding tab. For example, the physician will write treatment orders in the *Physician's Orders* section and notes about how the patient is doing in the *Physician's Progress Notes* section. A physical therapist would document his or her notes about rehabilitation strength training in the *Rehabilitation Therapy* section. However, while most other disciplines will make entries in only one or two sections, as a nurse you will document in multiple sections of the chart.

Typical Sections of the Source-Oriented Medical Record

Table 5-4 presents a list of the typical sections found in a source-oriented medical record. Note the sections marked with asterisks: those are the various areas in which you, the nurse, will document. Most of these section labels are somewhat self-explanatory as to the type of information that is located there, making it easy to locate specific data such as a new physician's order or the results of the chest x-ray, which is an advantage of this system. However, because there may be several members of other disciplines also caring for the patient, there may be information related to a patient problem spread out in several different sections of the medical record. If you have to scan the entire record in search of all of the data, it can be a time-consuming task,

Table 5-4 **Sections of Source-Oriented Medical Record**

Sections	Type Information
Admission Record *You may assist with record completion in certain circumstances.	*Demographic data,* including patient name, age, address, telephone number, religious preference; next of kin and contact information; occupation and employer's name and address *Personal identification data,* including birth date, social security number, photo ID; insurance data; permission to treat and permission to disclose patient medical data to insurance company and specified individuals; hospital identification number; admitting medical diagnoses
Advance Directive	Each patient must be asked if he or she has an advance directive such as a living will; any instructions regarding the extent to which the patient wishes to be provided medical care
*Surgical and Procedure Consents	Any signed consent forms for surgery or invasive procedures
Physician's Orders *You may write verbal orders.	Orders for treatments, medications, diet, procedures, care to be performed, activity level to be allowed
*Graphic Data	Vital sign graph, intake and output record, weights
*Care Flow Sheet	Form on which check marks or brief entries are made regarding: percentage diet consumed, type of bath, activity level, ROM exercise, repositioning intervals, number of bowel movements, Foley care, oral care, use of assistive devices, safety measures such as raised bed rails, height of bed, activation of bed brakes
*Care Plan	Plan of care identifying specific prioritized patient problems, interventions for them, and effectiveness of interventions; may include interdisciplinary contributions in addition to nursing's contributions
*Nurses' Notes	Chronological record of patient problems and condition along with the nursing care provided, the effectiveness of interventions
Laboratory Results	Results of laboratory tests run on blood or other body fluids or tissues
X-ray (or Radiological) Results	Results of x-rays
Consultation Reports	Reports by consulting physicians
History and Physical	Physician's initial assessment of body systems upon admission; includes medical diagnoses, past illnesses and surgeries, patient complaints and reason for seeking medical care, medications patient has been taking at home

Table 5-4   **Sections of Source-Oriented Medical Record** (continued)

Sections	Type Information
Surgical Reports *You will complete postanesthesia notes	Reports of all surgeries performed during this hospitalization, explaining anesthesia administered, description of actual surgical procedure, postanesthesia or recovery room record
Rehabilitation Therapy	Any physical, respiratory, occupational, or speech therapy administered along with patient's response and progress
*Medication Administration Record	Lists administered medications, dosages, route, date, time, and nurse who administered each; only the records for previous days are kept in the chart, while the current day's record is kept in a separate medication administration book
Physician's Progress Notes	Physician's notes regarding patient progress and responses to treatment
*Discharge Planning	Data from social services, case managers, home health care agencies, discharge planners

which is a distinct disadvantage. For example, a patient with diabetes admitted for treatment of pneumonia will most likely be receiving care or services from one or more physicians and nurses, as well as from respiratory therapy, radiology, the pharmacy, the laboratory, dietary services, and possibly physical therapy. When searching for information about the patient's gas exchange and whether it is improving, you would have to look in several sections of the record to locate all the data regarding the patient's gas exchange:

- **Nurse's Notes:** for latest assessment of breath sounds, characteristics of respirations, amount and color of sputum production, response to medications, frequency of use and effectiveness of supplemental oxygen
- **Physician's Progress Notes:** for latest report of improvement or decline of the patient's condition
- **Graphic Data:** for temperature, pulse, and respiratory rate trends; oxygen saturation levels
- **Rehabilitation Therapy:** for number of respiratory therapy treatments given and their effectiveness
- **Medication Administration Record:** for number of as-needed (prn) doses of cough medication that were required in the last 24 hours and which antibiotic has been administered
- **Laboratory Results:** for latest white blood cell count, hemoglobin level, and sputum culture and sensitivity results
- **X-ray Results:** for latest chest x-ray results

Problem-Oriented Records

Problem-oriented records differ from source-oriented records in that they are organized around the patient's individual problems rather than where the data came from, as in the source-oriented system.

Sections of Problem-Oriented Medical Record

The problem-oriented medical record will have four primary sections:

1. Database
2. Problem list
3. Plan of care
4. Progress notes

Additional forms such as a flow sheet or discharge summary sheet may be used according to facility policy. Table 5-5 provides an explanation of data to be included in each of these sections of the problem-oriented medical record.

The primary advantage of problem-oriented record keeping is that it encourages collaboration between all the disciplines providing care to the patient. All the health care providers contribute to the same database, problem list, plan of care, and progress notes. Working together, a plan of care is determined, listing the patient problems and potential patient problems chronologically as they are identified. Another advantage is that the list of these patient problems is kept at the front of the chart, where it is easily accessed without thumbing through the entire chart. The fact that all health care providers write their progress notes chronologically in the same *progress notes* section allows for quick retrieval of all of the involved disciplines' entries regarding the patient's responses to treatments.

Knowledge Connection

List the common sections of a source-oriented chart. Describe types of data that might be found within those sections. What are the four sections of a problem-oriented chart?

Table 5-5   Sections of Problem-Oriented Medical Record

Section	Type Data
Database	*Demographic data,* including patient name, age, address, telephone number, religious preference; next of kin and contact information; occupation and employer's name and address *Personal identification data,* including birth date, social security number, photo ID; insurance data; permission to treat and permission to disclose patient medical data to insurance company and specified individuals; hospital identification number; admitting medical diagnoses *Assessments,* including physician's history and physical, nursing's initial assessment Results of diagnostic tests, including laboratory tests and x-rays *Patient's current condition*
Problem list	Derived from the information in the database, a chronological (but not prioritized) list of potential and actual patient problems is developed; updated as problems resolve or worsen, or new problems appear; problems are numbered and kept at front of chart; these numbers are used to reference the specific problem when making an entry in the plan of care or progress notes
Plan of care	For each listed problem: physician's orders, nursing orders and plan of care, and interdisciplinary interventions are listed, including diagnostics, therapeutic plan, and teaching
Progress notes	Organized according to problem list; all disciplines chart on the same progress notes, numbering each entry to correspond with the problem list

Data to Document

The types of data that you will be expected to document will vary depending upon the facility in which you are working. In an acute care hospital setting, you would chart data for the following categories:

- Physical and emotional assessment
- Nutrition
- Hygiene
- Activity level
- Physician's visits
- Elimination (both bowel and bladder)
- All nursing care and interventions, including
  - Patient teaching
  - Discharge planning
- Patient's response to each intervention
- All patient complaints
- Safety issues
- Laboratory tests, x-rays, or other diagnostic tests that were done

Box 5-2 gives specifics to be charted for each category.

Knowledge Connection

Explain what types of daily activities should be documented in the medical record. List at least two examples of data that might be found in each of the 11 categories listed.

Methods of Charting

In this section we will discuss five of the most common methods of charting. The goal of all methods of charting is to provide an accurate picture of the patient's health status over a select period of time and treatment—one that clearly defines the patient's changing condition. The different methods of charting all employ the steps of the nursing process that you learned in Chapter 4. SOAPIER charting, PIE charting, and narrative charting can all be utilized with both documentation systems. However, focus charting and charting by exception may be used only with the source-oriented system.

SOAPIER Charting

SOAPIER charting may be used with either source- or problem-oriented systems, but is most frequently used in the latter and is typically used in the progress notes and nurse's notes. This method is one of the lengthier documentation formats, but it provides organization of entries. The acronym SOAPIER stands for:

- **Subjective data:** This is information verbalized by the patient, significant other, or family member. These data are influenced by the person's own personal experiences and perspective, which is what makes them subjective. You may summarize what was said or you may use the exact words and place them in quotation marks. There will not be subjective data for every entry; only chart them if they are pertinent, or related, to the problem.

Box 5-2

Specific Data to Be Charted Listed by Categories

Assessment
- Initial shift assessment done at the beginning of your shift to be used as a baseline.
- Any abnormal assessment findings that must be reassessed later in shift.

Nutrition
- Type of diet.
- How much the patient eats: such as 25%, 50%, 85%, or 100%. If 50% or less, include an assessment of why the patient ate such a small amount. Was there nausea or pain? Did the patient simply not like what was served? Was he or she simply *anorexic* (not hungry)? Did someone bring the patient a burger from the local drive-in?
- How was the diet tolerated: was there nausea, vomiting, indigestion, reflux, gas, or belching? Did the patient have difficulty swallowing? It is important to document if the patient required any assistance to eat.
- Did the patient consume any snacks during the shift? If so, what and how much?
- Is the patient drinking adequate fluids? Is the patient on intake and output? Was the patient instructed to record I/O?

Hygiene
- What type of bath was given: bed bath, partial sponge bath, tub bath, or shower?
- Did the patient require assistance, or was he or she able to bathe himself or herself?
- Was mouth care provided by you or performed by the patient? How often?
- Was a back rub performed?
- Was hair care, nail care, shaving, or skin care done?
- What was the patient's response to the hygiene? Did he or she state it made him or her feel better? Or did it make him or her more short of breath?
- Was the patient's skin clean, fresh, and intact? Any lesions or other problems noted?

Activity Level
- Is the patient on bedrest? Is he or she ambulatory without assistance or with assistance? If assistance is required, how many people are needed to ambulate the patient? Or can the patient only be gotten up for BRP or to sit in a chair?
- Was range of motion performed? Active or passive? To which extremities and how often?
- Was the patient logrolled? Or gotten up with the Hoyer lift? How did he or she tolerate the activity? Did the patient become short of breath? Did the pulse rate go from 66 to 110? Did the knees begin to buckle or did the patient become unsteady?

Physician Visits
- Did a physician see or examine the patient on your shift? If so, who?
- Did the physician remove clips from an incision? Were new orders written?
- Did you have to telephone or communicate data to a physician? If so, what information was reported and what orders were received?

Elimination
- Is the patient continent or incontinent of bowel? And bladder?
- When was the patient's last bowel movement? Voiding?
- What is the color, clarity, and amount (if on I/O) of urine?
- Did the patient have any complaints, such as burning or frequency?
- If there is a Foley catheter, additional information must be noted as well: is the Foley patent, is the catheter secured to the leg, and what is the total for the shift?
- What was the color, amount, and consistency of bowel movements? Were there patient complaints of gas (*flatulence*) or cramping?

Note: If there was no BM during your shift, a note indicating no BM should be made at the end of the shift. This makes it easier to track whether the patient has a bowel movement at least every 3 days.

Nursing Care (Implementation Step of Nursing Process)
Any care that you administer must be objectively documented, such as:
- Assisting to turn, cough, and deep breathe
- Changing an IV rate
- Inserting a Foley catheter
- Emptying a Jackson-Pratt drain
- Performing a back rub
- Providing mouth care or skin care
- Administering any one-time meds or prn meds
- Initiating an IV infusion
- Converting an IV line to a PRN lock
- Instilling a PEG tube feeding

Includes patient teaching and discharge planning, such as foot care or insulin administration for a diabetic patient; use of patient-controlled analgesia (PCA); wound or incision care; how to change a dressing.

Patient's Response to Interventions (Evaluation Step of Nursing Process)
How did the patient respond to your intervention, whether it was an assessment of vital signs or the insertion of a Foley catheter? For example, take the intervention of vital sign assessment. What was the patient's response? His pulse was 88, regular and distinct. His temp was 102.4°F. His BP was 138/76. These are his body's physical response to assessing these areas.

What might be an evaluation of insertion of a Foley catheter? It could be: "550 mL cloudy, amber urine returned—states she feels much better now" or "only 75 mL clear, light yellow urine returned."

If you turn, cough, and deep breathe a patient, the response might be something like "good cough effort, productive of large amount greenish-yellow sputum" or maybe "poor cough effort, cough is nonproductive, only performs coughing & deep breathing exercises when encouraged by nurse."

If you elevate the head of the bed to ease dyspnea, what might be a response from the patient? A couple of possibilities are: "respirations less labored when head of bed is elevated" or "color pink, respiratory rate 27/min, no complaints of shortness of breath." There is always a patient response to each intervention we perform, and we must chart them.

(box continues on page 98)

Box 5-2

Specific Data to Be Charted Listed by Categories (continued)

Safety Issues

Includes bed in low position, status of bed rails, suction machine available at bedside, call light within reach, and use of Hoyer lift with 3 assistants. Also includes such patient instructions as to call for assistance before getting out of bed because of possible unsteadiness due to medication, use of shower chair for taking a shower, and numerous other inventions taken to keep the patient from harm.

Laboratory and Diagnostic Testing

Document when a patient is taken to another department for tests or treatments. Include how the patient was transported: did

he or she walk, ride in a wheelchair, or go on a gurney? For example: "to radiology via W/C for a CXR." "Returned from MRI via gurney."

All Patient Complaints

This includes any complaints, such as pain, nausea, dizziness, anxiety, fear, tingling, itching, or does not like the ordered diet.

- **Objective data:** These are data that are related to the problem. Objective data must be something that you and others are able to discern with one of the senses.
- **Assessment data:** When used in the context of SOAPIER charting, assessment data refer to the problem you identify after you analyze the subjective and objective data. This step is very similar to the nursing diagnosis step, also known as the patient problem step, of the nursing process.
- **Plan:** This is the plan to resolve the patient problem or nursing diagnosis that you just identified. It is the plan of care.
- **Intervention:** This refers to the specific and measurable actions that you take to resolve the patient problem; it is how you actually carry out the plan you made in the previous step.
- **Evaluation:** This is identical to the evaluation step of the nursing process. It describes whether or not the interventions you just performed were effective by evaluating the patient's response. Did they help the problem? Did they achieve what you intended?

- **Revision:** There may or may not be a necessary revision for each problem. If the evaluation shows that the intervention you performed was effective in resolving the problem, then there is no need to revise the plan of care. If revision is not needed, write "none" or leave off the *R* step.

Figure 5-9 shows an example of SOAPIER charting.

PIE Charting

PIE charting is much shorter and documents fewer data than the SOAPIER charting style; however, because it only addresses the patient's problems, the concept of treating the patient holistically is lost. The PIE acronym stands for:

- **Problem:** This list is built from the collected data to identify the patient's problems, and as additional problems are identified, they are added to the original list.
- **Interventions:** These are the interventions you perform to address the patient's problems.
- **Evaluation:** This is your evaluation of the effectiveness of the interventions you performed.

Figure 5-10 shows an example of PIE charting.

Monett, Bradley #112484 Rm. # 651 BD 6-4-61 Admit 5-28-12		Mission Regional Hospital	
Date	Time	Nurse's Notes	
6-1-12	1350	S - C/O pain at IV site in lt. forearm. Describes pain as a 5	
		on scale of 0-10, burning and constant. -------------------------	
		O - 2 cm by 3 cm area erythema at IV insertion site, warm,	
		with slight edema. -------------------------------------	
		A - Developing phlebitis -------------------------------	
		P - Discontinue IV. Initiate new IV access. ----------------------	
		I - Catheter discontinued with tip intact. Restarted Rt.	
		dorsal wrist with 22 g with one attempt. ---------------------	
		E - IV fluids flow freely. Pump started. IV 1/2 NS infusing	
		at 125 mL/hr in Rt. dorsal wrist via Pump. No C/O	
		discomfort. Site clean, dry without edema. Instructed	
		to call if site begins to hurt. -------------------------------	
		R - None. ------------------------------------ K. Gann, LPN	

Figure 5-9 Sample documentation: SOAPIER note.

**Please note: below problem 2A is "activity intolerance related to impaired gas exchange."

Stephens, Christy #0621199 Rm.# 555 BD 6-21-80 Admit 6-21-12		Mission Regional Hospital
Date	Time	*Nurse's Notes*
6-23-12	0705	P - 2A ---
		I - Gotten up in chair with gait belt and 2 assists. O² off.
		E - Became SOB after 12 min. R-28 labored. P-101 C/O
		fatigue and weakness. SpO² 89%. O² reapplied at 3 L/min
		per NC. Lift used to return back to bed. After 5 min R-21
		and less labored. SpO² 93%. P-88. -------------- K. Gann, LPN

Figure 5-10 Sample documentation: PIE note.

Focus Charting

Focus charting is *focused* on the patient and patient concerns, problems, and strengths. There is not a constructed list of specific problems as there is in PIE charting. A common type of focus charting is DAR, which stands for:

- **Data:** This may contain objective or subjective data. For example, you might chart subjective information that the patient's son told you, or the patient's verbal complaint of pain. Objective data you might chart might include the result of pulse oximetry testing, vital signs, or a patient behavior that you observed. Any assessment finding that you detect through use of your visual, auditory, olfactory, and tactile senses would be noted under data. These entries represent the data collection and assessment stage of the nursing process.
- **Action:** Here you would chart your interventions. Examples might include teaching, repositioning, administering prn medication, changing a dressing, or notifying the physician of an abnormal laboratory result. These entries reflect the planning and implementation stages of the nursing process.
- **Response:** This refers to the patient's response to your interventions and reflects the evaluation phase of the nursing process.

Again, you can see that DAR charting is just another way to document the nursing process that occurs throughout your shift as you provide nursing care. Each entry you make does not require all three components unless it is appropriate for the entry. The order in which you chart the D, A, and R portions of the entry will depend upon the data and situation. A brief one- or two-word entry written in the column preceding the D, A, or R notes identifies the focus of the entry (Figs. 5-11 and 5-12).

Knowledge Connection

What does each letter stand for in the following charting method acronyms: SOAPIER, PIE, DAR? Under which initial in the acronym would a patient's complaint of pain be charted using the SOAPIER method? The PIE method? The DAR method? Where would you document the following information in each system: "States medication decreased pain from an 8 to a 3"? Where would administering Demerol IM be charted in each system? Where would you document the percentage (%) of clear liquid diet consumed?

Gann, Katie #021482 Rm. # 333 BD 2-14-82 Admit 6-21-12		Mission Regional Hospital
Date & Time	Focus	*Nurse's Notes*
6-22-12	Pain R/T	D - C/O bilateral chest soreness when coughing, a 7 on 0-10
0315	coughing	scale. Continues to have frequent non-productive cough.
		A - Cup of hot decaffeinated tea provided and drank. Then
		Gauifenesin syrup w/ Codeine 2 tsp given orally. Instructed
		to call for help before getting out of bed as med may make
		her sleepy and unsteady on feet. -----------------------------
		R - After 35 min. coughing decreasing in frequency. States
		discomfort totally gone. Drowsy. -------------- K. Gann, LPN

Figure 5-11 Sample documentation: DAR note.

Stelling, Lindsey #061186 Rm.# 1999 BD 6-11-86 Admit 6-29-12		Mission Regional Hospital
Date & Time	Focus	*Nurse's Notes*
6-30-12 0855	constipation	D - C/O abd. cramping. States no BM since 6-24. Bowel sounds hypoactive and abdomen slightly firm in all 4 quadrants. -- A - Dulcolax supp. administered rectally. Prune juice provided and drank. Encouraged to ambulate at least 4 times this shift in halls. ------------------------ B. Monett, LPN
6-30-12 1115	constipation	R - Has ambulated 2 times in hall. Had large, dry brown formed BM. States feels much better. ------------------------ -- B. Monett, LPN

Figure 5-12 Sample documentation: another DAR note.

Laboratory and Diagnostic Connection

Your Laboratory and Diagnostic Documentation Responsibilities

Even though you do not normally write the results of very many laboratory and diagnostic tests, you are responsible for monitoring the results of those tests ordered for your assigned patients and documenting whether or not you:
• Notified the physician of the results
• Explained the results to the patient
• Took any other action related to the test results

Because of this responsibility, you must be able to identify when results fall outside the normal range, making the result abnormal. You must also be able to differentiate when an abnormally high or low result has reached the *critical value level.* Your responsibility is not limited to monitoring and reporting results to the physician, however; you must be able to discern when a test result requires that you intervene, such as withholding a medication or treatment, even before you notify the physician. The documentation of performance of appropriate interventions and physician notification is important to protect you legally.

Charting by Exception

Charting by exception is quite different from all other types of documentation. All activities of daily living, vital signs, and assessment findings are charted on checklist-type flow sheets rather than writing them out as individual entries. Only variances from "normal," or what you would call *exceptions* to the rules, are written as entries. This method of charting is designed to drastically reduce your time spent completing paperwork, which is theoretically an advantage. However, there are varying opinions regarding the efficacy and safety of this method of documentation.

The primary disadvantage of charting by exception is the absence or omission of specific data that might be useful in defense of your actions or the patient's condition in a court of law. Testifying that certain data were not specifically charted because they fell within the realm of "normal" may

fail to provide convincing evidence that you acted appropriately or that the patient's condition was within normal limits. Our human nature often finds it easier to believe something that we can see, such as charted data, over something we say.

The facility whose policy is to document using the charting by exception method must develop and maintain its own written standards of nursing practice. This means that the facility needs to specify what it considers to be minimum criteria for patient care, which might include the following:

• Ranges of normal assessment findings for all age groups
• Ranges of normal and abnormal patient responses
• Descriptions of nursing skills and the specific steps of delivery to be used

Examples of specific nursing standards might include:

• The nurse will perform passive range-of-motion (ROM) exercises at least twice a day for patients who are on bedrest or limited activity.
• The nurse will provide oral care at least every 2 hours for unconscious patients and every 4 hours for patients who are NPO.

Then, when "mouth care" is check-marked on the flow sheet, it is assumed that it was performed accordingly.

Another disadvantage of charting by exception is that it makes it too easy to check off skills when they have not been done.

Narrative Charting

Narrative charting tells the story of the patient's experiences during the hospital stay. It is written in chronological order and relates the patient's health status from admission and through all changes in condition, up to and including his or her discharge status. It provides a continual description of the patient's condition, complaints, problems, assessment findings of all systems, activities, treatments, and nursing care provided, and the evaluations of effectiveness for each nursing intervention. The advantage is that it provides more details than most charting styles and a better time line of the patient's changing condition, especially during life-threatening emergencies such as cardiac and respiratory arrests. The disadvantage is the fact that it is time consuming. However, more experienced nurses who learned the narrative method and used it during many years of nursing practice often express the feeling that the time spent is well worth it because it provides the best protection.

Imagine you are working a 12-hour shift from 0700 to 1900 in a facility that uses the narrative charting style. After you have completed and documented the initial shift assessment, your next couple of entries might look something like this:

06-23-12   0755   C/O RUQ abdomen pain at 6 on scale of 0–10. Still NPO. 10 ½ NS 100 mL infusing per pump in

Lt. dorsal hand. Site without erythema or edema. C/O dry mouth. Mucous membranes pink, intact, dry. —————
————————————— Nurse's signature and credentials
06-23-12   0805   Demerol 100 mg IM administered Rt. ventral gluteal. Mouth care & lip moisturizer provided. Instructed to call for assistance before getting up R/T drug may cause drowsiness or dizziness. 2 rails up. Bed in low, locked position. Call light within reach. —————————
————————————— Nurse's signature and credentials
06-23-12   0845   Dr. Taylor here. New orders received to begin clear liquids & ambulate 4 times per day. ————
————————————— Nurse's signature and credentials

Box 5-3 presents an example of narrative charting for a typical 8-hour day shift.

Box 5-3

An Example of Narrative Documentation for a "Typical Day"

This is the verbal shift report you received at 0615 when you came on duty:

Luddy Julius, a 54-year-old male, a patient of Dr. Evans, was admitted at 0120 with a diagnosis of bacterial pneumonia and a secondary diagnosis of dehydration. He has a history of hypertension and gastroesophageal reflux disease. He presented in the ER with severe shortness of breath and stated that he had been coughing up quite a bit of thick yellow sputum for 3 days. He also stated he had been vomiting and unable to keep anything down for the past 24 hours and that he last urinated approximately 9 hours prior to admission. Admission vital signs were BP 102/58, temperature 102.6°F, pulse 105, respirations 33, and oxygen saturation 87%. Mucous membranes were pale and dry, and his lips were cracking. His skin was flushed, hot, and dry. Breath sounds were diminished in both lower lobes and almost nonexistent in the right lower lobe. Crackles were heard in the left upper lobe, and both crackles and inspiratory wheezes in the right upper and middle lobes. He was dyspneic and using accessory respiratory muscles. We applied oxygen 6 liters per minute via nasal cannula and oxygen saturation was up to 90% by 0155. Respiratory therapy gave him a handheld nebulizer treatment with Duoneb. His dyspnea improved, respiratory rate went down to 25. I started an IV of 1,000 mL of 0.45% normal saline with 20 mEq of potassium chloride in his left forearm with a 20-gauge intracath. It's infusing at 125 mL/hr via IV pump. At 0210, I gave him guaifenesin with codeine cough syrup 10 mL orally for his cough and Tylenol 650 mg orally for fever. At 0545 his temperature was 101.8°F and respirations 26. At 0615 his eyes were closed and respirations were regular but shallow at 25 per minute. He still has had no urinary output. His breath sounds were the same except with slightly less wheezing in the right upper and middle lobes, still minimal breath sounds in the right base.

The narrative documentation for the day shift might look something like this:

0720   BP – 136/74, T – 102.6, P – 92, R – 32, SpO₂ – 92% on O₂ 4 L/min per NC. Productive cough with yellow sputum at intervals. States he slept couple hrs after cough med. Tylenol 650 mg administered PO for fever. ————
————————— M. Monett, RN
0745   AAO×4, PEARL, skin pale, hot, dry, & nonelastic. Cool wet cloth applied to forehead. Conjunctiva pink. Mucous membranes pale & dry, lips cracking. Mouth care performed. Speech clear & appropriate. No neck vein distention.

Slightly dyspneic, using accessory respiratory muscles. C/O SOB but states it has improved since admission. Elevated HOB 30 degrees. Lungs auscultated, coarse crackles in all lobes except RML & RLL, where there are no breath sounds. O₂ at 4 L/min per NC. SpO₂ 92% Deep breathed & coughed ×10; productive of lg. amt. thick yellow sputum. Apical-radial pulse strong & equal at 92. Emptied urinal of 180 mL cloudy amber urine. States last BM was yesterday morning. Abdomen is flat, soft, and nontender to palpation. Active bowel sounds in all 4 quadrants. 10 1,000 mL ½ NS with 20 mEq KCl infusing Lt. forearm at 125 mL/hr per pump, site free of erythema, edema, & no ∆o tenderness at site. PPP strong & equal bilaterally ×4 extremities. Extremities pink & warm with brisk cap refill ×4, no edema. Strong hand grips bilaterally. Strong plantar & dorsal flexion bilaterally. No limitations of ROM detected. Call light within reach. Bed left in low position. Instructed to drink a glass of fluid every hour to help with rehydration and fever. Explained how to record I/O. Verbalized understanding. Requested a soft drink, provided. ————————— J. Ludwig, RN
0815   Ate 45% ADA diet without N/O. Drank soft drink, juice, & coffee. ————————— M. Monett, RN
0835   Dr. Imagod here to see pt. No new orders. ——— M. Monett, RN
0850   Assisted to bathroom, voided 120 mL cloudy, amber urine. A little weak and unsteady. Back to bed with 1 assist. Drank 240 mL. ——— M. Monett, RN
0930   C/O fatigue & not feeling good enough to take shower. Bed bath, mouth & skin care given. States feels "lots better after bath". Encouraged to drink. Requested coffee, provided & drank 150 mL. ——— M. Monett, RN
1010   To radiology via W/C for CXR. ——————— M. Monett, RN
1025   Returned from x-ray via W/C. No change in respiratory status. ———
————————— J. Ludwig, RN
1135   BP – 152/82, T – 101.4, P – 91, R – 23. C/O chest discomfort R/T coughing, 5 on scale of 0–10. Ibuprofen 400 mg given PO. Drinking fluids without N/O. ————————— M. Monett, RN
1225   States pain at 2. T – 100.6. Assisted to chair. Dp Br ×10, with good effort & productive of yellow sputum. 10 site unchanged. ——— M. Monett, RN
1245   Ate only a few bites reg diet. Drank 500 mL fluids. States is just "not hungry". No complaints of nausea. 10 site without erythema or edema. ———
————————— M. Monett, RN
1420   Assisted to bathroom, voided 180 mL clear, dark amber urine. Became dyspneic, R – 31 and slightly irreg. Assisted back to bed. O₂ reapplied at 4 L/min per NC. O₂ sats 89%. After 4–5 minutes, O₂ sats 92%, T – 100.6, P – 87 reg & strong, R – 29 shallow, states dyspnea better. Skin & mucous membranes pale. ————————— M. Monett, RN
1450   Eyes closed, resp shallow & reg. 10 site unchanged from 1245. In Total – 1,700 mL (10 – 950 mL, Oral – 750 mL); Out – 490 mL. Wife at bedside. Rails up ×2. Bed low position. ————— M. Monett, RN

Computerized Charting

Computerized charting, which means that you record your data with the use of a computer, is the trend in documentation, and if a hospital has not yet converted to computerized documentation, it is likely planning to transition to it in the near future (Fig. 5-13). Some government divisions recommend that electronic records be mandated for health care facilities that receive government monies, such as Medicare and Medicaid.

Many facilities have computer stations at various locations in each patient hall as well as at the nurse's station. Other facilities may use bedside terminals, and yet others provide handheld computers (Fig. 5-14). The handheld computers are designed to be carried while the nurse is making rounds, enabling entries to be made right at the bedside, which is a great advantage and helps to reduce documentation errors and omissions.

Computerized documentation resolves the problem of not being able to decipher physicians' and nurses' handwriting, another plus for patient safety. Also, having the patient's entire record in the computer allows multiple health care providers to access different portions of the chart at the same time and expedites the process of data retrieval. However, there are disadvantages. Some individuals are not computer literate and are intimidated by computer technology, but this is generally resolvable through facility-provided computer training and practice. Another drawback to computer

A

Figure 5-13 Most health care facilities are converting to computerized documentation.

B

Figure 5-14 Point-of-access computing. A, Handheld computer. B, Bedside terminal.

documentation is that most of the software programs provide you with a list of choices for each type of data that you need to document; these lists, however, limit your choices of words or phrases. Because of this limitation, you may be required to go the narrative section and type data using the specific wording that you need. Another disadvantage is the fact that computer systems can be hacked into illegally, putting patient confidentiality at risk if a hacker is successful in accessing the hospital's system.

Knowledge Connection
Explain what the current documentation trend is.

Long-term Care and Home Health Care Documentation

The documentation that is required by both long-term care and home health care seems quite different from that of an acute care hospital if you are attempting to compare *daily* documentation notes. The acute care hospital documentation would appear to be more inclusive and longer, and to represent the heavier workload, but this is misleading because neither long-term or home health care staff document on a daily basis for each patient. The reality is that both home health and long-term care have rigid and extensive documentation requirements for admission of each patient; often, the forms are even longer than those used in the hospitals.

Long-term Care

Charting requirements for long-term care are significantly different from those for acute care. The U.S. government regulates the documentation that is required in long-term care facilities, and those requirements vary according to the level of care required by the resident. Upon admission to the facility, in order to meet Medicare and Medicaid requirements for certification and reimbursement, the facility must complete an admission assessment document for each resident that is many pages in length.

Once the admission paperwork has been completed, there are differences in the amount and type of documentation that is performed on a more regular basis. When one considers the documentation that is needed and required in the long-term facility, it is important to remember that a long-term care facility is considered to be each individual's place of residence—his or her home, whether temporary or permanent. Rather than charting continually through each 24-hour day as with hospital documentation, an update regarding the patient's condition is only required to be documented once a week, or more often if problems or changes in condition occur. This update is known as the *weekly summary*. If a resident becomes acutely ill or suffers an accident or injury, documentation steps up to a daily recording of vital signs and assessments until it is determined that the resident has no need for continued daily monitoring.

Knowledge Connection
Explain how long-term care documentation differs from acute care documentation.

The Minimum Data Set for Resident Assessment and Care Screening

A federal law known as the Omnibus Budget Reconciliation Act (OBRA) mandates that an extensive assessment form called the *Minimum Data Set for Resident Assessment and Care Screening (MDS)* must be completed for each resident within 4 days of admission to the facility and updated every 3 months. The form consists of many assessments that must be made. A partial list of required assessments includes the following:

• Demographics
• Identification and background patterns
• Customary routines of the patient, including cycle of daily events, eating patterns, activities of daily living patterns, and level of involvement (with others)
• Communication and hearing patterns
• Cognitive patterns
• Vision patterns
• Psychosocial well-being
• Mood and behavior patterns
• Physical functioning and structural-related problems
• Continence of bowel and bladder
• Health conditions
• Disease diagnoses
• Medications the patient is taking

The entire government form may also be viewed and downloaded from the web at *http://www.cms.hhs.gov/ NursingHomesQualityInits/20_Downloads/MDS20MDSAll-Forms.pdf.*

Weekly Assessment Data

Because the long-term care facility is the home of the resident, some additional data are collected and documented in the weekly assessments mentioned above, along with the typical data found in a more traditional acute care assessment. This will include the following information:

• **Use of all prostheses:** such as glasses, dentures, hearing aids, or prosthetic limbs
• **Activity level:** whether the resident is bedridden or ambulatory, as well as the level of assistance that is required to perform the activity
• **Elimination control and habits:** whether the resident is continent or incontinent and if bowel training is performed
• **Nutrition versus malnutrition:** type of diet, percentage routinely consumed, type and frequency of supplemental nutrition, weight records
• **Ability to communicate:** if the resident is unable to speak, method utilized to communicate
• **Visitors and support system:** whether the resident has regular visitors or rarely receives guests; whether there is a strong support system for the resident

- **Social activities:** types in which the resident participates and frequency of participation
- **Ability to perform activities of daily living:** includes hygiene, dressing, nutrition and fluid intake

Medication Administration Records

Medication administration is charted each time medications are given, just as it is documented in the hospital. However, there is not a separate medication administration record (MAR) for each day as there is in acute care. On the MAR used in long-term care, administration of each drug is documented for the entire month on a single page. This must be done to decrease paper volume of charts that may extend over months and even years.

Knowledge Connection

Describe the types of data that should be included in weekly summaries in a long-term care facility. How is the long-term care MAR different from that found in a hospital?

Home Health Care

Home health care documentation is governed by the federal government agency known as the Health Care Financing Administration (HCFA). Certain criteria must be met to admit a patient to home health care, just as in long-term care; documentation of these data is part of the certification process. The admission forms must be extensive to provide adequate data to verify that the patient meets certification requirements. One example of an admission form is the *Outcome and Assessment Information Set,* known as *OASIS.* Figure 5-15 shows the first page of a 5-page admission form used by one agency. A copy of a complete OASIS form may be found at *http://www.cms.hhs.gov/oasis/.*

You must be an RN to perform this initial visit and assessment, as well as complete the OASIS form. Either RNs or LPN/LVNs may make subsequent visits. Each time you make a patient visit as a home health nurse, you will be expected to complete the organization's specified home health skilled nursing note form to document the visit (Fig. 5-16). It is important to show in your documentation that the patient is making progress toward specific goals. This documentation is regulated and audited by both the state health department and Medicare.

Five Documentation Mistakes That Carry Increased Risks

You will want to avoid all documentation mistakes, but particularly those for which the very nature of the mistake carries increased risks. This would include failure to document:

- Assessment findings
- Medications administered

- Pertinent health history
- Physician's orders

Documenting on the wrong chart or MAR also carries increased risks.

Failure to Document Assessment Findings

It is your responsibility to be competent in assessment and to determine if the findings indicate a change in the patient's condition. Because nurses are the only health care providers who provide patient care 24 hours per day, 7 days per week, it is most likely that it will be a nurse who is first present when there is a change in the patient's condition. Failure to identify and document even what may initially appear to be a minor change in condition may put the patient in jeopardy.

Some facilities have a policy stating that only the floor supervisors are to call problems in to physicians, meaning that problems must be reported to the supervisor when they are identified. If you are working under this type of policy and discover pertinent abnormal assessment findings, you may immediately go to your supervisor and report the findings, assuming that the supervisor will contact the physician and take care of the reported data. Avoid this line of thinking and method of performing. Even if the supervisor is responsible for notifying the physician, he or she is *not* responsible for documenting your assessment findings. You are responsible for documenting not only your abnormal assessment findings, but also the actions you took to address any actual or potential problems related to those abnormal findings. Never depend upon another individual to document your assessments or care. Be diligent to document all assessment findings.

Failure to Document Medications Administered

Follow your facility policy for administering and documenting medications. Always record the drug name, dosage, route of administration, and the correct time of administration as soon as possible. Failure to document administration of a medication carries the potential for another mistake to be made. If another nurse sees no documentation that the medication was given, he or she may give it again, thinking this to be the correct course of action for the patient and also thinking that he or she is doing you a favor as well. The patient has then received an extra dose, the significance of which is affected by several factors: the type of drug it was, the safe dosage range, the patient's age, the patient's liver and kidney functions, and the patient's response to the medication.

Failure to Document Pertinent Health History

This could include failure to document such things as the patient's allergies to a medication, food, or latex; a diagnosis of hemophilia; or a previous methicillin-resistant *Staphylococcus aureus* (MRSA) infection. An allergy that is not documented presents an opportunity for an allergic reaction to

PARKVIEW HOSPITAL HOME HEALTH ADMISSION								
HH #:		☐ New ☐ Readmit		Patient Name:				
Sex: ☐ M ☐ F	Date of Birth	Age	Marital Status S M D W	Race: ☐ White ☐ Black ☐ Hispanic ☐ Other		Social Security Number:		

Street Address		City		State	Zip	County	
Mailing Address							
Medicare	Medicaid		Insurance			Private Pay	
Pt. Phone #:		Emergency Contact:				Phone #:	
SOC Date:		Certification Period:					

Admit Source: ☐ Physician   ☐ HMO   ☐ Hospital   ☐ SNF   ☐ Other Facility
☐ Emergency Room   ☐ Court/Law Enforcement   ☐ Clinic   ☐ Not Available

Primary Physician:	Date Last Seen:	UPIN #:	
Address:			Phone:

Secondary Physician:	Date Last Seen:	UPIN #:	
Address:			Phone:

Pharmacy Name:	Phone #:
Travel Directions:	

Caregiver(s) in Home:

Diagnosis:

Start of Care Orders: ☐ SN   ☐ Aide   ☐ PT   ☐ OT   ☐ ST   ☐ MSW

Rehab/SNF:		Adm. Date:	Disch. Date:	
Hospital:		Adm. Date:	Disch. Date:	Surgery ☐ Yes ☐ No
Referred By:			Phone #:	
Nurse Receiving Verbal Order:			Referral Date:	
Team Leader:				
Initial Nurse:			Date:	

Figure 5-15   Portion of a home health OASIS admission form.

examination gloves or to a medication administered IV, both of which carry the potential to be life threatening. The safety measures that should be employed when caring for a patient with hemophilia may be overlooked if staff are unaware of the diagnosis, endangering the patient. A patient with a history of previous MRSA infection is at risk for repeat MRSA infection following surgical procedures. A physician would probably want to order a *prophylactic,* or preventive, dose of vancomycin or another antibiotic effective against MRSA to be administered prior to a scheduled surgery. However, if the history of MRSA is not documented, it may be overlooked, again endangering the patient.

Documenting on Wrong Chart or MAR

It is extremely easy to pick up the wrong chart or MAR and document about another patient. Patients can have the same last name, sometimes even the same first and last

**PARK VIEW HOSPITAL HOME HEALTH
SKILLED NURSING NOTE**

PATIENT SIGNATURE: _____

PATIENT NAME _____ **HIC #** _____ **DATE** _____

DIAGNOSIS _____

VS: AP _____ RP _____ reg-irreg   Temp. _____ o-r-ax-tym   Resp. _____ Wt. _____ ↑↓

BP: Rt arm   supine _____   Lt. arm   supine _____
              sitting _____   sitting _____   FSBS: _____
              standing _____   standing _____

BREATH SOUNDS: _____

PAIN: ☐ Yes   ☐ No   Location of pain _____ Intensity _____ (0=No Pain 10=Severe Pain)
Quality ☐ Aching ☐ burning ☐ Sharp ☐ Cramping ☐ Shooting ☐ Dull ☐ Stabbing ☐ Gnawing ☐ Throbbing
Type ☐ Continuous ☐ Intermittent
Relieved by _____

FOOD INTAKE: good - fair - poor - NPO - tube   **FLUID INTAKE:** good - fair - poor - NPO

Last BM: _____   ☐ No complaints   **Urinary:**   ☐ No Complaints
                          ☐ diarrhea   color _____   ☐ burning
                          ☐ constipation   ☐ cloudy
                          ☐ impaction   foley _____   ☐ strong odor
                          ☐ incontinent   ☐ freq./urgency
                          ☐ ostomy   ☐ nocturia
                                                               ☐ hematuria
BOWEL SOUNDS: _____   ☐ incontinence
SKIN: ☐ ostomy
color _____
     ☐ w/d   turgor: ☐ good   **OPEN AREAS** _____
     ☐ cool   ☐ fair
     ☐ clammy   ☐ poor   _____
     ☐ diaphoretic   ☐ tenting
     ☐ other _____   _____

EMOTIONAL STATUS: **MENTAL STATUS:**
     ☐ cheerful   ☐ flat affect   ☐ alert   ☐ disoriented
     ☐ depressed/crying ☐ other _____   ☐ oriented   ☐ lethargic
     ☐ anxious/nervous   ☐ forgetful   ☐ unresponsive

EDEMA: ☐ absent ☐ present ☐ describe _____

CONFIRMATION WRITTEN: ☐ yes   ☐ no
MEDICATIONS: ☐ no changes   ☐ changes   ☐ new _____

Reported to: ☐ RN   ☐ Physician: _____
_____ **DATE OF NEXT APPT.** _____

SUPERVISORY NOTE
	☐ Skilled Nursing		☐ Aide	
Staff person is providing appropriate care?	☐ Yes	☐ No	☐ Yes	☐ No
Staff person anticipates patient's needs?	☐ Yes	☐ No	☐ Yes	☐ No
Staff person has a good rapport with patient?	☐ Yes	☐ No	☐ Yes	☐ No
Plan of Care is being followed?	☐ Yes	☐ No	☐ Yes	☐ No
Plan of Care remains the same?	☐ Yes	☐ No	☐ Yes	☐ No

NURSE'S SIGNATURE _____ **DATE** _____
OK092932(FC3411FX)   Form# 90060 (Rev 3/05)

Figure 5-16 Sample of home health skilled nursing note form.

NURSE SIGNATURE _____ **DATE** _____ **TIME IN** _____ **TIME OUT** _____

SUBJECTIVE DATA: _____

_____

OBJECTIVE DATA: _____

_____

_____

_____

_____

_____

NURSING ASSESSMENT: _____

_____

_____

_____

_____

SKILLED INTERVENTION: _____

_____

_____

_____

PATIENT TEACHING: _____

_____

_____

PATIENT RESPONSE TO VISIT/TEACHING: ☐ tolerated visit/procedure w/o or min. difficulty

☐ difficulty tolerating visit/procedure   ☐ retains teaching w/o or min. difficulty
☐ need further teaching on _____
☐ retains teaching only with repetition x 2-3   ☐ unable to retain teaching
☐ caregiver present and retains teaching

HOMEBOUND STATUS: ☐ unable to leave home w/o assistance of _____
    ☐ dyspnea with minimal exertion .
    ☐ mobility limited due to _____

Next SNV _____   ☐ unable to walk more than ____ feet w/o extreme fatigue.
    ☐ unable to leave home due to open wounds.
    ☐ unable to leave home due to instability of condition per doctor's orders
    ☐ does not leave home, as indicated above, greater than_____ x _____
    ☐ only leaves home for medical reasons_____ x _____
    ☐ gradually increasing activity, but still homebound
    ☐ is no longer homebound

PLAN OF CARE: _____

Figure 5-16 cont'd

names, making it difficult to differentiate between their charts and MARs. Always check the chart and each page of the MAR for the patient's full name, room number, physician, and other identifiers as necessary, before documenting in or following the orders located in either the chart or MAR.

Real-World Connection

How Many Can There Be?

During a clinical day at a government hospital, one student nurse had a patient by the name of William Hershell May (not the patient's real name). All medical records were computerized, and the student was required, after entering her multiple pass codes, to type in the name of the patient for whom she needed to view the chart. She typed in "William May" and a medical record came up on the screen. The instructor was standing not far behind the student when she began to scan through the chart. The instructor stepped close enough to read over the student's shoulder, when a particular diagnosis caught his attention. The instructor asked the student if this was, indeed, the chart of her patient; the student replied that it was and began once again to flip through the various sections of the record. Immediately, the instructor noted another piece of information that did not make sense compared with the information he knew about the student's patient, so he asked the student to show him the room number on record in this particular chart. It was not the room number that the student had been going to during her nursing care, so the instructor requested that she pull up the social security number listed in the chart. She compared it to the last 4 numbers that they had been checking against on the MAR and they were not the same; the student was in the wrong chart.

When the instructor backtracked the steps the student had taken to pull up the chart, the instructor showed her that there was more than one patient with the same first and last names. The biggest surprise for the student came when she saw that the nurse had pulled up not only two patients with the name William May, but a total of seven patients named William May, two of whom also had "H" for the middle initial. Only two of the seven patients were currently in the hospital; the other five records were from previous admissions. The student was grateful that she had not had time to carry out any physician's orders from the wrong chart.

Failure to Accurately Document Physician's Orders

Once the physician writes an order for any type of treatment, test, procedure, medication, or interval frequency of any aspect of nursing assessment or monitoring, the orders go through a process known as *noting* or *transcribing* the order. This refers to the process of documentation that is required to ensure that the proper health care providers are notified of the order. This may include documentation in the Kardex; completion of requisitions; making computer entries; written or electronic notification to the pharmacy, dietary services, or physical, occupational, or respiratory therapy; scheduling of procedures or appointments; and various other forms of documentation. If the required documentation is not completed, physician-ordered diagnostics, treatments, and care will not be delivered. Because the physician's orders are the foundation of patient care, your accuracy in transcribing them serves as the scaffolding for delivery of patient care.

You will learn how to perform this skill at a later point in your education, probably after you begin attending clinicals. However, we mention it here because it is a vital area of documentation; a failure to accurately transcribe physician's orders can have harmful consequences and carries the potential to even be life threatening for your patients. In Chapter 6, we will address how to decrease risk of error while documenting verbal or telephone physician's orders. An example of a consequence that could occur as a result of failure to note a physician's order may be seen in Box 5-4.

Knowledge Connection

Explain the five types of documentation mistakes that carry increased risk.

Supervision/Delegation Connection

Must "You" Document Everything?

While most documentation must be completed by you, the licensed nurse, there are some portions that may be performed by a CNA or UAP who has been instructed in the proper manner to document the data. In a hospital, completion of such forms as the vital signs graphic sheet or a portion of the nursing care checklist or flowchart may be assigned to unlicensed personnel. As previously noted, a unit clerk or ward clerk may transcribe physician's orders, but you are still responsible to ensure that all required documentation for each order has been correctly completed. You are also responsible for signing the physician's order sheet, complete with date, time, and signature with credentials.

In long-term care, it is common to assign the CNA to document on designated records the following data:

- Date and type of bath given
- Intake and output shift totals
- Number of times resident is incontinent
- Number of bowel movements
- Percentage and type of nutritional supplements consumed

All other documentation remains your responsibility.

Box 5-4

The Importance of Accurate Order Transcription

The following scenario highlights why it is so vital to accurately transcribe physician orders:

The physician's order *"NPO at midnight for EGD (esophagogastroduodenoscopy) in a.m."* is overlooked by the nurse when the orders are being transcribed, so dietary is not notified. A breakfast tray is available for the patient the next morning and is served by the dietary aide. The patient eats, because the tray was served. A technician from the procedure room brings a wheelchair and takes the patient back for the

EGD. The patient receives conscious sedation. As the physician begins to insert the scope into the patient's throat, she vomits a moderate amount of undigested food. The procedure was cancelled at that point and rescheduled for another day. Luckily the patient did not aspirate and was fine.

This documentation oversight could have resulted in the patient aspirating and developing respiratory complications, all because one nurse missed one physician's order.

 Post Conference

Your clinical shift is almost over and you are giving the end-of-shift report to your instructor. You have a smile on your face because you are very pleased with your performance and the documentation that you had worried about so much. Immediately after you received the shift report about your assigned patient at the beginning of the shift, you quickly reviewed the facility's policy regarding confidentiality of medical records to determine who may be allowed access. You learned that the policy stated the patient may view his or her own chart simply by making a verbal request, but before allowing family members to view the chart, the patient must sign a written consent that lists the names of all individuals the patient is willing to allow to view his or her chart. You introduced yourself to the woman at the nurse's station who was requesting to view Minnie Whitefeather's chart and discovered that she was the patient's only daughter. Flipping through the chart, you located the signed consent that allowed the daughter to view her mother's chart. She read the laboratory reports that had been done the prior day and then handed the chart back to you, thanking you for assisting her.

After determining which type of documentation was used in the facility, you also reviewed your fundamentals textbook and then discussed it with your instructor before you began to chart. It all began to "come back" as you reviewed and talked with your instructor. You did quite well with that first day's charting; in fact, your instructor had only had a couple of minor recommendations for ways to improve it the next time you get to document. You left clinicals *almost* looking forward to the next opportunity.

KEY POINTS

- Documentation skills are equally important as highly technical nursing skills.

- Purposes of documentation include continuity of care; permanent record of patient's medical experiences; record of accountability for quality assurance, accreditation, and reimbursement; and legal record for both the patient and the health care providers.

- HIPAA guarantees confidentiality of the patient's medical record.

- Documentation should be done with blue or black ink, be legible, be signed, have the date and time at beginning of each entry, be in chronological order, be done in a timely manner, be succinct, have punctuation, and be accurate and objective.

- Use of correct spelling and approved abbreviations is vital.

- Incident reports are not to be filed in the patient's chart; they are kept separate.

- Corrections should be made by marking a single line through the wrong word and, above it, writing "mistaken entry" and your initials. It is never appropriate to scribble out an entry or use correction fluid or correction tape on a chart.

Review Questions

Select the answer that is most appropriate for each of the following questions. Some questions may have more than one correct answer. Check all that apply.

1. Which of the following phrases are written objectively?

   a. "Ate 45% full liquid diet. Did not act very hungry and acted like she should not have drunk all that she did."

   b. "Complaining of really severe pain and wants something for it."

   c. "Ambulated unassisted the length of hallway without complaints of fatigue or shortness of breath."

   d. "Does not feel good today. Angry and depressed."

   e. "Makes good eye contact, smiling. States feels 'much better today than yesterday'."

2. When using the focus method of charting known as DAR, you know that the R stands for what type of data?

   a. Any requests that the patient verbalizes

   b. The patient's responses to your nursing interventions

   c. Revisions that were made to the intervention

   d. The report data that you were given at the beginning of the shift

3. Which of the following times during a 7 a.m. to 3 p.m. shift would be appropriate times to document on the patient's chart?

   a. As soon as possible after the occurrence or event

   b. Once at the beginning of the shift, again about midway through the shift, and the last time at the end of the shift

   c. Before the physician makes morning rounds at 1015

   d. Following performance of physical assessments

   e. Not until all your patient care has been completed for the shift

   f. At least every 2 hours

4. Which of the following entries are good examples of succinct charting?

   a. "Bed bath was given and teeth were brushed. Hair was shampooed and tangles combed out. Soaked fingernails in warm soapy water for 20 minutes, then filed them and cleaned them using an orange stick. Legs were shaved and lotion applied to all pressure points and areas of dry skin. Gave her a back rub."

   b. "Sacral wound measures 2 cm × 4 cm with 1-cm depth. Wound bed pale and dry, with 1-cm black eschar center circumferenced by 0.5-cm dark erythema. No granulation noted. Moderate amount foul-smelling green purulent drainage."

   c. "Patient is having moderate amount of cramping in her abdomen. It seems to be from her uterus. When I inquired, the patient said it is time for her to start her menses. The patient also said she usually does not experience premenstrual cramping."

   d. "BP – 124/72, T – 98.8° orally, P – 64 strong & reg, R – 17 reg & even."

5. What type of documentation would you, as a nurse, be responsible for performing in the section marked *Physician's Orders*?

   a. The patient's plan of care to be followed

   b. The vital signs taken during your shift along with the intake and output totals

   c. Transcription date, time, and your initials

   d. When you noted the orders

   e. Verbal order given to you by the physician

   f. Nursing orders

Matching Questions

Match each section of the following source-oriented record with the data that would be found there. Do this by writing the letter of the corresponding piece of data in the blank of the source-oriented medical record section where it would be found. Use all pieces of data. More than one piece of data may be found in each section.

Section of Source-Oriented Record	Data Found in Record Sections
6. Graphic Data _____	a. nurse's physical assessment data
	b. physician's physical assessment data
7. Admission Record _____	c. respiratory therapy treatment notes
	d. patient's response to initiation of IV infusion
8. Nurse's Notes _____	e. notation of strength training exercise session
	f. voiced patient complaint
9. Advance Directive _____	g. living will
	h. report of chest x-ray results
10. Rehabilitation Therapy _____	i. consent for treatment
	j. 0800 vital sign results

CRITICAL THINKING EXERCISES

11. Using the narrative charting method, document the following data in the most complete, organized, and succinct manner you can:

It is 1400 and about ½ hour ago you started an IV of 1,000 mL D5W in the patient in room 1212. You left the bed in the low and locked position when you were done starting the IV. You had explained to the patient that, when she needs to get up to the bathroom, she should not go until she has called you and you have arrived to help her. You told her that it would be too hard for her to handle the tall IV pole with the heavy pump attached to it by herself. You set the pump to infuse the D5W at 80 mL each hour. It took you only 1 attempt to access the patient's vein. You put 2 rails up on the bed. The patient told you that she already had needed to call for assistance anytime she got up, and she certainly would need help now with the new IV.

Chart the data below using each of the three following specified documentation methods.

The patient in room 231 does not feel as good now (1115) as she did when you assessed her at the beginning of your shift. She says she aches all over and feels restless. You came on at 0700 and completed her assessment at 0740. Her temperature is currently 102.4°F orally and her pulse is 104, strong but irregular. You notice she is flushed over her face and neck. You decide to administer a prn medication, Tylenol 650 mg by mouth, since she has not had any in over 12 hours. When you touch her arm, you detect that it is hot and dry. You help to relieve discomfort by applying a cool cloth to her forehead and neck. Later, around 1255, you return to her room. She is no longer flushed. Her temperature is 100.2°F and pulse 84, regular and strong. Her eyes were closed and she was snoring softly, but awakened when you spoke her name. She tells you that she is not restless anymore. Now her skin is warm and slightly damp. She also says that the aching is beginning to improve.

12. Chart data using the PIE charting method.

13. Chart data using the SOAPIER charting method.

14. Chart data using the narrative charting method.

ADDITIONAL RESOURCES

For additional Resources, Questions, and Activities, please see:

 Student Resource Disk

 http://davisplus.fadavis.com

 Student Study Guide

REFERENCES

Brier J. Improved communication and collaboration using nursing documentation tools. *American Nurses Credentialing Center.* Available at: http://www.medscape.com/viewarticle/562951. Accessed August 12, 2009.

Brooks PS. Legal questions: "official" scribblings. *Nursing2007.* 2007;37(10):24.

Brous E. Documentation & litigation. *RN.* 2009;72(2):40-43.

Charting checkup: documenting telephone orders. *LPN2008.* 2008; 4(4):4.

Dortch T. Charting checkup: document it! The importance of accurate charting. *LPN2007.* 2007;3(4):25-26.

Ferrell KG. Documentation, part 2: the best evidence of care. *Am J Nurs.* 2007;107(7):61-64.

Hynes J. Charting checkup: don't be intimidated by Incident Reports. *LPN2009.* 2009;5(2):4-5.

Margolis M. Nursing management's visionary leader 2007. *Nurs Management.* 2008;39(1):16-19.

Melo D, Carlton KH, Thede LQ. CIN Plus: a collaborative model to ensure graduating nurses are ready to use the electronic health records. *CIN: Computers, Informatics, Nursing.* 2008;26(1):8-12.

Monarch K. Documentation, part 1: principles for self-protection. *Am J Nurs.* 2007;107(7):58-60.

Nurses Service Organization. *Special Report: How to Properly Document to Reduce Your Liability Risk.* 2008. Available at: http://www. accelacommunications.com/microsite/liability_center/nso-liability-center-special-report-aug08.pdf. Accessed August 24, 2009.

Rikli J, Huizinga B, Schafer D, Atwater A, Coker K, Sikora C. Implementation of an electronic documentation system using microsystem and quality improvement concepts. *Adv Neonatal Care.* 2009;9(2):53-60.

Rutherford MA. Standardized nursing language: what does it mean for nursing practice? *OJIN Online J Issues Nurs* [serial online]. 2008;13(1).

Communicating and Understanding

Communication and Relationships

Key Terms

Active listening

Aphasia

Body language

Communication process

Congruent

Connotative

Cultural sensitivity

Denotative

Empathy

Feedback

Nonverbal

Proxemics

Rapport

Shared meaning

Therapeutic

Verbal

Objectives

1. Describe the communication process.
2. List the factors that influence communication.
3. Describe the term *active listening.*
4. Compare therapeutic communication techniques with communication barriers.
5. Identify the preferred style of communication for nurses.
6. Describe how to communicate to manage conflict effectively.
7. Discuss effective methods of communicating with the health care team.
8. Define the term *empathy* and its role in patient-centered communication.
9. Identify effective communication techniques for patients with special needs.
10. Describe the interview process.

Clinical Connection:

Your Assignment: You have been assigned to care for a 54-year-old male patient with heart disease who has had coronary artery bypass surgery. In the report, you are told that he is very quiet and does not talk much with anyone. He is not married and has few visitors. You already feel uncomfortable about caring for him because you don't know what to say or how to get him to talk to you.

Your Actions: You have many concerns about the actions to take while caring for this patient. Should you ask him lots of questions, or is that prying? Should you just perform his care in silence if that is the way he wants it? How can you draw him out? You do not feel like you are good at making "small talk" with most people anyway. And does it even matter whether he talks or not, as long as you do a good job taking care of him?

You may be wondering whether communication is truly important in nursing. It is. Effective communication is the foundation of nurse-patient relationships: It helps establish the proper transfer of health care information, is essential in proper documentation practices, and is a key element when reporting information to other members of the health care team—all vital components of building relationships and carrying out professional responsibilities of caring for others. Yet, despite its importance, surveys tell us that nurses often feel unprepared for the wide range of communication skills that are necessary in clinical situations.

The Communication Process

Think of communication much like a gift exchange; you give a gift to a person and they give you one in return. Likewise, the **communication process** is an exchange of information, feelings, needs, and preferences between two people. When people are face-to-face, communication is not a passive one-sided event, like watching the news on television. It is not as simple as informing or telling. Rather, it is an active process that involves informing, or *sending,* and *receiving,* which includes listening, observing, processing, and comprehending in a reciprocal fashion. In face-to-face interactions, both parties will send and receive messages simultaneously by interpreting both the words spoken and the tone, body language, and inflection of the voice. To complete the communication process, the receiver will send **feedback**, or a return message, that indicates the message has been received, processed, and comprehended.

The goal of communication is to establish a mutual understanding of the meaning of a message, known as **shared meaning**, that indicates the message was communicated as intended. Figure 6-1 shows the receiver and sender in the communication process.

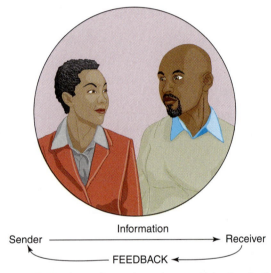

Figure 6-1   A sender and receiver participating in the communication process and offering feedback.

Types of Communication

The communication process consists of verbal and nonverbal language. **Verbal** communication is a conscious use of words, either spoken or written. An individual's choice of words may be dependent on age, education, developmental level, and culture. Verbal communication is more direct than nonverbal communication and is often used to give or receive specific information. Feelings can be expressed verbally by a speaker through changes in pitch, pace, and tone of voice.

Nonverbal communication is conveyed by **body language**—facial expressions, posture, body position, behavior, gestures, touch, and general appearance. Nonverbal communication is less conscious and more indirect than verbal communication; consequently, it often conveys more of what a person feels, thinks, and means than what is stated in words. It requires observation and forming a valid, or a true or intended, interpretation of the language. Verbal and nonverbal language should be **congruent**, or in agreement, to effectively meet the goal of shared meaning in communication.

Real-World Connection

Communicating With a Smile

One thing students can do to improve the nurse-patient relationship is to smile. Smiling has a positive effect not only for those receiving the smile but also for the person giving it. Smiling signals that you are friendly and approachable and that you are enjoying what you are doing. Young children, elderly individuals, and those with dementia respond especially well to smiling; it is a positive way of making a connection with them.

Factors That Affect Communication

Personal space, body position, language, culture, attitude, and emotions all contribute to the way people communicate. These are some of the factors that help to establish the norms of the communication process in a given situation.

Personal Space

The distance, or personal space, people place between themselves and others is called **proxemics**. It reflects feelings and attitudes and affects communication. Four personal space-distance zones have been identified for use in the United States:

1. **Intimate:** Ranging from physical contact to 18 inches
2. **Casual-personal:** 18 inches to 4 feet
3. **Social-consultative:** 4 to 12 feet
4. **Public:** 12 feet if possible

People who have a negative attitude toward a situation or who view a speaker as unfriendly will maintain a more distant position than someone with a more positive outlook. Generally, the more that people are acquainted with each other, the less personal space they place between themselves. Nurses are an exception.

You will most likely not be closely acquainted with those you care for, and yet, you must often be in close physical contact with them to provide effective care. Part of your job when caring for individuals within an intimate space range is to communicate to them that you respect that you are invading their personal space but that the closeness is necessary in order to help them at that moment.

When you care for patients from different cultures, it is very important to keep their comfort levels regarding touch and personal space in mind. More information about cultural aspects of nursing care can be found in Chapter 8. See Box 6-1 for information about personal space preferences within different cultures.

Box 6-1

Personal Space and Touch Preferences Within Cultures

As you work with patients from different cultures, it is important to keep in mind their preferences regarding personal space and touch.

- **Canada, United States, and Great Britain:** Require the most personal space, approximately 20 inches; tend to be physically reserved and do not touch others unless they have a close relationship.
- **Germany and Northern Europe:** Require a significant amount of personal and environmental space.
- **Caribbean and Latin America:** Prefer less personal space, 14 to 15 inches; also more touch friendly; stepping back from a person talking with you is considered insulting.
- **Africa:** Prefer less personal space and do not mind crowded public places.
- **Middle East:** Require the least amount of personal space; two Saudi men in conversation may stand only 9 to 10 inches apart; same-sex people stand very close together, whereas opposite-sex persons will stand further apart.
- **Mediterranean:** The most touch oriented; it is acceptable for two men to hold hands in public, but not two women.
- **Asia:** Most touch avoiding in eastern and northeastern Asia; it is considered quite rude to touch another person's head. In Japan, women may hold hands in public, but not men.

Body Position

A person's body position will communicate messages in several ways. For example, when a nurse stands over and peers down at a seated patient, it may demonstrate the desire of the nurse to maintain some distance physically or appear to have a position of authority. This may be perceived quite rightly by the patient as indicating that the nurse is not really concerned and does not care to listen. Slumping body posture may indicate disinterest or boredom. Folded arms may indicate a resistance to hearing a message. To demonstrate a willingness to communicate effectively with your patients, you need to communicate at eye level with the other person, lean slightly forward, and maintain an open body posture.

Language

Language or words convey our ideas to others when we communicate. Our choice of language is a factor in the success of the shared meaning of the message. Often there are misunderstandings in communication due to language choices. Nurses in particular need to ensure they use language that is clear; is unequivocal, meaning that the words have one meaning; and is free of bias.

You should avoid the use of medical jargon when communicating with patients to promote better understanding. Tailor your language to the patient's stage of development. When communicating with a person who speaks a language other than English, you may point to an object or use a picture board to communicate basic ideas. Arrange for an interpreter who speaks and understands the language your patient is communicating in to avoid any misunderstandings.

Culture

Culture consists of the shared values, beliefs, and practices of the majority within a group of people. It includes the attitudes, roles, behaviors, and religious or spiritual practices accepted by the group.

Culture influences communication to a great extent. **Cultural sensitivity** combines a recognition of and respect for the accepted patterns of communication in a culture. For example, a person is showing cultural sensitivity when he or she refrains from using language that would be deemed offensive or disrespectful by another culture when interacting with a person of that culture.

The most obvious cultural difference among people is language or verbal communication. If a patient does not speak and understand English, an interpreter who is familiar with health care practices can help to translate so misunderstandings and mishaps in treatment do not occur. Most health care facilities maintain a registry of employee interpreters or community agencies that provide interpreting services, and telephonic interpreting devices are available in most areas of the country.

As a nurse, you should also be aware that there are cultural variances in nonverbal communication patterns in your patients. Nonverbal communication, such as eye contact, personal space, the use of touch, and the meaning of gestures, may have varying significance in different cultures. Because these factors have a direct effect on communication meaning and will affect the quality of the care experience, observe your patients' nonverbal language to see what the cultural norms are for them and act based on those observations.

Attitude

Your choice of language and nonverbal behavior will be influenced by attitude. By definition, attitude is the manner, disposition, feeling, or position toward a person or thing. It is also defined as the position or posture of the body that is appropriate to or expressive of an action or feeling. An accepting, nonjudgmental attitude toward your patients and their situation is expressed by attentive language and open, focused nonverbal communication.

If you have a negative attitude toward your patient or situation, you may express it by disinterested verbal language, a stern expression, and a closed body stance and by maintaining a greater distance of personal space. As a nurse, you must be conscious of the attitude you display in your professional role and how communication of that attitude will affect your relationships with your patients and coworkers.

Emotion

Language has the ability to stir powerful feelings known as emotions. Language can inspire, give hope, and convey caring, but it can also generate negative feelings such as antagonism, fear, and prejudice. Problems occur when speakers use terms that seem objective but unknowingly hold an emotional bias.

Many words have two layers of meaning: The **denotative** meaning is the literal meaning, absent any interpretation. The **connotative** meaning refers to the emotional associations that can be attached to the word. Connotative language, whether used consciously or unconsciously, has the potential to shape a listener's attitude. Some words hold such strong emotional associations, so much like a trigger, that they may set off a storm of intense emotional reactions—good or bad. Words such as "love," "cancer," and "death" are emotionally charged words; they can elicit emotional responses that distract the listener because of past experiences, resulting in a message that is distorted and altered.

Knowledge Connection

List the three components of the communication process. Explain how body position and attitude are different and how they are similar in the way they affect communication.

Active Listening

Active listening techniques use all the senses to interpret verbal and nonverbal messages. In active listening, attention is paid to what the speaker is saying but also to what is not said. The mind focuses on the interaction and detects feelings as well as the spoken words. It takes real practice for the mind to tune out other intrusions and distractions and to focus on the speaker, then wait for the entire message to be delivered before interpreting what is said. With experience, you will be able to observe and interpret sensory stimuli to form a perception of what your patient may be feeling physically and emotionally but not verbalizing. Certain facial expressions, body postures, and movements can indicate what the patient is feeling.

To complete the process of active listening, you respond to the content heard in the message, share your perceptions, and state as feedback what you, as the listener, understood was said by the speaker. When you practice active listening as a nurse, you demonstrate to your patients that you are interested in their feelings, concerns, and needs. This interest helps build the foundation of a trusting relationship between nurse and patient that is critical to providing quality care. An example of this would be when a patient says, "I am so tired of all these treatments. They don't seem to do much good anyway." As an active listener, the nurse would respond by confirming that he or she understood what was stated and what was meant. A possible response might be, "It sounds as though you are getting discouraged about the treatments. It must be difficult to go through the radiation and not know if it is really helping." This gives the patient the opportunity to confirm the nurse's perceptions and discuss the patient's feelings further, or to correct any misperceptions the nurse may have.

Styles of Communication

Individuals develop a style or way of communicating that is based on their personality and self-concept. The three common types of style are passive or avoidant, aggressive, and assertive.

The *passive or avoidant* behavior style is characterized by the desire to avoid confrontation and the inability to share feelings or needs with others. Individuals with this style have trouble asking for help and allow others to take advantage of them, resulting in feelings of anger, emotional pain, and anxiety.

The *aggressive* behavior style is characterized by putting one's own needs, rights, and feelings before those of others. Individuals with this behavior style exhibit a superior attitude; they try to humiliate others and communicate in an angry, hostile way that does not acknowledge the feelings of others.

The *assertive* behavior style is characterized by standing up for one's self without violating the basic rights of others. Individuals with this behavior style show respect for others, express their own feelings in an honest and direct way, and act in a consistent manner that enhances self-worth.

Assertive communication is the most effective communication style for nurses to practice. An assertive style provides self-esteem and self-confidence and allows the nurse to care for others with a higher degree of commitment and respect. Unfortunately, many nurses do not consistently act or communicate in an assertive manner. Box 6-2 provides an explanation of the Describe, Explain, State, Consequences (DESC) method used to promote assertive communication.

Learning a New Communication Style

The style in which you communicate is a learned behavior, and it has surely been reinforced over time. We were all taught to "be nice" as children, but some adults take advantage of the nice behavior of others. Also, childhood experiences may have started a pattern of negative messages about self-worth. Additional comments or experiences while working in nursing may reinforce those negative messages of self-worth, especially if a nurse is fearful of repercussions from acting assertively.

It can be difficult to change behavior; it requires time, practice, and a conscious decision to change. To honor your own needs and to fulfill your responsibilities to your profession and patients, you will have to stick up for yourself in an assertive manner. Part of this is learning to avoid ambiguous language. Phrases such as, "Do you think you

---

Box 6-2
DESC Method

A communication method, abbreviated **DESC**, helps promote assertive communication. The four letters are used as a template to help the communicator to practice assertive communication.
- **D**escribe the behavior. Focus on what is observed or heard without a personal attack. Discuss the behavior, not the person.
- **E**xplain the impact of the behavior. Do not minimize the impact of the behavior.
- **S**tate the desired outcome. When you describe what you need from the other person, he or she does not have to guess and may be more likely to make changes.

  The first three elements of the DESC method may be sufficient to get the person to change behavior, but if not, then you must initiate the fourth step:
- **C**onsequences should grab the person's attention. You will need to restate your position and then ask the person something like,"What else do I need to do to get your attention?" or make the statement, "If you continue what you are doing, you and I will need to meet with the supervisor to resolve this." For most people, this will be the most difficult step to implement because nobody likes to go out of their comfort zone.

---

could," "Sort of," and "Maybe try..." are nonassertive and rarely get a person to change behavior. Practice using the DESC model until you gain confidence in communicating in that middle ground between passivity and aggression.

Knowledge Connection
Which style of communication do you use most often at school? At home? How can you change that style if it is not effective?

Therapeutic Communication

Therapeutic communication is patient-centered communication. The goal of therapeutic communication is to promote a greater understanding of a patient's needs, concerns, and feelings. When practicing therapeutic communication, the nurse helps patients explore their own thoughts and feelings, encourages expression of them, and avoids barriers to communication.

There are a variety of techniques a nurse can use to enhance therapeutic communication in a nurse-patient interaction. Over time you will probably become comfortable with a few of the techniques, but it is a good idea to become familiar with all the techniques and to try new ones periodically so you do not overuse certain techniques and come across as insincere. Also, be aware that some techniques, such as silence and reflecting, should be used in small doses because they may slow down communication. A list of therapeutic communication techniques and examples is found in Box 6-3.

Box 6-3

Therapeutic Communication Techniques

Practice using these therapeutic communication techniques with your friends and family as well as with your patients. You may be surprised at what you will learn.

- **Providing General Leads:** Encourages initiation or elaboration of a conversation. Some examples would be:
  - "I see what you are saying, and then what happened?"
  - "Tell me what treatment plan Dr. Smith talked to you about yesterday."
- **Using Silence:** Utilizes pauses or silence for up to several minutes without verbalizing. An example would be sitting quietly and waiting for the patient to explore thoughts and feelings.
- **Offering Self:** Shows concern and willingness to help. An example would be "What can I do to help you?"
- **Using open-ended questions or statements:** Encourages elaboration and discourages answering questions with one or two words. An example would be "Tell me more about..."
- **Using restatement:** Restates in different words the heart of what a patient said. Encourages further communication. Also conveys to the patient that you were actively listening. An example would be: *Patient:* "My daughter made me so mad yesterday!" *Nurse:* "Your daughter upset you yesterday?"
- **Seeking Clarification:** Helps to verify that the message sent was what was intended. This is necessary if the communication has detoured into many topics. An example would be "Are you saying...?"
- **Giving Information:** Provides relevant information. An example would be "You will need to report to the x-ray department at 8:00 a.m."
- **Using reflection:** Reflects same words back to the patient. This encourages verbalization of feelings. An example would be: *Patient:* "I'm so anxious about what my tests will show." *Nurse:* "You are anxious about your test results?"
- **Looking at Alternatives:** Helps patients explore options when making decisions about their care. An example would be "Have you thought about...?"
- **Summarizing:** Sums up the important points. An example would be "It looks like you've covered everything..."

Barriers to Therapeutic Communication

Many factors can contribute to unsuccessful communication. A sender may send a confusing or an incomplete message. A message may become distorted, misunderstood, or not received at all.

Factors that lead to unsuccessful communication are called blocks or barriers to communication. Everyone uses communication barriers from time to time, whether consciously or unconsciously. People may change the subject when they discuss uncomfortable topics, use clichés when they are unsure how to respond, or voice defensive comments when faced with a complaint. Nonverbal barriers to communication include looking distracted, turning away, or intimidating patients by standing over them when they are seated. Nurses should avoid using barriers when communicating with patients and learn ways to promote effective, therapeutic interactions. Other examples of barriers to communication include:

- **Asking questions that can be answered with a "yes" or "no" response:** "Do you feel better after talking to the doctor?"
- **Giving false reassurance:** "Don't worry, everything will be alright."
- **Asking too many personal, probing questions:** "Why do you think that?"
- **Giving advice:** "I think you should..." or "If I were you..."
- **Belittling a patient's feelings:** "There are other patients who need more help than you."
- **Expressing disapproval:** "I would never decide against chemotherapy."

Communication in a Crisis

In a crisis situation, things can happen suddenly and without warning, demanding that the nurse react quickly to ensure a good outcome for the patient. An important part of ensuring a good outcome in a crisis situation is the ability of the nurse to use effective communication tools to help manage the crisis. In such a situation, the nurse must use focused communication with language that is very clear and concise. A good communication tool to utilize in a crisis is called SBAR: Situation, Background, Assessment, Recommendation.

By following the SBAR guide, your communication will systematically be focused on the crisis situation, and use of SBAR can be adopted when you communicate with fellow staff nurses, supervisors, and physicians. Along with focused communication, your tone of voice should convey urgency but not panic. Likewise, your nonverbal behavior should display confidence and control, especially in front of your patients and their family members. Observing you communicate in a focused, controlled manner will help others cope with the crisis.

Anger or Hostility in Communication

Anger is a strong emotion that researchers say is often a cover-up for what a person is really thinking and feeling. Anger can be a signal or a message that we are being hurt, our rights are being violated, our needs are not being met, we are giving too much of ourselves, or we are not doing enough for ourselves. When we experience feelings of frustration, disappointment, or powerlessness, anger is never far behind.

There are two sides to anger. One side is guilt, which is directed inward at something we did or did not do. The other side is resentment, which is directed outward at others for what they did or did not do. Both guilt and resentment build up over time. If there is no change in the situation or resolution to the problem, a person may become consumed in the negativity of anger and end up harming relationships and hindering personal growth.

Anger expressed as hostility in communication can present in several forms, including screaming, sarcasm, rudeness, belittling comments or jokes, and direct personal insults. Conflict is a by-product of anger projected outward toward others. Conflict is common in health care because it is a highly emotional and people-oriented business. Patients are sick, confused, and frightened. Family members may feel helpless, sad, or guilty. Staff members are stressed by the daily physical and emotional demands of their work. As a result, conflicts may arise between patients and staff, families and staff, or members of the health care team. Conflict affects the quality of care and must not be allowed to continue unchecked! Box 6-4 presents tips for resolving conflict.

Knowledge Connection

Which therapeutic communication techniques come the most naturally to you? Which should you be careful not to overuse? Which barriers do you use most often?

Humor in Communication

Humor has a place in health care. It often helps to create an atmosphere that is relaxed and sociable. Research tells us that patients value informal, humorous social interaction because it allows them to step out of their sick role, helps establish rapport and trust, and passes the time, all while helping to relieve anxiety and tension. One study indicated that nurses who used humor appeared more approachable to the patients. Humor also makes anger more tolerable and can work to diffuse pent-up guilt and resentment if used appropriately.

While humor has its place, it is not appropriate when dealing with highly emotional or difficult issues. In addition, not all people who are ill may appreciate frivolous conversation or joking. When it comes to humor, you should be observant and take your cue from the patient before initiating humorous encounters or backing off from them.

Communication With the Health Care Team

Not only will you communicate with patients and families, you will communicate frequently with other members of the health care team. Whether you are communicating with your supervisor or coworker, it is important to approach the situation well prepared so that a clear message is given.

Upward Communication

The terms *upward* and *downward* communication refer to your placement on an organizational chart. Upward communication is the interaction with those in authority over you and is formal by nature. You will need to learn and utilize the channels of communication within your organization. If you are a team member, you will share information with your team leader. The team leader will share information with the unit manager, who in turn will report information to a supervisor, and so on up the chain of command. When you begin working, you will realize there are many layers of nursing between the bedside nurse and the nurses who have major decision-making responsibility for the entire facility. Those many layers can affect information flow. Box 6-5 offers tips for talking with your supervisor.

Box 6-4

Tips on Resolving Conflict

Conflict is very uncomfortable for most people. Some may try to avoid it or ignore it because they are unsure of what to do or say. These tips will help you positively confront and resolve conflicts.

- Speak privately with the other person. Remain polite and professional and thank him or her for taking the time to meet with you.
- When speaking, remain focused on the specific area of conflict. Do not focus on how you feel about the other person or how you think he or she should have acted.
- Be specific about what you perceive the problem to be. Express your feelings but do not be accusatory. Use "I" instead of "you" in your statements. This will allow you to take responsibility for your emotions and allow the other

person to explain his or her side of the story. For example, it is preferable for you to say "I am bothered by the comments you made the other day" instead of "You hurt my feelings the other day with your comments."
- Be prepared to hear how the other person feels toward you or the problem.
- Apologize for any misunderstandings.
- Ask the other person for ideas on how to resolve the conflict.
- It may be necessary to "agree to disagree." Try to focus on what you have in common, but you can civilly disagree on certain issues. Learning to respect another's beliefs and opinions is part of becoming a professional.

If you cannot satisfactorily resolve a conflict on your own, involve your supervisor.

Tips for Talking With Your Supervisor

It is important to communicate effectively when you need to talk with your supervisor about a problem.

- Keep your supervisor informed.
- If a problem develops, make an appointment to talk it over. Have specific information available, especially written documentation. Focus on problem-solving, not just problems.
- Show that you have important information to share and hold a sense of responsibility.
- Be careful which words you choose. Avoid blaming others, exaggeration, and overly dramatic expressions.
- Do not talk to your supervisor when you are angry, and do not respond with anger. Use "I" statements and explain what you are thinking.
- If you want to present a new idea, give your supervisor a written proposal, then meet to discuss it.
- Accept feedback and learn from it.

Never go above or around your supervisor. Always communicate directly with your supervisor before you go up the chain of command.

In grade school you probably played the whisper game, in which someone whispers a message to the next person and each person in turn repeats the message down the line. Often times, when the message reaches the end of the line, it is unrecognizable as the original message. Likewise, messages can get distorted when they travel through many people in an upward flow of communication. When communicating with supervisors, experts say it is important to state your needs clearly, explain the rationales for your requests, and suggest the benefits to others, not just you. Also, it is important for you to listen objectively to your supervisor's response because there may be good reasons for granting or not granting your request.

Communicating With Physicians

When the need arises, you may have to telephone a physician at his or her home or office. You may need to call a physician to clarify orders or to report on a change of patient condition; you may also need to call a physician if a patient has a special request or concern that cannot wait for regular rounds. You may even have to contact a physician who is on call for the primary physician. The way you communicate in all these circumstances is crucial to the continuity of care and safety of the patient.

Telephone and Verbal Physician's Orders

Communicating face-to-face with someone can sometimes be difficult; it is important to make certain that the sender's delivered message is received, interpreted, and understood by the receiver in the way the sender intended it to be. Getting your message delivered correctly or receiving the exact message that was intended becomes even tougher when the communication occurs over the telephone. Over the telephone, you cannot see the individual's eyes, facial expression, or body language, all of which contribute significantly to delivery of the true intended message. The other disadvantage of verbal communication is the lack of the sender's written word to use for clarification as needed.

When you need to telephone a physician regarding a patient's condition, be prepared by having the patient's chart and a pen to write down any orders the physician gives to you. It is a good idea to also have a pad or paper in case the physician gives you verbal orders on a different patient than the one about whom you are phoning.

Certain guidelines should be followed when contacting a physician. Before calling the physician, make sure you prepare:

- A quick assessment of the patient, reviewing the chart for history and background information
- A concise statement of the problem and why you are calling, making sure you have a list of all points you want to cover
- Current data, such as vital signs, laboratory results, diagnostic tests, surgeries, medications received, and allergies

Also try to anticipate what information the physician may need to make a sound decision.

When you call a physician, first identify yourself, where you are calling from, the name of the patient you are calling about, and the reason you are calling. Have the chart handy to refer to if necessary. Do not give your personal opinion unless asked to do so.

Writing Physician's Orders

Write the orders as the physician says them and always read them back to the physician, who should then verify that they are correct. Because it is easy to hear something different than what was actually said, this is a necessary step that should always be carried out. The Joint Commission's 2009 National Patient Safety Goals require all three steps under *Goal 2: Improve the effectiveness of communication among caregivers.* Be certain that the physician allows you time to ask any questions you may have regarding his or her orders, and to read back the orders as you wrote them, for verification. The ideal method for taking telephone orders is to have a second nurse listen on an extension to further verify what is said and co-sign the telephone order; however, this is not easily accomplished when you are busy or working short handed.

Refer to Box 6-6 for a list of data to include when writing a telephone or verbal order, and Figure 6-2 for an example of a correctly written telephone order.

All of these guidelines will take on greater importance if you need to call a physician during the middle of the night. Anticipate that you have awakened the physician and you should give him or her a moment to awaken and be able to listen attentively to your call. You will want to follow all the guidelines listed above and be especially concerned with clarifying information or orders that do not seem to be correct or are out of the ordinary. If you need to call a physician who is on call and probably does not know the patient, be prepared to give more background information to present a clear, concise profile of the patient.

Downward Communication

Nurses provide direction to and supervise other licensed and unlicensed assistive personnel. Communicating with those you supervise is called downward communication. When supervising, it is important to keep in mind that those you supervise have needs for satisfaction and self-esteem. Your method of supervision and communication should respect those needs. Even nurses who may have many years of experience may be still working on developing effective communication skills. New and inexperienced assistive personnel may need guidance to enhance their communication.

This focus on communication is especially important, as the trend in health care is to employ a culturally diverse work force and provide services to a culturally diverse population. Supervising nurses frequently use several types of downward communication techniques:

- **Job Instruction:** What to do or how to do it. The instruction should also include information about deadlines for job completion or other expectations about when to give any feedback of information.
- **Job Rationale:** Explanations about how one task relates to other tasks.
- **Practices and Procedures:** Information about what needs to be done, how it needs to be done according to the facility's policies and procedures, and possible benefits.

- **Feedback:** Information about how effectively a person is performing and outcomes or verification of instruction before a task is initiated, as well as during or after completion of a task.
- **Role Modeling:** Communicating in such a way that you demonstrate to assistive personal how to interact effectively and appropriately regarding the needs and care of your patients.

Shift-to-Shift Reporting

Ineffective communication is a major cause of medical errors. The Joint Commission concluded that, in the 10-year period from 1995 to 2005, ineffective communication caused 60% to 70% of the reported *sentinel events,* defined by The Joint Commission as unexpected occurrences involving death or serious physical or psychological injury, or the risk thereof. Hand-off or shift-to-shift reporting has been identified as an area in patient care that is vulnerable to ineffective communication. The *shift report* is the communication of the patient's condition and required nursing care by the off-going nurse to the oncoming nurse, a necessary step in preparation for the oncoming nurse to receive the patient into his or her care. The problem of ineffective communication has prompted experts to recommend standardizing the reporting process to make it more relevant and patient centered. The focus of end-of-shift reporting should be to pass along detailed, accurate, current information about the patient and changes in orders or plan of care, including changes that have already occurred and anticipated changes.

Shift Report

Each day when you report to work, especially if you work in a hospital, you will find that you need to know not only which patients you will be providing care for, but what type of care you must provide. Many methods of shift-to-shift reporting have been tried, but most of the time it has been decided that face-to-face reporting is the safest and most effective manner in which to communicate the information (Fig. 6-3). When you are the oncoming nurse, face-to-face reporting provides you with the opportunity to not only listen to the data reported to you by the off-going nurse, but to also ask questions. No one has a perfect memory, especially at the end of a work shift. When the oncoming nurse is given the opportunity to ask questions and clarify what the off-going nurse just said, the shift report becomes a safer and more effective communication tool. The Joint Commission's

William, Mayson #91208 Rm. # 804 BD 6-4-61 Admit 6-9-12	PHYSICIAN'S ORDERS
June 13, 2012 2125	Change IV fluids to LR 1000 mL @ 80 mL/hour
	T.O. Dr. Arthurs/B. Huntley, RN

Figure 6-2 This is an example of a correctly written telephone order.

Figure 6-3 This nurse is finishing her shift and giving the end-of-shift report to the oncoming nurse.

2009 National Patient Safety Goals also address this issue in Goal 2. They expect each health care providing organization to develop and maintain a uniform approach to improve the communication when turning over a patient's care to the next caregiver, specifying that it must include an opportunity to ask questions and receive responses.

Confidentiality of the Shift Report
Confidentiality as mandated by the Health Insurance Portability and Accountability Act (HIPAA) includes discussion of a patient's condition, such as during a shift report. Such discussions about patients must be conducted where privacy is ensured, not in the hallway or in the cafeteria where others may overhear.

Data to Include in a Shift Report
There is certain information that you must always include in your shift report, and there are times when it constitutes a tremendous amount of data, bringing up the issue of length of time spent in reporting. By the end of your shift, you will generally desire to report off and leave on time. Employers have a vested interest in you getting off duty in a timely manner to reduce overtime expenses. This requires you to be succinct while being thorough. If you select some sort of sequence or order in which to present each patient's report and use it consistently while you are learning how to give an end-of-shift report, you will develop a sequence that will become routine without having to think hard about it. Table 6-1 presents a list of specific items that should be included in a shift report. Box 6-7 provides an example of one nurse's shift report.

As soon as you begin the clinical portion of your training, start to develop your own format and order in which you present the information in your report. It will be helpful to use written documents to cue you about things you need to report, rather than relying totally on your memory. For example, if a Kardex is used at your facility, it is a good tool to use along with your "pocket-brains," or notes that you made during the shift. (See Chapter 5 for more information about the Kardex and pocket-brains.)

Table 6-1 Items to Include in Shift Report

Basic Patient Data		
Room number	Special safety issues such as:	Assistive equipment such as:
Patient name	Fall risk	Hearing aid
Patient age	Aspiration risk	Cane
Patient gender	Confusion	Walker
Physician	Paralysis	Prosthetic devices such as:
Admitting diagnoses	Tracheostomy	Eye
Other diagnoses	Inability to communicate	Arm
Allergies	Sensory deficits such as:	Leg
Frequency of VS	Blindness	
Diet order	Deafness	
Activity order		
Type bath		
Bowel/bladder status		
Any complaints		

Scheduled Procedures	Pertinent Diagnostic Results
Laboratory Tests	Normal results
X-rays	Abnormal results
Radiology Procedures	
Other Diagnostic Procedures	
Surgery	

Table 6-1 **Items to Include in Shift Report** (continued)

Abnormal Assessment Findings		
All findings outside of normal range Any changes in patient condition		

Interdisciplinary Therapies Ordered		
Respiratory Therapy Speech Therapy	Occupational Therapy Dietary Consult	Physical Therapy

Various Ordered Treatments		
Suction Antibiotic therapy	Dressing change Intravenous access	Wound care Telemetry monitoring

Shall We Chat?

The end-of-shift report is not a time for social conversation among coworkers. It is easy to fall into that trap, but it is important to remember that extraneous conversation is distracting and increases the risk of forgetting a piece of pertinent information that may affect the patient's care or condition. Be sure to save any conversation that is not patient centered for another time, such as when you are on break. This will save everyone time and decrease unnecessary time spent in shift reporting.

Written Communication

Nurses communicate not only with the spoken word but also with written language that is read by other members of the health care team. A good deal of communication that occurs in health care is in written form, and nurses in particular should develop the ability to write effectively. Written communication includes care plans, progress notes, memos, reports, and assignments.

Before you begin writing, know your audience, which is the person or group of people who will be reading what you write. It is important to know the audience because that will help define what writing style to use. You would use a more formal style for upward communication, making sure you utilize proper titles, format, grammar, punctuation, and spelling. You could use an informal style, more conversational, among your peers or those you may be supervising. In any case, do not let anything that you have written be sent out without first proofreading the material and making revisions if necessary.

Identify the purpose before you begin writing. Knowing the purpose will enable you to organize your thoughts around the "why" of your writing. Write what you mean. Choose words that are clear, specific, and concise. Use technical words appropriately, when the reader will understand the meaning. Keep sentences simple with one idea per sentence. Your reader should not have to guess what you are trying to say. A reader should be able to follow your thoughts easily without being diverted by unnecessary language. Finally, what you write will make a lasting impression and strongly influence how you are evaluated. People will make judgments about your credibility for a long time after you have written the words.

Box 6-7

Sample Shift Report

Nurses communicate with one another about patients all the time. Here is an example of a complete and detailed shift report between a nurse who is completing one shift and the nurse who will be relieving him.

Off-Going Nurse: "In room 1237 is Melissa Summers, a 37-year-old female patient of Dr. Holsted admitted this morning with an acute exacerbation of asthma. She also has diabetes mellitus type 2 that is under good control with diet and Januvia. She's allergic to penicillin, sulfa, and latex. On admit she was very hypoxic, pale with circumoral cyanosis, SpO$_2$ was 85%, respirations 44 shallow, irregular, and gasping, hardly able to speak. She improved rapidly with application of O$_2$, HHN treatment with Duoneb, and an IVPB of aminophylline. Her vital signs with SpO$_2$ are ordered every 4 hrs. SpO$_2$ was 90% with O$_2$ at 4 L/min per NC an hour ago. She had 100.4 oral temp and respiratory rate of 29 half an hour ago. Other vitals are within normal limits. She still has wheezes throughout all 5 lobes but no complaints of dyspnea at this time. Color is pale but no cyanosis. She's on a regular diet, up ad lib unless shortness of breath increases, and can take a shower using a shower chair and someone not in bathroom with her, but in the room on stand-by in case she becomes dyspneic. She has voided and had a BM this shift. Drinks lots of fluids without prompting. Her chest x-ray showed some infiltrate starting in both lower lobes, and another chest x-ray is ordered for in the morning. Doc started her on ampicillin IVPB every 6 hours."

Oncoming Nurse: "Did they do a WBC on her?"

Off-Going Nurse: "Oh, yeah. It was 16,500 and he wants it repeated in the morning."

A quick tip for written communication is KISS: **K**eep **I**t **S**hort and **S**imple!

The Nurse-Patient Relationship

It is extremely important for nurses and patients to develop **rapport**, or a relationship with mutual trust and understanding. It is your responsibility to take the lead in establishing the relationship with a patient, but it must be one that is based on trust.

Establishing Trust

When individuals become ill, they lose a measure of control of their environment and must rely on others to care for them until they recover. For nurses to be able to give care to patients, they must quickly establish a relationship with them. At the heart of the relationship is trust. You will establish a trusting relationship with your patients by what and how you communicate with them. Your nonverbal communication should convey that you are knowledgeable about their physical care needs and you are confident and competent when providing care. Your nonverbal behavior should also communicate that you are approachable and ready to listen. When you keep patient medical information confidential and do not discuss patients with friends and coworkers, you are also establishing trust.

Patients will look to you to provide emotional support, encouragement, and understanding. Fear of the unknown is emotionally upsetting to patients and may interfere with their treatment and recovery. When patients understand what is happening and have someone to trust, it helps empower them to face the emotional and physical demands of illness and allows them to participate more fully in their care.

You can provide emotional understanding and support by communicating empathy to your patients. **Empathy** is the ability to intellectually, not emotionally, identify with or experience the feelings, thoughts, or attitudes of others. You can understand and respect what a patient is experiencing without taking on the burden of experiencing it yourself. When you communicate empathetically, the patient knows that you acknowledge and respect his or her feelings and that it is safe to express these feelings to you.

As a nurse, you must keep some emotional distance and not allow the patient's problems to become your problems. You need that distance to think and act on behalf of the patient. Being empathetic will help you conserve your own emotional reserves so you can be available to all who need your care.

Patient-Centered Communication

Patient-centered communication has been defined as communication that encourages and empowers patients to participate in their care; it is an essential component to establishing a positive nurse-patient relationship. There are several ways a nurse conveys patient-centered communication as opposed to task-centered communication. One method is by demonstrating accessibility and readiness to listen through the use of attentive nonverbal behaviors. Attentiveness or attending behavior is considered a patient-centered form of communication, and it does require the nurse to display genuineness, warmth, and empathy. The nurse's behavior and communication must be perceived as real or genuine to the patient.

Verbal communication, such as language used and tone of voice, has also been identified as an important component of patient-centered communication. A friendly tone of voice will signal to patients that you have a genuine interest in and a willingness to listen to them.

Researchers say spending long periods of time with patients does not necessarily mean that a positive nurse-patient relationship will occur. What determines whether a positive relationship develops is not the quantity but the quality of the time spent and communication practiced.

Nurses often blame being short staffed or "not having the time" during a work shift for not practicing patient-centered communication. Focusing only on the task side of care is like putting blinders on and forgetting about the person beneath those tasks. When nurses are solely task centered, they may be very efficient in performing tasks, but they may then avoid therapeutic, patient-centered communication, which encourages and empowers patients to become partners in their care.

When you communicate with patients in a patient-centered way, you will keep the focus of the conversation on the patient, not on yourself. Even if patients ask you about your personal life, try to answer as briefly as possible and turn the focus back on the patient. For example, if the patient asks, "Are you married? Do you have children?" You could answer by saying, "Yes, I am and I have two kids. What about you? How long have you been married? Where do your children live?"

Communication During a Patient Interview

An interview is a more formal way of communicating. It is planned communication with a purpose. An interview is used to get or give information. Because this is a planned event, you will need to consider certain factors that will influence the interview. For instance, time, place, seating arrangement, and distance are some of the factors that will affect the interview. Also, the format of the interview should contain three major stages: the opening, body, and closing.

- The *opening* of an interview includes introducing yourself, explaining the purpose of the interview, and establishing rapport with the patient. For example, you might say, "My name is Jane Jones and I am going to be talking with you about the problems you have been having due to your heart condition."

- The *body* of the interview is the main part during which you will ask questions and obtain answers from the patient. It accomplishes the purpose of the interview.
- The *closing* of the interview occurs as you complete all the questions, offer the patient a chance to ask any questions he or she might have, and thank him or her for participating. It might include information about what will happen next. For example, you might say, "Dr. Jacobs will be in to see you shortly and she will order any tests needed to determine your diagnosis."

Interviewing is used extensively in the nursing process. Interviews can be conducted face-to-face or over the telephone. In all cases, the nurse uses two main types of interviewing techniques. The *directive interview* is structured and conducted to find out specific information. Close-ended questions are used to request specific data from a patient; they usually require a "yes" or "no" or a short response of specific, factual information. Close-ended questions begin with one of the following words:

- Who
- What
- When
- Where
- How
- Do
- Is

The patient gives information or answers questions without going into detail. The directive interview is used when time is limited or during an emergency.

Open-ended questions are used in the *nondirective* interview. The patient has much more input in the nondirective interview and is able to explore thoughts and feelings. An open-ended question states the broad topic that will be discussed and invites the patient to elaborate on responses. Open-ended questions are good questions for beginning an interview, changing topics, and drawing out attitudes. You will use close-ended questions as the interview progresses to obtain specific data, such as a health history. Nurses will use a combination of open- and closed-ended questions during an interview to obtain needed information.

Using Nonverbal Communication During the Interview

Nonverbal communication is another important consideration during the interview. Verbal communication can be easily manipulated by interview participants to create a selected impression. Nonverbal language can rarely be manipulated and most often reveals what is really going on with the interview participant. Body language should be observed for unstated feelings or behaviors. Also, be aware of your own body language and how it influences the effectiveness of the interview process.

The interview is an opportunity to assess an individual's health literacy. *Health literacy* is defined as the ability of an individual to obtain, process, and understand basic health information and services to make appropriate health decisions. Low health literacy has been linked to increased rates of hospitalizations, outpatient visits, health care costs, and noncompliance with instructions about chronic disease conditions. During the interview, the nurse must assess the patient's health literacy and communicate information in a way and language the patient will understand so he or she can become an active participant in his or her care.

Special Communication Needs

When you are working with patients with special needs, you will have to alter how you communicate with them to accommodate those needs. The following are effective communication techniques to use with patients with special sensory needs.

People Who Are Deaf or Hard of Hearing

When patients are hard of hearing, you must make an extra effort to be understood. Communication with patients who are deaf requires that you position yourself in front of them so they can see your lips. Other strategies for communicating with patients with a hearing deficit include:

- Finding out how the person communicates best—verbalizing, writing, lip reading, or signing
- Refraining from using an intercom and developing an alternative way of communicating
- Getting the person's attention before starting to communicate
- Facing the person
- Speaking clearly with adequate volume without shouting or mumbling
- Asking for clarification and feedback to make sure you have been understood
- Speaking to the patient, not the interpreter, if there is one present
- Verifying that the patient's hearing aid is inserted and is working properly, if appropriate; make sure batteries are checked frequently
- Eliminating background noise, such as turning down the television or other distractions

If the person reads lips:

- Speak in a normal way and not in an overly exaggerated manner.
- Use short, simple sentences.
- Do not block the view of your face with your hands.
- Do not chew gum.
- Make sure the lighting is good.

Other tips include the following:

- When someone asks, "What did you say?", avoid answering with comments such as "never mind" or "nothing." These comments are insulting and demeaning because they communicate that the person is not worthy of the effort of repeating yourself.
- Engage hard-of-hearing or deaf persons in one-on-one communication whenever possible, as they may struggle in large groups or when there are two or more speakers.
- Do not show impatience or exasperation when communicating, as this may cause the hearing-impaired person to shut down and back off from expressing needs.

People Who Have Speech and Language Impairments

Many people have difficulty with speech or language due to conditions such as deafness, cerebral palsy, cerebral vascular accident (CVA), head injury, multiple sclerosis, and ventilator dependency. Chances are you will encounter patients who have some form of a speech or language problem; you must have some understanding of how to best work with these individuals.

Two of the most important functions involving communication are language and speech. Language includes writing, listening, and reading skills. It also includes receiving information. Speech is the process by which language is communicated through sound. Combined together, speech and language, as well as nonverbal methods of communication, are the mechanisms through which humans share thoughts, feelings and information.

Aphasia is a general term for a dysfunction in language. A patient may have trouble processing language output, known as expressive aphasia, or may have difficulty understanding speech, known as receptive aphasia. Box 6-8 presents an explanation of different types of aphasias. Caregivers should not assume that a patient comprehends communication until the patient's actions indicate an understanding. A speech-language pathologist (SLP) will evaluate the patient for the type and level of impairment.

It will be your responsibility as the nurse to understand what speech and language deficits your patients may experience and to develop an appropriate plan of care for mutual understanding. You must also encourage them to communicate to the best of their abilities. Box 6-9 lists some techniques to use when working with patients who have aphasia. Other ways to help communicate with individuals who have aphasia are to use picture boards, write on paper, or utilize a computer or a telecommunication device for the deaf (TDD).

Box 6-8

Types of Aphasia

Patients who are unable to speak may have one or more types of aphasia.

Expressive aphasia, or Broca's aphasia, is a disturbance in speech planning and speech production. Persons with expressive aphasia cannot produce fluent speech. Their speech has been described as "halting." Expressive aphasia presents as:
- Single-word responses; inability to produce spontaneous conversation
- Slow, monotone utterances
- Inappropriate words
- Hearing, reading abilities are intact

Receptive aphasia (Wernicke's aphasia) is a deficit in auditory comprehension or with receiving information. The patient can hear but cannot understand what is said, or may be slow to respond, or may only understand a portion of what is said. Receptive aphasia presents as:
- Abnormal language
- Impaired reading and writing skill, as the person does not understand what is supposed to be accomplished
- Speech sounds with normal rhythm, rate, and fluency

Global aphasia (expressive and receptive) is a deficit of planning, production, and comprehension of language. Patients with global aphasia can speak and understand only a few words. Global aphasia presents as:
- Meaningless speech sounds
- Possibly *perseveration*, or the repetition of one word or thought

Communication with patients with aphasia is difficult. Patients with severe impairments may have to learn to read body language and gestures to communicate.

Box 6-9

Communication Techniques for Patients With Aphasia

It is possible to communicate with patients who are unable to speak or are unable to speak clearly. To do so, use these techniques:
- Make sure you have the patient's attention by touching him or her if necessary, and addressing him or her by name.
- Speak slowly.
- Use short sentences.
- Repeat what you said.
- Use gestures, demonstration, and facial expression if necessary.
- Speak in a normal tone of voice.
- Be respectful. The patient's social awareness and sensitivities are not impaired.
- Ask yes-or-no questions and write messages to help the patient understand.
- Listen carefully.
- Allow the patient to speak without interruption.
- Try to make the patient a "partner" in the communication.

Make no issue of the use of swear words or excessive jargon. A speech-language pathologist can make recommendations to deal with those behaviors.

Anatomy and Physiology Connection

The Nervous System's Role in Communication

The brain and nervous system directly affect our ability to communicate. Activities that precede, initiate, or support communication are controlled by the brain and nervous system. A variety of communication problems occur when there is a brain or nervous system malfunction. Parkinson's disease, CVA (also known as "brain attack" or stroke), and trauma cause damage to the brain and nervous system and often affect a person's ability to engage in the communication process.

The cerebral cortex of the brain has several areas that control voluntary muscle movement, sensory perception, and sensory interpretation—all of which are necessary in the communication process. The left frontal lobe contains Broca's motor speech area, which controls the movements involved in speaking. The left temporal and parietal lobes hold speech areas that are involved in thoughts that precede speech. The parietal lobes contain the general sensory areas where sensations such as touch are felt and interpreted. The occipital lobes contain visual areas that receive impulses from the eyes that allow us to "see" and interpret what is being seen. Deep within the cerebral hemispheres, gray matter called the basal ganglia regulates the use of accessory movements such as gestures when communicating.

Patients on Mechanical Ventilation

Attempting to communicate with patients who are intubated via an endotracheal tube and who cannot speak poses challenges for the nurse and causes high levels of patient anxiety and stress. Without the ability to speak, patients are unable to express thoughts, feelings, desires, and needs in the usual manner. The following are some guidelines to enhance communication when caring for the mechanically dependent patient:

• Place the patient in a comfortable position to communicate; this is usually with the patient sitting and positioned upright. Provide adequate pain relief if needed. Assess communication methods to determine what works best.

• Make sure the call light is within easy reach, and instruct the patient on how to use it. Reassure the patient that someone will come when the call light is activated.

• If the patient uses a hearing aid or glasses, make sure they are on or in place and in good working order. If the patient does not speak English, make sure a translator is available.

• Assess the patient for the ability to communicate by writing. Provide a tablet or a magic slate. Do not place an IV line in the patient's writing arm if possible.

• Instruct the patient that other ways he or she can call for attention include tapping the over-the-bed table or side rail, or using a bell or a clicking device.

• Evaluate the patient's ability to communicate without talking. Mouthing words may not be possible for every patient to

master. Communicate with the patient by asking yes-or-no questions and asking him or her to blink the eyes a certain number of times or shake or nod his or her head for a response.

• If available, use a portable text-to-speech communication device or a communication board.

• Encourage communication and reassure the patient often. If the patient is unresponsive, use therapeutic touch and stroke the patient to convey a sense of security. Continue to communicate with the patient using simple, conversational language and explain what you are doing. Instruct family members and visitors to do the same.

• Be sure to document your communication assessment and the communication strategies you developed. Also, ensure that successful communication strategies get passed along in the shift report so that all staff may successfully be able to communicate with the patient and the patient may benefit from the continuity of care.

Remember, being intubated is a highly stressful event for the responsive patient. Try to alleviate some of the stress by developing effective communication strategies with the patient and making them part of the care plan.

Patients Who Are Unresponsive

In a critical care environment, where the patients are very ill or need close observation, the nurse must be intensely focused on tasks related to their many physical needs. This often places communication with patients as a lower priority.

There is a strong relationship between patient responsiveness and the amount of verbal communication made by nurses. When patients are unconscious or connected to a ventilator, it is difficult for the nurse, especially nurses with little clinical experience, to engage in effective nurse-patient communication. Conversation is one-way—with no verbal response from the patient. Consequently, nurses who are working with sedated or unconscious patients will often "undervalue" the importance of talking with them. Inadequate nurse-patient communication in these instances has been shown to increase stress, anxiety, and social isolation for the patient.

Communication content with the unconscious patient is often more "informative" rather than conversational, meaning nurses will explain what tasks they will be performing or if a medical procedure is to be carried out. Informative language is important, but conversational language is also important because it conveys to the patient that you are taking the time to attend to the psychosocial needs that all humans require, as well as physical needs.

Most sedated or unconscious patients can still hear and comprehend verbal communication, and they respond emotionally to it. Do not speak about other patients while caring for a sedated or unconscious patient. It is a HIPAA violation, and also the patient may misinterpret and become distressed. Patients perceive nurses who do not make communication a high priority to be uninterested, unskilled, and not professional.

People and Places Connection

Communicating Across Developmental Stages

Language is part of a person's psychosocial and intellectual development, which occurs in varying stages over a lifetime. Knowledge of a patient's stage of development allows the nurse to tailor communication appropriately. Nurses care for patients in many stages of development from childhood to elderly patients, as well as mentally challenged patients, and you cannot take a cookie-cutter approach to communication. Adapt your communication strategies to coincide with the patient's stage of development. As a nurse, you will need to be aware of developmental stages and work within them to establish effective, patient-centered communication, including patient teaching.

Communicating With Older Adults

Older adults formed their values and beliefs at a time when society was very different than it is today. Their outlook is not always easy for a younger person to understand and vice versa. It is important for caregivers to bridge the generational gap with effective, therapeutic communication.

Active listening with all the senses is a necessary part of the process because older adults may have several physical changes that will alter their ability to perceive messages or communicate their needs. For example, an older adult may have hearing or vision impairments, chronic pain, or dementia. While hearing and vision are the main senses we use in communication, the other senses of touch, smell, and taste may also play a part when communicating with the older adult. Make sure you have the older adult's attention before speaking. Try to minimize environmental distractions such as a loud television.

 Post Conference

As you evaluated the care you gave your patient during post conference, you shared that at first it was difficult to talk to him and you found yourself chattering about inane things. Then, every time you asked him a question, he would respond just with a "yes" or "no." That is when you remembered to use open-ended questions. When you asked your patient open-ended questions, he responded better. You learned a little bit about his family. Eventually, you became a bit more comfortable with silence in the room. When his sister came to visit, she was very talkative and told you that her brother "never says more than two words to anybody." Hearing that made you smile, because you knew that, by using silence, asking open-ended questions, and establishing rapport, you had been able to communicate well with this patient.

KEY POINTS

- Communication is a reciprocal process that occurs simultaneously between two parties. It involves sending and receiving messages to arrive at a shared meaning.

- Communication occurs in two ways, verbal and nonverbal.

- Personal space, body position, language, culture, attitude, and emotions are factors that contribute to the way people communicate.

- Active listening techniques use all the senses to interpret verbal and nonverbal messages. The mind focuses on the interaction and listens for feelings as well as spoken words.

- Individuals develop a style of communicating that is based on their personality and self-concept.

- Therapeutic communication is patient-centered communication. The goal is to promote a greater understanding of a patient's needs, concerns, and feelings. There are defined techniques that promote therapeutic communication, such as empathy, and barriers we all use to block communication.

- Anger and/or hostility can lead to conflict. Conflict will affect the quality of care and must be managed.

- Communication with the health care team is accomplished in a variety of ways, verbal as well as written. It is important to respect the needs for satisfaction and self-esteem in those you supervise.

- Hand-off or end-of-shift reporting is an area of communication vulnerable to ineffective communication that increases the chances of medical errors.

- The interview is formal, planned communication designed to give or obtain information.

- The very young and elderly individuals have specialized communication needs that must be recognized and individualized.

REVIEW QUESTIONS

Select the answer that is most appropriate for each of the following questions. Some questions may have more than one correct answer. Check all that apply.

1. What is the term that indicates that a message was communicated as intended?

   a. Sending

   b. Receiving

   c. Comprehending

   d. Shared meaning

2. Factors that affect communication would include:

   a. personal space.

   b. culture.

   c. attitude.

   d. emotions.

3. Active listening involves:

   a. looking at a chart while the patient is speaking.

   b. pausing before speaking.

   c. checking your watch often during conversation.

   d. nodding your head in agreement.

4. An example of nonverbal communication that is congruent to the verbal statement by the patient "I'm having a lot of back pain" would be:

   a. smiling.

   b. reading a magazine.

   c. looking up at the ceiling.

   d. grimacing and rubbing his back.

5. An assertive behavior style includes:

   a. standing up for one's own self.

   b. putting one's own needs, rights, and feelings before others.

   c. showing respect for others.

   d. acting in a consistent manner that enhances self-worth.

6. You promote trust with a patient by:

   a. allowing family members to visit whenever they want.

   b. keeping medical information confidential.

   c. talking with her at length about her life.

   d. being sure to carry through when you say you will do something.

7. When communicating with people who are hard of hearing:

   a. set the intercom on high.

   b. speak in an exaggerated way.

   c. find out how the person communicates best.

   d. if the person uses an interpreter, speak to the interpreter.

8. Open-ended questions are good types of questions to use in what situations?

   a. Introducing broad topics during an interview

   b. Beginning an interview

   c. Changing topics in an interview

   d. Asking a patient about his or her feelings

CRITICAL THINKING EXERCISE

9. You are caring for Mrs. Etta Jones, a 79-year-old female who suffered a CVA 2 years ago that left her with an aphasic disorder. Mrs. Jones suffers from expressive aphasia and utters the word "yes" for all responses. What communication techniques would you use to ensure that Mrs. Jones' needs are being met and that she is being supported emotionally?

ADDITIONAL RESOURCES

For additional Resources, Questions, and Activities, please see:

 Student Resource Disk

 http://davisplus.fadavis.com

Student Study Guide

REFERENCES

Adamski PA. Implement a handoff communication approach. *Nurs Manage.* 2007;38(1):10, 12.

Alasald J. Communication with critically ill patients. *J Adv Nurs.* 2005;50:356-362.

Anderson M. *Caring for Older Adults Holistically.* 4th ed. Philadelphia: FA Davis; 2007.

Anderson M. *Nursing Leadership, Management, and Professional Practice for the LPN/LVN.* Philadelphia: FA Davis; 2005.

Benson E, Rippin-Sisler C, Jabusch K, Keast S. Improving nursing shift-to-shift report. *J Nurs Care Quality.* 2007;22(1):80-84.

Carter P. *Essentials for Nursing Assistants.* Philadelphia: Lippincott Williams & Wilkins; 2007.

Chitty KK. *Professional Nursing Concepts & Challenges.* 4th ed. St. Louis: Elsevier Saunders; 2005.

Cox S. Good communication: finding the middle ground. *Nursing2007.* 2007;37(1):57.

DeWitt SC. *Fundamental Concepts and Skills for Nursing.* 2nd ed. Philadelphia: Elsevier Saunders; 2005.

Kalisch BJ, Hurley P, Hodges M, Landers D, Richter G, Stefanov S, et al. PI tool patches broken communication. *Nurs Manage.* 2007;38(4):16, 18.

Leininger M, McFarland M. *Transcultural Nursing.* New York: McGraw-Hill Professional; 2002.

Markova T, Broome B. Effective communication and delivery of culturally competent health care. *Urol Nurs.* 2007;27:239-242.

Osborne, H. In other words...communicating with people from other cultures. Available at: http://www.healthliteracy.com/article.asp?PageID=3821. Accessed August 10, 2009.

Personal space around the world. Available at: http://www.realsimple.com. Accessed August 17, 2008.

Ramont RP, Niedringhaus DM. *Fundamental Nursing Care.* 2nd ed. Upper Saddle River, NJ: Pearson Prentice Hall; 2008.

Roberts D. Clear communication—accept nothing less. *MedSurg Nurs.* 2007;16:142, 148.

Sheldon LK, Barrett R, Ellington L. Difficult communication in nursing. *J Nurs Scholarship.* 2006;38:141-147.

Scanlon V, Sanders T. *Essentials of Anatomy and Physiology.* Philadelphia: FA Davis; 2007.

Wilkinson JM, Van Leuven K. *Fundamentals of Nursing.* Philadelphia: FA Davis; 2007.

Venes D, ed. *Taber's Cyclopedic Medical Dictionary.* 21st ed. Philadelphia: FA Davis; 2009.

Promoting Health and Wellness

Key Terms

Acute illness

Adaptation

Chronic illness

Continuum

Coping strategies

Dependency phase

Drug abuse

Exacerbation

Fight-or-flight response

Healthy People 2010

Obese

Overweight

Prodromal phase

Recovery phase

Remission

Risk factors

Seeking help phase

Stress

Symptomatic phase

Objectives

1. Define key terms related to health promotion and wellness.
2. Explain the wellness-illness continuum.
3. Describe two theories of wellness and illness.
4. Identify the two goals of Healthy People 2010.
5. Enumerate the 10 Leading Health Indicators of Healthy People 2010.
6. Identify risk factors for selected illnesses.
7. Define stress and adaptation.
8. Describe the symptoms of stress.
9. Describe the body's reactions during the "fight-or-flight" response.
10. Categorize coping strategies in response to stress.

Clinical Connection

Your Assignment: You are caring for a 45-year-old woman who is very healthy and is a long-distance runner. She has been diagnosed with gallstones and is scheduled for a *cholecystectomy,* the surgical removal of the gallbladder. She seems very anxious and tells you that she has never really been ill before. In fact, she tells you that she doesn't understand how she could get gallstones because she is such a healthy eater. She has many questions for you about her postoperative recovery and asks you, "Will I be well again after this surgery? Can I run again right away and eat my normal diet? I hate being sick. This was never supposed to happen to me."

Your Actions: As you actively listen to your patient, you might perceive that she sees being sick or ill as a failure on her part to live a healthy enough lifestyle. You might also perceive that, to her, "being well again" means being restored to her lifestyle without restrictions. Is that the meaning of illness or wellness? Does your patient grasp the fact that gallstones might or might not be due to her lifestyle? Is her thinking typical of most patients? What does it mean to "promote wellness" with this patient?

In our society, the idea of wellness covers a wide spectrum. Getting plenty of exercise, eating healthy foods, avoiding unhealthy activities, and perhaps taking dietary supplements may mean wellness to some people. To others, the quality of exercise is stressed above all else: 30 minutes of cardiovascular exercise and 30 minutes of weight training, followed by 15 minutes of floor exercise to cool down. Still others focus more on types of food and intake, with only a nod to exercise: Eat raw fruits and whole grains in the morning, lean protein and raw vegetables at lunch, and cooked vegetables with lean protein and whole grains for dinner, with snacks of nuts and dried fruits.

So, what is wellness? Is it what you eat or do not eat? Is it dependent on exercise? Or is it more than all of these things?

Theories of Wellness and Illness

To some individuals, a person is well when he or she is without a diagnosed illness. However, does that mean that, if a person has a well-controlled condition that is ongoing, such as hypertension, that person cannot be considered well? As nurses, we may see people with critical illnesses every day and, as a result, lose our perspective. We may think that anyone who is not in an intensive care unit is not actually ill. What about people whose lifestyle has been less than perfect? What about those who are overweight, do not exercise, eat unhealthy foods, or smoke tobacco? Are they guaranteed to become ill? Do they even deserve illness because they have not been actively trying to prevent it?

The above questions are difficult to answer, because illness means different things to different people. However, one popular definition of illness states that illness causes changes in a person's functioning, whether it be physical,

mental, spiritual, or emotional functioning. Some people have illnesses that affect their ability to function even though they appear perfectly normal, making it difficult for others to sympathize. Other people are visibly ill, such as the person who is very thin, weak, and pale, and the person who becomes short of breath with the slightest exertion.

The Wellness-Illness Continuum

Most of us are not completely well or completely ill at any given time. Rather, we move up and down along a **continuum,** or scale, with exceptional wellness at the top and severe illness at the bottom. Figure 7-1 shows such a

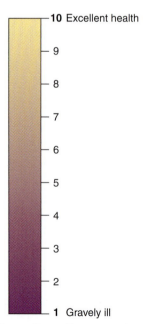

Figure 7-1 The wellness-illness continuum.

continuum. Even within a day, a person may move up or down on this continuum. For example, you may wake up with a sore throat and nasal congestion and you might consider yourself at 5 on the continuum. By afternoon, you are feeling better and may move up the scale to 7.

It is important to remember that physical health is not the only issue that is involved when discussing wellness and illness. A person may be well physically, but be depressed or have other mental conditions that would prevent him or her from being considered healthy. However, if a mental illness is being treated and managed well, the person moves closer to the exceptional wellness end of the scale.

Dunn's Theory of High-Level Wellness

In 1959, H. L. Dunn developed a theory about achieving high-level wellness. In his theory, he uses not only a continuum of health and wellness, referred to as the Health Axis, but also a vertical axis to represent the person's environment. In this theory, there are four quadrants to describe a person's condition based on the influences of wellness or illness and a favorable or unfavorable environment. Figure 7-2 shows the Health Grid developed by Dunn.

If a person with an ongoing health condition such as severe congestive heart failure is in a favorable environment with family, caregivers, needed medications, appropriate diet, and regular physician visits, on Dunn's grid this person would be identified as having "protected poor health." It is easy to see that a person with an illness such as tuberculosis who is homeless would be considered to have "poor health" on this grid.

Fitzpatrick's Rhythm Model

A nursing theory that deals with health and wellness is Dr. Joyce Fitzpatrick's rhythm model. One of the major concepts of Fitzpatrick's theory is that of wellness-illness.

Nursing is rooted in the promotion of wellness practices, the attentive treatment of those who are acutely or chronically ill or dying, and the restorative care of people during convalescence and rehabilitation. In this model, health is a dynamic state that results from the interaction of a person and his or her environment. A person's state of health can vary from wellness to illness, disease, or dysfunction, and it changes continuously throughout the person's life span.

Knowledge Connection
Where do you place yourself on the wellness-illness continuum today? Where would you have placed yourself yesterday? Where would you place yourself in Dunn's grid? What are the reasons for your choice?

Promoting Wellness

Concern regarding where our citizens fall on these types of continuums has led the U.S. government to establish an initiative for moving us all toward wellness. The current version of this initiative is known as *Healthy People 2010*.

Healthy People 2010

Through the office of Disease Prevention and Health Promotions, part of the Department of Health and Human Services, **Healthy People 2010** was established to improve prevention of disease and promotion of health in the United States. The stated goals of this program are to increase the quality and years of healthy life and to eliminate health disparities. In order to accomplish these goals, the initiative identified 28 *Focus Areas* for improvement. These focus areas are found in Box 7-1.

To track progress in meeting the Healthy People 2010 goals, 10 *Leading Health Indicators* have been identified.

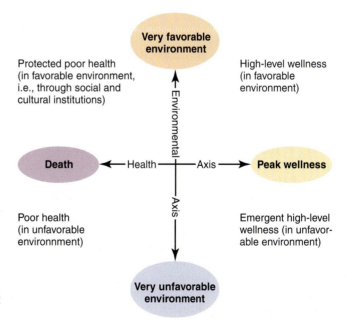

Figure 7-2 Dunn's Health Grid showing how a person's placement on the axes of health and environment influences outcomes.

Box 7-1

Focus Areas of Healthy People 2010

The 28 focus areas included in the Healthy People 2010 initiative are:

- Access to quality health services
- Arthritis, osteoporosis, and chronic back conditions
- Cancer
- Chronic kidney disease
- Diabetes
- Disability and secondary conditions
- Educational and community-based programs
- Environmental health
- Family planning
- Food safety
- Health communications
- Heart disease and stroke
- Human immunodeficiency virus (HIV)

- Immunization and infectious diseases
- Injury and violence prevention
- Maternal, infant, and child health
- Medical product safety
- Mental health and mental disorders
- Nutrition and overweight
- Occupational safety and health
- Oral health
- Physical activity and fitness
- Public health infrastructure
- Respiratory diseases
- Sexually transmitted diseases
- Substance abuse
- Tobacco use
- Vision and hearing

Resources for planning tools and details about programs regarding these 10 indicators are available at *www.healthypeople.gov* under "Resources for Action." These 10 indicators are:

1. Physical activity
2. Overweight or obesity
3. Tobacco use
4. Substance abuse
5. Responsible sexual behavior
6. Mental health
7. Injury and violence
8. Environmental quality
9. Immunization
10. Access to health care

These Leading Health Indicators are a reflection of the major public health concerns in the United States, and were chosen based on their ability to motivate people to take action. These indicators are used to illuminate individual behaviors, as well as the physical, social, and environmental factors that affect people in the United States.

Physical Activity

The importance of physical activity cannot be overemphasized in moving our nation toward wellness. Our society has become more and more sedentary over the past 150 years, especially as technology has advanced. Now we sit at a computer all day, e-mail information to an office next door, and print documents rather than walking to the copy machine. Television, movies, and video games keep us sitting when work is over. Exercise in our society often must be a conscious choice and an intentional effort.

Physical activity is associated with lower death rates for adults of any age, even when the person may engage in only moderate activity. When people start exercise programs, they reduce their risks of developing heart disease, diabetes, and colon cancer. Regular physical activity also increases muscle and bone strength, aids in weight control, enhances psychological well-being, and may even reduce the risk of developing depression.

Overweight or Obesity

Along with a sedentary lifestyle, our increased calorie intake has led to a nation of people who tend to be **overweight** (having an excess of body weight compared to set standards such as body mass index) and **obese** (having an abnormally high proportion of body fat). In Europe, Americans are sometimes referred to as "balloon people" due to our inflated size. Portion sizes have grown, making it difficult to stop eating once reasonable calorie amounts have been consumed at each meal. Most social events revolve around food, whether it is going to a ball game, a concert, the circus, or a movie, and these social events usually involve consuming unhealthy food. Busy Americans often do not take time to prepare meals and depend on "fast food" instead, which is often served in oversized portions and fried in oils. Excess weight, especially excess body fat, has been proven to contribute to a variety of illnesses and diseases, including heart disease, hypertension, diabetes, certain types of cancers, and osteoporosis.

Tobacco Use

While social and peer pressure and some local and state laws have helped decrease tobacco use, especially cigarettes, it is still a health concern. Smoking contributes to lung cancer and chronic obstructive pulmonary disease such as emphysema. Other types of tobacco, including smokeless tobacco, pipes, and cigars, are not without their own health consequences, as they can contribute to oral and lung cancers.

Smoking cessation aids are now available over the counter and can significantly increase a person's ability to quit smoking successfully. Patches, gum, and lozenges that release small amounts of nicotine are useful to ease withdrawal symptoms. Prescription medications, such as bupropion hydrochloride (Zyban), have also been helpful as an adjunct for smoking cessation by decreasing the desire to smoke.

It should be noted that nurses who smoke might have difficulty encouraging patients in cessation programs because they feel they are not good examples. We also need to remember that we serve as role models of behavior for people. If they see us smoke, the tendency is to think, "Well, if nurses smoke, it must not be too bad for you." In addition, nurses who smoke have been identified in the workplace as workers who take more breaks and structure patient care around taking breaks. They spend time washing their hands and brushing their teeth to remove the odor of smoke after a break, and coworkers who do not smoke can grow to resent this behavior. This resentment can make an already stressful workplace even more stressful for the smoker, which then increases his or her desire for more breaks, creating a vicious cycle.

Also, many hospitals no longer allow staff to smoke anywhere on the grounds or in hospital parking lots, making it that much more difficult for the smoker to get away for a smoke break. If you smoke, you may want to consider quitting while you are in school rather than to try to do so after you go to work.

Substance Abuse

While alcohol is socially acceptable and readily available, alcohol abuse is not without consequences. It can cause death, especially among teens and young adults, because it contributes to motor vehicle accidents, homicides, and suicides. In adults with lifetime patterns of abuse, it contributes to the development of diabetes, cancer, heart disease, and liver disease. Because it is a source of empty calories, it can add weight without providing nutrients. Alcohol abuse during pregnancy can cause fetal alcohol syndrome, which results in mental retardation and other health problems.

Use of drugs for purposes other than the reason they were prescribed, as well as the use of street drugs, is considered **drug abuse**. An accidental overdose of drugs can result in death. Abuse of drugs contributes to mental illnesses such as schizophrenia and paranoia. Damage to brain cells from drug use or abuse can leave people with the inability to support themselves, adding to the homeless population.

Nurses and physicians, as a group, are especially at risk for substance abuse. It is important to recognize the signs indicative of substance abuse not only in those around you, but in yourself as well. If you have a problem with drugs or alcohol, it is important for you to seek help, just like anyone else. Patient education about substance abuse is necessary to help patients identify the problem when it exists and to obtain appropriate treatment.

Responsible Sexual Behavior

The results of irresponsible sexual behavior are varied and dramatic, from a sexually transmitted disease that is easily treated with antibiotics to HIV, AIDS, and hepatitis B, all of which can cause death. In addition, unintended pregnancy brings about life-changing consequences.

As a nurse, you may provide information to patients with a diagnosis of sexually transmitted disease. People often trust nurses for correct information about sexual matters. Encouraging the use of condoms can help prevent sexually transmitted disease; however, condoms alone are not recommended as a reliable method of birth control, so other measures such as birth control pills should be encouraged.

Mental Health

Mental health is a state of successful performance of mental function, resulting in productive activities, fulfilling relationships with other people, and the ability to adapt to change and to cope with adversity. *Mental disorders* are health conditions that are characterized by alterations in thinking, mood, or behavior. *Mental illness* is the term that refers collectively to all diagnosable mental disorders.

The goal of Healthy People 2010 is to improve mental health and ensure access to appropriate quality mental health services. According to the World Health Organization (WHO), mental illnesses are on par with heart disease and cancer as a cause of disability. Mental disorders affect people across all aspects of life, regardless of age, gender, race or ethnicity, education level, or socioeconomic status.

It is important for you to recognize the impact of stress on your patients and to recognize their need for enhanced coping skills. *Coping skills* are positive adaptations that affect a person's ability to manage stressful events. To help patients who are struggling with mental illness, overwhelming stress, lack of coping skills, or addiction issues, encourage them to seek assistance from a qualified mental health professional. This can be a delicate subject due to the stigma that has been associated with mental disorders in the past, but you can help patients see the need for assistance in a kind and caring way. Hospitals have mental health staff readily available; however, a referral from the physician is usually needed. Ensure that patients know how to access mental health resources in their area.

Injury and Violence

Decreasing injuries from motor vehicle crashes and other accidents requires public education. Encourage the use of seatbelts when educating patients. Promote poison prevention measures when talking to parents of toddlers. Safety, first aid, and cardiopulmonary resuscitation (CPR) courses are available to the public. You may even be interested in becoming an instructor for these courses. Follow workplace safety requirements to protect yourself and your coworkers from on-the-job injuries.

Violence is prevalent in our society, and it often occurs during the commission of a crime. At other times violence may be due to the influence of alcohol and drugs, which impair judgment. In the emergency setting, a nurse may be the first person to encounter victims of domestic violence. It is important that nurses recognize the signs and symptoms of domestic violence and report it to the proper authorities, as required by law.

Environmental Quality

Americans are becoming more aware of environmental issues, including the quality of our air, water, and food production. In addition, we are more aware that exposure to chemical, biological, and physical agents can negatively affect our health. However, our concern must be focused worldwide, not just on the United States alone. Biological and chemical warfare is a very real threat anywhere in the world. In addition, illnesses that once would have affected perhaps just one or a few countries—for example, the bird flu—can now be transmitted quickly throughout the world via air travel and imported food products.

Immunization

The government mandates immunizations against a variety of childhood illnesses. In addition, optional vaccinations against adult-acquired viruses and other illnesses such as influenza, pneumonia, hepatitis, and human papillomavirus are also available. Children are required to have a total of 25 immunizations by the age of 6 to prevent:

• Diphtheria, polio, and pertussis (whooping cough)
• Tetanus and rotavirus
• Influenza and pneumonia
• Measles, mumps, rubella, and varicella (chickenpox)
• Meningitis and hepatitis A and B

These required immunizations are credited with obliterating most childhood illnesses. Some concern has arisen regarding the number of immunizations given to children at one time. For example, when there is a need to "catch up" on several missed immunizations, some individuals question whether multiple immunizations given at the same time will contribute to irreversible complications. A schedule for making up missed immunizations is available from the Centers for Disease Control and Prevention (CDC) and should be followed to prevent these complications.

Some parents are hesitant to have their children immunized due to the possibility of side effects or severe complications that have been attributed to the vaccinations. It is important to be nonjudgmental about their concerns. It is also important to help them clearly understand the benefits of the immunizations as well as the possible risks.

Access to Health Care

In the United States, the cost of health care insurance has spiraled out of control over the last 2 decades, making it impossible for some people to purchase. According to the Census Bureau, the revised estimate for the number of uninsured people in the United States in 2005 was 44.8 million, or 15.3% of the population. Because our health care system is insurance-driven, the lack of health insurance severely limits people's access to health care, which allows illness to go untreated. The cost of health care is so high that some people delay getting care in the hope that they will get better without treatment. By the time they do seek care, the illness may be very serious and require more resources to treat, therefore costing even more than it would have if the person had sought care earlier. In an effort to provide the needed health care for the very poor, the government instituted Medicaid, and for the health care needs of the elderly, Medicare.

In many situations, employers help pay for an employee's insurance. However, due to its high cost, employees often cannot even afford to pay for remaining family members. Insurance rates for smaller groups of people and for individual families exceed the rates for larger corporate groups. Because of this, contract workers and the self-employed often have great difficulty affording health insurance.

The number of uninsured people grows as people lose jobs and cannot afford individual insurance. Without insurance, when people become ill, they must seek health care where they will be accepted. Often they are required to pay before they can receive care. If they are unable to do so, they are referred to the few clinics and hospitals who will agree to treat them without payment up front.

The bottom line is that, without health insurance, an individual is unlikely to have access to quality health care, prenatal care, and preventative services. In addition to lack of insurance, some people are prevented from accessing care because of language barriers, or a lack of available health care professionals in their area.

Knowledge Connection
Which of the 10 health indicators do you see as most important? Why? What is the difference between being overweight and being obese?

Illness

In spite of efforts to promote wellness and decrease risky behaviors, people do become ill. Illness is not always due to the person's lack of effort to remain healthy. Some people do nothing to achieve a healthy lifestyle, engage in a number of risky behaviors, and are diagnosed with an illness, as expected. At other times, people work very hard at being healthy and are shocked when they develop a sudden severe illness. While cause and effect regarding lifestyle choices and illness have been proven to exist, sometimes illness occurs without previous risk factors. Therefore, it is important that you do not "blame the victim" when you care for patients who have been diagnosed with an illness or disease.

Just as it is difficult to know what caused an illness or why it happened to a particular person, it is also difficult to predict each person's response to illness. Some people seem to take even devastating diagnoses in stride, while others seem to panic over a diagnosis of a relatively minor, easily treated disorder.

Types of Illness

To some people, illness is defined as "not being able to do what I want to do." To others, illness could be defined as "any pain or discomfort because it means my body is not functioning normally." It is difficult to determine a single definition of illness because several types of illness exist and people perceive illness differently.

An **acute illness** strikes suddenly, and lasts for a limited time. An example of an acute illness would be food poisoning: you become very ill a few hours after ingesting contaminated food. You experience severe symptoms of nausea, vomiting, and diarrhea for 24 to 48 hours. Once your body rids itself of the offensive contaminants, you begin to feel better. Acute illness can also occur in situations in which hospitalization is required. For example, a patient is admitted with acute appendicitis and has an emergency *appendectomy,* or removal of the appendix. After surgery, the incision gradually heals and the patient eventually returns to normal activities.

A **chronic illness** is one that lasts for 6 months or longer and is characterized by intensifying or improving symptoms. Chronic illness may require treatment and medications or limiting a person's activities. An example of a chronic illness would be chronic obstructive pulmonary disease (COPD). People with COPD are often dependent on supplemental oxygen and have little energy reserve because of the effort required to breathe, thus limiting activities in which the person is able to participate.

Chronic illness is characterized by periods of either minimal symptoms or a complete absence of symptoms, called **remissions**, and periods of worsening symptoms, called **exacerbations**. Rheumatoid arthritis is an example of a chronic illness with periods of remission when joint pain lessens and mobility improves, and exacerbations when the opposite occurs.

Phases of Illness

Before a person develops symptoms of a specific illness, he or she may simply "not feel good," with generalized body aches and fatigue. This is referred to as the **prodromal phase** of illness.

As observable symptoms develop—for example, a sore throat and congestion, or a rash with a fever—the person enters the **symptomatic phase**. At this point, he or she makes a choice to either wait and see if the symptoms resolve, treat himself or herself with over-the-counter products or home remedies, or seek advice from friends and relatives.

Next comes the **seeking help phase**. The majority of people in our society seek help from a medical professional, such as a physician, physician assistant, or nurse practitioner. However, in some cultures, people may seek help from healers rather than physicians. Some seek out herbalists or other alternative practitioners. (See Chapter 11 for additional information on alternative medicine.)

Once a person has sought help, he or she must decide to follow the advice or recommended treatment, or to seek help elsewhere. In this **dependency phase**, a person relies on others for help in diagnosis and treatment. In many cases, the individual not only must depend on others for medical care, but may also be forced to rely on others to perform his or her work or family duties. Different people react in different ways to the dependent role. As the nurse, you are often the one whom patients must depend on during this phase of illness. Many patients adapt to this dependent role without difficulty, realizing it is a short-term situation; other patients react by becoming angry, fearful, or overly dependent, and still others may become manipulative.

The final phase is the **recovery phase**, when the person is slowly able to resume independence and regain his or her health. It should be noted that people with a chronic illness often remain in the dependency phase because complete recovery is not possible.

Knowledge Connection

Contrast acute and chronic illness. Contrast exacerbation and remission. List the five phases of illness.

Risk Factors for Illness

Researchers have identified **risk factors** for some illnesses. These are physiological, psychological, or genetic elements that contribute to the development of an illness or disease. Another type of risk factor is environmental elements, such as exposure to a chemical hazard that could lead to illness. Some risk factors can be modified or changed by alterations in lifestyle and nutrition. Other risk factors are non-modifiable, such as heredity, age, and gender. People who have risk factors for illnesses such as diabetes, heart disease, stroke, and cancer may be able to decrease their risk of developing the illness by modifying their diet and exercise routine, as well as managing their blood pressure and blood sugar. Table 7-1 lists modifiable risk factors for selected illnesses. An increasingly common modifiable risk factor for many illnesses is overwhelming stress and a lifestyle that lacks balance between work, play, and rest.

Cancer can have some familial tendencies, or be passed down in families, which is a non-modifiable risk factor. The American Cancer Society has identified seven warning signs of cancer; these are listed in Box 7-2. Knowledge of these warning signs can contribute to early detection and diagnosis.

Stress and Adaptation

According to Hans Selye, who developed the response-based model of stress, **stress** is identified as a nonspecific response of the body to any demand made on it. Any stress-inducing event is referred to as a *stressor,* and can include physical, emotional, pleasant, or unpleasant occurrences. How these stresses of daily life affect an individual depends largely upon the individual's ability to adapt. **Adaptation** is the ability to

Table 7-1 Modifiable Risk Factors for Selected Diseases

Risk Factor	Diseases
Obesity	Diabetes, heart disease, breast cancer, colon cancer
Diet high in trans-fatty acids, cholesterol, and triglycerides	Diabetes, stroke, heart disease
Hypertension	Stroke, heart disease, kidney disease
Smoking	Heart disease, bronchitis, COPD, stroke, lung cancer, and other types of cancer

Box 7-2

The Seven Warning Signs of Cancer

The first letters of each sign that a condition may be cancerous spell out the word CAUTION.
- **C** hange in bowel or bladder habits
- **A** sore that does not heal
- **U** nusual bleeding or discharge from any body orifice
- **T** hickening or a lump in the breast or elsewhere
- **I** ndigestion or difficulty in swallowing
- **O** bvious change in a wart or mole
- **N** agging cough or hoarseness

positively adjust to changes that occur in an individual's world. If one does not adapt to changes, the physiological and psychological responses can be harmful. Ongoing stress not only can result in illness and injury, but can lead to death if it is not relieved.

Anatomy and Physiology Connection

The Fight-or-Flight Response
When your brain perceives a threat to your well-being, it sends messages to the body to prepare to either *stay and fight* or *run away*. This innate protective response saved our ancestors from wild animals and other predators and is known as the **fight-or-flight response**. Your brain engages the sympathetic nervous system, which stimulates the endocrine glands to pump cortisol, adrenaline, and other hormones into the bloodstream, enabling you to hit harder, jump higher, see farther, and think or run faster. These

hormones cause the bronchial airways to dilate and the respiratory rate to rise, both helping to increase oxygen intake. The hormones also cause the heart rate to increase, blood vessels in the skin to constrict, and central blood vessels to dilate, in an effort to deliver more oxygen-rich blood to the brain, heart, and muscles needed for the fight-or-flight response. Glycogen is converted to glucose to provide additional fuel and energy. The pupils of the eyes dilate to allow better vision. The sense of hearing is heightened to detect warning sounds. Salivary glands decrease their secretions and peristalsis slows in the digestive tract in order to prevent the need for bowel elimination during this "emergency" or high-stress time. Arm and leg muscles tense in preparation for running or physical fighting. When the threat is removed, the parasympathetic nervous system dominates, and reverses these responses.

Selye's theory of stress and illness has probably been demonstrated at some time in your life, when you were in a situation of ongoing, unrelieved stress and then developed an illness. When we are stressed, our body responds with the fight-or-flight response described in the Anatomy and Physiology Connection. This is referred to as the *alarm phase.* If the stressor is removed in a relatively short period of time, our bodies return to normal. However, if the stressor continues in our life, and we do not find positive ways of relieving it, our bodies get stuck in that fight-or-flight response, producing high levels of cortisol and other stress hormones. The body works hard trying to resist the threats of stress and to keep working efficiently to prevent illness. Selye calls this the *resistance phase,* and it can continue for weeks, months, or years. Eventually, our bodies cannot keep up the pace of dealing with stressors and fighting off illness. This is the *exhaustion phase,* when the body's resources are depleted and we are most vulnerable to physical and psychological disease. Selye titled this the *general adaptation syndrome* (GAS) because it describes the body's attempts to adapt to the stressors we encounter.

Stress can be considered either negative or positive, but the body cannot tell the difference between the two. Negative stress has the potential to cause harm. Examples would be physical illness, disease, or death of a family member. Positive stress involves events that, while anticipated, may still be viewed as stressful. Examples would include an upcoming marriage, job change, or graduation.

People use different ways of coping to manage their stressors. The possible outcomes of stress and ways of coping are changing the stressor, adapting to the stressor by changing thoughts and behaviors related to it, or avoiding the stressor. If the stressor—or in many cases a variety of stressors—remains in place without the person adapting to it, the stressor eventually causes illness or even death.

When a person is dealing with several stressors at one time or a stressor that lasts for a long time, it is much more difficult for them to adapt. Your response to stressors depends on several factors:

- How do you view the stressor? Do you see it as something major or something that can be adapted to with increased time and energy?
- What is your current health status? Do you already have chronic illnesses such as diabetes or hypertension? Are you constantly in a state of exhaustion with few energy reserves?
- What are your support systems? Do you have friends and family who can help you with the details of life so you can use your energy to adapt to the stressor? Do you have people to listen to you when you need to talk about your stressors?
- What other factors are at play? Your age, life stage, and life experiences can influence your ability to adapt to your stressors.

The outcome of stress is that either you adapt to it or you develop a disease or illness. Our bodies use various feedback mechanisms to maintain *homeostasis,* or balance in the internal environment of the body. These are physiological responses and include GAS. The process of making changes, physical or psychological, in response to stress is adaptation.

The psychological response to stressors include feelings, thoughts, and behaviors. Common responses are fear and anxiety. Anxiety is a vague, uneasy feeling that is not centered on a specific source, and is emotional in nature. Fear is an identified danger or threat with a real or imagined source, and is cognitive in nature. One way we manage our fears and anxieties is by using *defense mechanisms,* which are unconscious reactions to decrease the stress. They help decrease tension caused by various stressors in our lives. Table 7-2 lists the types of defense mechanisms and examples of each.

Effects of Stress on Illness

When stress is continuous, it causes the sympathetic nervous system to go into "overdrive." Constricted blood vessels and increased heart rate can lead to hypertension and heart disease. Vasodilation in the brain may contribute to migraine headaches. Illness and hospitalization are also stressors that can worsen some conditions, such as diabetes. In fact, research has shown that simply being admitted to the hospital will increase most individual's blood glucose levels even though they do not have diabetes. Stress can also cause exacerbations in some chronic disorders, such as systemic lupus erythematosus, multiple sclerosis, fibromyalgia, arthritis, and asthma.

When a family member has a major illness, it inflicts stress on the healthy members of the family because of concerns over the cost of health care, as well as the care the patient is receiving, and fear of the ultimate outcome. It is vital that nurses be aware of all the stressors that both the patient and family members are facing.

Recognizing the Symptoms of Stress

How many times have you heard a coworker or fellow student say, "I am so stressed out"? It is a common phrase and it sounds as if we all know when we are stressed. However, that is not always the case. Some people do not realize that they are experiencing severe stress overload until they are very ill or have caused damage to relationships. Box 7-3 lists some symptoms of stress.

Stress Management

Coping strategies, the actions people utilize to combat stress, vary from person to person. It is important to note that both positive and negative coping strategies exist. Negative strategies cause harm to yourself or others—for example, drinking too much or kicking the cat. Positive strategies include those that are good for body, mind, and spirit. Examples of positive coping strategies for the body include:

- Eating regular meals with lower levels of fat and sugar
- Exercising regularly
- Sleeping an adequate number of hours every night
- Using deep breathing exercises to relax and relieve stress
- Listening to your body and giving it what it needs, such as extra rest when you are ill

Examples of positive coping strategies for the mind and spirit include:

- Saying "no" to people when necessary, preventing yourself from taking on more responsibility than you can handle.
- Taking time out to relax and have fun with family and friends.
- Laughing
- Reducing excesses in your life; getting rid of clutter both in activities and in possessions.
- Talking about your feelings with people you trust.
- Asking for help when you need it.
- Participating in worship services or spending time with nature.
- Taking a "mental vacation" from time to time. Close your eyes and picture a beautiful, relaxing place. Imagine yourself there. What are you doing? What do you see? What do you hear? What do you smell?
- Keeping a journal, either of daily life or of stressful events and your response to them.

Stress is a fact in our daily lives. It is not going to go away. We get to choose how we will respond to it. If you choose to use positive coping strategies, your life will not be ruled by stress.

Table 7-2   Defense Mechanisms

Mechanism	Description	Examples	Overuse Can Lead To
Denial	Unconscious refusal to see reality. Usually the first defense learned and used. Is not consciously lying.	The alcoholic states, "I can quit any time I want to."	Repression, dissociative disorders.
Repression (Stuffing)	An unconscious "burying" or "forgetting" mechanism. Excludes or withholds from our consciousness events or situations that are unbearable. A step deeper than "denial."	"Forgetting" a loved one's birthday after a fight.	
Dissociation	Painful events or situations are separated or dissociated from the conscious mind. Patients will often say, "I had an out-of-body experience" or "it happened to someone else, but it was as though it happened to me."	Patient who had been sexually abused as a child describes the situation as if it happened to a friend or a sibling. Police visit parent to inform parent of death of child in car accident. Parent tells police, "That's impossible. My child is upstairs asleep. You must have the wrong house."	One of the dissociative disorders, such as multiple personality disorder.
Rationalization	Use of a logical-sounding excuse to cover up true thoughts and feelings. The most frequently used defense mechanism.	"I did not make a medication error; I followed the physician's order." "I failed the test because the teacher wrote bad questions."	Self-deception.
Compensation	Making up for something we perceive as an inadequacy by developing some other desirable trait.	The small boy who wants to be a basketball center instead becomes an honor roll student. The physically unattractive person who wants to model instead becomes a famous designer.	
Reaction formation (Overcompensation)	Similar to compensation, except the person usually develops the *exact opposite* trait.	The small boy who wants to be a basketball center instead becomes an honor roll student. The physically unattractive person who wants to model speaks out for eliminating beauty pageants.	Failure to resolve internal conflicts.
Regression	Emotionally returning to an earlier time in life when there was far less stress. Commonly seen in patients while hospitalized. (Note: Everyone does not go back to the same developmental age. This is highly individualized.)	Children who are toilet trained beginning to wet themselves. Adults may start crying and have a "temper tantrum."	May interfere with perception of reality. May interfere with progression and development of personality.

	Definition	Example	Effect
Sublimation	Unacceptable traits or characteristics are diverted into acceptable traits or characteristics.	Burglar teaches home safety classes. Person who is potentially physically abusive becomes professional sports figure. People who choose to not have children run a day-care center.	The "socially accepted" behavior might actually reinforce the negative tendencies, and the person may still show signs of the undesirable behavior or trait.
Projection (Scapegoating)	Blaming others. A mental or verbal "finger-pointing" at another for the problem.	"I didn't get the promotion because you don't like me." "I'm overweight because you make me nervous."	Finds faults in everything and everyone. Fails to learn to take personal responsibility. May develop into delusional tendencies.
Displacement (Transference)	Transferring anger and hostility to another person or object that is perceived to be less powerful: the "kick-the-dog syndrome."	Parent loses job without notice; goes home and verbally abuses spouse, who unjustly punishes child, who hits the dog.	Loss of friends and relationships. Confusion in communication.
Restitution (Undoing)	Makes amends for a behavior one thinks is unacceptable. Makes an attempt at reducing guilt.	Giving a treat to a child who is being punished for a wrongdoing. The person who sees someone lose a wallet with a large amount of cash does not return the wallet but puts extra money in the collection plate at the next church service.	May send double messages. Relieves the "doer" of the responsibility of being honest in the situation.
Isolation	Emotion that is separated from the original feeling.	"I wasn't really angry; just a little upset."	Avoids dealing with true feeling; can increase stress.
Conversion reaction	Anxiety is channeled into physical symptoms. (Note: Often, the symptoms disappear soon after the threat is over.)	Nausea develops the night before a major exam, causing the person to miss the exam. Nausea may disappear soon after the scheduled test is finished.	Anxiety not dealt with can lead to actual physical disorders such as gastric ulcers and possibly some cancers.
Avoidance	Unconsciously staying away from events or situations that might open feelings of aggression or anxiety.	"I can't go to the class reunion tonight. I'm just so tired. I have to sleep."	

Box 7-3

Symptoms of Stress

When you are experiencing stress, you may have a few or a number of these symptoms:

- Frequent feelings of anger, helplessness, or hopelessness
- Headaches, back pain, and insomnia
- Hiding real feelings from family and friends
- Hurting loved ones with words or physical harm
- Constant worry, memory loss, and trouble thinking clearly
- Panic attacks with rapid heart rate, shortness of breath, and dizziness
- Isolation from friends and family
- Inability to make decisions
- Overuse of alcohol, drugs, or food to feel better

help patients manage the stress of hospitalization, encourage them to:

- Ask questions if they are unsure about a treatment, medication, or diagnosis. Be sure to explain what to expect before performing any procedure or treatment.
- Discuss their feelings with you or another health care professional if they are distressed about their diagnosis or care. Listen to the patient's concerns and provide reassurance when it is appropriate to do so.
- Ask for assistance if they are unable to sleep. Provide a back massage, warm drink, or other comfort measures to help the patient relax.
- Laugh at a funny story or movie. Use humor therapy when appropriate. Laughter increases endorphins and decreases residual effects of the fight-or-flight response.

Patient Teaching Connection

Patient Teaching to Decrease Stress

Hospitalization is a huge stressor. Your patients may need assistance from you to help cope with the experience. To

Knowledge Connection

Describe effects of the fight-or-flight response on the body. Which disease is listed as a result of all risk factors? How does stress affect a person who is hospitalized?

 Post Conference

At post conference, you reported on your clinical experiences. Once you were able to calm your patient and understand her concerns, you began to forge a strong nurse-patient relationship. You were able to explain to her what happens in gallbladder disease. You complemented her on her healthy lifestyle and established rapport. You put her mind at ease about what would happen after she recovered from her surgery, and cared for her postoperatively. You explained her activity orders for discharge: she should not lift anything over 5 pounds in weight for 2 weeks, and then she could return to her usual activities. You explored her feelings about wellness and illness, explaining the continuum concept, and helped relieve her anxiety both before and after surgery.

KEY POINTS

- The goals of Healthy People 2010 are to increase the quality and years of healthy life and to eliminate health disparities.

- Illness results for a variety of reasons and is not always the result of a poor lifestyle or taking risks.

- Illness can be acute or chronic and can mean different things to different people.

- The five phases of illness are the prodromal, symptomatic, seeking help, dependency, and recovery phases.

- Illness risk factors are modifiable or non-modifiable. Modifiable factors include exercise, diet, and lifestyle choices. Non-modifiable risk factors include heredity, age, and gender.

- Stress can be negative or positive, but the body cannot tell the difference and reacts in the same way to both.

- Stress causes a physiological reaction in the body called the fight-or-flight response.

- Frequent or unrelieved stress can lead to increased risk for illnesses.

- Positive strategies for coping with ongoing stress include limiting your obligations and responsibilities, spending time with people you enjoy, laughing, talking about your feelings, and asking for help when you need it.

REVIEW QUESTIONS

Select the answer that is most appropriate for each of the following questions. Some questions may have more than one correct answer. Check all that apply.

1. Acute diseases would include which of the following?

    a. Influenza

    b. Measles

    c. Hypertension

    d. Bacterial pneumonia

2. An individual has been to his physician for complaints of back pain and was informed that he has a herniated vertebral disk. He must now decide whether he wants to see a chiropractor for treatment, obtain a second opinion, or follow the instructions of the physician. This individual is in which of the phases of illness?

    a. Prodromal phase

    b. Dependency phase

    c. Seeking help phase

    d. Recovery phase

3. Which of the following could be classified as stressors?

    a. Getting married

    b. Receiving a promotion at work

    c. Losing a loved one

    d. Having a much-wanted baby

TRUE-OR-FALSE QUESTIONS

4. All risk factors for illness are outside of our control.

5. Five of the top 10 Leading Health Indicators of Healthy People 2010 are physical activity, tobacco use, amount of water drunk, whether one has ever been hospitalized, and whether or not one had all the normal childhood diseases.

6. A person is either well or ill at any given point in his or her life.

7. Illness means different things to different people.

8. One of the goals of Healthy People 2010 is to determine which ethnic group in the United States is the healthiest.

CRITICAL THINKING EXERCISES

9. Compare the physiological changes that may occur in each of the two following situations. Are they the same? If not, how are they different?

    • Situation #1: During the night you are home alone. You hear the breaking of glass at the patio entrance door and fear it is an intruder. Your body initiates the fight-or-flight response.

    • Situation #2: The physician has just told your patient some devastating news: she has advanced cervical cancer.

ADDITIONAL RESOURCES

For additional Resources, Questions, and Activities, please see:

Student Resource Disk

DavisPlus **http://davisplus.fadavis.com**

Student Study Guide

REFERENCES

Bandura A. Human agency in social cognitive theory. *Am Psychol.* 1989;44:1175-1188.

Centers for Disease Control and Prevention, U.S. Department of Health and Human Services. Immunization Schedules. Available at: http://www.cdc.gov/vaccines/recs/schedules. Accessed April 4, 2008.

Edelman CL, Mandle CL. *Health Promotion Throughout the Life Span.* 6th ed. St. Louis: Elsevier Mosby; 2006.

Office of Disease Prevention and Health Promotion, U.S. Department of Health and Human Services. *Healthy People 2010.* Available at: http://www.healthypeople.gov. Accessed May 3, 2008.

McEwen N, Willis EM. *Theoretical Basis for Nursing.* 2nd ed. Philadelphia: Lippincott Williams & Wilkins; 2007.

Reicherter E, Greene R. Wellness and health promotion: educational applications for older adults with the community. *Top Geriatr Rehabil.* 2005;21:295-303.

Scanlon V, Sanders T. *Essentials of Anatomy and Physiology.* Philadelphia: FA Davis; 2007.

Selye H. The stress concept: past, present and future. In: Cooper CL, ed. *Stress Research: Issues for the Eighties.* New York: Wiley; 1983:1-20.

Venes D, ed. *Taber's Cyclopedic Medical Dictionary.* 21st ed. Philadelphia: FA Davis; 2009.

Wilkinson JM, Van Leuven K. *Fundamentals of Nursing: Theory, Concepts & Applications.* Philadelphia: FA Davis; 2007.

Williams LS, Hopper PD. *Understanding Medical-Surgical Nursing.* 3rd ed. Philadelphia: FA Davis; 2007.

Ethnic, Cultural, and Spiritual Aspects of Care

Key Terms

Cultural awareness

Cultural competence

Cultural diversity

Cultural sensitivity

Culture

Discrimination

Ethnicity

Prejudice

Religion

Spiritual care

Spiritual distress

Spirituality

Stereotyping

Transcultural nursing

Objectives

1. Define key terms associated with cultural and spiritual nursing.
2. Explain why it is important to be aware of cultural differences.
3. Compare cultural awareness to cultural sensitivity.
4. Describe some of the ways in which cultural differences can affect nursing care.
5. Discuss at least five barriers to health care and how they prevent or lead to inappropriate health care.
6. Contrast the major religions and how they can affect health care of the patient.
7. Identify nursing interventions that you can employ to meet the spiritual needs of your patients.

🌐 Clinical Connection

Your Assignment: You are a female student nurse assigned to care for a male patient who is Muslim. He is recovering from surgery for prostate cancer and has a suprapubic incision. He is from Iran and has some difficulty speaking English. You know very little about the Muslim faith. You have been told that his wife is always at the bedside and she seems very nice. One nurse tells you that she cared for the patient yesterday and he has "something weird on a string around his neck."

Your Actions: It is important for you to familiarize yourself with Muslim beliefs as they affect health care. You have to determine if you, as a female, can be expected to care for a male patient of this faith. You also have to determine how best to meet his spiritual and cultural needs while you care for him. And maybe it would be good to find out about the item around his neck, too.

We are all different, and different in numerous ways. We may be different in the way we believe, think, speak, act, or live, but we are all individuals and deserve to be treated with respect and dignity, no matter what our ancestry, beliefs, or way of life. As a nurse, you will find it not only beneficial, but necessary, to broaden your awareness of the differences that may be found in others. This chapter discusses nursing care issues relating to the cultural and spiritual differences of the most common diverse populations.

Ethnicity and Culture

Ethnicity is the categorization of a group of people by a distinctive trait, such as the line of genealogy or ancestry, race, or nationality. **Culture** might be defined as the way of life that distinguishes a particular group of people from other groups. It is the whole of the learned behaviors of individuals within a specific group. It includes beliefs; values; symbols; art; music; morals; laws; customs; experiences; attitudes; religions; roles; concepts of space, time and the universe; belongings; communications; races; and ethnicities of an individual or group. Additional aspects included in the definition of culture are traditions, holidays, and specific celebrations and practices. These are addressed in the discussion of beliefs, religions, and spirituality later in this chapter.

Ethnicity and Culture in America

International migration to the United States has dramatically increased over the last 2 decades; this influx has contributed to the country's population explosion and heightened diversity. The Census Bureau report of 2000 indicated that minority groups, including Hispanics, African Americans, Asian Americans, and other people of color, comprised 25% of the population of the United States—and trends continue to show a steady increase in diversity (Fig. 8-1).

The emergence of these various cultural populations, with their many different beliefs and practices, continues to have an impact on the care that nurses provide. The Joint

Figure 8-1 Nurses commonly care for patients of different cultures than their own.

Commission, the primary evaluation and accreditation agency for health care facilities, has established that all patients have the right to receive medical care that is considerate of their culture, religion, and spiritual being. In August 2008, The Joint Commission began a project to develop proposed accreditation requirements for hospitals to advance effective communication, cultural competence, and patient-centered care, improving the safety and quality of care for all patients. The project, known as *Hospitals, Language, and Culture: A Snapshot of the Nation,* has helped to draw national attention to cultural competence and its effect on patient-centered care. Implementation of the proposed accreditation requirements for hospitals will be expected sometime after January 2011. You may read more about the project on the government's website at www.jointcommission.org/PatientSafety/HLC.

Therefore, as America becomes more diverse, nurses and other health care professionals will need to become culturally competent caregivers by increasing their knowledge of the various religious and spiritual beliefs held by people of different cultures within the country. **Cultural competence** requires that the nurse make a commitment to consider the cultural background of the patient and to provide appropriate care specific to the individual.

Transcultural Nursing and Cultural Competence

Transcultural nursing is care that crosses cultural boundaries or combines the elements of more than one culture. As America has grown in cultural diversity, the issues of transcultural nursing have increased in importance. Today, health care providers are being mandated to provide transcultural care by professional and governmental agencies. However, before the nurse can provide care that addresses the culture of the patient, there are several aspects of transculturalism that must be understood, including cultural diversity and cultural awareness.

Cultural Diversity

Cultural diversity is defined as the differences between groups of people in a certain geographical area, such as a city, state, or country; a specific place, such as a church or factory; or a conceptual community, such as the medical community. It is a way of identifying the group through the differences found between groups of people. Factors that determine the cultural diversity of a group might include the different ethnic groups, races, languages spoken, and religions within the larger group. Anything that is specific to the group that distinguishes the group from all other groups of people defines the culture of the group.

An example of cultural diversity found in a hospital would be the different ethnic groups represented among the hospital's employees, as a hospital might employee American, Mexican, Iranian, and Chinese doctors and nurses. Within each of these ethnic groups, a number of races may be represented, including Caucasian, Black, and Asian (Fig. 8-2). This group of doctors and nurses would speak English as well as their native languages.

Cultural Awareness

Transcultural nursing addresses:

• Cultural differences among patients
• Cultural differences among health care providers
• Culture of the individual nurse

The knowledge of various cultural beliefs and values is known as **cultural awareness**. Patients are different. Their beliefs are different. Their responses to illness and wellness are different depending on their cultural backgrounds—and even patients from the same cultural group may have differences in their health care beliefs and practices. Being culturally aware requires that you be culturally sensitive. **Cultural sensitivity** means that you provide care to the patient and

Figure 8-2 Diversity of ethnic backgrounds and cultures is common within the nursing profession.

show respect for and incorporate the patient's specific cultural beliefs and values into your nursing care. When patients feel that you are being culturally insensitive by ignoring their beliefs and values, they may delay or reject needed health care services.

Cultural Competence

Culturally competent care occurs when the nurse provides care to the whole patient, incorporating within that care the cultural context of the patient's beliefs and values. The nurse does not have to have expert knowledge of every culture or cultural group to be culturally competent. However, the culturally competent nurse chooses to be aware of the cultural differences and to become familiar with aspects of the patient's culture that impact and influence the patient's health and care. The nurse strives to understand anything that might influence the patient's health, including the patient's:

• Perceptions
• Expectations
• Behavior
• Decision-making processes

The nurse will work at identifying those cultural factors that will empower the patient to reach his or her full health potential. The culturally competent nurse conveys caring to the patient by showing respect for his or her beliefs and ideas and not assuming that the nurse knows what the patient is thinking or feeling. Providing care that is culturally competent will build trust between the nurse and the patient and promote cooperation.

Knowledge Connection

What does The Joint Commission say about patients from various cultures, religions, and spiritualities? List some of the factors or differences that might indicate cultural diversity. Describe the difference between cultural awareness and cultural sensitivity.

Real-World Connection

Meeting Rachael's Spiritual Needs

Rachael was an African American patient with terminal cancer in the small community hospital where she had worked as a nursing assistant for many years. The nurse caring for Rachael had carefully planned her delivery of care to include all hygiene, treatments, and medications that were ordered. Shortly after she began her shift, she headed to Rachael's room to perform her initial assessment and begin the delivery of her planned care. As she was completing her initial assessment, there was a knock on the door. Several family members and others had arrived and asked to see the patient. The nurse explained that she was busy giving nursing care, and asked if they could come back in about an hour. One of the family members took the nurse aside and explained that these were members from Rachael's small country church who believed that the laying on of hands and anointing of Rachael's body with oil could possibly cure her cancer. The ritual would last approximately an hour to an hour and a half. Even though it would interrupt the schedule of care that she had planned for the patient, the nurse knew that Rachael was a woman of strong faith and religious beliefs. Feeling that Rachael's spiritual needs were just as important as—maybe more important than—her physical needs, she told the family and church friends to take all the time they needed and to call her if they needed any assistance. The ritual took about 90 minutes, and the nurse had to re-prioritize her planned schedule, but she knew that she had done the right thing by allowing Rachael's spiritual needs to be met.

How Culture Affects Health Care

Many aspects of culture impact a patient's health, as seen in Tables 8-1, 8-2, and 8-3. Some cultural beliefs that affect health care include beliefs about food. For instance, patients who practice Hinduism may have difficulty following a protein-rich diet because Hinduism forbids the eating of beef and pork. The Jewish patient may find compliance with a high-protein diet a little easier than the Hindu patient; while pork is still prohibited in a Jewish diet, beef is not. Diet restrictions can even impact the medications a patient may take; for example, a Hindu patient may refuse to take medication that is packaged in a capsule because the capsule might be made from substances derived from beef or pork.

It is also important to be aware of the different beliefs about illness and wellness that may impact the patient's health and prognosis. Several cultures believe that health is the balance of the internal and external environments of the individual, incorporating the whole of the

Table 8-1   Beliefs About Illness

Principles of Beliefs	Basic Tenets of the Beliefs	Examples
Scientifically Based Beliefs, Biomedical		
Based on scientific research leading to best practices	If it can be proven scientifically, then it is accepted as truth and law. If it cannot be proven scientifically by research, it is an unfounded belief and myth.	Brushing teeth prevents tooth decay. Handwashing prevents the spread of disease. Immunization prevents disease.
Naturalistically or Holistically Based Beliefs		
A healthy state is one of balance and harmony. Examples include beliefs in yin and yang, or "hot" and "cold."	Yin and yang is an Asian belief that is upheld by many Asian Americans. The balance between yin and yang is what maintains and restores health. Yin and yang are compared to the sympathetic and parasympathetic nervous systems and the way they maintain balance in the body. Balance is maintained between hot and cold in order to maintain health. Some Hispanics and Asians believe that certain conditions are cold if they are manifested by vasoconstriction and decreased metabolism. Hot conditions or diseases are manifested by a high metabolic rate and vasodilation. The goal of treatment is to restore balance.	Cold diseases or states: menstrual cramps, rhinitis, colic. Hot diseases or states: hypertension, diabetes mellitus, pregnancy.

Table 8-1   Beliefs About Illness (continued)

Principles of Beliefs	Basic Tenets of the Beliefs	Examples
Religiously Based Beliefs		
Called *magico-religious*, the principle of these beliefs is that disease is caused by supernatural forces and health can be restored by supernatural forces. An example is voodoo.	Although many religions believe in prayer and the laying on of hands for healing, magico-religious beliefs indicate there is an added realm, the realm of magic. Magic can heal the illness as well as be the cause of illness; for example, those who believe in voodoo view the lion as a spiritual symbol of strength (Fig. 8-3). Parts of Africa and the Caribbean are known to practice voodoo. Others who practice magico-religion believe that illness is caused by some sinful act or by an actual demon spirit who is working against the individual. These patients may also believe that God is punishing them for sinful behaviors or lack of faith.	Depression is thought by some to be the result of sins. There is belief in the "evil eye," which is a term that means a look or an eye that can cast spells on individuals. Amulets, talismans, and rites are used to chase away bad spirits. Many herbs are used to heal.
Folk Healing		
Beliefs in practitioners of specific alternative therapies.	There are practitioners who promote the treatment and healing of disease who are not licensed as physicians or nurses or recognized by any certifying organization of higher learning. Many people seek assistance from herbalists, spiritualists, naturalists, and more. Other alternative practitioners provide therapeutic touch, iridology, naturopathic medicine, and reflexology.	The patient seeks a reflexologist, who performs massage of the sole of the foot to relieve the pain of a migraine headache.

Table 8-2   Ethnic Cultural Beliefs

Culture	Beliefs Affecting Health or Health Care	Nursing Care
African American	**Health** May feel mistrustful of others related to history of mistreatment. Often refuse advance directives and do-not-resuscitate status. May believe that healing is spiritual or religious in nature. May practice use of herbs. May believe in casting of spells. May have spiritual leader at bedside daily. May ask for laying on of hands. **Diet** Typically eat high-fat diet. **Domestic** Families are matriarchal. Numerous family members are apt to be present at the bedside.	Be accepting and respectful of beliefs. Document all refusals and discussions regarding refusals. Check to whom you should speak; the patient may desire that you speak to the oldest woman in the family (the matriarch) regarding the patient's health. Obtain written permission to provide medical details to her. Provide extra seating for visitors as needed. Provide time and privacy for rituals. Deliver nursing care around rituals whenever possible.

(table continues on page 152)

Table 8-2 **Ethnic Cultural Beliefs** (continued)

Culture	Beliefs Affecting Health or Health Care	Nursing Care
Asian Americans	**Health** Buddhists believe in karma of good and bad deeds; that illness and disease are results of karma; that illness has purpose (there are no accidents). Birth control is acceptable. Life support is not appropriate if there is dementia. **Diet** Buddhists are primarily vegetarian. Avoid intoxicating substances. May avoid intake of milk, cheese, and honey because they come from animals and insects. Forbidden items include coffee, alcohol, and tobacco. May not follow medically restrictive diets; believe it is sinful to waste food or refuse to eat what is offered to eat by others. **Domestic** Spiritual well-being requires a compassionate mind and willingness to suffer illness and death. Thus, they do not pray for healing. Rituals include prayers, beads, and images of Buddhist deities. Even though men and women are considered to be equal, mothers are thought to be more important than fathers. Buddhists believe in reincarnation. Abortion is forbidden. Killing of animals is forbidden. Wearing of fabrics from animals is forbidden, including fur, leather, and silk.	Discuss dietary restrictions and preferences to clarify individual beliefs, but realize patients may not follow dietary teaching. Provide a quiet atmosphere as much as is possible. Demonstrate respect and acceptance for beliefs and rituals. Consult with dietary service and inform unlicensed personnel caring for the patient to avoid providing the patient with forbidden items such as coffee.
Native American	**Health** Illness is considered to be a concern of the entire extended family; included in their concept of family is the extended family, blood, spirit, and tribe. May request the assistance of a shaman (medicine man with supernatural healing power). Many tribal healing rituals are considered sacred secrets and only shared with shamans from generation to generation. Believe in cleansing the ill with smoke of sacred plants. Some tribes have healing or purifying rituals that may be performed at the bedside. May include chanting, dancing, exorcisms, sand painting, or painting of body. May use amulets to ward off bad spirits or improve health. **Domestic** Either the patient or family members may make decisions regarding the patient's health. Extended family care for children, in health care setting may act as advocate for child and family.	Provide extra chairs for extended family if needed. Allow time and privacy for rituals as needed. Demonstrate respectful attitude toward beliefs and rituals.

Table 8-3 **Religious Cultural Beliefs**

Culture	Beliefs Affecting Health or Health Care	Nursing Care
Amish	**Health** Believe that the heart is the body's soul, therefore heart transplantation is forbidden. Ration end-of-life care to avoid wasting community resources; resources are more important for the living. Believe that health insurance is worldly and to purchase it would show a lack of faith. Do not believe in using hospital for birth or death; prefer these events to occur in the home; if hospitalization is necessary, patient must have consent of his or her church. Believe that, when a child is born with a disability, it is due to God's will. Generally do not fear death, but do fear disability. Surgery, dental work, anesthesia, blood transfusions, organ transplantation (except the heart) are acceptable when necessary.	Discuss health care decisions with both husband and wife; make joint decisions. If there is a potential for disability, inform patient or patient's family as soon as possible.
Catholic	**Health** The only accepted method of birth control is the rhythm method. Abortion and sterilization are forbidden. **Diet** No meat on special days, such as Fridays during Lent. Some desire to fast at designated times. **Domestic** A priest performs last rites before death. If no priest is available, anyone can perform baptism of the dying person.	Allow time for prayer if desired. Schedule nursing care accordingly. Respectfully ask the patient (or parents of a child) about desire for religious rituals, confession, communion, last rights, or infant baptism when patient is terminally ill or death is imminent. Show acceptance of beliefs and rituals. Contact the priest only with permission from the patient or parents.
Christian Science	**Health** Do not believe in traditional medical care. Provision of health care is considered to be specific Christian Science treatment or specific form of prayer. Believe healing is both physical and emotional. Believe that sickness is caused by lack of knowledge, fear, or sin and the individual will get well when the situation is corrected. Some believe that it is permissible to seek a physician's help with bone fractures and with childbirth. Physician is sought for delivery of baby. Whether contraception is permitted is up to the individual and family. **Diet** All drugs are prohibited as treatment of illness. Alcohol and tobacco are prohibited. Some do not believe in consuming coffee and tea.	Demonstrate active listening to encourage expression of feelings, as some may feel guilty about seeking medical care. Demonstrate accepting and respectful attitude toward beliefs and rituals.

(table continues on page 154)

Table 8-3 Religious Cultural Beliefs (continued)

Culture	Beliefs Affecting Health or Health Care	Nursing Care
Hindu	**Health** Believe in astrology. Require health care providers to be of the same gender as the patient. Believe that pain is due to the wrath of a higher power, so they must be stoic. Believe that all disease is caused by the supernatural when the three body humors (bile, phlegm, and wind) become unbalanced. Do not pray for recovery; take what is dealt to them. After hygiene measures (e.g., bath), they meditate and pray. Are known to self-medicate for certain problems. Use many medicinal recipes made of herbs. Women breastfeed newborns. Birth control may be used. Do not believe in abortion, circumcision, suicide, or euthanasia. **Diet** No beef, pork, or fowl allowed in diet. Do not use eating utensils in their native land, but can use them in the United States. Believe in fasting. Eat vegetarian diet only, but use a lot of spices. Yogurt and sweets are eaten at every meal. Avoid eating with left hand. **Domestic** Family relationships are important and generally close-knit. Dying patients may prefer to be alone with priest, family, or friends.	Exhibit respectful demeanor regarding their beliefs and rituals. Assign nurse of same gender as patient. Be careful to provide privacy and protect modesty during all nursing care. Avoid pressuring patient to take analgesics. Allow time and privacy for prayer and meditation at specified times during the day. Schedule nursing care around them. Face patient's bed north or east if possible.
Jehovah's Witness	**Health** Pray for healing. Blood transfusions are prohibited; can use only artificial blood expanders. Organ transplantation, sterilization, and abortion are prohibited. Birth control is permitted. Autopsy and cremation are permitted. **Diet** Alcohol, tobacco, and food with blood are prohibited.	Accept beliefs, be nonjudgmental. Verify with certainty that blood transfusions are prohibited by the patient. Talk to the patient to determine food preferences. Provide patient teaching related to nonblood plasma expanders.
Jewish	**Health** Good health is considered a prized possession. Belief in life is so strong that nothing may be done to hasten death, not even to relieve suffering. Rituals include sound vibration on prayer beads, prayer, meditation, and scripture reading. Do not put much faith in psychiatry. Perform ritual washing of hands. Circumcision and naming of male baby is performed on the 8th day. This is done by an official called the *mohel*. Believe the patient's feet should always be positioned toward the doorway exit from the room. Embalming is not performed and cremation is forbidden.	Demonstrate acceptance of beliefs and rituals. If movement of the patient may hasten death, avoid moving the patient at all. Try to plan for discharge before the Sabbath begins or right after it. Allow time for blessings and prayers before and after mealtimes. Do not schedule circumcision until the 8th day. Respect parents' right to not name baby until appropriate ritualistic time.

Table 8-3 **Religious Cultural Beliefs** (continued)

Culture	Beliefs Affecting Health or Health Care	Nursing Care
Jewish—cont'd	Believe that someone should be with the patient when death occurs and after death until burial has occurred. Believe body must be buried within 24 hours. Euthanasia, suicide, and assisted suicide are strictly forbidden. Product of conception is subhuman until birth of head or ¾ of body. **Diet** Perform blessings over food and again after eating it. Pork is forbidden. Dairy may not be consumed with meat. Even the utensils used to cook the two must be kept separate. Permitted to eat only meat from animals that are cloven-footed and cud chewing. Allowed to eat fish with scales and birds that are not predatory in nature. Immunization of children is not a popular belief. **Domestic** Most Jewish communities have an organization of volunteers who serve as the burial society, also known as the *chevra kaddisha,* who provide care for the deceased. The eyes of the deceased must be closed. The body will be cleansed and wrapped in a plain linen shroud, and may be laid on the floor. Abstinence and ritual cleansing required after menstruation. Husband will not touch his wife until after cleansing.	Position the bed so that the patient's feet are toward the doorway exit from the room. Communicate with dietary service regarding faith and dietary restrictions. Assess need for health screening. Provide patient teaching regarding health maintenance and risk reduction. Consult with the family regarding whether or not you may touch the body after death. Some families prohibit anyone other than the *chevra kaddisha* to touch the body after death.
Latter-day Saints (Mormons)	**Health** Sterilization is not permitted. Males may be circumcised for cleanliness and health, not religious reasons. Avoid cremation, unless it is required by law. Organ transplant is permitted. Abortion is prohibited. **Diet** Practice monthly fasts. Drug abuse is prohibited. Overeating, alcoholic beverages, smoking, coffee, cola, and tea are prohibited. **Domestic** Autopsy is okay if family agrees.	Exhibit nonjudgmental attitude toward beliefs. Remove undergarments only in emergency care situations. Provide time and privacy for prayers, meditation, and spiritual leader visits. Schedule nursing care accordingly.
Seventh-day Adventists	**Health** Pray for healing. Believe in healing associated with anointing with oil, which is done by the minister. Birth control is permitted. Abortions not to be done at will, but may be performed only when medically recommended. Death is just a form of sleeping. The soul and body remain until Christ comes again. **Diet** Alcohol, narcotics, stimulants, and caffeine are prohibited. Some are vegetarian.	Listen and offer presence to encourage verbalization of feelings. Be respectful of beliefs. Avoid trying to comfort the family of a deceased person by telling them that their loved one is in heaven, because they believe the soul and the body are still present and will remain until Christ comes again. If anointment has taken place, avoid bathing the patient for at least several hours.

Figure 8-3 During Carnival, a Haitian man's costume represents the lion's great spirit.

person, his or her physical, mental, social, and spiritual components. Some believe that the imbalance of these environments is the cause of illness. Chinese medicine is based on this belief.

The patient may believe that illness is caused by an imbalance between inanimate forces. Members of certain cultures, such as Hindus and some Hispanics, believe illness to be due to an imbalance between "hot" and "cold." As a result, a member of these cultures may only drink or eat hot foods when ill in an effort to restore balance and health. Due to fears that cold temperatures can cause illness, some Russians make efforts to stay warm at all times. For example, a Russian holding this belief might refuse to use an ice pack to treat an injured ankle. An Albanian woman who is ill may refuse to shampoo her hair due to fear of developing a headache or catching a cold.

Many traditional Chinese believe that illness is caused when there is an imbalance of the energy forms known as yin (cold) and yang (hot). In this belief system, the terms *hot and cold* do not refer to actual temperatures, but serve as descriptors of these energy forms, which exist not only in the individual's body, but also in foods, actions, and behaviors. India's practice of Ayurvedic medicine, which uses herbs, nutrition, cleansings, acupressure, massage, and yoga, is based on similar beliefs.

Knowledge Connection

Which foods are restricted in the Jewish culture? Hindu? Islamic? Asian? Which cultures eat yogurt or sweets with each meal? Which cultures avoid caffeine, including tea and coffee? Which culture always uses the right hand to eat?

Death and Dying

Although members of a specific culture normally develop and follow the beliefs of their culture, individual members develop their own beliefs, which may or may not be consistent with the beliefs or religion of their identified culture. Therefore, it is very important that the nurse provide care that is both culturally based and specific to the individual.

One of the common areas in which a patient's beliefs may differ with those of his or her culture is that of death and dying. There are many cultural aspects related to death and dying; it may be viewed by the culture as controlled by a supernatural force or purely as a scientifically based phenomenon. The individual, on the other hand, may hold the opposite view.

While members of some cultures prefer to die at home, others feel more comfortable in a controlled environment such as a hospital or hospice unit. Some cultures approve of life support; others do not permit mechanical means of prolonging life. Some feel that it is important to pray for the person's healing and recovery, while others believe that a person receives his or her just reward and that it is wrong to pray for a relief of his or her suffering. American members of the Hindu culture believe that remorse for the dead leads to more suffering of the soul and increases the soul's difficulty in leaving the earthy plane. Therefore, they prefer that those persons feeling the loss think only happy thoughts of the dead to facilitate their journey.

Some cultures, such as the Jewish culture, have specific persons who care for the body after death, and only those priests are to touch or prepare the body for burial. Others, such as the majority of Protestants in the United States, have no specific regulations or rites related to the care of the body, and the nurses will prepare the body for transfer to the funeral home, where the body will be prepared for burial.

Some cultures promote the presence of the family or the family and friends, while others prefer that the dying patient be given time alone for reflection and repentance. The more expressive cultures, such as the African American and the Hispanic American cultures, may exhibit loud moaning and chanting during the last hours of the patient's life as a means of providing comfort to the patient and family members. Other cultures, such as the Amish, may prefer a more quiet and peaceful environment. Some desire the continued presence of a spiritual leader, while others prefer the spiritual leader to come and anoint or pray for them and then leave.

While some patients may fear death, others may feel that there are things much worse than death. The Amish, for instance, fear disability more than death. Patient care should be directed toward data collection regarding the patient's beliefs and fears; misconceptions should be addressed during patient teaching. For further information regarding death and dying, as well as specific nursing interventions for dying patients, see Chapter 10.

Knowledge Connection

Describe the differences in beliefs regarding death and dying between Catholicism, Judaism, Hinduism, Christian Science, Buddhism, and Asian American religions.

Delivering Culturally Sensitive Care

When caring for patients from culturally diverse backgrounds, it is important to incorporate culturally sensitive care that conveys an attitude of caring. It is important to treat the patient with respect. It is not enough to go through the motions of providing care without communicating with the patient, even if the communication is difficult. Actively listening to the patient's expressions, permitting him or her time to express concerns, providing prompts when the words cannot be found, and providing presence all give the patient a sense of being cared for and respected.

Culturally sensitive caring requires awareness of the patient's actions as the nurse performs the care. The nonverbal response becomes most important when there is a language barrier that may prevent the patient from expressing himself or herself. If the care is cold or disrespectful, the patient may become resistive or have changes in his or her physical condition. If the patient becomes fearful or anxious, he or she may have changes in vital signs, such as an elevated heart rate and respiratory rate, an increase in blood pressure, or possibly development of a panic attack. If the patient feels he or she is being attacked or feels totally out of control of the situation, the patient may refuse care, become combative, or leave without the needed health care. In an effort to prevent these problems from arising:

- Allow the patient time to get his or her thoughts together.
- Use an interpreter if needed; if an interpreter is needed but one is not available, use prompts such as pictures or vocabulary cue cards.
- Be aware of the patient's nonverbal body language: It may alert the nurse to escalating tension and the need for a calm and quiet approach.
- Be aware that hand gestures mean different things in different cultures. For instance, a "thumbs-up" sign is a positive gesture for individuals of the dominant culture in the United States, but it has a vulgar connotation for individuals in Iran. The "okay" sign used in the U.S. culture means "zero" to individuals of Japanese culture.
- Understand that the patient may be able to speak English, but it may be broken or difficult to understand.

Barriers to Health Care

Several barriers to health care are specific to the individual. Some of the issues that may lead to lack of care or to the provision of inappropriate care include:

- Economics
- Education
- Geography
- Language
- Stereotyping
- Prejudice and discrimination
- Misunderstanding

Economics

For many, health care is obtained through individual insurance plans or private pay. Others obtain health care through public programs such as Medicaid, Medicare, and state programs. However, patients who have no private insurance and do not qualify for government assistance may not be able to afford health care and may wait until their condition or illness becomes life threatening before seeking care. *Note: There are currently discussions underway for a national health care plan as a possible additional option.*

You may find yourself caring for indigent and homeless patients. While others may look upon them as dirty, unpleasant, or even lazy, it is important that you see them as fellow humans deserving of dignity and respect.

Education

Research studies have shown that the higher a person's level of education, the more health care is obtained. The opposite is also true. Sometimes, even though families may be able to financially afford health care, individuals with less education tend to seek less medical help than those with higher educational levels. The level of education and literacy of a patient also plays a role in dictating how to provide patient teaching.

Geography

A patient's geographical area may have an impact on his or her ability to obtain health care. Many rural areas have limited access to health care providers and facilities, such as clinics or hospitals. Many low-income areas of larger cities have limited health care providers and facilities as well. Minority groups make up a greater percentage of low-income populations in the United States, leading to a decreased access to needed health care for those populations.

Language

A member of a minority group who speaks his or her native language but is not fluent in the common language of the population majority where he or she resides is at a distinct disadvantage. This language barrier can make it difficult for him or her to gain access to health care. For example, in the United States, minority group members for whom English is a second language sometimes find it difficult to determine where to go for various types of medical care. Even after the individual has successfully accessed the correct type of health care facility or provider, if the physician and the nurse do not speak the patient's native language, it can result in miscommunication, misunderstanding, increased anxiety, and frustration for both the patient and the caregiver. The caregiver may be unable to obtain information, or he or she may obtain incorrect information, leading to the provision of improper care and the planning of inappropriate treatment. Sometimes the patient will nod his or her head and indicate that he or she understands what you have said, when this is not true. Consequently, it is extremely important to use an interpreter when a language barrier exists.

The interpreter should be a trained interpreter and not be a family member or a small child due to the potential nature of the information that needs to be communicated. The possibility exists that the patient may be afraid to provide truthful information or be embarrassed to speak of the health care concern in the presence of the family member. With the increased emphasis on confidentiality and transcultural care, government mandates to provide trained interpreters are being put in place across the country. An example of a language barrier is noted in the story found in Box 8-1.

While understanding that language barriers make communication more difficult, it is important to keep in mind that a patient's limitations with the English language do not reflect limitations in the patient's intelligence.

Box 8-1

Breaking the Language Barrier: A Case Study

Read the case study about Anna and note how the simple act of taking time to ensure effective communication makes a difference in Anna's acquisition of medical care.

Anna, who spoke only Spanish, needed medical care and came to the free clinic looking for help. She came by herself with a small notebook that had a phone number in it. Upon arrival at the clinic, her distress was notable by her crying. The caregivers at the clinic could not speak Spanish and there was no interpreter in the clinic. Although the nurse practitioner did not speak Spanish, she was able to convey a sense of patience and caring, which helped to calm Anna. Anna indicated that the nurse should call the phone number written in her notebook, which she did, reaching an individual who spoke both English and Spanish. The interpreter would speak to Anna, then to the nurse, and then again to Anna. Although it took a while and required much work at communication, Anna was able to obtain the care that was needed for her diabetes. The interpreter offered to write a chart of Spanish words and the English equivalents for Anna to bring to future visits. Using this method, Anna came to the clinic several times over the next few months, each time with the chart and the name and phone number of the interpreter who would be available that day. She was able to obtain the medical care she needed to get her blood sugar levels under control again.

No matter which type of communication method you use, remember to deliver it in a respectful manner and avoid "talking down" to the patient.

It is useful to learn and use key words in the patient's language whenever possible. If an interpreter is not available, ask a family member or do research on the Internet and try to learn the terms for such words as "pain," "nausea," "hungry," "urinate," "medication," "feel good," "feel bad," "Can I help you?" and "Thank you." This demonstrates respect for the patient's language and helps to build rapport with the patient.

Stereotyping

Stereotyping may prevent individuals from seeking or obtaining the health care they need. Stereotyping is defined by many different disciplines, but essentially means that the person or group is looked at by another person or group through preconceived ideas and fixed impressions, or ideas that lead to prejudice and possibly mistreatment. The preconceived ideas may be based solely on the person's physical characteristics. Stereotyping occurs when the health care provider identifies the patient according to his or her understanding of the ethnic group or race to which the patient belongs and not as an individual with unique qualities and characteristics.

Most individuals are guilty of stereotyping at one time or another. Work to evaluate your own perceptions and beliefs regarding different ethnic groups or races. Remember that individuals within the same ethnic group or race may have different beliefs or behaviors. A culturally sensitive nurse must avoid categorizing patients simply by their looks, ethnic groups, race, language, or beliefs.

Prejudice and Discrimination

Prejudice is based on a preconceived idea about an individual solely based on physical appearance or a characteristic of his or her social or cultural group prior to determining or examining the facts related to the individual. **Prejudice** is a determination or judgment about a person or group based on irrational suspicion or hatred of a particular group, race, or religion. **Discrimination**, like prejudice, is a type of unfair treatment of one or more persons or groups. The discrimination is usually due to misguided and unfounded beliefs about the race, ethnicity, age, gender, or religion of the person or group. When a patient feels that he or she is being discriminated against, he or she will be reluctant to seek further assistance from the nurse, other health care provider, or profession.

Before a nurse can be successful in exhibiting sensitivity to those of different cultures, the nurse must examine and identify his or her own prejudices. Many individuals do not realize that they are prejudiced until they actively assess their feelings and beliefs. It is not necessary for a nurse to agree with differing beliefs, but it is paramount that the nurse be able to accept the patient's differences and deliver respectful nursing care in spite of the differences.

Even as you are trying to deliver culturally sensitive care, you may observe other staff members engaging in behaviors that demonstrate racial bias or cultural insensitivity. It is your responsibility to intervene in an appropriate manner on behalf of your patient's rights. That may require you to take the staff member aside and tactfully explain that the observed actions or words could be perceived by the patient as being insensitive and insulting, biased, or even discriminating. Relate the specific cultural beliefs held by the patient so the staff member will understand why his or her actions or words could have been offensive to the patient. If the staff member continues to persist in behaviors that are culturally insensitive, because you are your patient's advocate, it is your responsibility to report the problem to your supervisor so that resolution can be attained.

Misunderstanding

Misunderstanding is a barrier that is caused by a mistake of meaning or intention. When a misunderstanding arises between the patient and the health care provider, the patient may fear further encounters with the health care system. Fear of mistakes or retaliation may prevent the patient from seeking appropriate medication or diagnosis. Thus it is important that the nurse verifies the patient's understanding during all communication and patient teaching. You might ask the patient to tell you in his or her own words what he or she understood you to say. Avoid simply asking, "Do you understand?" Out of respect, many patients will automatically answer with a yes, whether they understood or not.

Knowledge Connection
Name at least five barriers to health care. Describe at least one way to overcome each of the five barriers. What are your own prejudices that you will have to overcome?

People and Places Connection
Respect the Beliefs of Others
While providing home health care to an individual of another culture, it is important to seek information regarding customs, expectations, acceptable behaviors, and courtesies that are unique to their culture. Providing nursing care in the patient's home is apt to involve even more adaptation in services than would be necessary in a hospital. You may have to remove your shoes before entering the home, abstain from wearing slacks during the home visits, avoid touching their prayer rug, or move the patient's bed so that it faces north. Some cultures may expect you to avoid prolonged eye contact, even while speaking directly to a person from that culture. Remember to show respect for the patient's beliefs, just as you would those of your own mother, father, or child.

Religion, Spirituality, and Creativity

Humans are more than the physical, and more than the sum of their parts. Humans are made up of body, mind, and spirit. The body is the physical, biological part of the person. As a nurse, you will learn about the physical body through the study of anatomy and physiology as well as the discussion of medical-surgical nursing. The mind is that part of the person that learns, thinks, communicates, makes decisions, and feels. The spirit is the essence of the person, the vital force or energy, distinct from the physical matter. Some people believe the soul and spirit to be interchangeable. In this textbook, the soul and the spirit are defined as being the essence of the person.

Religion, spirituality, and creativity are aspects of culture that provide the basis for the development of beliefs, values, morals, and ethical standards. **Religion** is the formal structured system of beliefs, values, rituals, and practices of a person or group, usually based on the teachings of a god or other spiritual leader. It is a belief in a higher power or supernatural being that the members of the religion revere and honor. A religion may incorporate a set of rituals that contribute to the worship of the higher power. For some people, religion may be based on a cause or principle that is sought after with fervent passion, rather than on the teachings of or belief in a higher power. Religions often have specific holidays or celebrate specific times as part of their belief systems. Table 8-4 presents a comparison of religious beliefs and practices.

Some cultures incorporate several different religions, while other cultures are known for one major religion. Some religions are monotheistic, believing in one god, while others are polytheistic, believing in multiple gods. Some cultures reject religion of any type, promoting the atheistic belief that there is no god. Regardless of the belief system, most believe there is a sense of humans that is beyond the tangible—a spirit, a sense of creativity, an essence of the supernatural that motivates, stimulates, and gives a sense of purpose and meaning to life. That intangibility is called spirituality.

Spirituality is the descriptive term that explains the spirit and the relationship of the spirit to the body, mind, and environment, including the patient's relationship to others. It is the spirituality of the person that gives meaning and purpose to life, making it the most important aspect of an individual. While spirituality usually incorporates religion, spirituality and religion may mean two very different things to a patient. For many, spirituality refers to the individual's expression (or living testimony) of his or her religious beliefs and represents the meaning of life, which includes a sense of involvement with the transcendent outside institutional boundaries. Others may believe that spirituality is completely separate from any formal religion and is simply the expression of who the individual is and how that individual relates to things of this world, such as nature.

Table 8-4 Major Religions and Their Tenets

Religion	Major Tenets
Buddhism	The main tenets of Buddhism are to avoid all evil and develop mankind through morality and purity; to awaken the mind to concentration and calmness for developing the ability to observe without reacting; and to do good by serving others. As one works to develop these states, one must have the right mental approach, mindfulness, concentration, intentions, and effort, as well as the right manner of speech, livelihood, and behaviors. The goal is to attain Nirvana, which is liberation and freedom from suffering. Revere Buddha as an example of a way of life (Fig. 8-4). Buddha teaches that birth, aging, illness, and death are suffering; that all suffering is caused by desiring pleasurable things and disliking or hating others; and that suffering will stop only when one is free of this aversion and attachment. Texts for beliefs: Hindu scriptures, holy writings of six Buddhist Councils, and the Tripitaka, which contains rules for monks, philosophical principles, and Buddha's sermons. Believe that happiness and good fortune are attainable by all, regardless of age, race, or background. Believe in meditation and reincarnation, meaning that humans go through many cycles of birth, life, death, and rebirth. Cycles of reincarnation will end when the individual is no longer attached to desire and the self.
Christianity Catholic	Believe in the Trinity (Father, Son, Holy Spirit), and that salvation comes through the blood of Jesus, the Son. The Pope and priests have eminence over the individual. Texts or sources for beliefs: Catechism of the Catholic Church and Roman Catholic Duoay Bible (includes Apocrypha). Sacraments include infant baptism, confirmation, penance, communion, anointing of the sick, holy orders, matrimony, and last rites. Any member of the faithful can be anointed with oil if they are in danger of loss of reason or of death from illness or old age. If the person has a new illness or becomes worse, he or she may receive the sacrament again.
Nondenomina-tionalism	The main tenets are to follow the commandments in the New Testament and to know that God is the creator and the holy heavenly Father of all. Text for beliefs: Holy Bible. The minister or preacher holds no eminent authority over the individual church members; only God and His word have authority. The major beliefs include searching the scriptures for truth, believing that the scriptures are the inspired word of God, repentance of sins, confession that Jesus is the Son of God, being baptized by immersion, and living a faithful life as a Christian.
Protestant	The authority of the individual is eminent over the authority of the priest or pastor. The mediator between God and man is Jesus. Texts for beliefs: Holy Bible and Books of Doctrine of specific religion, such as Lutheran, Baptist, and Methodist. The major beliefs include the belief in the authority of scripture, justification by faith, and the priesthood of the believer. Believe that Jesus' death on the cross redeems the individual and, along with God's grace, makes salvation possible.
Islam	The main tenets of Islam are the six articles of faith: Must follow Allah; texts to follow include Qur'an, Torah, Psalms (Qur'an is the only text that is unchanged by Christians or Jews); each person has two angels who are assigned to him or her; Allah used the prophets to deliver his messages and the last prophet was Muhammad (who was the greatest prophet of all time); life after death and hell; and Allah has all knowledge and control over everything. Texts for beliefs: Qur'an (Koran), Torah, Psalms. There are five pillars of faith: Allah and Muhammad are to be followed, no others; must pray in a position facing Mecca fives times daily; must help the poor and indigent; must fast during Ramadan; must travel to Mecca at least once in one's lifetime.

Table 8-4   **Major Religions and Their Tenets** (continued)

Religion	Major Tenets
Hinduism	The major tenet of the Hindu faith is the belief in Brahman, the underlying universal life force that encompasses and embodies existence. The goal of life is to be released from the karmic cycle of death and rebirth (reincarnation). Main gods are Shiva, Vishnu, and Shakti. Texts for beliefs: four Vedas. Believe in reincarnation, sacrifices, and use of spells against enemies. When ignorant of his or her Brahman, the self leads to the continuous karmic cycle of life, death, life, and death.
Judaism	The main tenet is that there is only one God who created the world and he is everywhere at the same time; is also all powerful and all knowing. Believe people have free will and are responsible for their own choices, decisions, and actions. Texts for beliefs: Torah and Old Testament. Believe that Old Testament law shows them how to worship and how they should treat others. The Torah has 613 commandments to follow, with the Ten Commandments serving as the most important teachings to institute in their lives. Believe when the Messiah arrives, he will not be Christ or any type of god, but will simply be a person from the lineage of King David, who will lead the world to unity and peace.

Research studies have found relationships between a patient's religious beliefs and practices, such as prayer, and his or her health. Findings indicate that expression of spirituality contributes to a healthier lifestyle; people who regularly participate in religious services tend to have a lower frequency of unhealthy behaviors and stronger support systems; and most research also finds improved emotional well-being in patients who claim to be religious. The health benefits of religion appear to be numerous: Religion can give meaning and purpose to the patient's life, empower the patient, and give the patient a sense of control. Religious beliefs tend to give hope and motivate people toward a better outcome.

Knowledge Connection

What are three health benefits generally found in patients with strong spiritual or religious beliefs or religious affiliation?

Spiritual Care

Spiritual care begins with an understanding of the differences between spirituality and religion, and an understanding of one's own spirituality, beliefs, and values. The nurse who provides spiritual care must understand his or her own purpose and goals related to providing spiritual care to the patient. The relationship of body, mind, and spirit is so closely interactive that an alteration in the body affects the mind and spirit, an alteration in the mind affects the body and spirit, and an alteration in the spirit affects the mind and body. An example of this interaction may be seen in the case study in Box 8-2.

Spiritual care addresses the possible effects of illness on the patient's belief system and spirituality. When a person faces the complications of illness, trauma, or any medical condition, he or she may begin to question his or her faith. The patient may believe that he or she is being punished by God, or the patient may accept a negative outcome, feeling that he or she deserves to be ill. The nurse

Figure 8-4 Buddha is revered as an example of the right way of life rather than a god.

Box 8-2

Spiritual Distress: A Case Study

In this case study about Mr. Govi, note how fear and other effects of spiritual distress can cause or increase physical signs and symptoms of illness.

Mr. Govi is a 42-year-old Caucasian male who is generally pleasant and self-assured. He is well educated and holds a doctorate in political science. He attended church regularly during his childhood, 20s, and 30s. He has not been attending church or living as he believes he should for some time now. His lack of spirituality has been on his mind and has begun to bother him. Today he began to feel short of breath and have pain in his chest. After an hour or so, he decided that he was having a heart attack. His wife phoned for an ambulance to take him to the local emergency room. In the ambulance, his pain was a 7 on a 0-to-10 scale, heart rate was 90 bpm, and respirations were 24 breaths/min. Upon arrival in the ER, he rated his pain as an 8, his heart rate was 96, and his respiratory rate was 24.

While the nurse connects Mr. Govi to a heart monitor and applies oxygen, his chest pain increases to a 9, his pulse rate increases to 110, and his respiratory rate increases to 29. He is now so distressed that he is having trouble thinking clearly. He feels weak and has a strong sense of doom. The sense of doom produces a fear that stimulates the sympathetic nervous system, causing the adrenal cortex to release adrenaline. It further raises the heart rate and blood pressure, increasing the workload of the heart and the need for oxygen. The nurse applies oxygen. While the nurse is gathering information from the patient, Mr. Govi makes the following statement, "I think I'm having a heart attack. God is probably punishing me!"

Eventually a heart attack is ruled out, and Mr. Govi is diagnosed with gastroesophageal reflux and treated with the appropriate medication. During his hospitalization, the nurse obtains permission from Mr. Govi to telephone his minister, requesting that he visit Mr. Govi.

At the time of his admission, Mr. Govi's data had included changes in his body and mind, as well as a feeling of abandonment or punishment by God. Physical changes in the body can be brought on by spiritual distress or emotional distress. When the distress is not addressed, it may lead to worsening spiritual distress, which can continue to feed and worsen the patient's health status.

caring for the patient in Box 8-2 had a choice to provide holistic care, which provides care to the whole person, including the body, mind, and spirit, or to ignore the spirit of the patient. It may be extremely helpful to the patient's condition to notify the patient's choice of clergy. Any spiritual stress that can be relieved will enhance the patient's physical health as well.

In 2007, another nursing diagnosis was added to the NANDA-I list that is related to spirituality, known simply as **spiritual distress**. Spiritual distress can occur at any time during a patient's life experiences. It may be seen during times of heavy financial stress, during major life changes such as divorce or death of a loved one, and during one's own illness or injury, especially if the illness is terminal. One example might be discontinuation of religious beliefs or practices under which the individual was reared: The individual may stop participating in the formal rites or rituals of his or her religion or worship, such as no longer attending church services or failing to pray on a regular basis. There may even be a questioning of or a total loss of faith, such as may occur with the death of a child. Others may find that, when their belief and value systems are challenged by disease, injury, or even nonmedical issues, they experience spiritual distress. Sometimes the patient may believe that, due to his or her having made a mistake or a bad choice, illness or intense suffering is a form of discipline by a higher being. The patient may even refuse to seek wellness if he or she believes that illness or death is deserved.

When the nurse identifies the patient as having spiritual distress, the nurse should not be judgmental or biased. It is important to realize that anyone can develop spiritual distress. Once the nurse identifies spiritual distress, the goals or outcomes of spiritual care are directed toward restoring the patient's comfort and relationship with himself or herself, others, fine arts and humanities, or God. The goals are specific to the patient and to the defining characteristics of his or her spiritual distress. An example of a goal is "the patient will express a feeling of hope for the future."

First, the nurse must determine the patient's current level of spiritual health by assessing for the characteristics listed in Box 8-3. If it is determined that the patient has spiritual distress, you can then determine the appropriate nursing care to provide. Nursing interventions will nearly always include:

- Offering presence, which means to give the patient time and attention.
- Providing opportunities for the patient to express his or her feelings.
- Using therapeutic communication techniques (see Chapter 6) to promote the expression of feelings.
- Contacting the religious or spiritual advisor of the patient's choice (only with the patient's permission).
- Providing for religious rituals as the patient desires, such as the practice of communion or the opportunity to pray.

When providing spiritual care, nurses must set aside their own beliefs to meet the needs of the patient. The nurse must show respect for the patient's cultural and religious beliefs and practices. As with all nursing care, the nurse must be nonjudgmental and unbiased.

Knowledge Connection

Describe at least three characteristics of spiritual distress related to the patient's connection to self. Name at least two characteristics of spiritual distress related to the patient's connection to God. List at least three interventions that might be appropriate when these characteristics are identified.

Box 8-3

Characteristics of Spiritual Distress

Characteristics of spiritual distress can be exhibited in various aspects of the patient's life, but you must be ever aware and alert to detect them.

Distress Related to Patient's Connection to Self
- Expression of anger
- Guilt
- Lack of acceptance
- Lack of courage
- Lack of forgiveness
- Lack of hope
- Lack of love
- Lack of meaning in life
- Lack of peace
- Trouble coping

Distress Related to the Patient's Connection to Others
- Expressing alienation
- Verbalizing a lack of a support system
- Refusal to interact with significant others or spiritual leaders

Distress Related to the Patient's Connection to Fine Arts and Humanities
- Lack of interest in nature
- Lack of interest or refusal to view spiritual literature
- Inability to express a state of creativity that was previously expressed

Distress Related to the Connections with God or a Greater Power
- A feeling of being abandoned
- Hopeless
- Suffering
- Anger toward God or a greater power
- Inability to experience the transcendent, participate in religious activities, pray, or be introspective
- Request to see or refusal to see a spiritual leader
- A change in spiritual practices

 Post Conference

At the end of your clinical day, you are tired but pleased with the outcome of your care for your patient, Mr. Habib. You have learned a great deal through this experience and look forward to sharing it with the other students. You learned that the item around his neck was an amulet that contained a portion of the Koran, the Muslim Holy Book. After reading about this, you knew to keep it dry and not to remove it. Mr. Habib was very nice, but very quiet. His wife would murmur information to you from time to time. Because he had a suprapubic incision, you asked another student, a male, to assess the incision for you. Mr. Habib was pleased with that arrangement, and you knew you had not offended him by assessing it yourself. At one point you were attempting to clear off his bedside table to set his tray down. You almost touched his Koran to move it out of the way, but his wife quickly stepped forward to move it. You remembered that you were not to touch it; only people who were "spiritually clean" could do that. When you removed the cover from his lunch tray, both you and the Habibs were distressed to learn that his green beans had been seasoned with bacon bits. You quickly offered to get him a new tray, and both he and his wife thanked you repeatedly for doing so. You knew he would be saying prayers at five specific times through the day, so you asked him when he wished to bathe and respected his wishes to prevent interrupting his prayer times.

KEY POINTS

- Every nurse will encounter multicultural patients and staff in the health care environments in which he or she works.
- The Joint Commission has established that patients have the right to considerate cultural, religious, and spiritual care.
- Culture is defined as the way of life of a group of people that distinguishes the members of one group or category of people from another.
- Religious beliefs, values, and the concept of spirituality are important cultural concepts.
- Cultural sensitivity means that the nurse provides care to the patient that shows respect for and

incorporates the patient's specific cultural beliefs and values.

• Cultural beliefs may affect health both negatively and positively.

• Nurses need to be aware of the patient's beliefs about prayer, suffering, death, and dying.

• Certain cultures and religions require that only members of their culture be allowed to touch the body of the deceased patient.

• Some cultures believe that it is wrong to pray for healing and recovery.

• In order to provide culturally sensitive care to a patient and significant others, the nurse must maintain a nonjudgmental attitude.

• Expression of spirituality is a healthy activity.

• Religion is the formal structured system of beliefs, values, rituals, and practices of a group based on the teachings of a spiritual leader who is revered and honored.

• The relationship of the body, mind, and spirit are so closely interactive that an alteration in any one of them may affect both of the other two realms.

REVIEW QUESTIONS

Select the answer that is most appropriate for each of the following questions. Some questions may have more than one correct answer. Check all that apply.

1. Which of the following is (are) responsible for the population explosion in America leading to an increase in the diversity of the citizens?

a. Tighter immigration laws

b. An influx of illegal aliens

c. Immigration

d. Adoption

2. Which of the following organizations has (have) worked to promote the patient's right to culturally competent care in U.S. hospitals?

a. U.S. Government

b. The Bureau of Immigration

c. The Joint Commission

d. American Association of Medical Workers

e. Patient Rights Committee

3. Nursing care that involves or combines the elements of more than one culture is called which of the following names?

a. Home care

b. Acute care

c. Hospice care

d. Transcultural care

e. Immigrant care

4. The patient has expressed the feeling that God has caused his illness. Which of the following would be most important for the nurse to consider when responding to the patient's feelings?

a. NANDA-I goals and nursing interventions for spiritual distress

b. The nurse's comfort with his or her own religious beliefs and background

c. That the patient has the right to his feelings, so no response is necessary

d. That the patient can rely on the family to give direction and support

e. That the resident priest should be contacted and a visit arranged

5. A patient who is bedridden is a member of the Muslim religion. Which of the following would be most important to the patient to provide her spiritual comfort?

a. Provide time for the patient to say the rosary.

b. Allow the patient to choose kosher foods from the menu.

c. Provide the patient with prayers for healing and decreased suffering.

d. Turn the patient's bed toward Mecca five times a day for prayer.

6. Muslim male circumcision is for which of the following purposes?

a. Establish personhood

b. Provide for cleanliness

c. Prevent cancer

d. Provide salvation

7. The nurse is assisting a patient of the Buddhist faith in planning meals for the day. Which of the following would be appropriate selections for a low-fat meal plan?

   a. Coffee with cream

   b. Steamed broccoli

   c. Grilled chicken breast

   d. Baked sweet potato

   e. Grilled cheese sandwich

   f. Spinach

   g. Biscuits with honey

   h. Beans

8. A patient is prepped for open-heart surgery and is asked to sign the permit for a blood transfusion, should it be deemed necessary. Although autotransfusion is generally practiced if the blood loss is great, a blood transfusion of another person's blood donation may be required. Which of the following patients might refuse the blood transfusion due to religious beliefs?

   a. Catholic nun

   b. Hindu man

   c. Amish woman

   d. Male Mormon

   e. Female Jehovah's Witness

TRUE-OR-FALSE QUESTIONS

9. For an Amish man, death is preferred over disability.

10. The nurse needs to be aware that the African American patient may fear signing a durable power of attorney for health care.

11. The nurse may promote the use of birth control pills as an acceptable method of birth control for the Catholic woman.

CRITICAL THINKING EXERCISES

12. Mr. Lambert is admitted with a kidney stone and is in severe pain. Ms. Radania, an African American practical nurse, enters his room to obtain his vital signs and give him his pain medicine. Mr. Lambert becomes very upset and tells her to leave. "I am not going to be touched by the likes of you," he screams. Describe the types of barriers to health care that are demonstrated in this situation. What could the practical nurse do that might improve the situation?

13. Mr. Miller and his family, which happens to be a large Amish family, have gathered together to wait for the doctor to tell them what is going on with Mr. Miller, the patient. There are several family members in the waiting room and at least five more in Mr. Miller's room. Why might Mr. Miller want the family with him when the doctor gives him his diagnosis and prognosis? If Mr. Miller requires surgery, who will make the decision whether or not to have the surgery? What financial considerations might be influential in the decision-making process?

ADDITIONAL RESOURCES

For additional Resources, Questions, and Activities, please see:

 Student Resource Disk

 http://davisplus.fadavis.com

Student Study Guide

REFERENCES

Andrews M, Boyle J. *Transcultural Concepts in Nursing Care.* 5th ed. Philadelphia: Lippincott Williams & Wilkins; 2008.

Aranda M. Relationship between religious involvement and psychological well-being: a social justice perspective. *Health Social Work.* 2008;33(1):9-21.

Asian Nation: Asian American History, Demographics, and Issues [Web site]. Available at: http://www.asian-nation.org/index.shtml. Accessed July 23, 2009.

At Health (2008). Why is there a compelling need for cultural competence? Available at: http://www.athealth.com/Practitioner/particles/compellingneed.html. Accessed July 23, 2009.

Campinha-Bacote J. A culturally conscious approach to holistic nursing. In: Program and Abstracts of the American Holistic Nurses Association Conference; June 16-19, 2005; King of Prussia, PA.

College of Registered Nurses of Nova Scotia. Position statement promoting culturally competent care. 2006. Available at: http://www.crnns.ca/documents/PositionStatementCultural06.pdf. Accessed July 23, 2009.

De D, Richardson J. Cultural safety: an introduction. *Paediatr Nurs.* 2008;20(2):39-43.

Hawter P. Death and dying in the Tibetan Buddhist tradition. 2005. Available at: http://www.buddhanet.net/deathtib.htm. Accessed July 23, 2009.

ISKCON Educational Services. The heart of Hinduism. Available at: http://hinduism.iskcon.com/index.htm. Accessed July 23, 2009.

The Joint Commission. Facts about the hospitals, language and culture: a snapshot of the nation (HLC). March 4, 2009. Available at: http://www.jointcommission.org/AboutUs/Fact_Sheets/facts_hlc.htm. Accessed July 23, 2009.

The Joint Commission. Hospitals, language, and culture. Updated June 2009. Available at: http://www.jointcommission.org/PatientSafety/HLC/. Accessed July 23, 2009.

Juckett G. Cross-cultural medicine. *Am Fam Physician.* 2005;72:2267-2274.

Kemp C. Asian cultures and health beliefs. 2002. Available at: http://personal.uncc.edu/macurran/2002/webproject/asi.htm#_Cambodian_Health_Beliefs. Accessed July 23, 2009.

Management Sciences for Health. The provider's guide to quality and culture: common beliefs and cultural practices. Available at: http://erc.msh.org/mainpage.cfm?file=5.3.0c.htm&module=provider&language=english. Accessed July 23, 2009.

McCormick T, Fish Mooney S. *Meditation: A Practical Guide to a Spiritual Discipline. Quiet Times for Forty Days.* Eugene, OR: Wipf & Stock; 2006.

NANDA International. *Nursing Diagnoses: Definitions and Classification, 2009-11 Edition.* Hoboken, NJ: Wiley-Blackwell; 2009.

Neff N. Folk medicine in Hispanics in the southwestern United States. Available at: http://www.rice.edu/projects/HispanicHealth/Courses/mod7/mod7.html. Accessed July 23, 2009.

Ngo-Metzger Q, August K, Srinivasan M, Liao S, Meyskens FL Jr. End-of-life care: guidelines for patient-centered communication. *Am Fam Physician.* 2008;77:167-174.

Rayman S, Almas K. Transcultural barriers and cultural competence in dental hygiene practice. *J Contemp Dent Pract.* 2007;8(4):43-51.

Rich TR. Judaism 101. Available at: http://www.jewfaq.org/toc.htm. Accessed July 23, 2009.

RN Central. Spiritual distress. 2007. Available at: http://www.rncentral.com/nursing-library/careplans/sd. Accessed July 23, 2009.

Snyder M, Lindquist R, eds. *Complementary/Alternative Therapies in Nursing.* 5th ed. New York: Springer; 2006.

Solari-Twadell P, McDermott M, eds. *Parish Nursing: Development, Education and Administration.* St. Louis: Saunders Elsevier; 2006.

University of Michigan Health System. Cultural competency: basic concepts and definitions. Available at: http://www.med.umich.edu/multicultural/ccp/basic.htm. Accessed July 23, 2009.

University of Virginia Health System. The meaning and practice of spiritual care. Available at: http://www.healthsystem.virginia.edu/internet/chaplaincy/whitepapersection1.pdf. Accessed July 23, 2009.

Walker, K. (2007). Cultural Proficiency. Available at: http://www.principalspartnership.com/culturalproficiency.pdf. Accessed July 23, 2009.

World Health Organization. Preamble to the Constitution of the World Health Organization as Adopted by the International Health Conference, June 19-22, 1946 (Official Records of the World Health Organization, no. 2, p. 100). New York: World Health Organization; 1946.

Yarbro CH, Frogge MH, Goodman M, eds. *Cancer Nursing: Principles and Practice.* 6th ed. Sudbury, MA: Jones and Bartlett; 2005.

Zerwekh J. *Nursing Care at the End of Life: Palliative Care for Patients and Families.* Philadelphia: FA Davis; 2006.

Growth and Development Throughout the Life Span

Key Terms

Ambivalent

Attachment

Cephalocaudal

Cognitive development

Development

Fontanels

Growth

Menarche

Moral development

Physical development

Proximodistal

Psychosocial development

Puberty

Reflexes

Regression

Spiritual development

Objectives

1. Define key terms associated with growth and development of humans.
2. Differentiate between growth and development.
3. Identify factors that affect growth and development.
4. Describe the stages of physiological development through the life span.
5. Describe the psychological development according to Erikson through the life span.
6. Describe moral development according to Kohlberg from toddler to older adult.
7. Explain cognitive development according to Piaget.
8. Describe spiritual development according to Fowler.
9. Identify safety concerns when providing nursing care at each developmental stage.
10. Describe health promotion activities for the nurse to utilize at each developmental stage.
11. Explain nursing implications for each developmental stage.

Clinical Connection

Your Assignment: You are assigned to care for José, a 16-year-old male with a newly diagnosed heart condition that was discovered after he collapsed on the basketball court. The family is very concerned, and someone is always with him. He has a 19-year-old sister with an infant son, and a younger brother who is 12 years old. His parents are in their late 40s. His 62-year-old grandmother is often at the bedside. All of them have many questions for you. You notice the infant appears underweight and fretful. The grandmother seems fragile and very pale.

   Your Actions: You must tailor your care to the developmental needs of an adolescent. You will need to review the nursing and health care issues of caring for an adolescent. When researching this information, you find that patient teaching, explanations of care, and preservation of modesty are major aspects of nursing care for an adolescent. In addition, the patient's family is involved in his care. You realize that they each have different needs regarding information and understanding of his care.

Often you will care not only for a patient, but for his or her family as well. Family members are concerned about the person who is ill, but they may also have health issues. It is not unusual for family members to ask nurses questions about their own health as well as about the care and health of the ill person. When responding to family concerns, it is important to remember the developmental needs and milestones of each age group. This chapter will help you learn how to meet the developmental needs of patients and their families.

Concepts of Growth and Development

Human beings are in a constant state of change from the moment of conception to death. Some of these changes are easily seen and others, though not visible, are occurring throughout the life span. These changes influence the health and nursing care needs of the individual. When nurses have an understanding of growth and development, they can plan and implement the most appropriate nursing care for each patient at his or her level of development.

   Growth is the term for the physical changes that occur in the size of human beings. During growth, the trunk of the body and extremities get longer and heavier. Bones become denser, and teeth erupt. Deciduous teeth appear first, then later fall out and are replaced by permanent teeth. Patterns of growth are similar for all people, but growth rates vary during different stages of development.

   Development refers to the increase in complexity of skills performed by a person. Development also refers to the behavioral aspect of growth and includes walking, talking, and meeting psychological benchmarks. Development is more difficult to measure than growth. Several theories about different aspects of development have evolved over time. In this chapter, we will discuss some of the more well-known theories of human development.

Principles of Growth and Development

Growth occurs in an orderly and predictable pattern, progressing from the head downward. This is referred to as a **cephalocaudal** pattern. Growth also occurs from the center of the body outward. This is referred to as a **proximodistal** pattern. Infants and children are evaluated by their growth and development patterns to determine developmental delays. Table 9-1 presents principles of growth and development and examples of each.

Factors That Influence Growth and Development

Many factors can influence growth and development. These factors can be loosely divided into biological and hereditary factors, environmental factors, and social factors. It is very important to realize how all of these factors can influence the growth and development of each individual.

- *Biological and hereditary factors* include the presence of physical or mental impairments that may delay or prevent a person from completing developmental tasks or growth benchmarks. Illnesses, whether genetic or due to other causes, can also delay progress through developmental stages. An example of a physical impairment would be a child who was born with cerebral palsy who cannot walk. An example of a mental impairment would be the child who experienced *anoxia,* or lack of oxygen, at birth and suffers brain damage. An example of an illness that delays progress through developmental stages would be the child born with a heart valve disorder who cannot exert himself or herself physically until the valve has been replaced. After that, the child quickly catches up with developmental expectations.
- *Environmental factors* include nutritional concerns and exposure to pollution and chemicals. Some children do not have nutritionally balanced food available to them, and this

Table 9-1 Principles of Growth and Development

Principle	Example
Growth and development follow an orderly, predictable pattern.	All children learn to sit before they walk.
Growth follows a cephalocaudal pattern.	Growth begins at the head and progresses to the chest and trunk; then, during the second year, the legs begin to grow rapidly.
Development starts in a proximodistal pattern.	The center of the body develops first, moving outward. Infants hold up their heads, then develop fine motor skills.
Simple skills are learned independently, then become part of complex skills.	Drinking from a cup requires hand-eye coordination, grasping, and hand-mouth coordination.
Development becomes more specific over time.	Infants react with their whole body when expressing pain or happiness. Toddlers react with tears or laughter.
Certain stages of growth and development are more critical than others.	The first trimester in pregnancy is when the fetus is most susceptible to the influence of drugs, chemicals, and viruses, which will cause congenital abnormalities.
Growth and development occur at an uneven pace.	There is slower physical growth in school-age children. In adolescence, there is rapid growth of legs and arms.

decreases their rate of development and growth. An example of this is the child who is given only cow's milk long after solid foods should have been introduced. Exposure to chemicals and heavy metals such as lead can affect the brain, leading to developmental delays. Pollution in the air can lead to respiratory illnesses such as asthma, decreasing physical development due to the inability to tolerate physical activity.

• *Social factors* are varied, but include cultural expectations, violence and abuse, resources and support systems, and parental influence. When infants are exposed to violence and abuse by caregivers, they are unable to develop healthy trust in those they innately turn to for help. This then affects their ability to complete future developmental tasks. Cultural expectations of behavior and abilities in young children may vary according to the culture. For example, the age at which a child in the United States is expected to be toilet trained and speaking may be very different than what is expected in another culture.

Theories of Development

Theories are used to describe and organize the growth and development experienced by all human beings. Since you will care for patients of all ages, it is important for you to know appropriate expectations of physical, psychosocial, cognitive, moral, and spiritual development when caring for your patients. In addition, you must tailor your care and patient teaching to the level of your patient. And, as always,

safety must be a primary concern as you care for patients of any age.

Physical development refers to the physical size and functioning of a person. Influences on physical development include genetics, nutrition, and function of the endocrine and central nervous systems. Table 9-1 provides a summary of the patterns of physical development.

Psychosocial development occurs throughout our lives in distinct stages, according to Erik Erikson, a psychoanalyst who pioneered this area of study. Each stage of psychosocial development requires that specific tasks be mastered. The stages and tasks for psychosocial development are described in Table 9-2.

Cognitive development refers to how we learn. Jean Piaget, a Swiss psychologist and theorist, studied his own children to help him understand how learning takes place as we develop. Piaget believed that cognitive development occurred from birth to adolescence in an orderly sequence of four stages. Based on this theory, we can see how human beings can adapt behaviors to the demands of a constantly changing environment. Piaget did not differentiate between cognitive development of the adolescent and the adult in his theories. Box 9-1 presents Piaget's four stages of cognitive development.

Moral development is the ability to think at higher levels and develop a value system that differentiates right from wrong. The theory of moral development was established by Lawrence Kohlberg, an American psychologist. He acknowledged that not all people reach all stages of moral

Table 9-2 Erikson's Stages of Psychosocial Development

Stage	Age	Task	Nursing Implication
Trust vs. Mistrust	Birth to 18 months	Learn to trust others	Provide consistent, affectionate care.
Autonomy vs. Shame/doubt	18 months to 3 years	Learn self-control and the ability to express oneself and cooperate	Increase independence by providing praise and encouragement.
Initiative vs. Guilt	3 to 6 years	Initiate activities and influence environment	Encourage creativity, answer questions. Do not threaten or label behavior as "bad."
Industry vs. Inferiority	6 to 12 years	Develop sense of social skills and self-esteem.	Keep realistic expectations for behavior and recognize accomplishments.
Identity vs. Role confusion	12 to 18 years	Seek sense of self and plan according to one's abilities	Assist with planning for future and help with decision making.
Intimacy vs. Isolation	18 to 30 years	Develop intimate relationships and choose career	Avoid criticizing relationships. Teach how to establish realistic goals.
Generativity vs. Stagnation	30 to 60 years	Become productive member of society and establish a family	Recognize accomplishments and provide emotional support.
Integrity vs. Despair	65+ years	Accept worth, uniqueness, and death	Review accomplishments made by person.

Box 9-1

Piaget's Four Stages of Cognitive Development

Piaget has divided his theory of cognitive development into four stages:

- **Stage 1, Sensorimotor:** from birth to 2 years; concept of cause and effect develops; learning through senses and use of body movement and language
- **Stage 2, Preoperational:** from 2 to 7 years; relates objects and events to self; begins to use symbolism, and imagination develops
- **Stage 3, Concrete operational:** from 7 to 12 years; concrete problem-solving and inductive reasoning develops
- **Stage 4, Formal operational:** from 12+ years; develops ability to analytically solve problems and engage in abstract reasoning

development. This is not truly a developmental theory, because progression through the stages may not be age related. All his research was based on males: He studied 84 boys over a period of 20 years to develop his theory. His theory is based on three categories:

1. **Preconventional level:** stages 1 and 2
2. **Conventional level:** stages 3 and 4
3. **Postconventional level:** stages 5 and 6

Box 9-2 gives more information about each of these stages.

Kohlberg is not without his detractors, however. Sharply critical of his work is Carol Gilligan, one of his former students. She feels that the moral development of females is not exactly the same as that of males. Her theory of moral development also has three stages:

1. **Preconventional:** focused on self
2. **Conventional:** interest and concern for others
3. **Postconventional:** focused on social responsibility for self and others

Her research has been criticized by some as limited, and her results are unable to be reproduced or validated.

Spiritual development theory has been described by James Fowler, an American developmental psychologist. He defines faith as a universal concern that is a process of developing trust. Fowler developed his six stages of spiritual development using information from Piaget and Kohlberg (Table 9-3).

Knowledge Connection

Explain how knowledge of normal growth and development is important when assessing patients. Which theories of development are based on ages and which are not?

Box 9-2

Kohlberg's Stages of Moral Development

Kohlberg's stages of moral development include three levels and six stages.

Preconventional Level—Ages 1 to 9 or 10; Focuses on Avoiding Punishment and Gaining Rewards

Stage 1. Punishment and Obedience Orientation
In this stage, to do right means not being punished, while doing wrong means punishment. The child obeys authority to avoid punishment. An example would be the child who tells on herself to avoid being punished when the wrong is found out.

Stage 2. Individualism and Relativism
In this stage, the child no longer takes one person as the authority and sees shades of right and wrong. The child focuses on what is fair rather than what might be best for a larger group, such as the family. An example is the child who wants a cat even though other family members are allergic to cat hair. The child sees the situation as completely unfair to him.

Conventional Level—Early Adolescence; Focuses on Conforming to Avoid Disapproval with Respect for Authority of Law and Order

Stage 3. Seeking Strong Interpersonal Relationships
In this stage, the young adolescent focuses on being good and helping others, not just to follow the rules but to feel good about his or her motives. An example might be a 13-year-old who helps an elderly neighbor with yard work without being paid to do so.

Stage 4. Law-and-Order Orientation
In this stage, the young adolescent follows laws for the greater good and due to respect for authority. An example of this stage might be an adolescent who participates in scouting or other civic clubs.

Postconventional Level —Postadolescence; Focuses on Behaving According to Internal Codes and Beliefs

Stage 5. Social Rules and Legal Orientation
In this stage, the adult's behavior is motivated by the desire to follow internal values and moral principles. For example, the adult will stop at a red light even though no one is watching and there is no other traffic.

Stage 6. Universal Ethical Principles
In this stage, the adult has concern for human rights and dignity, and desires an impartial interpretation of justice. Examples of this stage would include those people who work for justice and human rights throughout the world, such as Mother Teresa.

Table 9-3   Fowler's Stages of Spiritual Development

Stage	Age	Description
Undifferentiated	0 to 3 years	No concept of self or environment
Intuitive-projective	4 to 6 years	Imitates parents' behaviors about religion
Mythic-literal	7 to 12 years	Symbolism and stories explain religion and morals
Synthetic-conventional	13 to 17 years	While forming own identity, questions values and religious beliefs
Individuating-reflexive	18 to young adult	Referred to as "demythologizing stage" due to leaving home and developing one's own beliefs
Paradoxical-consolidative	30 years and older	Able to understand different views about faith; more interested in what is true than in what he or she might believe
Universalizing	Adult	Love and justice become tangible as he or she acts on beliefs about the importance of loving and caring for those who are unlovely

Stages of Child Development

In order to study the development of all aspects of children and adults as they grow, categories or stages of development have been identified. As you may have noticed, different theorists use different categories and age groupings. For the purposes of this textbook, we will use the following categories:

- **Infant:** birth to 1 year of age
- **Toddler:** 1 to 3 years of age
- **Preschooler:** 3 to 5 years of age
- **School-age child:** 5 to 12 years of age
- **Adolescent:** 12 to 19 years of age
- **Early adulthood:** 19 to 40 years of age
- **Middle adulthood:** 40 to 65 years of age
- **Older adulthood:** 65 years and older

Infant

Infants (birth through 1 year of age) are gradually becoming more aware of the world around them. In addition to survival skills of eating, sleeping, digesting, and breathing, infants are busy exploring what they can see and touch, including the faces of caregivers.

Physical Development

The first year of life is packed with physical growth and development. It is easy to see the cephalocaudal pattern of development in infants. First, they can hold up their heads at about 2 months of age, can sit up with help at around 6 months of age, and pull up to stand at nearly 1 year of age.

The principle of proximal-to-distal development is also observable in infants. Shortly after birth, they can grasp your finger by reflex. They can wave their arms and legs at approximately 3 months of age, and by 7 months they can reach for and pick up a toy using a pincer grasp.

Infants grow at a rapid rate, doubling their birth weight by 6 months of age and tripling it by 1 year. So the newborn who weighed 7 pounds 8 ounces at birth can be expected to weigh approximately 22.5 pounds when he or she is 1 year old. An infant's length increases at about 1 inch per month during the first year of life. An average length at birth is 18 to 20 inches, so an average height for a 1-year-old child would be 30 to 32 inches.

Newborns possess several reflexes to help them survive. **Reflexes** are automatic responses by the central nervous system and include:

- **Rooting reflex:** When the baby's cheek is gently touched, the infant will turn toward the stimulus and open his or her mouth to find milk (Fig. 9-1).
- **Sucking reflex:** When a nipple or finger is placed in a newborn's mouth, the baby begins to suck to obtain nourishment (Fig. 9-2).
- **Startle (Moro) reflex:** When babies are moved suddenly or jarred in some way, they extend their limbs outward and then pull them toward the trunk of their body to protect themselves from injury (Fig. 9-3).

- **Babinski's reflex:** When the sole of the foot on a newborn is stroked, the normal response is fanning of the toes while the great toe pulls upward (Fig. 9-4).

These reflexes slowly disappear as the child develops, all decreasing or disappearing by 6 months of age.

Each body system grows and develops more fully during an infant's first year of life. Head circumference is measured to determine brain growth and to detect any signs of problems with cerebrospinal fluid production. Indications of

Figure 9-1   Rooting reflex.

Figure 9-2   Sucking reflex.

Figure 9-3   Moro reflex.

Figure 9-4   Babinski's reflex.

normal growth patterns are that the head circumference will be 2½ times the birth circumference by age 1.

Fontanels are the spaces between the bones of the skull that are not yet fused together, sometimes called the *soft spots*. The brain is not protected by bone in these areas during the first year of life. The posterior fontanel, a triangular-shaped soft area found on the top of the head toward the back, closes first, at about the age of 4 months. The anterior fontanel, a diamond-shaped soft area found on the top of the head toward the forehead, closes last, at about 1 to 1½ years of age. Fontanels allow for rapid brain growth during the first year of life. Once the bones of the skull fuse together, there is no longer room for rapid growth.

Psychosocial Development

According to Erikson, the developmental task of the infant is developing trust. In normal situations, mother and baby bond shortly after the birth. The mother looks into the baby's eyes, checks his or her fingers and toes, talks to the newborn, and holds the baby close (Fig. 9-5).

In some situations, the baby has to remain in a special care nursery and is placed there immediately after

Figure 9-5   A new mother bonds closely with her baby.

birth. The mother should be encouraged to visit the baby, talking to and holding her newborn as often as allowed to promote mother-baby bonding, also called **attachment**.

If infants' needs for security, food, cleanliness, and love are met, they develop trust in their caregivers. When caregivers do not meet an infant's basic needs, the infant cannot develop trust and normal psychosocial development is negatively affected.

Cognitive Development

Cognitive development in the infant occurs through sensorimotor experiences (see Box 9-1 for Piaget's theory of cognitive development). For learning to occur, the infant must be allowed to have both sensory experiences, such as touching, tasting, seeing, and hearing, and motor experiences, such as moving, rolling, crawling, cruising, and walking. It is a common sight for an infant to pick up any item, then immediately put it in his or her mouth. This is the way the infant learns—through the sensations of touch and taste. Parents have to be vigilant to prevent unsafe items from going into the infant's mouth.

As newborns, infants respond to the environment through reflex action. As they grow older, they respond to repeated sensory and motor experiences by learning through repeated outcomes.

Moral Development

Infants do not possess a sense of right and wrong. They learn through gentle reprimand what behaviors are considered "right" and "wrong." At this age, they do not try to please others, but respond to the positive feelings of love and affection.

Toddlers

A toddler is a child from 1 to 3 years old. During this time, the child develops voluntary behaviors and gains control over certain motor skills. The family of the toddler is important in the development of the skills of the child, from toilet training to language development.

Physical Development

Toddlers gain 4 to 6 pounds per year, and their height increases at a rate of approximately 3 inches per year. At age 2, a child is generally about one-half of his or her adult height. So, an infant who is 18 inches long at birth and grows about 12 inches in the first year—or an average of 1 inch per month, as we have seen is normal during the first year of life—would be about 30 inches tall at 1 year old. By age 2, if the child grew another 3 inches, he or she would be 33 inches tall. Assuming that is half of his or her adult height, the child would reach 66 inches, or approximately 5 feet, 6 inches, as an adult.

By 2½ years of age, the toddler will have all 20 deciduous teeth. It is important that the child learn to brush his or her teeth or that the parents do so to prevent dental problems in later childhood.

As toddlers' muscles develop and mature, they begin to master additional skills. They learn to control sphincter muscles to master toilet training. Generally, toddlers develop anal sphincter muscle control first, and master bowel control. They develop urinary sphincter control during the daytime before they can stay dry during the night. Accidents and missed cues are common and do not indicate willful disobedience on the part of the child (Fig. 9-6).

Psychosocial Development

Erikson's developmental task for toddlers is autonomy versus shame and doubt. Toddlers struggle to establish their sense of self. Perhaps that is why they like the word "no" so much, because it gives them a sense of control over their daily activities. Toddlers need the opportunity to make decisions with limited choices. Too many choices will be overwhelming for a young child. For example, you might ask a toddler if he or she would like chocolate or vanilla ice cream; listing 14 flavors and asking a toddler to choose just one would be too overwhelming. It is important that toddlers be able to make choices without the parent questioning the decision. This helps them develop autonomy.

Another way to help toddlers master this developmental task is to allow them to perform and practice skills such as dressing themselves. Even though it would be easier and faster for a caregiver to do this, the child needs to be encouraged to accomplish these skills and to be praised for doing so. If a toddler gets his or her shirt on backward or his or her shoes on the wrong feet, he or she should receive gentle guidance rather than be shamed or ridiculed.

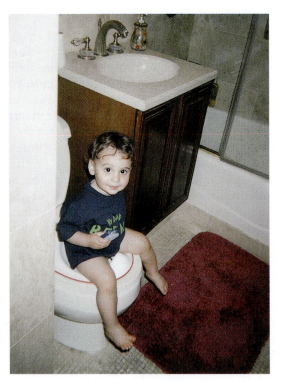

Figure 9-6 This toddler is mastering sphincter control and body cues to become toilet trained.

Toddlers are famous for throwing "temper tantrums" when they do not get their way or get their needs and wants met immediately. These tantrums are due to the child's frustration at not being in control. When such tantrums occur, it is best to remove the toddler to a quiet place away from the situation. For example, a toddler may have a temper tantrum in a store, demanding a toy that the parent has refused to purchase. If the parent picks up the child and removes him or her from the toy aisle, going to the restroom or the car, and speaks in a calm, controlled voice, the child will calm down. Then the parent can set firm limits with the child. It can be a challenge to remain calm and in control in such a situation. If the parent gives in and purchases the toy just to keep the child quiet, the child has learned to manipulate the parent using temper tantrums.

Cognitive Development

Piaget describes the cognitive development of a toddler and preschooler as being in the preoperational stage. The child at this age uses trial and error to master new skills and to achieve learning. During this stage of cognitive development, the child is the center of his or her world, or is *egocentric*. Toddlers have no concept of the needs or feelings of others. Their behavior is impulsive with no thought of how it will affect others.

Toddlers are also developing the concept of object permanence, meaning that they are learning that objects do not disappear when they can no longer be seen. When you play games such as peek-a-boo with toddlers, you are helping them learn this concept.

At this age, the child is also learning by imitation, watching a parent, caregiver, or older sibling and then imitating what they do. Toddlers like to pretend to cook, vacuum, and work with tools.

Moral and Spiritual Development

Again, toddlers imitate parents and caregivers in developing their moral values. As they learn right and wrong from parents and it is reinforced by family and caregivers, toddlers become more secure knowing the limits of acceptable behavior. It is important for parents and caregivers to model the moral behavior they expect from the toddler. For example, if a toddler uses the curse words he or she hears the parents use and then is punished for it, he or she does not understand the expected moral behavior.

At this age, toddlers begin to learn the spiritual beliefs of their parents and caregivers. For example, they may begin to say grace before eating a meal or hear stories that illustrate the family's spiritual beliefs.

Knowledge Connection

Explain the location and function of the fontanels. How can attachment occur if an infant is in a special care nursery? How tall will a child be as an adult if he is 35 inches tall at age 2? What are two ways to help the toddler develop autonomy?

Preschoolers

The preschool age group is from 3 to 5 years old. This is a time of rapid growth for psychological and cognitive development. The actual physiological growth of the child is not as rapid during these years as in the toddler years.

Physical Development

Lengthening of the trunk and body occur during the preschool years. The child starts looking taller. Preschoolers gain about 5 to 7 pounds per year and grow 2½ to 3 inches per year. They begin to lose some baby fat and look more slender, with extremities that grow quickly and may appear out of proportion with the rest of the body. They are steadier on their feet, with better balance and body control than toddlers. Deciduous teeth are all in, and preschoolers must be encouraged to brush often and well, as well as to choose healthy snacks rather than eating mostly sugary foods.

Four- and 5-year-olds can dress themselves without difficulty but may still need help tying their shoes. They can handle utensils well and can make their own sandwiches with supervision. They have mastered toilet training but may need reminders to wash their hands and wipe correctly.

Four-year-olds can climb and jump, but may overestimate their abilities, so they need to be supervised closely. Five-year-olds can begin more complicated physical activities such as skating and playing sports.

Psychosocial Development

The major development issue for preschoolers according to Erikson is initiative versus guilt. Children at this age need to be allowed to pretend, role-play, and explore an identity in the world and develop a sense of independence. They learn from parents and other adults about roles and initiative. Children in preschool often learn from adults in various positions, such as nurses, doctors, teachers, police, firefighters, and others who serve as role models.

Children at this age should be encouraged to explore within a safe environment. An example of this would be to allow a preschooler to be independent within a limited area in a playground, under the watchful eye of a caregiver. The child can explore and try new things with a caregiver nearby to ensure safety.

Cognitive Development

As discussed earlier, Piaget's stage for both toddlers and preschoolers is the preoperational stage. However, preschoolers have advanced to the point of being able to take turns, share toys, and obey rules. Preschoolers can respond to only one aspect of a stimulus, rather than being able to understand the whole situation. For example, if a preschooler sees an adult dressed in a mouse costume, complete with a mask covering the face, the preschooler is afraid, believing this is really a giant mouse. A child of this age cannot interpret the situation as an adult dressed up to look like a mouse.

At this stage, preschoolers can grasp concepts based on their previous experiences, rather than on their ability to formally reason. An example of this might be when a preschooler hears a parent arrange for a babysitter and becomes upset because it means his or her parents are going to leave for the evening.

Moral and Spiritual Development

The preconventional stage of moral development encompasses the preschool age. At this stage, children learn moral development from the adults in their lives. Examples set by parents and caregivers are imitated and lay the foundation for further moral growth. Preschoolers make moral decisions based on anticipated punishment for bad behavior.

This is the age when many children begin some type of church school or training. Preschoolers understand the concept of being kind and have the same beliefs as their parents. They have vivid imaginations and may misunderstand some spiritual concepts without support and explanation from their parents.

School-Age Child

At the ages of 5 to 12, the child begins to spend a significant part of each day at school away from family. There is less dependence on parents for activities on a daily basis. Children begin to spend time with school- and sports-related activities. Social groups expand, and children's understanding of the world deepens beyond the immediate family.

Physical Development

Children at this age have slow, steady growth of about 2 to 3 inches per year. They gain approximately 4½ to 6½ pounds per year. Limbs grow steadily at this age, which can cause "growing pains," especially at night. These pains are due to the stretching of muscles and ligaments in the arms and the legs. As school-age children enter puberty, they experience a growth spurt.

Young school-agers, 6- and 7-year-olds, begin loosing their baby teeth and replacing them with permanent teeth. When the permanent teeth come in, they may look big in the child's face until more growth occurs. During the school-age years, dental care is very important to detect and correct alignment problems and dental decay.

Psychosocial Development

School-age children have Erikson's developmental task of industry versus inferiority. They are industrious in various ways: schoolwork, sports, and developing new skills. They may have unrealistic expectations of their abilities and become easily frustrated when they do not perform as well as they thought they would. For example, a 10-year-old may be selected to participate in a spelling bee, study hard, and expect to take first place. He or she may be devastated due to misspelling a word in the third round. Parents and caregivers need to be encouraging and positive about how well the child did to make it to the spelling bee, rather than emphasizing the child's loss.

Children in this age group often enjoy sports and identify with a specific team. They also like learning and mastering new skills needed to improve in a sport, ride a bike, swim, and skate (Fig. 9-7). As they get older, school-age children learn skills needed to complete more complex tasks and projects. They need recognition and appropriate praise for their accomplishments.

At this age, children become more social and identify with peer groups. Friendships become very important to them and family becomes less important. They value their privacy, keep locked diaries in secret places, and become extremely distressed if their belongings are disturbed.

It is common for school-age children to be fearful. Younger children (ages 7 and 8) may be afraid of ghosts and being alone at night. Older children (ages 8 and 9) may be afraid that their parents will die or get a divorce, and 10- and 11-year-olds may be fearful of "bad guys" or of developing a life-threatening illness.

Cognitive Development

According to Piaget, young school-age children, up to age 7, are making the transition to concrete operational thought. By age 7, for example, the child no longer believes that an adult dressed in a mouse suit is a giant mouse. Now he or she knows it is just a person in a costume. Younger school-age children begin to understand cause and effect, and older children master this concept. For example, a 7-year-old may tease a dog several times to see what will happen, but an 11-year-old knows that teasing a dog will most likely result in the dog growling and possibly snapping at him or her.

At this stage, children spend a great deal of time in school, which may or may not be a comfortable place for the child. Issues such as bullying, relating to teachers and other children, and being successful in school influence the comfort level of each child. Parents need to be aware of school problems and be ready to act to help the child if needed.

Figure 9-7 This school-age child is improving his skills at baseball.

Moral and Spiritual Development

School-age children are moving to the conventional level of Kohlberg's stages. They are learning what it means to be thought of as a good person. By age 11 or 12, children begin to think of others and how to be fair, even if it means sacrificing something they want. Kohlberg refers to concern for others as *reciprocity*. Children at this age are beginning to learn how to regulate their own behavior to win the trust and loyalty of others. Moral beliefs are still based on the teaching of their parents and the behavior they model.

School-age children understand the concept of a God and begin to understand spiritual symbolism in stories, with guidance from their parents and religious teachers. They are learning to separate accepted spiritual facts from the fiction of their imagination.

Knowledge Connection

Why might a preschooler be afraid of a mascot at a baseball game? What causes growing pains in a school-age child? How can a parent help a school-age child accept a failure? How do school-age children grow in their understanding of cause and effect?

Adolescence

During the years from 13 to 19, teens undergo the change from childhood to adulthood. Both physiological changes and psychosocial adjustments occur. This time of transition is often as challenging for the parents as it is for the adolescent.

Physical Development

At the beginning of adolescence, there is a period of rapid growth referred to as a growth spurt. Boys grow 4 to 12 inches during the adolescent period, and girls grow 2 to 8 inches. Their weight increases in accordance with their height increase. Boys gain from 15 to 65 pounds during these years, and girls gain 15 to 55 pounds.

Puberty, the onset of the development of sexual characteristics and functions, occurs between the ages of 11 and 14. Females develop breasts and experience **menarche**, or the beginning of menstrual periods. Males develop facial hair and their voices deepen due to the enlargement of their vocal cords and larynx. The penis grows in length and diameter. In both sexes, pubic and axillary hair appears and hormone production increases.

After puberty, growth slows. Girls reach their adult height by 17 years of age, but boys continue to grow until they reach 18 to 20 years of age. Four more teeth erupt, the third molars or *wisdom teeth,* by about the age of 25. Often there is no room for these teeth and they have to be surgically removed.

Psychosocial Development

For adolescents, Erickson's developmental task is identity versus role confusion. The teen begins establishing his or her own identity apart from parents and family. It is important that teens test their values and compare them to those of others, then decide what they truly value and believe. In addition, older teens are facing the need to make decisions about their future: Will they continue with school or go to work? What kind of degree or career should they pursue?

Adolescents do want guidance and advice from their parents, but at the same time they want to be independent and make their own decisions. This is a time of conflict even in the best of situations. Wise parents expect older adolescents to pull away, to be somewhat critical of them, and to feel **ambivalent**, or to have opposing feelings, about their parents.

Some social issues facing adolescents today include sexually transmitted diseases, teen pregnancy, date rape, and substance abuse. As a nurse, you may be the person a teen turns to for information and help regarding these issues. They often do not want to go to their parents for assistance. Be open and matter of fact. Avoid acting shocked that the teen is involved in these kinds of situations. Provide factual information, answer questions, and be supportive as teens take positive steps to handle these issues.

Cognitive Development

According to Piaget, adolescents are shifting from concrete operational thinking to formal operational thinking. This means that teens are beginning to think logically with problem-solving skills. One example is being able to understand and apply the scientific process to problem-solving. Adolescents can begin to predict outcomes: if this happens, that will result.

In addition to this higher level of thinking, teens begin to have a wider view of the world. They may become interested in politics, environmental issues, and social justice. As their interests increase, adolescents learn about issues with global significance and ways that they can impact their world. You can see that cognitive development of the adolescent closely ties to moral development.

Moral and Spiritual Development

In this transition stage of moral development, teens believe they can make a difference in the world and wish to right the wrongs they see. No longer do they do the right thing simply to avoid punishment. Now they may question the moral rightness of some of their parents' beliefs and examples. They want to try out their own moral code at this age, sometimes without thoroughly thinking about the long-term results of their moral decisions.

This same type of questioning goes on in spiritual development as well. Teens begin to compare what they have always believed with the beliefs of other faiths. They may feel they find more similarities than differences. Adolescents may now be open to spiritual ideas that they have previously opposed. Often they are attracted to less formal worship settings rather than more traditional ones.

Knowledge Connection

At what age do girls reach their adult height? At what age do boys reach their adult height? Give an example of ambivalent feelings a teen might have about her parents.

Laboratory and Diagnostic Connection

Approaches to Procedures for Different Developmental Stages

While there are no laboratory or diagnostic tests for stages of growth and development, there are often common reactions of children to these procedures. It is very important to keep the age and stage of the child in mind when tests are ordered. Infants need to be held and comforted during and after such procedures. If a parent or family member is not available, you will want to provide this comfort. The same is true of toddlers and preschoolers. They are old enough to anticipate pain when they see a needle for drawing blood, or feel anxiety when they are separated from a parent. They may react in a panic. Speak to this age child in a calm, reassuring voice. Try to distract the child with a toy or book if possible. Again, be available to comfort the child if no one else can do so.

School-age children and adolescents may regress when they see a needle or if they have to be separated from a parent or caregiver for tests. At this age, it is important to give a brief explanation of what they will see, hear, and feel. Be honest about whether the procedure may hurt, but reassure them about what it feels like and that the discomfort will be brief.

Adults may be apprehensive about tests and blood draws as well, especially if they have had traumatic experiences in the past. It is important to remain calm and reassuring with adult patients too. You can distract them during a blood draw by asking questions about their lives and hobbies to keep their minds focused on other things. Answer questions about procedures and explain the purpose for what is being done.

Health Concerns for Infants, Children, and Adolescents

In addition to knowledge of normal growth and development patterns, it is important for you to be aware of safety issues for children of all ages. You may care for children who have been injured in avoidable accidents and need to do patient teaching with the family regarding ways to promote safety in the future. In addition, you may have the opportunity to answer questions from parents about ways to keep their children healthy. You may care for children in a hospital setting, so it is important to adapt your care to meet their needs.

Infants and Toddlers

It is part of your role as a nurse to promote safety and teach family members how to provide for the needs of infants and toddlers. It is also your responsibility to keep infants and toddlers safe while they are in your care.

Safety

When caring for infants and toddlers, it is extremely important to keep the following safety concerns in mind:

- **Prevent Falls.** Never leave an infant alone on an elevated surface. The danger of the infant rolling off and falling is too great. Examples include changing tables or high cribs with the side rails left down. *Safety: In these situations, keep one hand on the infant at all times. Toddlers like to climb, so keep side rails up and observe the child closely to prevent falls.*
- **Prevent Choking.** Children at these ages tend to put everything in their mouths as a means of exploration. Choking is an ever-present concern. *Safety: Never leave small objects within reach of infants and toddlers.*
- Nurses must use extra care not to accidentally leave needle covers, IV caps, or other small objects in the infant's or toddler's bed.
- **Prevent Drowning.** Infants and toddlers can drown in as little as 2 inches of water. *Safety: Never leave an infant or toddler alone in a bathtub.* Infants can be slippery when wet, so keep a firm grip on infants to prevent them from slipping beneath the surface of the water. Toddlers should never be left unsupervised around bathtubs or swimming pools, even small child-sized pools.

Health Teaching

In addition to teaching parents about safety, you may also teach about health issues. Proper nutrition is essential for young children and can be confusing for parents, who may hear conflicting advice from older generations versus current medical thinking. Support parents of infants in following the physician's guidelines for how long to stay on formula or breast milk alone, and when to begin adding cereals and other baby foods.

Toddlers are often finicky eaters, refusing all foods except certain preferred ones for several days in a row. Parents are often very disturbed by this. Encourage parents to provide a variety of healthy finger foods for the toddler to choose from. Examples might include small pieces of fruits such as banana, cheese pieces, pieces of cooked vegetables, and small sandwich pieces of peanut butter on bread. Avoid foods that could cause a toddler to choke easily, such as slices of hot dog. The child will usually choose enough foods to stay healthy.

Discipline is often a concern for parents of toddlers during those "terrible twos." Support parents in their choices for discipline, if possible. Provide gentle guidance with suggestions for options to try if you are asked for input. If "time-out" is used, a good guideline is to keep the toddler in the time-out location for 1 minute per year of age.

Parents must have realistic expectations of what an infant or toddler can accomplish. When parents and caregivers expect children to behave in a manner that only an older child could master, the parents may become frustrated. If this frustration mounts, it can lead to child abuse. When caregivers expect behavior that the toddler is incapable of

performing, the caregiver may end up harming the child. Many times a caregiver who abuses an infant gives as the reason, "He just would not stop crying."

Nursing Implications for Hospitalized Infants and Toddlers

Children of this age will want a parent or caregiver with them at all times. If that is not possible, you will need to offer comfort by holding and cuddling the infant or toddler. Remember the importance of meeting the needs of an infant so he or she will develop trust appropriately. When a hospitalized infant cries, if no parent or caregiver is with him or her, be sure that you meet the infant's needs.

Toddlers may respond well when you can take time to play with them. Build rapport by singing a child's song or reading a book to the toddler while you are in the room to perform routine care such as administering medications.

> ### Knowledge Connection
> How long should a 3-year-old be expected to sit in "time-out" when disciplined? What precautions will help prevent an infant from drowning?

Preschoolers and School-age Children

Preschoolers are unaware of unsafe situations and must be supervised closely while at play. School-age children may see themselves as invincible and dismiss potential for harm.

Safety

Safety issues for this age group include focusing on "stranger danger," playground safety, and water safety.

- **Stranger Danger.** Preschoolers must be taught to avoid talking to or trusting strangers. At this age, they believe what they are told and will often talk to anyone, sharing all kinds of information. It is important to teach this safety concept without making the preschooler fearful of everyone all the time. Be sure the preschooler knows it is acceptable to talk to a policeman or fireman to get help.

  School-age children need information about how to escape if abduction is attempted. This knowledge gives them confidence that they could handle such a situation. Several programs are available that provide this type of information.
- **Playground Safety.** Preschoolers may not think through the consequences of their actions and are therefore at risk for playground accidents. For example, they may walk in front of a swing while another child is swinging and be hit. Supervision is necessary to prevent them from attempting unsafe tricks such as jumping from the top of a slide.

  School-age children are very active and beginning to participate in sports. They must understand safety rules to prevent injury. They are less fearful than when they were younger and want to try out new skills without practicing them first. *Safety: Safety equipment is required and must be used in team sports, cycling, skateboarding, and other activities with potential for injury.*

- **Water Safety.** Preschoolers need to learn to swim to prevent accidental drowning. They still should not be left alone in water that is deeper than they are tall.

School-age children may participate in water sports and should be aware of safety rules to protect themselves and others in the water.

Health Teaching

Preschoolers need to have a bedtime routine that involves hygiene, such as brushing teeth and hair, dressing themselves, and some talking time at bedtime, such as with a bedtime story. They are often fearful of real or imagined things, such as a monster under the bed, and require repeated reassurance. Parents and caregivers need to be understanding and avoid impatience or belittling the preschooler.

School-age children need to have health screenings for common problems such as vision impairment, scoliosis, or hearing problems. It is important for them to be active and get exercise each day. Performance in school should be evaluated to help with early detection of learning disabilities or attention problems.

Nursing Implications for Hospitalized Preschoolers and School-age Children

When you care for preschoolers in a hospital setting, allow them to keep an object such as a blanket or stuffed animal with them for security (Fig. 9-8). A parent or caregiver should be encouraged to stay with the preschooler. To explain medical procedures to a preschooler, show him or her a stuffed animal or doll with a sling or cast to help explain

Figure 9-8   A preschooler clings to her stuffed animal and her mother for security.

what will happen. Allow the child to act out the procedure with the doll. Use words young children can understand. Remember that children at this age have many fears, so do all you can to help alleviate them. Use a night-light to help alleviate fear of the dark.

School-age children have a variety of needs due to the wide age range. Younger children, ages 6 to 8, may need frequent reassurance about what is being done because they have many fears about physical injury and bodily harm. Show them what to expect during procedures using a set of dolls created for the purpose. For example, use a set with a doctor doll, a nurse doll, and a patient doll, and then have the child tell you what will happen to be sure he or she understands.

Be honest if the child asks, "Will it hurt?" by replying openly: "It may sting for just a few seconds" or "We will give you medicine to make the hurt go away." Answer questions with enough information to satisfy the child, but without overwhelming him or her with information. **Regression**, or returning to earlier behaviors, may occur in school-age children when they feel insecure and threatened by treatments. You may see an 8- or 10-year-old crying, clinging to his or her parent, or having a temper tantrum. Remember to consider the illness and treatment from the child's view to understand the reaction.

Knowledge Connection

Why might a preschooler be at risk for injuries on the playground? At what developmental stage do children need routine health screenings? Give an example of regression in a hospitalized school-age child.

Adolescents

Teens tend to exhibit risk-taking behaviors in cars, motorcycles, and all-terrain vehicles. They often feel invincible and ignore safety rules, such as diving into water without knowing how deep it is. The part of the brain controlling judgment is not yet fully developed.

Safety

To help teens prevent accidents and injuries, caution them about the following safety issues:

- **Experimentation.** Teens may be willing to experiment with alcohol, tobacco, street drugs, and the prescription drugs of others as a way to demonstrate their independence. All of these activities put them at risk for life-threatening consequences.
- **Internet Social Networking.** Adolescents often meet others over the Internet. Many times they are simply meeting other teens who live in other places when they strike up friendships over the Internet. However, the possibility that they are communicating with predators cannot be ruled out. It is extremely important that adolescents not arrange to leave home to meet someone they have communicated with in this venue, especially if no one knows where they are going or why.

• **Firearms.** Even adolescents who have grown up around firearms for hunting and sport can be at risk for injury or death due to accidental or malicious shootings. Adolescents need to know how to handle firearms if those are kept in the home, and how to check that the "safety" is on before handling them. Alcohol and drug use with firearms is a lethal combination.

Health Teaching

While older adolescents often feel that they are very knowledgeable about most aspects of life, they may be operating on misinformation or partial information. It is important that they have complete and accurate information about such topics as sexually transmitted disease, birth control, and pregnancy. Teens may be hesitant to ask for information or be embarrassed about what they do not know. Give teens accurate, factual information in a nonjudgmental way.

Teens are often extremely distressed by the death of another teen, again because they tend to believe that they are indestructible, and the death of a peer contradicts that belief. Teens are easily influenced by others and their experiences. "Epidemics" of teen suicides have occurred when hopelessness or despair seemed to be contagious. Be supportive and caring when an adolescent experiences the suicide of a friend or even a mere acquaintance, and allow him or her to verbalize feelings without judging.

Nursing Implications for Hospitalized Adolescents

It is important to allow hospitalized adolescents to have some control over their schedules and environment. Keep in mind that the peer group is the most important to a teen, so the visitors they want to see will be other adolescents. Respect the teen's wishes to either have a parent present or not during examinations and procedures. Treat adolescents with respect and dignity. Avoid saying things that sound like you may be talking down to them. Ask what the adolescent patient knows about his or her illness before beginning any patient teaching.

Knowledge Connection
Why are teens likely to take risks? What are two things to consider when giving care to a hospitalized adolescent?

Supervision/Delegation Connection

Delegating the Care of Infants and Children
As a licensed nurse, you are responsible for all care given to patients who are assigned to you. You are also responsible for the supervision of unlicensed personnel whenever care or tasks are assigned to them. When delegating care of children to unlicensed personnel, you are responsible to ensure that the care provided is appropriate for the age of the patient. Ensure that the unlicensed health care provider is aware of any special actions and concerns for various age groups. For example, an infant should never be left unattended on a changing table.

Stages of Adult Development

Adults continue to develop, experiencing physical, psychosocial, cognitive, moral, and spiritual changes as they age. Adulthood is typically divided into three stages: young adult, middle adult, and older adult.

Young Adult

During this stage, between 19 and 40 years of age, people are often referred to as being "in the prime of their lives." This is due to the maturation of all body systems, the establishment of a career, and the search for meaningful relationships.

Physical Development

Body systems are fully developed and functioning at their optimal level, so many young adults often have no concern for their health. Yet during this time some may begin to experience an increase in cholesterol levels. Women between the ages of 20 and 30 are considered to be at the optimal age for childbearing. People in this age range are often in their best physical condition. The muscles are functioning at the greatest efficiency and coordination is at its peak, giving the young adult an advantage in sports and exercise.

Psychosocial Development

During young adulthood, intimate relationships develop. According to Erikson, the developmental task for this age group is establishing intimacy versus feelings of isolation. Young adults engage in productive work and begin to assume new roles as a husband or wife, and sometimes as parents. Figure 9-9 shows a young couple embarking on these new roles.

Emotional intimacy with family and friends is also a part of this developmental task. They must use introspection to know themselves and to be able to establish healthy relationships with others. Without this, adults of this age group become isolated and self-absorbed, leading to superficial relationships.

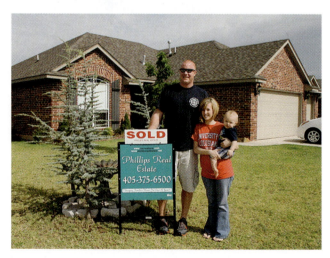

Figure 9-9 This young couple is taking on new roles, both as parents and as homeowners.

Cognitive Development

Young adults become less egocentric, valuing the input and opinions of others. They are able to reason and realistically problem-solve by drawing on experience and researching information. In the first part of young adulthood, they may have completed their basic schooling; however, in the later part of this stage, young adults may continue their education to obtain advanced degrees or certifications to be able to move up the career ladder.

Moral and Spiritual Development

Each adult develops a value system that is based on his or her beliefs and principles. This is how they define right and wrong. Young adults are able to see things within the context of setting rather than always in moral absolutes. This is the postconventional stage of moral development, according to Kohlberg. An example of this type of thinking would be that the young adult believes that injuring another person is wrong, but that to knock an intruder unconscious is not wrong because the person is protecting his or her family and possessions.

Young adults benefit from a spiritual support system that is based on their beliefs. During this time, they may return to the faith of their childhood, especially when they start their own family. They may feel a need to bring up their children with the faith of their family and roots.

Patient Teaching Connection

Teaching About Child Safety

Young adults starting families may need instruction on child safety. Teach parents of toddlers the importance of safety to prevent accidental deaths. You can do this in two ways: teach parents about the developmental stage of the toddler and about the causes of accidents so they can work to maintain their child's safety.

Motor vehicle accidents are one cause of injury and death among toddlers. Encourage parents to use car seats correctly. Teach them about the importance of vigilance when driving in areas where toddlers may be playing. It is very difficult to see a small child when you are backing up or pulling into a driveway. In addition, a child this age may dart out in front of a car without realizing it is dangerous.

Middle Adult

During the middle adult years, which are the years between 40 and 65 years of age, adults are concerned with being productive in both family life and work. Their accomplishments in these areas contribute to feelings of success and satisfaction.

Physical Development

During middle adulthood, the capacity for physical exertion decreases somewhat. It is still important for adults to engage in physical exercise to maintain cardiovascular health because the blood vessels lose some of their elasticity and blood pressure may elevate. During the late middle years, they may notice a decrease in the sensations of heat and cold. Gastrointestinal motility slows, which may cause constipation. There is loss of skin elasticity and subcutaneous tissue, which can lead to wrinkles. Hair begins to lose pigment and turn gray. There is a slight decrease in muscle tone and bone density. It is during middle age that women experience decreased production of estrogen and progesterone, resulting in menopause. Men have a decrease in testosterone, resulting in a decrease in viable sperm.

Psychosocial Development

Erikson's stage of development for this group is generativity versus stagnation. *Generativity* means serving the community, doing meaningful work, and influencing the family in a positive way. Middle adults who are comfortable with their successes generally feel good about themselves and their lives. They may volunteer and become active in the community. During this time, roles change within the family. Middle adults can find themselves caring for their aging parents as well as their adolescent children. They are often referred to as the "sandwich generation" for this reason. At this age, they may experience the "empty-nest syndrome" because their children leave home. However, they also may help raise their grandchildren. If they do not see themselves as achieving goals, they stagnate and focus only on themselves.

Cognitive Development

Middle-age adults reflect on the past and anticipate the future. They are able to learn new things, but their reaction time is slower. They need more time to learn complex tasks, but they are very accurate once the task is mastered.

Moral and Spiritual Development

Middle adults may reassess their values and beliefs. It may become important to help others live out their beliefs. Laws are obeyed because they protect the rights and welfare of others. According to Kohlberg, this is the postconventional stage of moral development.

Faith is a source of comfort as adults of this age seek meaning in their life experiences. They may find it easier to deal with illness and death in a framework of the significance of life.

Older Adult

Aging is a process that begins at birth and continues throughout the life span. Encourage older adults, those adults ages 65 years and older, to adopt a healthy lifestyle. It is important to understand that the changes brought about by aging are not indicative of disease.

Physical Development

Older adults experience a variety of changes in their physical condition due to the process of aging. They lose 2½ inches of height with each decade of life after age 30. The nose and ears continue to grow longer because they are made of cartilage and not bone. Table 9-4 describes changes that occur in each body system due to aging.

Table 9-4 Physical Changes in the Older Adult

System	Changes
Respiratory	The lung capacity is decreased due to the muscles of the respiratory system being less flexible and to changes in the skeletal structure of the rib cage. There is also a decrease in the effectiveness of the cough reflex.
Cardiovascular	The heart requires more time to recover after intense activity, and there is a decrease in cardiac output. The blood vessels have loss of elasticity, which can lead to hypertension.
Urinary	There is a decrease in the ability to filter waste from the blood. Bladder capacity decreases, and due to decrease of muscle tone, there is difficulty emptying the bladder completely and stress incontinence.
Gastrointestinal	The taste buds decrease in number. Choking and gag reflex decrease. Peristalsis of the gastrointestinal tract decreases. Liver function also diminishes, and the gallbladder is slower to empty.
Musculoskeletal	Muscles decrease in mass and tone. There is decrease in bone density. Degeneration of joints occurs due to "wear and tear" from use.
Neurological	The blood flow and oxygen use in the brain decrease. There are fewer neurons in the brain. Increased time is required to perform tasks that require speed, coordination, fine motor skills, and balance. Sleep disturbances occur. Short-term memory may decrease.
Sensory	The lens of the eye becomes less able to focus and the pupil does not accommodate as easily. There is also less lacrimal gland secretion. In the ears, there is a decrease in flexibility of the pinna and the number of neurons in the cochlea decreases.
Endocrine	The response of the endocrine organs to their target hormones decreases with age. The basal metabolic rate also decreases gradually. The body cells become less sensitive to the effects of insulin, causing an increased incidence of diabetes mellitus in older adults. Production of the sex hormones, estrogen and testosterone, also decreases.
Reproductive	With the decrease of estrogen, the pelvic organs decrease in size and elasticity. Breast tissue decreases. There is still a need for sexual intimacy and companionship for both men and women. In men, testosterone production decreases. There is a diminished size of the testicles. Sperm count decreases and the prostate gland may enlarge.

Psychosocial Development

As older adults reflect on their lives, it is important that they feel a sense of accomplishment. Erikson described this developmental task as integrity versus despair. As older adults think back over their lives, an activity known as *reminiscence,* they often experience feelings of satisfaction and worth. However, if they feel that their life has had little meaning, they tend toward despair. At this stage, older adults have wisdom to share with younger people and may focus on helping others and engaging in meaningful activities.

Cognitive Development

There is no decline in the older person's IQ. Reaction time slows and short-term memory recall decreases while long-term memory remains unchanged. Older adults can still learn new things, but it requires more time and repeated practice to master a new skill than when they were younger (Fig. 9-10).

Moral and Spiritual Development

Older adults base moral decisions on their own principles and beliefs. They can respect the values of others even though they differ. Older adults may feel more freedom to act on their beliefs.

As people age, they begin to see their friends and family members die. Older adults may experience the loss of many friends over the last years of their lives. Their spiritual beliefs often help them deal with the grief of losing friends and loved ones.

Health Concerns for Young, Middle, and Older Adults

When you care for adults, it is important to remember the challenges that they face in their own development. While we are unlikely to see a young adult as having the same concerns as an older adult, we often neglect to consider the issues of safety, health teaching, and nursing implications for adults.

Figure 9-10 These older people are learning new skills using the computer.

Safety

When you care for young adults, keep in mind that they may have concerns for their children while they are not at home to assume their usual roles. It is important for young adults to provide a safe environment in the home, which includes fire safety. Families need to have a plan for how they will escape and where they will meet in case of fire. The adults need to be sure there are working smoke detectors in the home. It is also important for them to model safe behavior for their children during play and recreational activities.

Middle adults may have more concerns about workplace safety. They know that they should follow all safety guidelines, but sometimes they neglect to do so, even when serious injury can occur. Other injuries at this life stage may be due to overexertion when they have not been very active. Damage to muscles and connective tissue may occur when middle adults take on a strenuous project even though they are not used to performing that kind of work.

Older adults are most at risk for injury from falls. This may be due to poor balance, poor vision, or some type of illness. They have very fragile skin that tears easily, leaving them at risk for infections. Adults in this age group may also be abused by caregivers. *Safety: Always be alert for signs of abuse and report them immediately.* Such signs would include unexplained bruises, unexplained fractures or old fractures that appear on x-rays that were never treated, burns that do not match the explanation of how they happened, and an overall fearful attitude by the older adult toward a caregiver.

Health Teaching

Encourage young adults to have yearly physical examinations and screenings for tuberculosis and other diseases. Teach breast self-examination to women and testicular self-examination to men. Encourage regular exercise for cardiovascular health and healthy lifestyle choices, such as staying at a healthy weight, making wise food choices, not smoking, and avoiding excessive alcohol use.

Monitor blood pressure and cholesterol levels of middle-age adults to detect and treat cardiovascular problems early. Encourage them to have vision screenings for *presbyopia* (farsightedness that develops with aging), cataracts, and glaucoma. Early treatment of some eye disorders can prevent

serious vision problems later. Encourage regular mammograms to detect breast cancer and regular blood tests to detect prostate cancer. Middle-age adults need to be screened regularly for the development of diabetes.

Many older adults have chronic illnesses that must be monitored, such as diabetes, heart disease, and lung disease. Encourage them to see their health care professionals on a regular basis for this. They need to obtain influenza vaccines each year and the pneumonia vaccine as well. Some older adults experience confusion, dementia, or Alzheimer's disease. This is not a normal part of aging but a disease process. It is important that they be diagnosed and followed closely to prevent possible injuries or dangers. Adults at this age have decreased kidney and liver function, which can lead to medication toxicity. They need to have blood work done on a regular basis to determine whether toxicity may be occurring.

Nursing Implications for Hospitalized Adults

When younger adults are hospitalized, you must meet their physical needs but you also need to realize that anxiety over finances, work, and care of their children can influence their recovery. Serious health issues are not as common in young adults, so hospitalization may cause great anxiety. Injury and accidents with lasting disability can devastate the entire family. Be very aware of the concerns and anxieties of young adult patients that you care for, keeping in mind their life stage and responsibilities.

Middle adults may have concerns about the care of elderly parents while they are hospitalized. They may experience a great deal of stress due to their inability to meet family responsibilities in addition to missing work. As a nurse, you can listen to their concerns and be a sounding board as they problem-solve about their situation. Encourage them to ask for help from other family members and friends when they are unable to meet those family responsibilities. Sometimes church members or other community groups are available to help so the patient's stress can be relieved and he or she can concentrate on getting well.

When older adults are hospitalized, they may be confused by the change in their environment and routine. They need reassurance frequently. If they are very confused, you can help them remember what is happening by reorienting them to their location, the date, and the time when you are with them. (See Chapter 32 for more information on caring for elderly patients.) While they are hospitalized, it is very important for you to keep them safe. Prevent falls by using bed and chair alarms and other alternatives to restraints. Protect older adults from injury by keeping the area around the bed free of clutter and equipment so they will not trip when they get out of bed. (See Chapter 13 for more information on safety.)

As a nurse who will be caring for patients of all ages, it is important to be knowledgeable about normal growth and development so you can assess patients of all ages and plan the most appropriate care for them.

While death can occur at any age, nurses often care for older patients who are close to death or who die in the hospital. See Chapter 10 for more information on caring for patients at the end of life.

People and Places Connection

Patient Populations in Home Health and Long-Term Care

Home health care and long-term care have typically been associated with the older adult. In the past, a major function of home health care was to help elders remain at home. Today, with shortened hospital stays, home health care is needed by patients of all ages to assist them with care they still need when they are discharged from the hospital. Home health care provides such things as dressing changes, IV medications, and care of drainage tubes.

This change from the past is also true of long-term care facilities. Today young and middle-age adults often stay in nursing facilities after they are discharged from a hospital. They may be there to recuperate from surgeries, injuries, or illnesses that require additional care, even though they can no longer remain in the hospital.

Real-World Connection

A School Nurse Supervisor's Experience

While working in a large urban school district in the southwestern part of the United States as a school nurse supervisor, I was responsible to ensure that children with complex nursing needs at the school were provided with appropriate care and for the training of the school nurses and staff. My biggest challenge was when I was asked to evaluate a 3-year-old female who was a quadriplegic and ventilator dependent and had a pacemaker. My job was to determine the care needed by this child so she could attend preschool 3½ hours a day. Assessing the nursing needs of this child was challenging since she continued to say "NO" to any question I asked her. She had been in the hospital for over a year, and her parents were very concerned about her entry into school. They needed detailed explanations about how her needs would be met at school. I arranged for the parents to visit the school and spend time in the classroom to increase their confidence that their child would be safe. A nurse was hired and trained specifically on the nursing needs of this child, as well as spending time interacting and playing with the child to establish a relationship and trust. The first day the child attended school, her parents spent time in the classroom. The time that I took to establish a relationship with this child and her parents, as well as the special training for the nurse and school staff, helped this child have a successful school experience for many years.

 Post Conference

In post conference, you had a lot to share. You felt good about the care you provided. Even though José is 16, he was terrified about having a heart problem. You recognized his moodiness as fear and feeling out of control. You were able to establish rapport with him, and he talked openly to you about his concerns: What would happen to his planned basketball career? Would he live a long life or a short one? The doctor gave him his answers. He is going to have to take medications, but he should be able to live a long and healthy life, including playing basketball.

His sister asked you a question about her baby, and that gave you the opportunity to teach her a bit about infant nutrition. His grandmother felt ill and you were able to encourage her to see her physician. His 12-year-old brother was crying in the hallway because he was afraid José would die, so you were able to reassure and comfort him. And now you understand better how a nurse responds to the needs of the whole family at varying stages of the life span.

KEY POINTS

- Growth of the body includes lengthening of the trunk and extremities and other physical changes in size.
- Development refers to the increasing skills and behavioral changes such as walking, talking, and meeting milestones in abilities.
- A variety of factors can delay or prevent growth and development. These include biological and hereditary factors, environmental factors, and social factors.
- Physical development occurs in an orderly, predictable fashion from the head down and the center of the body out. This is known as a cephalocaudal and proximodistal pattern.
- Psychosocial development requires the completion of specific tasks in each stage of life in order to move successfully to the next stage. This is based on the theory of Erik Erikson.

- Cognitive development involves the progression of learning throughout life, from learning cause and effect at an early age, to concrete problem-solving during the school years, to analytical problem-solving as an adult. This is based on the theory of Jean Piaget.

- Moral development refers to establishing a value system, distinguishing right from wrong, and the motivations for moral behavior. Lawrence Kohlberg has developed this theory of moral development.

- Spiritual development occurs as children first imitate their parents' beliefs and behaviors, learn about religion through symbolism and stories, then develop their own beliefs. James Fowler has developed this theory of spiritual development.

- Nurses need to know the principles of growth and development to assess patients for needs that relate to them. We can plan and implement care for all aspects of patient needs rather than focusing only on the physical needs.

- Infants and toddlers go through rapid changes in physical development. Their psychosocial development is geared to developing trust and autonomy. They develop cognitively through body movement and senses. They learn to do the right thing and avoid the wrong thing to avoid punishment.

- Preschoolers and school-agers grow taller with long limbs. They are learning how to participate in sports and other activities. School-agers master more complex motor skills such as riding bicycles and skating. They develop cognitively very quickly, grasping concepts based on previous experiences and using their imaginations. Morally, they begin learning shades of right and wrong. They learn from their parent's behaviors and through symbolism and stories.

- Adolescents have a growth spurt at the beginning of this life stage. Puberty also occurs at this time, as well as the beginning of sexual function. Adolescents struggle to establish their identity and independence. Cognitively, they are beginning to think logically and are developing problem-solving skills. Moral and spiritual development involves developing their own thoughts and beliefs rather than just accepting those of their parents.

- Adult stages of development include younger, middle, and older adults. The major tasks of these stages are establishing intimacy, generativity, and integrity. Cognitive development remains at the formal operational stage. Moral development focuses on behaving according to their

internal codes and beliefs. Spiritual development involves the ability to understand others' views about faith, with tangible forms of love and justice.

- Safety, health teaching, and nursing implications for patients of all ages must be addressed to provide optimum care for the whole person.

REVIEW QUESTIONS

Select the answer that is most appropriate for each of the following questions. Some questions may have more than one correct answer. Check all that apply.

1. Growth that progresses from the head downward is known as what type of pattern?

   a. Caudalocephal

   b. Cephalocaudal

   c. Proximodistal

   d. Distoproximal

2. When an infant cries, a caregiver comes to give comfort so the infant learns that her needs will be met. This is an example of:

   a. the theory of physical development.

   b. Piaget's theory of cognitive development.

   c. Kohlberg's theory of moral development.

   d. Erikson's theory of psychosocial development.

3. You are caring for a 10-year-old child who has had major surgery. When you get ready to change his dressing, he begins to scream at you and even tries to hit and bite you. This is an example of:

   a. lack of cognitive development.

   b. attachment behavior.

   c. regression.

   d. lack of moral development.

4. A 16-year-old girl comes to the clinic where you work. She is diagnosed with a sexually transmitted disease. She tells you she is worried that she might be pregnant. Which is the best response for you to make?

   a. "Would you like to have a pregnancy test and find out for sure?"

   b. "Do your parents know about this?"

   c. "If you are pregnant, I hope you don't plan to keep the baby!"

   d. "You should not be sexually active at your age."

5. Which of the following would be of concern to you when you assess a 3-month-old infant?

   a. Rooting reflex is absent.

   b. Sucking reflex is present.

   c. Posterior fontanel is closed.

   d. Infant does not move arms and legs.

   e. Infant grasps your finger and attempts to put it in his mouth.

   Identify which factor will cause a delay in growth and development for the following children. Write a B for biological/hereditary factors, an E for environmental factors, and an S for social factors.

6. A child born with spina bifida who is paralyzed from the waist down: ____

7. A child who has been sexually abused and does not behave appropriately around other children: ____

8. A child who was exposed to industrial-strength pesticide and suffered brain damage as a result: ____

CRITICAL THINKING EXERCISES

9. You are caring for a hospitalized 2-year-old. The toddler has a temper tantrum when you bring in his evening medications. Why is this happening? What will you do?

10. A 45-year-old woman is admitted to the hospital with extremely elevated blood pressure. She seems anxious, and you hear her on the phone telling her 17-year-old son to go check on his grandparents. You can tell the conversation did not go well. How can you help meet this patient's needs? What will you say?

ADDITIONAL RESOURCES

For additional Resources, Questions, and Activities, please see:

 Student Resource Disk

 http://davisplus.fadavis.com

Student Study Guide

REFERENCES

Centers for Disease Control and Prevention. Child development and public health. October 6, 2009. Available at: http://www.cdc.gov/ncbddd/child/development.htm. Accessed August 10, 2009.

Centers for Disease Control and Prevention. Health topics: childhood obesity. October 20, 2008. Available at: http://www.cdc.gov/healthyyouth/obesity/. Accessed August 10, 2009.

Centers for Disease Control and Prevention. Legacy for children. September 20, 2005. Available at: http://www.cdc.gov/ncbddd/child/legacy.htm. Accessed August 10, 2009.

Centers for Disease Control and Prevention. Using developmental screening to improve children's health. September 20, 2005. Available at: http://www.cdc.gov/ncbddd/child/improve.htm. Accessed August 10, 2009.

Daeg de Mott DK. Kohlberg's theory of moral reasoning. *Encyclopedia of Childhood and Adolescence* [serial online]. April 6, 2001. Available at: http://www.findarticles.com. Accessed August 1, 2009.

Dillon P. *Nursing Health Assessment: A Critical Thinking, Case Studies Approach.* 2nd ed. Philadelphia: FA Davis; 2007.

Erikson EH. *The Life Cycle Completed.* New York: Norton; 1997.

Feldman R. *Development Across the Life Span.* 5th ed. Upper Saddle River, New Jersey: Pearson Education; 2008.

Piaget J. *Origins of Intelligence in Children.* New York: Norton; 1966.

Polan E, Taylor D. *Journey Across the Life Span: Human Development and Health Promotion.* Philadelphia: FA Davis; 2007.

Wilkinson J, Van Leuven K. *Fundamentals of Nursing: Theory, Concepts and Application.* Philadelphia: FA Davis; 2007.

Loss, Grief, and Dying

Key Terms

Advance directive

Apnea

Circumoral cyanosis

Comorbidity

Do-not-resuscitate (DNR) order

Durable power of attorney

Euthanasia

Grief

Hospice

Living will

Mottling

Palliative care

Postmortem care

Respite

Role reversal

Objectives

1. Define key terms related to loss, death, and grief.
2. Explain the difference between curative care, palliative care, and hospice care.
3. Describe the function of each of the following documents: durable power of attorney, living will, do-not-resuscitate order.
4. Explain the traditional five stages of grief.
5. List at least five symptoms indicating end-stage disease.
6. Describe at least four beneficial effects of dehydration at the end of life.
7. Identify comments the patient might make indicating that he or she desires to discuss a terminal condition.

Skills

10-1 Postmortem Care

Clinical Connection

Your Assignment: You have been assigned to care for a 68-year-old woman with lung cancer that has *metastasized* (spread) to the brain. Your instructor pulls you aside when you arrive at clinical to explain that your patient is now actively dying. You ask for a different patient, but your instructor tells you that this patient needs your care, even if she is dying. You are terrified. You have never seen anyone die before, and you don't know what to expect.

Your Actions: Should you talk to this patient as you would other patients, or should you be silent because she is dying? Should you give her a bath? Or should you not disturb her for something as mundane as a bath? What if you are in the room with her when she dies? Should you call for help? What will you do after she dies? What will you say to her family, or should you say anything at all? What if you say the wrong thing?

Throughout your nursing career, many medical treatment decisions will become routine. Your patient will be sick. The physician will examine the patient, perform diagnostic studies and laboratory tests, and then prescribe treatment. The treatment plan will be followed, and your patient will get better.

However, as your patients become increasingly elderly and, subsequently, more ill, medical decisions and treatments can become more complex. Factors such as comorbidity (multiple diseases), dependence on others, and terminal illness can change the landscape of treatment choices open to them. As chronic illness takes a terminal trajectory, some medical treatments offer little benefit; others can even present potential harm.

In Chapter 3, we discussed the importance of ethics and patients' rights in the general field of nursing. In this chapter, we will provide you with an even deeper look at ethics and patients' rights: those of patients for whom there is no hope of a cure, those who have suffered great losses, and those who are grieving death. In preparation for these eventualities, we will guide you in determining what this means to you the nurse and how to better use the gift you are given when you have the opportunity to assist your patients and their families who are experiencing loss, grief, and even dying.

Dealing With the Terminal Patient

As your patients face difficult life situations, you must be prepared with skill and understanding to help them face serious illness, loss, and death. You must be able to provide them information and referrals to the resources that they will need to make the best decisions. In order to do this well, you will need to think through your own feelings on these issues. What are your attitudes toward aging, cancer, chronic illness, and the losses they represent? How do you feel about withholding treatment that may prolong life, but not improve the quality of that life? Providing or withholding artificial

nutrition and hydration can be controversial, even for health care providers. Naturally, these choices can be confusing and even frightening for patients and their families. Fearful patients may consider suicide or assisted suicide, or even ask you about euthanasia. Do not allow this to frighten you.

Professionals involved with end-of-life care feel strongly that, when fear is relieved, pain is managed, and needs for reconciliation are met, patients can approach loss and death without fear and with a sense of peace. When your patient understands that he or she will be honored and his or her dignity will be maintained, the issues of assisted suicide and euthanasia often become "nonissues." *However, it is important to note that, in Oregon, it is legal for the physician to write a mentally competent, terminally ill patient a prescription for a lethal dose of a Schedule II drug with which to commit suicide, once the patient has asked twice.*

Respect for human dignity is the fundamental principle when making your ethical decisions for practice. When you care for all patients, you are called upon to honor their values and beliefs, even if those values are not the same as your own. Although you do not agree, you are still expected to honor the patient's choices and see him or her as a person worthy of respect. When caring for patients who are dying, you will provide support to the patient, family, and significant others. You are expected to support the values and beliefs that the patient has exhibited in life even though they may be different from your own.

Medicating the Dying Patient

It is your responsibility to do everything you can to prevent a patient from needlessly suffering. Some patients worry that use of pain medications might result in addiction. Teach the patient that addiction is not a concern during the terminal stages of illness. Let the patient know that it is every individual's right to die with dignity and comfort. Teach the patient that pain is easier to control if medicated before it becomes severe. Encourage the patient to request pain medications as soon as he or she feels the need, that it is not necessary to try to *tough it out.*

Depending upon the cultural beliefs of the patient, use of pain medication may not be acceptable. Some cultures, such as Hindu and Asian American, feel that pain is to be suffered stoically. Tables 8-2 and 8-3 in Chapter 8 discuss further cultural beliefs that may affect your care of the dying. You will want to follow a code of ethics as you provide nursing care for various cultures with different beliefs:

The American Nurses Association Code of Ethics for Nurses: Provision I

"The nurse, in all professional relationships, practices with compassion and respect for the inherent dignity, worth, and uniqueness of every individual, unrestricted by consideration of social or economic status, personal attributes or the nature of health problems."

Source: Reprinted with permission from American Nurses Association, Code of Ethics for Nurses with Interpretive Statements, ©2001 Nursesbooks.org, Silver Spring, MD.

You may read all nine provisions of the code in Chapter 3, Box 3-1. You can find the entire American Nurses Association (ANA) Code of Ethics for Nurses With Interpretive Statements at *http://www.nursingworld.org/ethics/ code/protected_nwcoe813.htm#1.*

The ANA's Code of Ethics for Nurses clearly indicates that for a nurse to do anything to a patient with the purpose of ending his or her life is not an acceptable action, even if the nurse feels that he or she would be helping the patient or relieving the patient's suffering. In other words, it is not acceptable to assist a patient in suicide or to knowingly administer an unsafe dosage of medication that will most likely kill the patient, known as **euthanasia**. However, this does not relieve your responsibility to help provide as much comfort as possible and relieve fear and anxiety as death comes near. While most narcotic pain medications lower blood pressure and slow respirations, it is important that you remember that the disease process is what is killing the patient, not the normal doses of pain medication. Even so, if the patient already has low blood pressure and slower-than-normal respirations, you may have concerns about whether to give the pain medication. If you do have this concern, it must be overcome. If the patient has a do-not-resuscitate (DNR) order, according to the interpretive statements of the ANA Code of Ethics for Nurses, your first concern should be to relieve the patient's pain and dyspnea...yes, even if it could hasten respiratory or cardiac arrest.

Real-World Connection

To Give the Medication or Not?

A young RN had been providing nursing care for several months to a 32-year-old female patient in the terminal stages of breast cancer, with bone and brain metastases. She has a

DNR order. One morning as the nurse came on duty, she found the patient nonresponsive to verbal stimulus, but moaning in response to even gentle *tactile* (touch) stimulus. The patient was pale, clammy, restless, and dyspneic, with labored respirations at 10 to 12 per minute, and her Foley drainage bag was still empty, as it had been throughout the previous shift. Several family members sat quietly next to the bed, at times holding the patient's hand, stroking her brow, and whispering softly to her. One of the family members whispered to the nurse, "Please don't let her hurt. We just want her to be comfortable." The patient had been receiving small doses of morphine sulfate IV at 1-hour intervals, as needed, with good pain relief. The nurse administered the next dose of morphine and the patient's respirations eased, her restlessness calmed, and the moaning stopped. But within 30 minutes, the patient was once again restless, dyspneic with respirations 10 per minute, and moaning. So the nurse phoned the physician and asked if the morphine could be given more frequently than every hour. The physician gave the order to give the medication as often as every 30 minutes if needed to keep the patient comfortable. The nurse administered the morphine, which once again seemed to calm the patient's restlessness and ease her respiratory distress. But within 20 to 25 minutes the patient was having severe dyspnea, respirations were 8 per minute, her heart rate was irregular, and she was moaning continually with each breath. As the nurse administered the next dose of morphine, when about half of the dose was delivered, the patient's respirations dropped to 2 to 3 per minute, and then ceased. Without completing the administration of the morphine, the nurse got her stethoscope and auscultated for heart sounds and breath sounds. A few weak, irregular heartbeats were detected. As the nurse continued to listen with her stethoscope, her tears fell onto the patient's chest as the patient's heart sounds faded away completely.

It is time to do a little reflection before you go on: Have you examined your own feelings regarding terminal illness, dying, and death? How do your personal ethics impact your nursing practice in the areas of assisted suicide and euthanasia? What is your definition of death with dignity? For you, what would represent a dignified death?

Knowledge Connection

When you make your ethical decisions during nursing practice, what is the fundamental principle you must remember? Why should you honor patients' values and beliefs even when they are not the same as your values and beliefs? Explain what euthanasia is and how it differs from assisted suicide. What is the ANA's stance regarding assisted suicide and euthanasia?

Palliative Care and Hospice Care

You may think of nursing as *curative* or healing, and many aspects of nursing do fall within this realm. *Curative care* is that in which medications, treatments, and various therapies are provided with the intent of healing or curing a patient's illness. However, there are aspects of nursing care, known as palliative care and hospice care, that do not heal or cure the disease process; both are areas of growing specialty within the medical community. Hospice and palliative care offer a compassionate and humane approach to end-of-life care that maintains a patient's autonomy and dignity when facing what can be a very frightening time for the patient and his or her family.

Palliative care, or comfort care, is physician directed but is not intended to cure the patient's disease. It incorporates medication administration, nursing care, and other therapies that are performed to alleviate uncomfortable symptoms such as pain, nausea and vomiting, and dyspnea. Though this type of care may include advanced, aggressive interventions such as chemotherapy, surgery, and radiation, it is important to understand that these therapies are not performed as life-saving measures. For example, even though a patient may have cancer that is too advanced to be curable, surgery may be performed to debulk a large tumor to provide pain relief and alleviate other distressing symptoms. Whether at home, in acute care hospitals, or in long-term care facilities, patients who receive palliative care services *may* have a life expectancy of more than 6 months.

Hospice services are designed and available for patients in the later stages of terminal illness and do not commonly include measures meant to cure or stop the natural process of dying. Generally, hospice patients are thought to be in their final 6 months of life, and as with palliative care, the focus is more on comfort than on cure. Patient and family wishes are followed as the primary direction for care. The primary functions of the interdisciplinary hospice team include:

- Relieving patient pain and discomfort
- Lessening patient and family fears and anxiety
- Actively including the patient and family in both patient care and decision making
- Providing both the patient and the family emotional support through the various stages of the grieving process
- Providing respite for the caregivers

The family caregivers may be staying with the patient 24 hours a day, 7 days a week, which is extremely emotionally and physically draining. Providing **respite** means to make arrangements for provision of care in order that the family members may have a time to get away, rest, and rejuvenate without the strain and worry of continual caregiving. Even a period as brief as 3 to 4 hours can provide temporary relief for the family members.

As the team member at the bedside, you are often the coordinator of this team, playing the role of teacher, advocate, and manager to promote best practices for your patient. This is one of those times when you can have a profound impact on a life. By providing holistic patient-centered care and support, and by demonstrating your confidence, knowledge, and skills, you can help bring not only physical comfort, but also peace and a sense of life's quality to your patient at the end of his or her life.

Knowledge Connection

Explain what is meant by palliative care and hospice care. How do they differ from acute care nursing? What is meant by respite care?

Living Until They Die

Preparing for the eventuality of one's own death is not an easy task for most people in our society. But, given the time to consider the subject, most can tell you what they do not want at the time of their death:

- They do not want to die in pain.
- They do not want to die alone.
- They do not want to be a burden to their family.

Often included in this thought of "not wanting to be a burden" is the statement that they "would not want to be kept on machines" in a hopeless situation. Some will even go so far as to say that they would like to die at home, surrounded by the things and the people they love.

End-of-Life Documentation

Getting your patient to consider addressing end-of-life decisions is the first step. Once the decisions are made, however, some documentation is needed in order for there to be the assurance that these wishes will be carried out. When a competent individual documents these wishes ahead of time, it is known as an **advance directive** (Fig. 10-1). It can be accomplished with either a living will or a durable power of attorney (DPA).

Living Will

A **living will** is a written document prepared by a mentally competent patient, indicating which procedures and measures the patient does or does not want, should an end-of-life condition or disability occur. It may include surgeries, medications, intubation, ventilation, or other extraordinary life-sustaining measures. Many living wills also include instructions on whether or not to provide IV fluids or artificial methods of feeding such as feeding tubes if the patient becomes unable to eat and drink normally.

Durable Power of Attorney

While many people have wills in place so that their estates can be administered quickly and efficiently when they die, most individuals never think about who would make decisions for them should they become disabled or lose the ability to make health-related decisions.

A legal court document that grants the authority to make health care decisions and act as proxy for the patient should the patient become disabled is known as a **durable power of attorney**. This power is usually bestowed upon

Oklahoma Advance Directive for Health Care

If I am incapable of making an informed decision regarding my health care, I direct my health care providers to follow my instructions below.

I. Living Will

If my attending physician and another physician determine that I am no longer able to make decisions regarding my health care, I direct my attending physician and other health care providers, pursuant to the Oklahoma Advance Directive Act, to follow my instructions as set forth
below:

(1) If I have a terminal condition, that is, an incurable and irreversible condition that even with the administration of life-sustaining treatment will, in the opinion of the attending physician and another physician, result in death within six (6) months:

(Initial only one option)

_____ I direct that my life not be extended by life-sustaining treatment, except that if I am unable to take food and water by mouth, I wish to receive artificially administered nutrition and hydration.

_____ I direct that my life not be extended by life-sustaining treatment, including artificially administered nutrition and hydration.

_____ I direct that I be given life-sustaining treatment and, if I am unable to take food and water by mouth, I wish to receive artificially administered nutrition and hydration.

(Initial only if applicable)

_____ See my more specific instructions in paragraph (4) below.

(2) If I am persistently unconscious, that is, I have an irreversible condition, as determined by the attending physician and another physician, in which thought and awareness of self and environment are absent:

(Initial only one option)

_____ I direct that my life not be extended by life-sustaining treatment, except that if I am unable to take food and water by mouth, I wish to receive artificially administered nutrition and hydration.

_____ I direct that my life not be extended by life-sustaining treatment, including artificially administered nutrition and hydration.

_____ I direct that I be given life-sustaining treatment and, if I am unable to take food and water by mouth, I wish to receive artificially administered nutrition and hydration.

(Initial only if applicable)

_____ See my more specific instructions in paragraph (4) below.

(3) If I have an end-stage condition, that is, a condition caused by injury, disease, or illness, which results in severe and permanent deterioration indicated by incompetency and complete physical dependency for which treatment of the irreversible condition would be medically ineffective:

(Initial only one option)

_____ I direct that my life not be extended by life-sustaining treatment, except that if I am unable to take food and water by mouth, I wish to receive artificially administered nutrition and hydration.

_____ I direct that my life not be extended by life-sustaining treatment, including artificially administered nutrition and hydration.

_____ I direct that I be given life-sustaining treatment and, if I am unable to take food and water by mouth, I wish to receive artificially administered nutrition and hydration.

(Initial only if applicable)

_____ See my more specific instructions in paragraph (4) below.

Figure 10-1 Oklahoma's Advance Directive for Health Care.

(4) OTHER. Here you may:

(a) describe other conditions in which you would want life-sustaining treatment or artificially administered nutrition and hydration provided, withheld, or withdrawn,

(b) give more specific instructions about your wishes concerning life-sustaining treatment or artificially administered nutrition and hydration if you have a terminal condition, are persistently unconscious, or have an end-stage condition, or

(c) do both of these:

_____

_____

_____
Initial

II. My Appointment of My Health Care Proxy

If my attending physician and another physician determine that I am no longer able to make decisions regarding my health care, I direct my attending physician and other health care providers pursuant to the Oklahoma Advance Directive Act to follow the instructions of _____, whom I appoint as my health care proxy. If my health care proxy is unable or unwilling to serve, I appoint _____ as my alternate health care proxy with the same authority. My health care proxy is authorized to make whatever health care decisions I could make if I were able, except that decisions regarding life-sustaining treatment and artificially administered nutrition and hydration can be made by my health care proxy or alternate health care proxy only as I have indicated in the foregoing sections.

If I fail to designate a health care proxy in this section, I am deliberately declining to designate a health care proxy.

III. Anatomical Gifts

Pursuant to the provisions of the Uniform Anatomical Gift Act, I direct that at the time of my death my entire body or designated body organs or body parts be donated for purposes of:

(Initial all that apply)

_____ Transplantation therapy

_____ Advancement of medical science, research, or education

_____ Advancement of dental science, research, or education

Death means either irreversible cessation of circulatory and respiratory functions or irreversible cessation of all functions of the entire brain, including the brain stem. If I initial the "yes" line below, I specifically donate:

_____ My entire body

or

_____ The following body organs or parts:

_____ lungs		_____ liver
_____ pancreas		_____ heart
_____ kidneys		_____ brain
_____ skin		_____ bones/marrow
_____ blood/fluids		_____ tissue
_____ arteries		_____ eyes/cornea/lens

Figure 10-1 cont'd

IV. General Provisions

a. I understand that I must be eighteen (18) years of age or older to execute this form.

b. I understand that my witnesses must be eighteen (18) years of age or older and shall not be related to me and shall not inherit from me.

c. I understand that if I have been diagnosed as pregnant and that diagnosis is known to my attending physician, I will be provided with life-sustaining treatment and artificially administered hydration and nutrition unless I have, in my own words, specifically authorized that during a course of pregnancy, life-sustaining treatment and/or artificially administered hydration and/or nutrition shall be withheld or withdrawn.

d. In the absence of my ability to give directions regarding the use of life-sustaining procedures, it is my intention that this advance directive shall be honored by my family and physicians as the final expression of my legal right to choose or refuse medical or surgical treatment including, but not limited to, the administration of life sustaining procedures, and I accept the consequences of such choice or refusal.

e. This advance directive shall be in effect until it is revoked.

f. I understand that I may revoke this advance directive at any time.

g. I understand and agree that if I have any prior directives, and if I sign this advance directive, my prior directives are revoked.

h. I understand the full importance of this advance directive and I am emotionally and mentally competent to make this advance directive.

i. I understand that my physician(s) shall make all decisions based upon his or her best judgment applying with ordinary care and diligence the knowledge and skill that is possessed and used by members of the physician's profession in good standing engaged in the same field of practice at that time, measured by national standards.

Signed this _____ day of _____, 20____.

_____
Signature

_____
City of

_____
County, Oklahoma

_____
Date of birth (Optional for identification purposes)

This advance directive was signed in my presence.

_____
Signature of Witness

_____, OK
Residence

_____
Signature of Witness

_____, OK
Residence

Figure 10-1 cont'd

someone the patient trusts, such as a relative, a friend, or even a trusted financial institution such as the patient's bank. Without a durable power of attorney, health care decisions may be left to the legal hierarchy of family relationships, which usually is as follows:

• Legal guardian with health care decision-making authority
• Spouse
• Adult children of patient
• Parents of patient
• Adult siblings of patient

However, when there are no legal instructions dictating how to handle these situations, it can be left to the state courts to appoint a guardian to make these decisions, and the court may not select the person that the patient or family would choose. This can prove to be time consuming, expensive, and stressful for the patient's loved ones.

Do-Not-Resuscitate Order
A **do-not-resuscitate (DNR) order** is an order written by the patient's physician meaning that, should the patient's heart and respirations cease, no cardiopulmonary resuscitation or

other efforts to restart the heart and breathing should be performed—a serious and obviously life-ending measure with which you may find it difficult to comply.

History of DNR Orders

During the 1960s, researchers developed the techniques involved in cardiopulmonary resuscitation (CPR) as a means of rescuing victims of sudden death, when a person's heart or breathing stops. Originally, CPR was intended for use in situations such as drowning or electrical shock, or when an otherwise healthy person experienced complications of a heart attack, such as ventricular fibrillation. Early guidelines stated that there were certain cases when CPR should not be used. Researchers at the time felt it was clearly a violation of a person's right to die with dignity when resuscitation was attempted in cases of terminal, irreversible illness. Today, however, CPR has become the standard-of-care procedure for all patients in hospitals and nursing homes who experience respiratory or cardiac arrest, unless there are specific physician's orders stating "Do Not Resuscitate."

Following a DNR Order

In such conditions as advanced metastatic cancer or end-stage AIDS or renal failure, attempts at CPR are frequently futile. When CPR is successful in restoring breathing and circulation in a patient in an advanced stage of terminal disease, the patient is often revived only to suffer further pain and fear until death finally provides relief of suffering. Because the chain of events puts the start of CPR into motion, your patient could be placed on a ventilator even though he or she might not have wanted it. For many, this risk of prolonged survival "on machines" is a very serious burden. These rather grim thoughts should cause us to look at the ethical and compassionate considerations of performing such procedures on those who have life-limiting illness.

When caring for the patient with a life-limiting illness, it is important for you to remember that it is your responsibility to be an advocate for the delivery of dignified and humane care. Withholding CPR is medically justified when it is judged to be of no medical benefit. When fully informed of the potential benefits and risks of performing CPR, many patients choose the DNR option. You should always explain to your patient that having a DNR order does not mean that he or she will be neglected in any way; ensure the patient that care will still be provided and his or her comfort will remain a priority.

Documenting a DNR Order

A DNR order can be documented in three ways:

1. The patient may sign a "Do Not Resuscitate" form (Fig. 10-2).
2. The patient's health care proxy can sign the form.
3. The physician can write a DNR order on the patient's chart if he or she feels the clinical situation warrants. However, the physician does not generally write the order without consulting with the patient and family.

Knowledge Connection
When should a person execute a durable power of attorney? What preferences does an advance directive establish? When is CPR indicated, and when is it not?

Facing Loss

As human beings, we face different kinds of loss throughout the course of our lives. Despite the belief of many of us that things will never change and that situations and relationships will be consistent, change happens all of the time—and change usually means loss of one kind or another. Even something as minor as a little surgical scar can represent the loss of body image, so imagine the loss experienced with an amputation. Consider the loss of one's usual daily routine when twice-a-day insulin injections become necessary. Once a person has had cancer, even if cured, he or she is forever a "cancer survivor." One's sense of security and wellness is forever lost.

Illness and death bring all sorts of loss into a family: not only loss of that person, but the loss of all of his or her roles within the family. Many lose parents to Alzheimer's disease long before the parent actually dies. Children, even adult children, feel the loss of a parent comforter and advisor. **Role reversal** occurs when the children who are used to being cared for suddenly become the caregivers for their parents. Spouses lose lovers and companions. Losing the breadwinner of the family brings financial insecurity. When the family cheerleader and encourager dies, a spark of joy is extinguished, and with this loss comes grief and mourning. **Grief** is the mental and emotional distress and suffering that one experiences with death and loss, and is expressed in various ways by each individual.

Five Traditional Stages of Grief

Five emotional and psychological responses have been identified as being common in patients facing the ordeal of coping with loss and grief. Dr. Elisabeth Kübler-Ross was the first to document these findings in her groundbreaking book *On Death and Dying* in 1969. Although there are some differing opinions today on exactly how our patients and their families deal with loss, Kübler-Ross's five stages still provide a method of understanding how people cope with the prospect of dying as part of their life-threatening illness (Table 10-1).

It is also important to realize that there is no script for grief. Those who have experienced loss cannot expect to feel emotions in a particular set pattern. People work through and around these stages. Some experience all five stages, while others experience only a few or just one. Grief is as individual as those who feel it, and as varied as the circumstances that surround it.

The actual moment that life is lost to death is always troubling, to say the least. For the patient's loved ones, the separation and loss that accompany death are always sad and often difficult to cope with, let alone accept. However, as the nurse, you have the opportunity to improve the patient's

OKLAHOMA DO-NOT-RESUSCITATE (DNR) CONSENT FORM

I, _____, request limited health care as described in this document. If my heart stops beating or if I stop breathing, no medical procedure to restore breathing or heart function will be instituted by any health care provider including, but not limited to, emergency medical services (EMS) personnel.

I understand that this decision will not prevent me from receiving other health care such as the Heimlich maneuver or oxygen and other comfort care measures.

I understand that I may revoke this consent at any time in one of the following ways:

1. If I am under the care of a health care agency, by making an oral, written, or other act of communication to a physician or other health care provider of a health care agency;

2. If I am not under the care of a health care agency, by destroying my do-not-resuscitated form, removing all do-not-resuscitate identification from my person, and notifying my attending physician of the revocation;

3. If I am incapacitated and under the care of a health care agency, my representative may revoke the do-not-resuscitate consent by written notification of a physician or other health care provider of the health care agency or by oral notification of my attending physician; or

4. If I am incapacitated and not under the care of a health care agency, my representative may revoke the do-not-resuscitate consent by destroying the do-not-resuscitate form, removing all do-not-resuscitate identification from my person, and notifying my attending physician of the revocation.

I give my permission for this information to be given to EMS personnel, doctors, nurses, and other health care providers. I hereby state that I am making an informed decision and agree to a do-not-resuscitate order.

_____ OR_____

Signature of Person

Signature of Representative
(Limited to an attorney-in-fact for health care decisions acting under the Durable Power of Attorney Act, a health care proxy acting under the Oklahoma Rights of the Terminally Ill or Persistently Unconscious Act or a a guardian of the person appointed under the Oklahoma Guardianship and Conservatorship Act.)
This DNR consent form was signed in my presence

_____

Date

_____

Signature/Address of Witness

_____

Signature/Address of Witness

Figure 10-2 An example of the Oklahoma "Do Not Resuscitate" form.

Table 10-1 **Kübler-Ross's Five Stages of Grief in Death and Dying**

Stages		Key Phrases You Might Hear
Stage I	Denial	*Not me!* *This isn't happening to me!* *It can't be happening!*
Stage II	Anger	*Why is this happening to ME?* *Why me? It's not fair!*
Stage III	Bargaining	*I promise I'll be a better person IF...* *Just let me live to see my children graduate.* *If I could have one more chance.*
Stage IV	Depression	*I don't care anymore.* *I'm so sad, why bother with anything?*
Stage V	Acceptance	*It's going to be OK.* *I'm ready for whatever comes.*

Source: Kubler-Ross, E. *On Death and Dying.* New York: Macmillan; 1969.

dying experience or journey toward death, to make it as good as is possible, as well as easing the process for the family. This is accomplished by helping the patient and his or her loved ones overcome their fears of the dying process, providing adequate pain relief, providing support and understanding, and ensuring that dignity will be maintained.

To minimize some of the natural fears of dying, you will want to provide adequate information regarding the disease process, how it may progress, and that relief of pain and most symptoms is possible. It is helpful to assure the patient that he or she will have full control over his or her own plan of care and degree of pain and symptom control, including the right to refuse any aspect of treatment that may be offered. The holistic needs that must be met include knowing that the patient has control over whether he or she dies at home or in a health care facility, and who will be allowed to be present as death approaches. It is important to provide for the patient's spiritual needs and any religious rituals that might afford the patient comfort. Encourage the patient to make reconciliation wherever possible and with whomever there is discord. If your patient were dying at this moment, how comforting do you think it would be for the patient to hear the following promise, as stated by Dr. Ira Byock?

"We will keep you warm and we will keep you dry. We will keep you clean. We will help you with elimination, with your bowels and your bladder function. We will always offer you food and fluid. We will be with you. We will bear witness to your pain and your sorrows, your disappointments and your triumphs; we will listen to the stories of your life and will remember the story of your passing."

Source: With permission from Byock, I. *Dying Well: Peace and Possibilities at the End of Life.* 1997. Riverhead Trade.

As a nurse, you can assist the patient to die well by encouraging him or her to live life to the fullest extent rather than just waiting for death and by encouraging the patient to make time to say goodbye to family and friends in his or her own style.

Patients often seem to be able to exert an uncanny control over the timing of their death. Of course, their primary diagnosis, age, and overall health set a time frame for life expectancy. But a person may either consciously or unconsciously decide to stay alive for a specific event, to complete an important relationship, or to accomplish a special goal. It is a rare gift to your patient for you to recognize this and then offer the opportunity to hear and say the things that will help the patient to experience a peaceful death. Ira Byock, MD, suggested that five things need to be said as we approach the end of our lives:

1. "Forgive me."
2. "I forgive you."
3. "Thank you."
4. "I love you."
5. "Good-bye" and giving the patient permission to go.

These five brief statements represent reconciliation and closure, not only with family and friends, but often with the patient's concept of God and the spiritual. They may be viewed as peacemaking activities and are sometimes expressed in religious tones or seen as a spiritual experience. As human beings, many of us seek or look for eternal significance. Those with that faith often need the support of those around them to find the peace that their faith offers them. Table 10-2 describes religious and cultural differences in death and dying.

Table 10-2   Religious and Cultural Differences in Death and Dying

Religion	Handling of the Body	Special Considerations	Burial

Muslim
Faith is called Islam:
  Sunni (majority)
  Shia (minority)
Quran (Koran) is sacred book, containing guide on standards and ethics of leading a wholesome life.
Basic belief in God, the Prophet, the Koran, and the Final Day of Resurrection.
	Preferably by person of same sex.
	Modesty is of paramount importance.
	Keep body covered completely and placed, if possible, with feet toward Mecca.
	Autopsy is permitted to determine cause of death or for research for new remedies.
		Be aware of need for ablution and prayers five times daily.
		In some Muslim cultures the words "death," "dying," and "cancer" are considered taboo.
		Patient may wish to sit or lie with face toward Mecca.
		Prayer rug and Koran must not be touched by anyone ritually unclean, and nothing may be placed on top of it.
		Some wear an amulet that should not be removed and must remain dry.
			Burial is done promptly after first prayer after death.
			Cremation is forbidden.
			Burial is completely different from Christian customs. Some Muslims do not use a wooden coffin. The body is wrapped in a shroud.
			May desire for body to be returned to country of birth.

Roman Catholic
Belief in triune God:
  Father
  Son
  Holy Spirit
Intercession of Saints:
  Mary, Mother of God
  Apostles
	Funeral director
	Contact priest
		Rituals include administration of Holy Communion and Last Rites (or Prayer for the Sick).
		Priest is called before death—sacraments are given only to the living.
		Rosary is important—a mix of both voiced and silent prayer reflecting on the life of Christ and Mary, the Mother of Christ.
			Wake service.
			Prayer service.
			Funeral mass.
			Cemetery or tomb burial.
			Cremation has been forbidden, but is becoming accepted.

Protestant Christian
Belief in Trinity:
  Creator Father
  Savior Son, Jesus Christ
  Holy Spirit
	Funeral director
	Contact clergy of choice
		Some groups have liturgical traditions and religious practices of prayer, anointing oil.
		Death is considered entrance into eternal life of health, joy, and peace with God.
			Cremation is allowed.
			Cemetery burial.

Orthodox Belief in Creator God and Holy Trinity. Highly ritualized worship in Christian faith unchanged since fourth century.	Funeral director Parish priest	Body is considered to be highly sacred. In some ethnic groups, there is a high emotional reaction to death and dying. Family and friends play very important role in caring for patient.	Cremation is not permitted. Cemetery burial with body facing east. Orthodox funeral ceremony.
Buddhist Goal of practice is to develop the mind to its fullest potential, which involves the perfection of compassion and wisdom.	Contact Buddhist monk. Body is taken home for 1–3 days and not touched.	Believe in reincarnation. Death is extremely important since it is a transition point to the next life. Prayers are said, and sometimes a special text is read to the dying person.	Usually cremation is preferred. Ashes may be placed in local Temple below a photo of the deceased.

(table continues on page 198)

Table 10-2 Religious and Cultural Differences in Death and Dying (continued)

Religion	Handling of the Body	Special Considerations	Burial

Jewish
Branches of Judiasm:
  Orthodox
  Chasidic
  Reform Movement
  Conservative
  Movement
Belief in God as the single supreme being.
Holiness of the life of a person is placed above all else in medical decision making.
	Rabbi is consulted immediately upon death to help with very detailed preparations for the body and care of the family.
	Autopsies are permitted, if necessary, but all body parts must be buried.
	Organ donation is permitted.
		When nearing death, the patient is encouraged to unburden himself or herself of worries, fears, sense of guilt, and sense of wrongdoing.
		Attention from family and Rabbi is very important as the person should not go into death alone.
		Psalms are very important and should be read to patient.
		Rabbi or Hillel director can arrange for a quorum of 10 men, if patient is Orthodox, to be present for prayer.
			Cremation is discouraged.
			Bereavement cannot formally begin until body is buried.
			May request up to 4 days for preparation of the body for direct cremation or burial or for lying in honor before removal from the family home.

Your job, as the nurse, is to give your patient and his or her family the space, privacy, and time to explore their experiences and feelings about these issues. You may need to gently let them know these are tasks that they might want to address.

It is critical that you remember that these tasks are very individual, very different for each person. As a nurse, you must be careful *not* to define these experiences for your patients, but let them find their own way. Each person's age, life experiences, and religious background will guide him or her through his or her own unique journey at the end of life. Your own faith and confidence, and especially your presence—just being there if there is no family or friend prepared to do this—are a gift to your patient.

Knowledge Connection

How can being a cancer survivor represent a loss? How would you outline the stages of grief? Write your own list of things that you feel would help to make your own death a *good death*. What thoughts would you want to impart and to whom? What religious or cultural difference in your patient might cause you the most conflict in caring for him or her?

The Dying Process

Any description of the dying process must be considered as a very flexible list of events. Signs and symptoms of the changes that occur in the mind, spirit, and body as a person prepares to die do not always appear in the same order or in the same way. Death comes in its own time and in its own way and is as unique as each individual who experiences it. There are certain symptoms that you might expect to see when your patient begins to enter the end stages of his or her disease (Box 10-1).

Box 10-1

Signs and Symptoms of End-Stage Disease

These signs and symptoms are commonly present during end-stage disease. However, not all of them will be experienced by every patient; and some of the signs and symptoms may be present during earlier stages of certain disease processes.

- Anorexia
- Anxiety/fear
- Cachexia
- Confusion/delirium
- Constipation
- Diarrhea
- Dyspnea
- Fatigue
- Nausea and vomiting
- Pain
- Sadness/depression
- Weakness

These signs and symptoms begin to be exhibited with the patient's initial realization that what is happening is real, when the patient begins to have a true grasp of the idea that time is limited and that he or she is dying. One to 3 months before death, as the knowledge becomes real, your patient will likely begin to withdraw, at least for short periods of time. He or she will have less interest in current events, usual social activities, and sometimes even family members. This withdrawing is a turning in to one's self and can be a time of self-evaluation, life review, or spiritual exploration. It is very unique to each person and may occur in differing sequences or time lines. Box 10-2 presents an example of a typical calendar of events in the dying process.

Box 10-2

Typical Calendar of Signs and Symptoms of the Dying Process

This *calendar* of signs and symptoms of the dying process relates a *typical* timing of events only. It is important to understand that every patient will exhibit very different timing, an individualized schedule of his or her own body's design.

One to Three Months	One to Two Weeks	Last Days and Hours
Realization	Increased sleeping	Congestion and death rattle
Withdrawal	Weakness	Decreased urine output
Life review	Less communication with family	Glassy eyes/tearing
Spiritual exploration	Agitation	Edema of feet
	Anorexia	Mottling of feet and legs
	Changes in vital signs	Nonresponsiveness
		Vital signs: decreased blood pressure, weak and thready pulse, slow and shallow respirations

Psychological and Emotional Changes

As a patient get closer to death, it is common for the patient to review his or her life, sifting through memories, coming to terms with the fact that soon he or she will be leaving the physical body and entering into the afterlife. As your patient mentally processes his or her life, more time will be spent in introspection and reflection, or what appears to be day-dreaming, with the patient often not even answering when spoken to. Time spent in withdrawal and noncommunicative states may get longer and longer. As physical strength decreases, your patient may prefer to stay in bed, resting the physical body while the mind and spirit are working on a level that others cannot really see. Your patient will also have less need to communicate with family and friends. The patient may sleep more and more. It is hard to be "awake in this world" and "doing business in the next." Help your patient's loved ones understand this, because it can be very hurtful to them. Explain to them that external stimulation such as loud noises, bright lights, strong hugs, and face patting can be very distracting and distressing to the patient, and that slow, gentle touch and just being there for the patient take on more importance than long, more demanding conversation.

Another change your patient may undergo as death nears is a loss of interest in food. Liquids are generally more accepted than solids by patients who are dying, but even liquids may become too taxing for them to take in. If this happens to a patient who is in your care, remember that it is acceptable for your patient not to eat. Food is the fuel for the functioning body. It is not needed for the tasks the body now faces.

In the final 1 to 2 weeks prior to death, your patient may appear to be asleep much of the time, but he or she is easily awakened with gentle stimuli. However, keep in mind that it is *absolutely not necessary* to verify level of consciousness with a sternal rub or other painful stimuli you might use in assessing an unconscious patient in another situation. Gentle touch or quiet speech, when necessary, is all that is needed to communicate at this time. If your patient does not respond, respect this too.

Mental Changes

Your patient may experience what appears to be confusion and may talk to people about places and events that do not make sense to you or the family. He or she may pick at linens and have exaggerated arm movements. It is not necessary to restrict these activities; just protect the patient from injury on bed rails or equipment. Your patient may seem to be conversing with loved ones who have died before him or her. Avoid trying to correct or reorient the patient. This may agitate the patient and result in anxiety, restlessness, or erratic behavior.

Physical Changes

Numerous physical changes will be observed over the days and hours prior to death. It is important to remember that not all patients will follow the same pattern, and some changes will not be experienced by all patients.

Vital Signs

When a patient is dying, his or her blood pressure may be lowered. It is important to remember, however, that the taking of a patient's blood pressure can be somewhat painful to the patient and that, in the dying process, knowing the patient's blood pressure is secondary to the peace that you can offer by not interfering in his or her comfort.

It is quite noninvasive to check your patient's pulse, however. You can expect to see your patient's pulse increase up to 140 to 150 bpm, especially if he or she is febrile. Then, as the dying process continues, you can also expect to see the patient's pulse decrease. Just prior to death, the pulse rate may slow into the 30s and 40s.

Skin

Diaphoresis and clamminess will be noted along with skin color changes as the body begins to fail. Your patient may be flushed if he or she is feverish, or very pale with cyanosis of the nailbeds or around the mouth, known as **circumoral cyanosis**. Pallor increases very near the time of death.

Respiratory Changes

Respiratory changes also occur with approaching death. Your patient's respirations may increase to between 40 and 50 breaths/min before decreasing to 6 to 8 breaths/min. The breaths can be puffing or blowing, and there can be periods of **apnea** (no respirations) for 15 to 50 seconds. Breathing may be cyclic in nature, beginning with periods of shallow, slow breaths before respirations become progressively deeper until they peak as very deep breaths. The respirations then begin to progressively become shallower again, ending the cycle with a period of apnea. This breathing pattern is called *Cheyne-Stokes respirations* and is a strong indicator of nearing death. Observation for more than 1 minute is necessary to identify this breathing pattern accurately.

As death nears, fluids may accumulate in the trachea, causing a deep, moist rattling sound. Often referred to as the "death rattle," this sound does not indicate true respiratory distress for the patient, but it can be very distressing to the family. Suctioning is not the best solution as it tends to interrupt the patient's ability to breathe and stimulates the body to create more secretions, thus re-creating the problem. This symptom can be addressed with positioning and with medications to dry the secretions, such as scopolamine or atropine.

Physical Activity

In the last days and hours prior to death, the signs that have been present in the last few weeks can intensify. Restlessness can increase as your patient becomes more hypoxic. Short periods of restlessness do not necessarily require treatment. However, a condition of terminal restlessness that is severe and is a reflection of a lack of peace on the patient's part can and should be treated.

Fear and unfinished business are two big factors in determining how much resistance your patient may put into meeting death. Pain should be relieved. Hopefully, all emotional and spiritual issues have been resolved at this point, but occasionally you will have a patient who simply cannot find peace and who will require some kind of sedation.

Eyes

Your patient's eyes may remain closed, but they may also remain open or partly open. There is a glassy look to them and, because of conjunctival dryness and corneal irritation, there may be tearing. This is not the patient crying. It is important that you communicate this to the family.

Circulatory Changes

As death nears, peripheral circulation continues to fail and hands and feet become cold and cyanotic. As peripheral circulation fails, you may see **mottling** of the skin, or patches of varying colors of pallor and cyanosis in the feet, legs, hands, and dependent areas of the body. Mottling generally begins distally and progresses proximally. Peripheral pulses become difficult to feel. Because of decreased renal perfusion, urine output drops. As the muscles weaken, the patient may be incontinent.

Your patient will usually become nonresponsive sometime prior to death. You cannot awaken him or her with speech or touch. Again, painful stimuli are inappropriate at this time. The period of time from nonresponsiveness to actual cessation of vital signs varies widely from person to person.

Knowledge Connection

How would you differentiate starvation from the malnutrition and dehydration of the dying process? How would you respond to the question, "How long does mother have to live?" How would you respond if your patient told you he had been visited by a deceased relative? Differentiate between restlessness and terminal restlessness.

Nursing Care

Nursing care during the dying process is less about diagnostics, vital signs, and laboratory values and more about caring, touching, and providing presence or simply being there for the patient and family—the fundamentals of nursing that attracted us to the field in the first place (Fig. 10-3). While great skill, knowledge of the technical aspects of nursing, and understanding of the dying processes are needed, it is the basics of respect for your patient and the maintenance of his or her dignity, even in light of a possible dependence for activities of daily living, which are of the greatest value at this time in your patient's life.

Listening

Listen sensitively and carefully to your patient and to his or her family (Fig. 10-4). Take note of what they say and what they *do not* say. Anticipate needs and fears. This is unfamiliar territory for nearly everyone. Ask about the family and the patient's life, work, and interests. Give the patient your attention, and promise to try to remember.

Figure 10-3 Sometimes the most important thing you can do for a dying patient is to simply share a little of your time and compassion, just giving presence.

Figure 10-4 Encourage your patient and the patient's family members to express emotions and feelings, letting each individual know that these feelings are normal. This will help to build *rapport* (a trusting relationship) with your patient and family members.

Teaching

Using as little medical jargon as possible, gently tell the family what to expect, at the level at which they are prepared to hear this information. Two of the most difficult things that families face at this time are nonhealing wounds and poor appetite.

Wounds require adequate circulation and adequate nutrition in order to heal. In the terminal processes, usually neither is present. As with all palliative care, your goals with wounds must generally change from healing to comfort. In the event of a serious pressure ulcer, the best treatment is not usually going to be débridement, because granulation is not going to happen in a terminal patient. There is simply not adequate nutrition or body healing processes to heal a severe wound. Keep the area clean, and allow the wound to dry. Allowing it to form a self-sealing eschar over it actually helps to control pain and odor.

When the patient is diagnosed with a terminal illness, this is usually the time to throw out all the rules you have learned about nutrition and eating. With rare exceptions, such as renal failure or diabetes, it is usually time to encourage your patient to eat whatever foods he or she thinks sound and look appealing. Generally, you would offer high-protein and high-calorie foods. It is not the time to worry about salt or cholesterol intake. Eating three meals a day can be intimidating and nauseating to the patient with *anorexia*, or loss of appetite. Frequent, small snacks can be much more attractive.

At a later point in the illness, food will begin to have no appeal at all. Your patient's body will no longer want or need the physical energy that food gives. When that time comes, it is acceptable for your patient to eat as little as he or she wants. This is an extremely difficult time for most families.

When a loved one stops eating, the feelings of fear, anger, frustration, and sadness are often difficult to ease. The sense of loss may be most profound for the family member who had been the food preparer. We nurture by feeding loved ones special holiday meals, therapeutic diets, and their favorite foods. You might hear family members say, "I fix his favorite foods and then he won't eat them," or "He must eat if he is to get his strength back." This can be a terrific source of tension within the family, with the caregiver feeling angry and rejected and the patient feeling hurt and guilty. Helping all understand that the loss of appetite is related to the disease and is something over which the patient has no control may help the family shift the blame from the patient to the disease.

Patient Teaching Connection

Teaching Family Members How to Comfort the Patient
The patient's loved ones may struggle to find ways to help or comfort the individual who is so dear to them. They are often afraid to touch the patient for fear of inflicting pain. Some family members will have a need to physically demonstrate their love and caring. Help the family find nonfood ways of caregiving or nurturing:

- Reading to the patient
- Doing a manicure or pedicure
- Administering gentle massage of feet, hands, or head
- Gently brushing the patient's hair
- Singing softly to the patient, especially a song that might hold sweet memories
- Reminiscing about the good ole' days, and telling stories that might hold pleasant memories, allowing the patient to simply listen and drift in and out of recalled happy times
- Viewing old family photographs, especially those that bring particular joy to the patient

This is really teaching the family, but patient teaching needs include the family.

The issue of fluid intake has many of the same emotional attachments as does that of eating and feeding solid foods. The parent of an ill child has been encouraged to "give plenty of fluids." As nurses, we have been instructed in the benefits of "forcing fluids." And both the medical and lay communities consider dehydration to be a negative state, one that requires correction. However, dehydration is a normal part of the physiology of dying and can actually add to the comfort of your dying patient. The beneficial effects of dehydration include:

- Decreased urine output, resulting in less incontinence and less need for toileting
- Decreased production of gastric fluids, resulting in less nausea and vomiting
- Decreased pulmonary secretions, resulting in less need for suctioning and less respiratory distress
- Diminished edema and ascites
- Decreased pain perception

Dehydration and the malnutrition that goes along with the dying process are not starvation. Helping your patient's family understand this will be a tremendous gift to the process of providing peace and comfort to all involved.

Observation and Provision of Comfort

At the end of life, you will depend *less* upon laboratory values and measurements of blood pressures and pulse oximetry readings and *more* upon your skills of observation. Observe the patient closely for all aspects of comfort, including:

- **Pain and nausea:** Assess for pain and nausea; do not wait for the patient to find the strength to complain. If these are present, use medications and nonpharmacological methods to relieve them. Box 10-3 lists various nonpharmacological interventions for pain.
- **Gas exchange:** Is the patient dyspneic or cyanotic? If so, provide some oxygen. Is it really important that you know what the peripheral pulse oximetry reading is? No, it really is not.
- **Moisture of mucous membranes:** Are they dry? Then provide oral care. Dehydration is not uncomfortable for the dying patient, if you keep his or her mouth clean and lips moist. If the patient is still taking fluids, offer sips as often as every 30 to 60 minutes or as desired, but do not try to force the patient to drink.
- **Emotional or spiritual distress:** If you detect them, address them.
- **Positioning:** Is the patient restless? Make sure he or she is repositioned frequently, even if only small adjustments are made. It does not take complete side-to-side turning to change a pressure point. Apply lotion gently to pressure points and areas of dry skin. The use of an air-fluidized mattress or foam mattress overlay helps to relieve pressure on fragile skin and pressure points over bony prominences.
- **Elimination:** If there is a Foley catheter to drain urine, make certain the catheter is correctly secured to the thigh to avoid tension on the urethra, which is very uncomfortable. If the patient is incontinent, assess frequently and keep the bed clean and dry to avoid skin excoriation or breakdown. If there is no elimination, gently check for impaction or bladder distention as needed.

Seek help and support from other members of your team as needed for additional ideas and solutions. Offer a symptom management plan to the physician. The physician will rarely reject a well-thought-out plan of care with suggestions for solutions, rather than just presenting a list of problems. Contact your organization's chaplain or pastoral care department for assistance.

It is important to remember that your first goal at this time is comfort. Withholding narcotic analgesics out of fear of respiratory depression is not appropriate at the end of life.

Box 10-3

Nonpharmacological Interventions for Pain

Administration of pain medications is key in providing patient comfort, and these medications should never be ignored or administered sparingly. But there are many nonmedicinal interventions that have been shown to be as effective as, and sometimes even more effective than, the analgesics themselves. Learn to utilize all of these interventions as well as any others you or the patient and family might suggest, to enhance the comfort level of the terminal patient. If one intervention does not work for a patient, try another one, and still another one until you are successful in maximally relieving his or her suffering and distress.

- Distraction
- Heat/cold applications
- Massage
- Meditation/prayer
- Movement and range-of-motion exercises
- Music therapy
- Positioning
- Relaxation and breathing techniques

Your patient is dying of his or her disease process. It is natural and normal for respirations to decrease at this time. If narcotics have been part of the patient's medication regimen, dose levels to which he or she has been accustomed will not cause respiratory depression now. Even if narcotics are newly introduced at this time for pain, restlessness, or dyspnea, the small doses prescribed do not compromise your patient's respiratory status. Never withhold comfort medications because you are afraid.

If your patient becomes unresponsive, it is important to remember that research supports the idea that hearing is the last sense to go. It is helpful to discuss this with the family when the time comes, because two things commonly happen:

1. They forget that the patient may be able to hear them and discuss subjects that could be distressing to the patient.
2. They avoid speaking to the patient, because they do not know what to say and assume that the patient cannot hear them anyway.

Encourage the patient's family to nurture and comfort the patient even though there does not appear to be a response. You can model these behaviors for the family by continuing to interact with your patient as you would if you knew the patient could hear you, for he or she well might.

Knowledge Connection

What are the most difficult nursing issues that families face when changing from curative to palliative care? How can you help the family nurture the patient who is too ill to eat? What are the advantages of dehydration in palliative and hospice care?

Symptom Management

Assuring your patient that all symptoms of discomfort can be effectively managed, all the way to the point of death, addresses one of the greatest fears that people face as the reality of terminal illness descends. It is also one of the most frightening promises you will ever make. However, you can make these promises and you can make them with confidence:

• Pain can be relieved.
• Nausea can be managed.
• Respiratory distress can be eliminated.

On the rare occasion when symptoms cannot be completely eliminated, they can be brought to a level acceptable to the patient. No one need ever die while suffering in pain or gasping for air.

Pain Management

To effectively manage pain, you must first determine what type of pain your patient is experiencing. Accomplish this by asking the patient about the pain and listening closely to his or her answers. Your patient's words will tell you if the pain is visceral, osteogenic, neuropathic, or spastic. Each type of pain must be addressed in very specific ways in order to be effective. Good pain management includes not only medications, but also nonpharmacological measures. The different types of pain and pain management will be discussed more completely in Chapter 19. For a list of nonpharmacological interventions for pain, see Box 10-3.

Nausea

Controlling nausea is sometimes one of the greatest challenges of palliative and hospice care. As with pain, you must consider the source of the nausea to begin any effective treatment. Is it opiate induced? Is it caused by neurological problems? Are the symptoms coming from gastrointestinal events? Choices for appropriate medications will be based on these issues. Some examples of nonpharmacological interventions for nausea are listed in Box 10-4.

Box 10-4

Nonpharmacological Interventions for Nausea

As with pain, there are various nonmedicinal interventions that have been successful in alleviating nausea for some patients. Use some or all of these noninvasive, nonpharmacological interventions in addition to medications to prevent or relieve nausea.
• Cool compresses to face and forehead
• Deep breathing
• Meditation/prayer
• Music therapy
• Relaxation techniques
• Small sips of clear liquids at patient's temperature preference

Dyspnea

Dyspnea may well be one of the most frightening symptoms for your patient. Anyone who has experienced chronic lung disease has experienced air hunger and fears dying while gasping for air. You can be confident when you assure your patient that both pharmacological and nonpharmacological measures are very effective at the end of life to prevent this type of suffering.

Supplemental oxygen, bronchodilators, muscle relaxants, and judicious use of morphine can all contribute to your patient's peace and comfort at the end of life. The use of an electric fan to move the air around the patient is often very comforting to the patient experiencing dyspnea. Box 10-5 lists nonpharmacological treatments of dyspnea.

Knowledge Connection

What promises can you make to your patient about the care he or she will receive when dying?

Laboratory and Diagnostic Connection

Hypercalcemia

One laboratory result that requires immediate physician contact and possible treatment in hospice care is *hypercalcemia,* an excessively high level of calcium in the blood, usually the result of bony metastasis that is worsened by bedrest. There is a 50% mortality rate if the level is not reduced expediently. It may be evidenced by nausea, vomiting, confusion, constipation, lethargy, decreased deep tendon reflexes, polyuria, and extreme thirst. The common treatment is to increase fluid intake to help dilute the blood level of calcium, using IV fluids if necessary. Furosemide, a common loop diuretic, may be administered to increase urinary excretion of calcium. Calcitonin may also be ordered to lower the blood level by increasing resorption of calcium from blood to bones.

Box 10-5

Nonpharmacological Interventions for Dyspnea

There is nothing more frightening than the feeling that you cannot breathe! Do not hesitate to use every one of these interventions if needed, in addition to use of supplemental oxygen and appropriate medications such as bronchodilators, antianxiety drugs, sedatives, and opioids, which decrease fear and anxiety while providing pain relief. Teach these interventions to the patient and help him or her to optimize a sense of well-being that will help to relieve dyspnea. Take the time...it is so very important!
• Fan to move the air
• Meditation/prayer
• Positioning
• Pursed-lip breathing
• Relaxation techniques

Just Be There

Dying patients are experiencing an unfamiliar, but significant, event and usually feel the need to talk about what is happening to them. Though most people do not want to talk about death, your patient will often choose a single person with whom he or she can talk about dying. Most likely it will not be his or her physician. It is hard for doctors to acknowledge that all of their efforts have still failed and the patient is not going to survive. Death has won and medical science has been defeated. When death is the enemy, defeat is hard to accept.

It is also quite likely that the patient will not choose his or her family for discussion of these things. A dying patient's spouse, children, and even friends feel too much fear and pain, especially at first. It is too risky to talk with someone who does not want to face the grief and separation death will bring, let alone talk about it.

Nevertheless, people need to talk about what they are experiencing. You cannot choose that person for them, nor can you designate yourself as the chosen one, but you should be prepared to be the person with whom the patient feels the most secure and the most comfortable to talk about his or her own death.

Your patient is not likely to just open up and say, "I'm dying and I want to talk to you about it." You will have to listen carefully. The patient may almost talk in code. Statements may be more like, "I don't know what is going on," or "I don't think I'm going to make it," or "I don't know why God just doesn't take me," or even "I am just so tired." Any of these might be a request for conversation. Listen with a sensitive ear and heart or you might miss the opportunity to give and receive a wonderful gift.

Some of the most meaningful experiences in your nursing career may be sitting at the bedside of your dying patient, just being there. Not giving great words of wisdom, not having answers to every question, not even talking at all. Just being there, giving presence, helping with your fearlessness and your willingness to just listen. Perhaps you will even shed a tear. That's okay, too. Being willing to feel the patient's feelings and experience his or her emotions is a gift beyond measure.

So often when you are asked the question, "Why did you choose a career in nursing?", the answer is, "Because I want to help people." Well, here is an opportunity of unbelievable breadth, depth, and height. What greater honor could there be than to be present for the patient when he or she steps out of this world and into the next? As a nurse providing palliative or hospice care, you are there providing help for the patient at a most critical time of life for both the patient and his or her family. You have the opportunity to relieve pain, supply soothing comfort, provide respite, and allay fear, and the rewards for doing so are tremendous. There is not a greater or longer lasting feeling than the self-satisfaction that comes from knowing you helped make the dying process more meaningful, less frightening, and more comfortable for the patient and loved ones. Do not let personal fear cause you to shrink from even one such opportunity that is laid before you.

Knowledge Connection
What are your gifts to your dying patient? What are his or her gifts to you?

Postmortem Care

Postmortem care is the care provided after the patient's death. Even after the patient's respirations cease, the heart will sometimes continue to beat irregularly for 2 to 3 minutes. In the hospital or long-term care facility, notify the physician who is responsible for pronouncing death. If the patient is in hospice care, the physician still is notified, but the registered nurse generally makes this pronouncement. Document the time respirations and heartbeat ceased. Incontinence of bowel and bladder generally result with death. Ask the family if they would like to assist with bathing or care. Bathe the body and, if autopsy is not to be done, remove all tubings such as Foley catheters and IV lines. If there are dressings, leave them intact. Apply a clean gown and linens. Close the patient's eyes and mouth, place the hands across the chest, and elevate the head of the bed slightly. If the patient has dentures, they should be inserted. A rolled washcloth or small hand towel may be placed under the chin if the mouth will not remain closed. Unless the family prefers to be left alone, remain in the room with the family providing touch or support as needed. If they do not appear to need your physical touch, just remain unobtrusively in the room. Allow the loved ones as much time as they need. Skill 10-1 provides further information on postmortem care.

Skill 10-1 Postmortem Care

Assessment Steps

1. Safety: Verify identification of the patient.
2. Determine if there are family members and/or clergy that you must notify.
3. Determine whether an autopsy is to be performed or not. Has an autopsy permit been signed?
4. Determine if family members would like to assist in bathing the deceased loved one.

Planning Steps

1. Obtain necessary equipment and clean linens and gown.
2. If there is a roommate present, plan to assist him or her from the room.
3. Close the room door and privacy curtain.
4. Plan to handle the body with all due dignity and respect.

Implementation Steps

1. Safety: Don clean gloves to protect yourself from body fluids.
2. Raise the head of the bed slightly, between 20 and 30 degrees, to prevent discoloration of the face from pooling of blood.
3. Gently close the eyelids and mouth. Place a rolled washcloth or small towel underneath the chin if needed to hold the mouth closed.
4. *No autopsy:* Remove all tubing, such as oxygen, Foley catheter, drains, and nasogastric tube. Remove IV line and apply a bandage to prevent leakage. Apply clean dressings.
   With autopsy: Leave tubes in place, clamp them, then cut off at approximately 6 inches in length, fold over the cut end of the tubing, and tape it closed. Leave original dressings in place.
5. Leave or place dentures in mouth unless facility policy says to remove them. In this case, store in a denture cup and give to the mortician or keep with the body. Be sure to make a note in the chart indicating the disposition of dentures and any other prostheses.
6. Bathe the body to remove all body fluids, including blood, emesis, drainage, urine, or feces. Place a disposable pad under the hips to absorb any further drainage.
   Note: In certain cultures, this step must be omitted. Some religions strictly forbid washing and, in others, a special person must perform this task. In cultures in which the family's washing of the body is considered the last service that a family can give a loved one, the family should be given the necessary supplies and left alone in the room with the body.
7. Apply a clean gown and linens as needed.
8. Place the hands across the deceased's chest to prevent discoloration due to pooling blood.
9. Allow the family to view the deceased patient and to stay as long as they desire. Stay with them to offer emotional support unless they prefer to be alone.
10. When the family leaves, phone the mortuary if the body is to be transported to an independent mortuary.
11. Apply toe, ankle, or wrist identification band as per facility policy.
12. If policy dictates, secure the wrists together and the ankles together to make transport easier.
13. *If using shroud:* Place the body in supine position on a flat shroud or sheet. Fold the top and bottom ends of the shroud over the deceased's head and feet. Wrap the two sides of shroud or sheet around the body. Secure the shroud or sheet in place with straps placed around the chest, waist, and ankles. Apply a second identification tag to the ankle strap.
    If no shroud: Cover the body with a clean flat sheet to wait for the mortician.
14. Transport the body via gurney to the hospital morgue unless the mortician comes to the room to pick up the body.
15. Common courtesy dictates that all patient doors be closed before transporting the deceased down the hallway.

Evaluation Steps

1. Evaluate whether all documentation has been completed per facility policy, including postmortem care; disposition of personal belongings, assistive devices, and valuables; the time that the body was transported; and whether the body was transported to the facility morgue or to an independent mortuary.
2. Make certain that all family members' needs were met and that they have all left the facility.
3. Evaluate whether housekeeping has been notified regarding terminal cleaning of room.

Sample Documentation

3/5/12 0350 Body bathed by wife per her request. Son arrived as wife was completing bath. Informed son and wife to take all the time they needed. Coffee and ice water provided. ————
———————————— Nurse's signature and credentials

3/5/12 0420 Personal belongings given to wife. Itemized list signed and placed in chart. No valuables or personal medications in lock-up. Orderly assisted wife and son to transport belongings to private car. No further family members present. ————
———————————— Nurse's signature and credentials

3/5/12 0430 Postmortem care performed. No autopsy to be done. Saint Francis Mortuary notified. ————
———————————— Nurse's signature and credentials

3/5/12 0520 Body discharged to Saint Francis Mortuary personnel. Both upper and lower dentures were in mouth at time of transport. ———————— Nurse's signature and credentials

Post Conference

You share in post conference that this was one of the most amazing days you have had in clinicals. You cared for your patient by keeping her clean and comfortable. You talked to her and her family about her needs and how you would meet them. Her family was so kind to you. They were prepared for her death, but they were not ready to let her go. As her respirations grew slower and more erratic, they gathered around her bed. Each person said a good-bye in his or her own special way, and then she took her last breath. Everything was peaceful and calm. You were glad to help with postmortem care as a final act of reverence and dignity for this special lady.

KEY POINTS

- In order to assure the right to self-determination, also known as autonomy, the patient should be encouraged to complete an advance directive and durable power of attorney.
- Loss comes in many forms in our lives. All losses are grieved.
- Dying well is desirable and possible.
- Although flexible in timing and symptoms, the dying process does have a predictable pathway.
- Nursing care for the dying patient includes observation, listening, teaching, and symptom management.
- All symptoms of suffering can be managed or alleviated.
- Each life is significant.
- It can be one of the nurse's more rewarding roles to facilitate the passing of a life from this world to the next.

REVIEW QUESTIONS

Select the answer that is most appropriate for each of the following questions. Some questions may have more than one correct answer. Check all that apply.

1. Your patient can approach loss and death with a sense of peace when which of the following needs are met?

   a. Fear of the unknown is relieved by adequate knowledge.

   b. Pain and other signs and symptoms are effectively managed.

   c. Reconciliation with significant others is accomplished.

   d. The patient receives validation that he or she will die alone.

   e. Spiritual reconciliation is completed.

   f. Estate and financial matters have been settled.

2. Which of the following is *not* true of hospice care?

   a. Maintains patient autonomy and dignity

   b. Incorporates therapies to extend the patient's life

   c. Patient is thought to be in final 6 months of life

   d. Family wishes are primary direction for care

   e. Primary goals are relief of pain, lessening of fear, and provision of caregiver respite

3. The document that explains the patient's wishes regarding withholding or withdrawing life-sustaining treatments such as artificial nutrition and hydration is the:

   a. durable power of attorney.

   b. power of attorney.

   c. do-not-resuscitate order.

   d. living will.

4. When your patient states, "It's not fair that my cancer wasn't found sooner!", he is expressing emotions described as:

   a. denial.

   b. anger.

   c. bargaining.

   d. depression.

   e. acceptance.

5. "If I make it through the chemotherapy and radiation, then God will let me live," is an example of:

   a. denial.

   b. anger.

   c. bargaining.

   d. depression.

   e. acceptance.

6. In what religion is it particularly important to maintain the female patient's privacy/modesty by providing female caregivers?

 a. Buddhist

 b. Islam

 c. Protestant Christianity

 d. Judaism

 e. Catholicism

7. In what religious tradition is it particularly important to contact the religious leader or priest *before* death?

 a. Judaism

 b. Protestant Christian

 c. Roman Catholic

 d. Hindu

8. The dying process:

 a. is a flexible list of events.

 b. includes changes that are mostly physical and observable.

 c. includes a time of resting the physical while the mind and spirit are working.

 d. is amazingly similar for most patients.

 e. requires solitude.

9. Of the following symptoms, which is most indicative of imminent death? (Select either *a* or *b* for each of the following choices. You should have 6 answers when you have completed the question.)

a. tachycardia	or	**b.** bradycardia
a. circumoral cyanosis	or	**b.** peripheral mottling
a. tachypnea	or	**b.** periods of apnea
a. reaching out to family	or	**b.** withdrawal from family
a. pallor	or	**b.** flushing
a. unresponsiveness	or	**b.** agitation

10. When referring to the hospice nurse, the phrase "being there" means:

 a. being with the patient 24 hours a day, 7 days a week.

 b. being honest with patient and family.

 c. being willing to listen.

 d. listening for what the patient/family does not say.

 e. experiencing the emotions elicited during the dying process.

 f. conquering your own fears.

CRITICAL THINKING EXERCISES

11. How would you explain "CPR should not be the *standard of care* for the chronically ill resident of a long-term-care facility"?

12. Explain the difference between starvation and the malnutrition/dehydration of the dying process.

ADDITIONAL RESOURCES

For additional Resources, Questions, and Activities, please see:

 Student Resource Disk

 http://davisplus.fadavis.com

 Student Study Guide

REFERENCES

AGS Foundation for Health in Aging, American Geriatrics Society. Palliative care and hospice. Available at: http://www.healthinaging.org/agingintheknow/chapters_print_ch_trial.asp?ch=16. Accessed August 13, 2009.

American Nurses Association. ANA Code of Ethics for Nurses with Interpretive Statements. 2005. Available at: http://www.nursingworld.org/ethics/code/protected_nwcoe813.htm#1.1. Accessed August 13, 2009.

Byock I. *Dying Well—Peace and Possibilities at the End of Life.* New York: Riverhead Books; 1997.

City Hospice. *End of Life Decisions.* Available at: http://cityhospice.org/whyhospice.aspx. Accessed August 13, 2009.

Claessens P, Genbrugge E. Palliative sedation and nursing: the place of palliative sedation within palliative nursing care. *J Hospice Palliative Nurs.* 2007;9(2):100-106.

Fields L. DNR does not mean no care. *J Neurosci Nurs.* 2007;39:294-296.

Grossman S. Educating RNs regarding palliative care in long-term care generates positive outcomes for patients with end-stage chronic illness. *J Hospice Palliative Nurs.* 2007;9(6):323-328.

Karnes B. *Gone from My Sight—The Dying Experience.* Vancouver, WA: bkbooks; 2005.

Kübler Ross E. *On Death and Dying.* New York. Macmillan; 1969.

Lewis MA, Tamparo CD. *Medical Law, Ethics and Bioethics for the Health Professions.* Philadelphia: FA Davis; 2007.

Manning D. *Don't Take My Grief Away From Me.* Rev ed. Oklahoma City: In-Sight Books; 2005.

National Conference for Cardiopulmonary Resuscitation (CPR) and Emergency Cardiac Care (ECC): standards for PR and ECC. *JAMA.* 1974;227:864-866.

Smith R. Twelve principles of a good death. *BMJ.* 2000;320:129-130.

Taylor A, Box M. *Multicultural Palliative Care Guideline.* Eastwood, South Australia: Palliative Care Council of South Australia; 1999.

Ufema J. Insights on death and dying: protocol for peaceful death. *Nursing2008.* 2008;38(2):18.

University of Washington School of Medicine. Do not resuscitate orders. Available at: http://depts.washington.edu/bioethx/topics/dnr.html. Accessed August 13, 2009.

Zerwekh JV. Do dying patients really need i.v. fluids? *Am J Nurs.* 1997;97(3):26-30.

Complementary and Alternative Medicine

Key Terms

Acupressure

Acupuncture

Allopathic medicine

Alternative therapy

Chiropractic

Complementary therapy

Holism

Integrative health care

Massage therapy

Meridians

Yoga

Objectives

1. Differentiate between alternative therapy and complementary therapy.
2. Explain the concept of integrative health care.
3. Contrast CAM/Eastern medicine with Western medicine.
4. Describe the history, use, and effectiveness of chiropractic.
5. Discuss the types and benefits of massage therapy.
6. Explain the use of acupuncture and acupressure.
7. Enumerate six popular herbs and their uses.
8. Describe the purposes and benefits of yoga.
9. Explain how food and lifestyle changes can reverse some diseases.
10. Identify ways nurses can increase communication with patients regarding their use of CAM.

⊕ Clinical Connection

Your Assignment: You are assigned to care for a patient hospitalized for a hysterectomy and removal of the ovaries and fallopian tubes. She complains of back pain due to lying in a hospital bed for 2 days and nights, but she refuses to take pain medication. She listens to self-hypnosis CDs to help manage her postoperative pain. She tells you that she wants her chiropractor to visit her in the hospital to work on her neck and upper back to relieve her musculoskeletal discomfort. She urges you "not to tell," because her doctor does not believe in chiropractic, herbs, hypnosis, or other alternative therapies.

Your Actions: You must decide if this information needs to be passed on to the physician or charge nurse. You also must decide how to communicate with this patient in a way that does not convey disapproval, so she will not neglect to share information with you the way she withholds information from her physician. In addition, you need to know more about the types of complementary and alternative medicines she uses so you understand what helps her and why.

In a busy nursing unit, you may hear a coworker refer to a patient as "the gall bladder in room 209" or "the MI that went to CCU." This is not an acceptable way to refer to patients in any setting. Patients are people who have many aspects to their lives; being reduced to a medical diagnosis is neither an accurate nor an appropriate way to label them.

Yet, the health care system in the United States seems to look upon patients as a disease to be treated or a disorder to be repaired. This is partly due to the influence of 19th century philosopher René Descartes, who championed the idea that the mind and the body are not connected. At that time, medicine was first being pioneered, and the philosophy of Descartes had a huge influence on the way separate treatments were developed for physical illnesses and mental illnesses. Later, other philosophers challenged his ideas and thinking began to change, but such change has been slow to be reflected in Western medicine.

Alternative and complementary medicines, some of which originated in Eastern countries such as China and Japan, are at odds with this philosophy. A number of these therapies emphasize **holism**, or the relationships among all living things. Holistic health care, which includes the use of complementary and alternative medicine (CAM), emphasizes:

- Uniqueness of each individual
- Interaction between mind, body, and spirit
- Multiple factors as causes of illness and disease
- Patient's participation in treatment and healing

For many decades the Western and Eastern approaches to health care have been in conflict. In the past, if a patient took anything more than a multiple vitamin, the patient might not tell his or her physician for fear of being considered a "health nut." However, over the past 20 years, the use of CAM has become more and more mainstream. **Integrative health care** is a term that is used to describe the use of Western medicine and CAM in a coordinated way. Nurses

and other health care practitioners must learn about CAM and how its practices influence and assist traditional medicine. In addition, nurses must remain nonjudgmental about patients' choices to include CAM in their search for health and wellness. This integrative approach is true holistic health care. This chapter will help you understand different types of complimentary and alternative medicine and why they are helpful. It will also help you adopt a holistic approach to caring for your patients.

Alternative Therapy Versus Complementary Therapy

Alternative therapy and complementary therapy are technically different. **Alternative therapy** is a therapy used *instead* of conventional treatment, while **complementary therapy** is used along *with* conventional treatment. However, for many people, these two terms have become interchangeable, with a singular definition: treatment or therapies that are *different than* conventional treatment or therapies endorsed and used by the standard medical community.

Knowledge Connection
How is holistic health care different than your concept of health care? How can you as a nurse help contribute to integrative health care?

The Choice of Complementary and Alternative Therapies

Today's patients, many of whom access health care information by logging onto the Internet, are more knowledgeable than ever before. The more these patients learn about CAM, the more they become convinced that traditional medicine does not have all the answers; these are the people who eagerly seek out alternative theories and treatments. Other individuals utilize mainstream medicine but turn to alternative methods for what they believe to be health-enhancing measures. Patients also choose CAM because of issues surrounding:

- **Cost:** As traditional medical costs spiral out of control, patients view CAM as a cost-effective option.
- **Access:** In some communities, it is easier to access CAM than traditional medical care.
- **Self-determination:** Patients sometimes feel that the CAM practitioner encourages them to participate more in their own health care decisions; this is in contrast to the belief held by many patients that conventional medical practitioners have a tendency to direct care by telling patients what care will be provided.
- **Personal touch:** Some patients feel that CAM practitioners spend more time with them than conventional medical practitioners and are more apt to listen to their concerns. Also, CAM practitioners generally provide more of a hands-on approach; many types of CAM provide more physical contact and actual touching of the patient, although some do not involve touch.

Knowledge Connection
What is the difference between alternative therapy and complementary therapy? List some reasons why people might use complementary and alternative medicine.

Western Medicine

Allopathic medicine is a name used to describe traditional medicine, conventional medicine, or Western medicine. *Allopathic* refers to the treatment of disease by creating an environment that is antagonistic to the disease. The term *Western medicine* is used more commonly and will be used in this chapter to refer to allopathic medicine. One tenet of Western medicine is to prescribe drugs or treatments to kill foreign invaders, such as bacteria or viruses, which have made the body ill. These invaders must be eliminated for a return to health to take place.

Some practitioners of Western medicine tend to see health as the absence of disease, pain, or other symptoms of illness. Symptoms are disagreeable phenomena to be eliminated or suppressed. Prevention, until recently, was not a primary concern, and the mind and body were seen as separate, with no connection of the mind to the body and its function.

This is the type of health care with which most Americans are most familiar. You do not seek health care when you feel well, and when you have symptoms of an illness, you go to the doctor, who almost always writes a prescription for you. You then take the medication and hope that soon you are symptom-free, until the cycle repeats itself. For many people, at some point in their lives, an organ or system becomes so diseased that continuous medication is needed to stay symptom-free. And for many, surgery is necessary to repair or remove diseased organs. The Western medicine approach is that the correct medications and surgery will make you well.

Eastern and Alternative Health Care

Eastern medicine is often not what we think of as medicine at all. *Eastern* usually refers to ideas and practices from places such as Asia and India. The awareness and use of bioenergy, also called ch'i, prana, or life-force, is extremely important. From this flows a difference in definitions of health, illness, symptoms, and the role of physicians and of health care itself. These differences are often seen in CAM, as well.

In Eastern medicine, illness and disease are viewed as a disharmony, imbalance, or defect of energy in the body. Illness is a deviation from normal, healthy function. Symptoms are warning signs that the body is trying to heal itself but needs help; the symptoms are messages or signals about underlying issues of imbalance. The cause of illness is anything that interferes with the balance and movement of bioenergy: Diet, genetic makeup, lifestyle, trauma, negative thoughts, stress, and environmental toxins are all considered possible influences on health.

In Eastern medicine and some complementary and alternative medicines, illness progresses in this manner: An energy imbalance causes functional changes that can initiate a progression of chronic illness preceding pathological changes in tissue.

Personal responsibility is seen as a key to health. According to this philosophy, a person's lifestyle and emotional outlook can help prevent illness; this prevents the viewpoint that people are victims of disease.

A major emphasis in Eastern medicine is the prevention of illness. Humankind is seen as an ecosystem that, when working correctly, functions in harmony. Physicians, in turn, are viewed as assistants to help cultivate life and vitality. Mind and body are one, inextricably connected, each affecting the other and overall health.

Mind-Body Connections

Most all complementary and alternative medicines have as a basis the belief that the body has the inherent ability to heal itself, unless an illness or disease has progressed too far for this self-healing to occur. Also, rather than focusing on symptom relief and removal, CAM practitioners emphasize the need to treat the cause of illness. They also encourage preventive care rather than crisis care. A practitioner who follows these tenets and looks at the whole person rather than just the diseased part of the person would be closer to practicing holistic care than practitioners who practice using a more medical model.

Knowledge Connection
How does Western medicine view illness and disease? How does Eastern medicine view illness and disease?

Types of Complementary and Alternative Medicine

Many different types of complementary and alternative medicine and treatments exist, some more well-known in the United States than others. In this chapter, we will look in-depth at five of the more common practices:

- Chiropractic
- Massage therapy
- Acupuncture and acupressure
- Herbal supplements
- Yoga

In addition, we will provide general information about other types of CAM.

Chiropractic

Writings from China and Greece as long as 4,700 years ago mention spinal manipulation and the maneuvering of the lower extremities to ease low back pain. Hippocrates, who lived from 460 to 357 BC, wrote, "Get knowledge of the spine, for this is the requisite for many diseases."

In the United States, chiropractic was started as an art and science by D. D. Palmer in 1895. Palmer devised the name **chiropractic**, which is a combination of two Greek words meaning "done by hand." It refers to manipulation of the spine to relieve pressure on the nerves. Palmer was well read in the medical journals of the time and had knowledge of the developments that were occurring throughout the world regarding anatomy and physiology. Palmer theorized that the brain and nervous system controlled not only function and movement of the body, but also health or the lack thereof. Statistics show chiropractic to be one of the fastest growing forms of health care in America today, in terms of both patients and number of doctors.

The primary tenet of chiropractic is that natural and conservative methods of health care are preferable to invasive treatment and the use of drugs. Another important concept is that the nervous system plays a major role in health and disease. Doctors of chiropractic have a deep respect for the human body's ability to heal itself. They believe that, in many cases, surgery and drugs are not necessary and that, once nutrition and other lifestyle factors are improved and the person's nervous system is working at its full potential, the body is designed to correct itself. These doctors devote careful attention to the biomechanics, or movement, of the spine, as well as the anatomy and physiology of the spine and related structures. Additionally, they study the effects of the impulses through the spinal nerves on the musculoskeletal and neurological systems, and the role played by the proper function of these systems in the preservation and restoration of health.

Anatomy and Physiology Connection

The Spine, the Nerves, and Correcting Interference
The brain controls the functions of the body through a network of nerves that connect to the spinal cord. These spinal nerves connect with the cord inside the spinal column, where they are protected by the vertebrae, and each spinal nerve passes through openings between the vertebrae cushioned by the intervertebral disks. When pressure is applied to the spinal nerve as it exits the cord, the transmission of messages to and from the brain through that nerve are affected. The organs and muscles that the nerve *innervates* (connects with and passes messages to and from) are at risk for dysfunction due to nerve disturbance. In chiropractic, this is referred to as the *vertebral subluxation complex,* or VSC. If the nerve interference is corrected through manipulation of the spine or relaxation of muscle spasm, the messages to and from the brain are restored and correct function can be re-established.

Chiropractors regularly treat people with neuromuscular complaints such as headaches, joint pain, and neck and back pain. They also treat people with arthritis, tendonitis, and sprains and strains. Some chiropractors use only hands-on techniques when "adjusting" patients (Fig. 11-1). Others

Figure 11-1 A chiropractor treating a patient for upper back pain.

use equipment not unlike that found in physical therapy offices, such as ultrasound equipment, exercise areas, and traction tables.

Chiropractic may not be appropriate for all patients. Patients with certain health conditions such as osteoporosis and cancer and those who have had back surgery should share this information with the chiropractic practitioner so that he or she can administer appropriate treatment and avoid causing harm.

Massage Therapy

Massage has been in use for thousands of years. Writings from ancient Rome, Greece, Japan, China, Egypt, and India confirm this. **Massage therapy** is the application of stroking, pressure, friction, and kneading to muscles and other soft tissue to relax muscles and decrease stress (Fig. 11-2).

Massage first became popular in the United States in the mid-1900s, but in recent years it has gained even more in popularity. People seek massage therapy to relieve musculoskeletal pain, decreases stress, relieve depression and anxiety, increase relaxation, and promote an overall sense of

well-being. People also seek massage therapy because it feels good. Due to the stress-filled lives of many people, massage therapy has become extremely popular over the past decade.

Many varieties of massage are available. Some of the best known and most popular ones are:

- **Swedish:** This type of massage features long, flowing strokes; kneading; vibration; and compression. This is a calming massage shown to help relieve pain and joint stiffness.
- **Shiatsu:** This is a Japanese-style massage that uses thumb pressure to work along energy meridians, similar to acupressure.
- **Reflexology:** Practitioners of this type of massage use their thumb and fingers to stimulate pressure points on the feet. Practitioners believe that internal organs are associated with the nerve endings on the sole of the foot, based on the idea of energy pathways that are present in the body.
- **Deep Tissue:** This is a more vigorous, strenuous massage with focused pressure applied to tightened muscle areas and trigger points.

One of the advantages of massage therapy is its ability to relieve muscle tension and stress without using medications that may produce side effects. Another advantage for massage therapy is that it stimulates the circulatory system, which is advantageous to all the body systems. Massage therapy is also known for stimulating the body to produce endorphins, which are chemicals developed by the body that are useful in pain relief; they also help to provide a sense of well-being.

Individuals considering massage who have serious health issues should ask questions of their doctor and massage therapist before proceeding. Some conditions that could contraindicate massage include a history of blood clots in the legs or the lungs, a cancerous tumor that has not been removed, certain heart conditions, and severe osteoporosis (with vigorous massage).

Figure 11-2 A massage therapist performing massage.

importance of a diet rich in potassium, calcium, and magnesium if the client suffers from muscle cramping. She can explain how the body works and what the client can do to help the body work correctly. As a massage therapist, she can help relax muscle knots, soothe tense muscles, and stretch tight muscles. In addition, she helps the patient relax, rest, and cope with stress. She feels that this is truly integrative health care.

Acupuncture and Acupressure

Acupuncture is the ancient practice of inserting fine needles into carefully selected points located along **meridians**, or energy pathways, in the body. Classical Chinese medicine explains that channels of energy run in regular patterns through the body and over its surface. An obstruction in the movement of energy through these channels backs up energy like a dam would back up water in a river. It is thought that acupuncture stimulates the body's healing ability and corrects dysfunction. The practitioner places needles just below the skin's surface at various points along the meridians and twirls them to help remove the blockage. The existence of these meridians, the cause of disruption of energy through these pathways, and how the restoration of energy flow occurs have not been clearly identified. However, the National Institutes of Health (NIH) issued a statement for the use of acupuncture. This statement says that there is clear evidence that supports the effectiveness of acupuncture for the treatment of postoperative and chemotherapy-induced nausea and vomiting, nausea with pregnancy, and postoperative dental pain.

Acupressure is a blend of acupuncture and pressure and is a part of traditional Chinese medicine. All that is said and written about acupuncture is the same for acupressure, except that, rather than applying needles to parts of the body to affect the meridians' flow of energy, pressure is used.

In most states, medical doctors and chiropractors can receive extra training in acupuncture and practice it along with medicine or chiropractic. And in many states an individual can obtain a license to just practice acupuncture without also being a doctor.

Studies and stories abound in Asian countries about the use of and reliance upon acupuncture, although it has not become as popular in the United States. Many hospitals in Asia use acupuncture for most patients before and after surgery. These patients need very little, if any, pain medication. Interest in acupuncture soared in the United States after American visitors to China brought back firsthand reports of patients undergoing major surgery using acupuncture as the sole form of anesthesia.

Knowledge Connection

What is the explanation for the use of acupuncture to relieve pain or promote anesthesia? For which conditions does the NIH approve the use of acupuncture?

Herbal Supplements

Herbs have been used for at least 5,000 years by the Egyptians, Greeks, and Romans to promote healing and prevent illness. Today, herbs are widely used in Europe and are gaining popularity in the United States. The popularity of herbs in the United States may be due to several factors: one is that herbs often have fewer and less severe side effects than prescription medications. Another is that people can take a certain amount of control over their own health and try using herbs for conditions that health care professionals have not been able to successfully treat or for which their prescribed medication has been objectionable in some way. Often people choose to use herbs as a preventative for potential health problems. Some of the more popular herbs and their uses are found in Box 11-1.

Because some herbs can interact with medications and interfere with surgery and its outcomes, it is important that patients tell their health care providers about their use of herbs. Some people can become very confused about the effective use of herbal supplements, with the result that they take herbs that can interact with one another or cause undesirable outcomes. It is advisable to research herbs thoroughly or depend on the advice of a knowledgeable person such as a nutritionist or an herbalist. Some herbs that should be avoided during pregnancy or avoided altogether are listed in Box 11-2.

Yoga

Yoga is considered a mind-body intervention used to decrease the negative effects of stress through the use of breathing exercises, physical postures, and meditation. It evolved as a spiritual practice, but in the West it is viewed more narrowly as a form of exercise.

Yoga was first introduced to the United States in the late 1800s, but has been practiced for more than 5,000 years in the East. Yoga invokes ideas of harmony, health, and balance. It is believed to calm the nervous system and balance the mind, body, and spirit. It is thought by its practitioners to prevent diseases and illnesses by keeping the energy meridians open and flowing. Yoga has been used to lower blood pressure, lessen stress, and improve coordination, flexibility, concentration, sleep, and digestion. It has also been recommended by its proponents as supplementary therapy for conditions such as cancer, asthma, diabetes, and irritable bowel syndrome.

As an exercise, it has evolved into several subdivisions and variations. Hatha yoga is a common and popular form of yoga practiced in the United States. It prepares and conditions the body so that the mind can practice meditation without obstacles. It is slow paced and gentle, taking the practitioner through basic yoga poses. Ashtanga yoga is more fast paced and intense. It requires the practitioner to change quickly from one pose to another, always following the same order. Power yoga follows similar principles, but does not necessarily follow the same set of Ashtanga poses. Iyengar yoga emphasizes the use of props such as blocks,

Box 11-1

Popular Herbs and Their Uses

Many herbs and supplements are available. The list below includes some of the more popular herbs and the reasons they are used.

- **Aloe vera:** A well-known herb that is used alone and in many products for skin problems; some people drink it to promote overall health.
- **Capsaicin:** Used for tenderness and pain of osteoarthritis; some use it for fibromyalgia, diabetic neuropathy, and shingles.
- **Chamomile:** May be helpful for anxiety, to induce sleep, and to relieve stomach upset.
- **Echinacea:** Used as an antiviral agent to prevent or eliminate colds, flu, and other infections.
- **Feverfew:** Used as an anti-inflammatory; also used for migraine headaches, fever suppression, and menstrual cramps.
- **Garlic:** Helps reduce total blood cholesterol and low-density lipoproteins (bad cholesterol) over short periods of time, for example, 4 to 12 weeks.
- **Ginger:** Used to help relieve nausea and vomiting of pregnancy in recommended doses for short periods of time. Large doses of ginger may be unsafe for the developing baby, however.
- **Gingko:** Used for memory enhancement and dementia, and to help increase blood flow to the brain.
- **Ginseng:** Used to help lower bad cholesterol and protect the heart; also helps lower blood sugar in type 2 diabetes but not to dangerous levels; may help boost the immune system.
- **Peppermint:** Use of peppermint oil combined with caraway oil is helpful in treating heartburn; peppermint oil may improve irritable bowel syndrome and decrease spasms of the gastrointestinal tract before and after endoscopic procedures.
- **St. John's Wort:** Used for mild to moderate depression; studies have shown it to be at least as effective for this purpose as prescription drugs.
- **Saw Palmetto:** Used to treat enlarged prostate in men. Helps improve symptom of difficult urination, but does not actually shrink the prostate.
- **Soy:** Helps decrease cholesterol and low-density lipoproteins; helps improve acute diarrhea in infants, as in soy formulas; helps decrease menopausal symptoms such as hot flashes.
- **Valerian:** Used to treat insomnia; helps improve quality sleep and helps decrease the amount of time it takes to fall asleep.

straps, and blankets and is concerned with proper body alignment in each pose, as well as holding the poses for long periods of time. This emphasis helps prevent injuries and assists the body to obtain the maximum benefit from the exercise. Yoga is usually performed in classes with sessions conducted several times a week.

Additional Forms of Complementary and Alternative Medicine

A large variety of less common types of CAM are available, but these are used by a smaller portion of the population. While you may well encounter patients who use

Box 11-2

Cautions for Herbal Use

The U.S. Food and Drug Administration does not recommend the use of the herbs comfrey; ephedra, also known as ma huang; and kava:

- Comfrey contains substances that are toxic to the liver and can cause blood clots.
- Ephedra, or ma huang, causes increased blood pressure and causes stress to the circulatory system that can lead to heart attack or stroke.
- Kava also can cause liver toxicity, especially in those who already have liver disease.

It is also recommended that the following herbs be avoided in the first 12 weeks of pregnancy:

- Ginger in amounts of 9 grams or more.
- Ephedra and kava root, which can cause increased heart rate and shortness of breath.
- St. John's wort and echinacea, which have not been tested enough to risk possible effects on the fetus.

one or more of these therapies, you will probably hear more frequently about the types discussed earlier in the chapter. Box 11-3 provides explanations of additional types of CAM.

Lifestyle Changes That Reverse Disease

Another aspect of CAM is the belief that disease can be prevented or even eliminated by adopting a healthy lifestyle and eating whole foods that have not been processed or adulterated. Some studies have been done to validate these ideas.

Terry Shintani, a physician in Hawaii, found that obese patients who also had joint pain issues related to weight, as well as diabetes, lost weight and eliminated their diabetes and joint pain by following a diet of nearly unlimited vegetables, certain fruits, and a small amount of fish. Another physician, Dean Ornish, performed research on a way to reverse heart disease without drugs or surgery. This was accomplished by drastically changing the food intake and lifestyle of people with severe coronary artery disease. The subjects in the study actually reversed blockages in their coronary arteries by increasing their activity level and eating a controlled diet rich in vegetables, fruits, and whole grains, with very little meat.

While both of these physicians have shown how much food and lifestyle changes can truly reverse illness, many others feel that these changes are neither realistic nor attainable for the average American; therefore, surgery and medications must be employed. This is where Western medicine and CAM differ: While CAM seeks to find ways to avoid drugs and surgery, Western medicine sees no other viable choices.

Box 11-3

Additional Forms of CAM

There are numerous forms of CAM. Some of the more frequently used forms with their descriptions are listed here.

- **Aromatherapy:** Essential oils with strong fragrances are used to affect a person's mood or health; has been used for 6,000 years; some oils may cause irritation if applied directly to the skin; may be added to carrier oil for massage therapy.
- **Meditation:** A discipline in which the mind is focused on an object of thought or awareness, and usually involves turning attention to a single point of reference; many religions incorporate meditation; has been practiced for over 5,000 years; forms of meditation devoid of religious or mystic content have been developed in the West as a way of promoting physical and mental well-being.
- **Biofeedback:** Use of monitoring devices to help a person become aware of changes in heart rate, blood pressure, and muscle contractions so that they can be controlled using deep breathing and intentional relaxation.
- **Relaxation Therapy and Imagery:** Uses conscious awareness and visual images to relax muscles, lower respiration, and promote calm. Can ease stress and lower blood pressure.
- **Therapeutic Touch or Healing Touch:** An energy modality that encourages healing; practitioners place their hands near a patient to detect and manipulate the patient's energy fields, assisting in the natural healing process; developed in the United States and is endorsed by the American Holistic Nurses Association.
- **Phytonutrients:** Certain components of plants that are used to promote human health; fruits, vegetables, grains, legumes,

nuts, and teas are rich in phytonutrients; thought to protect against many diseases, including cancer.
- **Free radicals and antioxidants:** Oxidation produces free radicals, which begins a process that damages cells and causes aging; antioxidants are molecules capable of slowing the oxidation of other molecules.
- **Pet Therapy or Animal-Assisted Therapy:** Use of animals to help people who are ill; visits from animals can provide a welcome change from the routine, and can help lift depression and loneliness; research shows people who have had heart attacks and who have pets live longer, and that petting a dog lowers blood pressure.
- **Music Therapy:** Use of music to promote wellness, manage stress, express feelings, enhance memory, improve communication, and promote physical rehabilitation; used in many different settings, with patients of all ages; incorporated in therapeutic care of patients with psychiatric disorders, developmental disabilities, speech and hearing impairments, physical disabilities, and neurological impairments.
- **Play Therapy:** Used by licensed mental health professionals to communicate with children; Association for Play Therapy defines this therapy as "the systematic use of a theoretical model to establish an interpersonal process wherein trained play therapists use the therapeutic powers of play to help clients prevent or resolve psychosocial difficulties and achieve optimal growth and development"; usually used with children ages 3 to 11 to help them express thoughts and feelings.

Knowledge Connection

List three herbs and their uses. How can practicing yoga improve health? List four additional types of CAM and their uses. What is your response to the studies showing that food and lifestyle changes can actually reverse diabetes and coronary artery disease?

Nursing Care and CAM

When you care for patients who use CAM, it is important to respect their preferences and wishes. However, if the CAM modalities can interact negatively with medications or treatments prescribed for them, it is also important to be sure they understand this. In most nursing drug handbooks, you will find information about herbs that interact with the medication you are researching. Be sure to ask patients if they are taking any of the herbal supplements listed to prevent potential negative interactions. For example, St. John's wort and ginseng can decrease the effectiveness of warfarin, a blood thinner. Feverfew and echinacea, among others, can increase bleeding in patients taking warfarin.

When obtaining information for a patient's history, be sure to ask about alternative and complementary therapies. Do so in a nonjudgmental way, so the patient will be comfortable divulging the information to you. Record the information in the patient's nursing history without drawing conclusions. Remember, people use what they can find to help relieve their symptoms.

Patient Teaching Connection

Teaching About CAM and Medical Conditions

Use patient teaching to carefully caution patients about the use of CAM and interactions with their current medications or treatment. For example, a patient recently diagnosed with a compression fracture of the spine states that he goes to a chiropractor once a month. It is important for his chiropractor to know about this diagnosis and the exact location of the compression fracture before he is treated again. Instruct the patient to inform his chiropractor that he has a compression fracture of L3.

Post Conference

After caring for your patient for 2 days, you helped discharge her. It was amazing to see how well she did without traditional pain medication. When one of the nurses said to you, "She's kind of a nut, isn't she?", you found yourself defending your patient and her choices. This experience really opened your eyes to some aspects of complimentary and alternative medicine that you had never thought about before. While caring for your patient, you encouraged her to tell her doctor about all of her CAM use. He listened thoughtfully and did not judge her negatively for her choices. You also had the opportunity to teach her about some interactions between her natural supplements and her prescription medications that she did not know previously. So, you and your patient both learned from one another.

KEY POINTS

- Holistic health care involves treating patients as people who have many aspects to their lives, not just labeling them regarding their reason for hospitalization. Holistic care requires that we treat each patient as a unique individual with interactions between mind, body, and spirit.

- Complementary and alternative medicine (CAM) is being used more and more by our society, so nurses need to be aware and knowledgeable of it. It is more easily available and costs less than traditional medicine. In addition, CAM practitioners physically touch their patients, which increases its value to some people.

- Western, or allopathic, medicine bases its approach to disease and illness on the idea that foreign invaders, such as antigens, viruses, and bacteria, cause illness and must be treated with medications. Surgery may be required to remove or repair a diseased or malfunctioning organ.

- Eastern medicine, and many types of CAM, see disease or illness as a deviation from normal, healthy function and symptoms as warning signs of underlying imbalance. Illness is caused by anything that interferes with the balance and movement of bioenergy, including diet, lifestyle, trauma, environmental toxins, and stress.

- The mind, body, and spirit are all connected and must all be treated. Practitioners of CAM emphasize these connections and believe that the body has the inherent nature to heal itself if given the correct support.

- Chiropractic's primary tenet is that natural and conservative methods of health care are preferable and that the nervous system plays a major role in health and disease. Interference with nerve messages to and from the body and brain increases the likelihood of illness and disease. Chiropractors use manual adjustments and other equipment to correct this nerve interference.

- Massage therapy involves the use of stroking, pressure, friction, and kneading of muscles and other soft tissue. It helps decrease stress, relieve anxiety and depression, increase relaxation, and promote an overall sense of well-being.

- Acupuncture and acupressure have their roots in Chinese medicine and involve the use of long, thin, hollow needles inserted beneath the skin (acupuncture) or pressure on acupuncture sites (acupressure) to relieve blockages in the movement of energy through meridians throughout the body.

- Many different herbal supplements are used for a variety of reasons. They can interfere with medications, so question patients about their use of herbal supplements to determine potential interactions.

- Yoga is more than an exercise in Eastern medicine. It invokes harmony, health, and balance and can help calm the nervous system and balance the mind, body, and spirit.

REVIEW QUESTIONS

Select the answer that is most appropriate for each of the following questions. Some questions may have more than one correct answer. Check all that apply.

1. In holistic health care, the emphasis is on the uniqueness of each individual and the interaction between:

   a. health, environment, and disease.

   b. mind, body, and spirit.

   c. herbs, chiropractic, and massage.

   d. Western medicine, allopathic medicine, and CAM.

2. Which is true of alternative medicine and complementary medicine?

   a. They mean the same thing and are simply different than conventional treatment.

   b. They cost more than traditional medicine but may be more effective.

   c. Access to these medicines is limited, so few people can use them.

   d. Alternative medicine is used instead of complementary medicine.

   e. Complementary medicine is used with traditional medicine.

   f. Both d and e.

3. You see a patient while in clinical at a walk-in clinic. This patient has occasional abdominal pain of unknown cause, but otherwise is in good health. The doctor suggests blood work and a CT scan of the abdomen to diagnose the cause. The patient says he wants to wait, see his acupuncturist, and give his body the opportunity to heal itself. What is your response?

   a. Tell the patient that he MUST follow through with the doctor's orders.

   b. Express strong disapproval of this plan, both verbally and nonverbally.

   c. Encourage the patient to act quickly and return if the pain persists.

   d. Explain that the body cannot heal itself and requires a doctor's intervention to heal.

4. A patient says he wants to go to a chiropractor to see if it will help his low back pain because medical treatment has been ineffective. How might you respond?

   a. "Some studies have shown chiropractic to be an effective treatment for low back pain."

   b. "You would do better to stick with a real doctor."

   c. "I am not allowed to discuss alternative or complimentary medicine with you."

   d. "You need to ask your medical doctor for permission to do that."

5. A person with a tight, sore neck and headaches might use which of these CAM choices for relief?

   a. Echinacea

   b. Chiropractic

   c. Biofeedback

   d. Phytonutrients

   e. Massage therapy

   f. Acupuncture/acupressure

   g. Play therapy

   h. Ginko

   i. Relaxation therapy and imagery

SHORT ANSWER QUESTIONS

6. The cause and effect of illness according to Eastern medicine and most types of CAM follows this pattern: Energy imbalance _____ pathological tissue change.

7. A patient with nausea and vomiting due to chemotherapy for cancer might find relief from which type of CAM?

8. Which conditions could cause massage to be contraindicated for a patient?

CRITICAL THINKING EXERCISE

9. A patient is hospitalized with excessive bleeding after taking the blood thinner warfarin for 2 months. When you ask the patient about the medications she takes, she tells you that she started taking an herbal blend to prevent colds and flu about 6 weeks ago and she thinks it is helping her. What action will you take and why?

ADDITIONAL RESOURCES

For additional Resources, Questions, and Activities, please see:

 Student Resource Disk

 DavisPlus http://davisplus.fadavis.com

 Student Study Guide

REFERENCES

Barnes PM, Powell-Griner E, McFann K, Nahin RL. *CAM Use Among Adults.* Atlanta: National Center for Health Statistics; 2004.

Boon HS, Kachan N. Integrative medicine: a tale of two clinics. *BMC Complement Altern Med.* 2008;18(8):32.

Chou R, Huffman L. Nonpharmacological therapies for acute and chronic low back pain: a review of the evidence for an American Pain Society/ American College of Physicians clinical practice guideline. *Ann Intern Med.* 2007;147:492-504.

Chou R, Qaseem A, Snow V, Casey D, Cross JT Jr, Shekelle P, et al. Diagnosis and treatment of low back pain: a joint clinical practice guideline from the American College of Physicians and the American Pain Society. *Ann Intern Med.* 2007;147:478-491.

Drugs, Supplements, and Herbal Information. Medline Plus Web site. Available at: http://www.nlm.nih.gov/medlineplus/druginformation. html. Accessed August 24, 2009.

Haas M, Sharma R, Stano M. Cost-effectiveness of medical and chiropractic care for acute and chronic low back pain. *J Manipulative Physiol Ther.* 2005;28:555-563.

Haneline M. Symptomatic outcomes and perceived satisfaction levels of chiropractic patients with a primary diagnosis involving acute neck pain. *J Manipulative Physiol Ther.* 2006;29:288-296.

Herman PM, Craig BM, Caspi O. Is complementary and alternative medicine (CAM) cost-effective? A systematic review. *BMC Complement Altern Med.* 2005;5:11.

Hern JA. Use of complementary and alternative therapies in community-dwelling older adults. *Complement Med.* 2007;13:997-1006.

Horrigan BJ. New NHIS survey reveals that 38% of Americans use CAM. *EXPLORE.* 2009;5(2):7-13.

Lao L, Schyrer R. The status and future of acupuncture research: 10 years post-NIH consensus conference. *J Altern Complement Med.* 2008;14:859-860.

Manga Report. Ontario: Ministry of Health, Government of Ontario, Canada; 1993.

Massage Therapy as CAM. Bethesda, MD: National Center for Complementary and Alternative Medicine, 2006.

Mehta D, Gardiner P, Phillips R, McCarthy E. Herbal and dietary supplement disclosure to health care providers by individuals with chronic conditions. *J Altern Complement Med.* 2008;14:1263-1269.

Mitchinson A, Hyungjin MK, Rosenberg J, Geisser M, Kirsh M, Cikrit D, et al. Acute postoperative pain management using massage as an adjuvant therapy: a randomized trial. *Arch Surg.* 2007;142:1158-1167.

National Center for Complementary and Alternative Medicine. *Chiropractic: An Introduction.* NCCAM Publication No. D403. November 2007. Available at: http://nccam.nih.gov/health/chiropractic. Accessed August 14, 2009.

Natural Herbs. Available at: http://www.herbsguide.org. Accessed August 24, 2009.

Ornish D. *Dr. Dean Ornish's Program For Reversing Heart Disease.* New York: Random House; 1990.

Scanlon V, Sanders T. *Essentials of Anatomy and Physiology.* Philadelphia: FA Davis; 2007.

Shintini T. *Eat More, Weigh Less.* Kamuela, HI: Halpax; 1996.

U.S. Food and Drug Administration. Dietary Supplements. Available at: http://vm.cfsan.fda.gov/~dms/supplmnt.html. Accessed August 24, 2009.

Wilkey A, Gregory M, Byfield D, McCarthy P. A comparison between chiropractive management and pain clinic management for chronic low-back pain in a National Health Service outpatient clinic. *J Altern Complement Med.* 2008;14:465-473.

Williams L, Hopper P. *Understanding Medical Surgical Nursing.* 3rd ed. Philadelphia: FA Davis; 2007.

Patient Teaching

Key Terms

Auditory learning

Health promotion

Interpreter

Kinesthetic learning

Learning

Reinforce

Teachable moments

Visual learning

Wellness strategies

Objectives

1. Identify three primary learning styles.
2. Explain ways to address learning styles during patient teaching.
3. Describe factors that affect learning.
4. Discuss information to consider when arranging for an interpreter.
5. Discuss the importance of reinforcement of patient teaching.
6. Identify two primary purposes of patient teaching.
7. Define the concept of teachable moments.
8. Describe how to develop a teaching plan using the nursing process.
9. Discuss ways to implement a teaching plan.
10. Describe three ways to evaluate patient teaching.
11. Explain how to teach patients about Internet resources.

Clinical Connection

Your Assignment: You are assigned to care for a 42-year-old female with a new diagnosis of diabetes mellitus. She is overweight and sedentary, eats at restaurants most of the time, and knows very little about diabetes. She is very confused about the lifestyle changes she needs to make. She is scheduled to be discharged today on oral diabetes medication and with a glucometer.

Your Actions: To prepare to care for this patient, you must find out what she does know about her disease. You also need to find out how she learns best so you can provide her with appropriate learning materials. You will have to find a time and place to provide reinforcement for the learning that has already taken place. You will need to think about how she will get additional information and have her questions answered after she goes home. You also need to be sure she knows what medication she is to take, how to take it, and to be alert to side effects. She also will have to do her own finger stick blood sugar tests twice a day, so you will have to determine whether she can perform that skill once she is at home.

You may think of yourself as a student, not a teacher. Yet, you will be a teacher to your patients. Chances are good that you will not stand up in front of a class using a dry-erase board, but you will teach all the same. Every time you explain the purpose of a treatment or medication; show a patient how to care for a wound, drain, or tube; or answer a patient or family member's questions, you will be teaching.

Learning

One explanation of **learning** is that, when it occurs, behavior changes. True learning is not merely memorizing isolated facts or being able to recite a list of data. True learning is evidenced by applying new information. However, all people do not learn the same way.

Learning Styles

Although many different ideas exist about the ways in which people learn, the most familiar explanation of learning styles is also the first, developed in the 1970s. Known by some as VAK, the identified styles for learning are:

- **Visual learning**: learning by seeing, reading, and watching
- **Auditory learning**: learning by hearing and listening
- **Kinesthetic learning**: learning by touching and doing

People can learn in every style, but most people prefer one style when exposed to new information and ideas.

When you teach patients about their care, it is important that you address each style of learning. You may verbally explain information, but you need to provide written information and videos as well. If you are teaching a task, such as a dressing change, you will need to demonstrate what the patient is to do, then provide an opportunity for the patient to perform the task while you watch. This is referred to as a *return demonstration*.

Factors That Affect Learning

Not only do you need to address all three learning styles when teaching patients, you also need to consider the following factors that affect learning, including barriers that could delay or impede learning:

- **Environment:** Find a place that is quiet and free of distractions when you want your patient to learn new information.
- **Comfort:** Your patients will be unable to accomplish learning goals if they are in pain, drowsy from medications, too hot or too cold, or uncomfortable in other ways. Ensure the patient's comfort before you try to begin a teaching session.
- **Readiness:** It is difficult to learn anything if you are not ready to hear the information. Patients may be in the denial phase regarding their diagnosis, or they may feel that they do not need the treatment or medication you are explaining. Patients also may simply be too ill to hear and understand your teaching.
- **Language:** Patients cannot learn if the teaching is not provided in a language that they understand. If you do not speak the same language as the patient, arrange for an **interpreter**, or translator, to be present for patient teaching. (Box 12-1 provides information to consider when arranging for an interpreter.) Another language issue is that of using medical terminology and other terms that the patient may not understand. Be sure you are using general terms and not medical terms when you teach. If medical terms are necessary, be sure to explain the meanings of those terms.
- **Senses:** Patients cannot learn if they have visual or hearing impairments that interfere with their ability to see and hear the information being presented. Position yourself so that the patient can see your lips. Do not sit or stand in front of a window or light that causes a glare. Be sure the patients are wearing glasses or have in hearing aids if they wear them. Use larger print handouts for patients with visual impairments.

Box 12-1

Arranging for an Interpreter

When a patient does not speak English, it is necessary to have an interpreter present for patient teaching. Here are some ways to help you chose the best interpreter for the situation:

- Even if the patient can speak and understand some English, arrange for an interpreter who speaks the patient's primary language. During times of illness or crisis, the patient may be less able to speak and understand English.
- Whenever possible, use a professional or certified interpreter rather than a family member. The hospital or other facility will have a list of interpreters available to translate for you. You will need to plan ahead so you can arrange for an interpreter to be present during patient teaching.
- Arrange for an interpreter who has some understanding of medical terminology so that questions and answers can be translated correctly.
- Try to avoid using young children as interpreters for their parents. This may put the children in a culturally inappropriate situation if taboo areas of the body need to be discussed.

Repetition

It is not uncommon for patient teaching to be rushed, a last-minute task performed at discharge when the patient is anxious to leave the facility, but this is not the ideal time to attempt teaching. For learning to truly take place, information must be introduced, explained, and **reinforced**, or repeated several times. Ideally, you should begin teaching about the disease process, medications, and nursing care as they are introduced in the patient's care, preferably on the day of admission. You may feel that you are boring the patient when you repeat instructions or information, but you probably are not. While you are familiar with what you are teaching, the information is often completely new to patients. Hearing it repeatedly will help reinforce their learning.

One method of using reinforcement is to introduce the most important concept you want to teach first. Then return to that topic and teach it again last so the patient will remember it.

Knowledge Connection

Name the three learning styles. What should you keep in mind when arranging for an interpreter during patient teaching? What are five factors that affect learning?

Teaching About Health and Illness

Most information that you teach will focus on the patient's need to know about his or her own health and treatment of illness. Adult learners are motivated to learn in order to solve a problem or meet a need, so you will need to identify issues of care that the patient views as fitting this category. In addition, you will need to establish a realistic expectation of what patients are able to learn in the amount of time available for patient teaching.

Purposes of Patient Teaching

When you provide patient teaching, it will be primarily for two purposes:

1. To instruct patients on health promotion and wellness strategies
2. To explain disease processes, treatments, and care

Instruction regarding **health promotion** includes information about ways to stay healthy. Examples of this teaching include getting regular exercise, making healthy food choices, drinking enough water, and including adequate amounts of fiber, vitamins, and minerals in the diet. When you teach about **wellness strategies**, you will emphasize changing unhealthy practices. Examples of this include stopping smoking, losing weight if appropriate, using alcohol and sweets only in moderation, reducing stress, and lowering cholesterol levels.

Before you teach patients about disease processes, you may need to do some research because you want to be sure you are giving correct information to your patients. In the case of our Clinical Connection at the beginning of the chapter, you were assigned to care for a patient with newly diagnosed diabetes. You would need to include teaching about insulin and how it works in the body, and what happens when the body does not produce enough insulin or cannot use the insulin it does produce. It also includes teaching about the signs and symptoms of worsening diabetes, such as unstable blood sugar levels, as well as what to report to the health care provider and when to report it. It is also important to explain the potential complications of this disease, including poor circulation, delayed healing, heart disease, kidney disease, *neuropathy* (nerve damage), and *retinopathy* (retinal damage leading to possible blindness).

When you teach patients about treatments, medications, and self-care, you will help them understand how to care for themselves. Patients are more likely to comply with medication orders if they understand the purposes and effects of the medications they have been prescribed. Patients also follow ordered treatments better if they understand the purpose of the treatment and feel comfortable performing it. For example, in the situation of a diabetic patient, you might teach about the effects and side effects of oral medications to treat elevated blood sugar, how to perform a finger stick blood sugar measurement using a glucometer (Fig. 12-1), the signs and symptoms of high and low blood sugar levels, when to report finger stick blood sugar readings to the health care provider, and how to treat low blood sugar.

As you can see, nurses teach patients repeatedly as teachable moments present themselves throughout care. These **teachable moments** occur when:

- Patients ask you questions about their illness or treatment
- You hear or observe misinformation or an incorrect procedure and you give correct information
- You point out a cause-and-effect connection to the patient

Figure 12-1   A nurse is teaching a young child about finger stick blood sugar testing.

For example, you might explain that, when the patient bends his or her wrist, the IV pump starts to beep because the fluid cannot flow freely into the vein. Another teachable moment occurs as you administer medication with a glass of water, as it allows you to stress the importance of drinking a full glass of water with the medication so it will work better.

As you learn more about providing patient care, you will learn to identify many opportunities for patient teaching. Table 12-1 lists teachable moments in routine care.

Knowledge Connection

List four topics for patient teaching. What might you teach a patient when serving a meal?

Real-World Connection

The Focus of Patient Teaching

A patient with mild diabetes was brought to the hospital with chest pain. While she was in the emergency room, she had a heart attack. After a stent was placed, she recovered without complications and was sent home. The home health nurse visited the patient at home for follow-up assessment and teaching. She began to discuss diabetes and the patient's diet. The patient told the nurse, "I don't have to be on a diabetic diet. I had a heart attack, so I am on a heart healthy diet now." The patient teaching she received in the hospital focused completely on her cardiac problems, so the patient did not understand that she needed to follow a diabetic diet as well. Remember that patient teaching needs to be focused on all the patient's health issues, not just the primary reason for hospitalization.

Teaching Plans

When you have several people with the same teaching needs, it is cost and time effective to teach patients in small groups. When presenting to small groups, you will find it helpful to make a plan for your teaching. You may also use a teaching plan when instructing individual patients, especially when you have a great deal of information to present. Once a patient begins to ask questions in the teaching session, it is easy to lose your train of thought. Using a plan helps to ensure that you do not forget something pertinent.

Developing a Teaching Plan Using the Nursing Process

As you develop a teaching plan, you will employ the nursing process to help you make decisions about what to teach and how to teach it. When you develop care plans for patients

Table 12-1   Teachable Moments

During...	Teach About...
Bathing and personal care	How to perform skin care and foot care
Daily weights	When weight gain is caused by fluid, not food intake
Ambulation	The benefits of mobility for all body systems
Meals	Intake and output, benefits of water intake, and nutritional needs
Toileting	The benefits of fiber and water intake Intake and output Signs of constipation, dehydration
Treatments	The purpose of the treatment and expected outcome How to perform the treatment if appropriate
Medication administration	The reasons for the medication(s), possible side effects, when to report side effects

whom you care for in clinical, do not forget to include teaching as a part of your plan.

Assessment

To develop a teaching plan, you need to first identify your patient's learning needs. What does the patient already know? What is unclear? What information has yet to be presented? When you take steps to determine what your patient knows, you are assessing your patient's knowledge needs. It is helpful to determine if the patient prefers something visual, such as a video. Or, does the patient prefer to read about the topic before you discuss it?

It is also important to assess the patient's readiness to learn. For example, a patient who was just informed of a serious or life-threatening diagnosis is probably not emotionally ready to learn about treatment or how to take medication. Sometimes a patient may need some time to think about the news just received; other times, the patient may want you sitting quietly nearby. This provides support while allowing the patient time to develop questions.

Nursing Diagnosis

When you determine what the patient still needs to learn, you are establishing a nursing diagnosis. The two nursing diagnoses that deal with patient teaching are:

1. **"Deficient knowledge," with descriptors:** Used when the patient is lacking knowledge about the disease process or management of the disease, including diagnostic testing, medications, and treatment. Use this nursing diagnosis when planning care according to this example:

   "Deficient knowledge about antidiabetic medications related to new diagnosis of diabetes mellitus type II": Indicates that the patient is newly diagnosed with diabetes and has not learned needed information about antidiabetic medications, such as when to take them, what effects are expected, and potential side effects to report if they occur.

2. **"Readiness for enhanced knowledge," with descriptors:** Used when the patient has some basic knowledge about the illness, but is ready for further teaching. Use this nursing diagnoses when planning care according to this example:

   "Readiness for enhanced knowledge about signs and symptoms of hypo- and hyperglycemia related to new diagnoses of diabetes mellitus type 2": Indicates that the patient is newly diagnosed with diabetes and has had some exposure to the signs and symptoms of hypoglycemia and hyperglycemia, but is ready for further teaching on the subject.

   It is your responsibility to specify the topic of teaching.

Planning

After identifying patient teaching needs, you will decide how to teach about the topic. You will need to find resources for materials to use as handouts, select a time and place for teaching, and decide how to present the material based on the patient's learning preferences. In other words, you are developing a teaching plan. Box 12-2 has information on resources for handouts.

Implementation

When you sit down with your patient or patients and present the information in your teaching plan, you are performing the implementation portion of the nursing process. During teaching, be sure to:

- Establish a comfortable temperature in a room without distractions.
- Ensure that the patient is in a comfortable position, and not experiencing pain or discomfort.
- Involve the patient in your teaching by asking questions, asking for feedback, and allowing the patient to ask questions. Avoid lecturing to the patient.

Box 12-2

Resources for Patient Teaching Handouts

There are a number of different resources you can utilize when looking for specific patient teaching handouts. Some of the most prominent are:

- **Associations and Foundations:** Look for brochures or printed information about a specific disease and self-care for that disease from organizations such as the Arthritis Foundation, American Diabetes Association, and Multiple Sclerosis Society.
- **Health Departments:** City, county, and state health departments usually have patient education information available for health care professionals to distribute. Your health care facility may already have many of these handouts on file.
- **Patient Education Websites:** Check for information available on websites of universities and medical centers. Be cautious about printing and using any information that is not approved by associations or foundations. Be aware that many commercial websites that exist charge you to use their patient information.

You can also create your own patient teaching handout by using information from a variety of sources. However, be careful not to copy information word for word from a website or existing handout. You can summarize ideas and make bulleted lists to help patients remember key ideas. Keep your handouts at about a fifth-grade reading level so all patients can understand them. Write in short, simple sentences. When choosing handouts, remember the following criteria:

- Handouts need to be in simple language, without the use of confusing medical terminology. A fifth-grade reading level is most appropriate for all patients.
- If medical terms must be used, they should be clearly defined.
- Keep in mind that patients may need a translation of the handout in a different language. Ask an interpreter to do this so the information will be translated appropriately.
- Handouts should be short, between 1 and 2 pages, and in an easy-to-read type size (font). Use size 14 font or larger for patients with vision impairments.

- Explain why the patient needs to know the information. Adults learn best when they understand the relevance of the information presented.
- Have an interpreter present if needed so the patient can understand the teaching.
- Have patients wear eyeglasses or hearing aids if appropriate. Sit where the patient can see your lips as you speak. Avoid positioning yourself in front of a window or light with a glare.
- Speak clearly and distinctly, not loudly, if the patient wears hearing aids.
- Sit near the patient during teaching. Avoid standing over the patient.
- Present one piece of information at a time, allowing the patient time to absorb it before moving on.
- Arrange and present information in a simple-to-complex format.
- Explain how to perform a task, then demonstrate as you explain it a second time.
- Give frequent positive feedback to the patient. Say things like, "You are doing great." "I'm so glad you remembered that, it is important." "Show me again how well you can do that." Avoid saying anything that discourages the patient or would indicate that you thought the patient was ignorant.

Evaluating

Now you must determine if the patient has learned what you have taught. How will you tell? Have the patient restate the information you have shared. Ask questions covering the information you have presented. If you have taught the patient to perform a task, such as changing a dressing, have the patient perform the skill while you watch. You may need to give a few verbal cues as the patient performs the skill. Then have the patient repeat it again without the cues. Table 12-2 presents examples of ways to evaluate patient teaching.

Documentation of Teaching

It is very important for nurses to document the patient teaching they perform and the patient's response. This documentation is required by The Joint Commission, which is the accrediting agency for hospitals, and by third-party payers. Quality assurance departments will look for documentation reflecting topics of patient teaching and evaluation of learning. An example of documentation of teaching would be:

1620 Instructed on correct way to perform drsg change to
L great toe. Instructed to soak foot in warm water × 20 min as
ordered, pat foot dry carefully (including between the toes), apply
Neosporin to suture line with sterile swab, apply sterile 4 × 4,
and wrap foot with elastic bandage. Pt. returned demonstration,
had mild difficulty remembering to pat dry and to dry between
all toes before applying elastic bandage. To review again at 2000
dressing change. —————————————————
——————————————— *Nurse's signature and credentials*

Some hospitals have special patient teaching documentation forms so it is not necessary to write out the documentation in narrative format. Instead, you can fill in the columns with the topics taught; evidence of learning, either verbal or return demonstration; and documentation of any comments.

Knowledge Connection
What two nursing diagnoses apply to patient teaching? How will you position yourself during patient teaching?

People and Places Connection
Patient Teaching for Different Age Groups in Different Locations
Teaching Children
When teaching children, use age-appropriate information. Use a doll or teddy bear to represent the patient when explaining a procedure or treatment. Allow the child to perform the treatment on the doll or teddy bear as a return demonstration. By teaching a child what you are going to do next, you allow the child the opportunity to better understand, feel less stress, and be more compliant. Always tell the truth regarding whether or not the procedure or treatment will be uncomfortable. Take advantage of opportunities to speak at schools and day-care facilities. Emphasize a wellness or health topic such as when and how to wash your hands.

Teaching Elderly Patients
Have a caregiver or family member present during teaching if possible. Allow plenty of time for teaching so your elderly patient does not feel rushed. Be alert to cues that the elderly patient does not understand the teaching. He or she may put you off, saying, "I'll do it later" or "I already read it." This may be because the patient is confused or does not understand, but does not want to say so. Be very patient with elderly learners. Use plenty of repetition without getting frustrated.

Home Health Care Considerations
Patients who are to be discharged from the hospital but need more teaching can be referred to home health care for follow-up teaching. This requires a physician's order. Be alert to the need to ask for a referral for more teaching. A home health care follow-up can often prevent re-hospitalization if the patient has not mastered information needed for self-care.

Teaching Patients About Internet Resources

It is not uncommon to hear patients say that they, or a family member, have looked up their diagnosis on the Internet and then, when talking with them, discover that they obtained inaccurate or misleading information. In the information age, we can obtain an amazing amount of both information and misinformation. One of the newer roles of health care professionals is to educate patients not only about their disease process, self-care, health, and wellness, but also about how to obtain accurate information using the Internet.

Table 12-2   **Ways to Evaluate Patient Teaching About Foot Care**

Evaluation Technique	Example
Have the patient restate what has been taught	"Tell me what you learned about how to care for your feet because you are diabetic."
Ask questions to determine understanding	"What will you do about trimming your toenails when they grow too long?" "How will you wash and dry your feet?" "What type of shoes and house shoes will you wear?"
Ask the patient to give a return demonstration of a new task	"You change the dressing on your toe while I watch. I'll remind you of what to do if you need a hint."

Use the following guidelines to help your patients find accurate information from websites:

- Explain that preferred sites for health care information end in ".org," ".gov," or ".edu." Most other sites are for commercial use and often want to sell you something.
- Encourage patients to avoid reading blogs concerning disease processes or treatment. Explain that such entries are one person's experiences or opinions and are not the result of research or collective information.
- Encourage patients to use familiar sites with accurate information. For example, WebMD and PDRHealth are both sites with understandable and credible information.
- Urge patients to avoid using sites such as Wikipedia because anyone can post information on such sites, making it subject to opinion rather than fact.
- Explain that the authors' credentials and educational background should be clearly listed.
- Tell patients to check the date of the most recent posting to be sure they are not accessing outdated medical information.
- Explain that commercial websites promoting a product or products with extremely positive claims are not reliable sources of factual information and should be considered doubtful unless other corroborating factual information can be found.
- Give patients alternatives to the Internet for finding quick, accurate information. Encourage them to call their pharmacist if they have questions about medications. Encourage them to read the handouts and discharge information they were given by the hospital. If they continue to have questions or concerns, encourage them to notify their physician, another health care provider, or home health nurse.

Knowledge Connection

What types of websites would you encourage patients to avoid when they are seeking information about their disease or self-care?

Supervision/Delegation Connection

Patient Teaching and Delegation

It is not appropriate to delegate patient teaching in any circumstances. This is in the realm of a licensed nurse only. Assistive personnel are not educated in this aspect of care and, therefore, it is outside their scope of practice.

Post Conference

You completed caring for the patient who was newly diagnosed with diabetes. You had a great deal of new information to teach her. You remembered to assess her level of knowledge about diabetes and found that, because her mother is also a diabetic, she had some basic knowledge. You learned that her mother did not really follow diabetic diet recommendations, though. The patient told you that she is mostly a visual learner, so you provided her with handouts and pamphlets from the American Diabetes Association that you obtained from the diabetes educator. You were able to go over the information about diabetes, diet basics, and finger stick blood sugar tests with her during the afternoon when it was quiet. When you asked her questions about previous teaching the diabetes educator had done with her, she was able to answer them all correctly. Although she could perform a finger stick blood sugar test using a glucometer by the end of the afternoon, you recommended that she practice it again before being discharged. The diabetes educator is going to follow up with her after you leave today.

KEY POINTS

- Three common learning styles are visual, auditory, and kinesthetic.

- People generally prefer one learning style, but can learn in every style, so all three styles should be incorporated when teaching patients.

- Many factors affect learning, including the environment, patient comfort, patient readiness, primary language of the patient, and the patient's sensory impairments.

- Repetition and restating are good ways to reinforce patient teaching.

- Nurses teach patients throughout care during teachable moments.

- Purposes for patient teaching include teaching about health promotion, wellness strategies, disease processes, treatments, medications, and self-care.

- When you are teaching several patients together, or have a large amount of instruction for an individual patient, you will need to develop a teaching plan.

- Your teaching plan is developed using the nursing process and will be a part of your care plan.

- When you determine what patients need to learn, you are assessing knowledge deficits.

- Two nursing diagnoses are used for patient teaching needs: "Deficient knowledge" and "Readiness for enhanced knowledge."

- Planning for patient teaching includes obtaining appropriate handouts to give to patients.

- You will need to consider a number of implementation strategies before and during teaching.

- You can evaluate how well your patient learned by asking questions, asking for a summary of what he or she learned, and asking the patient to perform a return demonstration of a skill.

- Children learn best by using a doll or teddy bear as a patient and acting out procedures and treatments.

- When teaching elderly patients, be very patient and allow plenty of time. Be sensitive to signs that the patient is confused or does not understand your teaching, such as putting off learning or not answering questions.

- If patients need more teaching after discharge, consider asking for a home health care referral. Encourage patients to call appropriate health care professionals if they have questions.

- Reliable Internet sites for health care information generally end with ".edu," ".gov," and ".org." Blogs and commercial sites selling miracle products are not usually reliable sources of information.

REVIEW QUESTIONS

Select the answer that is most appropriate for each of the following questions. Some questions may have more than one correct answer. Check all that apply.

1. Your patient says that he is a hands-on learner, not a book learner. You understand his primary learning style to be:

   a. auditory.

   b. visual.

   c. mixed.

   d. kinesthetic.

2. Because you know the above patient's primary learning style, your teaching will be presented:

   a. verbally only; he will learn best if you just tell him what you want him to do.

   b. by video so he can see and hear the information as it is presented.

   c. in a variety of ways; verbally explain, give written information and videos if available, and demonstrate as you explain.

   d. as a demonstration only; he will learn best if you just show him what you want him to do.

3. As you prepare to teach your patient how to take his pulse, which of the following will be of concern to you?

   a. The television is on, visitors are talking, and someone is vacuuming in the hallway.

   b. The patient's primary language is not English.

   c. The patient is not wearing his glasses or his hearing aid.

   d. There is a large amount of clutter in the room.

   e. The patient is experiencing a significant amount of discomfort.

   f. The patient does not believe he needs any heart medications.

4. Which is an example of reinforcing previous teaching about a heart attack?

  a. Explaining for a third time to the patient about heart damage after a heart attack.

  b. Introducing information about the cause of a heart attack for the first time and leaving handouts for him to read.

  c. Asking the patient to explain to you what he wants to know about his heart attack.

5. A patient with no history of heart disease wants to keep his cholesterol at a healthy level. You will instruct him on foods high in cholesterol so he can avoid them. Which purpose of patient teaching does this exemplify?

  a. Health promotion

  b. Wellness strategies

  c. Explaining the disease process

  d. Explaining treatment for disease

6. Which nursing intervention is LEAST appropriate for teaching a patient about a low-salt diet?

  a. Explain why the patient needs to restrict salt in her diet.

  b. Present a short lecture on the effects of excess salt in the body.

  c. Discuss information in a simple-to-complex format.

  d. Frequently praise the patient or give encouraging feedback.

CRITICAL THINKING EXERCISES

7. An elderly patient refuses to watch a demonstration on using a glucometer and performing a finger stick blood sugar test. She tells you, "My husband used one of those. I know all about it." What might be occurring?

8. A patient with heart disease needs instruction on preventing cardiac complications due to high blood pressure. Which nursing diagnosis is appropriate for this patient?

9. A patient tells you that he has looked up his disease and its treatment on the Internet. As you teach, he argues with you about basic information, saying that he did not find that on the Internet. How would you handle his patient teaching?

ADDITIONAL RESOURCES

For additional Resources, Questions, and Activities, please see:

 Student Resource Disk

DavisPlus **http://davisplus.fadavis.com**

 Student Study Guide

REFERENCES

Chang M, Kelly A. Patient education: addressing cultural diversity and health literacy issues. *Urol Nurse.* 2007;27:411-417.

Doenges M, Moorhouse M. *Application of the Nursing Process and Nursing Diagnoses.* 5th ed. Philadelphia: FA Davis; 2008.

Fontane D, Ramon L. Nursing students access on-line teaching sheets: use could improve students' patient education skills. *Patient Educ Management.* 2007;March 1.

Freda M. Issues in patient education. *J Midwifery.* 2004;49:203-209.

Hohler SE. Hospital Nursing: Tips for better patient teaching. *Nursing2004.* 2004;34(7):32hn7-32hn8.

Kocent L, Szczepanik M. Create a paper trail to improve teaching, communication, and documentation. *Patient Educ Management.* 2005;February 1.

Koerling TM. Clinical Rounds: Patient teaching saves lives and money. *Nursing2005.* 2005;35(4):33-34.

Using technology to transform patient education. *RN.* 2004;67:26nm1.

Nursing Basics

Key Terms

Ambulate

Base of support

Body mechanics

Cardiopulmonary resuscitation (CPR)

Center of gravity

Chair or bed monitor

Code team

Fall assessment rating scales

Heimlich maneuver

Leg monitor

Mass casualty event (MCE)

Material safety data sheet (MSDS)

Rescue breathing

Restraint alternatives

Restraints

The Joint Commission

Objectives

1. Explain areas addressed by the National Patient Safety Goals.
2. Describe six factors that contribute to an unsafe patient environment.
3. Discuss the use of fall assessment rating scales and restraint alternatives in preventing falls.
4. Describe a situation in which restraints would be necessary.
5. Identify requirements for use of restraints and release of restraints.
6. Explain the acronyms RACE and PASS.
7. Describe three types of fires and extinguishers.
8. Determine actions to take when a patient is unresponsive.
9. Discuss the role of nurses in a mass casualty event.
10. Identify ways to use body mechanics to prevent injury when caring for patients.
11. Explain how lack of rest and substance use or abuse can contribute to unsafe patient care.
12. Describe ways to protect yourself from radiation hazards.
13. Discuss safe handling of chemicals and gases.
14. Identify the purpose of a material safety data sheet.
15. Explain ways to protect yourself from biological hazards.

Skills

13-1 Using a Bed/Chair or Leg Monitor

13-2 Applying Restraints

13-3 Using Body Mechanics

Clinical Connection

Your Assignment: You will be caring for Mrs. Lloyd, an 82-year-old female hospitalized for a stroke. While in the hospital, she tried to get up alone and fell, resulting in a left hip fracture. Two days ago, she had an open reduction and internal fixation (ORIF) on her hip, a surgery to repair the fractured portion of her femur and acetabulum. She is confused at times, especially at night. She nearly fell again yesterday when the bed monitor was accidentally left off of the bed and she attempted to get up. Her family is understandably very upset.

Your Actions: To prepare to care for this patient, you must know what her abilities and limitations are, especially regarding mobility. You already know she is at risk for falls. You must decide how you will keep this patient safe and avoid the possibility of further injury due to her confusion. You must determine that the bed/chair monitor is in the proper place at all times and carefully supervise the CNAs and UAPs who care for her to be sure that no further "accidents" occur.

Safety must be foremost in your mind when you care for any patient—not only the safety of the patient, but your own safety as well. In this chapter, you will learn a variety of ways to promote safety when caring for patients. Some nurses tend to grow complacent about safety as they work year after year. Please do not allow yourself to ever become indifferent to safety awareness.

Safe Environment for Patients

Patients come to hospitals expecting to be kept safe while they are treated for and recover from illnesses. You may have heard stories about situations that occur when that does not happen. Patients and families are devastated when additional injury or illness occurs during a hospitalization due to a lack of adequate safeguards for the patient.

At the same time, safety for nursing staff is also a major issue. Back injuries are one of the leading causes of disability among nurses. Nurses can be at risk for communicable disease and exposure to hazards such as blood and body fluids, as well as radiation. Health care facilities develop policies to promote safety and reduce illness and injury for patients and nurses alike.

National Patient Safety Goals

A national standard for patient safety has been established by **The Joint Commission**, the organization responsible for evaluating and accrediting health care organizations and programs in the United States. Their National Patient Safety Goals address specific safety problems in the hospital setting, such as identifying patients, communicating with caregivers, administering medication, reducing health care–associated infections, reconciling medications when patients are discharged or transferred, reducing falls, and improving recognition and response to changes in patients' conditions.

Requirements for meeting each goal have been established as well. It is up to each facility to determine ways to meet those requirements. In this book, we will emphasize safety throughout. Specific safety issues regarding medications will be discussed in Chapters 35, 36, 37, and 38.

Factors Contributing to an Unsafe Patient Environment

When patients are hospitalized, their entire environment changes. Nothing is familiar. As nurses, we view the hospital as a comfortable place; we see it laid out in an efficient and logical pattern. But for many patients, the hospital feels like a maze within a maze; the patient may feel confined to a tiny room miles away from anything familiar. Patients are also forced to wear a hospital gown and paper slippers, clothes that are nothing like what they are likely to wear at home. Privacy curtains that do not limit sound or smell do nothing to promote any feelings of true privacy. In addition to the strangeness of the hospital, many factors can contribute to creating an unsafe environment for patients.

Age and Ability to Understand

A hospital is threatening enough to adults, but for very young patients and elderly patients, it is an even more confusing place. It is difficult for children younger than age 10 to clearly understand what will happen and what is expected of them. If a parent can stay with the child, it helps him or her feel more secure. However, with family and work duties, that is not always possible. Elderly patients, especially those confused due to cognitive impairments, medications, or unfamiliar surroundings, are particularly at risk for falls. They may try to get up or walk without realizing they are attached to tubes and cords. Even though the nursing staff may explain these limitations, patients may not remember or clearly understand such deviations from normal.

Impaired Mobility

Patients who are unsteady on their feet or unable to bear full weight are at particular risk for injury if they attempt to **ambulate** (walk) without help. It is not uncommon for patients in the hospital to experience poor balance or general weakness after surgery or after being in bed for a prolonged period. Equipment, cords, and tubes are barriers to mobility in the hospital room, and these barriers are compounded by the patient's poor balance, weakness, or impaired mobility.

Communication

Patients who speak English as a second language may not grasp safety instructions. When you tell the patient to call for the nurse before getting up, the instruction may be unclear. Call on the telephone? Shout out? Be sure that your instructions are specific: "Press this button and tell us that you need to get up. Someone will come to help you." Sometimes patients do not want to bother the nurses and are hesitant to call for help. In some cultures, patients of one sex may not want a nurse of the opposite sex to assist with toileting and personal hygiene. Arrange for an interpreter when you give instructions if your patient does not understand English.

Pain and Discomfort

People in pain are generally irritable and anxious. They may disregard safety precautions in an effort to be more comfortable. For example, if a patient is in pain, he or she may attempt to get back in bed after sitting up in a bedside chair to relieve the pain and fatigue, even if he or she has been instructed to wait for help. Discomfort, such as a full bladder or rectum, is also a motivation for disregarding safety instructions. Patients who need to go to the bathroom may feel the need is urgent and attempt to go alone, especially if the call light is not answered promptly.

Delayed Assistance

A patient may ring the call light and then wait for assistance to the bathroom or elsewhere. But if no one answers, or no one comes to assist in a timely manner, the patient may attempt to go alone. *Safety: It is imperative that call lights be answered promptly and that assistance be quickly available to maintain a safe environment for patients.* While poor staffing patterns may contribute to delayed assistance for patients, nursing staff must make rapid response to requests for assistance a high priority.

Equipment

Hospital equipment is commonplace to nursing staff, who know its purpose and are familiar with its operation. However, to patients, the equipment can be upsetting. When alarms go off, patients and families often become anxious, feeling that something is terribly wrong. That anxiety can create an unsafe situation for the patient. Anxiety can lead to elevated blood pressure and heart rate; depending on the diagnosis, that can be an unsafe situation. Some patients attempt to get out of bed and go to the hallway to alert the nurses about an alarm because they are frightened by it. Even something as routine as side rails on the bed, often seen as a safety feature, can cause injury to some patients. Injuries and even deaths have resulted from entrapment of patients' heads and chests between the side rails and the bed, or between the upper and lower bed rails. Interestingly, researchers found that older, frail adults who experience confusion, pain, fecal impaction, and urinary retention are at highest risk for entrapment because they are more likely to move around in bed or try to get out of bed.

Knowledge Connection

How does a delay in answering call lights contribute to an unsafe condition for your patients?

Promoting Patient Safety

It is the responsibility of all health care staff to promote the safety of patients. Nurses have to be "on alert" at all times to detect potentially unsafe situations. It has been said that nurses make hypervigilant parents because they look at every situation and see what could happen and how injuries could occur. That is the result of protecting patients from potential harm.

Preventing Falls

One of the national goals for patient safety focuses on reducing the risk of patient harm from falls. The requirement for this goal is that each facility must have a fall reduction program, which includes ways to evaluate its effectiveness.

Fall Assessment Rating Scales

Many facilities have developed **fall assessment rating scales**, forms that, when filled out, give a numerical rating for each patient's risk for falls. The higher the number, the greater the patient's risk (Table 13-1).

Generally, the fall assessment rating scale is completed on every patient admitted to the hospital. Facility policy will determine which patients are considered "at risk." For those patients, a system for identification and precautions is put in place. For example, a patient is admitted and is rated a 65 on the fall assessment rating scale. Facility policy states that patients rated 50 or higher are at strict risk for falls. This patient is identified by flags or stickers on the chart, the Kardex, and the patient's door to serve as reminders to all staff. Some facilities use a specially colored armband on the patients themselves. Some controversy exists over how to identify patients in a confidential way, yet still alert staff to the risk of falls.

Restraint Alternatives

Patients identified as "at risk" for falls may need reminders to keep them from getting up when it is unsafe for them to do so. A number of products have been developed for this

Table 13-1 Morse Fall Scale

Item	Scale	Scoring
1. History of falling; immediate or within three months.	No 0 Yes 25	
2. Secondary diagnosis	No 0 Yes 15	
3. Ambulatory aid: • Bedrest/nurse assist • Crutches/cane/walker • Furniture	0 15 30	
4. IV/saline lock	No 0 Yes 20	
5. Gait/transferring • Normal/bedrest/immobile • Weak • Impaired	0 10 20	
6. Mental status • Oriented to own ability • Forgets limitations	0 15	

Total Score for Risk Level

Risk Level	Morse Fall Score	Action
Preventive fall precautions (Level I)	0–24	Implement Level I interventions
Modified fall risk (Level II)	25–50	Implement Level II interventions
Strict fall risk (Level III)	>51	Implement Level III interventions

Reproduced with the permission of Springer Publishing Company, LLC, New York, NY 10036.

purpose. They are not true **restraints**, which are vests, jackets, or bands with connected straps that are tied to the bed, chair, or wheelchair to keep the patient in one place. These **restraint alternatives** are less restrictive ways to help patients remember not to get up and try to walk, or to alert nursing staff that the patient is attempting to do so.

Monitors

One product used as a restraint alternative is the **chair monitor** or **bed monitor**, a pressure-sensitive device that generates an alarm when the patient's weight is no longer sensed, indicating that the patient is attempting to get up (Fig. 13-1a). A **leg monitor** is another type of chair monitor; it attaches to the patient's leg like a large bandage and generates an alarm when the leg is in a dependent position, indicating that the patient is attempting to stand (Fig. 13-1b). It

is important to continue to check frequently on patients at risk for falls. These monitors cannot anticipate possible falls. In addition, if the pressure-sensitive pad is not moved from the bed to the chair when the patient transfers to a chair, no alarm will sound when the patient attempts to stand. Skill 13-1 (page 247) provides more information on using a bed/chair or leg monitor.

Soft Devices

Often a simple reminder will prevent at-risk patients from trying to get out of the bed or chair. Soft devices are available that fit across the patient's lap while they are sitting in a wheelchair (Fig. 13-2). Other soft devices include bolsters that can be placed in the bed on either side of the patient to prevent him or her from slipping between or through the side rails.

Figure 13-1a This chair monitor alarm will sound when no weight is detected.

Figure 13-1b This leg monitor will sound an alarm when the patient is nearly vertical.

Figure 13-2 This lap guard keeps the patient from getting out of the wheelchair.

Strategies

A number of simple strategies may be used by nursing staff to help prevent falls in at-risk patients:

• Place a patient who is at risk for falls in a room near the nurse's station to make it easier for more people to see and check on him or her. Patients who are prone to falls may also benefit from sitting in a wheelchair near the nurses'

station, where they can see the activity and people, and where they are also easily visible.

• Stay with patients at risk for falls when they are in the bathroom or on the bedside commode. Do not leave them with the instruction to "Put on your call light when you are through," because often these patients will attempt to get up without calling for help.

• Keep the bed at the lowest level at all times except when the nursing staff is at the bedside. If there is a recurrent problem where the patient is unsafe due to repeated attempts to get out of bed, the mattress may even be placed on the floor to prevent injury to the patient.

• Place the over-bed table across the wheelchair like a tray to help patients remain seated in the chair. You can also use furniture or equipment to block areas that are off-limits to the patient so that he or she remains in a safe zone.

• Some patients who are at risk for falls seem to have a lot of energy and are looking for ways to stay busy. Try having them sit in a rocking chair near the nurses' station. Often the motion of rocking helps them relax as well as use pent-up energy. You can also give them simple but purposeful activities to do, such as folding washcloths or towels.

• Offer regular opportunities for the patient to go to the bathroom, have a snack, or have something to drink. Sometimes patients are attempting to do one of these things when they get out of bed unsafely.

• Assess your fall-risk patients frequently for subjective complaints such as nausea, pain, or other discomfort. These patients may be trying to get more comfortable but are unable to do so safely.

• Provide back rubs and distractions, such as music or television, to help patients be more comfortable and less restless. Use a night-light to decrease anxiety at night when surroundings are unfamiliar.

In spite of all best efforts, a fall may occasionally occur. Should you come upon a patient who has fallen, follow the steps in Box 13-1 to be sure you handle the situation appropriately.

Restraints

Other names for restraints are *protective devices* or *safety reminder devices.* Sometimes you will hear them called *Poseys* after the brand name of the first restraints on the market. Avoid using restraints if at all possible. Try all other options first, and try them more than once. Enlist the family to help, if they are available to do so. No one wants to feel "tied down" against his or her will. Elderly and confused patients, as well as those who are very young, often cannot understand the reason for this treatment. **Never** threaten patients with restraints. Instead, remind them about the purpose of the various lines, tubes, or restrictions and distract them by directing their attention to something else. For example, if a patient is pulling at his or her catheter, you could say, "I know that tube is uncomfortable, but it is necessary right now. Can I turn on the television for you?"

Actions to Take if a Patient Has Fallen

If a patient falls, it is important to know what to do. The following steps will guide you through the assessment and actions to take.

- Check the patient for obvious injuries. Look for bleeding, check level of consciousness, assess for signs of hip fracture (one leg shorter than the other and rotated outward), observe for deformities at any joint, and assess for paralysis or weakness on one side of the body.
- Call for help. It will take several staff members to move the patient off the floor. Follow facility policy for moving patients who have fallen.
- Take the patient's vital signs. The fall may be due to underlying cardiac or neurological problems such as an arrhythmia or a cerebrovascular accident.
- If the patient is not conscious, has unstable vital signs, or is not breathing or is without a pulse, call a Code Blue immediately.
- Assist the conscious patient to bed with the help of others, following facility policy.
- Notify the physician. Explain what occurred and give the patient's current condition. Be prepared to take orders for x-rays and other tests.
- Document the incident according to facility policy. An incident report must be completed. Charting should include details of finding the patient, vital signs, assistance to bed, and notifying the physician and orders obtained.

Students in nursing are sometimes confused about restraints. They may have seen situations on television or in movies where a patient in a mental health facility is out of control and is restrained in four-way restraints—one on each arm and one on each leg. This is a completely different situation than protecting a patient from injury or from pulling out tubes. Hospitals always use the *least restrictive environment* for patients, which means that patients are restrained only in the manner absolutely necessary to prevent harm.

In some situations, alternatives are not effective and all other options have been exhausted. If this occurs, the first step is to speak with the patient's physician. *You must have a physician's order for restraints.* The order should include the type of restraint and the specific period of time it is to remain in place. Generally the order will be for no more than 24 hours.

When an order has been obtained and the restraints are in place, nursing staff are required by the Health Care Financing Administration (HCFA) and The Joint Commission to follow these guidelines:

- Check on the patient every 30 minutes, making sure to check the skin for redness or chafing under the restraint and the extremities for warmth and color.
- Remove the restraint every 2 hours. While the restraint is off:
  - Offer fluids to the patient.
  - Assist with toileting as needed.

- Change the patient's position if in bed.
- Assess the extremities for edema, capillary refill time, sensation, and function.
- Assess skin over pressure points for integrity and erythema.
- Assist the patient to ambulate if that is appropriate.
- Stay with the patient the entire time the restraint is off.
- Document all actions on the appropriate flow sheet (Fig. 13-3).

There may be some variation of these guidelines from state to state due to specific laws and statutes. Facilities will have written guidelines regarding restraints, so be sure to know and follow your facility's policies.

Supervision/Delegation Connection

Delegation of Restraint Checks and Releases

When a patient has restraints applied, you can delegate the checks and releases to a CNA or UAP. However, you need to supervise your assistant by following up to ensure that checks are indeed being done and being documented on the flow sheet. It is very important that the patient is released from the restraints every 2 hours; otherwise you could be accused of false imprisonment. It is your responsibility to be sure that the checks and releases occur exactly as facility policy dictates.

Application of Restraints

It is important to use the correct restraint when you are carrying out a physician's order. Several types exist: vest or jacket, waist, wrist, and mitt. Table 13-2 presents descriptions and pictures of each type of physical restraint. Chemical restraints may also be ordered and used. These are medications prescribed to prevent restlessness and anxiety in the patient who may be in an unsafe situation without the medication. They are used judiciously by physicians. *Safety: No restraint, physical or chemical, is ordered or used unless absolutely necessary to keep the patient safe. They are never used for the convenience of staff.*

It is also extremely important that you know how to correctly apply restraints. You should be able to insert three fingers between the patient's body and the restraint to ensure that it is not too tight. Restraints are always tied in a quick-release knot. That way, if a patient needs immediate assistance, he or she can be quickly released from the restraint. If you struggle to master the quick-release knot, keep practicing. No other knot is acceptable when tying restraints.

Some patients have been injured or died when restraints were applied incorrectly. Most often, instances of severe injury or death were due to choking injuries when the vest or jacket restraint was put on the patient backward. The patient then slid down in the chair or wheelchair and the tight restraint compressed the chest or throat. *Safety: Always apply restraints according to facility policy and manufacturer's directions.*

RESTRAINTS Q 30 MINUTE CHECKLIST									DATE: _____			
	19:00	19:30	20:00	20:30	21:00	21:30	22:00	22:30	23:00	23:30	24:00	24:30
Siderails												
Oriented/ Disoriented												
Pulse/ Circulation												
Skin Condition												
Readjust Tension												
R.O.M.												
DATE:	01:00	01:30	02:00	02:30	03:00	03:30	04:00	04:30	05:00	05:30	06:00	06:30
Siderails												
Oriented/ Disoriented												
Pulse/ Circulation												
Skin Condition												
Readjust Tension												
R.O.M.												

Figure 13-3 Restraint Flowsheet.

Table 13-2 Types of Physical Restraints

Type of Restraint	Description of Use	Picture of Restraint
Vest	Used to protect a patient in danger of getting out of a wheelchair or chair. Placed on the patient with the crossover in front and the straps tied to the lower portion of the back of the wheelchair.	

(table continues on page 240)

Table 13-2   **Types of Physical Restraints** (continued)

Type of Restraint	Description of Use	Picture of Restraint
Waist	Used to protect a patient in danger of getting out of a bed or chair. Placed around the patient's waist, then the straps are tied to the movable portion of the bed or to the lower portion of the back of the wheelchair.	
Extremity	Used to protect a patient in danger of pulling out tubes or taking off monitoring devices. Placed around the patient's wrist, then tied to the movable portion of the bed.	
Mitt	Used to protect a patient in danger of pulling out tubes or interfering with treatments. Sometimes used to prevent scratching in patients with severe skin disorders. The patient's hand is placed within the mitt and the mitt is secured around the wrist. The straps can also be tied to the movable portion of the bed.	

Skill 13-2 (page 248) provides more instruction regarding the correct application of restraints.

Knowledge Connection

Name three alternatives to the use of restraints. How are restraints tied? What is the reason for tying them in this manner?

Responding to a Fire

Should a fire occur in a health care setting, it is imperative that staff know what to do and that they do it quickly and well. Fire drills are required periodically to be sure everyone practices the procedure to follow in case of an actual fire.

Each facility determines its own code word for a fire or fire drill. Common code words include "Code Red," "Code F," and "Paging Dr. Red." The code is usually announced via the intercom or paging system. If a fire occurs, the entire facility will respond. In some cases, if the fire is not in your wing or area of the hospital, your job will be to close patient room doors and stay within your area, sealed off by fire doors that automatically close.

If the fire is in your area, or you are the one to discover a fire, remember the acronym RACE and follow each letter:

- **Rescue:** Remove patients from immediate danger to a safer area of the hospital.
- **Alarm:** Sound the fire alarm according to facility policy. This may involve dialing an extension or pulling a fire alarm box. The fire department will automatically be notified.
- **Confine:** Confine the fire to one room or area. Close the doors according to hospital policy. Fire doors automatically close to help confine the fire to one wing of the hospital.
- **Extinguish:** You should only attempt to extinguish a small fire with a fire extinguisher. The fire department will extinguish larger fires. If you need to extinguish a small fire, obtain the nearest fire extinguisher and follow the acronym PASS:
  - **Pull** the pin found between the handles.
  - **Aim** the nozzle of the fire extinguisher at the base of the flames.
  - **Squeeze** the handles together to release the contents of the extinguisher.
  - **Sweep** the nozzle back and forth at the base of the flames to extinguish the fire.

The PASS acronym is just as important to remember as RACE. It is important to know what to do before a fire occurs so you can be ready to extinguish it in an emergency. You do not want to be trying to read the directions on the side of the extinguisher during a real fire.

Types of Extinguishers

It is always important to use the correct type of fire extinguisher when attempting to fight a fire. Different types of extinguishers have different contents, designed to quickly put out a specific type of fire. Fires are designated as type A, B, or C (Box 13-2), and fire extinguishers are labeled with these designations. Most fire extinguishers in health care facilities are combination extinguishers used for all three types of fires.

Knowledge Connection

When do you use the acronym RACE? When do you need to know the acronym PASS?

Patient Teaching Connection

Teaching Safe Oxygen Use in the Home
Teach your patients in home health care or a long-term care facility about using oxygen safely. Instruct them that no open flames can be present in the same room as the oxygen source. Explain that no one can smoke, burn candles, or use an open-flame heater, all of which can cause a fire. In addition, the patient should not use wool blankets or sweaters that could generate static electricity, or electrical appliances such as shavers that could cause a spark. The patient can use extension tubing to move around the house.

Responding to Individual Emergencies

As a student and a nurse, it is your responsibility to maintain your certification in **cardiopulmonary resuscitation (CPR)**, actions to restart the heart or breathing of an unresponsive victim without a pulse or respirations. Recertification is currently required every 2 years. Many changes in CPR have been implemented in the past 10 years as a result of research and technology. It is very important that you be current in your training and not rely on out-of-date information. Your CPR course will also include instruction and practice on the **Heimlich maneuver**, an action to relieve choking by thrusting just below a person's xiphoid process.

Some facilities may also require first aid certification, which must be kept current. Even if this certification is not required, you may wish to pursue it if you participate in community activities such as scouting, church groups, or sports teams, where injuries often occur. As nurses, we are used to having equipment and supplies at hand during an emergency or injury. A first aid course helps you be ready to use what is available, rather than what is ideal.

If, as a student, you come upon a patient who is unresponsive, it is appropriate for you to alert the emergency team. This is usually announced as a "Code Blue," but in some facilities it may be denoted as "Condition Blue" or a page for "Dr. Heart," followed by a room number. Follow your facility policy for initiating a Code Blue. It may involve dialing a certain extension number from the room or activating an emergency call light in the room.

Once you have called the code, begin CPR or **rescue breathing** (breathing for the patient in case of respiratory arrest when the pulse is still palpable), whichever is appropriate. Continue your efforts until the **code team**, a group of specially trained personnel designated to respond to

---

Box 13-2
Types of Fires and Extinguishers

Various types of fire extinguishers are available to fight different types of fires. It is important for you to obtain the correct extinguisher for the type of fire you are fighting.
- **Type A:** Paper, wood, fabric, trash
- **Type B:** Combustible liquids such as oil, gasoline and other petroleum-based products, and flammable gases
- **Type C:** Electrical fires such as shorts in wires, motor or equipment fires

Note: Most fire extinguishers are combination extinguishers that can be used to fight all three types of fires. However, each extinguisher is marked with the fires it should be used to extinguish.

codes throughout the hospital, arrives. The code team often consists of critical care nurses, respiratory therapists, and a resident or emergency physician. The code team will then take over the resuscitation efforts. When a Code Blue occurs in a critical care unit, it is not generally announced through the paging system. Instead, the critical care nurses carry out their code duties with limited assistance from other health care staff.

While the code team is working on the patient, make notes about the time you found the patient and exactly what you did so you can document them in the chart. Be aware of any family or friends of the patient who might be nearby during the emergency. Understandably, this is a frightening event and family members generally know something is terribly wrong. Try to assign a UAP or CNA to stay with the family. Offer them a private place to make phone calls, and offer water or coffee, and tissues if needed. Sometimes family members get overlooked during emergencies, yet they are in great need of someone to offer kindness, empathy, and emotional support.

It is possible that, if you are a staff nurse on break or at lunch and a Code Blue is called for your unit, you will be expected to return to the unit immediately to assist with other patients for the duration of the code.

Knowledge Connection

Name three actions to take if you come upon an unresponsive patient. List your actions in the order in which you would perform them.

Responding to Disasters

In our current world, the term *disaster* can refer to many things: bombings, fires, blizzards, floods, tornados, hurricanes, collapses of buildings, school shootings, bridge collapses, and anything causing mass casualties. The health care community is always front and center when it comes to dealing with these events, whether the 9/11 terrorist attacks of 2001 or Hurricane Katrina followed by the levee failures that flooded New Orleans in 2005. In some situations, the health care community's disaster plan was executed and all went relatively smoothly. In other situations, the planners did not anticipate all the complications that interfered with the arrival of help and supplies.

The Agency for Healthcare Research and Quality (AHRQ) defines a **mass casualty event (MCE)** as a public health or medical emergency involving thousands of victims. The office of the Assistant Secretary for Preparedness and Response, along with AHRQ and the U.S. Department of Health and Human Services, collaborated to establish guidelines for acceptable standards of care in an MCE. These guidelines help the health care community prepare in advance for various contingencies that could occur during an MCE. The normal standards of care must shift during disasters, and these shifts have to take moral, ethical, and legal implications into account.

Not all questions are answered by these guidelines, but some of the major points addressed include using a disaster triage model, treating first those victims who are most likely to survive, how to plan for any MCE rather than specific situations, and how to adapt the use of existing facilities for various needs.

Another type of MCE would be *bioterrorism,* the release of a biological or chemical agent into the air or water supply that could cause thousands of illnesses and deaths. In this situation, the health care community must be prepared not only to deal with the MCE, but to also have to deal with a potentially contaminated water supply and a highly contagious illness. In the case of bioterrorism, the first clue that the event has occurred may be several days later when people begin presenting at various emergency departments in the area with similar symptoms, such as rapidly progressing pneumonia. In many cases, by the time serious symptoms appear, the illness is severe and difficult to treat. As clusters of similar symptoms develop in an area, it is important that antibiotic treatment begin at once, without waiting for the usual laboratory confirmations.

Your responsibility as a student and as a nurse will be to know and follow your facility's disaster plan. Many different codes are used to indicate different types of disasters, so learn the codes used by your facility. Expect to be called in to work as an extra if a disaster occurs. It is appropriate for you to ensure the safety of your family first and then assist at your place of work. Some facilities have a plan for calling in extra help according to needs, rather than having a barrage of off-duty employees arriving at once.

Real-World Connection

Participating in a Disaster During Clinical Experience

When the Murrah Federal Building in Oklahoma City was bombed in 1995, an instructor and 11 practical nursing students were at a hospital eight blocks from the site. It was a typical clinical morning until 9:01.

When the bomb exploded, the hospital swayed. Windows shattered, and glass blew into the rooms and onto patients and nursing staff. The fire alarms sounded and the smell of smoke was everywhere. At first, the students thought something had happened just to the hospital building, but when they looked out the 11th-floor windows, a huge column of black smoke was visible where the federal building stood.

The hospital immediately went into its disaster plan. Students helped out by moving patients from damaged rooms to ones that were intact. As staff prepared for an influx of wounded, students assisted by administering routine medications, preparing supplies, and setting up additional areas for patient care if needed.

As the morning progressed, it became obvious that many had not survived the blast, and those who were more seriously injured would have to go to surgery before they came to the patient units. A young child from the day-care center was dead on arrival to the emergency room. Of course, she had no identification. A nurse described her simply by the color of her hair and the clothes she was wearing on the list of those who had perished.

The disaster plan worked exactly as it had been practiced. Everyone knew what to do and did their jobs with remarkable calm and professionalism. Each student who served that day was changed forever.

Since that time, many health care professionals have served in response to mass casualty events such as the World Trade Center attacks, hurricanes such as Katrina, and tornados and earthquakes. Be prepared, because you never know when it will happen in your world.

Safe Environment for Nursing Staff

Nursing staff in hospitals and other health care facilities provide much of the direct patient care and are therefore exposed to safety risks, including lifting and moving patients, working with medications and chemicals, and potential exposure to contaminated blood and body fluids.

These risks can be divided into three broad categories: physical, chemical, and biological hazards. Patients may be at risk for exposure to some of these hazards as well. Nursing staff are at risk for all of them. Box 13-3 describes examples of each of these types of hazards.

Minimizing Physical Hazards

One of the best ways to prevent physical injuries when lifting and moving anything is to use good posture and **body mechanics**, the movement of muscles of the body for balance and leverage. In addition, a number of devices are available to help move patients safely. It is important that you learn how to use these devices correctly and use them when it is appropriate so that you avoid potential injury. Chapter 16 includes more information on devices for moving patients.

Box 13-3

Types of Hazards to Nursing Staff

Various types of hazards exist when you are providing nursing care. It is important to be aware of these hazards so you can protect yourself.

- Physical hazards include injuries to back and joints; repetitive motion injuries such as carpal tunnel syndrome; exposure to lasers, which can injure the eyes if protection is not used; and exposure to radiation.
- Chemical hazards include exposure to cytotoxic medications and treatments, such as those used in chemotherapy; and exposure to other chemicals, including cleaning fluids.
- Biological hazards include blood and body fluids contaminated with HIV or hepatitis viruses, exposure to influenza viruses, and exposure to epidemics.

The American Nurses Association developed the Handle With Care program in 2004, which advocates the availability and use of equipment to help move patients safely and reduce the number of nurse injuries. Their goal is that nurses will eventually not need to lift patients manually at all.

Body Mechanics

Body mechanics involves using the joints and leverage of the body to your advantage, working with what your body is designed to do rather than working against it. Whether you are moving patients or boxes of supplies, certain guidelines still apply. To understand how to use proper body mechanics, you have to understand the location of your **center of gravity**. This is a middle point of the body, below the umbilicus and above the pubis, around which the body's mass is distributed. You must also understand the meaning of the **base of support**, which refers to your feet and lower legs. When you are lifting or moving a heavy object, this gives your body stability and balance. The wider your base of support, the lower your center of gravity. One way to establish a solid base of support is to keep your feet shoulder-width apart.

To use good body mechanics and prevent injury to yourself, follow these guidelines:

- Plan your work carefully. Think through how to do it safely.
- Elevate your work to a comfortable level. Raise the bed so you do not have to bend over to work, which will cause a strain on your back.
- Keep your feet shoulder-width apart, one foot slightly ahead of the other, when standing for long periods.
- Avoid twisting, which can cause strain or injury to the low back. Turn your whole body or pivot on one foot instead of twisting.
- When lifting heavy objects from a lower level, such as a low shelf or the floor, bend your knees, not your back. Squat to reach the object and keep your back straight as you flex your hip and thigh muscles to stand. In this way, you use the larger muscles of your body to support the load.
- When carrying an object, hold it close to your body with your elbows bent. If the weight is away from your body rather than close, your center of gravity shifts and your balance is affected. This increases the strain on your back muscles and also makes you more likely to lose your balance and fall.
- When possible, push, pull, or slide heavy objects rather than lifting them. Push rather than pull if at all possible to avoid extra strain on your back muscles.
- Get help when you need to move or lift a patient. Figure 13-4 shows a safety decision-making chart that can help you decide when assistance is needed.

Skill 13-3 (page 250) provides more information on the proper usage of body mechanics.

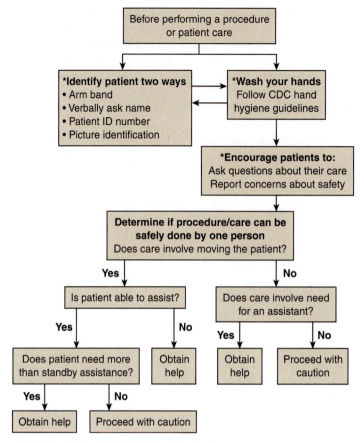

Figure 13-4 Safety Decision-Making Chart.

Adequate Rest and Appropriate Focus

Fatigue can contribute to conditions that result in injury. If you are exhausted, you may not think as clearly as you would if you were well rested. You are at risk for making an error that could hurt both you and a patient. It is important that you get enough rest to function safely as a nurse. When you are scheduled to work, make it a priority to be rested when you arrive. One reason mandatory overtime is such a major issue for nurses is that it can contribute to unsafe practice due to lack of rest.

Other influences that contribute to unsafe practice and poor decision making include abuse of alcohol, use of prescription medications such as narcotic pain relievers, and use of illegal drugs or prescription drugs in abusive amounts. Nurses have a high rate of drug use and abuse. If you are taking narcotic medications to treat an injury or illness, speak with your instructor before you go to your clinical facility. If you believe you may have a problem with overuse of alcohol or misuse of prescription drugs, speak with an instructor or school counselor to get help. If you suspect that a coworker or staff nurse is impaired, speak confidentially with your instructor so that this person can get help. Peer assistance programs are available to nurses for help with these types of problems. By speaking up, you may help prevent a dangerous situation for patients, for yourself, or for coworkers.

Radiation Hazards

Radiation, the emission of energy in the form of rays, waves, or particles, is used to diagnose and treat some diseases. When you care for patients treated with radiation, you may also be exposed. To prevent excessive radiation exposure, wear a lead apron during procedures involving x-rays and fluoroscopy. Wear a film badge if you work in a radiology area on a regular basis. This badge measures the amount of radiation to which you have been exposed over a period of time. If you are assigned to care for a patient with internal or implanted radiation, such as that used to treat certain cancers and thyroid conditions, limit the amount of time you spend with these patients to minimize your exposure. If you are pregnant, you should not care for these patients. Follow facility policy for alternative assignments in this situation.

Chemical Hazards

Nurses can be exposed to toxic chemicals when handling IV chemotherapy medications or other medications. Even cleaning supplies can pose hazards, especially if they spill or mix. Anytime you use chemicals, you should be aware of the hazards involved. Your facility is required to have a **material safety data sheet (MSDS)** on file for every chemical, which contains information about potential harm caused by exposure and directions for what to do if the product gets in your eyes, on your skin, or in your mouth. These sheets are available from the manufacturers of chemicals and cleaning products. It is your responsibility to know the location of the MSDS sheets (usually kept in a notebook) in your facility and to be aware of the hazards in the chemicals with which you work.

Gases are ever-present in the health care environment. Oxygen is generally piped into each patient unit in the hospital. Anesthetic gases are used in the operating suites. It is important to follow safety precautions when you are around gases. No smoking or open flame is allowed in the presence of oxygen. Even static electricity can cause a spark that could ignite a fire or cause an explosion. While oxygen is not explosive, it supports combustion. A fire burns faster and hotter in the presence of oxygen. Sheets and gowns saturated in oxygen burn very rapidly. If you work in the operating room, you will wear clothing and shoes that do not promote static electricity.

Biological Hazards

Nurses deal with the possibility of exposure to blood and body fluids containing serious, even fatal viruses. The Centers for Disease Control and Prevention (CDC), a federal agency involved in protecting patients and staff from the spread of disease, has developed guidelines to reduce this risk. These guidelines, called standard precautions and transmission-based precautions, help prevent the spread of blood-borne pathogens (see Chapter 14 for more information). Wash your hands before and after all patient contact and wear gloves when any risk of exposure to blood or body fluids is present.

Needle-stick injuries have been a major route for health care workers to be exposed to hepatitis B and HIV. Safer devices such as needleless access systems, while more costly for facilities, are designed to help decrease the risk of needle-stick injuries. Never recap a used needle, and always use puncture-proof, labeled containers (sharps containers) for disposing of used needles and other sharps. Chapters 14, 34, 37, and 38 present more information about safely handling needles and sharps. Always follow CDC guidelines to help protect yourself from biological hazards.

Safety is your responsibility. Be as vigilant about your own safety as you are about the safety of your patients. Anticipate potentially unsafe situations and take action to prevent them before they happen.

Knowledge Connection

Give one example of each type of hazard encountered by nursing staff. Explain one way to minimize each hazard you have identified.

Nursing Care Plan for Patients at Risk for Falls

Safety will be a part of the care plan for many of your patients. In this example, we focus strictly on the patient's risk for falls. In many care plans that you will write, the risk for falls will be just one of several safety-related nursing diagnoses for the patient.

Assessment

It is extremely important that you recognize safety concerns for each of your patients. One of the most common is that the patient is, or could be, at risk for falling. You cannot tell if this is the case by looking at the patient. Age is not necessarily a predictor for this risk.

Use a fall assessment rating scale or other assessment tool to determine the likelihood of fall risk (see Table 13-1). Follow facility policy for scoring the scale and alerting other staff to the fall danger.

Using a fall assessment rating scale for Mrs. Lloyd, the 82-year-old female patient in the Clinical Connection at the beginning of this chapter, you would identify her as a person at risk for falls because she has fallen previously, has more than one diagnosis, is weak on one side due to a stroke, and is confused at night. You would also need to assess her for other potential safety concerns such as choking because she has had a stroke and could have *dysphagia* (difficulty swallowing).

Nursing Diagnoses

Several nursing diagnoses relate to the safety of the patient. In assessing Mrs. Lloyd, we have determined that she is at risk for falls because of her left-sided weakness and confusion. If she does fall again, she could cause injury to her newly repaired hip fracture. To state this as a nursing diagnosis, you would word it as follows:

Risk for falls related to left-sided weakness and confusion
    You would not use "Risk for injury" as a nursing diagnosis in this situation because "Risk for falls" more correctly describes her problem.

(care plan box continues on page 246)

Nursing Care Plan for Patients at Risk for Falls (continued)

Planning

For Mrs. Lloyd, you need to find ways to prevent her from trying to get out of bed alone. Because of her confusion, left-sided weakness, and recently repaired hip fracture, you must determine interventions that will address these issues. You need some way to know when the patient is attempting to get out of bed. Some possible ways to alert staff to this situation might be:

- Apply a bed/chair monitor or leg monitor that will alarm if the patient tries to get up.
- Post reminders in the patient's room for the patient and family stating that the patient is to call for help before getting up.
- Frequently provide verbal reorientation for the patient. Tell her where she is, what has happened, and what you want her to do: "You are at All Saint's Hospital because you had a mild stroke. Then you fell and fractured your hip. You cannot safely get up by yourself, so push this button and ask for help when you need to get out of bed."

You also need to enlist the nursing staff in taking extra precautions for this patient's safety. Ideas for additional precautions are:

- Post fall precautions on the door to the patient's room, in the Kardex, and in the patient's chart according to facility policy.
- Answer her call light promptly so the patient will not tire of waiting for help and attempt to get up alone.
- Respond to the bed/chair/leg monitor alarms immediately to prevent a fall.
- Assist the patient to ambulate to the chair or the bathroom when needed.
- Do not leave the patient alone while in the bathroom or on the bedside commode. Stay nearby to assist the patient back to bed.

- Keep the call light within the patient's reach at all times.
- Keep personal items within reach so the patient does not injure herself by attempting to retrieve an item.
- Anticipate the patient's needs: Offer to assist her to the bathroom or bedside commode every 2 hours.
- Use half side rails, bumpers, or other restraint alternatives to remind the patient not to get up alone.
- Enlist the assistance of the family to stay with the patient at night if necessary.

In Mrs. Lloyd's situation, your expected outcome is that falls will be prevented. You also want a goal of no further injury occurring to this patient during her hospitalization.

Implementation

You can now implement the interventions that you have planned. Table 13-3 presents a summary of the care plan interventions.

Evaluation

To evaluate the effectiveness of your interventions, ask yourself the following questions:

- Were your interventions effective in preventing further falls?
- Did your patient avoid additional injuries during the rest of her hospitalization?

If the answer to both these questions is "yes," your interventions were successful in accomplishing your goals and outcomes. If you answered "no" to any of these questions, you must determine what went wrong and devise improved interventions for the future. (See Table 13-3 for a summary of the care plan evaluations.)

Table 13-3 **Care Plan for Patients at Risk for Falls**

Nursing Diagnosis: Risk for falls related to left-sided weakness and confusion
Expected Outcomes: Patient will be free from injury during hospitalization.

Interventions	Evaluations
Evaluate the patient's fall risk using Morse Fall Scale (see Table 13-1). Institute fall precautions: • Post fall precautions on the door to the patient's room, in the Kardex, and in the patient's chart according to facility policy.	Day 1: Patient was rated a 75 on Morse Fall Scale and was identified as a high fall risk. She was placed on fall precautions immediately after admission; signs were posted on her door to indicate this.
• Apply a bed/chair monitor that will alarm if the patient tries to get up. Respond to the monitor alarm immediately to prevent a fall. • Post reminders in the patient's room for the patient and family stating that the patient is to call for help before getting up. • Provide frequent verbal reorientation for the patient. Tell her where she is and what you want her to do. • Keep needed items within her reach.	Day 3: Patient had experienced no falls or other injuries.
Provide assistance to the patient to prevent falls: • Answer her call light promptly so the patient will not tire of waiting for help and attempt to get up alone. • Assist the patient to ambulate to the chair or the bathroom when needed. Offer toileting assistance every 2 hours. • Do not leave the patient alone while in the bathroom or on the bedside commode. Stay nearby to assist the patient back to bed.	Day 1: Patient was on bedrest and used the bedpan. Nursing staff checked on her every 30 min and she did not try to get up alone. Most of the time she would use the call light to ask for assistance, but occasionally she would call out to a staff member walking by her room. Day 2: Patient was able to get up to BR with assistance. She was still weak but less unsteady on her feet and understood that she was not to get up alone. Day 3: Patient was able to go to BR with standby assistance and was able to use her call light when she needed assistance.

Skill 13-1 Using a Bed/Chair or Leg Monitor

Assessment Steps

1. Determine the need for a monitor *to promote patient safety.* Follow facility policy regarding use of monitors.
2. Assess the need for further fall prevention measures. Avoid relying too much on the monitor alone.

Planning Steps

1. Obtain the pad for the bed/chair or the patch for the patient's leg, depending on the type of monitor to be used.
2. Check to be sure the alarm is working correctly *to prevent relying on faulty equipment.*

Implementation Steps

1. Follow the Initial Implementation Steps located on the inside front cover.
2. *For Bed/Chair Alarm:* Place the pad for the bed/chair alarm beneath the patient's buttocks. *The pad is pressure sensitive and will alarm if the patient tries to get up or if there is no weight on it for several seconds.*
   For Leg Alarm: Place the sensor patch on the patient's thigh. *It will alarm when the patient's leg is in a dependent position, indicating that the patient is attempting to stand.*

(skill continues on page 248)

Skill 13-1 (continued)

3. Attach control units to the monitor pads. For the bed/chair alarm, attach the control unit on the bed or the chair. For the leg alarm, the control unit attaches directly to the sensor patch. *The control units must be attached for the monitors to function.*

4. If possible, connect the control unit to the call light. Not all monitors are equipped with this function. However, when this function is in place, staff can respond more quickly *by both hearing the alarm and seeing the call light activated.*

5. Instruct the patient and family to call for assistance if the patient needs to get up. A nursing staff member will assist the patient and deactivate the alarm when needed. *This reduces the frequency of false alarms.*

6. Disconnect the alarm before assisting the patient out of the bed or chair, or before assisting the patient to stand. *This will prevent the alarm from sounding unnecessarily.*

7. If you assist the patient from the chair to the bed (or vice versa), be sure to move the alarm sensor pad first, so the patient will then be sitting or lying on the pad when in the new location. *This helps you avoid*

the possibility of forgetting to place the sensor pad in the new location.

8. Reactivate the alarm by reconnecting it to the sensor *to help prevent falls.*

9. Follow the Ending Implementation Steps located on the inside back cover.

Evaluation Steps

1. Determine the sensitivity of the alarm and adjust it to sound if the patient moves to get up. *This will alert you as soon as the patient begins to get up.*

2. Check on the patient frequently *to be certain that the alarm is functioning correctly and that the patient is safe.*

Sample Documentation

06/06/11 1120 Leg monitor applied to left thigh and connected to control unit. Alarm tested. Family and pt instructed to use call light for assistance before getting out of chair. ————————
———————————————— Nurse's signature and credentials

Skill 13-2 Applying Restraints

Assessment Steps

1. Assess the patient's response to restraint alternatives and previous attempts to prevent harm. *This will ensure the restraints are used as a last resort.*

2. Assess the need for restraints. Is the patient a danger to self or others? Are restraints necessary to perform a procedure or maintain tube or monitor placement?

3. Review the physician's order for type of restraint, indications for use, site of application, and duration of use of restraints. *This will help you avoid errors when carrying out the orders.*

Planning Steps

1. Obtain the appropriate restraint, *keeping in mind that the least restrictive restraint to prevent injury is required.*

2. Explain to the patient and family the need for restraint placement and the expected time frame for its use. *This will encourage patient and family cooperation.*

Intervention Steps

1. Follow the Initial Implementation Steps located on the inside front cover.

2. Place the restraint on the patient. For the *waist or belt restraint,* place the restraint around the patient's waist without wrinkles. For the *vest restraint,* place the vest on in such a way that the crossover is in the front. For the *wrist restraint,* place the padded portion around the wrist snugly enough to prevent it from slipping off, but not tight enough to impair circulation. For the *mitt restraint,* place the patient's hand inside the mitt with the fingers slightly flexed.

Correct placement prevents injury to the patient and increases the effectiveness of the restraint.

3. Ensure that the restraints are not too tight. You should be able to slide three fingers between the restraint and the patient when the restraint is applied correctly. *This amount of space prevents injury to the patient while keeping the restraint snug.*

4. Tie the restraint ties to the moveable part of the bed frame using a quick-release knot. A quick-release knot is also called a half-bow knot, and it will not come loose when the patient moves, but it will release completely when you pull on the loose end. *This allows you to release the restraints quickly in case of an emergency.*

Skill 13-2 Applying Restraints (continued)

To restraint

Pull to tighten

Bed frame

(A)

Hold here

Pull through and pull to tighten

(B)

Pull here to untie

(C)

5. **Never tie restraints to side rails.** When restraints are tied to the moveable portion of the bed frame, the patient will not be injured or uncomfortable when the head of the bed is raised. *Correct placement when tying restraints prevents injury to the patient when the bed position is changed.* When tying restraints to a wheelchair, cross the ties in the back, then tie them to the frame of the wheelchair *to prevent the patient from loosening the ties.*

6. Make any adjustments needed to the restraints *to prevent discomfort or impaired body alignment.*

7. Assess the patient in restraints every 30 minutes *to ensure that the patient is safe and not harmed by the restraint.* Check the distal pulses if the patient is in a mitt or wrist restraint *to ensure that circulation is not impaired.* Assess the skin in the extremity for warmth, color, and any complaints of numbness or tingling *to ensure that nerves are not being compressed.* Check the skin beneath the restraint for redness or chafing *to ensure that skin integrity is not being compromised.*

8. Release the restraints every 2 hours. Assist the patient to the bathroom, offer food and fluids, and give skin care, paying special attention to the skin under the restraints. Perform passive and active range of motion to the restrained extremities. *This allows the patient to have movement and activity while he or she is not restrained.*

9. Continue to use fall precautions for patients, even when restrained, *to prevent possible injury.*

10. Follow the Ending Implementation Steps located on the inside back cover.

Evaluation Steps

1. Determine the effectiveness of the restraints. Note whether the patient is comfortable and safe with restraints in place. Check to be sure the restraints are not causing circulatory impairment or skin breakdown. *This will help prevent any adverse effects due to the restraints.*

2. Determine the need for continuation of the restraints. Remove restraints when no longer necessary, *to promote the least restrictive environment for your patient.*

Sample Documentation

06/06/11 1510 Right wrist restraint applied per physician's order to prevent pt from pulling out NG tube and pulling off telemetry electrodes. Remains disoriented to time and place. Right radial pulse strong at 86/min. Hand warm, capillary refill 3 seconds, color pink. Assisted to drink a glass of orange juice. Watching TV with no complaints. —————————— Nurse's signature and credentials

Skill 13-3 Using Body Mechanics

Assessment Steps

1. Determine the best way to move the object: Can you push, pull, or slide, rather than lift it? *This will help you prevent injury.*

2. If necessary, determine whether you can use a lifting device. If not, determine how much help is required. *Obtaining assistance or using a lifting device will decrease the chance of injury while moving the patient or object.*

Planning Steps

1. Obtain the necessary lifting equipment if that is what you will use. Obtain assistance from nursing staff *to prevent injury to yourself and others.*

2. Determine how to use your assistant(s), if needed. Keep the safety of the patient and staff as your focus.

Implementation Steps

To Obtain an Item From a High Shelf

1. Use a step stool or other safe method to comfortably reach the object. *Trying to reach while on tiptoe can cause injury to your back.*

2. Tense your leg and arm muscles as you obtain the item *to avoid using your back muscles, possibly causing injury.*

3. Lower the item to waist level for balance.

4. Step down from the stool and carry the object close to your body at waist level with elbows flexed. *This is close to your center of gravity and keeps you balanced.*

To Obtain an Item From a Low Shelf or the Floor

1. Place your feet shoulder-width apart, widening your base of support *to give you stability.*

2. Flex your hips and knees, keeping your back straight and lowering your center of gravity. Avoid bending at the waist *as this puts strain on your back muscles.*

3. Lift the item with smooth, coordinated movements. *Jerky movements increase your chance of accident or injury.*

4. Hold the item close to your body as you straighten your hips and knees. The larger muscles of your legs carry the load, *which prevents injury to the smaller muscles in your back.*

5. Carry the item close to your body at waist level with elbows flexed. *This is close to your center of gravity and keeps you balanced.*

To Move a Patient up in Bed

1. Raise the bed to about your waist level *to avoid strain on your back muscles.*

2. Stand with your feet shoulder-width apart to widen your base of support, *which gives you stability.*

3. Turn your foot that is closest to the head of the bed so your toes point toward the headboard. *This helps you face the direction of movement so that you avoid twisting your back.*

4. On the count of 3, shift your weight from your lower foot to your upper foot as you move the patient up in bed. *This prevents any twisting movements that could injure your back.*

5. Lower the bed to its lowest level *for patient safety.*

Evaluation Steps

1. Determine the effectiveness of using good posture and good body mechanics. *The absence of back pain and injuries validates this.*

2. Determine if you used good decision making by getting help and/or using lift devices when appropriate.

Post Conference

When you review your care for Mrs. Lloyd, you have mixed emotions. She was not as confused as you thought she might be. She was oriented to person and sometimes to place, but not time. She recognized her family and learned your name quickly. She remained safe during your care and did not have any more falls, so you feel good about your care. However, the sensor pad for her bed/chair alarm was not always effective. Once when you took her to the bathroom, you forgot to turn it back on when you assisted her back to bed. Her daughter-in-law noticed that the alarm was off and called it to your attention. Fortunately, Mrs. Lloyd did not attempt to get out of bed during that time. It is now easier for you to understand how her earlier fall occurred, but you have also learned the importance of checking and double-checking for safety, even on patients who are being monitored.

KEY POINTS

- National Patient Safety Goals have been established to help decrease injury and harm to patients.

- Many factors can contribute to unsafe patient environments and must be addressed to promote patient safety.

- Several restraint alternatives and strategies exist and can be easily implemented to keep patients safer.

- If the use of restraints is unavoidable, a physician's order must be obtained first. Apply restraints correctly and check on the patient frequently. Release the restraints every 2 hours, allowing the patient to go to the bathroom. Offer food and fluids, and check for any signs of skin breakdown or bruising due to the restraints.

- If you delegate checks and releases of restraints to a UAP or CNA, you must be sure they are being done correctly and according to facility policy.

- It is extremely important to apply restraints correctly and to tie them with a quick-release knot to prevent patient injury or even possible death.

- If a fire occurs in your area, follow the acronym RACE—**R**escue patients from danger, sound the **A**larm, **C**onfine the fire, and **E**xtinguish the fire if it is small, or wait for the fire department if it is large.

- To correctly use a fire extinguisher to fight a fire, follow the acronym PASS—**P**ull the pin, **A**im the nozzle at the base of the flames, **S**queeze the handles together, and **S**weep the nozzle back and forth to extinguish the fire.

- If you come upon an unresponsive patient, initiate a Code Blue or its equivalent according to your facility's policies, and begin CPR or rescue breathing.

- During a mass casualty event, follow your facility's disaster plan and expect to be called in to work extra shifts.

- Nurses and nursing staff are regularly exposed to physical, chemical, and biological hazards, so it is important to know how to minimize these hazards and protect yourself.

REVIEW QUESTIONS

Select the answer that is most appropriate for each of the following questions. Some questions may have more than one correct answer. Check all that apply.

1. Which statement best describes the National Patient Safety Goals?

   a. They emphasize the importance of safe lifting and mandate hospitals to have equipment in place to phase out manual lifting.

   b. They address specific safety problems in the hospital setting and establish requirements for meeting each goal.

   c. They address needle-stick injuries and require hospitals to purchase needleless access devices.

   d. They identify specific communicable diseases and outline transmission-based precautions for each.

2. A newly admitted patient may be at risk for falls. While the patient is in the bathroom changing into a hospital gown, the admitting nurse would be <u>most</u> concerned about:

   a. ordering soft device bolsters for the bed.

   b. arranging for a bed monitor to be placed on the bed.

   c. staying near the bathroom to help the patient back to bed.

   d. determining whether to ask the doctor for an order for restraints.

3. A patient has been restrained to prevent him from pulling out his nasogastric tube. You assign a UAP to check on the patient. What directions will you give?

   a. "Check on him every 30 minutes and release him every 2 hours. Don't forget to document all your checks on the flow sheet."

   b. "Look in on the patient from the doorway every 2 hours. Make sure the tube is still in place."

   c. "Just to be extra careful, check on him every hour and ask if he needs to go to the bathroom."

   d. "Release him from the restraints every 30 minutes and document that you have done so."

4. You walk into a patient's room and find a fire involving the trashcan and curtains. What will you do <u>first</u>?

   a. Use the call light to tell the unit clerk to activate a "Code Red."

   b. Step into the hall and call for help, announcing a fire in this room.

   c. Use the telephone in the room to notify the fire department using a special code.

   d. Remove the patient from the room to a safer area of the hospital.

5. To use proper body mechanics, you need to be most concerned about:

   a. your center of gravity, your base of support, and using your leg muscles.

   b. obtaining lifting equipment, obtaining assistance, and keeping your feet apart.

   c. your center of support, base of gravity, and the position of your back.

   d. finding ways to avoid lifting and wearing a brace to protect your back.

6. During clinical, you think you see a staff nurse swallow a narcotic medicine she signed out for a patient. What will you do?

   a. Ask the staff nurse if she just swallowed that pill.

   b. Say nothing and watch the nurse to see if she acts different later.

   c. Tell a fellow student at break so you can both watch the nurse.

   d. Confidentially tell your instructor what you thought you saw.

7. While rinsing a used surgical instrument in a disinfectant called Cidex, some of the Cidex splashes on your lips and nose. Your <u>first</u> action is to:

   a. rinse your mouth and nose immediately with running water.

   b. consult the MSDS for Cidex to know what actions to take.

   c. induce vomiting in case you accidentally swallowed any of the chemical.

   d. wash the area immediately with surgical soap and water.

CRITICAL THINKING EXERCISES

8. A CNA that you supervise is consistently slow in answering patients' call lights. How will you emphasize safety when discussing this with him?

9. A mass casualty event has occurred in your area. You determine that your family is safe. What actions will you now take?

10. A patient falls when trying to get out of bed alone. You are to investigate possible causes for the fall. How will you go about your investigation?

ADDITIONAL RESOURCES

For additional Resources, Questions, and Activities, please see:

  Student Resource Disk

 DavisPlus http://davisplus.fadavis.com

Student Study Guide

REFERENCES

Chaffee MW. Making the decision to report to work in a disaster: nurses may have conflicting obligations. *Am J Nurs.* 2006;106(9):54-56.

Doucette JN. View from the cockpit: what the AIRLINE INDUSTRY can teach us about PATIENT SAFETY. *Nursing2006.* 2006;36(11):50-53.

Gustafson SE. Patient Safety: Assess for fall risk, intervene—and bump up patient safety. *Nursing2007.* 2007;37(12):24-25.

Mason DJ. Failure to Rescue: After Hurricane Katrina, assessing the heroisim and the breakdowns. *Am J Nurs.* 2005;105(10):11.

Protect Yourself: Avoiding back injuries. *Nursing2004.* 2004;34(2 Suppl Travel Nursing2004):24.

Rittenmeyer L. Disaster Preparedness: Are you ready? *Men Nurs.* 2007;2(3):18-23.

The Joint Commission. 2010 National Patient Safety Goals, Critical Access Hospital. Available at: http://www.jointcommission.org/PatientSafety/NationalPatientSafetyGoals.

Todd JF. Device Safety: Waking up to hospital bed entrapment risks. *Nursing2008.* 2008;38(1):14-15.

Veenema TG, Toke J. Hospital & Critical Care: When standards of care change in mass casualty events. *Am J Nurs.* 2007;107(9):72a-72f.

Walker-Cillo G. Bioterrorism! We put our plan to the test. *RN.* 2006;69(4):36-41.

Wilkinson J, Van Leuven K. *Fundamentals of Nursing: Theory, Concepts & Applications.* Philadelphia: FA Davis; 2007.

14

Medical Asepsis and Infection Control

Key Terms

Chain of infection

Direct contact

Disinfectant

Health care–associated infection (HAI)

Indirect contact

Localized infection

Medical asepsis

Microorganisms

Normal flora and fauna

Pathogens

Primary infection

Secondary infection

Septicemia

Standard precautions

Sterile technique

Sterilization

Surgical asepsis

Systemic infection

Transmission-based precautions

Vectors

Objectives

1. Define key terms related to medical asepsis and infection control.
2. Describe five types of pathogens.
3. Identify selected common illnesses caused by microbes.
4. Illustrate the chain of infection.
5. Differentiate types of infections.
6. Compare primary, secondary, and tertiary defenses against infection.
7. Explain factors that decrease the body's defenses.
8. Differentiate between the use of standard precautions and transmission-based precautions.
9. Compare medical and surgical asepsis.
10. Describe when and how to use hand hygiene.
11. Detail the use of standard precautions.
12. Compare the purposes and types of transmission-based precautions.
13. Explain ways to meet the emotional needs of patients who are isolated due to communicable disease.

Skills

14-1 Performing Hand Hygiene

14-2 Donning Personal Protective Equipment

14-3 Removing Personal Protective Equipment

Clinical Connection

Your Assignment: You are assigned to care for a patient who has an infection caused by methicillin-resistant *Staphylococcus aureus* (MRSA). You know this is a highly contagious infection that is resistant to all but one antibiotic. It frightens you to care for this patient because you are worried that you might catch the infection or take the microorganism home to your children.

Your Actions: One of the first things you do is look up this diagnosis to find out more about it. You learn that you need to protect yourself by using personal protective equipment (PPE) and by washing your hands frequently and thoroughly. You never thought much about how to wash your hands before, but now you want to be sure you are removing all microorganisms that could cause you or your family to become ill. You want to give good care to the patient, but protect yourself at the same time.

When you work in a hospital as a student or as a staff nurse, you are surrounded by some virulent germs. This can be very alarming if you do not understand the causes of infection or do not know how to protect yourself and your patients from disease-causing microorganisms. In this chapter, you will learn how to protect yourself as well as how to prevent the spread of disease-causing germs to other patients or your family.

Causes of Infection

Infections are caused by a variety of **microorganisms**. These are minuscule living bodies that cannot be seen without a microscope. Microorganisms that cause infection in humans are referred to as **pathogens**. They reproduce rapidly and can spread from one area of a person's body to another. Not all microorganisms are pathogenic, however. Many microorganisms live in and on our bodies, performing needed functions to protect us from harmful pathogens as well as helping us break down and digest food. These microorganisms are referred to as **normal flora and fauna**, which means the tiny plants and animals normally found in the human body.

Types of Pathogens

Pathogenic microorganisms are classified as bacteria, viruses, protozoa, fungi, or helminths.

Bacteria

Bacteria are one-celled microorganisms found virtually everywhere, including in the human body. It is only when they invade an area outside their normal location that problems result. For example, several bacteria live in the intestines to help the body digest food and absorb vitamins. They belong there. However, if those particular bacteria are introduced into the urethra and migrate to the bladder, they will cause a urinary tract infection.

Laboratory and Diagnostic Connection

Identifying Bacteria in the Laboratory

Bacteria are named and classified by their shape and identified in the laboratory. A specimen of drainage, sputum, stool, urine, or blood is obtained and sent to the laboratory. When it is examined under a microscope, the medical laboratory technologist identifies the bacterium by its shape (Fig. 14-1).

Cocci (*singular* coccus) are sphere-shaped bacteria. Sometimes they may be seen in clusters and are similar to grapes in appearance. These are known as *staphylococci.* They may also appear in chains, like a bead necklace, and are then referred to as *streptococci.* Or they may appear in pairs, like two balls side by side, which are described as *diplococci.* Bacilli (*sing.* bacillus) are rod-shaped bacteria. They have a log-like appearance and may vary in length. Spirilla (*sing.* spirillum) are long cells that spiral or coil, similar to a curl of long hair.

Another step in identifying which coccus, bacillus, or spirillum is under the microscope involves using a dark purple stain called Gram stain. The slide containing the microorganism is flooded with Gram stain, then rinsed with alcohol. It is counterstained with safranin and then rinsed with water. When it is viewed under the microscope again, the bacteria will have taken up the stain. Those that appear either purple or blue are known as gram-positive organisms. Those that appear pink or red are identified as gram-negative organisms. The amount and type of stain the bacterium retains is dependent on the composition of its cell wall. Different medications are most effective for different types of organisms and are prescribed based on their Gram stain response.

Rickettsia and chlamydia are types of bacteria, but they are different from most because they can only reproduce inside the cells of the host, similar to the way viruses must reproduce. Rickettsia and chlamydia are often spread through the bites of insects, such as ticks and mites, that are called **vectors**. The insects are carriers of the microorganisms, and when they bite a human, the human becomes ill due to infection from the rickettsia or chlamydia bacteria.

A Coccus   **B** Bacillus   **C** Spirillum

Figure 14-1   Bacteria identified by shapes (magnification × 2000).

Antibiotics are prescribed to treat infections caused by bacteria. There are many types of antibiotics, and each acts in a slightly different way to kill bacteria. (For more information about antibiotics and their actions, see Chapter 35.) It is important to note that antibiotics are effective against bacteria only, not against any other type of microorganisms.

Viruses

Viruses are not made up of individual cells, but rather are very tiny parasites that live within the cells of the host and reproduce there. They can only be seen with an electron microscope because they are too small to be visualized with a standard microscope. Unlike bacteria, viruses are not endemic to the human body, and all viruses potentially cause illness.

Few antiviral medications exist at this time, and their development is targeted on the viruses that cause the most severe illnesses. Many viral infections are mild and self-limiting, meaning that they will resolve in time without medication. Some individuals, when they are ill and seek medical attention, become upset if a health care provider does not prescribe antibiotics. However, antibiotics would not be effective against a virus. Sometimes prescribers will order antibiotics to prevent a secondary infection from occurring, but that is not necessary with every viral illness.

Protozoa

Protozoa are single-celled animals that live in water. They can be ingested by humans through water or food and, when that occurs, protozoa cause intestinal illnesses. Some protozoa are parasites that remain in the digestive tract. They are treated with antiparasitic drugs. Other illnesses are treated with anti-infectives specific for the causative protozoan.

Fungi

Fungi may be made up of one or more cells. Not all fungi require a microscope to be seen. For example, mold on bread and mushrooms growing in the yard are both examples of fungi. While fungi are present in the environment, they cause illness when they enter the human body through cuts or cracks in the skin. In immunosuppressed individuals, a fungal infection can become systemic, spreading throughout the entire body. Fungal infections are treated with antifungal medications available in creams, ointments, and oral and IV forms.

Helminths

Helminths are parasitic worms that can inhabit the digestive tract of humans. Some worms enter the body through the mouth, often through contaminated food. Once in the intestine, the worms may attach to the intestinal wall and absorb digested food, growing to great lengths. Other types of worms, such as pinworms, inhabit the intestines and lay eggs around the anus. The person feels intense itching in the anal area and when he or she scratches, the eggs lodge beneath the fingernails, making it easy to spread them to others or to self-reinfect if the hands are then around the person's mouth. These worms only grow to be about ½ inch long, but they can be very numerous—to the point that they can fill up the appendix and mimic appendicitis. Helminth infestations are treated with medication, known as anthelmintics or antihelmintics, designed to kill the specific parasitic worm.

Knowledge Connection
List three types of bacteria. How are viruses different from other microorganisms? Give examples of visible fungi.

Common Illnesses Caused by Microbes

Perhaps you have seen or experienced infection by some of these microorganisms. Table 14-1 provides a summary of some of the most common illnesses caused by these types of microorganisms.

Chain of Infection

In order for infection to spread from one person to another, a chain of events must occur. This chain of events is often referred to as the **chain of infection** (Fig. 14-2) and involves the following "links":

- An *infectious agent,* or causative organism
- A *reservoir,* or place the organism grows
- A *portal of exit,* or method by which the organism leaves the reservoir
- A *mode of transmission,* or vehicle by which the organism is transferred
- A *portal of entry,* or method by which the organism enters a new host
- A *susceptible host,* or person whose body the organism has entered

Table 14-1 Common Diseases Caused by Microorganisms

Microorganism	Disease	Treatment
Bacteria		
Staphylococcus aureus	Boils, toxic shock syndrome, osteomyelitis, MRSA—significant nosocomial infection	Antibiotics, although most strains are not killed by penicillin. MRSA can only be killed with one antibiotic, vancomycin, and is not affected by others.
Streptococcus group A (gram-positive coccus)	Strep throat, ear infections, scarlet fever, endocarditis; can lead to rheumatic fever, heart valve damage, transient kidney damage "Flesh-eating strep" is a rare strain causing necrotizing fasciitis that can lead to death	Antibiotics
Streptococcus group B (gram-positive coccus)	Neonatal infections, especially in premature births, causing pneumonia, meningitis, or septicemia in newborns	IV antibiotics
Clostridium perfringens (gram-positive bacillus; spore forming)	Gas gangrene in contaminated wounds—spores live in dead tissue and produce toxins that destroy more tissue, so bacteria spreads; the gas forms bubbles in the dead tissue	Amputation of affected limb
Clostridium difficile (gram-positive bacillus; spore forming)	Severe diarrhea; often develops with antibiotic therapy and is called psuedomembranous enterocolitis; this is a significant nosocomial pathogen	Only two antibiotics will treat this: vancomycin and metronidazole.
Escheria coli (gram-negative bacillus)	Normally found in the colon, but can cause infection if it enters the urinary tract or other parts of the body; a common cause of nosocomial infections	Antibiotics
Escheria coli 0157:H7 (gram-negative bacillus)	Infection of colon causing bloody diarrhea and kidney failure, known as hemolytic uremic "syndrome"; can be fatal, often due to consuming undercooked ground meat	Antibiotics, dialysis for kidney failure
Mycobacterium tuberculosis (bacillus)	Tuberculosis that destroys lung tissue, leaving large cavities; drug-resistant strains are becoming more common	Anti-tuberculosis medications
Borrelia burgdorferi (spirochete)	Lyme disease; spirochete transmitted by deer tick to human, causing flu-like symptoms, irregular heartbeat, and possible arthritis	Antibiotics
Rickettsia ricketsii (bacillus)	Rocky Mountain spotted fever spread by ticks; causes high fever, rash, and pneumonia and can lead to death	Antibiotics

Table 14-1   **Common Diseases Caused by Microorganisms** (continued)

Microorganism	Disease	Treatment
Viruses		
Herpes simplex	Type 1 causes fever blisters; type 2 causes genital herpes	Antivirals such as acyclovir
Herpesvirus 3 (varicella-zoster)	Chickenpox contracted first, then virus lies dormant in nerve endings; if reactivated in adults, causes shingles that result in painful blisters along nerve pathways	Antiviral: acyclovir
Influenza	"Flu" symptoms—aching muscles, fever, respiratory congestion, cough	Antivirals such as Tamiflu and Relenza Prevention: annual flu immunization
West Nile	Virus found in birds and spread by mosquitos; causes headache and confusion in some, but may be asymptomatic in others	No antiviral exists— supportive treatment
Fungi		
Microsporum epidermophyton	Ringworm, also known as tinea; can be found on the skin or scalp; causes itchy red, round patches Athlete's foot also caused by this fungus	Antifungals
Candida albicans	Yeast infections; called thrush when found in the mouth; often found in the vagina, and may be due to antibiotics that kill normal bacteria, allowing an overgrowth of yeast; can cause pneumonia and heart infections	Antifungals
Protozoans		
Entamoeba histolytica	Amebic dysentery, causes severe bloody diarrhea and can cause abscesses in body organs such as the liver, lungs, and brain	Amebicides and antibiotics
Giardia lamblia	Giardiasis, which causes diarrhea; often found in water but may also be spread through food prepared by people who have a mild case of the illness	Antibiotics
Plasmodium	Malaria; causes destruction of red blood cells and anemia; can lead to severe form that affects the brain	Antimalarials
Helminths		
Enterobius	Pinworms; look like white threads and grow in the intestine; most common parasitic worm in the United States	Antihelmintics
Taenia	Tapeworm; may enter humans through undercooked meat containing the worm cysts; head of worm attaches to wall of intestines with suckers and grows in segments; causes bloating, constipation, or diarrhea	Antihelmintics

Source: Adapted from Scanlon V, Sanders T. *Essentials of Anatomy and Physiology*. 5th ed. Philadelphia: FA Davis; 2007.

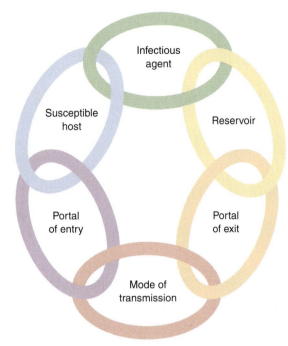

Figure 14-2 The links in the chain of infection, which must all be present for infection to spread.

The following example will help you understand the chain of infection.

A busy nurse is caring for eight patients in a hospital unit. It is a hectic day with many problems. The nurse assists the CNA in changing the linens in the room of Patient 1, who is hospitalized with severe diarrhea due to an infection caused by *Clostridium difficile*. The nurse wears gloves during this procedure, but is unaware of a tiny hole in the finger of one glove. After the procedure, the nurse neglects to wash his hands, but does use alcohol-based hand gel as he leaves the room. He then prepares oral medications for Patient 2 and delivers them to the room. Patient 2 swallows the medications and later develops a *C. difficile* infection as well. In this example, the chain of infection occurred in this manner:

- **Infectious agent:** *Clostridium difficile*
- **Reservoir:** Patient 1
- **Portal of exit:** bowel movement of Patient 1
- **Mode of transmission:** nurse's hands, because this organism is not killed by alcohol-based hand gel
- **Portal of entry:** Patient 2's mouth
- **Susceptible host:** Patient 2

Types of Infection

The example given above is an illustration of the chain of infection, but it is also an example of a **health care–associated infection (HAI)**, which is an infection that is acquired while the patient is being cared for in any health care setting, including home health care and long-term care. The former term for these types of infections was *nosocomial infections,* but they are now referred to as HAIs. The single most important way to break the chain of infection and to prevent HAIs is to perform hand hygiene (see Skill 14-1, page 271).

Infections may be **primary infections**, or initial infections caused by one pathogen only, or **secondary infections**, caused by a second, different pathogen. If a person has an infection in one area of the body (for example, in the lungs), it is described as a **localized infection**. If the infection then spreads from the lungs to other organs, it becomes a **systemic infection**, spreading through the bloodstream. When microorganisms are present and multiplying in the blood, it is referred to as **septicemia**. This condition is extremely serious, requiring aggressive treatment with IV antibiotics and support for the patient's inundated immune system. Infections may start as one type, then progress to another type. This does not mean that the causative organism changes, but rather that the type of infection progresses to become more severe.

Defenses Against Infection

The human body is designed to defend against invading pathogens. In fact, three "lines of defense" exist to help thwart infection. Most of us would suffer constantly with infections without this three-layer defense system, referred to as primary, secondary, and tertiary defenses.

Primary Defenses

The primary defenses include body systems, or portions of them, that block or trap invading pathogens.

- **Skin:** Intact skin protects the body from microbes that would cause disease in subcutaneous or deeper tissue. When breaks in the skin occur, such as cuts, scrapes, and burns, the resulting opening is a portal of entry for pathogens.
- **Mucous membranes:** These membranes produce sticky mucus to trap invading pathogens. In the respiratory tract, the mucus may be coughed up and expectorated or blown out of the nose, taking microorganisms with it.

  In the urinary tract, the urethra secretes mucus to trap pathogens that could enter the body through the urinary meatus. Then, the acidic urine washes the pathogens out of the body.

  In the vagina, mucus traps pathogens, preventing them from migrating into the uterus. The pH of vaginal secretions, along with the normal bacteria present in the vagina, are hostile to most microorganisms.
- **Gastrointestinal system:** The mouth provides entry into the gastrointestinal system and contains some bacteria. Saliva contains enzymes that help remove microorganisms

from the teeth. Normal flora helps prevent invasion by pathogens.

If any pathogens make it to the stomach, the strong hydrochloric acid found in digestive juices often kills them. Pathogens that enter the intestines, perhaps through food, meet with bile that breaks down and emulsifies fats, as well as killing microbes.

Secondary Defenses

The second line of defense occurs at the cellular level in reaction to toxins secreted by invading pathogens.

- **Inflammatory process:** This process is discussed in detail in Chapter 26, but a brief description is provided here. When an injury occurs, the W cells release histamine and other chemicals, which cause the blood vessels near the injury to dilate. This dilation results in redness and warmth in the area of injury. The blood vessels also become more permeable to allow an increased number of white blood cells, or *phagocytes,* into the injured area. These phagocytes surround the invading pathogens and consume them.
- **Elevated temperature:** The body responds to invading pathogens by creating an environment that is hostile to them. The increase of body temperature to 101°F or higher is too warm for most invading microorganisms to live and multiply. Certain microbes may take protection in spore form, but many will be killed.
- **Complement cascade:** When invading pathogens are detected in the body, complement is released. *Complement* is a group of specialized proteins that attack the pathogens by releasing chemicals that make their cell membranes rupture.

Tertiary Defenses

The third line of defense involves specialized white blood cells called *lymphocytes* that fight infection, either as B cells or T cells. These lymphocytes are found in lymph tissue, such as the spleen, thymus, lymph nodes, and tonsils. They are also circulating in the blood, searching for invading pathogens, which they identify by their surface proteins. When pathogens are found, the B and T cells signal phagocytes to destroy the invaders. The B and T cells have a major role in the antigen-antibody response.

Factors That Decrease Defenses

Have you ever noticed that you become ill more easily when you are tired and stressed? When the body is not healthy, well nourished, and well rested, the three lines of defense cannot function effectively. Box 14-1 describes factors that decrease the body's defenses against infection.

Knowledge Connection

List the links in the chain of infection. What are three components of primary defenses? What are three components of secondary defenses?

Box 14-1

Factors That Affect the Body's Defenses Against Infection

Many factors can influence the body's ability to defend itself against infection. They include:

- **Age:** Infants' and young children's immune systems are not well developed yet and cannot assist with defense against infection as well as the immune systems of older children and adults. In elderly individuals, the immune system gradually decreases in effectiveness, leaving them more vulnerable to invading pathogens.
- **Chemical Exposure:** Toxicity from chemicals impairs the body's defenses and ability to fight infection.
- **Chronic Illness:** The body's defenses are responding on a frequent basis to chronic illness and have no reserves to react effectively to a new infection.
- **Lack of Exercise:** Without adequate exercise, circulation slows and the flow of lymph and phagocytes decreases, interfering with their ability to destroy invading pathogens.
- **Lack of Rest:** The body needs adequate rest to repair damage and restore energy. Lack of rest increases the chance of infection occurring because the immune system cannot repair itself and function at its highest capacity.
- **Increased Stress:** When the body is frequently reacting to stressors, immune function can be impaired, which increases the risk of illness and infection (see Chapter 7).
- **Nonintact Skin:** Open wounds, such as surgical wounds, skin tears, and pressure ulcers, provide a portal of entry for microorganisms.
- **Poor Nutrition:** A diet that is lacking in fruits, vegetables, and certain dairy products negatively affects the body's defenses because it lacks vitamins and support for normal flora.

Preventing Infection

When you care for patients, it is very important to be aware of the potential for spreading infection. It is your responsibility to prevent the possibility of becoming a mode of transmission in the chain of infection, spreading microorganisms from patient to patient. It is just as important that you know how to prevent infection from spreading from a patient to you.

It is the responsibility of all health care workers to be vigilant about breaking the chain of infection. *Safety: The most effective way to break the chain of infection is to use appropriate hand hygiene.* The Centers for Medicare and Medicaid Services (CMS) have now ceased to pay for any costs related to three common hospital-acquired infections. These include urinary tract infections due to a urinary catheter inserted during hospitalization, infections in the blood due to central vascular lines, and infection in the chest incision after open heart surgery. When you use appropriate precautions and good techniques, you will not contribute to hospital-acquired infections.

Precautions for Preventing the Transmission of Pathogens

The Centers for Disease Control and Prevention (CDC) is a government agency within the U.S. Department of Health and Human Services that is responsible for tracking, regulating, and educating about public health issues. In order to protect patients and health care workers from the spread of pathogens in health care settings, the CDC has developed precautions to be used during patient care. These precautions were updated in 2007 and include both standard precautions, to be used in the care of all patients in all health care settings, and transmission-based precautions, to be used when caring for patients with communicable diseases.

Standard precautions are a group of safety measures performed to prevent the transmission of pathogens found in the blood and body fluids. This includes performing hand hygiene, wearing appropriate protective equipment if exposure is possible, and using cough etiquette. Standard precautions are performed with all patients, whether or not an infection has been diagnosed. They protect the health care worker from possible transmission of illnesses spread through contact with infected blood, such as hepatitis B, hepatitis C, and HIV. They also protect patients from the possible spread of pathogens from one patient to another. Further details for following standard precautions will be discussed later in this section. See Table 14-2 for information on personal protective equipment needed in standard precautions.

Transmission-based precautions are used to prevent the spread of known infection to patients or health care staff. They are used when a patient has a communicable illness that can be spread through contact, through respiratory droplets, or through the air. Gowns, gloves, masks, eye protection, and possibly head covers are used to prevent transmission of pathogens. Further details for following transmission-based precautions will be discussed later in this section.

Medical Asepsis

The term **medical asepsis** refers to practices performed to prevent the spread of infection. It is also sometimes described as using "clean technique." These practices, or techniques, include performing hand hygiene, maintaining a clean patient environment, using standard precautions, and using transmission-based precautions when necessary.

Medical asepsis is different than **surgical asepsis**, which refers to maintaining a sterile environment such as that found in operating rooms. **Sterile technique** means performing procedures in such a way that no pathogens will enter the patient's body when you insert tubes or give injections. You will learn abut surgical asepsis and sterile technique in Chapter 22.

The following is an example of a nurse using medical asepsis:

The nurse enters a patient's room to assist a patient who has used the bedside commode. The nurse washes his or her hands, puts on clean gloves, assists the patient in cleaning the genital area, then assists the patient into bed. The nurse then empties, rinses, and replaces the pan of the bedside commode. The nurse removes the gloves and washes his or her hands.

In this example, the nurse uses medical asepsis to protect himself or herself by performing hand hygiene frequently and wearing clean gloves, keeps the environment clean by emptying the bedside commode immediately, and protects the patient from possible infection by cleaning the genital area.

Clean Environment and Equipment

Maintaining a clean environment coincides with maintaining a safe environment for your patients. Clean up spills as soon as they occur for safety as well as to eliminate a breeding ground for bacteria. Wipe off dirty, dusty surfaces to decrease the possibility of microbial growth. Remove uneaten food from patient rooms to prevent possible growth of microorganisms that can cause illness.

When you clean surfaces in a health care setting, you will use a **disinfectant** cleaning agent, which will remove most pathogens. Some viruses and spore-forming bacteria are not killed by disinfection, however. **Sterilization** removes all pathogens using steam under pressure, heat, gas, or chemicals. It is discussed further in Chapter 22.

After you use equipment for one patient that can be reused for another patient (for example, an IV pump), it is very important that you disinfect it according to facility policy. If blood remains on a surface, even though the blood has dried, some viruses can still be present. Hepatitis B can live for up to 7 days on surfaces outside the body. In most cases, you will clean equipment after it is used and then send it to the central supply area of the hospital. It will be completely disinfected or sterilized there, and made ready for use by the next patient.

Real-World Connection

Who Is Responsible for Maintaining a Clean Patient Environment?

A nursing instructor noticed a smell in a patient room where two nursing students were caring for a debilitated patient. When she asked about it, the students replied that the patient had just used the bedside commode. The instructor told them to get some air freshener from the housekeeper's cart and use it in the room. Several hours later, the instructor returned and still noticed the smell. When she questioned the students again, they explained, "Housekeeping still has not come to empty the bedside commode." The instructor noted that this is a nursing task, not a housekeeping task. It is your responsibility to keep your patient's environment clean and free from potential pathogens.

Hand Hygiene

Nurses wash their hands repeatedly during patient care. You may not realize that there are correct and incorrect ways to perform hand hygiene. The way you are accustomed to washing your hands at home may not be the correct way to wash your hands in a health care setting. Sometimes students even feel a bit insulted that they are expected to demonstrate a skill as basic as handwashing. However, it is extremely important to be sure that all surfaces of the hands are cleaned thoroughly to dislodge and wash away all pathogens. When you care for patients, you should avoid wearing multiple rings on your hands. Many dress codes call for only one ring, such as a wedding band, and do not allow others. When you perform hand hygiene, it is important that you clean around your ring. It is possible for microorganisms to be present in and around the sets of your rings. Skill 14-1 details the steps of hand hygiene.

When to Perform Hand Hygiene
When working in a health care setting, the possibility of spreading pathogens on your hands is great. It is one of the most common methods of transmission in the chain of infection, so it is important to wash your hands in the following situations:

- After touching blood, body fluids, secretions, excretions, or contaminated items
- Immediately after removing gloves
- Upon entering a patient's room
- Before touching the patient or tubes connected to the patient
- Between caring for two patients in the same room
- When arriving on the nursing unit
- After returning to the nursing unit from breaks or meals
- After using the restroom
- Any time your hands are visibly dirty

Hand Hygiene Guidelines
In the 2007 hand hygiene guidelines from the CDC, the use of alcohol-based hand gels for cleaning hands is recommended because they can be used when handwashing with soap and water is not optimal. Additional highlights from the guidelines include:

- To use alcohol-based hand gels correctly, apply the product to the palm of one hand, then rub your hands together, covering all surfaces of the hands and fingers, until the hands are dry.
- Alcohol-based hand gels should be used before and after care of each patient, just as gloves should be changed before and after each patient.
- If the hands are visibly soiled, they should be washed with soap and water.
- Hand hygiene does not eliminate the need for gloves, nor does using gloves eliminate the need for hand hygiene. Gloves reduce hand contamination by 70% to 80%, prevent cross-contamination, and protect patients and health care personnel from infection.
- Health care personnel should avoid wearing artificial nails and keep natural nails less than ¼ inch long if they care for patients at high risk for infections.

Safety: It is important to know that alcohol-based hand gels do not kill spores and are not recommended when caring for patients infected with Clostridium difficile.

In 2009, the World Health Organization (WHO) established Guidelines for Hand Hygiene in Health Care. These guidelines are very similar to the CDC's recommendations. Box 14-2 presents additional information on the WHO guidelines.

Patient Teaching Connection

Incorporating Hand Hygiene in Patient Teaching
Avoid making the assumption that every patient knows how to correctly perform hand hygiene. When you are teaching a patient a skill, such as how to do a finger stick blood sugar test, be sure to include the correct way to wash hands in your teaching. Also, it is important to inform patients that they have every right to ask every health care worker who enters their room to perform hand hygiene before touching the patients' wounds or tubes. If this is not automatic on the part of the health care worker, then it is appropriate to remind the worker to clean his or her hands.

Box 14-2
Additional Information on WHO Guidelines for Hand Hygiene in Health Care

In addition to the CDC, the WHO has also made recommendations regarding hand hygiene in health care. Because it is a worldwide organization, their guidelines encompass situations that could be encountered in underprivileged countries as well as the United States.
- No artificial nails or nail extenders (tips) should be worn by those having direct contact with patients.
- Natural nails should be kept short, with tips less than 0.5 cm long.

In some situations, soap and clean water may not be readily available to perform a surgical scrub. The following recommendations are for using an alcohol-based hand rub instead of a surgical scrub prior to going into surgery.
- When using alcohol-based hand rub before going into surgery, wash hands first with plain soap and water to remove any visible soil. Then place 5 mL (the equivalent of three doses) into your left palm. Use the elbow of your right hand to press the dispenser.
- Dip the fingertips of your right hand in the gel for 5 seconds to decontaminate the nails.
- Then smear the hand rub up your right forearm to the elbow, using circular movements around the forearm until the rub evaporates.
- Repeat for the other arm.
- Then put 5 mL of hand rub in your left palm, again operating the dispenser with your elbow. Rub both hands together up to the wrists, covering all hand surfaces until the hands are dry.
- Total hand prep with hand gel should last 3 to 5 minutes.
- When the hands and forearms are completely dry, apply sterile gloves.

CDC Guidelines for Standard and Transmission-based Precautions

Another part of medical asepsis involves following the requirements established by the CDC for the prevention of transmitting communicable pathogens. The first form of protection is standard precautions, which are to be used with all patients, regardless of diagnosis or suspected diagnosis. The second form of protection is the use of transmission-based precautions, which requires the use of specific protective equipment when caring for patients with illnesses that are communicable through contact, respiratory droplets, or the air. It is very important to note that transmission-based precautions are always used *in addition to* standard precautions.

Standard Precautions

When you perform hand hygiene, then put on gloves before touching anything that is contaminated with blood or body fluids, such as when you go to empty a patient's drain, you are following standard precautions. If there was danger that the blood or body fluids in the drain could splash when it was emptied, you would wear a face shield, mask, and gown, again following standard precautions. You will take these precautions for all patients, not just those diagnosed with hepatitis or HIV. Table 14-2 shows the components of standard precautions to be used in the care of all patients in all health care settings. It is very important to know the correct order in which to put on the protective equipment and the correct order for removing it, to prevent contamination of surfaces and of yourself. Skill 14-2 (page 272) describes the correct way to put on personal protective equipment, and Skill 14-3 (page 274) describes the correct way to remove personal protective equipment.

Wearing gloves is a major part of standard precautions. As a nursing student and a nurse, you will put on and remove innumerable pairs of gloves each day. For medical asepsis, including standard and transmission-based precautions, you will wear clean gloves. You use a different technique for putting on sterile gloves, which are worn for sterile procedures. Donning a sterile gown and sterile gloves as well as performing sterile procedures are covered in Chapter 22.

Gloves made of latex can cause allergic reactions in both health care workers and patients. Most health care

Table 14-2   Standard Precautions for the Care of All Patients in All Health Care Settings

Component	Use
Hand Hygiene	Wash hands for 20 seconds using soap and water or use antibacterial hand gel unless hands are visibly soiled. Avoid using hand gel if caring for a patient with illness caused by spore-forming microorganisms.
Personal Protective Equipment Gloves	Wear when touching blood, body fluids, secretions, or items contaminated with them. Wear for touching patient's mucous membranes and nonintact skin.
Gown	Wear when performing procedures and patient care if there is a possibility of your exposed skin or clothing coming in contact with blood, body fluids, secretions, or excretions.
Mask, eye protection, face shield	Wear during patient care procedures that could cause splashing of blood, body fluids, or secretions. Examples would be suctioning and endotracheal intubation.
Needles and other "sharps" (anything that could puncture a trash can liner)	Never recap a used needle; do not bend or break needles; use safety needles whenever possible; place all used sharps in a puncture-resistant sharps container.
Respiratory hygiene/cough etiquette	Cover your mouth and nose with a tissue when sneezing or coughing; if tissue is unavailable, cough into your upper sleeve, not your hand. Use hand hygiene immediately after coughing or sneezing. Also, any person entering a health care facility with a cough, congestion, or increased respiratory secretions is to follow these recommendations.

facilities offer non-latex gloves for patient care to prevent these reactions. However, it is important to be aware of latex reactions and whether you or your patients have them. The signs and symptoms of latex reactions can be found in Box 14-3.

Transmission-based Precautions

Infection control is everyone's responsibility in the hospital setting. However, most hospitals have an infection control department or nurse who is responsible for following patients diagnosed with communicable diseases. The infection control nurse will set up the protective equipment supplies and post the appropriate precautions for all staff and visitors to follow. You are responsible for following the posted guidelines and ensuring that visitors and staff from other departments do so as well.

Airborne Transmission

Airborne transmission occurs when infectious particles are so small and lightweight that they can float in the air and be spread through air currents. A person entering the room could possibly inhale these particles. When you care for a patient who has a suspected or confirmed communicable disease transmitted through the air, such as tuberculosis or chickenpox, additional precautions are required. In addition to standard precautions, the nurse will wear a specific type of face mask called an N95 respirator (Fig. 14-3). These respirators must be fitted to each individual to ensure that no air leaks exist. In this way, all of the air breathed by the nurse while he or she is in the room is filtered to remove airborne microorganisms.

In addition, patients with illnesses that can be transmitted via the airborne route are placed in special rooms, called *airborne infection isolation rooms,* which have a lower pressure gradient than the hallway. These rooms, formerly known as *negative pressure rooms,* are designed to

Figure 14-3   A nurse wearing an N95 respirator mask, which is required for the care of patients with certain respiratory illnesses.

prevent microorganisms from floating from the patient's room into the hallway.

Droplet Transmission

Some diseases can be transmitted from the respiratory system of one person to another through the small droplets that occur when a person coughs, sneezes, or talks. Another person could then inhale or swallow such droplets and contract the illness. It is recommended that you keep a distance of 3 feet between yourself and patients with droplet-transmitted illnesses unless you are wearing protective equipment. If two patients must share a room and one has a droplet-borne illness, the beds should be at least 3 feet apart and the curtain should be kept closed to prevent droplet spread.

When you care for a patient who has been diagnosed with a communicable disease that is spread through respiratory droplets, you would wear a mask over your mouth and nose, as well as following standard precautions. Illnesses that require this kind of protection include influenza (flu), bacterial meningitis, certain types of pneumonia, and certain streptococcal (strep) infections. In addition, you would instruct the patient to cover the mouth and nose with a tissue when coughing or sneezing. The tissue must then be discarded in a biohazard bag, not left on surfaces such as the over-bed table. The patient should perform hand hygiene after coughing or sneezing.

Direct and Indirect Contact Transmission

The most common path of microorganism transmission is by **direct contact**. This means that the microorganism spreads from one person directly to another, usually on the hands. For example, a health care worker's hands become contaminated with a respiratory microorganism while he or she picks up a patient's used tissue. Then the worker puts his or her hands around his or her mouth, inhaling the microorganism, which then causes illness in the health care worker. **Indirect contact** occurs when microorganisms leave one person (reservoir) and contaminate an object such as a blood pressure cuff (mode of transmission), which is then used on another patient (susceptible host). The second patient becomes ill due to contact with the same microorganism. Remember that you touch many surfaces in a day, including elevator buttons, door handles, and telephones, and if your hands are not clean, you can easily spread microorganisms to those surfaces that will then be touched by susceptible people.

When you care for a patient who has been diagnosed with an illness that can be transmitted by contact with infected material or surfaces touched by infected material, you will wash your hands, put on gloves, and put on a gown as you enter the room. You will wear gloves when you touch the patient's skin, even if it is intact, or when you touch items or surfaces close to the patient, such as the side rails or over-bed table. Table 14-3 summarizes the appropriate protective equipment necessary and indications for the use of transmission-based precautions.

precautions are being followed correctly. To do that, you will need to observe the staff members carefully and evaluate them for any problems or breaches in technique. Then you will need to kindly point out any errors in technique so that your staff members will be safe from pathogens.

Psychological Aspects of Transmission-based Precautions

An important aspect of caring for patients with illnesses requiring special precautions is to be aware of the psychological impact of being isolated from the general population. These patients often have multiple-drug-resistant organisms (MDROs), such as methicillin-resistant *Staphylococcus aureus* (MRSA), vancomycin-resistant enterococcus (VRE), or *Clostridium difficile,* that sound frightening to their family and friends. Then, the visitors are required to put on gowns, gloves, and perhaps masks just to be allowed into the room.

It is your responsibility to explain to patients and their visitors the importance of following the CDC's guidelines for transmission-based precautions. You must also enforce the precautions for everyone who enters the room to help prevent the spread of pathogens to others.

Patients diagnosed with communicable diseases and who are on transmission-based precautions tend to have less staff contact than other patients. This may be due to the fact that putting on PPE is time consuming, so nursing staff perform all care possible while they are in the room, then leave for long periods of time. Another contributing factor is that the isolated patient cannot leave the room to walk in the hall. These patients may be lonely, feel neglected, and

Table 14-3   Transmission-Based Precautions

Type	Required PPE	Indications for Use
Contact	**Put on gloves and a gown when entering the room**; wear gloves when touching patient's intact skin and the surfaces and articles in close proximity to the patient, such as side rails and medical equipment. **Plus standard precautions**	To prevent transmission of pathogens spread by direct or indirect contact; use in the presence of excessive wound drainage, fecal incontinence, and when the patient is infected with multiple-drug-resistant organisms, such as MRSA, vancomycin-resistant enterococci (VRE), and *Clostridium difficile.w*
Droplet	**Put on a mask when entering the room.** NOTE: If the patient has H1N1 flu, an N95 respirator is required. Instruct patient to follow respiratory hygiene/ cough etiquette. **Plus standard precautions**	To prevent transmission of pathogens spread through close contact with respiratory secretions or mucous membranes. Examples include influenza (flu), group A streptococcus, bacterial meningitis, rubella (German measles), and *Mycoplasma* pneumonia.
Airborne	**Put on a fit-tested N95 or higher respirator when entering the room.** Patient must be placed in an airborne infection isolation room with negative pressure. **Plus standard precautions**	To prevent transmission of pathogens small enough to be suspended in the air and spread through air currents. Examples include tuberculosis, rubeola (measles), chickenpox, and severe acute respiratory syndrome (SARS).

have fewer visitors than patients who are not in isolation. Some ways to help alleviate these feelings of seclusion include:

- Spending time talking with the patient while you are in the room. Avoid accomplishing all your tasks and then leaving immediately.
- Asking the patient if you can bring him or her anything to pass the time, such as newspapers or magazines. Many times items in the isolation room must be destroyed when the patient is discharged, so newspapers and magazines are good choices.

- Avoiding expressing distaste regarding the patient's diagnosis or having to enter an isolation room. Patients may feel rejected or unclean because of their diagnosis. Remember that the patient is a person first, and that the diagnosis is secondary to his or her human needs.

Knowledge Connection

When will you use standard precautions? When will you use transmission-based precautions? How can you help a patient under tansmission-based precautions to feel less socially isolated?

Nursing Care Plan for a Patient with a MRSA Infection

When you plan care for patients with infections, you will need to focus not only on the type of infecting microorganism and transmission-based precautions necessary for that situation, but also on ways to support the patient's immune system to promote healing.

Assessment

You have determined that the patient is diagnosed with a MRSA infection. This is an MDRO requiring contact precautions, as it can be spread by direct or indirect contact. MRSA can be found in the skin, causing boils and abscesses; in a surgical wound; or in the respiratory tract. If it is in the respiratory tract, the patient will also be placed on droplet precautions.

As you gather data about this patient by reading the history, you learn that he is a 59-year-old male and has a surgical wound infected with MRSA. He had a left total knee replacement about 1 month ago and less than a week after discharge developed redness, pain, and edema in his left knee. He also had *purulent,* or pus-filled, drainage oozing from the incision. He was readmitted to the hospital, where a wound culture showed a MRSA infection, and he was placed on contact precautions.

What do you assess regarding the presence of infection?

- Assess the wound for signs and symptoms of infection, such as redness, edema, or swelling, and the appearance of wound drainage. (See Chapter 26 for more information on wound assessment.) Your findings are redness of the anterior aspect of the left knee with widespread edema and a small amount of thick yellow drainage on the dressing.

- Assess vital signs, especially for elevated temperature. If the temperature is elevated, it is not uncommon for the pulse and respirations to be elevated as well. Your findings are blood pressure of 145/92, temperature of 101.9°F, pulse of 98, and respirations of 24.
- Do not forget to assess the sixth vital sign, pain. When tissue is infected, the inflammatory response often results in edema and pressure on pain receptors. Remember to assess pain using a pain scale. (See Chapter 19 for more information on assessing vital signs and pain.) In this case, the patient rates his pain at a 6 on a scale of 0 to 10.
- Assess the nearby lymph nodes. The lymph nodes enlarge as part of the body's response to infection. Your findings are enlarged, tender lymph nodes in the groin.
- Gather information from laboratory reports. Monitor the white blood cell count because it rises above normal with a bacterial infection. Your findings are that this patient's white blood cell count was elevated, but is decreasing with antibiotic therapy using vancomycin.
- Assess the patient's response to isolation due to transmission-based precautions. The patient tells you that he is angry that he has this infection and feels that he got it while in the hospital for his knee surgery. He feels "shoved off and ignored."

Nursing Diagnoses

In this situation, the nursing diagnoses should reflect issues regarding infection, pain, and isolation, which you identified in your assessment. Look at the NANDA-I list to help you identify the most appropriate diagnoses. Your selections should include the following and be ranked in order of priority.

(care plan continues on page 268)

Nursing Care Plan for a Patient with a MRSA Infection (continued)

To address the MRSA infection:

- Risk for (spread of) infection related to presence of MRSA in knee wound
- Impaired skin integrity related to open knee incision
- Hyperthermia related to infection

To address the patient's pain:

- Acute pain related to recent knee surgery and infection and edema of knee

To address the contact precautions:

- Social isolation related to contact precautions manifested by the patient's complaints of loneliness and frustration

If you thought of additional nursing diagnoses that could apply to this situation, such as impaired mobility and nutritional needs, you are certainly correct. In this chapter, we have focused specifically on nursing diagnoses that relate directly to infection. See Table 14-4.

Planning

For the nursing diagnoses of "Risk for infection related to presence of MRSA in knee wound" and "Impaired skin integrity related to open knee incision," what actions do you need to take?

- Maintain contact precautions and standard precautions to prevent the spread of MRSA to other sites and to other people.
- Wear a gown and gloves when you enter the room.
- When changing the knee dressing twice daily, inspect the wound for signs of improvement in the infection, such as decreased redness, decreasing edema, decrease in the size of the wound, and decreased drainage (see Chapter 26).
- Monitor the body's response to the IV antibiotic vancomycin by tracking laboratory values, specifically white blood cell levels.
- Notify the health care provider if signs or symptoms of worsening infection occur, including fever, increased drainage, and increased pain.

Interventions for the nursing diagnosis of "Acute pain related to recent knee surgery and infection and edema of knee" would include:

- Ask the patient about his pain level every 2 hours and have him rate his pain on a 0-to-10 scale (see Chapter 19).

- Administer pain medications as ordered and needed. Avoid making the patient wait for more than 5 minutes for requested pain medications.
- Teach the patient to ask for pain medication before pain becomes severe, because waiting makes it more difficult to alleviate the pain.
- Determine the effectiveness of the ordered pain medication. Do the positive effects last 3 to 4 hours? If not, does the patient need something stronger? Are the side effects manageable? Notify the prescriber if changes are needed (see Chapters 36 and 37).
- Use techniques such as distraction to help relieve pain (see Chapter 19).

To address the nursing diagnosis of "Social isolation related to contact precautions manifested by the patient's complaints of loneliness and frustration," you can do the following:

- Ensure that the patient understands the purpose of contact precautions.
- Spend extra time with the patient after your nursing tasks are finished, talking with the patient about his concerns, fears, and frustrations.
- Bring in distractions for the patient as requested and allowed, such as newspapers, magazines, puzzle books, and playing cards.
- Encourage visitation by teaching the patient's family that the contact precautions should not prevent them from making visits, that it is safe to visit their loved one.
- Encourage family members and friends to employ methods of distraction, such as joining the patient to watch sports events on television or play cards or board games.

You will plan toward positive outcomes for this patient. These include:

- Resolution of the MRSA infection without spread from the knee wound to other body sites, and without spread to other people
- Management of the patient's pain to keep the rating at a 3 or below

Implementation

You can now implement the interventions that you have planned. Table 14-4 presents a summary of the care plan interventions.

Nursing Care Plan for a Patient with a MRSA Infection (continued)

Evaluation

To determine the effectiveness of your nursing interventions, ask yourself the following questions:

- Was the MRSA contained to the patient's knee wound?
- Was his pain managed to the degree that he was comfortable most of the time (consistently kept below a 4)?
- Were contact precautions maintained by staff and visitors?

If you can answer "yes" to these questions, you have met the outcomes goals for which you planned. If you answered "no" to any of these questions, you must determine what went wrong and devise improved interventions for the future. (See Table 14-4 for a summary of the care plan evaluations.)

Table 14-4   Care Plan for a Patient with a MRSA Infection

Nursing Diagnosis: Risk for (spread of) infection related to presence of MRSA in knee wound
Expected Outcomes: Patient will identify actions to reduce risk of spread of infection by discharge from the hospital. Patient will have a healed wound within 1 month and will be free of redness and edema and be afebrile.

Interventions	Evaluations
Maintain contact precautions and standard precautions to prevent the spread of MRSA to other sites and to other people. Wear a gown and gloves when you enter the room.	Day 1: All staff maintained contact precautions. Family and other visitors were instructed about wearing a gown when entering the room and gloves if they touch the patient. Day 2: Visitors needed reminders of appropriate PPE, but complied without problems. Staff continued to maintain precautions. Day 6: All visitors and staff maintain appropriate precautions. No evidence of spread of MRSA.
When changing the knee dressing twice daily, inspect the wound for signs of improvement in the infection, such as decreased redness, decreasing edema, decrease in the size of the wound, and decreased drainage.	Day 1: Mod amt of malodorous purulent drainage on dressing; wound margins reddened; edema of knee apparent. Wound open just above patella, measuring 3 cm × 2 cm and 2 cm deep Day 4: Mod amt of serosanginuous drainage noted on dressing; no odor detected. Knee less edematous. Wound above patella smaller in size, 2 cm × 1.5 cm and 1.5 cm deep.
Monitor the body's response to IV antibiotic vancomycin by tracking laboratory values, specifically white blood cell (WBC) levels.	Day 1: WBC count was 15,966. IV vancomycin administered q 12 hr as ordered. Day 4: WBC count was 12,854, indicating positive response to vancomycin Day 6: WBC count was 11,220, continuing to fall in response to IV antibiotic.
Notify the health care provider if signs or symptoms of worsening infection occur, including fever, increased drainage, and increased pain.	Day 1: Patient complained of pain rated a 7 on a 0–10 scale. Pain relieved to a 5 with administration of ordered narcotic analgesic. Oral temp ranged from 100.6°F to 99.9°F. Day 4: Afebrile. Patient rated pain a 6 before pain medication and a 3 after medication. Day 6: Continues afebrile. Rates pain at a 4 prior to pain medication and at a 1 or 2 after medication.

(table continues on page 270)

Nursing Care Plan for a Patient with a MRSA Infection (continued)

Table 14-4   Care Plan for a Patient with a MRSA Infection (continued)

Nursing Diagnosis: Acute pain related to recent knee surgery and infected wound as evidenced by rating pain a 7 on a 0–10 scale, grimacing with movement, and diaphoresis
Expected Outcomes: Patient will rate pain at a 3 or below within 72 hours. Patient will verbalize understanding of pharmacological regimen for antibiotics and pain medication prior to discharge.

Interventions	Evaluations
Ask the patient about his pain level every 2 hours and have him rate his pain on a 0–10 scale Administer pain medications as ordered and needed. Avoid making the patient wait for more than 5 minutes for requested pain medications.	Day 1: Patient complained of pain rated a 7 on a 0–10 scale consistently prior to pain medication. Pain relieved to a 5 with administration of ordered narcotic analgesic. Day 4: Afebrile. Patient rated pain a 6 before pain medication and a 3 after medication. Day 6: Continues afebrile. Rates pain at a 4 prior to pain medication and at a 1 or 2 after medication.
Teach the patient to ask for pain medication before pain becomes severe, because waiting makes it more difficult to alleviate the pain.	Day 1: Patient c/o of mod to severe pain when medicated with narcotic analgesic. Instructed regarding need to ask for medication before the pain becomes severe. Verbalized understanding. Offered pain med after 4 hr and patient took it, rating the pain at a 6. Day 4: Patient taking pain medication every 4–5 hr and states he is more comfortable when he does not wait too long. Day 6: Requires pain medication only every 5–6 hr to remain comfortable.
Determine the effectiveness of the ordered pain medication. Instruct patient regarding the effectiveness of antibiotic in helping to relieve pain as well.	Day 1: Pain medication effectiveness lasted only 3–4 hr, but did reduce pain during that time. Day 4: Patient complains of nausea after taking pain medication. Instructed to take it with a cracker or other food so it is not taken on an empty stomach. Day 6: Nausea relieved by taking med with food. Pain med continues to effectively manage his pain. Day 7: Patient verbalizes understanding of role that antibiotics play in resolving infection and therefore decreasing pain.
Use techniques such as distraction to help relieve pain.	Day 1: Patient distracted from pain only during visit from family. As soon as they left, he complained of increased pain and was again medicated. Day 2: Encouraged patient to watch TV, read, and do crossword puzzles to help distract him from the pain. He agreed to try. Day 3: Pain is resolving some and patient is using different things to distract himself from it.

Nursing Diagnosis: Social isolation related to contact precautions as evidenced by patient's complaints of loneliness and frustration
Expected Outcomes: Patient will participate in available social interactions during contact precautions. Patient will occupy time with allowed activities during contact precautions.

Interventions	Evaluations
Ensure that the patient understands the purpose of contact precautions.	Day 1: Patient verbalized concerns about family members being exposed to MRSA. Explained the purpose of contact precautions and patient verbalized understanding.
Spend extra time with the patient after your nursing tasks are finished, talking with the patient about his concerns, fears, and frustrations.	Day 2: Patient expressed boredom and loneliness due to contact precautions. Brought in newspapers and magazines for patient.

Nursing Care Plan for a Patient with a MRSA Infection (continued)

Table 14-4   Care Plan for a Patient with a MRSA Infection (continued)

Interventions	Evaluations
Bring in distractions for the patient as requested and allowed, such as newspapers, magazines, puzzle books, and playing cards.	Day 3: Nursing staff spending extra time as available with patient to decrease feelings of isolation. Patient states he feels less bored and alone than earlier. Day 4: Patient playing cards with friends for most of the evening.
Encourage family members and friends to employ methods of distraction, such as joining the patient to watch sports events on television or play cards or board games.	Day 1: Family has visited only once and seems hesitant to go in the room. Nursing staff explained contact precautions and answered questions. Day 4: Patient playing cards with friends for most of evening. Family visits often and watches TV with patient.

Skill 14-1 Performing Hand Hygiene

HANDWASHING

Assessment Steps

1. Determine when to perform handwashing: before and after donning gloves, entering and leaving patient rooms, returning to the unit after breaks and meals, coming on duty, and after using the restroom *to prevent the spread of microorganisms.*

Planning Steps

1. Be sure that soap in a dispenser is available. *Safety: Do not use bar soap as it harbors bacteria.*
2. Obtain paper towels *for drying your hands.*
3. Push up your watch and sleeves, if necessary, *to prevent them from getting wet.*

Implementation Steps

1. Turn on the water and adjust it to a comfortable temperature. *Water temperature that is too hot can cause dry, cracked skin; water temperature that is too cool may not kill microorganisms.*
2. Wet your hands under running water, being careful not to touch the dirty sink with your fingertips *to avoid contamination of your hands.*

3. Obtain a quarter-size amount of soap in the palm of your hand and work into a lather *for ease of distribution over your hands and wrists.*
4. Rub the palms together using friction. Place one hand on top of the other and rub with fingers interlaced, then reverse hands and repeat. *Friction helps dislodge soil and remove microorganisms.*

5. Rub the fingernails against the palm of the opposite hand to work the lather around and under the nails *to loosen and remove soil around and under the nails.*
6. Lather around each wrist *to clean them as well as the hands.*
   Note: It is recommended that you wash for at least 20 seconds—the length of time it takes to sing "Happy Birthday" twice.
7. Rinse the hands with your fingers pointed downward, *to allow water to run from the cleanest area downward.* Again, avoid touching the dirty sink with your hands *to prevent contamination.*
8. Obtain a clean paper towel and dry hands.
9. Obtain another clean paper towel and turn off the faucet. *This prevents you from touching the dirty faucet handles with your clean hands.*
10. Drop the paper towels in the trash can without touching it.

(skill continues on page 272)

Skill 14-1 (continued)

Evaluation Steps

1. Determine whether your hands touched any contaminated surfaces after you washed them. If so, repeat the handwashing procedure *to ensure that your hands are no longer contaminated.*

USING HAND GELS

Assessment Steps

1. Determine when it is appropriate to use hand gels. The indications are the same as for handwashing except that *you must wash your hands with soap and water if they are visibly soiled or if contamination by spore-forming microbes is likely.*

Planning Steps

1. Locate gel dispensers in patient rooms, hallways, and the nurse's station *so you are aware of availability when the gel is needed.*

Implementation Steps

1. Hold one hand under the dispenser and obtain the manufacturers recommended amount of product in the palm of your hand *for maximum effectiveness.*

Safety: Different manufacturers recommend different amounts of product for maximum effectiveness.

2. Rub your hands together so that the product covers all surfaces of the hands and fingers *to help remove microorganisms from all areas of your hands.*

3. Continue rubbing your hands together with the fingers interlaced until the hands are dry *to remove and kill microorganisms.*

Evaluation Steps

1. Determine that your hands are completely dry and that the gel was spread over all surfaces of the hands and fingers *to ensure that microorganisms from all surfaces have been killed.*

Skill 14-2 Donning Personal Protective Equipment

Assessment Steps

1. Determine the type of PPE required to maintain standard and/or transmission-based precautions. *This will ensure that you take the proper precautions for the situation.*

Planning Steps

1. If allergic to latex or powder, locate latex-free or powder-free gloves *to prevent local or systemic reactions.*

2. Obtain necessary PPE for the task. Be sure you obtain the correct size of nonsterile gloves; they are generally available in small, medium, large, and extra large. *Correct glove size prevents open areas around the wrists where microorganisms or fluids might enter.*

3. Remain outside the patient's room or in the anteroom when donning PPE if the patient is on transmission-based precautions *to prevent contact with fluids, air, or droplets before you have on the appropriate PPE.*

Implementation Steps

1. Perform hand hygiene. *Hand hygiene is necessary before donning gloves or other PPE.*

Donning Gown

1. Hold the gown by the shoulders and allow it to unfold *to prevent contaminating the outside of the gown.*

2. Slip your arms through the gown's sleeves.

3. Pull the gown up onto your shoulders by grasping the inside of the gown at the shoulders *to prevent touching the outside of the gown with your ungloved hands.*

Skill 14-2 (continued)

4. Fasten the gown in the back at the neck, then at the waist, *to keep your back covered.*

Donning Mask or Respirator

1. Place the mask over your mouth and nose and tie the upper ties above your ears first, then tie the lower ties at your neck, *to protect your mouth and nose from airborne microorganisms. Safety: Do not bring lower ties up on the head. This causes gaps at the side of the mask, allowing microorganisms to enter.*

2. Bend the flexible band across the bridge of the nose for a snug fit *to prevent microorganisms from entering gaps in the mask.*

3. Pull the bottom edge of the mask down so it is below the chin *to cover the entire mouth and nose area.*

4. If using a respirator, check to be sure it is fitted against your face on all sides *to prevent microorganisms from entering any areas that gap.*

Donning Eye Protection

1. Put on goggles or face shield and adjust to fit *to protect your eyes from splashing of blood or body fluids.*

Note: Face shields are usually attached to the mask.

Donning Gloves

1. Pull the sleeve edges of the gloves down over the proximal half of the hand portions before donning gloves. This will help to keep the glove cuff over the gown sleeve, *which will prevent gaps through which microorganisms may enter.*

2. Pull the first glove onto your nondominant hand, *making it easier to put on the second glove.*

3. Pull the cuff edges of the glove up over the wrist of the isolation gown *to prevent gaps through which microorganisms may enter.* After adjusting the glove cuff, the gown sleeve may be pulled up slightly if necessary, but be certain to keep your wrists securely covered *so that movement will not pull the glove and sleeve apart, exposing the wrists to contamination.*

4. Repeat for the dominant hand.

5. Change gloves if they become torn or heavily soiled, and use hand hygiene before regloving *to prevent contamination of your hands with blood or body fluids.*

Evaluation Steps

1. Evaluate your technique for donning PPE *by determining if all steps were followed correctly.*

Skill 14-3 Removing Personal Protective Equipment

Assessment Steps

1. Determine where you will remove the PPE. Remain just inside the patient's room at the doorway *to prevent taking contaminants into the public hallway.*

Planning Steps

1. Determine the order in which to remove PPE: gloves, goggles, gown, then mask or respirator *to prevent contamination during removal.*
2. Treat the outside or front side of all PPE as contaminated *since it has been exposed to contaminants.*
3. Locate appropriate trash receptacle for disposing of all PPE *to prevent having to carry contaminated PPE to another location.*

Implementation Steps

Removing Gloves

1. Grasp the outside of the glove on your nondominant hand with your dominant hand and pull downward to remove. *This prevents contact of your clean hands inside the gloves with the outside of the gloves.*
2. Hold the removed glove in your dominant (and still gloved) hand. Slide the fingers of your ungloved hand under the glove on your dominant hand at the wrist. *This protects your ungloved hand from contact with the soiled gloves.* Safety: *Do not touch the outside of the glove with your bare fingers.*
3. Peel the remaining glove off from the wrist toward the fingers. As it turns inside out, the first glove will remain within the second glove, *allowing the soiled outsides of both gloves to be contained within themselves. You will only touch the clean inside portion of the gloves.*

4. Drop the gloves into the appropriate waste receptacle without touching it *to prevent contamination of your hands.*

Removing Eye Protection

1. Touch only the earpieces of the goggles or the headband of the face shield with your bare hands. *The remaining portions are contaminated.*
2. Remove the goggles or face shield.
3. Drop the goggles or face shield into the appropriate waste receptacle.

Removing Gown

1. Unfasten the gown ties at the neck, *being careful not to touch any part of the front of the gown, which is contaminated.*
2. Unfasten the ties at the waist *to allow removal of the gown.*
3. Lean forward to remove the gown. *This helps to keep the contaminated gown from contaminating your uniform.* Remove the gown by peeling it from one shoulder toward the hand, then the other shoulder toward that hand. The gown will turn inside out, *keeping the soiled portions on the inside and preventing contamination.*

4. Hold the gown away from your body *to prevent accidental contact with any soiled area of the gown.*
5. Roll the gown with the front exterior portion of the gown wrapped inside the rest of the gown. *This prevents the external contaminated side of the gown from contaminating your uniform or skin.*

6. Drop the gown into the appropriate waste receptacle.

Skill 14-3 (continued)

Removing Mask or Respirator

1. Touch only the ties or elastic of the mask or respirator. *Safety: Remember that the front of the mask/respirator is contaminated.*
2. Always untie the bottom ties first, then the top ties. *This prevents the contaminated side of the mask from contaminating your neck during removal.*
3. Discard in the appropriate waste receptacle.

Perform hand hygiene immediately after removing all PPE *to remove any microorganisms that you may have touched.*

Evaluation Steps

1. Determine that all PPE is in the appropriate waste receptacles *to ensure that it is not a reservoir for microorganisms.*
2. Evaluate your technique for removing PPE *by determining if all steps were followed correctly.*

 Post Conference

During the conference after clinicals, you were relieved that your day had gone so well. It took you a little while to get comfortable putting on the gown and gloves before you went into your patient's room, and removing them as you left his room. However, it was not long before you stopped worrying so much about the infective organism, MRSA. You must have washed your hands or used hand gel at least 50 times today, but you felt certain that you had not contaminated anything. You will go home tonight without concerns that MRSA is somehow on your clothes or hands. After being in a gown and gloves all day, plus washing your hands so much, you know you are protected and will not be taking anything infectious home with you.

KEY POINTS

- Bacteria, viruses, protoza, fungi, and helminths are classifications of microorganisms that cause human illnesses.
- The chain of infection illustrates how an infectious agent is transferred from a reservoir through the portal of exit via a mode of transmission to the portal of entry of a susceptible host.
- Several types of infections exist. Health care–associated infections (HAIs) are preventable by using appropriate hand hygiene and precautions.
- The body possesses a three-layer defense system: primary defenses involving the skin, mucous membranes, and gastrointestinal system; secondary defenses involving the inflammatory process, elevated temperature, and complement cascade; and tertiary defenses involving the B- and T-cell lymphocytes.
- Ways to prevent infection in the health care setting include hand hygiene and use of standard and transmission-based precautions.

- Medical asepsis involves the use of clean technique, performing hand hygiene, maintaining a clean patient environment, and the use of CDC precautions.
- It is extremely important to know when, why, and how to perform correct hand hygiene.
- Standard precautions are established by the CDC to prevent the transmission of pathogens in blood and body fluids. They require health care workers to wear gloves when caring for all patients to prevent any contact with blood-borne pathogens. They also require staff to wear a gown, mask, and goggles if they risk touching or being splashed by blood or body fluids.
- Transmission-based precautions address three types of microbial spread: contact, droplet, and airborne. Transmission-based precautions are always used in addition to standard precautions.
- When caring for patients on transmission-based precautions, it is very important to address their emotional needs due to social isolation.

REVIEW QUESTIONS

Select the answer that is most appropriate for each of the following questions. Some questions may have more than one correct answer. Check all that apply.

1. When you learn that your patient's infecting bacterium is identified as a gram-positive streptococcus, you know this means that:

   a. it appears in rod-shaped pairs and cannot be treated by antibiotics.

   b. it appears in sphere-shaped clusters and stains red in the laboratory.

   c. it appears as a long, coiling cell and stains blue in the laboratory.

   d. it appears in sphere-shaped chains and stains purple in the laboratory.

2. A patient complains that he feels ill and the doctor told him it was a virus, but would not give him any antibiotics. He is upset with the doctor. What is the reason for the physician's action?

   a. Most viruses are immune to antibiotics.

   b. Antibiotics only kill bacteria, but do not kill viruses.

   c. Only the newest, most expensive antibiotics will kill viruses.

   d. Antibiotics are not necessary unless the viral infection is severe.

3. The **most effective** way to break the chain of infection is to:

   a. isolate all infected patients from remaining patients and assign only one staff member to each room.

   b. wear gowns, gloves, masks, and protective eyewear when entering every patient's room.

   c. perform effective hand hygiene according to CDC guidelines.

   d. use an N95 respirator for entering the room of any infected patient.

4. Which is true of performing hand hygiene?

   a. Use before and after a snack in the break room.

   b. Do not perform hand hygiene if you will be donning gloves.

   c. Use hand gel if your hands are visibly dirty.

   d. Use hand hygiene between providing care for two patients in the same room.

   e. No need to use hand hygiene if you leave a patient's room to obtain clean supplies and return immediately.

   f. Use soap and water instead of hand gel if the hands could be contaminated with spore-forming microbes.

5. A patient is placed on droplet precautions. You know his wife needs more teaching about what PPE to use when she says:

   a. "I don't need to wear a mask if I stay a foot away from him."

   b. "I will wash my hands and put on a face mask before I go into his room."

   c. "I will remove the mask just inside the door of his room."

   d. "This disease is spread through small droplets that spray out when he talks, coughs, or sneezes."

SHORT ANSWER QUESTIONS

6. A patient on airborne precautions tells you he feels like a leper and that people who come in his room look like aliens with those face masks on. How could you respond?

7. How does lack of rest decrease the body's ability to defend itself against infection?

CRITICAL THINKING EXERCISES

8. Create a scenario to illustrate the chain of infection. Identify each link of the chain in your scenario.

9. A patient is on droplet precautions. You are going in the room to suction her tracheostomy, which could cause splashing, and you could have contact with respiratory secretions. What PPE will you need?

ADDITIONAL RESOURCES

For additional Resources, Questions, and Activities, please see:

Student Resource Disk

 http://davisplus.fadavis.com

Student Study Guide

REFERENCES

Barclay L, Lie D. MRSA screening may not reduce infections in surgical patients. Medscape Medical News, March 11, 2008. Available at: http://cme.medscape.com/viewarticle/571251. Accessed September 18, 2008.

Barclay L, Vega C. Probiotic may reduce sick days from work. Medscape Medical News, November 14, 2005. Available at: http://cme.medscape.com/viewarticle/516801. Accessed September 18, 2008.

Barlam T, Kasper D. Common contamination of gloves and gowns with methicillin-resistant *Staphylococcus aureus* and vancomycin-resistant enterococci during routine patient care. Available at: http://www.medscape.com/viewarticle/581407. Accessed October 10, 2008.

CDC Infection Control Guidelines Updated—standard precautions now include respiratory hygiene and cough etiquette. Available at: http://www.modernmedicine.com/modernmedicine/Infectious+Disease/CDC-Infection-Control-Guidelines-Updated/ArticleNewsFeed/Article/detail/505915. Accessed September 13, 2008.

Centers for Disease Control and Prevention. Guideline for Hand Hygiene in Healthcare Settings—2002. Available at: http://www.cdc.gov/handhygiene/index.html. Accessed August 10, 2009.

Centers for Disease Control and Prevention. Infection Control Guidelines. Available at: http://www.cdc.gov/ncidod/dhqp/guidelines.html. Accessed August 10, 2009.

National Institute for Occupational Safety and Health. Latex Allergy: A Prevention Guide. NIOSH Publication 98-113. Available at: http://www.cdc.gov/niosh/98-113.html. Accessed August 10, 2009.

Premier Safety Institute. Education Critical to Implement 2008 CMS Hospital-Acquired Conditions Rule. Available at: http://www.premierinc.com/safety/safety-share/02-08-full-txt.jsp#story-04. Accessed August 10, 2009.

Scanlon V, Sanders T. *Essentials of Anatomy and Physiology.* Philadelphia: FA Davis; 2007.

Shaver-McRae H, McRae G, Jas V. Environmentally safe health care agencies: nursing's responsibility, Nightingale's legacy. *OJIN Online J Issues Nurs.* 2007;12(2).

Siegel JD, Rhinehart E, Jackson M, Chiarello L, and the Healthcare Infection Control Practices Advisory Committee. Guideline for Isolation Precautions: Preventing Transmission of Infectious Agents in Healthcare Settings 2007. Available at: http://www.cdc.gov/ncidod/dhqp/gl_isolation.html. Accessed August 10, 2009.

Stanton C. CDC issues updated isolation guideline. *AORN Managers* [serial online]. Available at: http://www.aorn.org/Managers/July2007Issue/CDCIssuesUpdatedIsolationGuideline/. Accessed August 12, 2009.

Tarrac SE. Application of the updated CDC isolation guidelines for health care facilities. *AORN J.* 2008;87:534-542.

Wilkinson J, Van Leuven K. *Fundamentals of Nursing: Theory, Concepts and Application.* Philadelphia: FA Davis; 2007.

World Health Organization. WHO Guidelines on Hand Hygiene in Health Care. Available at: http://whqlibdoc.who.int/publications/2009/9789241597906_eng.pdf. Accessed August 10, 2009.

Key Terms

Activities of daily living (ADLs)

Assisted care

Bath blanket

Draw sheet

Excoriation

Hygiene

Lesion

Leukoplakia

Lice

Maceration

Mitered corner

Mottling

Nits

Ocular prosthesis

Seborrhea

Self-care

Special mouth care

Tinea capitus

Total care

Venous return

Objectives

1. Define key terms associated with personal care.
2. Categorize personal care tasks performed at particular times during the day.
3. Describe the benefits of bathing patients, both for the patient and for the nurse.
4. Explain factors to consider when planning patient care and bathing.
5. Enumerate three categories of personal care.
6. Identify types of baths and their purposes.
7. Contrast back massage with applying lotion to the back.
8. Discuss key aspects of providing oral care to unconscious and conscious patients.
9. Describe assessments to make during oral care, hair care, and nail care.
10. Explain how to remove jewelry from piercings and circumstances that could make removal necessary.
11. Discuss how to remove contact lenses, artificial eyes, and hearing aids.
12. Explain how to clean and insert an ocular prosthesis and hearing aids.
13. Identify ways to minimize noise, odors, and clutter in the patient's environment.
14. Differentiate between open, closed, and surgical beds.
15. Describe nursing responsibilities when making occupied and unoccupied beds.

Skills

15-1 Administering a Complete Bed Bath
15-2 Administering Perineal Care
15-3 Administering a Back Massage

(skills continue on page 280)

Skills (continued)

15-4   Administering Oral Care for an Unconscious Patient
15-5   Administering Oral Care for a Conscious Patient
15-6   Providing Denture Care
15-7   Shaving a Male Patient
15-8   Providing Nail Care
15-9   Shampooing Hair With the Patient in Bed
15-10 Making an Unoccupied Bed
15-11 Making an Occupied Bed

🌐 Clinical Connection

Your Assignment: You are a male student assigned to care for a female patient who requires a bed bath. This is your first female patient, and you are nervous and a little embarrassed about the bath. A fellow student who has been a CNA for several years tells you that you shouldn't have to do the bath, that an aide should do it instead. She says she thinks the instructor does not like you and that is why you received the assignment.

Your Actions: You have a choice between speaking to your instructor about your assignment or performing care for this patient with a good attitude. Assuming you decide to perform care as assigned, you will need to plan to provide privacy and maintain the patient's dignity during the bath.

So whose job is it anyway? Is it beneath a nurse to bathe patients? Is bathing a patient an ineffective use of a nurse's education? Some student nurses in the United Kingdom's Royal Academy of Nurses wanted a resolution saying that they should not be required to give baths. One student was quoted as saying, "I do not wash bottoms. There are other people to do that." The resolution was soundly defeated. In this chapter, you will learn some reasons why that happened.

Routinely Scheduled Care

Most facilities have established specific times for routine care to be given. This helps to prevent missing an aspect of care. Routine care may be delegated to a certified nursing assistant (CNA) or to unlicensed assistive personnel (UAP), but it is your responsibility to be sure the care is completed. An example of generally used routine care follows:

- **Early Morning (Early a.m.) Care:** Assist with toileting. Give the patient a warm, wet washcloth to wash the hands and face. Assist with oral care if desired. Some people prefer to do oral care after they have eaten breakfast, while others prefer it before eating. Provide fresh water if allowed.

- **Morning (a.m.) Care:** This is done after breakfast. For many patients, this will include assisting with a bath. For all patients, this includes toileting, oral care, back massage, shaving, hair care, and dressing or changing the gown. Assist the patient to get out of bed if he or she is able to do so. Have the patient sit in the chair while you straighten or change the linens.

- **Afternoon (p.m.) Care:** After lunch, patients may need assistance to be comfortable to rest or to receive visitors. Assist the patient with toileting, then straighten the bed, and assist the patient to a position of comfort. Provide the patient's preference of oral fluids unless contraindicated.

- **Bedtime (h.s.) Care:** Assist the patient to prepare for sleep. Assist with toileting. Offer the patient's preference of oral fluids, such as a glass of milk or juice, unless the patient is NPO or on a restricted diet or fluid allowance. Brush the teeth or remove dentures. Remove glasses and hearing aids. Give a back massage. Place needed items within reach, such as the call light, fresh water, and urinal. Straighten the room, putting away items not being used. If the patient is ambulatory, arrange furniture so there is a clear path to the bathroom, to reduce fall risk. Straighten the linens and obtain an extra blanket if needed. Dim the lights or turn them off and provide a night-light, according to the patient's preference.

Knowledge Connection
What times of the day and evening are appropriate for providing a bath? Why is routine care an important part of individualized nursing care?

Bathing

Hygiene is a term used to describe keeping oneself clean and well-groomed. When each of us prepares for the day, the activities involved—such as bathing, washing and styling hair, brushing and flossing teeth, dressing, and shaving—are referred to as **activities of daily living (ADLs).**

When people are healthy, they perform these activities themselves. When they are weak, in pain, emotionally distraught, confused, or lacking mobility, they need partial or complete assistance to accomplish ADLs.

Assisting patients with hygiene and grooming gives you the opportunity to learn a great deal about your patient as well as provide comfort. Bathing a patient offers benefits to both the patient and the nurse.

Benefits of Bathing Patients

As you provide personal care for your patients, you have the opportunity to make multiple assessments that you might otherwise miss. The following paragraphs detail the benefits of bathing to the patient and provide examples of observations to make while performing this skill.

Cleanses the Skin

As you wash, you remove dirt, bacteria, dead skin cells, sweat, and odors. Bathing is helpful not only in making the skin clean, but in making it smell fresh and clean, as well as helping to prevent infection.

Provides an Opportunity for Skin Assessment

Bathing the skin gives you the opportunity to observe skin problems that are not obvious. Look for redness, cracking, and **maceration**, which is softened skin due to continuous exposure to moisture. This often occurs in skin crevices such as under the breasts and scrotum, in the axilla and groin areas, between the toes, and between the buttocks. Look for **excoriation**, or scrapes on the skin, that may be due to scratching or that may occur during care. Performing a bed bath also allows you to assess skin temperature to determine whether it is hot and dry, normal, or cool and clammy. In addition, you have an opportunity to notice any skin breakdown over bony prominences at its earliest stage, which could be a reddened area that does not return to normal color after pressure is removed.

Increases Circulation

During a bed bath, you will wash from distal to proximal to improve blood return from the extremities back to the heart. This is referred to as **venous return**. Assess for indications of pooling of blood, such as redness in the hands and feet; a red, warm area in the calf of the leg; or **mottling**, a purplish blotching of the skin when circulation slows greatly. While bathing the patient, you have ample opportunity to flex and extend all joints and extremities, which further stimulates the circulation and aids in preventing stiffness of joints.

Increases Sensation

If the patient is comatose or neurologically impaired, the bath provides sensory input for the brain to process, including friction from the washcloth, moisture and warmth from the water, olfactory stimulation from the clean, soapy smell, and the silky, slippery feeling of soap and suds. Even patients without neurosensory deficits tend to have decreased sensation when lying in a hospital bed. Observe for evidence of pain or discomfort during the bath, such as grimacing, pulling away from you or pushing your hand away, moaning, or verbalizing pain by saying "Ouch" or "Stop."

Provides Comfort and Relaxation

The feeling of cleanliness is conducive not only to comfort and relaxation, but also to rest and sleep, all of which are important to healing and restoration of health. When patients do not feel well and have to remain in a lumpy hospital bed, they soon become weary of lying there: muscles ache and joints become stiff. Remaining in the same gown or pajamas more than a day is unpleasant as well. They may begin to smell, wrinkle, and become uncomfortable. Assess the patient for muscle tension in the back and shoulders as you bathe the back and perform a back massage. Talk with patients about their cares and concerns. This may be when you learn that an elderly patient who lives alone is worrying about his cats, or that a patient with three children is not sleeping because she is concerned about how her children are getting to and from school.

Provides Improved Self-esteem

All of us feel better when we look and smell fresh. After bathing the patient, style the hair in the way the patient prefers. Assist male patients to shave or trim the beard and moustache. Assist female patients to shave the legs or axillae or apply makeup if desired. Listen as patients talk during this care. Assess the effect of illness, injury, treatment, or surgery on the person's ability to feel good about himself or herself. For example, a patient who has had a mastectomy may make comments about not being a real woman anymore, or a patient who has facial scarring may make comments about scaring small children. Such comments give you an opportunity to further explore the patient's feelings and self-esteem issues. Concerns about self-image are not uncommon when patients have had body-altering surgeries.

Contributes to the Establishment of the Nurse-Patient Relationship

Providing a bed bath is one of the most effective ways you can establish trust and rapport with your patient. There are few things that are more intimate than personal hygiene. If you demonstrate respect, preserve the patient's modesty, and show caring and compassion all while making the patient "feel so much better," you make great strides toward a stronger nurse-patient relationship. During the bath, the nurse spends an uninterrupted block of time with the patient. The patient may feel more comfortable bringing up a subject that requires extended conversation, or the patient may give hints for you to pursue further. This type of conversation does not occur easily when the nurse comes into the room to quickly change an IV or hand the patient medications to swallow. More time with the patient doing hands-on care translates into the opportunity to hear what the patient is feeling and thinking.

Knowledge Connection

How does bathing a patient benefit the patient? How does it benefit the nurse?

Anatomy and Physiology Connection

Hair, Nails, and Glands

The hair and nails are considered appendages of the skin. Hair grows from the root at the base of the follicle. In the matrix of the hair root, new cells are formed and produce keratin. As they die, they are incorporated into the hair shaft, so when you comb and brush a patient's hair, you are actually caring for dead keratinized cells. The hair functions to keep the head from losing body heat by providing insulation.

In the same way, nails grow from the nail root contained within nail follicles. The new nail cells produce a different, stronger form of keratin. When the cells die, they are incorporated into the nail. Beneath the nail is living tissue. Nails function to protect the ends of the fingers and toes, and to increase the ability to pick up small objects with the fingers. When you trim a patient's nails, you are cutting off dead and keratinized cells.

The sebaceous glands secrete *sebum* (oil) onto the skin surface or into hair follicles to keep the skin and hair lubricated. Because skin is the first line of defense against invading pathogens, it is important that sebum keeps it moist and protects it from drying and cracking, which would leave an entryway for pathogens. That is why, when you bathe patients, you need to assess the skin for any open areas or cracking, and why it is important to lubricate dry skin with lotion.

The sweat glands, especially the apocrine sweat glands located in the axillae and genital areas, produce sweat during stressful and emotional circumstances. The eccrine sweat glands are found over the rest of the body, but are concentrated in the palms of the hands, upper lip, and forehead. They produce sweat in response to heat and exercise. When the sweat from the apocrine sweat glands remains on the skin, bacteria begin to break it down. By-products of this breakdown cause the smell we call *body odor*. When you bathe patients, you remove this sweat so that the bacteria do not have the opportunity to break it down.

Patient Preferences and Abilities

When planning personal care and bathing, you need to determine patients' preferences regarding the time and type of bath. It is important to take the patient's cultural influences into account regarding bathing. It is also necessary to determine the patient's abilities to assist, and whether or not you will need additional nursing staff to complete the bath.

Timing

Patient care in the acute care setting tends to follow an established pattern: baths are part of morning care and are therefore done in the morning. However, not all patients want to bathe in the morning. Consider the patient who slept poorly during the night and who wants to sleep until lunchtime, or the patient who works nights and sleeps days, or the patient who normally bathes just before going to bed at night. It is important for you to consider the patients and their preferences regarding the time of their bath.

Students are sometimes hesitant to discuss when a patient would prefer to bathe. Some are timid and wait for the patient to ask to clean up. Others are insistent that the patient allow a bath early in the shift so their work will flow according to the usual pattern of morning care. Some students do not really want to perform personal care, so they take any hesitancy on the part of the patient as a refusal of care.

It's All in the Approach

Most patients are ready for a fresh gown and straightened sheets in the mornings at the very least, as well as personal care such as oral hygiene and grooming. If you are hesitant as a student, your patients may decide that you do not really want to help them with bathing and dressing. If you say, "You don't want me to help you with your bath now, do you?" it is clear that you would rather not perform this task. It is important to be positive and warm in your approach to bathing and other ADLs. Avoid giving the appearance that you are really busy or are in a big hurry. Exhibit the attitude that you would desire to be shown to your own mother, father, or child. As a nursing student and as a nurse, it is your job to see that personal care needs are met. An approach to the patient who seems to delay or put off bathing is to say, "Would you like help with your bath now, or would you prefer that I come back in an hour?" This gives the patient a choice and allows for the patient to be somewhat in control of his or her own care.

Culture

In addition to considerations regarding the timing of the bath, make sure to include cultural influences. Remember that in some cultures it is not appropriate for a person to be bathed by a member of the opposite sex. Ask if it is acceptable to the patient for you to help with the bath. If it is not, arrange for someone else to do the bath. For example, if you are female and have a male patient who is from a culture that does not allow a female to bathe a male, you could ask a male nurse to give the bath to your patient. Be sure to offer to do a bath for him on one of his patients in return. It may be acceptable if a family member is present during the bath. Be respectful of cultural taboos.

In some cultures, people do not bathe daily or even every other day. Instead, weekly baths are the norm. This may be due to restricted water supplies in the country of origin, or may be due to beliefs that more frequent exposure to water is unhealthy. Although in America we consider it offensive if we smell body odor on others, in some countries body odor is completely acceptable. Again, be sure to ask permission to bathe a patient or assist with bathing.

Abilities

When determining if a patient can help with the bath, you must consider the patient's abilities. It is helpful to assess his or her ability to:

- Understand and follow directions
- Move and turn enough to assist with the bath
- Tolerate the physical demands during a bath, including whether the patient is too weak, too ill, or in too much pain to participate

Knowledge Connection

How do you individualize personal care?

People and Places Connection

Personal Care Considerations for Children, for the Elderly, and in Special Settings

When providing personal care to children, be sure to consider the modesty in school-age children and adolescents. Be respectful of their need for privacy by placing a sign on the room door stating that a bath is in progress so patients will not be embarrassed by interruptions. Always knock before entering the room.

In older adults, the sebaceous and sweat glands produce less oil and sweat. It is not necessary or desirable to bathe daily. Their skin requires frequent application of lotion to prevent dryness. They also chill easily due to decreased circulation, so keep the environment warm when you are bathing elderly patients.

In the home health care setting, it is very important to respect the client's preferences regarding bathing. It is often difficult for clients to get in and out of home showers or tubs, so you may have to adapt equipment for this purpose. For example, you can use a rustproof lawn chair for the client to sit on in the shower. You can place a similar type of chair in the bathtub and use a hand-held sprayer attached to the bathtub faucet to bathe the patient. In home health care, it is often necessary to make do with what is available, even if it means pumping water from a well and then heating it on the stove in order to bathe the client.

In long-term care, a resident's bath or shower is routinely scheduled for two or three times per week because the skin of an older person tends to be dry and fragile. However, the residents should be clean at all times. If they are incontinent, it is important to provide frequent and thorough perineal care to prevent skin breakdown and odor. They should also be assisted to wash up before and after meals.

Assistance

Nurses must evaluate patients' ability to participate in care, as well as how much assistance they require. It is important to encourage the patient to do as much as possible, but also to accurately determine what the patient is capable of doing. Sometimes this may vary from one day to the next. If the patient rested poorly during the night, is in pain, is short of breath, or is excessively fatigued, he or she may be unable to do as much as on a previous day. Box 15-1 describes types of care that patients may need.

One problem encountered often in the care of hospitalized patients is that the nursing staff may think the patient can do more than is really possible. So, the staff member places a pan of water with soap in front of the patient and disappears. When the staff person returns, they assume the bath has been done and put it all away. The patient may not have really had a bath.

To give thorough nursing care, you must stay close, see how the patient tolerates the activity of bathing, and help as needed. In this way, you will be sure that good nursing care is truly delivered, and your patient has truly been bathed.

Supervision/Delegation Connection

Determining Delegation of a Bed Bath

How do you decide when to delegate a bed bath? While the bath is time consuming, you should perform it when the patient's condition is unstable, when you need more information about a patient's skin condition, when you need to evaluate the patient's capabilities to assist with personal care, or when you need to develop or strengthen the nurse-patient relationship.

Box 15-1

Types of Care

Personal care is performed in different ways: by the patient, by the staff, or a combination of both.

- **Self-care** refers to patients who are able to perform ADLs without assistance. Most patients in hospitals or care facilities require at least some assistance.
- **Assisted care** refers to the need for some assistance with ADLs. This may mean needing another person to wash hard-to-reach areas such as the back, feet, and lower legs; assistance in helping a patient out of the tub or shower; or help obtaining necessary items for care, such as a bath basin with water.
- **Total care** means that patients are able to do very little or nothing for themselves.

Types of Baths

A bath in a hospital is different than a bath at home when a person is well. The exertion of bathing can be quite exhausting for a person who is ill. The type of bath used can be tailored to the needs of the patient (Box 15-2). When you determine which type of bath to perform, it is important to consider the patient's energy level, ability to tolerate standing or sitting for the duration of the activity, and respiratory status to tolerate steam and exertion. The physician may order a specific activity level, such as complete bedrest. In that case, you must assist the patient with a complete bed bath.

A complete bed bath or towel bath requires the least effort on the part of the patient. Skill 15-1 (page 294) provides more information on administering a complete bed bath. A partial bath or help bath requires a minimal amount of activity by the patient. When you perform a bed bath, you will need to follow certain guidelines to prevent contamination of clean areas and to keep your patient comfortable:

- Cover the patient with a **bath blanket**, a large lightweight flannel blanket, during the bath to prevent exposure.

Uncover only the area of the body that you are washing, leaving the rest of the body covered. This also prevents the patient from becoming chilled during the bath.

- Fold the washcloth into a mitt around your hand (see Skill 15-1) to prevent trailing cold edges of the washcloth over the patient as you bathe him or her. This takes a bit of practice but is worth the effort to make your patient more comfortable.
- Wash from the cleanest areas to the dirtiest areas to prevent transferring bacteria from a dirty area to a clean area.
- Wash extremities from distal to proximal, which helps return blood to the heart. While patients lie in bed, blood tends to pool in the extremities. Using the distal-to-proximal motion helps move the blood in the veins back to the heart (*venous return*). This is important because when blood pools in the extremities, it increases the risk that a *thrombus*, or blood clot may form.
- When washing extremities, start with the arm farthest away from you, then wash the nearer arm. This prevents you from reaching across an arm you have washed to reach the far arm. Your scrubs are considered dirtier than the arm

---

Box 15-2

Types of Baths

Baths given in the health care setting may be referred to in different ways, depending on the amount of help required by the patient or the type of bath being given.

Complete Bed Bath

The patient is unable to be out of bed, so the bath is accomplished using a basin of water at the bedside. All parts of the body are washed. Generally the patient is too ill to help and the nurse performs all care.

Assisted or Help Bath

May be done in bed or with the patient sitting up in a chair. The patient participates as much as he or she is able. If the patient becomes fatigued or short of breath, or develops pain, the nursing staff finishes whatever the patient cannot reach or complete.

Partial Bath

Only selected areas of the patient are bathed. This type of bath may be done when the patient is in pain or nauseated to prevent moving him or her more than is comfortable. Generally, a partial bath includes washing the face, hands, axilla, buttocks, and perineal area, or the parts of the patient that would cause odor if not washed.

Tub Bath

In this type of bath, the patient sits in a tub of water that may or may not include whirlpool action. All of the patient's body is washed while he or she is in the tub. It is difficult for some patients to bend enough to sit down in and get out of a tub. The danger of slips and falls exists. Newer tubs are designed with doors in the side that open for entry and exit, making them less dangerous for patients.

Shower

The patient can sit on a bench or shower chair or stand under the spray of a shower. It is possible to turn the spray off while applying soap to the patient, then turn it back on to rinse. Use caution not to chill the patient. You can usually wash the patient's hair during the shower with little difficulty.

Therapeutic Baths

This is usually a tub bath given for a specific reason. It may be a whirlpool bath to remove infected or necrotic tissue from wounds. It may also involve having the patient soak in the tub with medication added to the water to soothe itching or skin disorders.

Towel or Blanket Bath

This type of bath is done with the patient in bed. It may be commercially prepared or created by the nursing staff. It includes a bath blanket, washcloth(s), and towel(s) in a large bag. The linens are saturated with a no-rinse skin cleanser. The entire bag is then heated in the microwave and taken to the bedside. The patient is covered with a regular bath blanket, which is replaced with the heated moistened bath blanket from the feet up. The patient is massaged through the warm blanket. The heated washcloths are used for the face and the heated towels are used to cleanse the back, buttocks, and perineum.

Bag Bath

This type of bath is similar to the towel bath, but contains 12 to 15 washcloths that are saturated with no-rinse skin cleanser and heated in a bag in the microwave. Each washcloth is used to wash one area of the body, then discarded to prevent cross-contamination and contamination of wounds with dirty bath water. The disposable version is expensive, but the idea can be duplicated with reusable washcloths in a zip-type plastic bag.

you have just washed, and reaching across a clean area could possibly contaminate it. If you wash the far arm and leg first, then wash the nearer arm and leg, contamination will not be a concern.

• Change water anytime it becomes dirty, soapy, or cool. Always change the water after bathing the feet and again after bathing the buttocks and rectal area. For some patients, even tap water for a bath may be unsafe. Patients who have had surgical openings of the sternum to access the heart and lungs, known as *sternotomies,* and those with impaired immune systems may become infected from the bacteria found in most tap water. In these cases, you may have orders to bathe the patient with sterile water or a commercially prepared towel bath (Fig. 15-1). Box 15-2 includes an explanation of a towel bath.

• Perform perineal care during the bed bath and anytime a patient has been incontinent. You can use soap and water for this care. Some commercial perineal washes are available as well. Skill 15-2 (page 296) provides more information on administering perineal care.

• Some patients are able to perform their own perineal care during the bed bath, and would prefer to do so. When the bath is completed except for perineal care, it is appropriate to give the patient the washcloth and provide privacy for washing the genitals. If you say, "Now you can finish your bath," be sure the patient knows what you expect. It may be necessary to be more specific and say something like, "I will step out so you can wash your private areas."

Tub baths, showers, or therapeutic baths require the most effort because the patient must be able to sit or stand for the duration of the bath, usually 5 to 15 minutes, as well as be able to get in and out of the tub or shower. The heat of a shower or bath can cause *vasodilation,* or widening of blood vessels. This, in turn, causes a lowering of the blood pressure. As a result, it is not unusual for patients to become light-headed or dizzy, or even to faint, during a bath or shower. *Safety: Stay with the patient during the first bath or shower after a surgery or illness in case he or she becomes dizzy or feels faint.* You can provide privacy by working in the room while the patient is in the bathroom, but stay

very near in case the patient needs help. You can delegate the responsibility of staying near and assisting the patient to a CNA or UAP, but be sure to emphasize the importance of checking on the patient often during the bath or shower, and listening for the patient to call for help.

Nursing Responsibilities During Bathing

Whether a patient can assist with the bath or not, the nurse must be responsible for a variety of concerns during the bath. Your responsibilities include:

• Assessing the skin for rashes, breaks in integrity, bruising, and lesions.

• Completing the bathing process in a timely manner. Avoid leaving the patient with no gown, with a pan of water that cools off, or in the shower or tub waiting for help to get out.

• Being alert to signs of patient fatigue so you can assist as needed. If the patient becomes short of breath or begins experiencing pain, be prepared to assume the responsibility for the bath.

• Intervening in ways to conserve the patient's energy during the tub bath or shower. Patients with respiratory illness or heart conditions may become extremely fatigued before the end of a shower or tub bath. Some ways to help conserve energy while bathing include:

  • Having the patient put on a terrycloth robe immediately after the bath or shower. This prevents the need for using energy to dry off with a towel.

  • Using a bench in the shower if the patient is unable to stand for the duration of a shower. The patient can sit during the shower and save the energy required to bend over to wash the legs and feet.

  • Using a chair or bench in the tub if the patient cannot sit all the way down in the tub and easily get back up. Use a sprayer attached to the tub faucet or showerhead to wash the patient's body.

Patient Teaching Connection

Teaching About Antibacterial Soaps

A patient insists that you use antibacterial soap during the bath because "it kills more germs than that soap you have." Antibacterial hand soaps are extremely prevalent in homes and public places. However, these antibacterial soaps have *not* been proven to be any more effective than regular soap for the prevention of infections by a U.S. Food and Drug Administration advisory panel. Some research studies seemed to indicate that antibacterial soaps could contribute to antibiotic-resistant bacteria, but that has not been proven outside the research setting. Teach your patients to use regular soap and water unless they have been instructed to use antibacterial soaps by their health care provider, but to wash their hands often since handwashing has been proven to decrease transmission of bacteria and viruses.

Figure 15-1   This nurse is administering a towel bath.

Grooming

In addition to hygiene, you will assist patients with oral care, hair care, applying deodorant and lotion, dressing or putting on a clean gown, shaving, and nail care, all of which is referred to as grooming. As female patients begin to feel better, you may assist them with applying makeup as well. All of these aspects of ADLs are important to the patient's self-esteem.

Back Massage

During the bath and during evening care, perform a back massage for the patient. Not only does it help relax the patient, it also stimulates circulation. It is necessary to use lotion or oil during a back massage to prevent excessive friction on the patient's skin. Lotion rubs into the skin and is absorbed, necessitating reapplication to keep skin friction at bay.

It is important to massage the muscles, not just apply lotion to the skin (Fig. 15-2). Use the flat side of your fingers rather than you fingertips as you stroke the back to prevent uncomfortable pressure. Use the sides of the thumbs to massage the muscles. Be sensitive to tight, firm areas of muscle tension and work over those areas a bit longer than elsewhere to try to relax the muscles. Pay special attention to the area from the neck to the top of the shoulders. These trapezius muscles tighten in response to anxiety and stress. Do not neglect the lumbar and sacral areas. For many, these lower back areas fatigue quickly and receive little support while the patient lies in bed. Massage in this area also helps increase circulation and prevent pressure ulcers.

Back massages may not be indicated if the patient has certain heart conditions, as it can stimulate the vagus nerve and slow the heart rate. If the patient has fractures of the ribs or vertebrae, a back massage would not be appropriate because it could increase pain and put pressure on the fractured area.

Back massage is quickly becoming a lost art among nurses. They often feel that they do not have enough time to provide this care. But back massage takes very little time and is of great benefit to the patient. Skill 15-3 (page 298) presents more information on how to provide a back massage.

Figure 15-2 Correct technique for back massage.

Oral Care

Providing oral care for patients not only freshens the mouth, but also allows you to assess the mouth for problems that could be affecting the patient's nutritional and health status. Look for decaying, broken, or missing teeth. Observe for reddened or bleeding gums, ulcerations of the mucosa, and coating of the tongue. White patches on the tongue or oral mucosa, known as **leukoplakia**, can be precancerous lesions.

Oral Care for the Unconscious Patient

When you care for a patient who is unconscious, it is still necessary to give oral care. *Safety: You must be careful to minimize any chance of aspiration of fluids. To do this, position the patient on either side with the bed flat. In this way, fluids can run out of the mouth instead of down the throat. Keep a suction device ready for use.* Assess the mouth for lesions and dried mouth secretions known as *sordes*. When you clean the mouth, use the least amount of fluid possible, usually 5 mL or less, to prevent aspiration. You will use a small amount of toothpaste and a brush, as well as sponge swabs to clean the mouth and teeth. Lemon-glycerin swabs are not recommended for cleaning the lips or inside of the mouth because they cause drying of the oral mucosa. If they are used over a long period of time, they may cause damage to tooth enamel. Apply water-soluble lip balm to keep the lips moist. Skill 15-4 (page 298) presents the steps of oral care for the unconscious patient.

Special mouth care is the term used for oral care for patients whose conditions result in a need for more frequent care and who need assistance for this care. Such conditions include being unable to take food or fluid by mouth (NPO), receiving oxygen by cannula or mask, having a nasogastric or feeding tube in place, and being unconscious. Special mouth care is usually performed every 2 hours, but follow the facility's policy. When the patient is unconscious, a natural reflex causes the jaw to bite down on anything inserted into the mouth. Make a padded tongue blade by wrapping several gauze squares around one end of a tongue blade and taping them in place. Then insert the padded end of the blade into the patient's mouth and turn it vertically to hold the mouth open while you perform oral care.

Oral Care for the Conscious Patient

Conscious patients may or may not be able to perform their own oral care. If the patient is unable to brush his or her own teeth, assist by putting a small amount of toothpaste on the brush and brush the teeth at a 45-degree angle to the gums. Move the brush in small circles on the inside and outside of the teeth, and with back-and-forth strokes across the biting and chewing surfaces of the teeth. Assist with flossing the teeth by gently sliding a 6- to 10-inch piece of dental floss between the teeth, moving it in a backward-and-forward motion. Avoid going deeper than the gum line, as this can damage the gums and cause bleeding.

If the patient is able to perform oral care, assist by setting the needed items on the patient's over-the-bed tray.

Safety: Remain with the patient if any danger of choking exists, such as with a patient who has swallowing difficulties. Skill 15-5 (page 299) presents the steps of providing oral care for a conscious patient.

Denture Care

Patients may have full dentures or partial dentures, known as a *bridge.* Partial dentures replace one or more missing teeth and are often removable for cleaning. Dental implants also replace missing teeth, but they are not removable. When cleaning full or partial dentures, be sure to handle them carefully. They are custom-made for each person, so they are expensive. They can break if they are dropped. Line the sink with a towel so that, if the dentures slip while you are cleaning them, they will land on a soft surface (Fig. 15-3). Use cool water to clean the dentures, as hot water can damage them. Store dentures overnight in a denture cup and water. Add a cleaning tablet if the patient desires. Avoid treating partial dentures with metal parts with a cleaning tablet; instead, place them in water overnight. Skill 15-6 (page 300) presents the steps in performing denture care.

Knowledge Connection

What are the benefits of back massage? Why is positioning important when you perform oral care for an unconscious patient?

Shaving

Both male and female patients may require assistance with shaving. Most men shave daily, and if the beard is allowed to grow for 2 or 3 days before shaving, it may become very uncomfortable. *Safety: Patients taking anticoagulant medications, which delay blood clotting, should only be shaved with electric razors and not with blades of any kind, as this could cause excessive bleeding if the patient were accidentally cut.*

Figure 15-3 Correct cleaning technique for dentures. Note the towel in the sink to prevent breakage.

When you shave a male patient with a disposable razor, always shave in the direction of hair growth to prevent causing razor burn and ingrown whiskers. When you shave a male patient with an electric razor, move the razor in circular motions over the beard for the closest shave. It is also important to clean an electric razor when you are finished shaving the patient. If the razor becomes clogged with cut whiskers, it will cut poorly and be uncomfortable for the patient. To clean the razor, follow the manufacturer's instructions. Usually this involves removing the head of the razor and brushing the recesses and blades to remove debris, then replacing the head. Skill 15-7 (page 301) provides more information on shaving a male patient.

For female patients, generally the axillae and the legs are the areas shaved. Some women may need assistance to shave or pluck stray hairs on the chin or upper lip. Be aware that, in many cultures, women do not shave their legs or axillae, so it would not be appropriate to offer shaving assistance to them.

Nail Care

Before performing nail care, you should assess the nails for discoloration, ridges, and redness where the skin and nail meet. Patients who are diabetic easily develop infections around nails, so look closely at both fingernails and toenails. Thick, yellowed toenails often have that appearance due to a fungal infection. Prescription medications are available to treat this, so the patient should be advised to consult a podiatrist.

Clean under the fingernails using a small wooden stick (orangewood stick) or file designed for this purpose. When you care for patients' nails, always clip them straight across, then file off any sharp corners. Clipping toenails deeply at the corners can lead to ingrown toenails. *Safety: If the patient is diabetic, file the nails rather than clipping them to prevent accidentally clipping toe tissue. Because patients with diabetes have poor circulation, such an injury could lead to severe infection and even amputation.*

Skill 15-8 (page 302) presents more information on providing nail care.

Knowledge Connection

Under what circumstance must a patient be shaved with an electric razor? How can you help prevent ingrown toenails when performing nail care? What is important to remember regarding patients with diabetes and nail care?

Hair Care

In addition to helping patients look and feel better, performing hair care gives you the chance to assess the patient's scalp for potential problems. Inspect the scalp and hair root area for the presence of **lesions**, or open areas. A round area of hair loss with a lesion may indicate ringworm or **tinea capitis**, which is a fungal infection that can affect any part of the body and can be spread from one person to another.

Dry, flaky skin on the scalp may be dandruff. The patient may need to use a special shampoo to relieve the itching and flaking that can accompany dandruff. Thick, oily scales on the scalp may be due to **seborrhea**, or an overproduction of sebum. When this occurs in infants, it is sometimes called *cradle cap.*

Inspect the hair close to the scalp for the presence of tiny parasites called **lice**. Clear bumps affixed tightly to the shaft of the hair are the **nits**, or eggs, of lice. An infestation of lice causes intense itching of the scalp as the lice burrow in to obtain nourishment. Lice are easily transmitted to others by sharing hats, combs, or brushes, or with close contact. Outbreaks of head lice are common occurrences in day-care facilities and elementary schools. Treatment with specific shampoo is required. In addition, the nits must be removed with fine combs so they do not hatch into more lice. For this reason, the shampoo treatment is repeated approximately 1 to 2 weeks after the first treatment. Lice- and nit-treating shampoos can be toxic, so follow package instructions carefully.

African American patients who need hair care assistance require specialized hair treatment. The natural hair can mat or tangle easily and should be combed and brushed daily. It is important to apply oil to the hair and scalp, which also tends to be dry. Mineral oil or moisturizing hair cream can be used to lubricate the scalp and protect the hair. If the hair has been chemically treated with straighteners or relaxers, it can also be dry and easily broken and requires special care when you comb, brush, and shampoo it. If the hair is styled in cornrows or braids, you can shampoo it in that style. Cover the hair with a stocking cap first and then shampoo through the cap.

Shampooing Hair

Patients may require assistance to keep hair clean during an illness or injury. If possible, wash the hair while the patient is in the tub or shower. Have the patient protect the eyes by holding a washcloth over them. Rinse with the patient's head tilted back to keep the shampoo from running into the eyes. If the patient cannot take a tub bath or shower, another option is using a special shampoo that does not need to be rinsed. This type of shampoo is applied to the hair, combed through, and then the hair is dried. It is not as effective as hair washing, but it does help clean the oils out of the hair.

The patient's hair can also be washed while the patient remains in bed (Fig. 15-4). Skill 15-9 (page 303) provides more information on shampooing the hair with the patient in bed. To do this, special equipment is used to contain the water and shampoo. An inflatable head cradle or rigid shampoo board is placed beneath the patient's head and neck. A large bag is filled with clean warm water, and a hose is attached to the bag that ends with a sprayer nozzle. Or a basin can be used to hold the warm water, which is then scooped out with a pitcher and poured over the hair. The hair can be washed and rinsed using the water from the bag or pitcher. The inflatable head cradle contains the water and is emptied upon completion of the procedure. If the rigid

Figure 15-4 Shampooing the hair while the patient is in bed.

shampoo board is used, the water runs out of the board into a trash can lined with a garbage sack, which is emptied after the procedure.

Styling Hair

Style hair according to the patient's preference. Avoid using hairstyles that are not age appropriate, especially for older patients. For example, do not style a 72-year-old woman's hair in pigtails or a ponytail as you would for a young child. This is demeaning to an older woman, who deserves respect.

Caring for Piercings

Body piercing is becoming more and more popular, so you will most likely encounter patients with jewelry in piercings other than in their ears. Common piercing sites include the nose, lip, eyebrow, tongue, nipples, navel, and genitalia.

Piercings that are new must be kept clean and monitored for infections. If your patient with a piercing is unable to do this, you will need to assist. Follow instructions provided by the patient for piercing care. Soap, water, and alcohol are generally used for care of piercing sites. Assess for redness, swelling, pain, or drainage from the site, which would indicate potential infection.

Sometimes it is necessary to remove jewelry from a piercing if it could interfere with surgery; *intubation,* which involves passing a tube through the mouth to the trachea; diagnostic testing, such as magnetic resonance imaging (MRI); or catheterization. If the jewelry is made of nonmagnetic stainless steel or titanium, similar to materials used for joint replacements, it would not have to be removed for an MRI. Some piercings close quickly over a period of just a few days, so the patient may prefer that jewelry remains intact if at all possible.

Removing jewelry from piercings is not always a simple task. Kits are now available to hospitals that contain tools for removal of jewelry from piercings, along with descriptions of each of the common types of jewelry, how they are inserted, and how they should be removed. Table 15-1 provides descriptions of different types of jewelry for piercings and how to remove them.

Eye and Ear Care

Some patients wear glasses or contact lenses and may require assistance with them. Clean patients' glasses with warm water and a soft cloth. Avoid using paper towels or tissues because they can scratch the lenses. Be sure the patient knows where you have put the glasses if he or she is not wearing them. Place them within easy reach, as some patients need their glasses to read or watch television.

Contact Lenses

Most patients wearing contacts will be able to remove and insert the lenses themselves. However, if it is necessary for you to remove contact lenses, follow these steps:

A. Wash your hands and put on gloves.
B. Pull down on the lower lid and place one finger across the top of the upper lid, applying gentle but firm pressure.
C. Ask the patient to blink.
D. Hard lenses will pop out between your fingers. A soft contact lens will wrinkle off the eye, and you can grasp it with your fingers. If the soft contact is not easily grasped in this manner, pull the bottom eyelid down and the top eyelid up. Then gently use your gloved finger to pull the contact down off of the *iris* (colored part of the eye) to be grasped and removed. *Safety: Do not slide the lens down the iris with pressure as this can scratch the cornea.*

E. Hold the lens gently and carefully while you place it in the appropriate well of the lens case, either left or right. *Safety: Be sure you put the lenses in the correct side of the case so the patient will not insert them into the wrong eye.*
F. Fill the wells, covering the lenses with saline or special soaking solution, according to the patient's routine.

Artificial Eyes

An artificial eye may be used in two different situations. The eye may have been *enucleated,* or complete removed, leaving only the socket. In many of these cases, a globe is implanted in the socket to restore the shape of the eye. The other situation occurs when the eye is intact but is blind, perhaps from birth or due to disease. This is referred to as a *blind globe.*

One type of artificial eye is called a *scleral cover shell.* It is like a thick contact lens that fits flush against the implanted globe or blind globe. It is made of opaque acrylic and covers the whole eye area, not just the iris. The color of the *sclera* (the white part of the eye), iris, pupil, and minute blood vessels are hand painted to match the patient's other eye. Because it is fitted over the globe, which is attached to muscles, this type of artificial eye moves in tandem with the sighted eye.

If no ocular implant is in place, the socket is flat and somewhat deep. The **ocular prosthesis** (artificial eye) is custom made to fit the socket and is also hand painted with great detail to match the existing eye. This type of artificial eye does not move.

Table 15-1   Removing Piercing Jewelry

Name of Jewelry	Description and Removal
Barbells	Jewelry with round knobs on each end. Some knobs are removable and some are not.
Vertical Barbell	A straight shaft with round knobs on each end. At least one knob, sometimes both, will unscrew; when the knob is removed, the shaft will slip out of the piercing.
Curved Barbell	A curved shaft with round knobs on each end. Only one knob will unscrew; the other is fixed. To remove, unscrew the movable knob and slide the curved shaft out of the piercing.
Circular Barbell	A circular shaft with two round knobs. Both may unscrew or only one. Unscrew the removable knob and carefully slide in a circular motion to remove from the piercing.
Captive Ring	A circular shaft with two ends meeting inside a single ball. To remove, use very small needle-nose type pliers. Insert them in the ring and gently separate the handles to widen the ring. As the ring ends spread open, the single ball is released. Then slide the shaft out of the piercing. *If it is difficult to slide the shaft from the piercing, apply a small amount of water-soluble lubricant to the shaft.*
Prince Albert	This is essentially a curved barbell placed in a piercing of the penis. The barbell enters through a piercing in the lower portion of the head of the penis and exits through the urethra. In a reverse Prince Albert, the barbell enters the urethra and exits through a piercing in the top of the glans. Remove as you would a curved barbell.

To care for these eye prostheses, follow the patient's usual care routine. If the patient is unable to remove the artificial eye for cleaning, you will need to assist. A small suction cup on a hollow handle is used to move the prosthesis to and from the orbit. While squeezing the handle of the suction cup, place it on the prosthetic eye and then release the handle. It will remain attached to the prosthesis.

To remove the prosthesis when no implanted globe is present, only an ocular prosthesis, follow these steps:

A. Wash your hands and put on gloves.
B. Dip the end of the suction cup in saline.
C. Lift the upper eyelid.
D. Squeeze the suction cup and place it on the iris of the prosthesis.
E. Stop squeezing.
F. Use the handle of the suction cup to lift the prosthesis out of the socket.

To remove the prosthesis when a natural or implanted blind globe is present, follow these steps:

A. Wash your hands and put on gloves.
B. Dip the end of the suction cup in saline.
C. Squeeze the suction cup and place it on the iris of the prosthesis.
D. Stop squeezing.
E. Raise the upper eyelid.
F. Tilt the prosthesis out from under the upper lid.
G. Lift the prosthesis out. When dealing with a natural blind globe be careful not to touch or press on the cornea, which is very sensitive.

Cleanse the prosthesis with sterile water or saline, according the patient's routine. Irrigate the eye socket with eye irrigating solution. Small amounts of mucus may gather in the socket. Assess for large amounts of thick yellow or green mucus that would indicate infection.

To replace the artificial eye, follow these steps:

A. Wash hands and put on gloves.
B. Dip the suction cup in saline.
C. Squeeze the suction cup handle and attach it to the iris of the prosthesis.
D. Stop squeezing the handle of the suction cup.
E. Ensure that the prosthesis is wet with saline or lubricating solution.
F. Lift the upper eyelid, making a gap between it and the blind globe or implant.
G. Slide the top of the prosthesis beneath the upper eyelid and release the lid.
H. Pull down on the lower lid and slide the prosthesis behind the lower lid.
I. Release the lower lid.
J. Squeeze the handle of the suction cup; it will release from the prosthesis.
K. Return the suction cup to its appropriate storage place.

Hearing Aids

A number of older patients use hearing aids and may require assistance to insert, remove, and store them. In recent years, hearing aids have become more sophisticated through the use of computer technology. Rather than magnifying all sounds, including background noises, newer types of aids can magnify voices while not increasing extra noises. Some of the newer aids must be carefully protected from moisture, including being kept in a special moisture-absorbing medium when not in use. Figure 15-5 shows different types of hearing aids.

Cleaning Hearing Aids

If the earmold can be separated from the hearing aid (for example, in the behind-the-ear model), turn off the aid and detach it. Clean the earmold with warm soapy water. The

Figure 15-5 Three different types of hearing aids: a, Behind-the-ear hearing aid; b, In-the-canal hearing aid; and c, In-the-ear hearing aid.

in-the-canal style of hearing aid may have a screen or filter to block wax. If so, spread a clean cloth on a hard surface and gently tap the aid against the cloth to remove wax from the screen or filter. Clean other types of aids by wiping them with a damp cloth and cleaning the opening with a pipe cleaner, cotton-tipped applicator, or toothpick to remove any wax buildup.

To remove a hearing aid, follow these steps:

A. Turn off the hearing aid.
B. Turn the earmold slightly toward the nose and lift out.
C. Store the aid in its case or moisture-control container.

To insert a hearing aid, follow these steps:

A. Check the battery by turning the hearing aid on to full volume and listening for it to whistle, which indicates that it is working.
B. If you do not hear a whistle, check the battery and replace as needed.
C. Turn off the hearing aid and lower the volume.
D. Insert the hearing aid into the ear and adjust the volume as needed.

Knowledge Connection

Under what circumstances should jewelry be removed from a body piercing? How can you tell if the battery in a hearing aid is working?

Managing the Environment

Another aspect of patient care is making the environment comfortable and conducive to rest. This is not always easy to do given all the noise and activity found on a nursing unit.

The Patient Room

Most hospitalized patients spend the majority of their time in the patient unit or hospital room. This may be a private or semiprivate room. When a roommate is present, it is very important to provide privacy whenever you give care. This can be achieved by pulling the curtain separating the two beds and speaking in a soft voice when discussing health care issues with the patient. If further privacy is needed, it is appropriate to move the patient to a conference room or examination room for discussion of sensitive topics.

Furniture

The hospital bed is a special type of bed designed to be placed in a variety of positions, which will be discussed later in this chapter. Both the head and the foot of the bed can be elevated. In addition, the area under the knees can be raised to prevent the patient from sliding down in the bed when the head of the bed is elevated. The mattress is covered with water-repellent material and is firmer than many home mattresses. The bed usually has rails on either side that can be raised as a safety measure to prevent falling or for the patient to grasp when turning from side to side. Often the controls for the television and the nurse call light are built into the side rails so they are always within easy reach.

The over-the-bed table is designed to be placed alongside the bed or across the bed. It is wheeled for ease of movement and may have a movable top that pushes back to reveal a small storage area that is convenient for glasses, combs, and brushes. Generally it contains a mirror that the patient can use for shaving or applying makeup. Food trays are placed on this table, and it is then placed across the bed so the patient can eat. It is important to remove any unpleasant sights and smells from the tabletop before placing the food tray on it. Remove anything from the over-the-bed table that you would not want sitting on your kitchen table during a meal, including toilet tissue, a dirty emesis basin, a urinal, trash, soiled tissues, and soiled drinking glasses or dishes from previous meals.

The bedside stand usually contains three drawers and can be used for supplies, personal items, and clothing. It is difficult for the patient in bed to reach for items in the drawers, so generally infrequently needed items are stored there. When a patient leaves the room due to transfer or discharge, it is important that you empty all the drawers and ensure that personal belongings are sent with the patient. Usually a small closet is built into the area across from the bed so clothing may be stored there as well.

Environment

The patient may have many concerns about the hospital environment that the nurse may not notice because the concerns are commonplace in the hospital. However, they are not commonplace for the patient. Some problems and ways to manage them include:

- **Noise.** Keep the patient's door closed or nearly closed to help block out hallway noise and activity. Avoid shouting or calling out in the hallways or from the nurse's station. If the patient wishes, keep the television or radio on for soft background noise. Answer call lights and extinguish alarms on equipment promptly.
- **Odors.** Remove and empty bedpans, urinals, bedside commodes, and emesis basins promptly. Use sprays to neutralize odors, but avoid perfumed sprays that could cause reactions in patients with respiratory disorders such as asthma. *Safety: The health care staff should not wear perfumes, colognes, aftershave, or scented body lotions while caring for patients. Some patients with respiratory disorders can react strongly to such scents, causing an asthma attack or difficulty breathing.*
- Sometimes food odors can be unpleasant if the patient is nauseated. Remove food trays promptly if the patient does not wish to eat. Keep the tray warm in the kitchen or other

appropriate location if the patient may want it later. Empty trash promptly to prevent lingering odors in the room.

- **Clutter.** It does not take long for over-the-bed tables and bedside stands to become crowded with the patient's belongings and patient care supplies. In addition, patients sometimes keep food from their meal tray to eat later. The water pitcher, drinking glass, and straw should be within the patient's reach. Many hospital rooms have a plant shelf where you can put cards, vases, and potted plants. Do not remove personal items from within reach without the patient's permission. Try to arrange needed items so that they are within reach and move less frequently used items to the drawers in the bedside stand.

- **Equipment.** Hospital rooms become cluttered quickly with equipment, supplies, and visitors' belongings. It is extremely important to keep pathways from the bed to the bathroom clear for the patient. Ensure that cords are out of the way to prevent tripping. Assist the patient in and out of bed to ensure that the IV lines and other attached tubing do not get pulled or kinked. Keep equipment against the walls if possible and out of walkways. Promptly remove equipment that is not in use.

Bedmaking

In the acute care setting, linens are changed frequently. Follow policy at your facility for routine changes and also change the linen if the bed is soiled. When making beds, several options exist, for both the unoccupied bed and the occupied bed.

Unoccupied Bed

The bed is considered unoccupied when the patient is out of the bed while the linens are changed. The patient may be sitting up in the chair or may have left the patient unit for therapy or diagnostic tests. Several types of unoccupied beds may be made:

- **Open bed:** This type of bed is made with the top linens fanfolded to the foot of the bed so the patient can easily slip into the bed and pull them up.
- **Surgical bed:** This type of bed is made with the top linens fanfolded to the side of the bed (the side away from the door). When the patient returns on a stretcher, he or she can easily be moved into the bed without the top linens being in the way. The patient can quickly be covered without his or her feet getting tangled in the linens. The top sheet and blanket are spread over the patient, then tucked at the foot of the bed. Not all facilities use the surgical bed, but it is a good way to keep linens out of the way during a transfer from stretcher to bed.
- **Closed bed:** In acute care, the closed bed is only used when the patient is discharged. The room is terminally cleaned and the bed is made with fresh linens. The top linens are spread to the head of the bed to keep the bed clean. This will be converted to an open bed when staff are alerted to a patient admission.

Skill 15-10 (page 304) provides more information on making an unoccupied bed.

Occupied Bed

The bed is considered occupied if the linens are changed while the patient remains in the bed. This is done when the patient is unable to be out of bed. The patient is turned to one side while soiled bottom linens are loosened and fanfolded to the middle of the bed, beneath the patient. A clean fitted sheet and draw sheet are applied to the bed up to where the patient is lying. Then the patient turns to the other side, rolling over the "hump" of soiled and clean linens. The nurse goes to the opposite side of the bed and removes the soiled linens, then spreads out and tucks in the clean linens. With the patient lying on his or her back, the top soiled linens are removed and the clean ones applied. Skill 15-11 (page 306) provides more information on making an occupied bed.

Nursing Responsibilities in Bedmaking

Bedmaking is often delegated to a CNA or a UAP. Whoever makes the bed, it is very important to make the bed tightly without wrinkles. Wrinkles in a poorly made bed can contribute to the development of pressure ulcers as well as patient discomfort.

Making the bed in a hospital is different than making beds at home. The number one concern is patient safety. *Safety: Make certain the bed rails are raised on the opposite side of the bed from where you are working. Remember to raise the rails on the working side of the bed before going around the bed to the other side.* Some facilities use mattress covers to make the plastic mattress more comfortable. Then you will most likely use a fitted sheet for the bottom sheet. Next, you will apply a **draw sheet** or turn sheet. This type of sheet is narrower than a flat sheet. Also, a flat sheet has a wide hem at the top and a narrow hem at the bottom. A draw sheet has two narrow hems on each end. Some draw sheets are wide enough to fold in half lengthwise, and some are designed to be a single layer. The draw sheet is positioned horizontally across the bed with the top edge aligned at the patient's shoulders and the bottom edge at the patient's knees.

The edge of the draw sheet is tucked between the mattress and springs on one side of the bed. When you go to the other side of the bed, grasp the draw sheet firmly in the middle with both hands. Pull the sheet tightly across the mattress and down to tuck it between the mattress and springs. Next, pull the draw sheet at the edge near the top and tuck it; follow by doing the same at the edge near the bottom. Smooth out wrinkles. A tight, smooth draw sheet is the secret to a comfortable bed.

Draw sheets are used to protect the bottom sheet from minor soiling and to help lift and turn heavier patients. A disposable or washable incontinence pad may be used to protect the bottom sheet and draw sheet from soiling. Then only the pad has to be changed instead of having to change the whole bed.

When you apply the top linens to the bed, turn the top sheet so the seams are away from the patient and spread the sheet and blanket smoothly across the bed. Then tuck them *together* at the foot of the bed. This prevents loosening the top sheet when tucking the blanket. Go to the side of the bed and form a **mitered corner** (slanted corner) as you tuck both the sheet and blanket together. (See Skill 15-10 for details on how to form a mitered corner.) The purpose of this type of corner is to anchor the linens more firmly than if they were only tucked at the foot of the mattress.

Whether you make an occupied or unoccupied bed, it is important to cuff the top sheet over the blanket or spread to prevent rough fabric edges from irritating the skin of the patient's face and neck. Sheets and blankets are laundered in the hospital laundry or at a commercial facility and may be more stiff and scratchy than linens at home.

When making an occupied bed, the process of tucking the top linens under the foot of the mattress causes *plantar flexion* of the patient's feet (toes pointed downward). This can result in pressure ulcers on the toes or contribute to *footdrop,* where the foot remains in a permanent state of plantar flexion. Footdrop impairs the patient's ability to walk again. This is also uncomfortable for the patient and can be easily remedied by grasping the top linens above the patient's toes and pulling upward an inch or two, making room for the natural foot position.

Another consideration when making an occupied bed is that you will be placing a clean fitted sheet and draw sheet beneath soiled existing sheets. If necessary, you can place a disposable pad between the clean and soiled linens to prevent contamination.

Bed Positions

Another issue regarding the patient's environment is positioning the bed for patient comfort or for therapeutic reasons. It is important for you to be familiar with bed positions and to be able to place the bed in various positions quickly. In some situations, positioning of the bed and patient can help prevent severe shortness of breath or shock. Table 15-2 provides descriptions and uses of common bed positions.

Knowledge Connection

How can you control odors in a patient's room? What bed position is used for a patient in shock? How do you keep a draw sheet tight and smooth?

Table 15-2 Common Bed Positions

Position	Diagram	Use
Flat	 Flat position	Used for resting or sleeping and after certain procedures such as lumbar punctures and back surgery.
Fowler's	 Fowler's position	Knees slightly elevated to prevent sliding down; used when patients want to sit up to watch TV or converse with visitors.
Semi-Fowler's	 Semi-Fowler's position	Used for patients on continuous tube feedings to prevent aspiration and for comfort when patient does not wish to be completely flat.

(table continues on page 294)

Table 15-2 **Common Bed Positions** (continued)

Position	Diagram	Use
Trendelenburg	Trendelenburg position	Used for patients who have very low blood pressure (shock) to return blood to the brain and vital organs. Keeping the head of the bed flat with the feet elevated is the preferred bed position for patients with breathing difficulty or head injury.
Reverse Trendelenburg	Reverse Trendelenburg position	Used to elevate the patient's head without bending at the waist for patients who have returned from procedures requiring that the legs be kept straight at the groin, such as a cardiac catheterization.

Skill 15-1 Administering a Complete Bed Bath

Assessment Steps

1. Review the patient's chart for activity orders and position restrictions.
2. Assess the patient's ability to turn, follow directions, and remain in one position.
3. Determine the need for assistance during the bed bath.
4. Determine the patient's status: Is there pain, fatigue, or shortness of breath? Are there cultural issues to address?
5. Determine the type of bath most appropriate for this patient.

Planning Steps

1. Gather needed equipment and supplies: bath basin, towels (two or three), washcloths (two or three), soap, bath blanket, clean gown or pajamas (obtain a snap-shoulder gown if the patient has an IV line), laundry bag, clean linens for occupied bed change.
2. Plan to give the bed bath at the time the patient prefers.
3. Plan for privacy throughout the bath by placing a "Bath in Progress" sign on the door.

Implementation Steps

1. Follow the Initial Implementation Steps located on the inside front cover.
2. Prepare the patient and the room: provide privacy, adjust the room temperature, and offer the bedpan or urinal. *This prevents interruptions during the bath.*

3. Fill the bath basin approximately two-thirds of the way full with warm water (105°F). Test the temperature by applying water to your inner wrist to determine that it is not too warm. *This prevents discomfort from water that is too hot or too cool.*
4. Place the basin on the over-the-bed table and position the table parallel to the bed.
5. Lower the side rail nearest you. Assist the patient to move closer to you.
6. Remove the blanket or bedspread. Spread the bath blanket over the top sheet. Ask the patient to hold on to the bath blanket while you remove the sheet from beneath it. *This prevents exposure and keeps the patient warm.*
7. Untie the patient's gown and remove it. If the patient has an IV infusion that is not on a pump, slide the gown down the arm, then remove the IV bag from the stand and slide the bag through the sleeve in the same direction as the patient's hand *to prevent the IV tubing from becoming tangled in the gown.* If the IV infusion is on a pump, a gown with snaps or other closure on the shoulder must be used. *Safety: Do not disconnect IV tubing to change patient gowns because this can lead to infection.*
8. Place a towel under the patient's head to protect the pillow.
9. Fold a washcloth into a mitt around your hand. To do this, dampen the cloth. Then wrap it around your hand, holding it in place with your thumb. Fold the remaining portion of the cloth over your fingers and tuck it under the edge in your palm.

Skill 15-1 (continued)

10. Wash one eye using a corner of the bath mitt. Wash from the inner *canthus* (corner of the eye) to the outer canthus *to prevent spreading pathogens across the eye.*

11. Repeat with the opposite eye and a different corner of the washcloth.

12. Wash the face without soap. Use any special facial cleanser the patient may provide. Wash the neck and ears. Rinse the face, neck, and ears and pat dry.

13. Expose the arm farthest from you by folding the bath blanket away from the arm, but keeping the rest of the patient covered.

14. Remove the towel from beneath the patient's head and place it lengthwise beneath the far arm.

15. Wash and rinse the far hand and arm using long strokes from the hand to the axilla *to promote venous return. Safety: Support the arm joints as you lift the arm to prevent possible injury to the elbow or shoulder.* Pat the arm dry using the towel beneath it.

16. Repeat for the near arm.

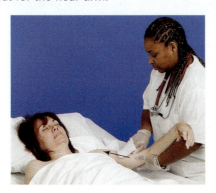

17. Apply deodorant to the axillae according to the patient's preference.
Note: If the towel has become damp, obtain a new towel. If the water is cool or dirty, empty the basin and obtain fresh water.

18. Place the towel horizontally across the patient's chest. Fold the bath blanket back to the patient's waist. *This protects the patient's modesty and keeps patient warm while allowing access to the chest area.*

19. Fold the towel toward the waist while you wash and rinse the chest. For female patients, lift each breast to wash and rinse beneath it. Assess for skin breakdown, as it often occurs in skinfolds. Dry thoroughly beneath each breast.

20. Replace the towel over the chest and fold upward to expose the abdomen. Wash, rinse, and dry the abdomen. *Safety: If abdominal incisions are present, wash gently around dressings or tape.*
Note: If the towel has become damp, obtain a new towel. If the water is cool or dirty, empty the basin and obtain fresh water.

21. Replace the bath blanket over the chest and fold back to expose the far leg. Place the towel lengthwise under the leg.

22. Wash and rinse the far leg, using long strokes from ankle to hip.

23. Assist the patient to bend the knee and place the foot flat on the bed. Bring the basin to the bed and place it by the patient's foot. Assist the patient to place the foot into the bath basin and allow it to soak. *This helps soften and remove dead skin buildup on the foot and helps clean thoroughly between the toes.*

24. Wash the foot carefully. Wash between the toes and inspect for reddened areas or skin lesions.

25. Remove the basin to the over-the-bed table. Pat the foot and leg dry using the towel beneath the leg.

26. Repeat the procedure with the near leg.
Note: If the towel has become damp, obtain a new towel. If the water is cool or dirty, empty the basin and obtain fresh water.

27. Assist the patient to turn onto his or her side so the back is facing you. Place a dry towel lengthwise along the back. *Safety: The far side rail should be up to prevent falling when the patient turns on his or her side.*

(skill continues on page 296)

Skill 15-1 (continued)

28. Fold the bath blanket up to expose the patient's back. Wash and rinse the back, then pat it dry with the towel. Perform a back massage (see Skill 15-3).

29. Wash the rectal area. Separate the buttocks and clean the area well. Assess for skin breakdown in the gluteal folds. *Safety: Wear gloves to prevent exposure to body fluids and pathogens.*

30. If the patient has been incontinent of stool, clean the area with toilet tissue first, then wash with the washcloth. *Safety: Always wash from front to back to prevent contamination with fecal matter or bacteria.*

31. Wash, rinse, and dry with towel placed along the back earlier. Cover any soiled area on the sheet with a towel or bed protector until the bath is completed and the sheets can be changed.

32. Change the water. Rinse out the basin and wipe it clean if needed. *This prevents contamination from the basin and water when you perform perineal care.* Obtain a clean washcloth and towel.

33. Assist the patient to turn onto his or her back and position the patient for perineal care.

34. Perform perineal care (see Skill 15-2) and remove gloves. Wash hands.

35. Reposition the bath blanket. Assist the patient into a clean gown or pajamas. If an IV infusion is present, obtain a gown with shoulder snaps or closures. If the IV infusion is not on a pump and no snap gown is available, put the IV bag through the gown sleeve first, then put the patient's arm through the sleeve.

36. Change the occupied bed (see Skill 15-10).

37. Follow the Ending Implementation Steps located on the inside back cover.

Evaluation Steps

1. Evaluate the condition of the patient's skin. Note any red or open areas or signs of pressure.

2. Evaluate the patient's condition during the bath. Did the bath tire the patient excessively? Is the patient in pain or short of breath?

3. Evaluate the patient's comfort. Is the patient clean and comfortable after the bath?

Sample Documentation

Personal care is often not documented except on a flow sheet. If abnormal findings are present, they are documented in the nurse's notes as shown below.

9/17/10   0940   *Complete bed bath given. 3-cm reddened area noted on coccyx. Occlusive dressing applied. Positioned on right side.*
———————————————— *Nurse's signature and credentials*

Skill 15-2 Administering Perineal Care

Assessment Steps

1. Assess the need for perineal care if the procedure is not part of a complete bed bath.

2. Assess the need for clean sheets if the ones on the bed are soiled.

Planning Steps

1. Gather needed equipment and supplies: washcloths, towel, bath blanket, toilet tissue, incontinence pad, clean sheets as needed.

2. Determine the need for assistance of another staff member to complete perineal care.

Implementation Steps

1. Follow the Initial Implementation Steps located on the inside front cover.

2. Position the patient on his or her back. Remove the blanket or bedspread and cover the top sheet with a bath blanket. Have the patient hold on to the blanket while you remove the top sheet from beneath it.

For a Female Patient

3. Turn the bath blanket so it is in a diamond shape across the patient, with a point toward the head, one toward the feet and the two others at the sides.

4. Ask the patient to bend her knees and place her feet flat on the bed. Grasp one of the side points and wrap the blanket around the patient's leg and foot. Repeat with the other side. This leaves the lower point of the diamond between the patient's feet, where it can be lifted up and folded back. *This provides warmth and privacy for the patient during perineal care. Safety: Wear gloves to prevent exposure to body fluids and pathogens.*

Skill 15-2 (continued)

5. Use toilet paper to clean any fecal material from the perineal area, wiping from front to back. *Safety: Always wash from front to back to prevent contaminating the vaginal and urethral areas with E. coli.*

6. Dampen the washcloth and apply soap or periwash. Make the washcloth into a mitt as in the procedure for a complete bed bath (see Skill 15-1).

7. Spread the patient's labia with your nondominant hand and use a different part of the washcloth to clean the far side, near side, and middle of the vulva, washing from front to back. Continue to wash the outer labia and perineum until clean.

For a Male Patient

3. Place the bath blanket over the patient's chest and fold the bed linens down to expose the perineal area.

4. If the patient is uncircumcised, retract the foreskin. Wipe in a circular motion from the tip of the penis around the glans. Repeat using another area of the washcloth. Rinse and pat dry. Replace the foreskin. *Safety: It is necessary to replace the foreskin to prevent constriction of circulation and possible edema and necrosis of the glans penis.*

5. If the patient is circumcised, wipe in a circular motion from the tip of the penis around the glans. Repeat using another area of the washcloth. Rinse and pat dry.

6. Rinse washcloth and reapply soap or periwash.

7. Wash shaft of the penis and scrotum. Rinse and pat dry.

For Both Male and Female Patients

8. Assess skin for excoriation or maceration. *If the patient is incontinent, the skin may break down due to exposure to urine and feces.*

9. If the patient has a catheter, clean as above, then use the washcloth to gently wipe the catheter from the insertion site away from the body. *Safety: Hold the catheter so no traction is placed on the tubing as you wash to prevent causing trauma to the urethra.*

10. Turn the patient to the side and clean the rectal area if you are not continuing a complete bed bath. Again, wash from front to back, rinse, and pat dry (see Skill 15-1).

11. Change the linens and bed protector as needed.

12. Follow the Ending Implementation Steps located on the inside back cover.

Evaluation Steps

1. Evaluate the patient's skin condition and frequency of incontinence.

2. Evaluate the need for skin barrier cream such as Desitin ointment.

3. Evaluate the patient's tolerance of the procedure. Did it cause shortness of breath, pain, or fatigue?

Sample Documentation

Personal care is often not documented except on a flow sheet. If abnormal findings are present, they are documented in the nurse's notes as shown below.

9/17/10   1440   *Incontinent of urine and sm amt pasty brown stool. Perineal care completed. No redness, excoriation, or maceration noted. ———————— Nurse's signature and credentials*

Skill 15-3 Administering a Back Massage

Assessment Steps

1. Review the patient's diagnoses for contraindications to back massage, such as heart conditions, bradycardia, pulmonary emboli, and musculoskeletal disorders or fractures of the ribs and vertebrae.

2. Inspect the skin for rashes or lesions. Avoid massaging over open areas or rashes.

Planning Steps

1. Gather needed equipment and supplies: skin lotion or oil and a towel.

Implementation Steps

1. Follow the Initial Implementation Steps located on the inside front cover.

2. Position the patient on his or her side or stomach and untie gown *to provide access to the full back.*

3. Apply lotion or oil to your hands to warm it and to avoid startling the patient by applying it directly to the back.

4. Place your hands on either side of the spine at the patient's waist with your palms and fingers flat.

5. Rub gently with continuous pressure up to the neck. With fingers flat against the patient's skin and moving in large circles, stroke from the neck to the waist.

6. Repeat Steps 3 and 4 three times, covering all of the area of the back from the spine outward.
   Safety: Do not massage directly over vertebrae to prevent possible injury to the patient.

7. Use consistent pressure that is comfortable to the patient. *Too much pressure can cause pain or discomfort. Too little pressure can tickle the patient.*

8. Massage from the neck to the shoulder, keeping your fingers flat and sliding them down the side of the neck and along the trapezius muscle. Repeat on the other side. Note muscular tightness in this area and repeat strokes to relax the tightness.

9. Apply lotion again to reduce friction on the skin.

10. Use the sides of the thumbs, alternating between the left and right thumb, to massage around each scapula. You should feel the discreet edges of the bone without tight muscle or your thumbs bumping over muscle attachments. If this is felt, work gently but firmly over the areas to try to release them. Do not work so deep as to cause pain or discomfort to the patient.

11. Massage with the sides of the thumbs from near the spine outward, alternating between your left and right thumb to cover from the low back to the shoulder. Repeat on the other side.

12. Massage over the low back in small circles using the flat part of your fingers.

13. Massage with long strokes from the low back to the neck with your hands flat. Then make large circles outward on either side of the spine, moving back down to the low back. Repeat three times.

14. Wipe off any excess lotion or oil.

15. Follow the Ending Implementation Steps located on the inside back cover.

Evaluation Steps

1. Evaluate your patient's level of relaxation and comfort. Offer to lower the lights and provide quiet for rest after massage.

2. Evaluate the need to work on a particular area further if the patient complains of continued tightness.

Sample Documentation

Personal care is often not documented except on a flow sheet. If abnormal findings are present, they are documented in the nurse's notes as shown below.

9/17/10 2140 *Back massage given. Pink area noted on L scapula, which disappeared after massage. States she is "relaxed and ready to sleep."*
—————————————————————— *Nurse's signature and credentials*

Skill 15-4 Administering Oral Care for an Unconscious Patient

Assessment Steps

1. Assess the condition of the mouth to see if there are any bridges, dentures, broken teeth, or lesions.

2. Assess gag reflex by placing a tongue blade on the back of the tongue. If gag reflex is present, it is safe to proceed. If gag reflex is not present, do not put liquids in the patient's mouth. Use only sponge swabs to clean the lips, mouth, and tongue.

Planning Steps

1. Determine the type of oral care devices to use.

2. Gather needed equipment and supplies: sponge swabs, towel, suction equipment, padded tongue blade, bed protector, emesis basin, water or dilute mouthwash, and irrigation syringe.

Skill 15-4 (continued)

3. Determine the need for personal protective equipment. Obtain gloves and mask with face shield and gown if there is risk of splashing of body fluids.

Implementation Steps

1. Follow the Initial Implementation Steps located on the inside front cover.

2. Put the bed in the flat position unless contraindicated.

3. Turn the patient on his or her side with a bed protector and towel under the head and the emesis basin at the cheek. *Safety: Attach the oral suction device to the suction tubing. Turn on the wall suction to "regular," not "intermittent," and test it to be sure it is in working order.*

4. Moisten the sponge swab with a small amount of water and squeeze out excess *to prevent aspiration of water.*

5. Insert the padded tongue blade and turn it vertically between the teeth to hold the mouth open. *It is a natural reflex to bite down when something is placed in the mouth.*

6. Use the sponge swabs or a soft toothbrush with a small amount of toothpaste to brush all surfaces of the teeth and tongue. Use the swabs to clean between the cheeks and gums where mucus may collect. Use separate swabs for different parts of the mouth *to prevent cross-contamination.*

7. Irrigate the mouth with approximately 10 mL of water or dilute mouthwash using the irrigation syringe. Allow the fluid to drain into the emesis basin or suction it out if necessary.

8. Apply water-soluble lip balm to the lips. *Safety: Do not apply petroleum-based products to lips. If the patient is on oxygen, it can cause burns. If the patient aspirates it, it can cause pneumonia.*

9. Remove the basin and dry the patient's face. Empty and rinse the basin and toothbrush if used. Return to appropriate storage location. Dispose of sponge swabs in biohazard trash.

10. Follow the Ending Implementation Steps located on the inside back cover.

Evaluation Steps

1. Evaluate the cleanliness of the patient's teeth and mouth. Examine the condition of the mouth after care for evidence of trauma or bleeding.

2. Evaluate the need to provide oral care more frequently due to mouth breathing and drying of mucous membranes.

Sample Documentation

Personal care is often not documented except on a flow sheet. If abnormal findings are present, they are documented in the nurse's notes as shown below.

9/17/10 0815 Oral care given. Gag reflex intact. 1-cm red area with 1-mm yellow center noted on left cheek. Physician notified.
——————————————— *Nurse's signature and credentials*

Skill 15-5 Administering Oral Care for a Conscious Patient

Assessment Steps

1. Assess the mouth for lesions, broken teeth, gum disease, sordes, and color of mucous membranes.

2. Ask the patient about his or her usual oral care. Does the patient use mouthwash, floss, or whitening products?

Planning Steps

1. Gather needed equipment and supplies: toothbrush, toothpaste, dental floss, emesis basin, towel, drinking glass, water, and mouthwash if desired.

2. Determine the need for personal protective equipment. Obtain gloves and mask with face shield and gown if there is risk of splashing of body fluids.

Implementation Steps

1. Follow the Initial Implementation Steps located on the inside front cover.

2. Assist the patient to sit upright in a chair or the bed.

3. Place emesis basin, water in glass, toothbrush, and toothpaste on the over-the-bed table.

4. Place a towel across the patient's chest.

5. Moisten the toothbrush in the water and apply a pea-sized amount of toothpaste on the toothbrush.

6. Hold the emesis basin under the patient's chin, or have the patient do this if he or she is able.

7. If the patient is able to brush his or her teeth, hand the patient the toothbrush and stay near in case he or she needs assistance or becomes choked.

(skill continues on page 300)

Skill 15-5 (continued)

8. If the patient is unable to brush his or her own teeth, begin brushing by holding the bristles at a 45-degree angle to the teeth. Brush in small circles over all the inner and outer tooth surfaces. *Safety: Allow the patient to spit out mouth contents as often as needed to prevent choking. Have suction apparatus available if aspiration is a concern.*

9. Brush the biting and chewing surfaces of the teeth in a back-and-forth motion.

10. Ask the patient to stick out the tongue and gently brush it to remove debris. *This makes it less likely to stimulate the gag reflex when you brush the tongue. Food and bacteria on the tongue are the usual cause of bad breath.*

11. Hand the patient the glass of water for rinsing the mouth.

12. Assist the patient to floss between the teeth. Use 6 to 10 inches of dental floss. Wrap the ends around the middle fingers of each hand or use a floss holder.

13. Slide the floss between the teeth and move back up. Avoid going too forcefully and injuring the gums. Bend the floss around each tooth to floss all sides.

14. Offer diluted mouthwash if desired.

15. Assist the patient to wipe the mouth with the towel. Remove, empty, and clean the toothbrush and emesis basin. Return them to the appropriate storage area.

16. Moisturize the lips.

17. Follow the Ending Implementation Steps located on the inside back cover.

Evaluation Steps

1. Evaluate how the patient tolerated the procedure. Did the patient complain of pain, fatigue, or shortness of breath?

2. Evaluate the appearance of the teeth and gums. Are they clean, and is the mouth fresh?

3. Evaluate for any trauma or bleeding due to brushing teeth or possible gum disease.

Sample Documentation

Personal care is often not documented except on a flow sheet. If abnormal findings are present, they are documented in the nurse's notes as shown below.

9/17/10 0815 *Assisted with oral care. Able to rinse own mouth but not brush teeth. Gums pink and mucous membranes moist and pink. C/O fatigue at end of procedure.* ————————
——————————— *Nurse's signature and credentials*

Skill 15-6 Providing Denture Care

Assessment Steps

1. Determine the type of dentures the patient wears. Are they full plates or partials? Upper and lower plates?

2. Inspect the inside of the mouth for lesions or evidence of poorly fitting dentures.

3. Inspect dentures for cracks, or loose or broken teeth.

Planning Steps

1. Gather needed equipment and supplies: denture cup, toothbrush, toothpaste or denture cream, towel, mouthwash if desired, and gauze 4x4s.

2. Determine the need for personal protective equipment. Obtain gloves. Also obtain a mask with face shield and gown if there is risk of splashing of body fluids.

Implementation Steps

1. Follow the Initial Implementation Steps located on the inside front cover.

2. Line the sink with a towel *to prevent damage if dentures accidentally slip.*

3. Don gloves. *Safety: You will be exposed to body fluids that could contain pathogens.*

4. Remove the upper dentures by using a gauze 4x4 to grasp them. *The gauze keeps the dentures from slipping in your gloved hands.*

5. Rock the dentures gently from side to side to loosen, then pull them down and out. If necessary, place one gloved finger above the upper plate against the gum and press downward to break the suction so you can remove the dentures.

Skill 15-6 (continued)

6. Remove the lower plate by grasping it with a gauze 4x4 and lifting up and out.

7. Place the dentures in a denture cup and take to the sink.

8. Rinse with cool water. *Hot water can damage or warp dentures.*

9. Squeeze a small amount of toothpaste or denture cream onto the toothbrush.

10. Brush the tooth surfaces and all other surfaces of the upper dentures. Repeat for the lower dentures. *Food can become trapped between the gums and the dentures, so all surfaces must be thoroughly cleaned.*

11. Rinse the dentures again with cool water. Do not dry them because *dentures are easier to insert if they are moist.*

12. Have the patient rinse his or her mouth with water or dilute mouthwash *to remove any food trapped between the gums and the cheeks.*

13. Apply denture adhesive to the inner surfaces of the plates if the patient wishes.

14. Replace the upper denture by sliding it into the mouth and pushing up with the thumb on the palate of the denture to obtain a good seal.

15. Replace the lower denture by tilting it slightly, sliding it into the mouth, and pressing it gently downward into place.

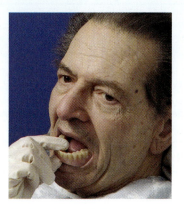

16. Place the towel in the dirty laundry and return the denture cup, toothbrush, and toothpaste to the bedside stand.

17. Follow the Ending Implementation Steps located on the inside back cover.

To Store Dentures for the Night

Follow the steps above to remove and clean the dentures. Place them in the denture cup and cover them with cool water. If the patient wishes, place a denture tablet in the water first and allow it to dissolve, then add the dentures. Assist the patient to rinse his or her mouth with water or dilute mouthwash.

Evaluation Steps

1. Evaluate the condition of the patient's mouth without the dentures. Were there any lesions or reddened areas?

2. Evaluate the dentures themselves. Are they in good repair? Does the patient need to consult a dentist?

Sample Documentation

Personal care is often not documented except on a flow sheet. If abnormal findings are present, they are documented in the nurse's notes as shown below.

09/17/10   1020   *Dentures removed, cleaned, and placed in denture cup for the night. Dark pink crusted area noted at the left corner of the mouth. Denies pain or discomfort.* ————
————————————————— *Nurse's signature and credentials*

Skill 15-7 Shaving a Male Patient

Assessment Steps

1. Assess the beard area for lesions, eczema, or ingrown whiskers.

2. Determine the type of razor to use. Check the chart to see if the patient is on anticoagulants. If that is the case, you must use an electric razor.

Planning Steps

1. Gather needed equipment and supplies: disposable razor, shaving cream, towel, washcloth, basin of water, and aftershave if desired *or* the patient's electric razor with cleaning tools, preshave lotion, and aftershave if desired.

2. Determine the need for personal protective equipment. Obtain gloves. Also obtain a mask with face shield and gown if there is risk of splashing of body fluids.

Implementation Steps

1. Follow the Initial Implementation Steps located on the inside front cover.

For Using a Disposable Razor

2. Fill the basin with warm water. Moisten the washcloth and place it on the beard for 1 to 2 minutes. *This helps soften the beard and lift the whiskers.*

3. Apply a liberal amount of shaving cream to your hand. Spread the cream over the patient's beard and moustache area.

4. Rinse and dry your hands.

5. Don gloves. *Safety: You will be exposed to body fluids that could contain pathogens.*

6. Remove the cover from the disposable razor. Begin shaving on the cheeks. Shave in the direction of hair growth *to prevent irritation and ingrown hairs.*

(skill continues on page 302)

Skill 15-7 (continued)

7. Shave the moustache area if patient desires. Have the patient pull his upper lip over his teeth *to increase access to the area between the nose and lip.*

8. Shave chin from lower lip downward. Use caution shaving the contour of the chin as it is easy to nick.

9. Shave the neck in an upward direction *to prevent causing ingrown hairs or irritation to the skin.*

10. Wipe the patient's face with a wet washcloth. Pat dry with towel. Check for any missed areas and touch up if needed.

11. Apply aftershave lotion if desired.

12. Follow the Ending Implementation Steps located on the inside back cover.

For Using an Electric Razor

2. Apply preshave lotion *to lift the whiskers.*

3. Turn the razor on and shave the cheeks using a circular motion. You may need to go over an area more than one time.

4. Shave the moustache area in a downward motion.

5. Shave the neck in a circular upward motion *to prevent causing ingrown hairs or irritation to the skin.*

6. Apply aftershave lotion if desired.

7. Clean the razor by removing the head and brushing out debris with the small brush supplied with the razor. Replace the head and return the razor to the appropriate storage area.

8. Follow the Ending Implementation Steps located on the inside back cover.

Evaluation Steps

1. Evaluate the closeness of the shave. Is there razor burn or nicks?

Documentation

Personal care is often not documented except on a flow sheet. If abnormal findings are present, they are documented in the nurse's notes.

Skill 15-8 Providing Nail Care

Assessment Steps

1. Assess the condition of the nails: the length, redness around nails, splitting or cracking of nails, thickness or discoloration.

2. Review the chart for a diagnosis of diabetes or peripheral vascular disease. *Safety: For these diagnoses, file nails only. Do not clip or cut due to the risk of damaging tissue that might not heal.*

Planning Steps

1. Gather needed equipment and supplies: a basin with warm water, an orangewood stick, lotion, nail clippers, and an emery board.

2. Plan to do nail care for both hands and feet unless it is contraindicated.

3. Determine the need for personal protective equipment. Obtain gloves if needed. Also obtain a mask with face shield and gown if there is risk of splashing of body fluids.

Intervention Steps

1. Follow the Initial Implementation Steps located on the inside front cover.

For Fingernails

2. Assist the patient to sit up in bed or a chair.

3. Place the patient's hands in the basin of warm water one at a time for 5 minutes to soak and soften the nails and cuticles. Perform nail care on the first hand after it has soaked, while the other hand is soaking.

4. Have the patient lay his or her hands on the towel spread on the over-the-bed table.

5. Using the pointed end of the orangewood stick, clean beneath the nails. Use the flatter end to push back the cuticles.

6. Clip the nails (unless contraindicated) straight across. *Nails that are rounded are more likely to ingrow.*

7. Use the emery board to file the corners *so they are not sharp to prevent scratching.*

8. Apply lotion to the patient's hands and forearms and massage into the skin.

For Toenails

2. Assist the patient to bend the knees and soak the feet in the basin one at a time for 5 minutes. Perform nail care on the first foot after it has soaked, while the other foot is soaking.

3. Place a towel on the bed and have the patient put his or her foot on the towel.

4. Clip the toenails (unless contraindicated) straight across. File straight across with an emery board to prevent scratching.

Skill 15-8 (continued)

5. Dry the feet well, paying special attention to the areas between the toes *to prevent maceration of the skin.*

6. Apply lotion to the feet but not between the toes.

7. Clean and return equipment to its appropriate storage location.

8. Follow the Initial Implementation Steps located on the inside back cover.

Evaluation Steps

1. Evaluate the appearance of the fingernails and toenails. Are there any ingrown nails or infected or inflamed areas? Report as appropriate.

2. Evaluate the effectiveness of the nail care. Does the patient need to be seen by a podiatrist?

Sample Documentation

Personal care is often not documented except on a flow sheet. If abnormal findings are present, they are documented in the nurse's notes as shown below.

09/17/10   1530   *Nail care given for hands and feet. Left foot has 2-mm reddened area between 2nd and 3rd toes. Physician notified.* —————————— *Nurse's signature and credentials*

Skill 15-9 Shampooing Hair With the Patient in Bed

Assessment Steps

1. Check hair for mats, tangles, and any scalp lesions.

2. Review the chart for any contraindications to shampooing the hair in bed, such as a head or neck injury. In that case, chose to use a rinse-free product instead.

Planning Steps

1. Gather needed equipment and supplies: shampoo board or inflatable head cradle, shampoo, water for rinsing in a bag with a nozzle or in a basin with a pitcher, towels, washcloth, bed protectors, plastic trash bag, trash can to contain water.

2. Ask the patient's preference in how to shampoo and products to use.

3. Determine the need for personal protective equipment. Obtain gloves if needed.

Implementation Steps

1. Follow the Initial Implementation Steps located on the inside front cover.

2. Assist the patient to the supine position (lying on back) with the bed flat unless contraindicated.

3. Comb through hair to remove tangles.

4. Place a plastic trash bag inside the trash can if you are using a shampoo board. Position the trash can to receive the water from the sleeve of the board. If you are using an inflatable head cradle, place the plastic trash bag beneath the cradle to protect the bed.

5. Place bed protectors beneath the patient's head and shoulders after removing the pillow. Place a rolled towel at the patient's neck and pad well if using a shampoo board.

6. Position the shampoo board or cradle beneath the patient's head and neck.

7. Fill the basin or bag with warm (105°F) water.

8. Give the patient the washcloth to hold over the eyes during the procedure *to prevent shampoo or water from getting in the eyes.*

9. Use a pitcher or the bag with the nozzle to wet the hair thoroughly.

10. Apply a small amount of shampoo to your hands and rub it through the hair, lathering well.

11. Massage the scalp with your fingertips during shampooing *to stimulate circulation in the scalp.*

12. Rinse with the pitcher or bag with nozzle. Rinse thoroughly *to prevent itching.*

13. Apply conditioner if desired by the patient. Rinse out if appropriate.

14. Remove the board or cradle and wrap the hair in a towel. Blot the hair dry, do not rub it. *Rubbing hair and scalp with a towel can cause breakage of hair.*

15. Comb gently through the hair. Remove tangles by working from the ends of the hair toward the scalp *to prevent pulling.*

16. Use a hair dryer if desired by the patient, or allow to air dry. Style according to the patient's wishes.

(skill continues on page 304)

Skill 15-9 (continued)

17. Remove towels, empty the water from the trash can or inflatable cradle, and replace all equipment.
18. Follow the Ending Implementation Steps located on the inside back cover.

Evaluation Steps

1. Evaluate the condition of the scalp and hair. It should be soft and clean without flakes or oil.
2. Evaluate how the patient tolerated the activity. Did it cause fatigue, pain, or shortness of breath?

Sample Documentation
Personal care is often not documented except on a flow sheet. If abnormal findings are present, they are documented in the nurse's notes as shown below.

09/17/10   2045   *Hair shampooed, rinsed, and dried. Bedrest maintained. Tolerated activity but became SOB as hair was being dried.* ———————— *Nurse's signature and credentials*

Skill 15-10 Making an Unoccupied Bed

Assessment Steps

1. Assess the patient's ability to be out of bed during the linen change. Review the chart for activity level.
2. Determine linens needed for the bed change.

Planning Steps

1. Plan to change linens when the patient will be out of bed, either sitting up in a chair or off of the unit for therapy or a procedure.
2. Gather needed equipment and supplies: mattress pad (if needed), fitted sheet, draw sheet, bed protector (if in use), flat sheet, blanket or spread (if needed), pillowcase, and laundry bag or hamper.
3. Determine the need for personal protective equipment. Obtain gloves if needed.

Implementation Steps

1. Follow the Initial Implementation Steps located on the inside front cover.
2. Remove the spread or blanket. If it is not soiled, fold it carefully and place it over the back of a chair to be put back on the bed. If it is soiled, place it in the laundry hamper or bag.
3. Fold soiled top linens to the center of the bed. Check for any personal belongings that might have been left in the bed, such as glasses, a gown, or a book.
4. Loosen fitted bottom sheet and fold it to the middle of the bed. Remove the pillow from the pillowcase and place the pillow in a chair.
5. Place all soiled linen in a laundry bag or hamper. *Safety: Do not allow the soiled linens to touch your scrubs to prevent contamination.* NEVER put soiled linen on the floor *because this spreads microorganisms.*
6. If the mattress is damp or soiled due to incontinence, spray with a disinfectant spray and wipe with a clean washcloth *to prevent contaminating the clean linens.*
7. Unfold the fitted bottom sheet to cover the half of the mattress closest to you, and slide the corners over the mattress corners.
8. Unfold the draw sheet and center it so that it will cover an area from the patient's shoulders to his or her knees. *This keeps the patient centered on the draw sheet for turning and moving.*
9. Tuck the draw sheet between the mattress and springs.

10. Go to the other side of the bed and spread the bottom sheet over the remainder of the bed. Slide the corners over the corners of the mattress.
11. Spread the draw sheet across the bed. Grasp the draw sheet in the middle and pull tightly across and down. Tuck it between the mattress and the springs. Grasp the draw sheet near the upper edge, pull, and tuck. Repeat near the lower edge of the draw sheet.
12. Unfold the top sheet to cover the half of the mattress closest to you. *This keeps you from walking around the bed several times during the procedure, conserving your energy.* Ensure that the seams (rough edge of hem) are up, or away from the patient, *to prevent scratching of the patient by the rough edges.*
13. Unfold the blanket or spread to cover the half of the mattress closest to you. Position so that the blanket is approximately 4 inches below the top edge of the flat sheet *to make a cuff over the rough edges of the blanket.*
14. Tuck blanket and sheet together under the foot of the bed, between the mattress and the springs. *This prevents you from loosening the sheet when you tuck the blanket separately.*

Skill 15-10 (continued)

15. Make a mitered corner by grasping the sheet and blanket together at a 45-degree angle to the foot of the bed. Lay the angled portion on the bed and tuck the lower edge of the blanket and sheet under the mattress. Then let the angled portion of the blanket and sheet hang freely. You should have a tight, slanted corner at 45 degrees from the end of the mattress. *This keeps the sheet and blanket from pulling out as the patient moves and turns.*

16. Repeat Steps 13-15 on the other side of the bed.
17. Cuff the top sheet over the blanket at the head of the bed. All seams and rough edges should be away from the patient.
18. Replace the pillowcase by holding the pillow lengthwise and pinching the bottom corners together. Slide the pillow into the case while it is lying on the bed. Release the corners when they are aligned with the pillowcase corners. *This prevents you from holding the pillow next to your scrubs or under your chin, which could cause contamination.*

19. Place the pillow so that the opening of the pillowcase is away from the door.

For an Open Bed
Follow Steps 1-19 above, then fanfold the top linens to the foot of the bed *to make it easier for the patient to get into the bed.*

20. Assist the patient into bed and ensure comfort.
21. Follow the Ending Implementation Steps located on the inside back cover.

For a Surgical Bed
Follow Steps 1-13 above, then fanfold the top linens to the side of the bed away from the door. *This allows a patient returning on a stretcher to be easily moved into the bed.* Once the patient is in the bed, you will tuck in the top sheet and blanket together at the foot of the bed and make mitered corners at each side.

14. Assist the patient into bed and ensure comfort.
15. Follow the Ending Implementation Steps located on the inside back cover.

Evaluation Steps

1. Evaluate the bed for smooth, tight linens and corners.

Documentation

This type of information is generally documented only on a flow sheet.

Skill 15-11 Making an Occupied Bed

Assessment Steps

1. Review the patient's chart for activity level. Those on bedrest will need an occupied bed change.

2. Assess the patient's ability to remain on his or her side while you change the bed.

Planning Steps

1. Determine if another staff member is needed to help during the bed change. It is not uncommon for this procedure to take two staff members.

2. Gather needed equipment and supplies: fitted sheet, draw sheet, bed protector (if in use), flat sheet, blanket or spread, pillowcase, and laundry bag or hamper.

3. Determine the need for personal protective equipment. Obtain gloves if needed.

Implementation Steps

1. Follow the Initial Implementation Steps located on the inside front cover.

2. Remove the spread or blanket. If it is not soiled, fold it and place it over the back of a chair to be put back on the bed. If it is soiled, place it in the laundry hamper or bag.

3. Leave the top sheet in place unless it is soiled. If it is soiled, replace it with a bath blanket and place it in the laundry hamper or bag.

4. Assist the patient to move to the far side of the bed and to turn away from you. *Safety: Be sure that the far side rail is up to prevent the patient from falling.*

5. Ensure that no tubes or wires are tangled in the linens.

6. Lower the side rail closest to you and loosen the bottom linens. Tightly fold the linens toward the patient and tuck them next to him or her.

7. Unfold the clean fitted sheet and slip the corners over the mattress corners. Unfold the draw sheet and tuck it under the mattress, positioning it from the patient's shoulders to his or her knees. *This keeps the patient centered on the draw sheet for turning and moving.*

8. Fanfold the fitted sheet and draw sheet toward the patient. Tuck them beneath the tightly folded soiled linens. *Safety: If there is a danger that the soiled linens are wet or could contaminate the clean ones, place a towel or waterproof pad between the clean and dirty linens.*

9. Put up the side rail and assist the patient to turn to the other side of the bed. Warn the patient that he or she will be rolling over the "hump" of both clean and used linens. Place the pillow beneath his or her head for comfort.

10. Go to the other side of the bed and lower the side rail. Pull the soiled linen off of the bed and put it in the laundry bag or hamper. *Safety: Do not allow the soiled linens to touch your scrubs to prevent contamination.* NEVER put soiled linen on the floor *because this spreads microorganisms.*

11. Spread the fitted sheet and draw sheet across the bed. Slip the corners over the mattress corners. Smooth the draw sheet by grasping the middle and pulling tightly across and down. Tuck it between the mattress and springs. Repeat with the top and bottom edges of the draw sheet. *This helps make a tight bed with fewer wrinkles, which is more comfortable for the patient.*

12. Assist the patient to turn onto his or her back in the center of the bed.

13. Unfold the clean top sheet so it is centered on the bed. Be sure the seams are away from the patient.

14. Remove the bath blanket by pulling it from beneath the clean top sheet. Put it in the laundry bag or hamper and avoid touching it to your scrubs.

15. Replace the blanket or spread so it is centered on the bed and the top edge is approximately 4 inches lower than the top edge of the sheet.

16. Tuck the sheet and blanket together at the foot of the bed. Make a mitered corner (see Skill 15-10).

17. Go to the other side of the bed and tuck the sheet and blanket together at the foot of the bed. Make a mitered corner.

Skill 15-11 (continued)

18. Grasp the top linens over the patient's feet and pull up approximately 3 inches. *This prevents plantar flexion of the foot leading to footdrop.*

19. Cuff the top sheet over the edge of the blanket *to prevent any rough edges from being against the patient's skin.*

20. Change the pillowcase (see Skill 15-10), and replace the pillow.

21. Ensure that the patient is comfortable.

22. Follow the Ending Implementation Steps located on the inside back cover.

Evaluation Steps

1. Evaluate the patient's level of comfort in the bed. Is it free of wrinkles?

2. Evaluate the patient's tolerance of the procedure. Are there any complaints of pain, fatigue, or shortness of breath?

Documentation

Personal care is often not documented except on a flow sheet. If abnormal findings are present, they are documented in the nurse's notes.

Post Conference

As you attended post conference after clinicals, you thought about all the things you learned about your patient during her bath today. She really opened up to you about some of her health problems and concerns. In fact, she was thrilled to have you take care of her today and was not upset at all that you were a male nursing student. Also, during the bath, you noticed a fine raised rash on her back that you showed to your instructor. It turned out to be a reaction to an antibiotic that could have gotten much worse if you had not noticed it. When you evaluate your nursing actions, you feel good about caring for this patient and meeting her needs, even the most basic needs of bathing and grooming. You do not at all feel that you wasted your valuable time by bathing this patient.

KEY POINTS

- Providing personal care for patients gives you the unique chance to make multiple observations about their skin, hair, and mouth as well as an unparalleled opportunity to establish the nurse-patient relationship.

- When you plan personal care, it is extremely important to learn about the patients' preferences regarding timing of care, their cultural influences, and their capabilities to assist with care.

- There are many ways to bathe patients, from a complete bed bath for a helpless patient to a shower with minimal assistance. Different types of baths require various amounts of participation on the part of the patient. It is the nurse's responsibility to know the appropriate way to bathe a patient based on each person's individual needs.

- Back massage has many benefits for the patient, including promoting relaxation, relieving muscle tension, and stimulation circulation. Back massage is far more than rubbing lotion on a patient's back. Nurses should make every effort to provide this care for their patients.

- When you provide oral care for unconscious patients, it is very important to prevent aspiration. Keep the patient positioned on the side during oral care and be prepared to use suction to remove fluids if it is necessary.

- Assess the hair and scalp for contagious conditions such as tinea capitus (ringworm) and lice. Give special care for the hair of African American patients, both in combing and in shampooing.

- Expect to care for patients with body piercings. Be prepared to remove jewelry from piercings only if necessary due to infection or possible interference with surgery, intubation, catheterization, or diagnostic testing.

- Nurses may need to remove, clean, and insert contact lenses, ocular prostheses, and hearing aids, and need to know the steps involved in each procedure.

- Minimizing negative aspects of the patient's environment such as odor, noise, and clutter as well as providing clean, fresh bed linens is a valuable part of patient care.

REVIEW QUESTIONS

Select the answer that is most appropriate for each of the following questions. Some questions may have more than one correct answer. Check all that apply.

1. The circulatory effect of venous return is accomplished by bathing:

   a. the back along the trapezius muscles.

   b. the extremities in a distal-to-proximal direction.

   c. the arm furthest away from you first, then the nearer arm.

   d. the extremities in a proximal-to-distal direction.

2. The staff nurse says that your patient refused her bath yesterday and really needs one today. The patient says she is too exhausted to have a bed bath and just wants to sleep. Your best response would be:

   a. "That's fine. Sleep is more important than a bath anyway."

   b. "I will do your bath first, then you will sleep better."

   c. "I have other patients to care for, so we need to do your bath now."

   d. "You rest now and I will come back in about an hour to do your bath."

3. You are giving evening care to your patient. What care will you provide?

   a. Assist with toileting.

   b. Give a warm, wet washcloth for washing hands and face.

   c. Change the gown.

   d. Offer a back massage.

   e. Straighten the linens and get an extra blanket.

   f. Brush or comb hair.

   g. Remove glasses, dentures, and hearing aids.

   h. Ensure that needed items for the night are within reach.

4. In which situations would it be inappropriate for the nurse to delegate the patient's personal care to a CNA or UAP?

   a. A patient whose vital signs are unstable

   b. A patient who required total care

   c. A patient whose capabilities to assist with personal care are unknown

   d. A patient who is from a different culture

   e. A patient who has a worsening skin condition

5. You know a patient with diabetes needs more teaching about nail care when he says:

   a. "My daughter can cut my toenails so they are rounded without any sharp edges."

   b. "I won't clip my toenails anymore. I will just file them."

   c. "Any reddened area on my feet can be a problem, so I will tell the doctor if I see any."

   d. "I don't want to risk even a small cut on my toes or feet."

CRITICAL THINKING EXERCISES

6. A patient is returning from the cardiac catheterization laboratory and has orders to keep his leg straight for several hours. Because of this, he cannot sit up or bend at the groin. Which type of bed will you make for him, and what bed position would be most appropriate?

7. You are giving special mouth care to a semiconscious patient. She keeps biting down on the toothbrush. What action will you take?

8. A patient with severe respiratory disease becomes very short of breath. What environmental issues could contribute to this situation?

9. A CNA that you supervise tells you that a female patient from India refuses to take a bath. The CNA whispers to you that the patient has strong body odor and needs to shave her armpits. How will you handle this situation?

ADDITIONAL RESOURCES

For additional Resources, Questions, and Activities, please see:

 Student Resource Disk

 http://davisplus.fadavis.com

 Student Study Guide

REFERENCES

Boyles S. Plain soap as good as antibacterial. *WebMD Health News* [serial online]. August 17, 2007. Available at: http://www.webmd.com/news/20070817/plain-soap-as-good-as-antibacterial. Accessed March 10, 2008.

Clark AP. Nosocomial infections and bath water: any cause for concern? *Clin Nurse Specialist.* 2006;3:119-123.

Flori L. Healthier Aging: Don't throw in the towel: tips for bathing a patient who has dementia. *Nursing2007.* 2007;37(7):22-23.

Huiras R. Piercing prognosis. *NurseWeek Heartland Ed.* 2007;May/June.

Mager & Gougleman, Inc. Eye care. Available at: http://www.artificial-eyes.com/eye_care.htm. Accessed March 20, 2008.

Meneses M, Castillo DH. Our magnetic moments: the oral care committee, past, present, and future. American Nurses Credentialing Center, My Magnet Story Essay Series. MedScape Web site. March 5, 2008. Available at: http://www.medscape.com/viewarticle/570937. Accessed March 2, 2008.

Olesen EM. Issues in Nursing: Are you too posh to wash? *Nursing2004.* 2004;34(11):57.

Scanlon V, Sanders T. *Essentials of Anatomy and Physiology.* Philadelphia: FA Davis; 2007.

Wilkinson JM, Van Leuven K. *Fundamentals of Nursing: Theory, Concepts & Applications.* Philadelphia: FA Davis; 2007.

Moving and Positioning Patients

Key Terms

Contractures

Dorsiflexion

Footdrop

Fowler's position

Lateral position

Logroll

Orthopneic position

Orthostatic hypotension

Plantar flexion

Position of function

Prone position

Semi-Fowler's position

Shearing

Sims' position

Supine position

Syncope

Transfer

Trochanter roll

Objectives

1. Define key terms associated with moving and positioning patients.
2. Describe the effects of immobility on seven body systems.
3. Enumerate nursing measures to prevent complications of immobility for these body systems.
4. Describe the psychological effects of immobility and nursing measures to prevent psychological complications.
5. Discuss the importance of positioning patients correctly and performing frequent position changes.
6. Identify commonly used patient positions.
7. Explain the purpose of the Handle With Care campaign established by the American Nurses Association.
8. Describe devices available to increase safety and ease of transferring patients.
9. Enumerate guidelines for performing a manual patient transfer.
10. Contrast types of specialty beds and their purposes.
11. Summarize the importance of assisting a patient to dangle prior to transfer or ambulation.

Skills

16-1 Performing Passive Range-of-Motion Exercises

16-2 Positioning Patients

16-3 Moving a Patient Up in Bed

16-4 Turning a Patient in Bed

16-5 Transferring a Patient from Bed to a Stretcher, Chair, or Wheelchair

16-6 Transferring a Patient With a Mechanical Lift

16-7 Assisting a Patient to Dangle

16-8 Assisting With Ambulation

Clinical Connection

Your Assignment: You will be caring for a 56-year-old male patient who is paralyzed in both legs as the result of a spinal cord injury after a motor vehicle accident. He is a patient in the rehab unit. He is unable to turn himself in bed and spends part of each day in a motorized wheelchair. The nurse tells you in report that skin breakdown is a major concern and that he has a Clinitron bed to help prevent it. The nurse also tells you that the patient has had difficulty adjusting psychologically to his limited mobility. As you leave the room, the nurse says, "Come and get me when you are ready to transfer him to the wheelchair. We use a battery-operated lift for him."

Your Actions: You are rather confused after report because you don't know anything about the patient's specialty bed or a battery-operated lift. In fact, it sounds like the patient has far more challenges than you were expecting when you were assigned to work on the rehab unit. And you find yourself wondering how you can help him avoid skin breakdown when he cannot turn or move around in a wheelchair very well.

The human body is intended to move in order for a person to remain healthy, and every organ in the body depends on movement for optimal function. Physiological and psychological changes can result as consequences of immobility. This chapter will help you determine what to do for patients with mobility problems and how to help prevent further complications from immobility.

Effects of Immobility

Immobility occurs as a result of lack of activity and movement, which may occur when a person is ill and less active than usual. When movement is restricted, body systems immediately react—and they continue to react as long as immobility persists. When a patient is placed on prolonged bedrest, for reasons such as coma, multiple trauma, long intensive care stays, severe weakness, and overwhelming infection, even more complications can result. However, it is important to recognize that complications resulting from bedrest and immobility, while numerous, are preventable.

It has been recognized for many years that immobility and prolonged bedrest have adverse affects. As early as 1947, an article about the dangers of immobility was published in the *British Medical Journal.* In 1967, the *American Journal of Nursing* published the often-cited article, "The Hazards of Immobility," detailing the effects of immobility on each body system. Prior to these publications, it was common for medical authorities to prescribe strict bedrest for many days or even weeks. Now we know that, the longer a patient remains inactive, the more his or her chances of developing complications increase. Such complications include:

• Blood clots
• Pneumonia
• Bone demineralization
• Kidney stones
• Constipation
• Pressure ulcers
• Urinary retention
• Depression

You, as a nurse, have an important responsibility for ensuring that the complications resulting from immobility are minimized and for maintaining patient mobility when possible.

Physiological Effects

It is essential that individuals remain active to maintain optimal functioning of all body systems. As a nurse, you will be responsible for anticipating and minimizing the effects of inactivity and immobility on your patients. Table 16-1 summarizes the effects of immobility on various body systems.

Effects of Immobility on the Musculoskeletal System

When a patient is unable to move about, he or she can suffer from *muscle atrophy,* which means that muscle decreases in size, tone, and strength as a result of disuse. Along with the muscle tissue, connective tissue such as ligaments and tendons undergoes structural and functional changes after 4 to 6 days of immobility. These changes lead to decreased joint flexibility, decreased range of motion, and **contractures,** or shortening and tightening of the muscles due to disuse. This is why your muscles feel weak when you have been ill and have remained in bed for several days.

Osteoporosis is a condition that occurs due to loss of bone minerals; it leads to an increased risk of skeletal fractures. Immobility increases the risk of osteoporosis because a lack of activity and weight bearing results in a loss of calcium from the bones. This bone demineralization can begin

Table 16-1 Effects and Complications of Immobility

Body System	Effects of Immobility	Potential Complications
Musculoskeletal system	Decreased muscle strength and muscle mass; shortening and tightening of connective tissue; calcium leaves the bones, resulting in weakness and brittleness	• Muscle atrophy • Footdrop • Contractures • Osteoporosis
Cardiovascular system	Decreased cardiac output; pooling of blood in the extremities, increased cardiac workload	• Orthostatic hypotension • Blood clots in extremities • Blood clots traveling to lungs, heart, and brain
Respiratory system	Decreased respiratory muscle strength and decreased lung expansion; impaired oxygen and carbon dioxide exchange; pooling of respiratory secretions	• Atelectasis • Hypoxemia • Hypostatic pneumonia
Gastrointestinal system	Decreased peristalsis; decreased appetite; increased intestinal gas	• Constipation • Flatulence • Distention
Urinary system	Pooling of urine in the renal pelvis; incomplete emptying of the bladder; increased calcium in the blood to be filtered by the kidneys	• Urinary tract infection • Renal calculi
Integumentary system	Decreased oxygen and nutrients to tissues; skin and capillaries compressed between the bed and bony prominences	• Pressure ulcers
Neurological system	Decreased oxygenated blood circulating to nerves trapped between the bed and bone; decrease in normal cues and activities; decreased balance when initially out of bed	• Compression neuropathy • Impaired level of consciousness • Confusion
Psychological effects	Decrease in normal social interaction; decrease in independent activity	• Depression • Anxiety • Impaired sleep

as early as 2 to 3 days from the onset of immobility. The calcium leaves the bones and enters the bloodstream, placing the patient at an increased risk for kidney stones as the excess calcium in the blood must then be filtered out by the kidneys.

Nursing Measures to Prevent Musculoskeletal Complications

The most basic nursing measure to prevent musculoskeletal complications is to maintain proper body alignment, which means to keep the head, trunk, and hips positioned in a straight line. The legs should be positioned so that the toes always point the same direction as the anterior or ventral side of the body. This is accomplished by preventing the legs from rotating in the hip sockets either medially or laterally. The arms should be maintained in correct alignment with the shoulders and trunk and not allowed to fall forward in a "slump-shouldered" position, which causes the thorax to curve in an unnatural manner. Correct body alignment should be maintained in the supine position, all variations of side-lying positions, and even while sitting. When lying in the supine position, the patient's ankles should be flexed approximately 90 degrees so that the toes point toward the ceiling. This is referred to as **dorsiflexion** of the foot. If the toes are allowed to fall toward the foot of the bed, the proper dorsiflexion of the ankle is lost and permanent plantar flexion of the foot develops, a condition known as **footdrop**. This condition will be discussed further later in this chapter.

One common nursing measure that is used to combat the physiological effects of immobility is the use of *range-of-motion (ROM) exercises,* which are a series of activities designed to move each joint through all of its natural actions. To decrease the incidence of muscle atrophy and contractures, it is necessary to maintain muscle mass and healthy bones. Use these actions to help prevent muscle contractures and osteoporosis:

- Perform ROM exercises every 8 hours to maintain muscle strength and flexibility as well as joint flexibility. These may be active or passive exercises (Box 16-1).
- Ensure that you support the weight of the extremity at the joints during passive ROM exercises (see Skill 16-1, page 327).
- Apply any supportive or therapeutic devices for maintaining proper body alignment, such as a trochanter roll or foot board, correctly and follow orders for their use exactly. A **trochanter roll** is a rolled towel or cylindrical device placed snugly against the lateral aspect of the patient's thigh to prevent the leg from rotating outward. A *foot board* is a board placed at a 90-degree angle to the foot of the bed so the patient's feet will be supported in a normal flexed position to prevent footdrop. It must be placed against the plantar surface of the patient's feet for it to be effective (Fig. 16-1). Some facilities use *footdrop boots,* a splint-like padded device that supports the foot in proper plantar flexion and suspends the heel over a small pocket of air, thereby also reducing the risk of pressure ulcer development on the heel.
- Assist patients out of bed and with ambulation as soon as orders permit to limit the demineralization of bones.

Figure 16-1   A foot board holds the patient's feet in a functional position.

Effects of Immobility on the Cardiovascular System

Bedrest results in a 50% reduction of blood flow to the legs and contributes to *venous stasis,* or pooling of blood in the veins of the lower legs. When a patient is lying down rather than sitting or standing, the heart actually has to work harder to pump blood throughout the body. This is because the muscles in the legs normally contract as you walk, sit, and stand, helping return venous blood from the lower extremities to the heart. When those skeletal muscles are not in use, the heart must work harder to pump blood throughout the body, increasing its workload. This is also a contributing factor to the pooling of blood in the legs, which can lead to blood clots.

When a patient is confined to bed, he or she may develop a blood clot, which may then dislodge and travel through the vein. One type of blood clot is called deep vein thrombosis (DVT), which is a clot that develops in the deep veins of the legs. These types of clots can impair circulation in the limb. Other clots may develop in the more superficial veins of the legs but are less of a threat to limb circulation.

Any stationary clot or clot fragment may dislodge and enter the circulation. It is then referred to as an *embolus,* or a traveling blood clot. The clot breaks away from the vein wall in the leg and travels through the bloodstream. As the embolus travels through the venous system back to the heart and lungs and into the arterial blood flow, there is a risk that it will become lodged in a small arterial capillary that supplies blood to vital organs, such as the lungs, heart, and brain. Once the embolus becomes lodged so that it blocks blood flow to a portion of a vital organ, oxygen and nutrients are prevented from reaching the tissue, resulting in the death of the affected cells. When it occurs in the lungs, it is referred to as a *pulmonary embolus* (PE); in the heart it is known as a *myocardial infarction* (MI), or *heart attack;* and when it occurs in the brain it is termed a *cerebrovascular accident* (CVA), commonly known as a *stroke.* An embolism to any of these three vital organs may result in death. An

Box 16-1

Active Versus Passive Range-of-Motion Exercises

Range-of-motion exercises are used in a variety of situations. They may be active or passive, depending on who is moving the extremity.
- Active range-of-motion exercises are performed by the patient without physical nursing assistance. The nurse may remind or encourage the patient to perform the exercises, but the patient is able to move all extremities independently.
- Passive range-of-motion exercises are done with the nurse performing the exercising of the patient's joints while providing proper support to the patient's extremity. Passive exercises are indicated when a patient is too weak to move his or her own extremities or when one or more extremities are paralyzed.

embolism has been identified as the most preventable cause of death during hospitalization.

Orthostatic hypotension, also known as *postural hypotension,* is a decrease in blood pressure that occurs when a patient changes from a reclining or flat position to an upright position, such as sitting or standing, and is common after being restricted to bedrest. Due to slow or insufficient vasoconstriction once the patient becomes vertical, blood pools in the lower extremities and abdominal organs, which results in a drop in the blood pressure and inadequate circulation to the brain. This can cause the patient to become dizzy, pale, clammy, or nauseated because the blood pressure drops more than normal and the heart rate increases more than normal in an effort to pump blood to the head. If the blood pressure falls too far, the patient may experience **syncope**, or *fainting.* If the patient exhibits any of these signs upon standing, assist him or her to a sitting or reclining position.

The patient is most likely to experience orthostatic hypotension the first few times he or she gets up after a surgery or any other procedure requiring bedrest for several hours. This is why it is extremely important for you, the nurse, to be with any patient the first time he or she gets out of bed. If dizziness or syncope occurs, you will be there to prevent injury to the patient.

Nursing Measures to Prevent Cardiovascular Complications

To prevent the formation of venous thrombosis, it is important to keep the blood from pooling in the legs, where clots most commonly form. To do so, follow these guidelines:

- Encourage movement of the extremities. If the patient is unable to do so, you will perform passive ROM exercises (see Skill 16-1)
- Apply ordered devices to prevent pooling of blood in the legs. These include *antiembolism stockings,* which are close-fitting elastic stockings that usually cover the whole leg, and *sequential compression devices* (SCDs). SCDs are air-filled sleeves that are wrapped around the patient's lower legs and connected to a pump that inflates and deflates each area of the sleeve in a sequence designed to move blood in the legs toward the heart. (See Chapter 33 for more information about antiembolism stockings and SCDs.)

To help decrease the workload of the heart and prevent orthostatic hypotension, it is important to gradually move the patient from a lying position to a sitting or standing position. Use these actions to prevent orthostatic hypotension:

- Encourage movement of the extremities, especially dorsiflexion and plantar flexion of the feet, which will cause muscle contraction that will help push the blood in the veins back to the heart. If the patient is unable to move his or her extremities, perform passive ROM exercises to promote muscular pressure on the veins to assist the flow of blood back to the heart.
- Change the patient's position frequently to improve blood return to the heart from the rest of the body.

- If possible, change the patient's position from horizontal to vertical. Elevate the head of the bed as much as possible or allow the patient to sit in a chair if permissible.
- Remain with the patient the first few times he or she gets out of bed. Follow procedures for assisting the patient to dangle (see Skill 16-7, page 337) before allowing the patient to stand.

Knowledge Connection

Describe an adverse effect on the musculoskeletal system of the patient with limited mobility. Identify two nursing measures to assist in maintaining joint flexibility and muscle strength of the patient with limited mobility. What is orthostatic hypotension?

Effects of Immobility on the Respiratory System

When the patient is unable to move about and take deep breaths, the result is a decrease in lung expansion and respiratory muscle weakness. As an individual rests in bed, he or she tends to take shallow breaths that limit the expansion of the lungs. Pneumonia and *pulmonary emboli,* or blood clots in the lungs, are adverse respiratory conditions that can occur in immobilized patients. They are preventable, so it is extremely important for you to use appropriate nursing measures discussed in this chapter.

Hypostatic pneumonia is a type of lung infection that occurs when a patient is immobile. Secretions pool in the lungs, and the warm, dark, moist environment is ideal for bacterial growth, resulting in an infection. Health care–associate infections (HAIs), once called *nosocomial infections,* are preventable in today's health care settings. (See Chapter 14 for more information on HAIs.) Because such illnesses are preventable, some insurers are refusing to pay costs related to certain HAIs. It is extremely important that you know what to do to prevent such illnesses and utilize your nursing knowledge to be proactive.

Atelectasis, the collapse of lung tissue affecting part or all of a lung, can occur due to the inability of the lung to fully expand. It may also occur when a patient does not take full, deep breaths to keep the alveoli open. When the alveoli collapse, oxygen and carbon dioxide exchange is impaired, resulting in lowered oxygen in the blood, or *hypoxemia.*

Nursing Measures to Prevent Respiratory Complications

To prevent atelectasis and pneumonia, it is necessary to increase lung expansion, strengthen respiratory muscles, improve oxygen and carbon dioxide exchange, and improve the effectiveness of coughs. Use these actions to prevent respiratory secretions from pooling in the lungs:

- Turn the patient from side to side at least every 2 hours to permit lung expansion.
- Elevate the head of the bed 45 degrees or more to promote lung expansion (see Table 16-3 later in this chapter).
- Encourage cough and deep breathing exercises every hour while awake (Box 16-2).

Turning, Deep Breathing, and Coughing

Assisting a patient to turn, deep breathe, and cough is a frequent nursing intervention. This important action helps prevent respiratory and circulatory complications of immobility.

- **Turning:** Turn the patient from side to side at least every 2 hours and make him or her comfortable. This stimulates circulation to help prevent blood clots and prevents stasis of fluids in the lungs.
- **Deep Breathing:** Instruct the patient to take a long, slow, deep breath and hold for 3 seconds, then exhale slowly. This should be repeated at least five times. This serves to expand the lungs and increase gas exchange.
- **Coughing:** Instruct the patient to inhale using long, slow, and deep breaths. Hold for 3 seconds, then cough forcefully on the third or fourth expiration. Repeat at least five times. This also helps to prevent stasis of fluid in the lungs.

- Encourage the patient to use an incentive spirometer, taking 10 to 20 deep breaths every hour to expand the lungs in an attempt to reach a preset level of inspiratory volume (see Chapter 28). An incentive spirometer is a device used to encourage patients to take deep breaths because it provides visual feedback. The spirometer consists of one to three chambers, with a small ball or platform in each one. As the patient inhales, expanding the lungs, it causes the ball or platform in the chamber to rise. The greater the volume of air that is inhaled, the higher the number of balls or platforms that rise, and the further they rise (Fig. 16-2).

Effects of Immobility on the Gastrointestinal System

When patients are not able to be physically active, they may have a decreased appetite. However, because they are healing

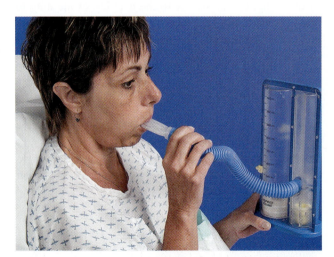

Figure 16-2 A patient using an incentive spirometer to expand her lungs and prevent respiratory complications of immobilization.

from illness or injury, good nutritional intake is extremely important (see Chapter 23). The major effect of immobility on the gastrointestinal system is the lack of *peristalsis,* or natural movement of the intestines. Again, without activity, the smooth muscle of the intestines is less active. This generally results in constipation, flatulence, and distention, and may also cause indigestion and lack of appetite.

When peristalsis slows, food moves more slowly through the gastrointestinal tract, allowing the colon to absorb too much water. When too much water is absorbed from the food, the result is dry, hard feces.

Nursing Measures to Prevent Gastrointestinal Complications

To help prevent constipation, intestinal gas, and lack of appetite, it is important that you encourage appropriate food and fluid intake. Muscle contraction and exercise help to stimulate peristalsis, making it important to ensure as much movement and physical activity as allowed, even when the patient is ordered to be on bedrest. Use these measures to help prevent gastrointestinal discomfort for your patients:

- As soon as the physician's orders allow, assist the patient to get up in a chair or ambulate at least three to four times daily. Encourage the use of a bedside commode or getting up to the bathroom rather than using a bedpan.
- While the patient is on bedrest, ensure that the patient repositions at least every 2 hours and encourage active ROM exercises or provide passive ROM to all joints at least once every 8 hours.
- Place the patient in a sitting position to defecate on the bedpan or bedside commode, allowing gravity to assist in the elimination process. (See Chapter 30 for more information about digestive elimination.)
- Inquire about the patient's food likes and dislikes.
- Help the patient select well-balanced, nutritious meals from the menu.
- Encourage the patient to choose foods with fiber to help prevent constipation. Include fresh fruits and vegetables, raw if possible, to add fiber.
- Encourage fluid intake of 8 ounces or more every 2 hours to help prevent constipation unless the patient is on a fluid restriction. Be sure to offer and bring fluids that the patient likes to drink.
- Instruct the patient to avoid drinking fluids through a straw if intestinal gas is a problem. Each time the patient swallows a sip of fluid, he or she also swallows a strawfull of air.
- Assess and document the activity level of bowel sounds and the frequency and characteristics of bowel movements. (See Chapter 30 for more information on assessing the digestive system.)
- If a patient has not had a bowel movement in 3 days, administer a laxative or enema according to the physician's orders. If there is no order, you need to obtain one. The exception to this situation would be when the patient's normal elimination routine at home is less frequent than every 3 days.

• Provide a laxative or stool softener as needed, according to the physician's orders.

Effects of Immobility on the Urinary System

The patient who is lying in bed is at risk for a urinary tract infection because urine can pool in the renal pelvis of the kidney. Normally urine moves from the renal pelvis into the ureters, and then to the bladder, when the person is upright. Bedrest interferes with this normal movement of urine. In addition, the patient is at risk for developing kidney stones, or renal calculi, because excess calcium in the blood is filtered out by the kidneys.

When a patient must void on a bedpan or use a urinal while remaining in bed, he or she is less likely to completely empty the bladder, resulting in urinary retention. This retained urine provides an excellent medium for bacteria to proliferate, possibly causing a bladder infection that can spread to the remaining urinary tract.

Nursing Measures to Prevent Urinary Complications

To avoid urinary stasis and prevent urinary tract infection and renal calculi, use these measures:

• Provide adequate fluid intake to avoid concentrated urine. Again, offer beverages of the patient's choice and encourage intake of 8 ounces or more every 2 hours unless he or she is on a fluid restriction.
• Assist the patient to urinate in a sitting position to encourage full empting of the urinary bladder. Male patients may be able to urinate best if they are allowed to stand at the bedside. Be sure to obtain a physician's order allowing this activity if the patient is on bedrest.
• Assess the patient's output. He or she should void at least every 8 hours. If the patient who is properly hydrated is unable to void, he or she may need to be catheterized to drain the bladder.

Effects of Immobility on the Integumentary System

When a patient is immobile and consistent pressure is applied to the same area of the body, the blood flow to that area is reduced or is stopped entirely; when this occurs, the skin and underlying tissue dies. This is referred to as a *pressure ulcer,* also called *skin breakdown* or a *decubitus ulcer.* The area may be red at first, but the skin will continue to deteriorate if the circulation to the area does not improve. Shearing of the skin will further destroy the integument. **Shearing** occurs when the skin layer is pulled across muscle and bone in one direction while the skin slides over another surface, such as a bedsheet, in the opposite direction. This shearing and friction on the skin can cause abrasions and open areas.

Patients on prolonged bedrest are especially at risk for developing pressure ulcers. (See Chapter 26 for more information on pressure ulcers.) Special support surfaces and specialty beds have been developed to help alleviate this risk. Air-fluidized beds, low air-loss beds, and combination beds were all designed for this purpose.

It can be difficult to turn patients with multiple trauma and other musculoskeletal conditions. As a result, some beds have been developed that turn from side to side so the patient has less chance of developing respiratory and cardiovascular complications while on bedrest. Table 16-2 provides information about different types of support surfaces and specialty beds.

Nursing Measures to Prevent Integumentary Complications

To prevent skin breakdown and to maintain skin integrity, use these guidelines:

• Provide adequate nutrition because tissue cannot repair itself without proper nutrients (see Chapter 23).
• Reposition patients at least every 2 hours in bed and every hour in a wheelchair if they are unable to turn or shift their own weight
• Inspect bony prominences for redness at least every 2 hours. If you find areas of redness, massage around the area but not on it. (See Chapter 26 for more information about pressure ulcers and their treatment.)
• Use mild soaps for cleansing the skin, followed by gentle but thorough drying to help maintain skin integrity.
• Provide an appropriate surface for the patient, such as mattress overlays, specialized mattresses, and specialty beds.

Effects of Immobility on the Neurological System

When a patient is immobile, several neurological complications may result. The patient may become less mentally alert, and the vision may be less clear. Balance and coordination will decrease as immobility persists. In addition, if the patient is not turned and positioned appropriately, nerves may be compressed between the bones and the firm surface of the bed, resulting in impaired nerve function called *compression neuropathy.* The most common site for compression neuropathy in the lower extremities of the immobile patient is the peroneal nerve at the fibular head. Compression of this nerve can result in footdrop, which causes the foot to point in the downward position of **plantar flexion**. This condition can be permanent, and will prevent the patient from being able to walk normally when he or she is able to ambulate. Footdrop may also be caused by injury, paralysis, and weakness of the muscles and nerves of the foot.

Table 16-2 **Support Surfaces and Specialty Beds**

Surface/Bed	Description	Figure
Support Surfaces Mattress overlays	Applied to the top of the mattress; may be filled with air or gel, or made of foam	 Eggcrate mattress
Specialized mattresses	Mattresses containing special foam, such as "memory foam" or chambers containing air that can be controlled with a dial	 Synergy® Air Elite mattress
Specialty Beds Air-fluidized bed	Bed frame without a true mattress; instead, encased area is filled with small round beads coated in silicone to prevent clumping; air is pumped through the bed, which causes the beads to mimic liquid; patient rests on a thin sheet within the air-fluidized compartment	 Clinitron® II Air Fluidized Therapy System
Low air-loss bed	Bed frame lined with a pocketed air mattress; each pocket is filled with air that can be inflated or slightly deflated to prevent pressure on any one area; can be customized for the needs of each patient	 Envision® E700 Low Air Loss Therapy System

Table 16-2 **Support Surfaces and Specialty Beds** (continued)

Surface/Bed	Description	Figure
Combination air-fluidized and low air-loss bed	Combination bed in which the lower part is an air-fluidized type and the upper section is a low air-loss type	Clinitron® Rite Hite® Air Fluidized Therapy System
Continuous lateral-rotation bed	Special type of bed frame which allows the entire bed to turn from side to side; mattress is low air-loss and bed can be programmed to turn by degrees at set intervals	TotalCare® SpO2RT bed

Nursing Measures to Prevent Neurological Complications

To prevent adverse effects of immobility on the neurological system, it is important to take measures to maintain alertness, visual acuity, and balance. Use these measures to promote normal neurological function:

- Determine the patient's level of consciousness by asking specific questions related to person, place, and time. (See Chapter 21 for more information on assessment of level of consciousness.)
- Use a foot board or high-topped tennis shoes to keep the patient's feet in a natural position, to promote the ability bear weight and walk normally.
- Perform neurological checks to determine changes in the patient's neurological status. (See Chapter 21 for details on how to assess the patient's neurological condition.)
- Provide clues to the correct date and time in the room. Keep a calendar and clock within the patient's line of vision. Open the curtains to allow the patient to observe the weather and the season.
- If the patient is confused about time, place, or person, gently reorient him or her by supplying the correct information. For example, if the patient thinks it is Tuesday, you

might say, "Today is Thursday. You have been here for two days now," to help the patient reorient to time.

Psychological Effects of Immobility

Psychological effects of immobility will differ with each individual. Depression, anxiety, hostility, and fear are common adverse effects of immobility. Restricted mobility affects the patient's self-image, independence, and ability to meet his or her own needs. If a person has always taken care of himself or herself and now must rely on others for simple activities such as washing his or her face, the patient may be frustrated or embarrassed. In addition, he or she may be concerned about finances, work, and family issues. The patient may also feel isolated due to limited social interactions. He or she may feel rejected or forgotten because others do not come to visit as often as desired.

Sensory deprivation may also occur when a patient must lie in bed all day and all night, especially if the patient is alone in the room. With decreased sensory stimulation, the patient may experience auditory or visual hallucinations.

It is also possible that patients will have difficulty sleeping when they are unable to be out of bed and active. They may be restless and irritable, and they may take out their frustrations on you. Should this occur, do not take any outburst by the patient as a personal attack. Try to put yourself in the patient's place and empathize with his or her feelings. Then use your nursing skills to help the patient find ways to occupy time and to sleep better. (See Chapter 19 for more information about promoting rest and sleep.)

Nursing Measures to Prevent Psychological Complications

To help prevent depression, anxiety, and fear, and to promote feelings of self-worth, use these nursing measures:

- Minimize sensory deprivation by ensuring that the patient has distractions to keep himself or herself occupied. These include television, radio, books, magazines, newspapers, and puzzles.
- When you are with the patient, try to involve his or her senses with pleasant smells, tastes, sounds, and sights.
- Help improve sleep patterns by encouraging patients to remain awake and alert most of the day. Keep window curtains or blinds open in the daytime to allow natural light into the room.
- Encourage and allow the patient to do as much as possible for himself or herself during patient care, such as helping with the bath, performing active ROM exercises when able, and making decisions about his or her care.
- Allow the patient to express concerns. Encourage the patient to talk about the things that are worrying him or her. Be kind and listen without giving advice. Take steps to involve other professionals, such as the social worker, pastoral care, or home health care, if appropriate.
- Encourage visits with family and friends. Try to schedule care around visitors if the patient has few guests. Allow visitors to participate in care if they wish to do so and the patient wishes them to be involved.

Knowledge Connection

How can you help prevent footdrop? How can you promote mental alertness in an immobilized patient? What are some common psychosocial effects of immobility?

Positioning Patients

When patients are unable to move independently, you will need to provide assistance in position changes to prevent complications that are associated with immobility. Traditionally, the gold standard for frequency of position change of immobile patients has been every 2 hours, although some patients may need to be repositioned more frequently.

Assisting Patients With Position Changes

It is important to maintain good body mechanics when positioning patients to prevent injury to the patient and staff. (See Chapter 13 for more information on body mechanics.)

Safety: For safe patient handling, always lock the wheels of the equipment. Elevate the bed to a comfortable working height for you. Following patient care, place the bed in the lowest setting with the wheels locked to prevent possible injury when the patient gets out of bed.

As a general rule, patients who need assistance with positioning will need position changes at least every 2 hours when on bedrest. If the patient is confined to a wheelchair and cannot shift position independently, you will need to adjust his or her position in the wheelchair every hour. Patients who are at risk for skin breakdown may need even more frequent position changes. This includes patients who are thin, dehydrated, malnourished, or immobile. In most situations, you will position all extremities so that they will maintain their function and flexibility.

The term **position of function** means placing the extremities in alignment to maintain the potential for their use and movement. Positioning for function will help prevent undue pressure on nerves and help prevent discomfort, pain, and nerve damage. Many simple positioning devices are available for use to help maintain good alignment and prevent excessive pressure on joints and nerves. Positioning devices include pillows, hand rolls, arm boards, and foot boards. When you are placing a patient's extremity in the position of function, avoid direct pressure over bony prominences, compromised tissue, or pressure ulcers. You may need to use additional padding on positioning devices to prevent pressure.

Patient Teaching Connection

Explaining to Promote Cooperation

When you care for patients who have mobility problems, always make a point to explain what you will be doing for the patient. Many patients who will require positioning assistance may be sedated from surgery, or have decreased levels of understanding from a CVA, head injury, or dementia. When you give instructions as to how the patient can help with the position change, be sure they are at an appropriate level of understanding for the patient. (See Chapter 12 for more information on patient teaching.) The patient will be more cooperative and less likely to resist during repositioning when he or she understands what is to be done. It is important to remember that, no matter how well a patient is positioned, it is necessary to reposition at least every 2 hours and possibly more frequently if the patient is unable to move himself or herself.

Selecting Appropriate Positions and Positioning Devices

In many situations, you will decide which position to use for procedures and to promote comfort for your patients. Specific positions are used for specific purposes. Table 16-3 identifies the common patient positions, describes each, and lists the purposes for which they are used.

When you position patients, it is very important that you support the limbs and areas of the body not in contact

Table 16-3   Common Positions and Their Purposes

Position	Description	Purposes
Supine	Lying on the back with arms at sides	For physical examination, resting in bed, undergoing anesthesia
Dorsal recumbent	Lying on the back with arms at sides, legs apart, knees bent, and feet flat on the bed	For physical examination of abdomen and genitalia, perineal care, examination during labor
Trendelenburg	Lying on back with arms at sides, bed positioned so foot is higher than the head	During some abdominal surgeries to shift abdominal contents upward
Reverse Trendelenburg	Lying on back with arms at sides, bed positioned so that head is higher than foot, but with no flexion at waist	After certain angiography procedures, allows head of bed to be elevated without causing pressure on the femoral artery During certain abdominal surgeries to shift abdominal contents downward
Lateral	Lying on the left or right side, supported behind back and between knees and ankles with pillows, in good body alignment	For patient comfort and to promote lung and cardiac function To relieve pressure on bony prominences of the coccyx and sacrum
Sims'	Lying on left side in semiprone position with right leg flexed and drawn up toward the chest; the left arm is positioned along the patient's back	For rectal examinations and for administering enemas
Fowler's	Semi-sitting position with various degrees of head elevation with knees slightly elevated	Purposes vary based on elevation
Low Fowler's	Head of bed elevated 30 degrees	To prevent aspiration during tube feeding
Semi-Fowler's	Head of bed elevated 45 degrees	To comfortably watch television or converse with visitors After abdominal surgeries to relieve tension on incision To assist patients who have difficulty breathing
High Fowler's	Head of bed elevated 90 degrees	To eat and drink without risk of choking To assist patients who have difficulty breathing
Orthopneic	Sitting upright with head of bed elevated 90 degrees or on the side of the bed with feet flat on the floor; patient leaning slightly forward with arms raised and elbows flexed, supported on an overbed table	To assist patients in severe respiratory distress, by allowing chest to expand to maximum capacity for moving air in and out of the lungs

(table continues on page 322)

Table 16-3 **Common Positions and Their Purposes** (continued)

Position	Description	Purposes
Prone	Lying on stomach with head turned to the side	To improve oxygenation in patients with acute respiratory distress. To relieve pressure on the back, coccyx, and hips
Lithotomy	Lying on back with knees flexed above the hips and legs supported in stirrups	For vaginal examinations, delivery of neonate, pelvic and gynecological surgery and procedures

with the bed. You will accomplish this by using pillows and other positioning devices. The placement of these devices is discussed in Skill 16-2 (see page 331). Table 16-4 describes commonly used positioning devices, their purposes, and their placement. Box 16-3 describes how to make these positioning devices out of common items.

Knowledge Connection
What is the gold standard for frequency of position change of the immobile patient while on bedrest? Frequent repositioning of the immobile patient can prevent which complications? What is the first thing the nurse does after approaching the patient prior to repositioning?

Moving and Lifting Patients

An enormous task required of the nursing staff is the safe handling and movement of patients. Nursing has one of the highest rates of musculoskeletal injuries related to the work environment compared to other occupations, resulting in a number of nurses leaving the profession. And many nurses who remain in the profession have left bedside nursing due to the physical demands of direct patient care. Researchers suspect that many musculoskeletal injuries that occur to nursing staff are unreported. It is very important that you learn how to protect yourself from injury by using proper body mechanics (discussed in Chapter 13), and how to safely lift and move patients.

Table 16-4 **Positioning Devices**

Positioning Device	Purpose	Placement
Pillow	Used to keep the head in proper alignment with the spine and reduce excessive pressure on nerves caused by stretching of the neck	Under the head and shoulders when in a supine position
	Used to relieve pressure on the lumbar spine and increase comfort	Under the knees in a supine position
	Used to maintain proper alignment of the hips and legs, and to pad bony prominences	Between the knees and ankles in a lateral position
	Used to reduce rotation of the spine and maintain proper spinal alignment	At the back in a lateral position
Arm board	Used to prevent flexion of a joint, such as when an IV catheter is near the joint	Wrist or elbow
Blanket roll	Used to support the back or soles of the feet	Place blanket roll firmly at the patient's back or at the soles of the feet

Table 16-4   Positioning Devices (continued)

Positioning Device	Purpose	Placement
Hand roll	Used to maintain a position of function of the hand and fingers of a patient with decreased movement of the hand and fingers	In the palm of the hand
Foot board	Used to maintain a position of function of the feet in relation to the legs of a patient with decreased movement and strength of the lower extremities	Against the soles of the feet
Stirrups	Positioning for vaginal surgery, pelvic examination, or delivery of infant	Place feet in the stirrups to position the lower legs and feet in a lithotomy or dorsal recumbent position
Trochanter roll	Used to prevent external rotation of the legs	At the lateral side of the hip and thigh

Box 16-3

Making Positioning Devices From Common Objects

You can make positioning and supportive devices out of common objects that may be available in a home health care client's home. These work as well as a more expensive commercial alternative.

- **Arm board:** You can cover a piece of balsa wood with foam or a washcloth for padding and make an arm board. To increase comfort, add a wrist roll fashioned like a hand roll from a washcloth folded in half. Place under the patient's wrist to support the wrist and increase comfort. Use this to keep the arm straight if an IV is inserted near a joint.
- **Blanket roll:** To make a blanket roll, roll a small blanket into a firm roll. Use this to keep the patient lying on his or her side.
- **Hand roll:** You can make a hand roll by folding a washcloth in half, then rolling it into a log shape. Tape the ends in place to prevent unrolling of the hand roll. Use this in the palm of the hand to prevent contractures of the fingers.
- **Foot board:** It is possible to improvise and fashion a foot board, to prevent footdrop, by placing a blanket roll at the patient's feet. You can make a blanket roll by rolling a small blanket into a firm roll approximately the width of the patient's feet.
- **Trochanter roll:** You can make a trochanter roll by tightly rolling a sheet or blanket securely and placing it against the lateral side of the thigh to prevent outward rotation of the hip and leg.

Safe patient handling is of great concern not only to nurses, but to their employers and their professional organizations. In the workplace today, there is a new emphasis on ways to replace manual lifting with equipment designed to assist nursing staff with lifting and moving patients.

The American Nurses Association (ANA) has instituted the Handle With Care campaign in response to the significant number of musculoskeletal disorders reported by nurses. The purpose of the campaign is to build an industry-wide program in health care to prevent musculoskeletal injuries. Many health care facilities are instituting "no lifting" programs to relieve nursing staff of the need to lift patients, instead using lifting equipment such as sit-to-stand lifts, hydraulic lifts, and battery-operated lifts. It is your responsibility as a nursing student and later as a nurse to learn how to correctly use such equipment. While it might at times seem faster to move patients manually, the saved time is not worth the risk of a debilitating injury caused by lifting more weight than your body can tolerate.

Devices for Lifting and Moving Patients

Various types of equipment are available to assist in the movement of patients, including transfer belts, nylon friction-reducing devices, slide boards, and partial or full weight-bearing assistive devices, including sling-type battery-operated patient lifts. Overhead ceiling lift devices are becoming the equipment of choice in new hospital construction and remodeling.

Moving Patients in Bed

When patients are unable to move or turn themselves in bed, the nursing staff must do this for them. An overhead *trapeze bar*, a triangular device suspended above the patient on an overbed frame, allows the patient to lift some or all of his or her weight off of the bed, which is helpful when moving the patient up in bed or turning the patient (see Skill 16-3, page 332).

Turning a Patient

Draw sheets are helpful to move and turn the patient in bed. A draw sheet can be untucked and used for turning the patient. Before turning a patient on his or her side, it is recommended to move the patient toward the side of the bed opposite of the direction in which you will turn the patient. For example, if you wanted to turn a patient onto his or her left side, you would first move the patient toward the right side of the bed. Then, when the patient is turned, he or she will be positioned in the center of the bed, rather than at the edge (see Skill 16-4, page 333).

Logrolling a Patient

When a patient has had spinal surgery or a spinal injury, it is necessary to turn his or her body as one unit. This procedure is known as a **logroll** because the patient is turned in the same way a log would be rolled. Three nursing personnel are required to correctly logroll a patient. One stands at the patient's head, one stands at the waist, and one stands at the thighs. The staff member standing at the head controls the turn. He or she will give directions and count to 3 before the move occurs. *Safety: It is very important that all three staff members turn the patient at the same time. Failure to do so can cause damage to the patient's spine, which could potentially result in paralysis.* When the count is given, all three staff members will move the patient to the side of the bed opposite the direction in which he or she will be turned. Then the two staff members not standing at the head of the bed will move to the opposite side of the bed to turn the patient toward them. Again, the person at the head will direct the turn. He or she will support the patient's head and neck during the turn. On the count of 3, the patient is turned as one unit, using a draw sheet to keep his or her neck, shoulders, and hips in alignment during and after the turn (see Skill 16-4).

Transferring Patients

You will often assist patients out of bed to sit in a chair, or to move from the bed to a stretcher or wheelchair for transport to another area of the hospital. It is very important that you know the correct way to **transfer**, or move patients from one place to another, in a way that is safe both for you and for the patient.

Before attempting to transfer a patient, you will need to know how much assistance the patient will require. If the patient can stand, but is unsteady on his or her feet, you will provide only minimal assistance. However, if the patient cannot stand on both feet, perhaps because one side is paralyzed, you will need to provide a great deal of assistance to prevent the patient from falling to his or her weak side. If the patient is unable to bear weight, you

will transfer the patient using a lift. To accomplish this, you will need the assistance of one or more people. If you are transferring a patient from the bed to a chair or wheelchair, always place the chair or wheelchair on the patient's strong side. For example, if the patient has left-sided weakness, place the chair or wheelchair on the patient's right side. When you assist this patient from the wheelchair to the bed, place the wheelchair so that the patient is transferring toward his or her strong side. In other words, the bed should be on the patient's right side.

Transfer Belts

Once you know the amount of assistance the patient will need, you will then determine which assistive devices might be useful for the transfer. If the patient can fully or partially bear weight, you will need to use a transfer belt, also called a gait belt. This device is constructed of strong webbed fabric that is placed around the patient's waist during transfers or ambulation. It provides a place for you to grasp the patient without holding onto clothing that could tear or come loose if the patient loses his or her balance.

Slide Sheets

Slide sheets are nylon friction-reducing devices made of thin webbed nylon sheets slightly smaller than the surface of the hospital bed (see Skill 16-4). A slide sheet is placed beneath the patient, allowing the patient to move easily from the bed to a stretcher or up in the bed (Fig. 16-3). Always use caution, as these nylon devices are intended to require minimal staff exertion. Skill 16-5 (see page 335) provides the steps needed to use a slide sheet to move a patient from the bed to a stretcher.

Slide Boards

Slide boards, also called transfer boards, are another method used to transfer a patient from the bed to a stretcher or a stretcher to the bed. A slide board is a hard, thin, flat plastic board that can be used with a draw sheet or plastic trash bag to help reduce friction (Fig. 16-4). The patient is turned using the draw sheet, and the board is placed on the bed next to the patient, spanning the space between the bed and the

Figure 16-3 Once the slide sheet is positioned under the patient, two nurses stand on the far side of the stretcher and pull the patient from the bed to the stretcher.

Figure 16-4 This patient is being moved with a slide board and draw sheet, which decreases the workload on the nurses as well as preventing friction on the patient's skin.

stretcher. The patient is turned onto the slide board and the health care providers use the sheet to simultaneously slide the patient across the board from the bed to the stretcher.

Sit-to-Stand Lifts

Partial weight-bearing assistive devices, also known as sit-to-stand lifts, are useful when transferring a patient who is in need of assistance, such as those who are weak, elderly, or recovering from surgery. These devices may be used to transfer the patient from the bed to the chair, the bedside commode, or the bathroom. The patient is assisted to a standing position on the locked device (Fig. 16-5). Some devices may have seats, while others provide slings to support the patient during the transfer. The device is unlocked for transport. The patient is then wheeled to the

Figure 16-5 A sit-to-stand lift is used to move the patient from a sitting to a standing position.

chair, bedside commode, or bathroom. The device is then locked and the transfer is made.

Lifts

Sling-type battery-operated patient lifts are used for the patient who is non–weight bearing. The patient is rolled to the side and a sling constructed of a thin webbed material is positioned beneath him or her according to the manufacturer's recommendations. Several different types of slings are available, and proper training is critical for safe use of all transfer assistive devices. The sling is then attached to the battery-operated lift device that raises the patient into a sitting position above the level of the bed. The lift is stabilized with a wide base of support and moved to the desired location. During this time the patient is sitting in the sling, and then he or she is gradually lowered to a chair or wheelchair. When the patient has been transferred from the bed to a chair and will require assistance for transfer back to the bed, the sling is left in place beneath the patient. When the patient is later transferred back to the bed, the sling is then removed. Sling-type battery-operated patient lifts are the device of choice if a patient has fallen to the floor and requires assistance to be returned to the bed or a chair. Using this device after a patient has fallen reduces the chance of staff or patient injury.

Battery-operated lift devices are preferred because the nursing staff does not have to lever the patient's weight. Older models of lifts are not battery operated, but operate using hydraulics. While these require some effort to lever weight on the part of the nursing staff, they are far preferable to lifting a patient without assistance (Fig. 16-6). These lifts operate in the same way as discussed previously except that, once the patient is centered in the sling and it is attached to the lift, you must pump a lever to lift the patient into a sitting position above the bed surface. Once the

Figure 16-6 A mechanical lift is used to transfer patients who cannot easily be transferred by the nursing staff.

patient is transferred to the desired location, a valve is turned that releases air, gently lowering the patient into the chair or wheelchair (see Skill 16-6, page 336).

Overhead ceiling lift devices are becoming more popular in the safe patient handling campaign. These devices require tracks in the ceiling for patient lifts. These lifts are being incorporated into new hospital construction or remodeling. A sling is placed under the patient and attached to the lifting device prior to transfer. Overhead ceiling lifts require even less staff exertion than battery-operated models, which require health care providers to push the device supporting the patient during the transfer.

Real-World Connection

Safety Tips for Stretchers

An elderly patient was in the radiology department after completion of a CT scan. The patient was to be moved from the CT scan table to the stretcher. The stretcher was placed against the CT scan table and locked. A second nurse was unaware that the stretcher had been locked; she pressed the foot lock and inadvertently unlocked the bed. The patient fell between the CT table and the stretcher during the transfer when the stretcher moved unexpectedly. *Safety: Always verify that the stretcher or bed wheels do not roll by physically attempting to move the stretcher or bed.*

Manual Transfers

Although the use of assistive devices is recommended in the ANA's safe patient handling initiative, such devices may not

always be available. *Safety: If you must transfer a patient without an assistive device (called a manual transfer), you must use proper body mechanics.* Proper body mechanics includes using a wide base of support and standing close to the object being moved, keeping your back straight, and avoiding twisting your torso. Use your thigh muscles instead of the muscles in your back. (Again, see Chapter 13 for a review of proper body mechanics.) Remember to explain to the patient what you will do and instruct him or her about what to do during the transfer (see Skill 16-5).

When you perform a manual transfer to move a patient from a bed to a stretcher, a draw sheet or bath blanket is helpful. First, assess the situation to determine the number of staff members required to safely transfer the patient. Consider the patient's weight, level of consciousness, and physical ability. For patients who can assist with the transfer, use a draw sheet. Roll the patient and place the draw sheet under the patient, extending from the shoulders to the thighs. If the patient is unable to assist with the transfer, you can use a bath blanket under the patient from the head to the feet, then grasp the bath blanket to move the patient to the stretcher.

Knowledge Connection

What is the primary purpose for using patient lift devices? What is the first thing a nurse does when preparing to use a patient lift device?

Supervision/Delegation Connection

Safety in Numbers

When you are manually moving or transferring patients, it is imperative to carefully assess each situation. Be sure that you have the proper number of staff available to assist with the move. While you can delegate transferring patients to UAPs and CNAs, it is important that you are aware of the patient's abilities. If the patient is unsteady, heavy, or weak or paralyzed on one side, then at least two members of the nursing staff should assist with the transfer. It may be necessary to delegate additional nursing staff to assist with safe patient movement or transfer to avoid patient or staff injury.

Assisting With Ambulation

Patients needing assistance with ambulation should move from the supine position to the standing position in stages to avoid possible dizziness, orthostatic hypotension, and syncopal episodes. To safely move a patient from the supine to the standing position, raise the head of the bed, then assist the patient to sit on the side of the bed to be sure that the patient is able to tolerate the change in position. The patient's feet should be firmly on the floor or a footstool. This process is referred to as *dangling* (see Skill 16-7, page 337). If the patient becomes dizzy while dangling, assist him or her back to the Fowler's or semi-Fowler's position on the bed. If the dizziness continues, lower the head of the bed to the low Fowler's position if it is not contraindicated for this patient. Once the dizziness has passed, return the patient to the Fowler's position. Check the patient's pulse and blood pressure prior to attempting to assist the patient to dangle again. Next, allow the patient to dangle for 1 to 3 minutes, and then check the pulse and blood pressure. If the patient does not experience dizziness and the pulse and blood pressure do not change significantly, allow the patient to proceed to a standing position with staff support available. However, if the pulse rate increases more than 20 bpm, the blood pressure drops more than 10 mm Hg, or the patient experiences dizziness, assist the patient back to a sitting position, lift the legs onto the bed, and lower the head of the bed slightly. Remain with the patient. In 1 to 3 minutes, recheck the pulse and blood pressure. Notify the physician of the patient's vital signs and response to dangling.

After the patient is able to dangle without adverse reactions, you will assist him or her to a standing position. *Safety: Be certain that the patient is wearing nonskid footwear.* Place your feet in front of the patient's feet and your knees against the patient's knees to provide stability when he or she is moving from a sitting to a standing position. A transfer belt may be helpful as it provides a place to grasp hold of the patient. If the patient experiences dizziness, assist him or her back to a sitting position. When the patient is able to stand without dizziness, proceed with ambulation. Stand at the patient's side for support. If a transfer belt is used, hold the belt tightly near the patient's body. If a transfer belt is not used, provide support by securely placing one arm around the patient at the waist, and grasping the patient's forearm that is nearest you with your other hand. Begin by slowly ambulating the patient short distances, such as to the bedside commode, bathroom, or door of the patient's room, as the patient tolerates. Take into consideration that the patient will need enough stamina to ambulate back to the bed (see Skill 16-8, page 338).

If the patient begins to fall, pull him or her toward your body and allow the patient to slide down your leg to the floor. As you lower the patient, bend your knees. Keep your back straight as you lower the patient to the floor. *Safety: Do not attempt to hold a patient upright if he or she loses consciousness or is falling. This will only injure you and possibly injure the patient.*

Lifting and Moving Obese Patients

Some patients are *obese,* which means that they are more than 30% overweight. When you lift and move these patients, you must take care to protect yourself and the patient from injury. Be sure to use equipment approved for the weight of the patient. Enlist the help of coworkers to move large patients and to prevent injuries. It may be necessary to obtain specialized equipment designed to lift and move patients who weigh in excess of 300 pounds (136 kg).

Protecting Yourself and Your Patients

Your knowledge of transfer techniques, body mechanics, and the use of transfer devices is key to protecting yourself and your patients from injury. In addition, one mark of a good nurse is the ability to anticipate possible problems and to then take steps to prevent those problems. For example:

A female patient puts on her call light and asks to use the bathroom for the first time after having abdominal surgery. Nurse A is busy and sends a UAP to assist the patient with no particular instructions. The patient becomes dizzy and nearly faints on the way to the bathroom. Nurse B thinks through the patient's situation, realizing that her blood pressure is running a bit low and she has not been out of bed for over 24 hours. Nurse B, although busy, goes in with the UAP and they first assist the patient to dangle, then assist her to the bathroom, carefully monitoring her responses.

Which nurse would you rather have caring for your loved one? Which nurse would you rather be?

Skill 16-1 Performing Passive Range-of-Motion Exercises

Assessment Steps

1. Check the chart for any contraindications to full range-of-motion (ROM) exercises.
2. Assess the patient for complaints of pain, nausea, and the need for toileting before beginning exercises. If the patient complains of pain or nausea, medicate and wait 30 minutes before performing ROM exercises. Assist with toileting as needed before starting the exercises.

Planning Steps

1. Obtain a bath blanket or use the top sheet and blanket to cover the patient during exercises. Keep all parts of the patient covered except the limb you are exercising *to preserve dignity and keep the patient warm.*
2. Ensure that equipment is away from the bed to allow enough space for abduction of the limbs *to prevent injury during exercise.*

(skill continues on page 328)

Skill 16-1 (continued)

3. Plan to repeat each exercise 5 to 10 times. Plan to move each joint to the maximum extent of its motion. *Safety: If you meet resistance during exercise, stop at that point. Do not force a joint nor exercise a joint beyond the point of pain.*

Implementation Steps

1. Follow the Initial Implementation Steps located on the inside front cover.
2. Exercise the neck:
   a. Place your hands on either side of the patient's head and gently move the chin to the chest, then return it to a neutral position *to flex the neck muscles.*
   b. Lift the patient's head so the chin is pointed toward the ceiling and return it to a neutral position *to extend the neck muscles.*
   c. Turn the patient's head to the left side and return it to a neutral position; then turn it to the right side and return it to a neutral position *to rotate the neck.*

b. Move the patient's arm away from his or her body to a 90-degree angle *to abduct the shoulder.*

d. Tilt the patient's head to the right side, moving the ear toward the shoulder. Repeat for the left side. *Safety: Move the neck gently and carefully as bone spurs can be dislodged and cause neurological damage if neck motion is forced.*

3. Exercise the shoulder:
   a. Place your hands so one is above and the other is below the patient's elbow. Keeping the patient's arm straight, lift it up until the inner elbow is even with the patient's ear and return it to the patient's side. *This will extend the shoulder.*

c. Return the patient's arm to the side of his or her body *to adduct the shoulder.*
d. With the elbow slightly bent, move the patient's hand to his or her opposite shoulder *to internally rotate the shoulder.*
e. Return the patient's arm to the side of his or her body with elbow flexed *to externally rotate the shoulder.*

4. Exercise the elbow:
   a. With your hands still in place, bend the patient's elbow, moving the patient's hand toward his or her shoulder to flex the elbow.
   b. Return the patient's hand to the side of his or her body to extend the elbow.

Skill 16-1 (continued)

c. Turn the patient's lower arm so the palm is upward *to supinate the arm.*

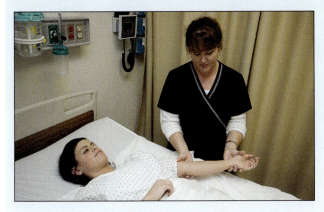

d. Turn the patient's forearm so that the palm is downward *to pronate the arm.*

5. Exercise the wrist:
   a. Place one of your hands above and the other below the patient's wrist. Bend the patient's wrist so the palm is at a 90-degree angle to the forearm to flex the wrist. Return the wrist to the neutral position.
   b. Then gently bend the wrist so the palm is facing upward to hyperextend the wrist. Return to the neutral position.

c. Tilt the wrist to the thumb side *to perform radial deviation* and return it to the neutral position.
d. Tilt the wrist to the little finger side *to perform ulnar deviation* and return it to the neutral position.

6. Exercise the fingers and thumb:
   a. Grasp the patient's fingers and separate each from the adjacent ones *to abduct the fingers.*
   b. Bring each finger close to the adjacent ones *to adduct the fingers.*
   c. Place your hand over the patient's hand and close it into a fist *to flex the fingers.*
   d. Straighten the patient's fingers to extend the fingers.
   e. Touch each fingertip to the thumb tip *to perform opposition of the thumb.*
   f. Move each finger and the thumb in a circular motion *to circumduct the fingers and thumb.*

7. Exercise the hip and knee:
   a. Place one hand under the patient's calf just below the knee and the other under the heel of the patient's foot. Slowly bend the hip and knee, keeping the lower leg parallel to the bed, *to flex the hip and knee.* Return to the resting position.

b. Keeping the patient's upper leg, knee, and lower leg straight, place one hand beneath the knee joint and the other hand under the lower leg and move the leg from the midline of the body outward to the side as far as is comfortable to abduct the hip. *Safety: If the upper leg and lower leg are not kept straight, slight rotation occurs at the knee joint and may injure the anterior cruciate ligament (ACL).*

(skill continues on page 330)

Skill 16-1 (continued)

c. Move the leg back to the midline and cross it over the other leg *to adduct the hip. Safety: Do not bring the leg beyond the midline of the body if the patient has had a total hip replacement as this could cause dislocation of the artificial hip.*

d. Maintain your hand positions and roll the leg inward until the great toe touches the bed *to internally rotate the hip. Safety: If the upper leg and lower leg are not rolled as a single unit, you may injure the ACL.*

e. Maintain your hand positions and roll the leg outward until the little toe touches the bed *to externally rotate the hip. Safety: If the upper leg and lower leg are not rolled as a single unit, you may injure the ACL.*

8. Exercise the ankle and foot:

a. Place one of your hands above the patient's ankle and one on the sole of the patient's foot. Gently push the foot back so that the toes are pointing toward the patient's head *to plantar flex the foot.*

b. Gently pull the patient's foot forward so the toes are pointing toward the foot of the bed *to dorsiflex the foot.*

c. Turn the sole of the foot inward toward the midline *to invert the foot.*

d. Turn the sole of the foot outward toward the outside of the body *to evert the foot.*

e. Gently move the foot in a circular motion *to circumduct the ankle.*

f. Separate the toes from the adjacent ones *to abduct the toes.*

g. Bring the toes together with the adjacent ones *to adduct the toes.*

h. Place your hand over the patient's toes and bend them downward to flex the toes and straighten them *to extend the toes.*

9. Follow the Ending Implementation Steps located on the inside back cover.

10. Document and report any abnormal range of motion to the charge nurse or physician.

Evaluation Steps

1. Determine whether any joints were resistant to full ROM movement. If so, note which joint(s) and at what degree was resistance found.

2. Evaluate how well the patient tolerated the exercise. Did he or she complain of pain or discomfort? If so, during the exercise of which joint(s)? Did the patient grimace or show any other sign of discomfort?

Sample Documentation

4/9/2011 1630 *Passive ROM performed to all joints. Grimaced when left shoulder extended and internally rotated. Resistance met when left shoulder extended to approx 140°. No resistance noted when left shoulder internally rotated. ―――――*
―――――――――― Nurse's signature and credentials

Skill 16-2 Positioning Patients

Assessment Steps

1. Determine the position the patient has most recently been in, then determine the position to use next, or determine the position most appropriate to the patient's needs.
2. Determine if any positions are contraindicated for this patient.
3. Determine the number of people needed to change the patient's position. If the patient is heavy or unable to help, obtain assistance and use an assistive device.

Planning Steps

1. Obtain slide sheets or other type of assistive device if needed.
2. Enlist the assistance of one or more nursing personnel as needed.

Implementation Steps

1. Follow the Initial Implementation Steps located on the inside front cover.

For the Supine Position

2. Assist the patient to turn onto his or her back *into a position for sleeping or resting.*

3. Place pillows beneath the patient's head, arms, and knees *for comfort and to support the joints. Safety: Slightly elevate only the forearms, not the upper arms. Elevation of the upper arms will pull the shoulders out of correct body alignment.*
4. Elevate the head of the bed slightly if it is more comfortable for the patient.
5. Follow the Ending Implementation Steps located on the inside back cover.

For the Fowler's Position

2. Assist the patient to the supine position.
3. Elevate the head of the bed:
   • 45 to 60 degrees for the Fowler's position *for watching television or talking with visitors.*
   • 30 to 45 degrees for the low Fowler's or semi-Fowler's position *for reading or resting.*
   • 60 to 90 degrees for the high Fowler's position *for eating meals or to facilitate easier respirations.*

4. Place pillows behind the patient's head and under his or her knees *for comfort and to support the joints. Safety: Elevate the knees only slightly because pressure against the back of the knees may restrict circulation to the lower legs and increase risk of thrombus formation.*
5. Follow the Ending Implementation Steps located on the inside back cover.

For the Lateral Position

2. Assist the patient to turn onto his or her right or left side *to relieve pressure on the back, sacral, and coccygeal area. Safety: When turning patients, it is helpful to flex the patient's knees first. If the patient cannot assist with this, flex his or her knees yourself. Once you begin to turn the patient, the flexed knees will extend beyond the patient's body and help to pull the weight of the legs during the turn. This action decreases the amount of effort required to turn the patient.*
3. Flex the knee of the upper leg and rest it on a pillow placed between the patient's legs *to prevent pressure areas from developing on the knees and ankles.*
4. Place a pillow under the patient's head and pull the lower shoulder just *slightly* forward *to prevent pressure on the joint and nerves.*
5. Fold a pillow lengthwise and place it at the patient's back. Tuck the edges of the pillow beneath the patient's back. *This keeps the patient on his or her side. If the patient leans backward, the pillow will stay tucked behind him or her.*

6. For the *lateral oblique position*, follow the steps above except place the top leg behind the body *to prevent pressure on the trochanter.*

7. Follow the Ending Implementation Steps located on the inside back cover.

For the Left Sims' Position

2. Assist the patient onto his or her left side, then move the patient so that he or she is lying partially on his or her stomach. Turn the patient's head to the right *for comfort.*
3. Flex the right arm at a 90-degree angle at the elbow and support it with a pillow *for comfort and to support the joint.*
4. Flex the right leg and place the thigh on a pillow, keeping the left leg resting on the bed with the knee slightly flexed. *This allows access to the rectal area and the sigmoid colon for rectal examinations and administration of enemas.*

(skill continues on page 332)

Skill 16-2 (continued)

5. Pull the left shoulder slightly back so it is not under the patient *to prevent pressure on the joint and nerves.* The left arm will rest along the patient's back *for comfort.*

6. Follow the Ending Implementation Steps located on the inside back cover.

For the Prone Position

2. Assist the patient to the lateral position, then onto the abdomen, with his or her head turned to the side *for comfort.*

3. Move the arms to a 90-degree angle at the elbow and support them on pillows *for comfort and to support the joints.*

4. Place a small pillow or folded towel beneath the patient's abdomen *to relieve pressure in the low back.*

5. Follow the Ending Implementation Steps located on the inside back cover.

Evaluation Steps

1. Determine if the patient is in good body alignment after being positioned. Make any changes needed to support the body and joints in good alignment.

2. Evaluate the patient's level of comfort. If the patient is not comfortable, make adjustments to promote comfort, such as moving pillows or joints.

3. Evaluate how well the patient tolerated the position change and note any complaints of pain or discomfort. Take steps to relieve pain if it persists after the position change.

Sample Documentation

4/11/11   1830   *Assisted to rt lateral position and supported with pillows. C/o discomfort in left arm and shoulder, relieved by pillow placement.* ———— *Nurse's signature and credentials*

Skill 16-3 Moving a Patient Up in Bed

Assessment Steps

1. Determine which assistive device would be most appropriate to decrease the chance of injury to your patient, your coworkers, and yourself.

2. Determine how much the patient can assist you.

Planning Steps

1. Obtain the appropriate assistive device, such as a slide sheet.

2. Enlist assistance from a coworker if needed.

Implementation Steps

1. Follow the Initial Implementation Steps located on the inside front cover.

2. Lower the head of the bed to as flat as the patient can tolerate. *It is easier to move the patient on a horizontal plane than to move him or her uphill.*

3. Remove the pillow from under the patient's head and position it vertically next to the headboard *to protect the patient's head when moving him or her up in bed.*

Moving the Patient with a Draw Sheet Only

4. Stand on one side of the bed with a coworker on the opposite side. Both you and your coworker should follow these steps:

   a. Roll the draw sheet up until it is close to the patient's body to more easily lift and move the patient.

   b. Grasp the draw sheet near the patient's shoulders and hips to help you move the patient's center of gravity.

   c. Instruct the patient to flex his or her neck, bend the knees, and place his or her feet flat on the bed. Ask the patient to grasp the trapeze bar over the bed if one is available. Tell the patient to push against the bed with his or her feet on the count of 3. *In this way, the patient can assist with moving his or her body, reducing strain on you and your coworker.*

   d. Stand with your front foot pointed toward the head of the bed and your back foot pointed toward the side of the bed *to use the correct body mechanics and reduce the possibility of injury.*

   e. On the count of 3, shift your weight from your back foot to your front foot while lifting the patient with the draw sheet and moving him or her up in bed. *This uses the muscles in your legs, not your back, to move the patient.*

5. Follow the Ending Implementation Steps located on the inside back cover.

Skill 16-3 (continued)

Moving the Patient with a Slide Sheet

4. Turn the patient to one side and place a slide sheet or large plastic bag beneath the draw sheet, positioned so that it reaches from the patient's shoulders to below the hips. *This helps you move the patient's center of gravity.*

5. Turn the patient to the opposite side and smooth the slide sheet evenly beneath the draw sheet.

6. Stand on one side of the bed with a coworker on the opposite side. Both you and your coworker should follow these steps:
   a. Roll the draw sheet up until it is close to the patient's body to more easily lift and move the patient.
   b. Grasp the draw sheet near the patient's shoulders and hips.
   c. Instruct the patient to flex his or her neck, bend the knees, and place his or her feet flat on the bed. Tell the patient to push against the bed with his or her feet on the count of 3. In this way, the patient can assist with moving his or her body, reducing strain on you and your coworker.
   d. Stand with your front foot pointed toward the head of the bed and your back foot pointed toward the side of the bed to use the correct body mechanics and reduce the possibility of injury.
   e. On the count of 3, shift your weight from your back foot to your front foot while lifting the patient with the draw sheet and moving him or her up in bed. This uses the muscles in your legs, not your back, to move the patient.

7. Turn the patient from side to side to remove the slide sheet. Remember to flex the patient's knees prior to turning the patient.

8. Follow the Ending Implementation Steps located on the inside back cover.

Evaluation Steps

1. Determine if the patient is positioned in good body alignment after moving him or her up in the bed.

Documentation

Personal care is often not documented except on a flow sheet. If abnormal findings are present, they are documented in the nurse's notes.

Skill 16-4 Turning a Patient in Bed

Assessment Steps

1. Determine the amount of assistance needed. *Safety: When logrolling a patient, you will need three staff members—one at the patient's head, and yourself plus another coworker at the patient's body.*

2. Determine onto which side you will turn the patient, based on previous positions.

Planning Steps

1. Obtain a slide sheet, large plastic bag, or plastic film to use as a friction-reducing device.

2. Enlist the assistance of another person if needed.

Implementation Steps

1. Follow the Initial Implementation Steps located on the inside front cover.

2. Place the patient in the supine position with the head of the bed lowered *to allow you to work with gravity when turning the patient.*

Turning with a Draw Sheet

3. Turn the patient to one side and place a slide sheet or large plastic bag beneath the draw sheet, positioned so it reaches from the patient's shoulders to below the hips. *This helps you move the patient's center of gravity.*

4. Turn the patient to the opposite side and smooth the slide sheet evenly beneath the draw sheet.

5. Move the patient to the right side of the bed if you are turning him or her onto his or her left side. *This gives room for the patient to be turned and remain in the center of the bed, not up against the side rail. Reverse this step if you are turning the patient to his or her right side. Safety: Remove the plastic bag or plastic film from beneath the patient at this point to prevent it from holding moisture against the patient's skin.*

6. Flex the patient's knees to help pull the body weight into the turn. Or you may move the patient's right leg over his or her left leg if you are turning the patient to the left *to help keep the patient's weight in the center.* Reverse this if you are turning the patient to his or her right side.

7. Move his or her right arm across the chest *to keep the weight of the patient in the center.* Again, reverse if turning in the opposite direction.

(skill continues on page 334)

Skill 16-4 (continued)

8. Position his or her left shoulder so that it is abducted and externally rotated *to prevent it from becoming trapped under the patient during the turn.*

9. Stand with your feet shoulder-width apart *to provide a wide base of support.* Place one foot more forward than the other *so you can shift your weight as you move the patient.*

10. Grasp the draw sheet with one hand near the patient's shoulders and just below his or her hips *to allow you to move the patient's center of gravity.* Use the draw sheet to turn the patient.

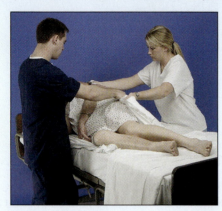

11. On the count of 3, bend your knees and hips and shift your weight from the back foot to the front foot. Your coworker on the opposite side of the bed will shift his or her weight from the front foot to the back foot as the patient comes toward him or her. *This allows both you and your coworker to use good body mechanics while smoothly moving the patient.*

12. Reposition the patient's left shoulder slightly forward *to prevent pressure on the joint and nerves.* Reverse this if the patient is being positioned on the right side.

13. Position with pillows as described for positioning the patient in the lateral position in Skill 16-2.

14. Follow the Ending Implementation Steps located on the inside back cover.

Logroll the Patient

3. A slide sheet should already be in place beneath the patient *to facilitate turning the body as a single unit.*

4. Have one coworker stand near the patient's head *to be responsible for keeping the head and shoulders in alignment with the rest of the body.*

5. Stand even with the patient's waist and have your remaining coworker stand at the patient's thighs *to ensure that the patient's body remains aligned during the turn.* Lower the side rail closest to you.

6. Instruct the patient to cross his or her arms across the chest *to keep them protected during the turn.*

7. All three coworkers now grasp the slide sheet closely to the patient's body. On the count of 3, move the patient toward you and your coworker as one unit. *Safety: Do not allow different parts of the spine to move at different times as this can cause damage to a spine that has been injured or*

surgically repaired. This allows the patient to be in the center of the bed once turned.

8. Raise the side rail. You and your coworker now move to the opposite side of the bed. Lower the side rail nearest you. Place a pillow between the patient's legs and, if allowed, replace the pillow under his or her head without moving the head out of alignment with the spine.

9. You and your coworker will face the patient, standing with your feet shoulder-width apart, one foot slightly ahead of the other. While placing your weight on your forward foot, bend at the hips, flex your knees, and grasp the draw sheet on the opposite side of the patient.

10. The coworker who is controlling the patient's head and shoulders will count to 3. On the count of 3, each staff member moves the patient using the draw sheet in one fluid motion *to prevent twisting or torque on the patient's spine.* The patient's head and hips should be kept in a straight line at all times *to prevent damage to the spinal cord.*

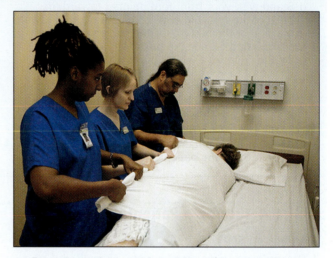

11. Prop the patient on his or her side using a pillow or rolled blanket. Keep the head and hips in a straight line. It is usually necessary to place a pillow between the patient's knees and ankles to prevent the top leg from pulling forward, causing the hip to be out of alignment.

12. Follow the Ending Implementation Steps located on the inside back cover.

Evaluation Steps

1. Determine if the patient remained in a straight line during the turn.

2. Evaluate the effectiveness of the three staff members working together.

3. Evaluate the position and comfort of the patient.

Sample Documentation

5/12/12   1915   Logrolled to left side without do discomfort or pain. Body alignment maintained. ————————
———————————— Nurse's signature and credentials

Skill 16-5 Transferring a Patient from Bed to a Stretcher, Chair, or Wheelchair

Assessment Steps

1. Assess the patient's ability to help with the transfer.
2. Determine the need for assistive devices such as a slide sheet.
3. Determine the need for coworker assistance.
4. Assess the patient for complaints of pain, discomfort, or nausea. Administer ordered medications as appropriate.
5. Assess the patient for weakness on one side of the body.

Planning Steps

1. Obtain needed equipment, such as a transfer belt and a friction-reducing device (slide sheet or slide board), and a gown or robe and nonskid slippers if you are transferring the patient to a chair or wheelchair.
2. Enlist the assistance of coworkers as needed.
3. Determine the number and types of tubes and equipment attached to the patient. Plan to protect them during the transfer *to prevent tangling or pulling loose of tubes or equipment.*
4. If the patient has a weak side, position the chair or wheelchair on the patient's strong side. *This allows the patient to bear weight on his or her strong side during the transfer, reducing the chance for loss of balance and falls.*
5. Prepare the equipment as needed for transfer via stretcher or wheelchair. For example, unplug the IV pump or obtain a rolling IV pole, obtain an E-cylinder of oxygen if the patient is on continuous oxygen, and disconnect suction.

Implementation Steps

1. Follow the Initial Implementation Steps located on the inside front cover.

Transferring to a Stretcher

2. Lock the wheels on the bed and lower the head of the bed.
3. Turn the patient from side to side to place the slide board, slide sheet, or a large plastic bag beneath the draw sheet.
4. Move the patient close to the side of the bed where the stretcher will be placed, keeping a sheet or blanket over the patient *to preserve modesty and provide warmth.*
5. Lower the side rail and position the stretcher firmly against the bed. Raise or lower the bed so that it is the same height as the stretcher. *Safety: Lock the wheels on the stretcher to prevent possible injury to the patient and the nursing staff.*
6. *Safety: If the patient has a Foley catheter, avoid raising the catheter drainage bag above the level of the patient's bladder, which can result in backflow of urine into the bladder, increasing the risk of urinary tract infection.*
7. Stand on the far side of the stretcher with a coworker. Lean against the stretcher as an added measure to ensure that the stretcher does not move away from the bed during transfer.

8. Pull the patient onto the stretcher using the slide sheet or slide board.
   - If using a slide sheet, lay the straps of the sheet across the stretcher. Both you and your coworker will grasp the straps of the slide sheet and, on the count of 3, pull steadily. *This will move the patient across to the stretcher with minimal effort since friction is reduced.* You can leave the slide sheet in place until the patient returns to the bed, then remove the slide sheet by turning the patient from side to side.

   - If using a slide board, have the patient flex his or her neck to keep the head up. Pull on the draw sheet, moving the patient across the slide board and onto the stretcher. Remove the slide board.

Safety: To secure the patient on the stretcher, reach across the patient and grasp the draw or slide sheet. Pull it snugly across the patient's trunk and pelvis, similar to a cocoon. Secure the stretcher's lap belt across the patient's pelvis and raise both stretcher rails, ensuring that the patient is covered.

9. Follow the Ending Implementation Steps located on the inside back cover.

Transferring to a Chair or Wheelchair

2. Assist the patient into a robe or a second gown with the opening to the front *to cover the patient's exposed back and protect modesty.* Apply nonskid slippers to the patient's feet *to reduce risk of falling.*
3. Apply a transfer belt to the patient *to provide a way to hold onto the patient during the transfer.*
4. Raise the head of the bed to a sitting position *to prevent the patient from having to move himself or*

(skill continues on page 336)

Skill 16-5 (continued)

herself to the sitting position. Place one hand on either side of the patient and grasp the transfer belt. *Safety: Lock the wheels on the bed and lower it to the lowest position to prevent injury to the patient.*

5. Explain exactly how you are going to get the patient up, instructing him or her how to assist in the process. *This helps to reduce anxiety and increase cooperation during the transfer.*

6. Stand facing the bed with one foot forward of the other. Maintain a wide base of support. Flex your knees and hips. *This gives you a wide base of support and maintains good body mechanics for the transfer.*

7. On the count of 3, move the patient to a sitting position on the side of the bed with his or her feet resting on the floor. Ensure that the patient is not dizzy or nauseated and is ready to proceed. Assist the patient to put on nonskid footwear and a robe.

8. Stand facing the patient with your feet against his or her feet, and your knees against his or her knees *to keep the patient's feet from slipping or the knees from buckling.*

9. Flex your hips and knees as you grasp the transfer belt on either side of the patient's waist. *This gives you the ability to hold the patient near his or her center of gravity.*
   Note: If two people are assisting, each one grasps the transfer belt at the patient's waist and places one foot and knee against the patient's foot and knee.

10. Instruct the patient to hold onto your shoulders, not your neck, *to prevent injury to your neck or upper back.* Straighten your knees and hips and bring the patient to a standing position.

11. Wait briefly for the patient to adjust to a standing position. Turn the patient to align with the wheelchair or chair. *Safety: Ensure that your feet and the wheelchair footrests are out of the way to prevent the patient from tripping.*

12. Have the patient step back until he or she feels the chair or wheelchair against the back of the knees, then grasp the chair arms and gently lower him or her into the chair. Keep your back straight, flexing your hips and knees as the patient sits in the chair, *to use your leg muscles, not your back muscles, and prevent possible injury.* Ensure that the patient's hips are positioned against the back of the chair *so that proper body alignment is maintained.*

13. Place the patient's feet on the footrests and cover the patient's lap with a sheet or blanket *to protect modesty and provide warmth.*

14. Follow the Ending Implementation Steps located on the inside back cover.

Evaluation Steps

1. Determine if the transfer occurred safely and smoothly. If not, what problems occurred and how could they be prevented?

2. Determine how well the patient tolerated the activity. Did he or she become frightened, anxious, or dizzy?

Sample Documentation

11/4/11   2040   Transferred to chair with assist of one. Pivoted on R leg and maintained balance well. Resting comfortably in chair, call light within reach. ———— Nurse's signature and credentials

Skill 16-6 Transferring a Patient With a Mechanical Lift

Assessment Steps

1. Determine where the patient is to be moved.
2. Determine the need to move furniture and equipment to have a clear pathway for the lift.
3. Assess the patient for concerns regarding use of the lift and movement out of bed.

Planning Steps

1. Obtain the lift and sling.
2. Enlist the assistance of at least one coworker. *Safety: Always have at least two members of the nursing staff operating the lift and moving the patient.*

Implementation Steps

1. Follow the Initial Implementation Steps located on the inside front cover.
2. Roll the patient side to side and place the sling beneath the patient so it starts at the shoulders and ends at the knees. *Safety: Position the sling carefully so the patient is completely supported when being lifted and moved.*
3. Fasten the sling around the patient's legs according to manufacturer's instructions.
4. Position the lift at the side of the bed with the wheels in widest position *to increase the base of support.*

Skill 16-6 (continued)

5. Attach the sling to the lift. **Note:** The shorter chains attach to the top openings of the sling and the longer chains to the lower grommets. *This pulls the patient up to a sitting position when the lift is activated.*

6. Activate the lift to slowly raise the patient. This may involve pushing a button or pumping a lever.

7. Slowly pull the lift away from the bed, once the patient is above the level of the bed. *Safety: Two members of the nursing staff are required; one person holds onto the patient in the sling and guides him or her, and the other person pushes the lift.* The person guiding the patient in the sling explains each movement that is about to occur *to prevent increasing fear and anxiety;* he or she also makes frequent eye contact with the patient, observing for signs of fear, and offers reassurance.

8. Push the lift to the desired location and align it so the patient is over the chair.

9. Release the valve that slowly lowers the lift, while your coworker guides the patient into the chair. Ensure that the patient's hips are positioned against the back of the chair *to ensure proper body alignment.*

10. Detach the sling from the lift and store the lift in the designated area *to prevent blocking traffic ways.*

11. Leave the sling in place beneath the patient until he or she is returned to the bed. Then turn the patient side to side and remove the sling.

12. Follow the Ending Implementation Steps located on the inside back cover.

Evaluation Steps

1. Determine the effectiveness of the transfer: Was the patient safely positioned in the sling? Were you able to move the patient with a minimum of swaying? Was the patient aligned well with the chair or bed before being lowered into it?

Sample Documentation

10/14/11 1135 Transferred via lift from bed to wheelchair. C/O anxiety as lift was raised. Reassured by UAP and guided throughout transfer. Resting comfortably in wheelchair. Call light within reach. ————— Nurse's signature and credentials

Skill 16-7 Assisting a Patient to Dangle

Assessment Steps

1. Check the physician's order for the patient's activity level.

2. Assess the patient for complaints of pain rated a 5 or above on a 10-point scale prior to dangling. If this is the case, medicate the patient according to the physician's orders and wait until the pain decreases to assist the patient to dangle.

3. Assess the patient's pulse and blood pressure while the patient is in the supine position.

Planning Steps

1. Enlist the assistance of a coworker if help is needed.

Implementation Steps

1. Follow the Initial Implementation Steps located on the inside front cover.

2. Elevate the head of the bed until the patient is in a sitting position. *This prevents the patient from having to move from a lying to sitting position prior to dangling.* Apply a transfer belt *to give you something to hold onto as you assist the patient to dangle.*

3. Place one hand on either side of the patient and grasp the transfer belt.

4. On the count of 3, move the patient to a sitting position on the side of the bed. Ensure that the patient is not dizzy or nauseated and is ready to proceed.

5. Lower the bed so that the patient's feet rest on the floor. *Allowing the feet to rest on the floor prevents pooling of blood in suspended lower extremities, which would occur if the feet were not supported.*

(skill continues on page 338)

Skill 16-7 (continued)

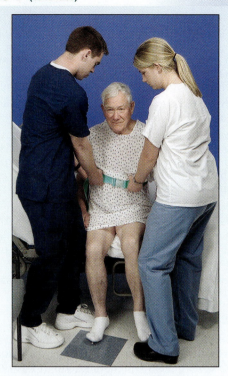

6. Assess the patient's pulse and blood pressure for an increase or decrease of more than 20 bpm or 30 mm Hg. Assess the patient for complaints of dizziness, nausea, or pain. *Safety: If the vital signs are outside these parameters, or if the patient complains of these symptoms, immediately assist the patient to Fowler's or low Fowler's position to prevent possible syncope and injury. If the dizziness continues, lower the head of the bed until the dizziness passes. Then return the patient to the Fowler's position and repeat steps 4–6.*

7. Remain with the patient while he or she dangles for 1 to 3 minutes and assist the patient to put on his or her robe and nonskid footwear. If the patient tolerates this process, it is safe to proceed with transferring the patient to a chair or wheelchair (see Skill 16-5) or to assist the patient with initial ambulation if there is a physician's order to do so (see Skill 16-8).

8. When the dangling process is complete, return the patient to bed and assist him or her to a supine position.

9. Assess pulse and blood pressure again, comparing them to your findings when the patient was supine and sitting.

10. Follow the Ending Implementation Steps located on the inside back cover.

Evaluation Steps

1. Evaluate the patient's response to dangling. Did the pulse and blood pressure remain stable with position change? Did the patient complain of pain, dizziness, or nausea?

Sample Documentation

11/4/11   1935   Assisted to dangle on side of bed. P – 66, BP – 112/76 in supine position. P – 74, BP – 120/80 when dangling. Denies do nausea, pain, or dizziness. Remained on side of bed for 6 min, then assisted to supine position in bed. P – 76 and BP – 122/78 after return to bed. ————————
———————— Nurse's signature and credentials

Skill 16-8 Assisting With Ambulation

Assessment Steps

1. Check the physician's orders for activity level.

2. Assess the patient for complaints of pain, discomfort, nausea, or dizziness. Take appropriate action if complaints exist, and delay ambulation if needed.

3. Determine the need for coworker assistance during ambulation.

Planning Steps

1. Obtain a transfer belt according to facility policy.

2. Obtain the patient's robe and nonskid footwear.

3. Prepare the equipment as needed for ambulation. For example, unplug the IV pump or obtain a rolling IV pole, obtain an E-cylinder of oxygen if the patient is on continuous oxygen, and disconnect suction.

Implementation Steps

1. Follow the Initial Implementation Steps located on the inside front cover.

2. Assist the patient to dangle (see Skill 16-7). *If the patient is able to tolerate dangling, you can then proceed with ambulation. If not, follow the procedure in Skill 16-7.*

3. Assist the patient to put on his or her robe and nonskid footwear *to prevent possible slips and falls.*

4. Fasten a transfer belt around the patient's waist. *Safety: The belt should be snug without being too tight. You should be able to insert three fingers between the belt and the patient to prevent injury to the patient.*

5. Assist the patient to a standing position. Stand slightly behind and next to the patient, holding the transfer belt on the patient's far side and near side. *Safety: This gives you control of the patient if he or she should start to fall.*

Skill 16-8 (continued)

10. Call for assistance. *Safety: Do not attempt to get the patient back up by yourself.*

11. Obtain a set of vital signs *to determine if the patient has a lowered blood pressure or pulse rate.*

12. Assist the patient back to bed using a lift or other equipment *to prevent injury to yourself and the patient.*

13. Follow the Ending Implementation Steps located on the inside back cover.

Evaluation Steps

1. Determine the effectiveness of your preparation: Did you use a transfer belt with the correct fit? Did you grasp it in the correct manner?

2. Evaluate ambulation. Did the patient tolerate it without problems? Were you focused on the patient at all times? Did equipment or tubes get in the way during ambulation?

3. Evaluate your response to a fall. Did you protect the patient from actually falling? Did you lower him or her gently to the floor? Did you protect yourself from injury in the process, using good body mechanics?

Sample Documentation

11/12/12   1720   Assisted to ambulate in hallway, gait belt in use. Amb approx 14 feet. C/O of dizziness and began to sag. Lowered gently to floor by nurse without hitting floor or walls. BP – 88/60, P – 116, R – 28. ————————————

———————————— Nurse's signature and credentials

11/12/12   1735   Assisted from floor via lift and returned to bed. BP – 100/68, P – 100, R – 24 when returned to bed. Physician notified. ———————— Nurse's signature and credentials

---

6. Walk with the patient, ensuring that tubes and equipment are out of the way of the patient's feet and legs to prevent tripping. A second person may be needed to assist with the IV or a catheter drainage bag.

7. Observe the patient during ambulation for shortness of breath, fatigue, complaints of dizziness, or increasing pain. *These symptoms indicate intolerance of ambulation.*

8. Return the patient to the bed or chair after ambulating the prescribed distance or if the patient becomes symptomatic.

Breaking a Fall

9. If the patient begins to fall or faint, pull him or her toward you. Lower yourself and the patient to the floor. *Safety: Do not attempt to keep the patient upright. Do not bend your back; rather, bend your forward leg and allow the patient to slide down the inner aspect of your leg to the floor. Avoid letting the patient's weight slide down the front of your lower leg, as this can hyperextend your knee joint and cause injury.*

Post Conference

Your clinical experience in the rehab unit was very educational. You shared with your clinical group in post conference that you now know how to use a battery-operated lift and that you understand the use of a Clinitron bed to help prevent pressure ulcers in patients at risk for skin breakdown. You described how the bed works to blow air through the microbeads within it to reproduce a fluid-like surface for the patient. You shared that your patient was very depressed about his paralysis and would barely interact with you. While you found this frustrating, you also understood his reactions. By the end of the second day, he was a little more responsive, but you agreed with the staff nurse that he would need counseling to deal with the changes in his life.

KEY POINTS

- Immobility negatively affects every body system, causing complications such as blood clots, kidney stones, bone demineralization, pressure ulcers, pneumonia, urinary tract infections, constipation, confusion, and depression.

- Nurses must anticipate such complications and be proactive by implementing measures to prevent them. These nursing interventions include performing passive range-of-motion exercises, turning the patient frequently, encouraging the patient to cough and deep breathe often, applying antiembolism stockings and sequential compression devices as ordered, assisting the patient to dangle and ambulate, using therapeutic devices correctly, encouraging food and fluid intake, preventing urinary retention, and utilizing specialty beds and mattresses.

- Positioning patients correctly requires knowledge not only of the position but the appropriate supportive devices and their correct locations. Positioning patients to maintain function is extremely important to the patients' recovery.

- Nurses must use good body mechanics when moving and positioning patients to prevent injury to themselves and injury to the patients. They must also know about available assistive devices for lifting and moving patients, including how to use them to decrease the risk of musculoskeletal injury.

- Assistive devices for lifting and moving patients include slide sheets, transfer or gait belts, slide boards, sit-to-stand lifts, battery-operated lifts, and overhead ceiling lifts.

- When performing manual transfers, the nurse must be ever-vigilant to keep the patient and himself or herself from injury. Always set up the transfer so that the patient is moving toward his or her strong side.

- Before a patient stands to transfer to a chair or to ambulate for the first time after a surgery or procedure, assist him or her to dangle on the side of the bed and check the pulse and blood pressure for changes.

- Always take the time to assist patients who are getting out of bed for the first time or if complications during transfer or ambulation are possible. Anticipate potential problems and be proactive in preventing them.

REVIEW QUESTIONS

Select the answer that is most appropriate for each of the following questions. Some questions may have more than one correct answer. Check all that apply.

1. Which of the following would not be considered a consequence of immobility affecting the musculoskeletal system?

   a. Decreased muscle strength

   b. Muscle atrophy

   c. Skin breakdown

   d. Contractures

   e. Pressure ulcers

   f. Increased bone weakness

2. Number the following steps for assisting a patient to dangle in the correct sequence.

   a. The patient becomes dizzy while dangling.

   b. Take the patient's vital signs and document.

   c. Raise the head of the bed.

   d. Explain to the patient what you are going to do.

   e. Assist the patient to a resting position on the bed.

   f. Assist the patient to a dangling position.

3. For the safest patient transfer, which devices are best to use?

  a. Transfer belt

  b. Wheelchair

  c. Webbed nylon sheets

  d. Stretcher

  e. Overhead ceiling lift

4. The Handle With Care campaign is supported by the American Nurses Association, and its purpose is to:

  a. require all hospitals to install ceiling lifts for every patient.

  b. increase awareness of musculoskeletal injuries to nurses and establish a fund for their care.

  c. compile research about the types and frequency of injuries that occur to nurses during their working life.

  d. prevent injuries to nurses by increasing the use of assistive devices for moving and lifting patients.

5. A male patient in the supine position is:

  a. lying flat on his back with legs extended and arms to the side.

  b. resting in bed with the head of the bed elevated 45 degrees.

  c. lying on his side with legs flexed.

  d. resting in bed with the head of the bed elevated 90 degrees.

6. The ideal method for transferring a patient includes:

  a. assessing the situation and the environment.

  b. ensuring that one of the transfer team members is a strong male.

  c. properly using transfer or lift devices.

  d. using the appropriate number of staff members.

  e. explaining the procedure to the patient.

    1. a, b, e

    2. a, c, d, e

    3. a, c, e

    4. a, b, c, e

7. The purpose of dangling is to:

  a. check for changes in vital signs with position changes.

  b. determine the patient's response to being suspended in a lift sling.

  c. prevent possible syncope and injury.

  d. place the patient in position so he or she will be in the center of the bed after being turned.

  e. determine the patient's ability to bear weight on both legs during a transfer.

  f. determine if it is safe for the patient to ambulate or transfer.

CRITICAL THINKING EXERCISES

8. You are caring for a patient who had a heart attack 2 days ago. You are assisting her to walk in the hallway. She expresses a desire to walk all the way to the end of the hall. This is only the second time she has ambulated outside of her room. How will you respond?

9. While you are walking, the patient suddenly gasps and loses consciousness. What will you do?

ADDITIONAL RESOURCES

For additional Resources, Questions, and Activities, please see:

 Student Resource Disk

DavisPlus **http://davisplus.fadavis.com**

 Student Study Guide

REFERENCES

ANA receives award for safe patient handling education. *South Carolina Nurse.* 2008;Oct-Dec.

Asher R. The dangers of going to bed. *Br Med J.* 1947;4:967-968.

Bartley MK. Keep venous thromboembolism at bay. *Nursing2006,* 2006;36(10):36-41.

Baumgarten M, Margolis D, Localio A, et al. Pressure ulcers among elderly patients early in the hospital stay. *J Gerontol A Biol Sci Med Sci.* 2006;61:749-754.

Bridges N, Jarquin-Valdivia A. Use of the Trendelenburg position as the resuscitation position: to T or not to T? *Am J Crit Care.* 2005;14:365-368.

Clark M. Pressure ulcer prevention. In: Morison MJ, Rijswijk LV, eds. *The Prevention and Treatment of Pressure Ulcers.* New York: Elsevier Mosby; 2001:78-80.

de Castro A. Handle With Care®: the American Nurses Association's campaign to address work-related musculoskeletal disorders. *Orthop Nurs.* 2006;25:356-365.

Denholm B, Downing D. Clinical issues: lithotomy position [serial online]. *AORN J.* 2008;87:429-438.

de Vega R, Iglesias B, del Ray G, Ferrer G, Rey A. (2007). Effect of Sims modified position over the rotation and foetus progress down on women on their first birth with epidural anaesthesia [in Spanish]. *NURE Investig.* 2007;4(31):6.

Dierker E, Steffes A, Tidwell S. (2007). Safe patient handling curriculum content. *Kansas Nurse.* 2007;82(3):8-9.

Drake D, Baker G, Keehner M, et al. Challenges in caring for the morbidly obese: differences by practice setting [serial online]. *Southern Online J Nurs Res.* 2008;8(3).

Engst C, Chhokar R, Miller A, Tate B, Yassi A. Effectiveness of overhead lifting devices in reducing the risk of injury to care staff in extended care facilities. *Ergonomics.* 2005;48:187-199.

Fletcher K. Immobility: geriatric self-learning module. *J Med-Surg Nurs.* 2005;14(1):35-37.

Galiatsou E, Kostnati E, Svarna E, et al. Prone position augments recruitment and prevents alveolar overinflation in acute lung injury. *Am J Respir Crit Care Med.* 2006;174:187-197.

Holm D, Hendricks C. Immobility and bone loss in the aging adult. *Crit Care Nurse Q.* 1989;12(1):46-51.

Hospital designs for safe patient handling [serial online]. *Hosp Employee Health.* 2008:58-59.

Kolecki P, Menckhoff CR. *Shock, hypovolemic: treatment & medication.* [E-Medicine from Web MD.] March 24, 2009. Available at: http://emedicine.medscape.com/article/760145-treatment. Accessed August 31, 2009.

Kottink A, Nene A, Groothuis-Oudshoorn C, Ijzerman M. Therapeutic effects of an implantable peroneal nerve stimulator in subjects with chronic stroke and footdrop: a randomized controlled trial. *Phys Ther.* 2008;88:437-438.

Nelson A, Baptiste A. Evidence-based practices for safe patient handling and movement. *Orthop Nurs.* 2006;25:366-379.

O'Connell M. Positioning impact on the surgical patient. *Nurs Clin North Am.* 2006;41:173-192.

Olson E. The hazards of immobility. 1967. *Am J Nurs.* 1990;90(3):43-48.

Parameswarden K, Todd D, Soth M. Altered respiratory physiology in obesity. *Can Respir J.* 2006;13(4):203-210.

Powell-Cope G, Hughes NL, Sedlak C, Nelson A. Faculty perceptions of implementing an evidence-based safe patient handling nursing curriculum module [serial online]. *OJIN Online J Issues Nurs.* 2008;13(3).

Rauen C, Chulay M, Bridges E, Vollaman K, Arbour R. Seven evidence-based practice habits: putting some sacred cows out to pasture. *Crit Care Nurse.* 2008;28:109-114.

Rothrock J, Smith D, McEwen D. *Alexander's Care of the Patient in Surgery.* 12th ed. St. Louis: Mosby Elsevier; 2003.

Safe patient handling: it's the law [serial online]. *Minnesota Nurs Accent.* 2007:8-9.

Sobieraj D. Development and implementation of a program to assess medical patients' need for venous thromboembolism prophylaxis. *Am J Health Syst Pharm.* 2008;65:1755-1760.

Thomas P, Paratz J. Is there evidence to support the use of lateral positioning in intensive care? A systematic review. *Anesth Intensive Care J.* 2007;35:239-255.

Timmerman R. A mobility protocol for critically ill adults. *Dimensions Crit Care.* 2007;26(5):175-179.

Walick K, Kragh J Jr, Ward J, Crawford J. Changes in intraocular pressure due to surgical positioning: studying potential risk for postoperative vision loss. *Spine.* 2007;32:2591-2595.

Whitney J, Phillips L, Aslam R, et al. Guidelines for the treatment of pressure ulcers. *Wound Repair Regen.* 2006;14:663-679.

Winslow E. High Fowlers won't always ease breathing. *Am J Nurs.* 1996;96(2):59.

Yanazume S, Yanazume Y, Iwamoto I, et al. Severe leg compartment syndrome associated with dorsal lithotomy position during radical hysterectomy. *J Obstet Gynaecol Res.* 2006;32:610-612.

Key Terms

Afebrile

Apnea

Biot's respirations

Bradycardia

Bradypnea

Cheyne-Stokes respirations

Diastolic pressure

Dyspnea

Eupnea

Febrile

Hypertension

Hypotension

Hypothermia

Pulse deficit

Pulse pressure

Sphygmomanometer

Stridor

Systolic pressure

Tachycardia

Tachypnea

Objectives

1. Define key terms associated with assessment of the six vital signs.
2. Describe the six vital signs, their significance, and their normal ranges.
3. Identify times when vital signs should be assessed.
4. Summarize the guidelines for vital sign assessment.
5. Outline the four circulatory qualities and how they determine blood pressure.
6. Relate at least six factors that affect blood pressure, temperature, pulse, and respiration.
7. Contrast the effects of hypertension and hypotension on the body.
8. Describe how and where to assess peripheral pulses.
9. Distinguish how the body regulates each vital sign.
10. Describe how to assess pain.

Skills

17-1	Assessment of Blood Pressure
17-2	Assessment for Orthostatic Hypotension
17-3	Assessing Body Temperature by Various Routes
17-4	Assessing the Radial and Apical Pulses
17-5	Assessing Peripheral Pulses
17-6	Using Doppler Ultrasound to Assess Nonpalpable Pulses
17-7	Assessing Respirations
17-8	Assessing Oxygen Saturation

Clinical Connection

Your Assignment: While caring for your patient in clinical, you take his vital signs with an automatic vital sign machine at 8 a.m. and get BP – 126/74, T – 98°F, P – 64, SpO$_2$ – 98% on room air. Your patient has a good morning and is sitting up in the chair reading when you take his vital signs with the same machine at noon. The readings are BP – 94/46, T – 96.6°F, P – 51, and SpO$_2$ – 70% on room air. When you repeat vital signs with the machine, you get similar readings.

Your Actions: Because these midday vital signs are below normal adult ranges, you are concerned. Should you assist the patient to bed and notify the physician regarding his abnormal vital signs? Should you push the emergency call light? Or should you look at the patient and evaluate whether or not the vital sign readings could be inaccurate. Would it be beneficial to take the vital signs manually, rather than relying on the machine? What should your next course of action be?

The human body responds physiologically to all stimuli, both internal and external. External stimuli include air, sunshine, environmental temperature, sound, electricity, and any number of stimuli found outside the body itself. Internal stimuli include hormones, enzymes, electrical conduction of impulses along nerve pathways, gases, and pH. To provide appropriate nursing care to a patient, the nurse must know how the patient's body is physiologically responding. One of the basic ways to determine this is to assess the patient's vital signs. In this chapter, you will learn not only how to assess vital signs but how to relate them to vital physiological functions of the body. You will learn the implications of abnormal readings and the appropriate nursing care to provide.

The Six Vital Signs

Vital signs, the fundamental measurement of life signs, include five objective measurements:

1. Blood pressure (BP)
2. Temperature (T)
3. Pulse (P)
4. Respirations (R)
5. Oxygen saturation (SpO$_2$)

There is also a sixth subjective measurement: pain.

The five objective vital signs tell how certain systems are functioning, provide data regarding the patient's overall condition, and provide a baseline against which you can measure even subtle changes. Though subjective, the assessment of pain is important because this feeling of distress can have effects on the blood pressure, pulse, and respirations and serves as a warning that tissues are actually being injured or about to be injured. In fact, pain is one of the primary reasons individuals seek medical care, and it gives us insight as to what may be wrong with the patient's health.

You will *assess,* or measure, vital signs often because it is a quick and efficient way to monitor a patient's physiological condition, identify new problems, and determine if

an intervention should be performed or if prior interventions were effective. It is important to remember that vital signs are only of value when they are accurate. The inaccurate measurement of vital signs can result in a range of serious problems, from failure to detect deterioration in condition all the way to death.

It is also important to understand that vital signs must be evaluated in conjunction with the patient's overall condition. Even though vital signs are one of the most important and frequent assessments that you will make, they do not always reflect changes occurring in the patient's condition. For example, a patient with a serious respiratory illness such as pneumonia may still have a respiratory rate within the normal range. Therefore, further assessments such as breath sounds and chest x-ray are required to detect deviations in function. Remember to always look at the whole patient, not just his or her vital signs.

Supervision/Delegation Connection

There Are Times When You Should Not Delegate Vital Signs

Vital sign assessment is commonly delegated, but because the skill of measuring vital signs is simple to perform and is performed many times a day, day after day, it is possible to take the process and the delegation of vital sign assessment for granted and to become totally dependent upon unlicensed personnel for their measurement. Though it is appropriate in most cases to delegate this task to CNAs or UAPs, keep in mind that vital sign assessment is ultimately your responsibility. You are responsible for analyzing the vital sign findings and for determining when further action is necessary, whether you take the vital signs yourself or not. These are the *vital signs of life* that indicate when your patients' conditions begin to change.

There are times when you should assess a patient's vital signs or reassess them after someone else has already taken them, including:

• After administration of IV medications that may affect the vital signs

- With a change in level of consciousness
- When the patient is in an unstable postoperative condition
- If there is uncontrolled bleeding
- When the patient has pale, cold, and clammy skin
- Anytime you suspect shock, stroke, pulmonary embolism, heart attack, or any other serious condition

Occasionally there are times when you cannot identify a patient's problem, but something just does not seem right with his or her condition. Never ignore those feelings. It has been proven that we can subconsciously detect subtle changes in a patient's condition without being able to consciously identify the change. It is always better to repeat vital sign assessment and find nothing out of the ordinary than to miss a problem because you did not reassess. Learn to trust your intuitive instincts that tell you the vital signs should be reassessed. Your patient's condition may be dependent upon it.

There are designated times to assess vital signs. Most hospitals have a routine schedule of once every 8 hours, unless the physician orders it more frequently or the nurse determines that there is sufficient reason to measure them at shorter intervals. It is standard to measure vital signs when a patient is admitted to the facility, and they are considered part of the initial shift head-to-toe assessment. Box 17-1 lists other times to assess vital signs.

Further guidelines for assessment of vital signs include:

- Using an organized and systematic approach to assessment of vital signs. For example, if using an oral non-mercury thermometer, place it in the mouth first, then assess the other vital signs while waiting on the temperature reading.
- Using the appropriate equipment for each patient, such as using a child's BP cuff for a child or a large adult cuff for an obese patient.
- Being familiar with normal ranges for different ages.
- Always comparing vital signs with previous vital sign ranges for that specific patient.

- Knowing the patient's medical history, medications, and therapies, as these can sometimes have predictable effects on vital signs.
- Understanding and interpreting the vital sign findings.
- Recording and communicating significant vital sign changes to the physician, as well as to the nurse on the next shift.
- Minimizing environmental effects on vital signs, such as waiting 15 to 30 minutes after the patient has a cold drink to assess oral temperature.

Knowledge Connection
List at least five times or situations when you should assess vital signs rather than delegate them. List at least five guidelines regarding the assessment of vital signs.

Blood Pressure

Blood pressure is the measurement of the pressure or tension of the blood pushing against the walls of the arteries in the vascular system. The amount of pressure is determined by a combination of the following four circulatory qualities:

1. Strength of the heart contraction, or pumping action of the heart
2. Blood viscosity, or thickness
3. Blood volume
4. Peripheral vascular resistance, or elastic recoil ability of the blood vessel walls

The stronger the contraction of the heart, the greater the volume of blood pumped out of the heart into the arteries. The amount of blood ejected from the heart in one contraction is known as the *stroke volume*. The volume of blood pumped from the heart in a full minute is termed the *cardiac output*. The greater the cardiac output, the higher the blood

---

Box 17-1

When to Assess Vital Signs

Every facility will have designated or set times to assess vital signs, such as a specific time on each shift. However, there are many additional situations and circumstances in which it is important that you assess a patient's vital signs. It is your responsibility to identify when it may be necessary to perform this common but important assessment. Additional times to assess vital signs include, but are not limited to, the following:

- On admission to the hospital
- At each visit to a clinic or emergency room
- At each home health or hospice visit
- Every 8 hours or according to hospital policy
- According to physician's orders if more frequent than hospital policy
- Anytime a patient complains of feeling unusual or different
- When you suspect a change in condition

- Before, during, and after administering medications or treatments that affect any of the physiological controls of temperature, pulse, respiration, or oxygen saturation
- Before, during, and after blood product transfusion
- Before, during, and after a surgical procedure or invasive diagnostic procedure
- At least every 4 hours whenever one or more vital signs is abnormal
- A second time, or more, when a vital sign assessment finding is significantly different from the last assessment
- Every 5 to 15 minutes when the patient's condition is unstable, such as after delivery, surgery, or trauma

Note: Vital signs are routinely only assessed once a week or once a month in long-term care, depending upon facility policy.

pressure will be. Conversely, the lower the cardiac output, the lower the pressure will be.

When the heart contraction is weaker or the blood volume is decreased, such as in dehydration or hemorrhage, the blood pressure will decrease. Some conditions that will decrease the heart's contraction strength include congestive heart failure and myocardial infarction (commonly known as a heart attack), which ultimately damage the heart muscle, rendering the contraction of the muscle weaker.

Pregnancy, on the other hand, increases the blood volume, and when there is a higher fluid volume within the vascular system, BP will naturally rise. During exercise, the heart beats faster in an effort to help meet the increased demand for oxygen, and as a result raises BP. When the arterial walls are nonelastic or constricted, the blood pressure will increase. An example of this would be *arteriosclerosis,* otherwise known as hardening of the arteries, which is a gradual process that happens to everyone as they progress through the life span.

Laboratory and Diagnostic Connection

Hematocrit Impacts Blood Pressure

When there is a higher proportion of red blood cells (RBCs) to blood plasma, the viscosity of the blood is increased, which causes the blood pressure to rise. A diagnostic test known as the *hematocrit* is a measurement of this concentration of RBCs in the plasma. Loss of fluids, such as in dehydration, results in a higher hematocrit, while overhydration decreases the hematocrit percentage. Normal ranges are as follows:

- **Newborns:** 49% to 54%
- **Children:** 35% to 49%
- **Adult females:** 37% to 47%
- **Adult males:** 40% to 54%

Factors Affecting Blood Pressure

The patient whose family has a history of hypertension (elevated blood pressure) or other circulatory system problems is more likely to develop hypertension than the patient who does not have a family history of circulatory problems. Diseases such as diabetes and kidney disease also can affect BP. Other factors that affect one's blood pressure include:

- **Age:** The average systolic pressure in newborns is around 40 mm Hg. BP gradually increases throughout the life span.
- **Race:** Hypertension tends to have a higher incidence in African Americans, especially males.
- **Exertion or exercise:** Both cause the heart rate and cardiac output to go up, which then raises the BP.
- **Rest:** When a person is at rest, the parasympathetic system is stimulated and lowers the BP.
- **Circadian rhythm:** BP naturally lowers during sleep, increases with waking until peak is reached in the afternoon, and begins to lower during the evening.
- **Anxiety, stress, and emotions:** These stimulate the sympathetic nervous system, raising BP.

- **Medications:** These can directly or indirectly lower or raise BP.
- **Nicotine and caffeine:** Nicotine can raise BP long term, while caffeine only raises BP for a short interval.
- **Obesity:** BP is higher in some overweight and obese individuals.
- **Level of hydration:** Dehydration, which leads to volume loss, tends to lower BP; overhydration, which leads to volume increase, tends to raise BP.
- **Hemorrhage:** Loss of volume lowers BP.
- **Increased intracranial pressure:** This raises BP.

Components of a Blood Pressure Reading

The measurement of BP involves assessment of two values:

- **Systolic pressure**, which is the measurement of the force exerted by the blood against the walls of arteries during contraction of the heart ventricles. This is when the pressure is the highest.
- **Diastolic pressure**, which is the measurement of the pressure exerted by the blood on the artery walls while the heart ventricles are not contracting; this is the lower of the two pressures. During diastole the ventricles are at rest.

There is a simple word association you can use to help you remember which pressure term relates to the resting state of the heart ventricles: When the ventricles are not contracting, the heart is resting or having down time. *Diastolic* pressure equates with *down* time.

Blood pressure is measured in millimeters of mercury (mm Hg) and is written as a fraction. If the systolic pressure is 120 mm Hg and the diastolic pressure is 72 mm Hg, the blood pressure is written as 120/72 mm Hg, or just 120/72. The systolic pressure will always be the highest reading and is documented as the top number of the fraction, with the diastolic pressure being written as the bottom number.

Pulse pressure is the measurement of the difference between the systolic and diastolic pressures (subtract the smaller number, the diastolic, from the larger number, the systolic) and is normally between 30 and 50 points. A pulse pressure less than 30 or greater than 50 is considered abnormal. An example of a normal pulse pressure of 40 is seen in a blood pressure of 112/72 mm Hg.

The normal range for adult blood pressure is between 90/60 and 120/80 mm Hg. When the systolic pressure rises above 120, it is considered to be *pre-hypertension* (Table 17-1). **Hypertension** is the term used to describe a systolic reading consistently above 140 or a diastolic reading consistently over 90.

To make the medical diagnosis of hypertension, the elevation must be documented on at least two or more separate occasions.

Blood Pressure Equipment

Blood pressure is assessed using a stethoscope and a BP cuff, otherwise known as a **sphygmomanometer** (pronounced *sfig'-moe-man-om'-et-er*), which comes with an aneroid or electronic pressure manometer, or gauge.

Table 17-1 **Categories for Blood Pressure Levels in Adults Over 18 Years of Age***

Category	Systolic (mm Hg)	Diastolic (mm Hg)
Normal	Less than 120	Less than 80
Pre-hypertension	120–139	80–89
High blood pressure[†] – Stage I	140–159	90–99
High blood pressure – Stage II	160 or higher	100 or higher

*This is for individuals who are not on medicine for high blood pressure, are not having a short-term serious illness, and do not have other conditions, such as diabetes or kidney disease.

[†]There is an *exception* to this definition of high blood pressure. A blood pressure of 130/80 mm Hg or higher is considered high blood pressure in people with diabetes and chronic kidney disease.

Source: National Institutes of Health, April, 2006. Retrieved from http://www.nhlbi.nih.gov/health/dci/Diseases/Hbp/HBP_All.html. Accessed August 10, 2009.

Sphygmomanometer

The aneroid sphygmomanometer consists of an inflatable rubber bladder that holds air, a cloth cuff that covers the bladder and is long enough to wrap around the extremity, rubber tubing from the bladder to the gauge to indicate the pressure, and rubber tubing from the air bladder to a bulb that is used to pump up the air bladder. A screw valve is attached proximally to the squeezable bulb, and allows you to fill and empty the air from the bladder as you observe the pressure manometer. The aneroid gauge must be calibrated every 6 months to remain accurate, so make certain the needle is on zero before using a cuff.

An electronic sphygmomanometer has a transducer that uses sound waves to determine the pressure and a digital gauge to provide the readout, and it automatically inflates and deflates. There is neither a squeezable bulb nor a need for a stethoscope when using an electronic cuff.

The sphygmomanometer may be mounted on the wall above the patient's bed or on an automatic vital sign machine, or it is available as a smaller, portable cuff unit. Box 17-2 provides additional information regarding automatic vital sign machines, and Figure 17-1 shows the different BP cuff types.

The cuffs also come in different sizes, and the correct size must be used to accurately assess the blood pressure: If it is too large the reading will be erroneously low, and if it is too small the reading will be erroneously high. The width of the blood pressure cuff should cover approximately two-thirds of the upper arm. Figure 17-2 shows a BP cuff containing an inflatable bladder.

Stethoscope

A stethoscope has a sound-transmitting chest piece consisting of a bell and a diaphragm that attaches to rubber tubing that leads to two hollow metal tubes (binaurals) with earpieces attached to the ends. The earpieces are placed in the ears corresponding to the angle of the ear canals and should point toward the face when the stethoscope is in place. The chest

Box 17-2

Automatic Vital Sign Machines

Automatic vital sign machines have the capability to assess multiple data simultaneously, including:
- BP
- Temperature
- Pulse rate
- SpO_2

Some machines are capable of displaying trends in vital signs. You can preset intervals at which the machine is to measure the vitals, as well as set automatic high and low alarms to warn of abnormal findings. You can print the vital signs for posting in the patient record. These machines are convenient for frequent vital sign assessment schedules, such as postoperative and blood product transfusion schedules. *Safety: Manually assess vital signs as needed to validate machine accuracy.*

Figure 17-1 *Front row, left to right:* a digital sphygmomanometer, an automated vital signs monitor, and an aneroid manometer and cuff. *Back center:* A wall-mounted aneroid manometer and cuff.

Cuff

Valve

Bulb

Tube to sphygmomanometer

(a)

|← Bladder length →|

Cuff

Bladder

Bladder width

(b)

Figure 17-2 A blood pressure cuff showing placement of the inflatable bladder within the cuff.

piece is placed against the patient's skin: The bell is used to auscultate the lower pitched sounds such as the heart sounds and BP (Fig. 17-3), while the larger flat side, known as the diaphragm, is used to auscultate high-pitched sounds such as the lung sounds. Note that some stethoscopes do not have a bell, thus requiring that the diaphragm be used.

Figure 17-3 A stethoscope. *Top:* The concave side, known as the bell, is used for auscultating heart sounds and other low-frequency sounds. *Bottom:* The flat side, known as the diaphragm, is used for auscultating higher pitched sounds, such as breath sounds and blood pressure.

Assessment Sites

Blood pressure is normally assessed with the cuff around the upper arm and the stethoscope over the brachial artery at the antecubital site, on the inner aspect of the elbow. It can also be performed on the lower arm by wrapping the cuff around the lower arm and placing the stethoscope over the radial pulse. However, certain conditions prevent you from using these sites, including:

• Amputation of the arm
• Mastectomy on the selected side
• Presence of a shunt for renal dialysis on the selected side
• Casts, braces, or dressings
• Recent vascular surgery or trauma on the selected side
• In some cases, the presence of an IV infusion on the selected side

When conditions prevent you from assessing BP on either arm, it can be measured on the leg by wrapping the correct-size cuff around the midthigh (Fig. 17-4), with the cuff bladder on the posterior aspect of the thigh and the tubing exiting the cuff distally (toward the knee), and placing the stethoscope over the popliteal artery behind the knee. The systolic pressure may register 10 to 40 mm Hg higher in the leg than in the arm, but the diastolic pressure should be about the same.

Korotkoff's Sounds

Upon inflation of the cuff and accompanying compression of the artery, the flow of blood is not audible with a stethoscope. As you begin to deflate the cuff and allow the return of blood flow, you will hear the tapping sounds representing this blood flow. These are known as *Korotkoff's sounds,* named after the Russian physician who first described the sounds heard over an artery during cuff deflation. There are five Korotkoff's sounds:

• **First sound:** clear, rhythmic tapping sound gradually increasing in intensity
• **Second sound:** soft, swishing or murmuring sound representing turbulent blood flow

Figure 17-4 Position the cuff bladder on the posterior aspect of the thigh with the bottom edge 1 to 2 inches (2.5 to 5 cm) above the popliteal fossa, centering the arrow on the cuff directly over the popliteal artery. Wrap the cuff snugly around the thigh.

- **Third sound:** sharper, crisper rhythmic sound
- **Fourth sound:** softening or muffling of rhythmic sound
- **Fifth sound:** silence

You may or may not hear all five of the sounds that represent different stages of returning blood flow, but the first sound heard is documented as the systolic pressure and the point at which you last hear any sound is documented as the diastolic pressure.

Measurement of Blood Pressure

After selecting the site for assessment and determining the correct size cuff, bare the arm, and wrap the cuff around the extremity about 1 to 2 inches above the auscultation site for your stethoscope. While palpating the arterial pulse distal to the cuff, close the screw valve and squeeze the bulb to rapidly pump the inflatable cuff up to 70 mm Hg for an adult. Now continue to slowly pump the pressure up about 10 mm Hg at a time, until you can no longer feel the pulse, noting the point at which you lose the pulse. Then deflate the cuff and wait 15 to 30 seconds. Place your stethoscope over the arterial pulse and keep the chest piece of the stethoscope flat against the bare skin. Pump the cuff up to approximately 30 mm Hg above where you last felt the pulse. For example, if you last felt the pulse at 116 mm Hg, pump the cuff up to 146 mm Hg. It is uncomfortable for the patient and may cause erroneous readings to pump the pressure up to 180 or 200 mm Hg when pressure is not that high. Slowly unscrew the valve to release air from the cuff bladder at 2 to 3 mm Hg per second, while listening for Korotkoff's sounds. Record the number at which you hear the first Korotkoff sound and the number at which you hear the last sound. Write it as a fraction, such as 118/76. If you hear the sounds all the way to zero on the manometer, record the number at which the sound decreased in amplitude as well as the zero, such as 126/74/0. Further description of blood pressure assessment is found in Skill 17-1 (see page 364).

Auscultatory Gap

When assessing the blood pressure in patients with hypertension, you may detect the first Korotkoff sound and then lose the sounds for 20 to 30 mm Hg, before the sounds return. This silence and return of sounds is known as an *auscultatory gap.* If you do not adequately inflate the cuff while palpating, this gap can be missed and an erroneously low blood pressure reading recorded. An error of this nature might result in failure to identify an elevated blood pressure that requires treatment. Use caution to palpate carefully and then inflate to 30 mm Hg above that point. If an auscultatory gap is detected, record the number at which it began and ended, for example: BP – 162/74 with auscultatory gap 158 to 138.

Hypertension

Normally, the arterial walls are elastic, with stretch and recoil abilities to accommodate the changing volume of blood in the cardiovascular system. However, as arteriosclerosis progresses through the years, the gradual loss of elasticity in the arterial walls results in less stretch and recoil. The heart has to work harder to pump the blood through the cardiovascular system as the rigidity of the artery walls increases. The rise in blood pressure that occurs as a result is known as *primary* or *essential hypertension.* When there is a renal or endocrine disease process that results in elevation of BP, it is termed *secondary hypertension.*

Hypertension is a widespread health problem in the United States, and because there are frequently few or no symptoms, it often goes untreated. Thus, it is important that you educate your patients and encourage them to have annual blood pressure screenings. Also teach your patients the risk factors that contribute to the occurrence of hypertension (Box 17-3).

Treatment of Hypertension

Treatment of hypertension usually involves a number of lifestyle changes, such as reducing dietary intake of salt and fat, weight loss, smoking cessation, reduction or cessation of excessive alcohol intake, stress reduction, and increasing physical activity and exercise, as well as the use of medications when lifestyle changes are not adequate. Left untreated, hypertension can result in permanent damage to the following:

- Brain, in the form of a stroke
- Heart, in the form of congestive heart failure or myocardial infarction (heart attack)
- Kidneys, resulting in kidney failure
- Retinas of the eyes, resulting in loss of vision

Hypotension

When BP suddenly falls 20 mm Hg to 30 mm Hg below the patient's normal BP or falls below the low normal of 90/60 mm Hg, it is considered **hypotension**. However, it is important to note that some perfectly healthy individuals normally run blood pressures in the lower ranges, such as a person with a small body build or an athlete in good physical condition. This is one reason it is necessary for you to always be familiar with your patient's normal range of vital signs. What would be abnormal for one patient, and require treatment, might be normal for another patient, with no need for treatment.

Box 17-3

Risk Factors for Hypertension

It is important to identify an individual's risk factors for development of hypertension. Common risk factors include:
- Positive family history of hypertension
- Smoking
- Chronically high stress level
- Moderate to heavy alcohol consumption
- Obesity
- Elevated cholesterol levels in the blood

Normally, the peripheral arteries have enough elasticity and recoil to constrict and provide for a slight increase in blood pressure to counteract the forces of gravity upon arising from a lying position to a sitting or standing position. In older adults, much of this elasticity has been lost, thus slowing or reducing the constriction of the arteries, allowing the blood to pool in the lower extremities upon standing. As a result, BP drops, sometimes enough to result in dizziness and *syncope* (fainting). When position changes result in a systolic pressure drop of 15 to 25 mm Hg or the diastolic pressure falls 10 mm Hg, this is known as orthostatic hypotension, also known as *postural hypotension*. Patients who are dehydrated, have anemia, or have been limited to bedrest for extended periods of time, and those who are receiving medications such as narcotic analgesics, sedatives, and anesthesia medications, are more prone to orthostatic hypotension. Skill 17-2 (see page 366) provides information on the assessment of orthostatic hypotension.

It is advisable to teach these patients to slowly sit up from a reclining position, and then to sit on the edge of the bed for several minutes to allow their blood pressure to balance before standing up. After he or she has stood up, you should encourage the patient to stand for several seconds before walking away from the bed to make sure that he or she is not going to faint.

If a patient becomes faint due to hypotension, the initial treatment is to lay the person in a *modified Trendelenburg* position. This is a supine position with the feet elevated above the level of the heart. This increases the blood flow to the brain. A *full Trendelenburg position* involving further positioning to lower the head below heart level is no longer recommended.

An extremely serious condition results when hypotension is due to hemorrhage or shock. Immediate medical intervention is necessary to provide adequate blood supply and oxygen to the life-sustaining organs.

Body Temperature

Body temperature is the difference between the amount of heat the body produces and the amount of heat that is gained or lost to the external environment. The core temperature, the temperature of the deeper structures and tissues, is normally slightly warmer than that of the more superficial body tissues. The core temperature is the most important measurement to maintain as it determines the conditions in which the brain, heart, and other internal organs must survive.

Measurement of the true core temperature is accomplished with a sterile thermometer probe inserted into the pulmonary artery, heart, or urinary bladder. However, in most circumstances it is adequate to measure the body temperature using a clinical thermometer and less invasive methods, which are presented in this chapter. The body's surface, or skin, temperature is typically assessed by laying your hand on the skin to determine if it is warm, hot, cool, or cold, as well as whether it is dry or moist.

Scales of Temperature Measurement

Health care providers measure body temperature using either the Fahrenheit scale or the centigrade scale, also known as the Celsius scale. Figure 17-5 shows a comparison of the two scales, and Box 17-4 presents a conversion formula.

Thermogenesis

The production of heat is known as *thermogenesis.* One of the ways the human body produces heat is through the processes occurring after ingestion of food: digestion, absorption, breakdown, and synthesis of proteins. Because the intake of food results in the increase of these metabolic functions, the production of heat increases. In other words, body heat is a by-product of metabolism. More heat is produced as metabolism speeds up and less is produced when metabolism slows down. The *basal metabolic rate (BMR)* is the amount of heat produced by the body when at total rest. Because an increase in metabolism results in more heat production, any physical activity that increases the metabolism will also increase heat production. Muscle contraction normally produces about 25% of body heat in the resting state. Shivering, an involuntary skeletal muscle response, can raise heat production to four to five times normal. Depending upon the level of exertion, exercise can increase the metabolic rate up to 50 times normal, thus explaining why you feel so "hot" when performing moderate to heavy exercise.

Numerous other factors influence heat production, including the hormones thyroxine, produced by the thyroid gland; epinephrine and norepinephrine, secreted by the adrenal medulla; and adenosine triphosphate (ATP), which is an energy source produced in all cells during cellular respiration. The liver is always metabolically active and produces 15% to 20% of body heat in the resting state.

People and Places Connection

Newborns Cannot Shiver

As you know, adults and children begin to involuntarily shiver when body temperature differences develop. However, newborn infants, especially premature infants, cannot shiver. They are born with a limited supply of vascular brown adipose tissue, which is primarily metabolized for heat production. That is why providing external sources of warmth, such as controlled environmental temperature, radiant warmers, incubators, caps, and blankets, is so important for maintaining the newborn's body heat.

Older adults may also have a difficult time maintaining normal body temperature due to the limited amount of subcutaneous fat cells available to insulate their internal organs. If they have any type of circulatory impairment, this inhibits the vasoconstriction and vasodilation aspects of controlling body temperature.

Body temperature

Temperature regulation by the hypothalamus

Upper limit of survival? — 114°

112°

110°   44° — Temperature regulation is seriously impaired

Heat stroke or high fever — 108°   42°

106°

104°   40°

Strenuous exercise or fever — 102°   38° — Temperature regulation is efficient

100°   37°

Usual range of normal — 98°   36°

96°

94°   34°

92°

90°   32° — Temperature regulation is impaired

Hypothermia (cold weather or immersion in cold water) — 88°

86°   30°

84°   28°

82°

80°   26° — Temperature regulation is lost

78°

76°   24°

74°

72°

70°

68°

Lower limit of survival? — 66°

°F   °C

Figure 17-5 Ranges of normal and abnormal body temperatures in degrees Fahrenheit and degrees Celsius.

Thermoregulation

Thermoregulation, or regulation of body temperature, is primarily controlled by the part of the brain known as the *hypothalamus.* When the hypothalamus functions correctly, it maintains a comfortable core temperature known as the *set-point.* When this set-point is exceeded, signals are sent causing the body to sweat and the blood vessels to dilate. This vasodilation brings more blood to the skin's surface for increased heat loss through radiation, resulting in reduction of temperature. The sweat helps to reduce temperature through evaporation. When the sweat production is high enough to be seen on the skin, it is termed *diaphoresis.*

The hypothalamus also has capabilities to increase heat production by causing muscles to shiver and to conserve body heat by constricting vessels in the body's outer surface layers and extremities. This vasoconstriction helps to redirect the majority of blood flow to the vital organs, primarily the brain and heart, to maintain adequate core temperature.

Factors Affecting Body Temperature

Many internal and external factors affect body temperature. Some of the common factors are environment, time of day, gender, physical activity and exercise, medications, food or liquid intake, stress, and illness.

Environment

The climate and temperature of the environment affect the body temperature accordingly. If the environment is hot, the body temperature will tend to be higher, and when the environmental temperature is cold, the body temperature will tend to be lower.

Time of Day

The body has a "time clock" or rhythm of its own, known as the *circadian rhythm*. The body's physiological functions vary somewhat over the 24-hour day. Most individuals' body temperature will drop 0.5°F to 1°F lower between midnight and dawn and raise 1°F to 2°F in the late afternoon and evening, thus explaining why children always seem to get "sicker" after the typical physician's office closes in the afternoon.

Gender

Only slight differences are found in the ranges of normal vital signs for men versus women. However, women tend to have a slight rise in body temperature during ovulation. This is due to the rising level of progesterone, a hormone that prepares the uterus for pregnancy.

Physical Activity and Exercise

During activity and exercise, muscles require fuel in the form of glucose to metabolize or burn for energy. As mentioned earlier in the chapter, the more metabolism increases, the more heat the body produces. Thus, exercise raises the body temperature and inactivity lowers it.

Medications

Various medications affect the body temperature. Stimulants such as ephedrine increase the body's metabolism and, thus, raise body temperature. Other medications such as acetaminophen will cause an elevated temperature to lower.

Food Intake

Because calories are burned, providing fuel for metabolism, the amount, type, or lack of food ingested can directly affect the body temperature. Hot and cold fluids can have mild effects on the oral temperature reading for 15 to 30 minutes after ingestion.

Stress

Individuals who are anxious or stressed may tend to have a slightly higher body temperature due to the stimulation of the sympathetic nervous system. This results in production of excessive amounts of hormones such as epinephrine, which will raise the body's metabolic rate, including the temperature.

Illness

Various diseases and injuries can directly affect the hypothalamus, resulting in changes in body temperature. Common conditions affecting body temperature include inflammatory processes and infections caused by bacteria or viruses, fluid loss, central nervous system tumors, head injuries, and heat stroke.

Knowledge Connection

Explain what is meant by set-point. Identify at least five factors that can affect body temperature. Describe how the body regulates its temperature.

Types of Thermometers

Various types of clinical thermometers may be used to assess the body temperature, including a glass or plastic non-mercury thermometer, disposable chemical-strip thermometer, electronic thermometer, tympanic thermometer, and temporal artery thermometer (Fig. 17-6). Glass and plastic non-mercury thermometers have either an elongated tip with a blue indicator or a rounded tip with a red indicator. The rounded tip and red color indicate the thermometer is for rectal use. The elongated tip with a blue indicator may be used for oral and axillary temperature measurement only. Some disposable chemical-strip thermometers are designed for topical application to the skin and others are designed for oral or axillary use. Electronic thermometers may be used to assess oral, axillary, or rectal temperatures. The tympanic

Figure 17-6 Types of thermometers. *(a)* Non-mercury thermometer. *(b)* Tympanic thermometer. *(c)* Electronic thermometer. *(d)* Digital-tape or other paper strip thermometer.

thermometer is used only for measurement of the temperature of the tympanic membrane in the ear. Temporal artery thermometers are used to scan the temporal artery of the head for blood temperature.

Disposable thermometer sheath covers should be used each time a glass or plastic non-mercury, electronic, or tympanic thermometer is used to prevent cross-contamination. Before using non-mercury thermometers, they must be shaken down so the temperature reading is below 95°F (35°C).

Routes of Temperature Assessment

Body temperature is most accurate when measured at sites where there is a rich blood supply. The common routes used to measure temperature are the oral, axillary, tympanic, skin,

temporal artery, and rectal routes. The *axillary route* consists of placing the thermometer under the arm, in the armpit. The tympanic route requires the use of a special thermometer designed to fit into the ear canal and measure the temperature of the tympanic membrane. A scanning thermometer may also be used to measure the temperature of the blood by scanning the temporal artery.

For continuous, noninvasive monitoring of body temperature, a temperature probe or chemical-strip thermometer may be applied to the skin. In intensive care units, it is sometimes important to continuously monitor the patient's core temperature by inserting a sterile catheter probe into the pulmonary artery. Each route has advantages and disadvantages that are listed in Table 17-2. Skill 17-3 (see page 367) covers how to assess body temperature by various routes.

Table 17-2 Advantages and Disadvantages of Temperature Assessment Routes

Route	Advantages	Disadvantages
Oral	Convenient and easily accessible route. Simple. Does not require position change.	Risk of body fluid exposure. Affected by smoking, drinking hot or cold liquids, and oxygen administration. Not for infants, small children, or confused or unconscious patients.
Skin	Convenient, safe, easily accessible, and comfortable route for patient. Provides continual assessment to reflect changes quickly. Easy and does not require position change. Good for use with newborns. Unaffected by eating, drinking, or smoking.	Affected by perspiration. Reflects surface rather than core temperature. Affected by severe environmental temperatures.
Tympanic membrane	Convenient and easily accessible route. Good for use with newborns. Quick (less than 5 seconds). Good for patients with difficulty breathing or on supplemental oxygen. Often can be performed without disturbing a sleeping patient. Comfortable for patient. Unaffected by eating, drinking, or smoking.	Inaccurate if probe is not pointed directly at the tympanic membrane. The walls of the ear canal are cooler than the tympanic membrane. Correct placement is difficult in children's ear canals. Affected by environmental factors such as radiant heaters or incubators. Cannot be used for patients with ear infections or after ear surgery. Higher cost of equipment.
Temporal artery	Quick (less than 5 seconds). Easy, noninvasive, and comfortable. Good for use with small children. Does not require positioning. Unaffected by eating, drinking, or smoking.	Affected by perspiration. Inaccurate if hair is thick on forehead. Higher cost of equipment.

(table continues on page 354)

Table 17-2 **Advantages and Disadvantages of Temperature Assessment Routes** (continued)

Route	Advantages	Disadvantages
Axillary	Safe and noninvasive. Can be used with unconscious patient.	Takes 5–8 minutes. Temperature will be at least 1° F less than core temperature. Changes in temperature are slower to be reflected. Must be continually held in place by nurse.
Rectal	Provides core temperature. Reflects temperature changes quickly.	Source of embarrassment for patient. Requires positioning of patient. Risk of body fluid exposure. Risk of rectum perforation, especially in newborns. Cannot be used for patients with diarrhea, severe hemorrhoids, or rectal surgery.
Internal catheter probe	Most accurate. Provides core temperature. Continual monitoring.	Most invasive. Requires sterile technique. Risk of vessel perforation and infection.

Oral

To accurately measure an oral temperature, you must make certain the patient has not eaten, drunk, or smoked within the last 15 to 30 minutes. After applying a disposable thermometer cover sheath, the thermometer should be placed deep into the sublingual pocket under the tongue. Make sure the patient is able to hold the thermometer in place with his or her tongue. If not, select another route for temperature assessment.

If a non-mercury thermometer is used, it should be left in place for 3 minutes. Single-use oral paper thermometers vary in length of time required, so read the instructions carefully before using them. An electronic thermometer will only be left in place until it signals the assessment is complete, usually in less than 1 minute. Again, read the instructions for use first.

Axillary

The axillary route is used for patients who cannot hold the oral thermometer in place or for patients for whom the oral route might pose a safety risk, such as a patient who is having seizures. The thermometer should be inserted into a disposable plastic thermometer cover and placed under the arm in the axilla for 5 to 8 minutes. Make sure the thermometer bulb is encased within the axilla and does not protrude behind the arm. Either a non-mercury or an electronic thermometer may be used when assessing temperature using the axillary route. If an electronic thermometer is used, leave it in place only until it signals the temperature has been read, usually less than 1 minute.

Tympanic

The tympanic thermometer is an infrared device used with a disposable cover over the tip of the speculum. Gently pull the pinna up and back on an adult and down and back on a small child younger than 3 years. The speculum should be inserted gently into the ear canal, pointing the tip toward the mandible on the opposite side of the face, and making a seal between the ear and the speculum. After pushing the indicated button on the device, it takes only 1 to 2 seconds to read the temperature.

Skin

If using a disposable topical chemical-strip thermometer, peel the backing off and apply the sticky side of the thermometer directly to clean, dry skin. If using a special thermometer with a skin probe, tape the probe to the skin and observe the continual temperature readout. *Safety: If the skin probe is part of a radiant heating device such as those used on newborns, make certain to set the temperature alarms so the infant is not at risk of being overheated to dangerous levels.*

Rectal

You may use a non-mercury thermometer or an electronic thermometer with a separate rectal probe that is usually marked with red to indicate it is for rectal use. Insert the thermometer into a disposable plastic thermometer cover sheath and lubricate the tip of the thermometer with a water-soluble lubricant. Wearing gloves, insert the thermometer into the rectum approximately 1 to 1½ inches for an adult, ½ to 1 inch for a child, and ½ inch for an infant. The thermometer is left in place for 2 minutes unless it is electronic, which will take less than 1 minute. *Safety: Due to the risk of intestinal perforation, this route is not recommended as the route of choice.*

Temporal Artery

A special thermometer is used to scan the temporal artery temperature. While pressing the scan button with your thumb, the probe is placed on a dry forehead and moved slowly across the width of the forehead and temple. The probe is then lifted off the skin and touched to the neck just behind the earlobe.

Normal Body Temperatures by Selected Routes

The normal range for core temperatures varies from 97°F to 99.6°F (36.1°C to 37.5°C), with the average being 98.6°F (37°C). The oral, tympanic, and temporal artery routes are the most common routes used to measure the temperature and should provide close to the same readings, within about 0.5° (Table 17-3). The rectal route provides the closest to the core temperature and is approximately 1°F higher than the oral temperature. The axillary route will be approximately 1°F lower than the oral.

Elevated Temperature

Various terms are used to indicate an elevated body temperature, including *fever, pyrexia,* and *hyperthermia.* The term **febrile** is used to indicate the state of having a fever and **afebrile** is used to indicate the state of being without fever. *Hyperthermia* is more commonly used to describe serious elevations above 105°F or 40.5°C.

Fever is the body's natural way of protecting itself from bacteria, viruses, other microorganisms, and foreign bodies that invade the body and threaten its state of health. After these invaders enter an area of the body in which they do not belong, the body stimulates specialized white blood cells whose purpose is to ingest the invaders. These specialized blood cells, known as *phagocytes,* secrete pyrogens, which stimulate secretion of prostaglandin hormones. The prostaglandin hormones trigger the hypothalamus to raise the set-point for body temperature in an effort to prevent replication of the offending microorganisms—in other words, to raise the temperature high enough to inhibit microorganism reproduction. To assist in raising the temperature, the body tries to conserve body heat through surface vasoconstriction. This can cause the patient to feel chilled or cold. Muscles may begin to involuntarily contract, known as *shivering,* as the body attempts to increase its metabolic rate to reach the new temperature set-point. As the new set-point is attained, the fever also stimulates production of interferon, which is the body's natural defense mechanism against invading viruses.

Because fever is the body's natural defense against infection, it is accepted practice to allow the fever to accomplish its purpose unless it becomes too high. Most physicians will not attempt to reduce fever until it elevates above 102°F (38.9°C). Elevations above 105°F (40.5°C) can result in damage to body cells. Fever may occur and be constant, or it may come and go in differing patterns.

Signs and Symptoms of Fever

Every patient with a fever will not present in the same manner. Some of the common signs and symptoms that may indicate fever include:

- Flushed, warm skin
- Dry mucous membranes
- Glassy or droopy eyes
- Increased irritability or restlessness
- Photophobia, which means the eyes have increased sensitivity to light
- Thirst
- Headache or myalgia
- Lethargy or drowsiness
- Diaphoresis
- Anorexia
- Confusion, especially in children and elderly
- Seizures in infants and children

Nursing Care for Patients with Fever

When caring for a patient with fever, you will want to perform the following:

- Assess all vital signs at least every 2 hours, and more often depending upon the degree of abnormality.
- Provide allowed fluids frequently, and measure intake and output as soon as fever is detected, as it is important to remember that your patient will have an additional need for adequate fluid intake (up to 3 liters per day) to allow for proper cell function and to prevent dehydration. If you detect signs that the patient is dehydrating or not taking adequate oral fluids, it is your responsibility to notify the physician for possible IV fluid orders.
- Take extra care to offer foods the patient likes, and offer five to six smaller feedings rather than the routine three meals per day. This will provide your patient with the nutritional needs necessary to accommodate his or

Table 17-3   Normal Temperature Equivalents by Sites

	Oral	Tympanic	Rectal	Axillary
Fahrenheit (°)	98.6	98.6	99.6	97.6
Celsius (°)	37	37	37.5	36.4

her increased metabolic rate. It will also provide proper nutrition for febrile patients, who often experience anorexia.

- Provide mouth and skin care to prevent dryness. Apply petroleum jelly to lips and lotion to skin. A cool washcloth may be applied to the eyes, forehead, or neck. A tepid sponge bath may be given to ease the patient's discomfort, as long as you are careful to avoid chilling the patient and causing shivering, which will actually raise the temperature.
- Encourage limited activity and rest to reduce the amount of heat produced through physical activity.
- Encourage the patient to use minimal covers unless shivering occurs. Then a blanket may be used in an attempt to prevent shivering.
- Apply cloth-covered ice packs to the forehead or neck, axillae, and groin for high fevers, making sure to avoid causing shivering.
- If the patient is perspiring, keep gown and linens clean and dry to avoid chilling.
- Administer *antipyretic,* or fever-reducing, medications as ordered. Common antipyretics used include salicylates, acetaminophen, and ibuprofen.
- In higher fevers, it may become necessary to provide supplemental oxygen to meet the body's increased metabolic needs.

Knowledge Connection

Describe how and why the body raises its temperature during illness. List at least four signs and symptoms of fever. Explain at least three nursing actions you should take when a patient exhibits fever.

Patient Teaching Connection

Children With Viruses: No Aspirin!

It is important to educate your patients regarding the proper medications to use for fever reduction in children. Avoid all salicylate use, including aspirin, in children less than 15 years of age due to the increased risk of Reye's syndrome. Reye's syndrome is an acute and potentially fatal childhood disease, affecting the central nervous system and liver, that has been associated with administration of aspirin to children with viruses.

Hypothermia

Hypothermia, or body temperature below 96°F (34.4°C), slows body metabolism. Though hypothermia may be induced deliberately to reduce the body's need for oxygen during neurological or cardiac surgeries, prolonged or severe periods of hypothermia can result in death. Mild hypothermia is treated with warm clothes or blankets and ingestion of warm drinks such as broth or soup. *Safety: Because up to 40% of body heat can be lost through* *the head, coverings such as a hat or scarf can dramatically help reduce heat loss.* More severe hypothermia generally is treated with additional measures such as heating blankets, hot water bottles, warmed IV fluids, or warm baths. Patients with severe hypothermia should be brought up to normal temperature slowly due to the risk of irregular heart rhythm and shock.

Pulse

The heart's four chambers rhythmically contract and relax. With each contraction of the ventricles, oxygenated blood is forced out of the left ventricle through the aorta to be delivered to the body's arteries. The amount of blood discharged from the left ventricle with each contraction is known as the *stroke volume.* This pumping action of the heart results in a fluid wave of blood that travels through the arteries as they rhythmically expand and contract. This arterial fluid wave can be palpated as a gentle pulsing, tapping, or throbbing sensation at various points over the body; this is called the *pulse.* The pulse corresponds to the contractions or beats of the heart and is counted by the number of beats per minute (bpm). The volume of blood pumped from the heart in 1 minute is known as the *cardiac output.* The average adult heart pumps approximately 5 liters per minute.

The central or primary pulse site, the *apical pulse,* is located over the apex of the heart where the contraction is the strongest (Fig. 17-7). The apex of the heart, the cone-shaped end of the left ventricle, actually touches the anterior chest wall at or near the fifth intercostal space. This spot is known as the point of maximum impulse (PMI) and is

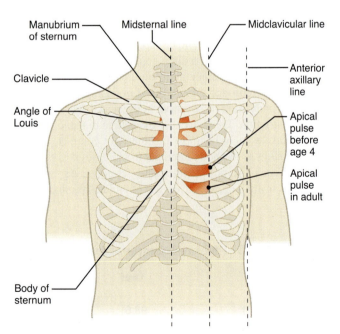

Figure 17-7 Location of apical pulse for adults and children.

located 3 to 4 inches to the left of the sternum, in the fifth intercostal space, at the midclavicular line. In a child, it may be found in the fourth or fifth intercostal space. You should be able to feel the PMI with your fingertips. The PMI is the site over which you will place your stethoscope to auscultate, or listen to, the apical pulse.

Though less convenient to assess, the apical pulse is the most accurate pulse because both heart sounds can generally be heard and it provides information about the valves and contraction of the atria and ventricles that cannot be detected when assessing peripheral pulses. The apical pulse can be auscultated even when peripheral pulses cannot be detected. It is assessed for a full minute to listen for irregularities. When auscultating the heart sounds, you normally hear two sounds called the S_1 and S_2, or "lubb-dupp." Together, these two sounds represent one complete heartbeat. If both the S_1 and S_2 or lubb-dupp sounds are heard clearly and distinctly, the volume or strength of the apical pulse is described as *distinct* or *strong*. If both heart sounds cannot be heard distinctly, it is described as *distant* or *muffled*.

The apical pulse should be the same rate as the peripheral pulses, but when the heart does not pump effectively, this may result in a blood flow that is not strong enough to consistently deliver a fluid wave to the more distant pulse sites from the heart. Often this occurs when the pulse is irregular, resulting in an apical pulse rate that is faster than the radial pulse. When the radial pulse is slower than the apical pulse, this is known as a **pulse deficit.** For example, the heart rate may be 83 bpm but the radial pulse is only 77 bpm. This would be a pulse deficit of 6 bpm, and should be recorded and reported. The number of the pulse deficit, 6 in the previous example, represents the number of heartbeats in which the force of the heart's contraction fails to produce a pulse wave strong enough to be felt at, or *perfuse* to, the radial pulse site. Beats that do not perfuse are ineffective in circulating the blood. Skill 17-4 (see page 369) presents more information on assessing the radial and apical pulses.

Anatomy and Physiology Connection

What Makes the Heart Beat?
Though contraction of the heart is a function of the cardiovascular system, the rate of contraction is regulated by the medulla oblongata, located in the brainstem of the central nervous system. In a normal healthy heart, contraction of the heart, or the heartbeat, initiates in the sinoatrial (SA) node in the top of the right atrium in the form of an electrical impulse. The impulse is conducted through the atrium on the electrical conduction pathway, causing the atria to depolarize and contract. The impulse continues on the electrical conduction pathway through the atrioventricular (AV) node in the right ventricle. From there, the impulse is transmitted through the bundle of His and the Purkinje fibers throughout both ventricles. Once the impulse has been transmitted through both ventricles, the ventricles depolarize and contract. As the ventricular contraction begins, the AV valves, also known as the *tricuspid* and *bicuspid valves,* slam shut, causing the first heart sound: the longer, lower pitched sound known as the S_1 or "lubb." As soon as the ventricles begin relaxation, the semilunar valves, also known as the *pulmonary* and *aortic valves,* close, causing a shorter and sharper sound: S_2 or "dupp." Thus the pattern of normal heart sounds is a rhythmic "lubb-dupp,… lubb-dupp,…lubb-dupp."

Peripheral Pulse Sites

There are various other pulse sites where the pulse may be palpated by applying gentle fingertip pressure over the artery against the underlying bone. These sites are known as the *peripheral pulses* (Fig. 17-8). The peripheral pulse sites include the following:

- **Temporal:** can be used when radial pulse is not accessible
- **Carotid:** used in cardiac arrest and cardiopulmonary resuscitation (CPR)
- **Brachial:** used to measure BP, can be used to assess pulse rate in small children
- **Radial:** routinely used for pulse rate assessment

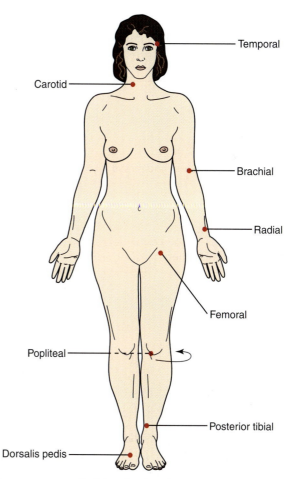

Figure 17-8   Peripheral pulse sites.

- **Femoral:** used to determine circulation to the leg, cardiac arrest
- **Popliteal:** used to determine circulation to the lower leg
- **Posterior tibialis:** used to determine circulation to the foot
- **Dorsalis pedis:** used to determine circulation to the foot

The temporal pulse can be felt over the temporal bones on the sides of the head. The carotid pulse is located on the sides of the neck between the trachea and the sternocleidomastoid muscle. The brachial pulse is found in the medial elbow crease of each arm, known as the antecubital space. The radial pulse runs parallel to the radius bone on the thumb side of the wrist. The femoral pulse can be palpated along the groin crease at the top of the thigh. The most difficult pulse to locate is the popliteal, found behind the knee. It will help to have the patient slightly flex the knee before palpating. To feel the dorsalis pedis pulse, place your fingertips at the space between the great toe and the second toe. Move the fingers proximally until they rest over the metatarsals of the foot. The posterior tibialis pulse is located by laying your fingertips on the medial aspect of the ankle, directly behind the medial malleolus bone.

Any of the peripheral pulses can be used to assess the heart rate, but the easily accessible radial pulse is the most commonly used site; if it is weak or cannot be felt, then the apical pulse is auscultated. Use the apical pulse for assessing pulse rate in children under the age of 3, when the radial pulse is weak or has irregular rhythm, and prior to administering heart rate–altering medications such as digoxin. The peripheral pulses are generally assessed for strength or volume, comparing the right and left sides for equal strength. During CPR, the carotid artery is easily palpated to determine the presence of a pulse. *Safety: Never palpate both carotid pulses at the same time, as this can drop the pulse and blood pressure.* Skill 17-5 (see page 370) presents more information on assessing peripheral pulses to detect circulation.

Pulse Assessment

As a nurse, you will assess three characteristics of the pulse:

1. Rate
2. Rhythm
3. Volume (strength)

The normal range of pulse rate for adults is 60 to 100 bpm. If the pulse is less than 60 bpm, it is known as **bradycardia**; a pulse greater than 100 bpm is termed **tachycardia**. Numerous factors can affect the pulse rate (Table 17-4).

The rhythm is determined by comparing the intervals between the beats. If all the beats are evenly spaced, the

Table 17-4   Factors Affecting Pulse Rate

Factor	Effect
Age	Newborns: 120–160 bpm 1–2 years: 90–120 bpm 3–18 years: 80–100 bpm Adults: 60–100 bpm
Emotions, hormones, and stress	Stimulate sympathetic nervous system, increasing pulse rate.
Medications	Can either speed or slow pulse rate. Drugs such as digitalis or propranolol slow the rate, while epinephrine and theophylline speed up the rate.
Caffeine and nicotine	Speed the rate.
Exercise	Speeds the rate during activity. Long-term training and conditioning, such as in athletes, will slow the rate. A well-conditioned athlete may have a pulse rate less than 60 bpm.
Meditation, rest, and sleep	Lower the pulse rate.
Circadian rhythm	Pulse rates are slowest from predawn hours to dawn and faster as the day progresses toward evening.
Blood volume: Decreased, as in hemorrhage and dehydration	Hemorrhage and dehydration will increase the pulse rate in an effort to more quickly transport the oxygen carried by red blood cells to the body tissues.

Table 17-4 **Factors Affecting Pulse Rate** (continued)

Factor	Effect
Increased, as in fluid overload	Fluid overload will cause pulses to be full and bounding, sometimes faster.
Body temperature	As body temperature increases, each degree Fahrenheit results in speeding the heart approximately 10 bpm. As the body cools, each degree results in slowing the pulse 10 bpm.
Hypoxia	Increases the pulse rate.
Cardiovascular disease	Different diseases can raise, lower, or make the pulse irregular.
Increased intracranial pressure	Typically lowers the pulse rate and may cause it to be irregular.

rhythm is described as regular. If there are differences in the interval lengths, the pulse is termed *irregular.* If peripheral pulses are palpated with each cardiac contraction, the blood fluid wave is reaching the pulse points, or is said to be *perfusing.* Volume or strength of a radial pulse is somewhat subjective in its description. A scale of 0 to 3 is generally used to assess pulse volume (Table 17-5). If the palpated

Table 17-5 **Scale for Measuring Peripheral Pulse Volume**

Description of Pulse	Scale and Terms
Pulse feels very strong and full and is easily counted. Does not obliterate even with moderate pressure.	3+ or Bounding
Pulse is easily detected, feels strong, and is easily counted. Can be obliterated with moderate pressure. Considered the normal finding.	2+ or Strong
Pulse feels weak and can be obliterated with slight pressure.	1+ or Weak
If the pulse is so faint and weak that it is difficult to feel it long enough to count the rate, an additional descriptor may be used.	*Thready*
Pulse is not detectable.	0 or Absent

pulse is easily detected, it is generally described as strong or 21. This would be considered a normal finding. A pulse that is faint and difficult to feel is categorized as weak or 11. If the pulse is so weak that slight fingertip pressure on the pulse site results in the pulse disappearing, the pulse is classified as *thready* or *feeble.* A thready pulse disappears, or *obliterates,* due to an inadequate volume of blood ejected from the heart with each contraction. In other words, the pumping action of the heart is too weak to deliver an adequate blood fluid wave to the peripheral pulse sites. The result of this problem is decreased delivery of oxygen and nutrients to the tissues, thus preventing optimal functioning of tissues, organs, and systems. A pulse that is very strong and does not disappear, even with moderate pressure, would be classified as a full, *bounding,* or 31 pulse.

If a pulse is not detectable by palpation, it is termed *absent* or rated as a 0. If this occurs, your next step is to palpate for the next *proximal* pulse in that extremity. If you cannot feel the next proximal pulse either, proceed up the limb to the next proximal pulse until you detect the peripheral pulse that is farthest away from the heart. For example, if you cannot palpate the dorsalis pedis pulse, palpate for the posterior tibialis pulse and if unable to feel it, palpate for the popliteal pulse, and finally the femoral pulse. While assessing for these pulses, there are further assessments you should perform on the extremity *distal* to the pulse site, including skin color, skin temperature, sensation, and capillary refill time.

• Is the color a healthy pink or is it pale or cyanotic, indicating impaired circulation?
• Is the temperature of the skin warm, as it should be? Or is it cool or cold, again indicating impaired circulation?
• Does the patient have adequate sensation in the distal aspect of the extremity? Can he or she differentiate between dull and sharp sensations as you apply the stimuli to the distal portion of the extremity? You may use something soft such as a gentle brush of your fingertip or a tissue

across the patient's skin. You can use some like a pencil eraser or the side of the barrel of your ink pen. Use something that is relatively sharper, such as a pin or the pointed tip of a pencil or ink pen, to provide a sharp stimulus.

• What is the *capillary refill time?* This is assessed by gently squeezing a nailbed of the extremity to empty the capillaries of blood. The nailbed will turn pale until you remove the pressure, after which it should return to a pink color as the capillaries refill with blood. Normally this will occur within 3 seconds in an adult and within 5 seconds in an elderly patient. If it takes longer to refill, this is an indication that there is circulatory impairment. In a patient whose nails are thickened and yellowed or one who is wearing nail polish, you may press the tip of the finger or toe to assess capillary refill.

After assessing the extremity for proximal pulses and other signs of adequate circulation, obtain a *Doppler ultrasound machine*, a device that uses sound waves to determine if blood flow is present. Listen for the most distal peripheral pulse that you were unable to palpate, to confirm that there is adequate arterial blood flow to the site. Skill 17-6 (see page 372) describes the use of Doppler ultrasound to assess nonpalpable pulses.

Knowledge Connection

List eight peripheral pulse sites. Name three characteristics of the pulse you should assess. What would be your concern if you found the femoral pulse to be weak or absent? Explain how to assess capillary refill.

Respiration

Respiration is the interchange of oxygen (O_2) and carbon dioxide (CO_2) between the atmosphere and the body and involves both external respiration and internal respiration. *External respiration* is the exchange of these gases between the lungs' alveoli and the blood found in the capillaries that surround the alveoli. *Internal respiration* is the process of exchanging gases between the circulating blood and the tissue cells that make up the body. The movement of air into and out of the lungs is known as *ventilation.* The mechanics of respiration involve the act of breathing in, termed as *inhalation* or *inspiration,* and breathing out, described as *exhalation* or *expiration.* Although the act of breathing is a function of the respiratory system, it is regulated by the central nervous system—specifically by the medulla oblongata and the pons, two structures of the brainstem, and by chemoreceptors in the carotid and aortic bodies. The *carotid body* is a section of the carotid artery wall and the *aortic body* is a section of the aortic arch wall, both of which contain chemical receptor sites that detect decreases in the blood level of O_2, known as hypoxemia. When hypoxemia is detected, electrical impulses are generated and sent via nerves to the medulla, which will then increase the respiratory rate or depth as needed to correct the hypoxemia.

Inspiration

To effect inspiration, the medulla sends an impulse via the phrenic nerves to the diaphragm muscle and along the intercostal nerves to the intercostal muscles telling the muscles to contract. The contraction of the diaphragm causes it to flatten and move downward, while the contraction of the intercostal muscles results in pulling the ribs upward and outward, enlarging the chest cavity.

Expiration

Once the medulla stops sending the motor impulses to inhale, the intercostal and diaphragm muscles begin to relax, once again shrinking the thoracic or chest cavity to the smaller, pre-inhalation state and compressing the lungs. The elastic connective tissue of the alveoli recoils somewhat like a rubber band, forcing the air that is mostly CO_2 out of the alveoli so it can be exhaled and returned to the atmosphere.

Assessing Respiration

The only equipment required to assess respiration is a watch with a second hand. Assess respiration for:

• Rate per minute
• Depth
• Rhythm
• Pattern
• Respiratory effort

Because individuals can voluntarily control their breathing for short intervals of time, it is best to assess the respirations without the patient's awareness. This may be accomplished by positioning the patient's arm across his or her chest or abdomen. Feel for the radial pulse and hold the pulse site while you assess first the respirations and then the radial pulse. It will appear that you are simply taking the patient's pulse, and this will help to distract the patient from concentrating on his or her breathing. While pressing two fingers against the pulse site, count the respiratory rate for 30 seconds and multiply times two for a 1-minute rate, and then continue to palpate the radial pulse site to assess the pulse rate. If the patient is very ill or respirations deviate in any manner from the norm, assess for a full minute.

Rate

Each respiration consists of one inspiration and one expiration. Observe the rise and fall of the chest or abdomen to count the rate. The normal rate for adults is between 12 and 20 bpm. When the rate, depth, rhythm, pattern, and respiratory effort fall within normal parameters, the term **eupnea** is used to describe the respirations. **Bradypnea** describes a respiratory rate below 12 respirations per minute; when the rate exceeds 20 respirations per minute, the term is **tachypnea.**

When the breathing rate slows, it results in a decreased intake of O_2 that can result in a deficiency of O_2 in the tissues and cells. When respirations cease or are absent, this is known as **apnea**. You have only a brief window of 3 to 5 minutes in which to restore respirations before brain damage and death occur.

Because the heart and lungs work together to provide circulation of nutrients and oxygen, the factors that affect the heart rate generally affect the respiratory rate as well. For example, as fever raises the pulse rate, it will also increase the respiratory rate. Breathing speeds up in an attempt to meet the body's increased metabolic needs and to remove excess heat. For every 1°F rise in body temperature, the respiratory rate increases approximately four breaths per minute. Table 17-6 presents further factors that affect the respiratory rate.

Depth

The depth of respiration is observed by the amount of chest expansion with each breath and is related to the volume of air that is inhaled. The average amount of air inhaled in one breath is between 300 and 500 mL and is known as the *tidal volume*, which can be assessed with special equipment. Without special equipment, you can only observe the rise and fall of the chest to provide a subjective measurement of the depth, usually described as shallow, normal, or deep.

Rhythm and Pattern

The rhythm of normal respirations is one that is regular, or has evenly spaced intervals between the respirations. When the intervals are not consistent, you assess them as irregular. When the rhythm is irregular, further assess the respirations to determine if the respirations fall into certain patterns, as described in Table 17-7.

Respiratory Effort

Respiratory effort refers to the amount of work required to breathe. Normally, the act of breathing is effortless and is performed unconsciously. An individual who is having labored or difficult breathing is said to be having **dyspnea**. The severely dyspneic patient will usually appear frightened, anxious, or worried. The first thing you may notice when you look at the patient is a "wide-eyed" or startled appearance. This may be indicative that the impaired gas exchange has progressed to the point of hypoxemia or hypoxia. *Hypoxemia* is the term used to denote a decreased oxygen level in the blood. If hypoxemia is not relieved, hypoxia, or decreased delivery of oxygen to the tissues and cells, occurs.

Often the patient does not appear to have dyspnea until he or she begins to exert energy, which increases the body's metabolic demand for oxygen. Exertional dyspnea only occurs during activities such as speaking, eating, repositioning, or ambulating. Another sign of difficult

Table 17-6 **Factors Affecting Respiratory Rate**

Factor	Effect
Age	Normal rates: Newborns: 30–60 Infants: 20–40 Children: 20–30 Adolescents: 14–25 Adults: 12–20
Smoking	Increase
Environmental temperature	Heat: Increase Cold: Decrease
Exercise or exertion	Increase
Rest, sleep, and meditation	Decrease
Pain, anxiety, stress, and fear	Increase
Medications, such as narcotics and sedatives	Decrease
Drug overdose, such as aspirin	Increase
Respiratory diseases, such as asthma and emphysema	Increase
Metabolic acidosis, such as caused by diabetes	Increase
Metabolic alkalosis, such as caused by severe vomiting	Decrease
Increased intracranial pressure	Decrease

breathing is use of the accessory respiratory muscles: the neck and abdominal muscles. It is important to assess which activities result in exertional dyspnea, document findings in the patient's record, and report such findings to the RN supervisor.

Some patients find it too hard to breathe unless positioned in an upright position, such as sitting or standing. This condition is known as **orthopnea**. More information about nursing care of the patient with orthopnea can be found in Chapter 28.

Table 17-7 Abnormal Respiratory Patterns

Pattern	Explanation	Graph of Pattern	Associated With
Cheyne-Stokes respirations	Respirations begin shallow, gradually increase in depth and frequency to a peak, then begin to decrease in depth and frequency until slow and shallow; this is followed by a period of apnea lasting from 10 to 60 seconds. Pattern is repetitious.		Children: may be a normal pattern Adults: usually ominous—coma, heart failure, head injury, drug overdose, impending death
Kussmaul's respirations	Respirations are increased in rate and depth, with long, strong, blowing or grunting exhalations.		Diabetic ketoacidosis or renal failure
Biot's respirations	Respirations are faster, deeper, and irregular, with periods of apnea.		Meningitis and central nervous system disorders

Related Characteristics

Other respiratory assessments go hand-in-hand with those previously detailed, including the audible sounds during ventilation and the breath sounds that are auscultated with a stethoscope:

- **Stertorous** breathing refers to noisy, snoring, labored respirations that are audible without a stethoscope.
- **Adventitious sounds** are abnormal sounds that may be heard when auscultating the lungs with a stethoscope, and include wheezes, rales or crackles, rhonchi, and stridor.
  - **Wheezes** are musical, whistling sounds and may be audible without a stethoscope or heard only during auscultation.
  - **Rales,** or **crackles,** are adventitious sounds that may be auscultated with a stethoscope and are due to air moving over secretions in the lungs. Rales are short, choppy, popping, snapping, or raspy sounds that may resemble the sound made by rubbing strands of hair between your thumb and index finger. Rales may be classified as fine or coarse depending upon their characteristics.
  - **Rhonchi** are continuous, low-pitched, rattling or bubbling, snoring or sonorous wheezing sounds that can be auscultated when there is partial obstruction of the larger airways due to secretions or tumor.
  - **Stridor** is an audible high-pitched crowing sound that results from partial obstruction of the airways.

You will learn more about auscultating breath sounds in Chapter 21. Skill 17-7 (see page 372) provides additional information on assessing respirations.

Oxygen Saturation

When oxygen enters the blood, it binds with hemoglobin in the RBCs to be transported to and made accessible to the cells of the body. Normally, 96% to 100% of the hemoglobin in arterial blood is bound with oxygen molecules. This saturation level is measured with an electronic pulse oximeter by attaching the plastic clip sensor to the fingertip, the earlobe, the bridge of the nose, or, when circulation is adequate, the toe. Special sensor probes can be applied to the forehead, the palm, or the sole of the foot of an infant. The LED (light-emitting diode) emits light and then calculates the measurement of the reflected light waves to monitor the pulse saturation, known as the SpO_2. A digital readout displays the results. The pulse oximeter can be applied and read intermittently or it can be applied for continual monitoring.

The selected assessment site should have adequate blood flow and be clean and dry, as moisture interferes with accuracy. Artificial nails do not allow accurate assessment because the LED cannot read through them. Remove dark fingernail polish to allow for accurate readings. Patient movement also interferes with accuracy. Finger probe assessment findings are produced in less than 30 seconds, and earlobe sensors deliver results in less than 15 seconds. If the results are below 90%, the RN supervisor should be notified. For further instructions regarding assessment of oxygen saturation, see Skill 17-8 (page 373).

Pain Assessment

Acute pain is pain that has a sudden onset, may have severe symptoms, and runs a shorter course than *chronic pain,* which is of longer duration or ongoing with little change or progression. Pain has only been considered as one of the vital signs for a few years, but acute pain can have such dramatic effects on the pulse, respirations, and blood pressure that it is important to assess pain along with the rest of the vital signs. Chronic pain does not affect the other vital signs in the same manner that acute pain can. The characteristics of pain that should be assessed include:

- Site or location
- Characteristics, such as sharp, dull, constant, intermittent, stabbing, cramping, or burning
- Severity based on a pain scale

Site or Location

It is important to inquire where the pain is located. It is easy to assume that a patient who has had a surgical procedure performed on the left leg is having pain in the left leg, when the fact may be that the patient has a headache, a backache from lying in the bed, or abdominal pain related to intestinal gas. Always ask the location of the pain.

It is also important to know that patients may use terminology differently than you do. For example, a patient may deny pain when asked if he or she "has any pain." Further inquiry may find that the patient is having "discomfort," "cramping," or "tenderness." Some patients feel that "pain" is something that is intolerable, therefore thinking their discomfort does not really qualify as pain. Be thorough when assessing pain and use more than one term. You might ask, "Are you having pain or discomfort anywhere?"

Characteristics

When the patient indicates he or she is having pain, ask for an additional description of the type of pain. Is it sharp or dull? Is it cramping or stabbing? The patient's description sometimes helps you to differentiate between conditions or possible sources of the pain. For example, a complaint of "heaviness" in the chest or the patient stating "it feels like an elephant is standing on my chest" describes a different and potentially more serious type of pain than might be expected if the patient were to say "It is only tender when I cough or sneeze."

Pain Scale

Use a pain scale, such as a scale of 0 to 10 with 0 being "no pain" and 10 being "worst pain you can imagine," when assessing the patient's pain. Because pain is a subjective matter for the patient, use of the numerical scale allows for introduction of a certain amount of objectivity. After pain medication has been given, it is important to reassess the patient's pain using the same pain scale used prior to treatment of the pain so that you can objectively determine whether the medication was effective or not. This is part of the evaluation phase of the nursing process. For young children or patients with impaired cognition, you will probably use the Wong-Baker FACES Pain Rating Scale, consisting of a picture of a series of faces that show varying degrees of comfort, from smiling, to frowning, to crying (Fig. 17-9). The child can point to the picture that matches his or her pain level (Fig. 17-10).

Documenting Vital Signs

Vital signs are generally documented on a graphic sheet designed solely for this purpose (Fig. 17-11). This allows one to see the trends at a glance and identify highs and lows quickly. Most facilities also require that vital signs also be documented in the nurse's notes.

Wong-Baker FACES Pain Rating Scale

0	1	2	3	4	5
No hurt	Hurts little bit	Hurts little more	Hurts even more	Hurts whole lot	Hurts worst

Figure 17-9   Wong-Baker FACES Pain Rating Scale. Source: From Hockenberry MJ, Wilson D. *Wong's Essentials of Pediatric Nursing.* 8th ed. St. Louis: Mosby; 2009. Used with permission.

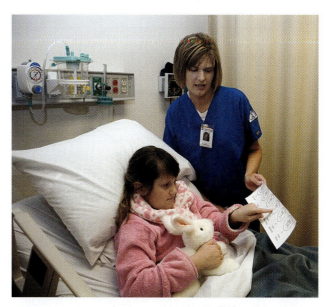

Figure 17-10   A nurse using the FACES pain rating scale for pain assessment in a child.

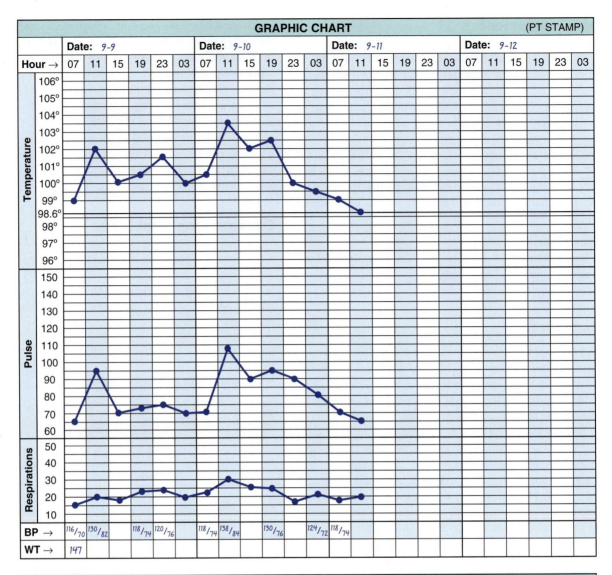

Figure 17-11 A sample graphic chart.

Skill 17-1 Assessment of Blood Pressure

Assessment Steps

1. Determine when and how frequently to take the patient's blood pressure.

2. *Safety: Assess if there is a contraindication to taking the blood pressure on either arm.* If the patient has had a mastectomy, has had removal of lymph nodes, or has a hemodialysis shunt or an IV infusion on either side, that side should not be used for blood pressure assessment. If both arms are contraindicated, assess the blood pressure in the thigh using a thigh cuff.

3. Assess which size blood pressure cuff is needed. *It should cover two-thirds of the arm circumference (distance around the arm) to obtain an accurate blood pressure.*

Skill 17-1 (continued)

4. Review the range of blood pressure readings recorded in the patient's chart. *This shows the blood pressure trend, which helps to indicate how high to inflate the cuff.*

Planning Steps

1. Gather supplies: sphygmomanometer with cuff and stethoscope. *Safety: Clean the stethoscope earpieces with alcohol and the cuff with the facility's approved disinfectant to prevent cross-contamination. Being prepared saves time and effort.*
2. Unless it is an emergency, plan to allow at least 5 minutes of inactivity and at least a 30-minute interval between smoking or consumption of caffeine and blood pressure assessment. *This allows the blood pressure to stabilize after the hemodynamic changes caused by physical movement and stimulants such as caffeine or nicotine.*

Implementation Steps

1. Follow the Initial Implementation Steps located on the inside front cover.
2. Support the patient's arm at the level of his or her heart with palm facing upward. *The BP may erroneously increase by as much as 20 mm Hg if the arm is not supported.*
3. Roll or push the sleeve of the patient's gown up to expose the bare upper arm *for more accurate placement of the cuff.*
4. Snugly wrap the cuff around the upper arm, centering the inflatable bladder over the brachial artery. If using the forearm, center the arrow over the radial artery. Position the bottom edge of the cuff approximately 1 inch above the antecubital space in an adult, and less than 1 inch in a child. Make certain the gauge is attached to the cuff or positioned at the same height as the cuff. *The center of the cuff bladder must be positioned over the brachial artery to obtain an accurate reading. Placing it 1 inch above the antecubital space leaves room for placement of the stethoscope diaphragm. The gauge position can affect the accuracy of the reading.*
5. Close the screw valve by turning it clockwise *to direct the air into the cuff bladder.* If this is the first assessment of blood pressure on this patient, use the palpation step to determine how high to inflate the cuff. If recent measurements of BP were recorded in the chart, the palpation step is not required, unless the BP is variable.
6. Palpate the brachial pulse with two fingertips, while rapidly compressing the bulb to inflate the cuff to 70 mm Hg. Then slowly continue inflating the cuff 10 mm Hg at a time until the pulse is no longer palpable. Make a mental note of the number at which the pulse was lost so you will know how high to inflate the cuff when you assess the BP, which will be 30 mm Hg higher than the point where you could no longer palpate the pulse. Then screw the valve counterclockwise and quickly deflate the cuff. *This helps to indicate how high to pump the cuff.*

7. Wait 15 to 30 seconds before reinflating the cuff, allowing arm veins to refill.
8. Place the stethoscope earpieces into your ears with the angle of the earpieces pointing toward your face. *This positions the earpieces correctly within the ear canals so sounds can be heard more clearly.* Place the bell or flat diaphragm over the brachial artery. If using the bell, apply gentle pressure to hold the stethoscope in place. If using the flat diaphragm, press more firmly until a seal is made with the skin. *This makes it easier to hear Korotkoff's sounds.*

9. Screw the valve clockwise to close it; *this allows air to enter the cuff bladder.* Compress the bulb until the cuff is inflated to the desired number.
10. Slowly turn the screw valve counterclockwise, letting the cuff deflate 2 to 3 mm Hg per second while listening for the first Korotkoff sound. *If you deflate the cuff too rapidly, you may miss the first sound, causing the blood pressure to appear to be lower than it really is.*
11. Make note of the number at which the first sound is heard and continue to listen as the cuff slowly deflates. Note the number at which the last sound is heard. Make certain that there are no further sounds for 10 to 15 mm Hg.
12. Deflate the cuff rapidly and completely. *This allows restoration of circulation to the arm.*
13. Remove the cuff and straighten the patient's gown.
14. Record in your pocket notes the BP and any auscultatory gap detected. Transcribe it to the chart as soon as possible.
15. Follow the Ending Implementation Steps located on the inside back cover.
16. Document BP on a graphic sheet in the nurse's notes, and in the patient's care plan. *By graphing the BP, trends may be identified as well as any abnormal values.*

(skill continues on page 366)

Skill 17-1 (continued)

Evaluation Steps

1. Evaluate if BP is within the patient's expected range. Is the BP elevated? Dangerously low?

2. Report abnormal BP findings according to facility policy.

Sample Documentation

8/3/10   1600   BP – 114/66 *in left arm, supine.* ————
———————— *Nurse's signature and credentials*

Skill 17-2 Assessment for Orthostatic Hypotension

Assessment Steps

1. Review the range of BP readings recorded in the patient's chart so you will know how high to inflate the cuff. *This helps to indicate how high to pump the cuff and whether the patient requires assessment for orthostatic hypotension.*

2. *Safety: Assess if there is a contraindication to taking the BP on either arm.* If the patient has had a mastectomy, has had removal of lymph nodes, or has a hemodialysis shunt or IV infusion on either side, that side should not be used for blood pressure assessment. If both arms are contraindicated, assess the blood pressure in the thigh using a thigh cuff.

3. Assess which size BP cuff is needed. Make certain the inflatable bladder width covers two-thirds of the upper arm. *A cuff that is too small will produce a falsely elevated reading, and one that is too large will result in a falsely low pressure.*

Planning Steps

1. Gather supplies: sphygmomanometer with cuff and stethoscope. *Safety: Clean the stethoscope earpieces with alcohol and the cuff with the facility's approved disinfectant to prevent cross-contamination. Being prepared saves time and effort.*

2. Unless it is an emergency, plan to allow at least 5 minutes of inactivity once the patient is placed in the supine position and at least 30 minutes following smoking or consumption of caffeine before assessing blood pressure. *This allows stabilization of blood pressure after the hemodynamic changes that occur with movement and stimulants such as caffeine and nicotine.*

Implementation Steps

1. Follow the Initial Implementation Steps located on the inside front cover.

2. Place the patient in the supine position and wait 5 minutes before taking BP. *This allows the pressure to stabilize after activity.*

3. Support the patient's arm at the level of his or her heart with the palm facing upward. *Positioning the arm above or below the heart level may cause an inaccurate BP measurement.* Avoid allowing the patient to hold his or her own arm up; *tensing of the arm muscles will raise the systolic pressure.*

4. Roll or push the sleeve of his or her gown up to expose the bare upper arm. *This provides better visualization of the antecubital area for placement of the stethoscope. The blood pressure reading is also*

more accurate when performed directly on bare skin as opposed to taking it over layers of fabric.

5. Snugly apply the cuff to the upper arm as for assessment of BP. *A cuff applied too loosely will result in a false elevation in the blood pressure measurement.*

6. Close the screw valve by turning it clockwise. *This prevents air from escaping from the cuff as the bulb is pumped.*

7. Palpate to locate the patient's brachial pulse. *Placement of the stethoscope diaphragm directly over the brachial pulse produces a louder, clearer blood pressure.*

8. Rapidly inflate the BP cuff approximately 30 mm Hg above the point at which you can no longer palpate the brachial pulse. *The artery is now occluded, preventing blood from flowing into the distal arm.*

9. Slowly unscrew the valve, allowing the cuff to deflate. Note the reading at which you once again are able to feel the brachial pulse. *This is known as the palpated systolic pressure, which should be slightly lower than the auscultated systolic pressure.* Then rapidly deflate the cuff completely. *This allows the blood trapped in the veins to be released and restores arterial circulation to the distal arm.*

10. Place the stethoscope earpieces in your ears directed toward your face. *Sound is better transmitted when the earpieces follow the direction of the ear canals.*

11. Place the stethoscope bell or flat diaphragm over the brachial artery. *The bell allows better hearing of the lower pitched Korotkoff's sounds.* Make certain the stethoscope hangs free from your ears and does not touch the bed or linens. *Allowing the stethoscope to rub against the bed or linens causes noise that can prevent the hearing of Korotkoff's sounds.*

12. Screw the valve clockwise once again *so the cuff will hold air.*

13. Compress the bulb until the cuff is inflated to approximately 30 mm Hg above the palpated systolic pressure. *This helps to ensure detection of the initial Korotkoff sound.*

14. Slowly turn the screw valve counterclockwise, letting the cuff deflate 2 to 3 mm Hg per second while listening for Korotkoff's sounds.

15. Make note of the number at which the first Korotkoff sound is heard and continue to listen as the cuff slowly deflates. Note the number at which the last Korotkoff sound is heard. Continue to listen for more sounds, allowing the gauge to drop another 10 to 15 mm Hg. *This helps to ensure accuracy.*

Skill 17-2 (continued)

16. Deflate the cuff rapidly and completely. *This allows circulation to resume to the arm.*

17. Leave the cuff in place on the arm.

18. Record the BP and patient's position to be documented in the chart after completion of assessment.

19. Lower the bed and have the patient sit up on the side of bed with the feet flat on the floor for 1 minute.

20. Retake the BP while the patient sits upright. *Normally the pressure should increase just slightly as the cardiovascular system works a little harder to pump blood to the head, which is now higher than the heart.*

21. Write down the BP and the patient's position to be documented in the chart after completion of assessment.

22. Assist the patient to stand at the side of the bed and wait for 1 minute. *Safety: Observe for dizziness and assist the patient to bed should it occur.*

23. Retake the BP while the patient is standing.

24. Have the patient sit down on the side of the bed and remove the cuff.

25. Write down the standing BP to be documented in the chart after completion of assessment.

26. Clean the cuff and wash hands. *This helps to reduce cross-contamination. BP cuffs have been shown to carry significant levels of microorganisms.*

27. Follow the Ending Implementation Steps located on the inside back cover.

28. Document BPs on a graphic sheet in the nurse's notes, and in the patient's care plan *to inform other nurses and staff members.*

Evaluation Steps

1. Evaluate if the BP showed a normal pattern of increase:
   • Sitting BP slightly higher than supine BP
   • Standing BP slightly higher than sitting BP
   Or if the BP dropped 15 to 20 mm Hg, showing an abnormal pattern of decrease:
   • From supine BP to sitting BP
   • From sitting BP to standing BP

2. *Safety: If orthostatic hypotension is indicated, instruct the patient to call for assistance before attempting to get out of bed.*

3. Report abnormal findings according to facility policy.

Sample Documentation

> 3/27/10   1230   Assessed for orthostatic hypotension. Supine BP – 122/76, Sitting BP – 110/68, Standing BP – 98/58. C/O dizziness upon standing. Assisted back to bed. Dizziness abated within 1 minute. Instructed to call for assistance before getting out of bed to avoid falls. Verbalized she would be sure to call for help. Bed rails raised times two. Call light within reach. Bed in lowest position. ———— Nurse's signature and credentials
>
> 1250   Dr. Know-it-all phoned with results of BP assessment. New order received to assess BP supine, sitting, & standing every 4 hours. ———— Nurse's signature and credentials

Skill 17-3 Assessing Body Temperature by Various Routes

Assessment Steps

1. Determine which route will be the most appropriate to use with this patient.

2. Review the patient's chart to determine his or her range of temperature.

3. Determine which type of thermometer would be best for use with this patient.

Planning Steps

1. Obtain supplies: thermometer and thermometer sheath or disposable probe cover; tissue, lubricant, and gloves if assessing temperature via the rectal route.

2. If using an electronic or tympanic thermometer or automatic vital sign machine, check the low battery light.

Implementation Steps

1. Follow the Initial Implementation Steps located on the inside front cover.

2. If assessing temperature by the *oral route,* determine whether the patient has had anything hot or cold to drink or has smoked within the last 15 minutes. If so, wait another 15 minutes before assessing temperature. *This helps to ensure accuracy.*

3. Position the patient appropriately. *For the oral, axillary, temporal, or tympanic routes,* position the patient in a sitting or supine position. *For the rectal route,* position the patient in the Sims' or lateral position. Be certain to provide privacy if assessing temperature by the rectal route.

4. If you are using an individual non-mercury thermometer, check the reading and shake it down, bringing the reading down below 95°F (35°C). *This prevents a false elevated temperature.* Then apply the appropriate thermometer sheath or probe cover. *This prevents cross-contamination.*

(skill continues on page 368)

Skill 17-3 (continued)

5. **Oral route:** Place the thermometer under the tongue, deep into the sublingual pocket, and leave in place for 3 minutes. Make sure the patient closes his or her lips. *This helps to prevent falsely low temperatures.*

Axillary route: Place the thermometer in the axilla, making certain the tip of the thermometer is covered by the arm posteriorly. Leave in place for 5 to 8 minutes. *The blood supply under the arm is not as abundant as under the tongue, requiring a longer length of time to ensure accuracy.*

Temporal route: Making sure the skin is dry, place the probe lightly against the forehead skin and scan the thermometer across the forehead and left or right temple area. Lift the probe and briefly touch it to the area just behind the ear.

Tympanic route: Apply the probe cover. While pulling the pinna upward and back in an adult, or downward and back in a small child, gently insert the probe into the ear canal, pointing the probe toward the mandible on the opposite side of the face. Depress the button on the handheld unit and read the temperature readout.

Rectal route: *Safety: Apply gloves.* Lubricate the tip of the thermometer sheath or probe cover with water-soluble lubricant. *This makes insertion easier. Safety: Carefully insert the thermometer 1½ inch into the rectum of an adult, taking care not to perforate the rectum.* Hold in place for 2 minutes. An exception occurs when using an electric thermometer, as it will only be left in place until it beeps.

6. Remove the thermometer, then remove the sheath and dispose of it. Read the temperature. If using an electronic or tympanic thermometer, eject the probe cover into the trash and return the thermometer to the charger.
   Rectal route: Wipe the anus with tissue to remove excess lubricant. Remove gloves.

7. Write down the temperature and route.

8. Follow the Ending Implementation Steps located on the inside back cover.

9. Document temperature and route on a graphic sheet and in the nurse's notes in the following manner:
   Oral route: 98.6°F
   Tympanic route: [T] 98.6°F
   Axillary route: [ax] 98.6°F
   Rectal route: [R] 98.6°F

Evaluation Steps

1. Compare the temperature reading with previous readings.

2. Compare the temperature route with the equivalent oral route.

3. Evaluate if the temperature correlated with any signs and symptoms displayed.

Skill 17-3 (continued)

4. If the temperature is abnormal, decide what nursing action may now be necessary.

5. Report abnormal findings according to facility policy.

Sample Documentation

9/18/10 0800 T– ᵃˣ 98.6°F. ————————
————————— *Nurse's signature and credentials*

Skill 17-4 Assessing the Radial and Apical Pulses

Assessment Steps

1. Review the patient's chart to determine previous pulse rate and site obtained.

2. Review the medication administration record for any medications that may affect pulse rate or assessment site. *Some cardiac medications require assessment of an apical pulse.*

3. Determine which pulse site is to be assessed.

Planning Steps

1. Be certain a watch or clock with a second hand is available. Obtain a stethoscope if assessing the apical pulse. *Being prepared saves time and effort.*

2. Plan to wait 5 minutes if the patient has recently ambulated. *This allows the rate to return to its resting rate.*

Implementation Steps

1. Follow the Initial Implementation Steps located on the inside front cover.

Radial Pulse

2. Rest the patient's forearm comfortably across the abdomen if supine, or on the arm of the chair if sitting in a chair, with the palm facing down. *The pulse is easier to detect if the patient's arm muscles are relaxed. The palm-down position allows you to place your hand on top of the wrist and easily curve your fingers around the radius to access the radial pulse.*

3. Gently grasp the wrist, placing the first and second fingertips over the radial artery. Apply slight pressure until a recurring pulse is felt.

4. While observing the second hand of your watch, count the pulse for 60 seconds, noting any irregularity and volume or strength of pulse. *Safety: An*

experienced nurse can count the rate for 15 seconds and multiply times 4, or count the rate for 30 seconds and multiply times 2. However, as a student, you should always assess the pulse for a full minute until you have more experience. This will help to prevent errors due to subtle irregularities that may not be detectable to an inexperienced student. Even experienced nurses should count the pulse for a full minute if there are any irregularities.

5. Follow the Ending Implementation Steps located on the inside back cover.

Apical Pulse

2. Elevate the head of bed or have the patient sit upright unless contraindicated, *to better position the heart against the anterior chest wall for easier auscultation.*

3. Being careful to preserve modesty, loosen the patient's gown to allow access to the left side of the chest. Palpate the fifth intercostal space on the left side of the sternum. Do this by palpating the angle of Louis (felt as a prominence between the top of the sternum and the body of the sternum, just below the suprasternal notch). Move a fingertip to the left of the sternal prominence, into the second intercostal space. Placing a finger in each space, count down to the fifth intercostal space. Walk your fingers laterally to the midclavicular line. Palpate for the point of maximal impulse (PMI).

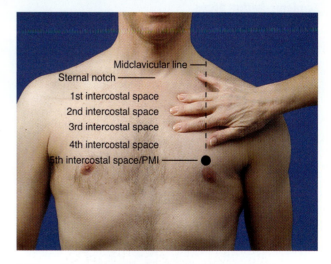

4. Place the bell or flat diaphragm of the stethoscope directly on the skin, over the PMI. *This is the point where the heart contraction is felt, making it easier to hear the apical pulse clearly.*

(skill continues on page 370)

Skill 17-4 (continued)

5. Listen to determine that both S_1 and S_2 are detected, and note the strength or volume of both sounds by determining whether the S_1 or S_2 sound is muffled, distant, or distinct. Also note any third or fourth extra sounds. Listen to the rhythm, noting any irregularities and whether they are "regular irregularities," such as a skip every fifth beat.

6. Count the rate for a full minute. This is always the length of time used when auscultating the apical pulse. It helps to better detect any arrhythmias.

7. While continuing to auscultate the apical pulse, palpate the radial pulse with your free hand. Feel and listen concurrently for another minute to determine that the radial and apical pulses are the same, without a pulse deficit. If there is a difference in the two pulse rates, solicit help from a second nurse. One nurse then counts the apical pulse while the second nurse counts the radial pulse concurrently for 1 minute, using the same watch second hand. You would then document both rates and the amount of the difference (pulse deficit).

8. Rearrange the patient's gown and position for comfort.

9. Record pulse rate, rhythm, and strength or volume for use in later documentation.

10. Follow the Ending Implementation Steps located on the inside back cover.

11. Document pulse rate and characteristics on a graphic sheet and in the nurse's notes.

Evaluation Steps

1. Evaluate whether the findings are consistent with condition and any expected therapeutic effects of prescribed medications.

2. Determine if further action needs to be taken.

3. Report abnormal findings according to facility policy.

Sample Documentation

5/17/10   2215   AP – 84, regular and distinct. No pulse deficit.
———————— Nurse's signature and credentials
6/11/10   1430   AP – 76, regular and distinct. Radial pulse 69, irregular and weak. Pulse deficit of 7 beats per minute. ——————— ———————— Nurse's signature and credentials

Skill 17-5 Assessing Peripheral Pulses

Assessment Steps

1. Review the patient's chart for previous findings and any record of disease process that may affect the strength and equality of peripheral pulses.

Planning Steps

1. Plan to use Doppler ultrasound if any pulse is not palpable.

Implementation Steps

1. Follow the Initial Implementation Steps located on the inside front cover.

2. As you palpate each pulse, be sure to palpate both left and right pulses and compare the strength.
   a. *Temporal pulse:* Using two fingertips, palpate over the temple area, lateral and superior to the eye. Some facilities do not require that the temporal pulse be assessed as part of the peripheral pulses.

   b. *Carotid pulse:* Using two fingertips, gently palpate to the side of the trachea, in the depression between the trachea and sternocleidomastoid muscle on the side of the neck. *Safety: NEVER palpate both carotids simultaneously or press hard enough to impair blood flow to the brain, as this has been known to result in a stroke.*

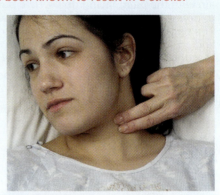

   c. *Brachial pulse:* Using two fingertips, palpate the brachial artery in the antecubital area.

Skill 17-5 (continued)

d. *Radial pulse:* Using two fingertips, palpate the radial pulses in both wrists.

Note: If assessing peripheral pulses only to determine adequate circulation to the extremities, it may not be necessary to count the rate. There may not be a need to palpate the more proximal brachial pulses if the more distal radial pulses are both strong.

e. *Femoral pulse:* Using two or three fingertips, palpate firmly in the midline of the groin crease. *This pulse is deeper than most pulses.*

f. *Popliteal pulse:* Using two or three fingertips, palpate behind the knee in the middle of the popliteal fossa.

g. *Posterior tibialis pulse:* Place two or three fingertips on the medial aspect of the ankle, just below the malleolus.

h. *Dorsalis pedis pulse:* Place two or three fingertips gently on the dorsal aspect of the foot, on a line extending from between the great toe and the second toe. Follow the groove between the extensor tendons proximally until the pulsation is felt over the dorsal surface of the foot.

Note: If assessing peripheral pulses only to check circulation to the extremities, there may be no need to palpate the more proximal femoral and popliteal pulses if the more distal dorsalis pedis or posterior tibialis pulse is strong.

3. Record pulse rhythm and equality of strength for use in later documentation. *This improves accuracy in documentation.*
4. Follow the Ending Implementation Steps located on the inside back cover.
5. Document pulse characteristics on the flow sheet or in the nurse's notes as soon as possible.

Evaluation Steps

1. Evaluate if distal peripheral pulse findings were within the patient's range of normal and consistent with the patient's condition.
2. Report abnormal findings that are inconsistent with the patient's condition.

Sample Documentation

5/3/10   1730   *Radial and pedal peripheral pulses strong and equal bilaterally.* ———————— *Nurse's signature and credentials*

Skill 17-6 Using Doppler Ultrasound to Assess Nonpalpable Pulses

Assessment Steps

1. Assess the need for use of Doppler ultrasound. *If pulses are palpable, the use of Doppler is not required. If pulses are not palpable, Doppler is used to determine adequate circulation to an extremity.*

Planning Steps

1. Obtain a Doppler ultrasound machine and transmission gel. Check the low battery light on the Doppler. *Being prepared saves time and effort.*

Implementation Steps

1. Follow the Initial Implementation Steps located on the inside front cover.

2. Apply a small dab of transmission gel over the pulse site to be assessed or to the transducer probe on the Doppler. *This improves the clarity of sound.*

3. Turn on the Doppler.

4. Using only light pressure, hold the transducer probe against the skin over the pulse site. Move the transducer probe only enough to locate the strongest pulse sound.

5. After assessing the pulse, clean the gel from the patient's skin and from the transducer probe with a dry cloth or tissue. Then clean the transducer probe surface with a damp cloth only. *Harsh chemicals will damage the transducer.*

6. Follow the Ending Implementation Steps located on the inside back cover.

7. Document the pulse and that Doppler ultrasound had to be used in the nurse's notes.

Evaluation Steps

1. Evaluate if the pulse findings were within the patient's range of normal and consistent with the patient's condition.

2. Report that a pulse was obtainable only with Doppler ultrasound.

Sample Documentation

1/14/10   1845   Unable to palpate left pedal pulse. Doppler used to obtain rate of 80. Left foot pink & warm, with 3-second capillary refill. ——————————— Nurse's signature and credentials

---

Skill 17-7 Assessing Respirations

Assessment Steps

1. Review the patient's chart for the previous range of respirations and disease conditions that might influence respiratory efforts.

Planning Steps

1. Plan to wait 5 minutes after physical activity to begin assessment.

Implementation Steps

1. Follow the Initial Implementation Steps located on the inside front cover.

2. Position the patient in the supine or sitting position. Grasp his or her wrist as you would if you were assessing the radial pulse. Position the arm across the patient's abdomen or chest. *This distracts the patient from your assessment of his or her respirations.*

3. While observing the passage of 1 minute on your watch, observe the rise and fall of the chest, counting an inhalation and expiration as one complete

Skill 17-7 (continued)

breath. Count the rate of respiration for 1 full minute, noting rhythm, depth, and effort. *Safety: An experienced nurse can count the rate for 15 seconds and multiply times 4, or count the rate for 30 seconds and multiply times 2. As a student, you should always assess the respirations for a full minute until you have more experience. This will help to prevent errors due to subtle irregularities that may not be detectable to an inexperienced student.*

4. Write down the rate, rhythm, depth, and effort for use in later documentation.
5. Follow the Ending Implementation Steps located on the inside back cover.

6. Document respiratory rate on a graphic sheet and the rate, rhythm, depth, and effort in the nurse's notes.

Evaluation Steps

1. Evaluate if respiration findings were within the patient's range of normal and consistent with the patient's condition.
2. Report abnormal findings according to facility policy.

Sample Documentation

12/3/10   0315   R – 16 regular, shallow, effortless. Skin pink. SpO_2 – 97% on room air. —— Nurse's signature and credentials

Skill 17-8 Assessing Oxygen Saturation

Assessment Steps

1. Review the patient's chart for the previous range of SpO_2 and disease conditions that might influence respiratory gas exchange. Assess the patient's hemoglobin level. *A low hemoglobin reduces the oxygen-carrying capacity of the blood.*
2. Assess whether the patient has a physician's order for supplemental O_2.
3. Determine which site will be used for the next assessment: fingertip, earlobe, nose, toe, or forehead.

Planning Steps

1. Obtain a pulse oximeter with appropriate sensor to be used for the selected site. Check the low battery light. *Being prepared saves time and effort.*
2. Plan to assess the SpO_2 with O_2 on (if applicable) or on room air if no supplemental oxygen is being delivered.

Implementation Steps

1. Follow the Initial Implementation Steps located on the inside front cover.
2. If using an extremity, assess the finger or toe for adequate capillary refill to assure adequate circulation to the site to be assessed. *A digit without adequate circulation would not provide an accurate oxygen saturation level.*
3. Prepare the site. The site should be clean and dry. Remove nail polish if using a finger or toe. *Polish interferes with accurate measurement.*
4. Apply the appropriate sensor to the site that was selected for assessment.

5. Turn on the oximeter and check that preset alarms for high and low SpO_2 are set.
6. Read the digital readout and record for later documentation.
7. Remove the sensor if this is a one-time assessment. If assessment is to be continual, leave the sensor in place. *Safety: Inspect and change locations of the sensor every 2 hours to avoid tissue necrosis from prolonged pressure.*
8 Follow the Ending Implementation Steps located on the inside back cover.
9. Document SpO_2 on a graphic sheet or flow sheet and in the nurse's notes.

Evaluation Steps

1. Evaluate if SpO_2 findings were within the patient's range of normal and consistent with the patient's condition.
2. Report abnormal findings according to facility policy.

Sample Documentation

12/9/10   0845 SpO_2 – 94% on room air via NC. ——
—— Nurse's signature and credentials
12/11/10   0900 SpO_2 – 97% with O_2 on @ 2L/min via NC.
—— Nurse's signature and credentials

🌐 Post Conference

You provided care for your patient who, according to the automatic vital sign machine, had abnormal vital signs. In evaluation of your nursing care, you review the actions you took:

- You further assessed the patient and found him to be awake, alert, oriented, and smiling; skin pink, warm, and dry; oral mucosa and nailbeds pink; respirations normal depth, regular, and effortless at 19 breaths per minute; and radial pulse regular at strong 69 bpm.
- You reviewed the 8 a.m. vital signs: BP – 126/74, T – 98°F, P – 64, SpO_2 – 98% on room air.
- You compared the 8 a.m. vital signs to those obtained at noon, which were BP – 94/46, T – 96.6°F, P – 51, and SpO_2 – 70% on room air, indicated dramatic differences from those obtained at 8 a.m.
- You performed manual reassessment of vital signs with an aneroid blood pressure cuff and portable pulse oximeter, with the following results: BP – 122/78, AP – 69, R – 10, SpO_2 – 96%.
- You determined that the automatic vital sign machine was inaccurate and removed it from use until repairs and calibration could be completed.

This event reinforced in your mind the importance of looking at all of the assessment data and performing manual assessment, rather than always depending on automatic vital sign machines or looking at just one piece of data.

KEY POINTS

- There are six vital signs: blood pressure, temperature, pulse, respirations, oxygen saturation, and pain assessment.
- The normal ranges for blood pressure in adults are systolic pressure between 90 and 120 mm Hg and diastolic pressure between 60 and 80 mm Hg.
- The normal range for core temperatures varies from 97°F to 99.6°F (36.1°C to 37.5°C), with the average being 98.6°F (37°C).
- The normal range for the adult pulse is 60 to 100 bpm.
- The normal range for adult respirations is 12 to 20 per minute.
- Normal SpO_2 range is between 96% and 100%.
- The peripheral pulse sites include temporal, carotid, brachial, radial, femoral, popliteal, posterior tibialis, and dorsalis pedis (pedal).
- Pain should be assessed using a pain scale of 0 to 10 for adults and a scale using a series of facial expressions for children.

REVIEW QUESTIONS

Select the answer that is most appropriate for each of the following questions. Some questions may have more than one answer. Check all that apply.

1. In which of the following situations would it be inappropriate to delegate the vital sign assessment?

   a. Routine vital signs on a patient with pneumonia

   b. A patient whose level of consciousness has gone from alert to responding only to pain stimuli

   c. A teenager admitted with influenza A whose temperature 2 hours ago was 100.6°F orally

   d. A confused and lethargic patient brought to the emergency room after being involved in an automobile accident

   e. An adult patient who becomes diaphoretic and pale and complains of sudden onset of severe left chest pain while ambulating in the hallway

2. Which of the following vital signs, all taken on adults, have one or more components that fall outside of typical normal ranges?

    a. BP – 118/66, T – 99.2°F, P – 74 regular and strong, R – 17

    b. BP – 98/62, T – 98.2°F, P – 98 regular and strong, R – 20

    c. BP – 142/88, T – 98.4°F, P – 62 regular and bounding, R – 14

    d. BP – 120/74, T – 100.6°F, P – 86 regular and strong, R – 24

3. Uncontrolled hypertension can result in permanent damage of which organs?

    a. Heart and eyes

    b. Pancreas and spleen

    c. Large intestine and skeletal structures

    d. Brain and kidneys

    e. Urinary bladder

4. You must assess the temperature of an 89-year-old female who is confused, hostile, and combative. Which route would be most appropriate to use?

    a. Rectal

    b. Oral

    c. Temporal

    d. Axillary

5. Upon assessing the vital signs of a 56-year-old male, you find that he has an apical pulse of 88 bpm and a radial pulse of 71 bpm. Which of the following numbers would be correct to document as the pulse deficit?

    a. 0

    b. 7

    c. 15

    d. 17

    e. 159

SHORT ANSWER QUESTIONS

6. List the characteristics of a pulse to include in your vital sign assessment.

7. Describe how to assess pain in an adult.

8. Explain what is meant by *systolic pressure* and *diastolic pressure*.

9. Explain how to assess a patient for orthostatic hypotension.

CRITICAL THINKING EXERCISES

10. Enumerate possible vital signs and other findings that might indicate a patient has impaired circulation.

ADDITIONAL RESOURCES

For additional Resources, Questions, and Activities, please see:

 Student Resource Disk

 http://davisplus.fadavis.com

Student Study Guide

REFERENCES

Cuddy M. Treatment of hypertension: guidelines from JNC 7. *J Practical Nurs.* 2005;55(4):17-21.

D'Arcy Y. Assessing pain with pain-rating scales. *LPN2007.* 2007;3(6):13-16.

D'Arcy Y. Pain management by the numbers: using rating scales effectively. *Nursing2007.* 2007;37(11):14-15.

Dillon PM. *Nursing Health Assessment: A Critical Thinking Case Studies Approach.* 2nd ed. Philadelphia: FA Davis; 2007.

Hart A, Davidhizar R. What the nurse should know about the pulmonary system. *J Practical Nurs.* 2006-2007;56(4)-57(1):6-7, 11-13.

Joint Commission. (2008). *2008 National Patient Safety Goals.* Available at: http://www.jointcommission.org/PatientSafety/NationalPatientSafetyGoals/08_npsg_fact. Accessed October 18, 2007.

Maddox T. Don't let hypertension sneak by you. *Nursing Made Incredibly Easy!* 2006;4(1):9-11.

National Institutes of Health. What is high blood pressure? April, 2006. Available at: http://www.nhlbi.nih.gov/health/dci/Diseases/Hbp/HBP_All.html. Accessed March 16, 2008.

Rhoades J, Meeker BJ. *Davis's Guide to Clinical Nursing Skills.* Philadelphia: FA Davis; 2008.

Rushing J. Assessing for orthostatic hypotension. *Nursing2005.* 2005;35(1):30.

Smeltzer S, Bare B. *Brunner & Suddarth's Textbook of Medical-Surgical Nursing.* 11th ed. Philadelphia: Lippincott Williams & Wilkins; 2008.

Wilkinson JM, Van Leuven K. *Fundamentals of Nursing: Theory, Concepts & Applications.* Philadelphia: FA Davis; 2007.

Williams LS, Hopper PD. *Understanding Medical-Surgical Nursing.* 3rd ed. Philadelphia: FA Davis; 2007.

Key Terms

Aquathermia pad

Cellulitis

Contraindications

Deep venous thrombosis

Edema

Hemostasis

Hypothermia

Indications

Interstitial space

Metabolism

Mottling

Orthostatic hypotension

Pallor

Permeable

Phagocytosis

Phlebitis

Rebound phenomenon

Tepid

Vasoconstriction

Vasodilation

Vessel lumen

Objectives

1. Define key terms related to applying heat and cold.
2. Contrast the physiological effects of local heat and cold applications.
3. Identify at least four uses for heat therapy.
4. Explain how application of heat can support healing.
5. Detail the nursing assessments to make prior to, during, and after application of heat therapy.
6. Describe three uses for cold therapy.
7. Compare the methods of heat and cold application.
8. Summarize the nursing assessments pertinent to cold applications.
9. Teach a patient how to make a simple cold pack using only a washcloth and a zip-type plastic bag.

Skills

18-1 Application of Dry or Moist Heat

18-2 Application of Aquathermia Pad (K-pad)

18-3 Administering a Sitz Bath

18-4 Application of Cold Packs

🌐 Clinical Connection

Your Assignment: You will be caring for a 72-year-old female who has developed sepsis due to a bladder infection. She has an overwhelming infection in her bloodstream. Her temperature has been spiking to 103.8°F (39.8°C). The physician has ordered a hypothermia blanket to be applied when her temperature exceeds 104°F (40.0°C).

Your Actions: To prepare for this assignment, you will need to research how to correctly apply a hypothermia blanket. You will need to know how to monitor the patient's temperature while she is on the blanket and what parameters you should use when maintaining the blanket. You will also need to know how to tell if the patient is becoming too cold, or if the cold therapy is causing injury to the patient's skin.

The terms *heat* and *cold* probably seem basic and nonthreatening to you. The concepts behind the terms are simple, but the effects that heat and cold can have on the body tissues and their functions are dramatic.

When we refer to environmental heat and cold, meaning the effects of weather, excessive exposure can result in severe trauma or death. In smaller, controlled doses, heat and cold are used as therapeutic applications to specific parts of the body for both local and systemic effects. The local effects of heat and cold applications impact the body's cutaneous layers where the heat or cold is applied, including the underlying subcutaneous tissue, muscles, and vascular structures, as well as their functions. Systemic effects of heat and cold involve more than a specific area and can affect entire body systems. An example of this would be raising body temperature with application of warm packs or a warm bath.

In this chapter, you will develop a better understanding of the uses and benefits of these therapies and the complications that can result if safety measures are not carried out. You will also learn how to correctly apply various heat and cold therapies and to make appropriate assessments pertinent to each.

Heat Therapy

The local application of heat to an area of the body results in **vasodilation** of the vessels underlying the area (Fig. 18-1). This means there is an increase in the size of the cavity or opening inside the vessel, known as the **vessel lumen**, allowing for an increased flow of oxygenated and nutrient-rich blood to the site. The pores in the capillary walls also become more **permeable**, which means they open wider. This allows increased passage of plasma, oxygen-carrying red blood cells, nutrients, and white blood cells from the capillaries into the spaces between cells, known as the **interstitial spaces**, and to the cells themselves.

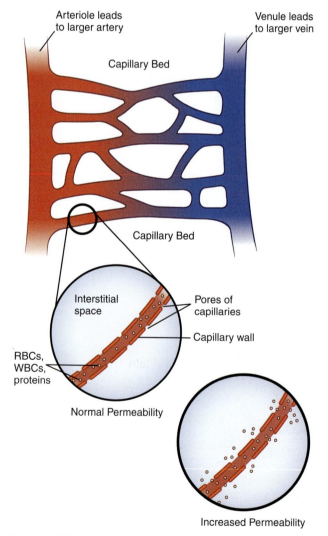

Figure 18-1 Vasodilation and increased permeability.

Indications for Heat Therapy

Most circumstances require a physician's order for application of heat therapy. Some facilities provide standing physician's orders allowing nurses to apply a warm compress in specific situations, such as inflammation of a vein due to IV therapy, a condition known as **phlebitis**. It is your responsibility to be familiar with your employer's policies and procedures regarding heat application. Unless there is a standing order or protocol for the procedure, be certain to obtain an order from the physician.

There are numerous **indications** for heat therapy, or situations in which it should be used, including:

• Relaxation of muscle spasms
• Pain relief
• Support of the healing process
• Reduction of edema once it has stabilized (stopped increasing)
• Elevation of body temperature.

Relaxation of Muscle Spasms and Pain Relief

Heat therapy relaxes muscles in spasm, such as tight or tense muscles that might result from driving an automobile for a long distance or standing for a long period of time, such as in hospital nursing. At the end of the day, use of a hot tub or whirlpool bath often relieves the tired and sore muscles of a snow skier on a once-a-year vacation.

Support of the Healing Process

When heat is applied to an inflamed site, the resulting increased blood flow delivers adjunct *phagocytes,* which are defensive white blood cells, to the wound site. These defensive white blood cells perform **phagocytosis**, meaning they surround, engulf, and digest the offending microorganisms and debris in the cells and exudate, which helps to prevent infection. The increased blood flow delivers the extra oxygen and nutrients that are needed to support the increased **metabolism**, or the chemical and physical processes required to build and maintain body tissues. Without the increased metabolism, the tissue does not heal properly in a timely manner.

Reduction of Edema

Sometimes an acute injury results in a large amount of edema, such as you might see with a sprained ankle. **Edema** is the term for swelling that occurs when excessive fluid leaves the vascular system and remains in the interstitial spaces. This presence of extra fluid in a space where it does not normally reside increases the pressure on nerve endings, resulting in pain and discomfort. Applying heat at this stage of inflammation will simply increase the amount of swelling and, therefore, is contraindicated. After 48 to 72 hours, once the edema stabilizes, heat may then be applied to dilate the capillaries and veins so they can carry away the excess fluid, thus reducing the edema.

Elevation of Body Temperature

Application of heat is helpful in raising the body temperature for comfort as well as for patients with **hypothermia**, a condition that occurs when an individual's core temperature drops below 95°F (35°C). Warm packs, hot water bottles, and hypothermia blankets may be used to help the patient feel warmer and raise lowered body temperatures. In extreme cases of hypothermia, the physician may even order intravenous infusion of warm normal saline to help raise the body temperature.

Contraindications for Heat Therapy

Though heat is appropriate therapy for the above-listed indications, there are certain **contraindications** for heat therapy, or situations in which heat should not be used. If heat is used in a situation in which it is contraindicated, it may result in harm or damage. For example, if heat is used on new injuries, it will result in more edema than would normally occur with the injury. Thus heat is contraindicated and should never be used on new trauma or damage to tissue. Further contraindications for heat therapy are listed in Box 18-1.

Knowledge Connection

Explain the physiological effects of local heat application. Describe how application of heat can support the healing process.

Methods of Heat Application

Heat can be delivered as dry or moist heat (see Skill 18-1, page 385). Because water is a better conductor than air, moist heat penetrates quicker and deeper into the tissues

---

Box 18-1

Contraindications for Heat Applications

Heat applications should be used judiciously, as there are specific situations and conditions in which it is unwise or actually detrimental to apply heat. This list is not all-inclusive.

• **Suspected appendicitis:** The use of heat therapy to the right lower abdomen during acute appendicitis could cause enough increased blood flow to the area that it results in a ruptured appendix.
• **Bleeding wound or injury:** Applying heat to a bleeding wound or injury would dilate the vessels, increasing the bleeding.
• **Newly injured joints:** Heat increases edema, making joint mobility more difficult.
• **Large areas of the body in certain cardiac patients:** Extensive heat application can result in massive vasodilation to the superficial skin and subcutaneous layers, depriving the major organs, such as the brain, heart, lungs, and kidneys, of adequate blood supply, which can cause serious damage.

than dry heat. There are numerous methods of delivering heat therapy, including:

- Hot water bottles
- Commercial heat packs
- Heating pads
- Aquathermia pads
- Hypothermia blankets

All of the above applications methods can be used dry or with a wet towel for moist heat, except the hypothermia blanket, which is dry. Other methods of applying moist heat include:

- Hot compresses
- Soaks
- Sitz baths
- Whirlpool baths

Safety: Never use microwaves to heat compresses because of the danger of burns.

Local heat application is generally used just long enough for maximum vessel dilation to occur, which is 20 to 30 minutes, and heat is reapplied every 2 to 3 hours as ordered. Leaving heat packs in place longer than 45 minutes can cause constriction of vessels instead of dilation. This is known as **rebound phenomenon**. In other words, the treatment results in a worsening of the original condition rather than improving it.

Hot Water Bottles

Fill hot water bottles two-thirds full with warm water and expel the remaining air. Secure the closure device and place a cloth cover or small towel between the bottle and the patient's skin to prevent burns.

Commercial Heat Packs

Many companies manufacture easy-to-use heat packs, activated by squeezing, striking, or twisting the plastic package. *Safety: Again, be certain to place some type of cloth barrier between the patient's skin and the heat pack.*

Heating Pads

Electrical heating pads are rarely used in hospitals and long-term care facilities due to the risk of burns. Most facilities require signing a release of responsibility form before allowing a patient to use his or her own heating pad from home. If you do use a heating pad, make sure to use only low and medium temperature settings to prevent burns. *Safety: Never place heating pads under the patient because the heat cannot dissipate and may result in a severe burn. Do not apply a heating pad to an infant or a sleeping or confused patient.*

Aquathermia Pads

An **aquathermia pad** (K-pad) is a device with a small, electrically heated water storage tank and two tubes connected to a network of tubing within a disposable pad. The

warmed, distilled water is pumped from the storage tank and circulates back and forth between the water tank and the pad (Fig. 18-2). These pads can be used continuously because they can maintain a specific temperature.

The temperature of the water is controlled by the temperature dial on the tank and can be set between 90°F (32.2°C) and 110°F (43.3°C). The most common temperature setting used is 105°F (40.5°C). *Safety: A key must be used to set the temperature dial to avoid inadvertent changing of the temperature.*

Some K-pads are designed to be used dry; others are made moist by wetting the absorbent outside layer of the pad. The most common uses for a K-pad are to treat blood clots in the lower leg, a condition known as **deep venous thrombosis**, and inflammation and infection of the skin and underlying tissue, a condition known as **cellulitis**. Make certain that the physician's order includes the temperature setting, whether it should be moist or dry, and how long the application is to remain in place.

Skill 18-2 (page 386) presents more information on applying an aquathermia pad.

Hypothermia and Hyperthermia Blankets

There are numerous types of heating and cooling blankets, including forced-air warming blankets and water-circulating blankets. Some of these blankets have a temperature setting to gradually raise or lower body temperature as needed.

The most common uses for hypothermia blankets are to warm the body either during surgery or postoperatively and to raise the body temperature of an individual exposed to environmental conditions, such as snow, cold temperatures, or submersion in cold lake water. When used as a hyperthermia blanket, the temperature is set to a cooler temperature to reduce high fevers from disease or heat stroke. Depending on their design, hypothermia and hyperthermia blankets may be able to be placed underneath or over the patient, while others are designed to be placed both under and over the patient at the same time. *Safety: The patient's vital signs and core temperature are constantly monitored while the blanket is in use.*

Figure 18-2 Aquathermia pads circulate water in the interior of the pad to create a constant temperature.

Real-World Connection

How Much Good Can Application of Heat Really Accomplish?

In the 1980s, in the midst of a freak blizzard in Oklahoma, an ambulance radioed a small rural hospital that they were bringing in a 32-year-old female patient who, the night before, had been beaten unconscious and thrown out of a car into a deep snow drift, where she had lain in single-digit temperatures for approximately 10 to 12 hours, wearing only jeans, a shirt, oxford tie shoes, socks, underwear, and a medium-weight parka. Her clothes were snow-laden and frozen solid. Her pulses were not palpable and respirations were barely discernible. Her apical pulse was faint and irregular. There was no audible or palpable blood pressure, and her temperature registered "below 86°F (30°C)" on the rectal core temperature probe. Her skin was gray and mottled.

Though it was believed that there was little hope for her survival, the nurses and physician teamed up to do everything they could. After removing her frozen clothing, the physician ordered warmed blankets, as this was before hypothermia blankets were widely available, and warmed and humidified oxygen. He also ordered hot water bottles placed on the top of her head, under both axillae, on each inguinal area, and on both feet. The nurses monitored her level of consciousness, vital signs, and electrocardiogram (EKG) monitor strips continually. The patient remained unresponsive even as her body temperature slowly rose over the next 4 hours to 91°F (32.7°C) and then 92°F (33.3°C). Within 6 hours, her core temperature finally reached 95°F (35°C) and she was speaking coherently. She suffered some minor frostbite on her fingers, earlobes, and toes, but otherwise recovered fully within 72 hours. Once she was awake and alert, the nurses learned a fact that probably played an important role in her survival: She was a full-blooded Eskimo who had lived all her life in Alaska. She was just in Oklahoma visiting friends when she suffered the life-threatening event.

Hot Compresses

Dip gauze or a cloth in a hot solution (type and temperature ordered by the physician), wring it out, and apply to an inflamed area. Use sterile gloves, supplies, and technique if the skin is not intact. Otherwise, simple clean technique is adequate. (See Chapter 22 for information regarding sterile technique.)

Warm Soaks

For warm soaks, submerge the patient's body part in a pan of warm water or use a whirlpool with water between 105°F and 110°F (40°C to 43°C). Warm soaks are useful for increasing the circulation to the extremities to aid healing, as is needed with infection of the foot.

Sitz Baths

The sitz bath is a source of comfort, increases blood flow to support healing, and cleanses to aid in prevention of infection. They are commonly used for patients recovering from vaginal childbirth or hemorrhoid surgery. A special plastic basin is filled with warm water and set on the toilet. The bucket or bag is filled with warm water between 105°F and 110°F (40°C to 43°C) and hung 18 to 24 inches (45.7 to 60.9 cm) above the patient's hips. The water drains via tubing that extends to the basin and snaps in place in the bottom of the basin (Fig. 18-3).

After the patient sits down on the basin in the toilet, the tubing is unclamped, allowing warm water to flow into the basin, causing a gentle swirling of warm water to bathe the patient's perineum. This is usually continued for 10 to 15 minutes. The nurse must stay in close proximity the first time the patient uses the sitz bath, as the vasodilation in the perineal area causes blood to pool in the pelvic region. *Safety: When the patient stands after completion of the sitz bath, close monitoring is required to make certain the patient does not suffer a drop in blood pressure upon standing.* This is known as **orthostatic hypotension** and results in decreasing blood flow to the brain, causing the patient to become faint or fall.

Skill 18-3 (page 386) provides more information on administering a sitz bath.

Whirlpool Baths

Generally, whirlpool baths are administered by physical therapy, but some facilities such as long-term care facilities delegate use of the whirlpool to nursing. A *whirlpool* is a large stainless steel or porcelain tub with powered jets that circulate the water around the patient. The tub must be filled with water above the level of the power jets before turning on the pump, or water will be sprayed everywhere. They are very relaxing and can be used for routine bathing, wound care and débridement, or relaxation and loosening of tight muscles and stiff joints prior to physical therapy treatments. *Safety: Children and elderly, confused, or sedated patients must NEVER be left alone in a whirlpool tub, as the depth of water makes drowning a real risk.*

Figure 18-3 A sitz bath soaks the patient's perineal area.

Knowledge Connection
What are the risks of different methods of heat application?
Which type of heat penetrates the deepest, dry or moist?

Nursing Care During Heat Therapy

Safety: The safety of the patient must be your primary concern during heat therapy. Assess the patient's age and cognitive level of function, orientation, sedation, sensory impairment, and impairment of circulation. Certain diseases such as diabetes and peripheral vascular disease impair circulation to the extremities. Patients with these conditions may be more susceptible to burns. Before application of any type of heat therapy, you must assess the skin for temperature, color, sensation, edema, and integrity. Remember that sterile technique must be used for broken skin when applying hot compresses.

People and Places Connection

The Skin of Seniors and Children Is Fragile
Two populations require extra caution when applying heat therapy: elderly individuals and children. Elderly patients often have reduced tactile sensation due to the loss of touch receptors. Their skin is also thinner and drier, making it easier to damage the tissues. *Safety: The temperature of the heat application should be lowered to a setting between 95°F and 100°F to reduce risk of tissue injury. The skin condition should be assessed more frequently, every 5 to 10 minutes.*

Be aware that the very young child or cognitively impaired older adult may not have the communication skills to relate problems to you. The warm packs, for instance, could be too hot and be burning the skin and these patients may not know how to tell you. For this reason, it is recommended that these patients be attended throughout heat therapy.

Safety: If using electrical equipment, assess the condition of the equipment and the electrical cord for defects. Do not use frayed cords or those with the insulation layer scratched, allowing wires to show. Make sure the plug is securely attached to the cord. Make certain that electrical cords are placed where they will not cause someone to trip over them. Advise patients to use heating pads only while awake and for no longer than 30 minutes at a time.

Carefully check the temperature of the heating device before applying it to the patient. Make certain the temperature setting is in accordance with the physician's order, usually around 105°F (40.5°C). Instruct the patient to notify you quickly if the heat application becomes too warm. After initiation of the heat therapy, reassess the area and surrounding skin within 5 minutes, noting if the skin is bright red or blistering. Check the site every 10 to 15 minutes until treatment is completed. Skin should be pink or light red, but never bright or dark red. Place the patient's call light within reach before leaving the room. When a K-pad is ordered continuously, assess the site at least hourly.

Before placing a patient in a whirlpool tub, disinfect the tub thoroughly to avoid cross contamination from the previous patient. *Safety: Use a lift to transfer patients in and out of the tub, helping to prevent falls. Check the temperature of the water and make sure it is not too hot before lowering the patient into the tub.* Again, never leave elderly patients, children, patients with diminished mental capacity, or sedated patients alone in a whirlpool tub. Take care to heat the environment to a comfortable temperature to avoid chilling your patient. Use a bath blanket or towels to appropriately drape your patient during transfer; this provides for modesty as well as warmth preservation.

If using a hypo/hyperthermia blanket, be certain to place the blanket either over or under the patient as instructions indicate. Observe the patient temperature monitoring device closely to avoid raising or lowering the temperature too quickly. Monitor vital signs, level of consciousness, and condition of skin at least every 30 minutes. An EKG monitor is generally applied to observe heart rhythm during systemic heating or cooling.

Always reassess the skin after removal of the heat source to evaluate the patient's response. Ask the patient if the therapy helped. Was the treatment effective? Did it do what you intended? Did it help to reduce discomfort? If it was a whirlpool for wound care, did it débride the wound of all slough and debris? Evaluation of the effectiveness of treatment is always necessary to provide data for use in determining if the plan of care needs modification or not.

Patient Teaching Connection

Heating Pad Use Carries Risk
In the home setting, it is more common to use heating pads as the primary source of heat therapy. The patient and family should be taught how to safely apply and monitor the heating pad. Points to include in teaching are:

- *Safety: Inspect the cord and pad for fraying or bare wires.*
- Assess the site for color and warmth to touch.
- *Safety: Set a timer for no longer than 20 to 30 minutes.*
- Use low or medium setting. *Safety: Avoid the highest setting.*
- Check the skin under and around the heating pad every 10 minutes for excessive redness or signs of blistering.
- *Safety: Never lie on top of the heating pad or sleep while using it.*
- Avoid use of petroleum products on the skin during heat application.
- Avoid use of a heating pad on a new injury or trauma and bleeding wounds.
- Avoid use on areas that continue to swell.

Cold Therapy

Local application of cold to a site causes **vasoconstriction**, or narrowing, of the veins and capillaries. The pores in the capillary walls become less permeable to the passage of fluid from the vessels to the interstitial space. These processes result in decreased blood flow to the area. When used systemically, cold lowers the body temperature, which slows metabolism. Cooling the body below normal temperature has been used in cardiovascular and neurosurgery to decrease the tissue oxygen demand. This helps preserve heart and brain cells that might otherwise die from lack of oxygen, known as *ischemia,* at normal body temperature and metabolic rate.

Indications for Cold Therapy

A physician's order is required for application of most cold therapies, though it is generally accepted that cold packs may be applied to new localized injuries seen in the emergency room. You should check your facility's policy before using cold therapy without an order. Cold packs are used for prevention of edema, control or stoppage of bleeding, pain relief, numbing of sensation, reduction of muscle spasm, and reduction of fever. Table 18-1 compares and contrasts the effects of cold applications versus those of heat applications.

Prevention of Edema

Application of cold therapy is generally the treatment of choice for injuries that tend to swell, such as a sprained ankle or bone fractures, or overuse of a joint, such as in tennis elbow. It is commonly used after joint surgeries and neck and throat surgeries. The vasoconstriction reduces the amount of fluid that leaves the capillaries and leaks into the interstitial space, which results in less edema. Cold therapy is recommended for the first 48 to 72 hours after an injury that can result in swelling.

Hemostasis

The vasoconstriction caused by application of cold also helps to stop active bleeding, or produce **hemostasis**. Cold therapy is useful after trauma, dental surgery, and tonsillectomies, and to stop nosebleeds.

Pain Relief

Cold applications are helpful when applied to painful sites such as hemorrhoidectomy or skeletal surgery incisions, perineal lacerations and episiotomies due to childbirth, the forehead and occipital areas for headaches, and the face for sinus congestion pain. Much of the pain relief effects result from the prevention of edema, which causes increased pressure on nerve endings. Many physicians have found ice packs effective to help relieve migraine headaches, facial pain from temporomandibular joint (TMJ) problems, and chronic back and neck muscular spasms when medications do not.

Numbing Sensation

Application of cold therapy is useful to numb a particular area, such as to relieve itching of insect bites or allergic rashes. It is also used to relieve the stinging or burning sensation of minor burns such as sunburn.

Table 18-1 Effects of Local Heat and Cold Applications

Heat	Cold
Vasodilation	Vasoconstriction
Increases blood flow to site.	Decreases blood flow to site, decreasing bleeding.
Increases inflammatory response. Delivers increased number of red and white blood cells, oxygen, and nutrients to aid healing.	Decreases inflammatory response. Slows bacterial growth.
Increases capillary permeability.	Decreases capillary permeability.
Increases cellular metabolism.	Decreases cellular metabolism.
Will *increase* edema if used during the first 48 hours following trauma. Will *decrease* edema if used after edema has stabilized.	Helps prevent edema.
Relaxes muscles.	Relaxes muscles.
Decreases pain.	Decreases pain. Numbs sensation.

Reduction of Muscle Spasm

It used to be thought that only heat applications would relieve muscle spasms, but we now know that cold applications also help to interrupt the cycle of muscle tension and spasms. Cold therapy is the treatment of choice if the spasm is acute.

Fever Reduction

When an individual has a fever, the body's metabolism increases and, as a result, more calories and oxygen are required to maintain the increased metabolism. Once the fever becomes so high that the body cannot provide adequate supplemental calories and oxygen, the brain may suffer permanent damage if the fever is not reduced quickly.

One of the most effective and noninvasive methods of reducing high fever in both children and adults is to apply cold therapy. Ice packs may be placed on the forehead, in the axillae, and on the inguinal areas. The packs cool the blood as it courses through the major vessels to the extremities and through the abundant vascular supply to the face and head. A tepid tub or sponge bath, with water at 90°F (32.2°C), may also be used, but chilling should be avoided. When the patient is chilled too rapidly, he or she will begin to shiver, which can raise body temperature rather than lower it.

In extremely high fevers that do not come down with either of the above methods, the physician may order cold water irrigation, known as *lavage,* of large body cavities such as the stomach or colon. Intravenous infusion of cold normal saline may also be given in an effort to reduce the fever.

Figure 18-4 Cold applications. From left to right: (a) refreezeable gel pack, (b) disposable refillable ice pack, (c) small glove-filled ice pack, and (d) instant chemical cold pack.

children. Use some type of barrier between the ice bag and the skin to prevent tissue damage.

Refreezable Commercial Cold Packs

These commercial packs are generally filled with a gel-like substance that hardens while remaining malleable when chilled in the freezer. They warm with use, necessitating refreezing after 20 to 30 minutes. The advantage is their ease of use.

Chemical Cold Packs

Chemical cold packs may be smaller than refillable ice bags and must be activated. Instructions for activation are printed on the container and usually require squeezing or twisting the bag until the chemicals mix and become cold. They are only good for one application before disposal.

Cold Compresses

Cold compresses can be made by wetting a folded washcloth, placing it in a zip-type plastic bag, and placing it in the freezer for a short period. Or you may use a bowl of ice water and simply dip the washcloth into the water, wring it out, and apply the washcloth to site. If the skin is not intact, the compress should be made using sterile water and sterile dressings such as gauze 4x4s.

Tepid Baths

Tepid (cool, but not cold) baths are used mostly for reduction of body temperature when use of medication is undesirable or ineffective. Either a tub bath or pan of water for sponging the patient can be used. Avoid chilling the patient to the point of shivering, which raises body temperature.

Nursing Care During Cold Therapy

Assessment of the skin is done prior to application of the cold therapy, noting integrity, sensation, temperature, and color of skin. *Safety: Always use a thin cloth barrier*

> ### Knowledge Connection
> What are five uses of cold therapy? How does local application of cold help with hemostasis? What does systemic cooling of the body do to the basal metabolic rate?

Methods of Cold Application

Cold applications include refillable ice bags or collars, refreezable commercial cold packs, chemical cold packs, cold compresses, and tepid baths (Fig. 18-4). Cold, like heat, can be applied dry or moist. Moisture increases the depth and rate of cold penetration. Skill 18-4 (page 387) provides more information on application of cold packs.

Refillable Ice Bags, Collars, and Gloves

The refillable ice bags may be made of rubber or waterproof paper, with clamp or foldable closures. Bags should be filled one-half to two-thirds full with ice and some water. Do not overfill the bag or it will be difficult to mold it to the appropriate body part. Then expel the remaining air from the bag and hook the closure.

Some facilities use disposable rubber gloves and fill them with ice. They are secured by tying the glove opening in a knot, as you do a balloon. These smaller ice packs are good for use on the perineum, fingers, and nose and on small *between the ice pack and the patient's skin to prevent frostbite and damage to the tissues.* Leave cold packs in place no longer than 20 to 30 minutes. When cold therapy is left in place too long, the vasoconstriction continues, depriving tissues of oxygen and nutrients to the point of injury and necrosis. The patient may complain of pain or a burning sensation. If left in place until skin temperature drops to 60°F, rebound phenomenon may be seen: vasodilation occurs in an attempt to prevent the tissue damage. *Safety: Assess the skin for pallor or mottling every 10 to 15 minutes during therapy.* **Pallor** appears pale or white; **mottling** occurs in irregular blotches, usually blue or purplish-blue. When using cold therapy for local effect only, the patient may require a blanket to cover the rest of the body or the room temperature may need to be raised a few degrees to prevent chilling discomfort. Limit time in a tepid bath to 10 to 15 minutes to prevent overcooling to the point of shivering.

Evaluate the effects of the cold therapy. Did it achieve the intended results? Has the bleeding stopped? Did it relieve the pain or reduce the fever? Always assess the patient's response to cold therapy for untoward effects, as individuals sometimes react differently than expected. When using cold to reduce fever, be certain to assess the body temperature after 10 minutes of tepid bathing or ice packs.

Knowledge Connection

Describe the assessments you should make prior to application of cold. How do they differ from assessments during the treatment? What assessments do you make to determine the effectiveness of the cold therapy?

Skill 18-1 Application of Dry or Moist Heat

Assessment Steps

1. Review the physician's order and nurse's note on the last heat application. *This will help to determine the type of heat delivery device to use and how the patient tolerated the previous treatment.*
2. *Safety: Assess the patient's age and cognitive level of function, orientation, sedation, sensory impairment, and impairment of circulation to determine if there are any contraindications.*
3. *Safety: Assess the site where heat is to be applied, noting the appearance, color, presence of edema, temperature of site and surrounding skin, integrity of skin, and any discomfort. This provides a baseline against which you can measure the effects of the application.*

Planning Steps

1. Obtain the correct type of heat delivery device, such as a hot water bottle, commercial gel, or chemical pack, and a barrier or protective covering such as a towel. *Planning saves time and effort.*

Implementation Steps

1. Follow the Initial Implementation Steps located on the inside front cover.
2. **If using a hot water bottle:** Fill the bottle one-half to two-thirds full with hot tap water. Fold the top of the bottle over to remove extra air and fasten the closure securely. *By not filling the bottle too full, you allow it to conform to the site to which it is applied.*
   If using a commercial gel pack: *Safety: Follow instructions on gel pack for heating.*
   If using a disposable commercial chemical pack: *Safety: Activate the chemical pack according to pack instructions.*
3. *Safety: Check the temperature against your wrist and allow the patient to test it against his or her wrist to make certain it is not too hot.*

4. *Safety: Apply the heat delivery device to the appropriate site using a dry protective cloth covering or barrier device to prevent burns.* If moist heat is ordered, apply a warm moist towel to the skin. Lay the heat delivery device on the moist towel, making certain it does not directly touch skin, and *cover the device with a dry towel to help maintain the heat.*
5. After 5 minutes, reassess the site for bright redness of skin to make certain it is not too hot. *Safety: Continue to reassess skin every 10 to 15 minutes, asking the patient about discomfort. If skin becomes dark red or bright red or the patient complains that it is too hot, remove the heat pack immediately.* Otherwise, leave the heat pack in place for the ordered length of time.
6. Follow the Ending Implementation Steps located on the inside back cover.
7. Document the condition and each assessment of the skin along with the heat application in the nurse's notes.

Evaluation Steps

1. Remove the heat pack after the appropriate length of treatment. Assess the site for objective data such as color, temperature, and edema.
2. Assess the subjective data related to effectiveness of the heat application by asking the patient about any change in discomfort/comfort level at the site.

Sample Documentation

12/03/10   14:30   Complained of sacral discomfort rated a 7 on a scale of 0 to 10. Described it as muscle "tightness." Dry heat applied using disposable chemical pack wrapped in towel to sacral area for 30 minutes as ordered. Skin intact, pink, without edema, warm to touch. States heat seemed to relieve much of the muscle tightness & discomfort down to a 2. ——————
——————————— Nurse's signature and credentials

Skill 18-2 Application of Aquathermia Pad (K-pad)

Assessment Steps

1. Review the physician's order and previous nurse's note. *This provides needed data, such as temperature setting and the patient's response to the last treatment.*

2. *Safety: Assess the patient's age and cognitive level of function, orientation, sedation, sensory impairment, and impairment of circulation to determine if there are any contraindications.*

3. Assess the patient's discomfort level and assess the site for color, temperature, edema, and integrity of skin. *This provides a baseline against which to measure effectiveness of treatment.*

4. Examine the K-pad pad and cord for defects. *This helps to reduce accidents.*

5. *Safety: Review the manufacturer's instructions for use of the K-pad.*

Planning Steps

1. *Safety: Make certain there is an electrical outlet that can be reached in such a manner that the cord will lay where it will not cause falls.*

2. Obtain the disposable pad that attaches to the K-pad unit and distilled water to fill the tank. *Preparation saves time and effort.*

Implementation Steps

1. Follow the Initial Implementation Steps located on the inside front cover.

2. Fill the tank to the indicated level with distilled water. Do not overfill.

3. Attach the disposable pad by connecting the two tubes on the pad to those extending from the K-pad unit. *This allows water to flow from the K-pad unit into the pad.*

4. *Safety: Using the designated key, set the temperature dial to the ordered setting, usually 105°F (40.5°C). This helps to prevent burns.*

5. Allow 10 to 15 minutes for the unit to heat the distilled water that is circulating through the maze of tubes inside the pad. If the physician has ordered "moist" heat, carefully pour several ounces of water on the absorbent side of the pad until the surface is completely moistened. Otherwise, leave the pad dry. *Moist heat penetrates deeper and quicker than dry heat.*

6. Place the pad on the appropriate body part. If it is ordered on an extremity, secure with ties or wrap it with a towel to help hold it in place. *Safety: Do not use pins. Pins will make holes in the tubes inside the pad.*

7. *Safety: Assess the site every 10 to 15 minutes, noting any changes in the color and temperature of the skin. Ask the patient about any discomfort to make certain it is not too hot.*

8. Follow the Ending Implementation Steps located on the inside back cover.

9. Document the condition and each assessment of the skin along with the heat application. Include the temperature at which the K-pad is set.

Evaluation Steps

1. After completion of treatment, evaluate for effectiveness. Did it achieve the desired results? Did it help the problem for which it was applied? Reassess for objective data, including color, temperature, edema, and integrity of skin. Assess subjective data: Did the heat make a difference in how the site felt?

Sample Documentation

4/13/10   08:30   Dry K-pad to left lower leg for 30 minutes, temp @ 105°F. Skin intact, mildly pink, warm to touch, midcalf measures 17.5 cm compared to right @ 17 cm. States the calf still aches, a 3 on a scale of 0 to 10. Pedal pulses strong and equal bilaterally. Capillary refill 5 seconds in left and 3 seconds in right foot. —————— Nurse's signature and credentials

---

Skill 18-3 Administering a Sitz Bath

Assessment Steps

1. *Safety: Determine if this is the patient's first sitz bath or a subsequent sitz bath. If patient has had a previous treatment, review the nurse's note regarding the prior bath to determine how the patient responded. You will need to know if the patient became faint afterward.*

Planning Steps

1. **If using a regular tub:** Prepare the tub by disinfecting it *to prevent cross-contamination.*
   If using a disposable portable sitz bath: Gather needed equipment and supplies: sitz bath tub, clean gown, two towels, washcloth, any other personal items the patient may need. *Preparation saves time and effort.*

2. Heat the bathroom *to prevent chilling.*

3. *Safety: Review the manufacturer's instructions for use.*

Implementation Steps

1. Follow the Initial Implementation Steps located on the inside front cover.

2. **If using a regular tub:** Fill the tub approximately 4 to 5 inches deep with warm water between 105°F and 110°F (40.5°C and 43.3°C). *The water must be deep enough to adequately cover the perineum. Safety: Water hotter than 110°F (43.3°C) can burn the patient.*
   If using a disposable sitz bath: *Safety: Fill the water container with warm water between 105°F and 110°F and prime the tubing to remove air from the line.*

Skill 18-3 (continued)

Clamp the tubing. Hang the container on a hook or IV pole to a height approximately 18 to 24 inches above the toilet seat. Insert tubing from the water container through the designated opening in the sitz basin and snap it into grooves in the bottom of the basin. Place the basin on the toilet rim. *Safety: Fill the basin with warm water between 105° and 110°F.*

3. **For regular tub:** *Safety: Assist patient to get into the tub. This reduces risk of falls.*
   For disposable sitz bath: Assist patient to sit on the toilet and basin with the perineum immersed in the water. Unclamp the tubing and allow water to drain from the water container into the basin. As the basin fills, the excess water will drain through the overflow opening and into the toilet.

4. Make certain the patient does not become chilled. A bath blanket or towel may be draped around his or her shoulders *for added warmth.*

5. *Safety: Inform the patient to avoid standing unassisted after completion of the sitz bath. Make certain the patient can reach the call light. If this is the first time her or she has used the sitz bath, remain close enough to the bathroom door that you can be summoned if the patient begins to feel faint.*

6. After the completion of the sitz bath, assist the patient to stand and dry off as needed.

For regular tub: *Safety: Disinfect the tub to reduce risk of cross-contamination.*
For disposable sitz bath: Clean the basin, dry it, and return it to its storage area. Rinse the water container with cool water. Unclamp the tube and hang it in the shower to drain. *This leaves the basin ready for the next use.*

7. Follow the Ending Implementation Steps located on the inside back cover.

8. Document the sitz bath in the nurse's notes or on the flowsheet.

Evaluation Steps

1. Assess the perineal area for edema, color, and drainage, and ask the patient about discomfort level.

Sample Documentation

6/24/10 2100 Assisted with portable sitz bath. Water 107°F. Treatment lasted 10 minutes. Dried and assisted back to bed. Perineum still slightly edematous with no bruising. Episiotomy with good approximation and light red edges. States the sitz bath "sure did feel good." No complaints of weakness or pain. ———
————————————— Nurse's signature and credentials

Skill 18-4 Application of Cold Packs

Assessment Steps

1. Review the physician's order and previous nurse's note on the last cold application. *This will help to determine the type of cold delivery device to use and how the patient tolerated the previous treatment.*

2. *Safety: Assess the patient's age and cognitive level of function, orientation, sedation, sensory impairment, and impairment of circulation to determine if there are any contraindications.*

3. Assess the site where cold is to be applied, noting the appearance, color, presence of edema, temperature of site and surrounding skin, integrity of skin, and any discomfort. *This provides a baseline against which to measure the effects of the application.*

Planning Steps

1. Obtain the correct type of cold delivery device, such as a reusable ice bag, collar, or glove or a commercial gel or chemical pack, and a barrier or protective covering such as a towel. *Being prepared saves time and effort.*

Implementation Steps

1. Follow the Initial Implementation Steps located on the inside front cover.

2. **If using ice bag, glove, or collar:** Fill one-half to two-thirds full of ice. Remove excess air and close the device. *This allows the ice bag to conform to the application site.*

If using commercial gel pack: Remove the gel pack from the freezer.
If using disposable commercial chemical pack: Activate the chemical pack according to pack instructions, usually by striking, twisting, or squeezing the container.

3. Apply cold delivery device to the appropriate site using a *dry* protective cloth covering or barrier device *to prevent tissue damage.* If *moist* cold is ordered, apply a moist towel to the skin. Lay the cold pack on top of the moist towel, making certain it does not directly touch skin, and cover it with a dry towel. *Moist cold penetrates faster and deeper than dry cold.*

4. *Safety: After 5 minutes, reassess the site for pallor or mottling of skin to make certain it is not too cold. Continue to reassess skin every 10 to 15 minutes, asking the patient about discomfort.* If skin becomes pale or mottled or the patient complains it is too cold, remove the cold pack immediately to prevent frostbite. Otherwise, leave the cold pack in place for the ordered length of time.

5. Follow the Ending Implementation Steps located on the inside back cover.

6. Document the skin assessment and cold application.

Evaluation Steps

1. Remove the cold pack after the appropriate length of treatment. Assess the site for objective data such as color, temperature, sensation, and edema.

(skill continues on page 388)

Skill 18-4 (continued)

2. Assess the subjective data related to effectiveness of the cold application by asking the patient about any change in discomfort/comfort level at the site. Did it help the pain?

for 20 minutes as ordered. Ankle skin intact, pink with bruising, 1+ pitting edema, toes warm to touch with brisk capillary refill, pedal pulses equally strong. States the cold pack reduced pain to a 3. ———————— Nurse's signature and credentials

Sample Documentation

3/3/10   12:30   Complained of right ankle discomfort rated a 6 on a scale of 0 to 10. Described pain as throbbing. Applied dry cold pack using disposable chemical pack wrapped in towel to right ankle

 Post Conference

You cared for your patient with sepsis and a highly elevated temperature. When you evaluated how you did on this assignment, you found that you did pretty well and were pleased with your performance. You had remembered to read the accompanying instructions to the hypothermia blanket and applied the blanket accordingly. You also located and read the facility policy for this skill and found there were no discrepancies between the manufacturer's instructions and the facility policy. You reviewed the specific parameters of the physician's order as well. By remembering to assess the patient's skin before, during, and after the treatment, you were able to determine that no injury occurred. You knew to remain with the patient so that you could assess the vital signs at the frequency dictated by facility policy, and monitor the patient for signs of excessive cold, level of consciousness, and condition of skin at 10 minutes and then every 30 minutes thereafter until the fever was adequately reduced. You were relieved that the patient responded appropriately and did not exhibit any problems. To document the care, you recorded the patient's vital signs on the graphic sheet in the chart and charted your assessment findings in the nurse's notes according to facility policy.

KEY POINTS

- Local application of heat results in vasodilation and increased permeability of capillaries.

- Indications for heat therapy include relaxation of muscle spasms, pain relief, reduction of inflammation, support of the healing process, reduction of edema once it has stabilized, and elevation of body temperature.

- Application of heat increases metabolism.

- *Safety: Contraindications for use of heat therapy include suspected appendicitis, bleeding wound, new injury or trauma, and application of heat over large areas of the body in certain cardiac patients.*

- Local cold applications result in vasoconstriction and decreased permeability of capillaries.

- Indications for use of cold therapy include prevention of edema, hemostasis, pain relief, numbing of sensation, muscle relaxation, and reduction of fever.

- Risks for injury from cold therapy include tissue damage, frostbite, and hypothermia.

- *Safety: Nursing assessments pertinent prior to heat and cold applications include: patient's age and cognitive level of function, orientation, sedation, sensory impairment, impairment of circulation, appearance, color, presence of edema, temperature of skin, and whether or not there is discomfort.*

- *Safety: Nursing assessments pertinent during and after heat and cold applications include: appearance, color, presence of edema, and temperature of skin, and whether or not there is any change in the patient's comfort or discomfort level.*

REVIEW QUESTIONS

Select the answer that is most appropriate for each of the following questions. Some questions may have more than one correct answer. Check all that apply.

1. A patient has an erythematous area at the site where you just discontinued an IV infusion. There is no edema, but the patient complains of the site being very tender. The treatment of choice would be which of the following?

   a. Telling the patient the tenderness will subside without treatment

   b. Administering a sitz bath

   c. Applying an ice pack

   d. Applying a warm pack

2. Which of the following treatments would possibly help relieve a patient's discomfort from a muscle spasm in her lumbar area?

   a. Immersion in a whirlpool

   b. Administration of a tepid sponge bath

   c. Application of a warm pack

   d. Application of a cold pack

3. A child has a minor cut on her scalp that continues to ooze blood after the wound is cleansed. Which type of heat or cold application would be appropriate in this situation?

   a. Examination glove filled with ice

   b. Sterile warm compress

   c. Tepid sponge bath

   d. Warm K-pad

   e. Cooling blanket

4. During a heat application, which of the following assessment findings would indicate the heat pack should be removed immediately?

   a. Skin is pale pink.

   b. Skin is dark red.

   c. Temperature of the site is slightly warmer than surrounding skin.

   d. Patient denies discomfort.

   e. Skin is starting to look "bubbly."

   f. Skin is hot to touch.

5. During a cold application, which of the following assessment findings would indicate the cold pack should be removed immediately?

   a. Skin is pink.

   b. Skin is white.

   c. Skin is mottled.

   d. Patient complains of a "burning" sensation.

   e. Skin is very cool to touch.

   f. Patient states the itching from the rash site is decreasing.

SHORT ANSWER QUESTIONS

6. The physician has written the following order: "Apply K-pad to left lower leg." What further information must you get from the physician before carrying out this order?

7. Explain how local application of heat will support the healing process.

CRITICAL THINKING EXERCISES

8. Melonie Jones, a 68-year-old female, is diabetic and suffers with the complication of neuropathy and impaired peripheral vascular circulation. As a result, she has poor circulation to and decreased sensation in her feet. She has fractured her left ankle so badly that she will require a cast once the edema has gone down. The physician has ordered ice packs to the left ankle for 30 minutes every hour. What precautions must you take and what assessments are pertinent for you to make before, during, and after each cold application? Explain your answer.

9. A 19-year-old male sprained his right ankle while playing basketball yesterday. He tells you that it has swollen to nearly double its size since he went to bed last night. He wants to apply a heat pack to help the edema resolve so he can play in the game tomorrow. What do you tell him?

ADDITIONAL RESOURCES

For additional Resources, Questions, and Activities, please see:

 Student Resource Disk

 http://davisplus.fadavis.com

 Student Study Guide

REFERENCES

Bahrt G. Cooler heart, better odds: induced hypothermia. *Nurs Manage.* 2009;40(7):22-29.

Beattie S. In from the cold. RN [serial online]. 2006;November. Available at: http://www.rnweb.com/rnweb/content/printContentPopup.jsp?id=382181. Accessed January 2, 2008.

Brown PW. Evaluation focuses on tendons, nerves, and vessels: pointers for managing common hand injuries. *J Musculoskel Med.* 2007;24(8):354.

Day MW. Action STAT: frostbite. *Nursing2008.* 2008;38(1):72.

Day MW. Keeping your cool when heat stroke strikes. *Nursing2009 Crit Care.* 2009;4(4):30-33.

Guide to care for patients: back pain. *Nurse Pract.* 2006;31(4):57-58.

Gulick D. *Sport Notes: Field & Clinical Examination Guide.* Philadelphia: FA Davis; 2008.

Harvey CV. Spinal surgery patient care. *Orthop Nurs.* 2005;24:426-440.

How hot is too hot? *Men Nurs.* 2009;39(5):8-11.

Johns Hopkins School of Medicine. Topical heat therapy reduced pain intensity, increased relief, and improved disability scores. *Biotech Week.* 2006;486(Feb).

Koran Z. Therapeutic hypothermia in post-resuscitation patient: the development and implementation of an evidence-based protocol for the emergency department. *J Trauma Nurs.* 2009;16(1):48-57.

Michlovitz SL, Bikab TP. *Modalities for Therapeutic Intervention.* 4th ed. Philadelphia: FA Davis; 2008.

Miller NC, Askew AE. Tibia fractures: an overview of evaluation and treatment. *Orthop Nurs.* 2007;26:216-223.

Pullen RL, Edwards T. Caring for a patient with rheumatoid arthritis. *LPN2009.* 2009;4(4):28-34.

Rand SE, Goerlich C, Marchand K, Jablecki N. The physical therapy prescription. *Am Fam Physician.* 2007;76:1661-1666.

Rhoads J, Meeker BJ. *Davis's Guide to Clinical Nursing Skills.* Philadelphia: FA Davis; 2008.

Scanlon V, Sanders T. *Essentials of Anatomy and Physiology.* Philadelphia: FA Davis; 2007.

Thompson HT, Kirkness KJ, Mitchell PH, Webb DJ. Fever management practices of neuroscience nurses: national and regional perspectives. *J Neurosci Nurs.* 2007;39:151-162.

Treas LS, Hauschildt J, eds. *Fundamentals for Nursing Review Module Edition 5.0.* Overland Park, KS: Assessment Technologies Institute; 2005.

Venes D, ed. *Taber's Cyclopedic Medical Dictionary.* 21st ed. Philadelphia: FA Davis; 2009.

Wilkinson JM, Van Leuven K. *Fundamentals of Nursing: Theory, Concepts & Applications.* Philadelphia: FA Davis; 2007.

Williams L, Hopper P. *Understanding Medical-Surgical Nursing.* Philadelphia: FA Davis; 2007.

Pain Management, Rest, and Restorative Sleep

Key Terms

Acute pain

Adjuvant

Analgesics

Chronic pain

Circadian rhythm

Controlled substances

Cutaneous pain

Effleurage

Endorphins

Holistic

Intractable pain

Neuropathic pain

Nociceptors

Patient-controlled analgesia (PCA)

Phantom limb pain

Prostaglandins

Radiating pain

Referred pain

Restorative sleep

Substance P

Visceral pain

Objectives

1. Define key terms related to pain management, rest, and restorative sleep.
2. Explain the gate control theory.
3. Identify the expert regarding the level of a patient's pain.
4. Describe the role that endorphins play in pain perception and relief.
5. Compare the different types of nociceptive and neuropathic pain.
6. Outline the factors that affect pain and pain perception.
7. Paraphrase how to thoroughly assess pain.
8. Correlate acknowledgment and acceptance of pain to treatment of pain.
9. Identify at least three nonpharmacological methods of pain relief.
10. Differentiate between classifications of analgesics.
11. Characterize restorative sleep.
12. Enumerate sleep requirements for different age groups.
13. Name six specific factors that affect sleep.
14. Describe interventions you might use to promote sleep.

Skills

19-1 Application of TENS Unit

> ## 🌐 Clinical Connection
>
> **Your Assignment:** You are assigned to care for a patient who had a left above-the-knee amputation 3 days ago. He has been restless and has not slept well. Today he is very tired and irritable, especially with his wife, who earlier in the day voiced frustration with her husband's moodiness and went home in tears. He has difficulty rating his pain when you try to evaluate it and finally tells you, "I must be nuts because what really hurts is my left foot—only it isn't there!"
>
> **Your Actions:** To care for this patient, you will need to:
> - Educate him about phantom pain
> - Use interventions to relieve his pain
> - Help him understand the need for restorative sleep
> - Assist him to rest and sleep
>   How will you meet all of these needs?

The management of pain and discomfort are imperative for one to truly rest and experience restorative sleep, that which helps the body to regain strength and return to a healthful state. In this chapter, you will learn different methods to decrease and relieve your patient's pain and provide comfort, as well as ways to help the patient to experience beneficial rest and sleep.

Pain

Pain serves as a warning sign indicating that actual damage has occurred or that the potential exists for damage of tissue. Pain can be a sensory and or emotional experience, is complex with many components, and means different things to different people. The human response to pain varies not only from culture to culture, but from individual to individual. As you learned in Chapter 17, pain is so important it is known as the fifth vital sign.

Nature and Physiology of Pain and Its Transmission

Pain can have negative effects on and even destroy numerous aspects of a patient's life. Pain can make it difficult to:

- Perform activities of daily living
- Rest and experience restorative sleep
- Eat
- Perform normal body movements and exercise
- Maintain family relationships
- Work or maintain a job
- Have a social life or maintain friendships
- Maintain cognitive abilities
- Focus on spiritual beliefs

Thus, it is important to develop an understanding of pain and how you can assist your patients with pain relief and development of coping skills for dealing with unrelieved pain. Your beliefs regarding pain will affect how you respond to patients and, as a result, impact your patients' lives. We encourage you to open your mind and begin to view pain **holistically**, which includes viewing the physical, mental, social, and spiritual aspects of a person as parts of the integrated whole being. This will prepare you to best meet your patients' pain relief needs.

One of the core things to remember about a patient's pain is that pain is always *what the patient says it is*. If the patient says the pain level is an 8 on a scale of 0 to 10, with 10 being the worst pain one can imagine, then the pain is an 8. It does not make a difference if the patient *does not appear* to be in pain or if you think the source of the pain should not cause *that much* pain. *It is what it is* to the patient, and that is what you will want to treat.

Gate Control Theory

In the 1960s, researchers proposed a theory that helps to explain the transmission and perception of pain and how even nonpharmaceutical interventions can relieve the pain. The theory purports that the transmission of pain impulses to the central nervous system is controlled by a "gate," which opens and closes in response to sensory input. The gate must be open for the pain impulse to be transmitted to the brain and interpreted as pain. When the gate is closed, the nerve impulse for pain is blocked from transmission.

It is thought that the thalamus can open and close the gate in relationship to stress and anxiety: An increase in stress can cause the gate to open, while decreased stress and anxiety can close the gate. Stimulation of the broad nerve fibers is thought to close the gate, while stimulation of the narrow nerve fibers is thought to open the gate. The broader nerve fibers are stimulated by such things as exercise, heat, cold, massage, and transcutaneous electrical nerve stimulation (TENS). The smaller, narrow nerve fibers are directly stimulated by injury and damage to the tissues. Thus, when tissue damage or injury stimulates the narrow nerve fibers, it makes sense when a person naturally begins to rub the painful site in an effort to relieve some of the pain. An example is when you bang your elbow against the corner of a cabinet, the first reaction is usually to grab the elbow and rub it vigorously. This helps to relieve the pain.

Thoughts and emotions are also believed to have an effect on opening and closing the gate, by stimulation of endorphin production. **Endorphins** are natural body chemicals produced by the brain in response to pleasant thoughts or feelings, exercise, laughter, sex, and massage. They act similarly to morphine and produce feelings of euphoria, well-being, and pleasure. They bind to the opiate receptor sites, which help to close the gates and block the transmission of pain to the central nervous system. Long-distance runners sometimes experience what they describe as "hitting the mark" or a "runner's high" that allows them to continue running more miles without experiencing any discomfort or pain. Think of a time when you and a friend or relative have gotten tickled about something, began laughing, and just could not stop laughing for several minutes. Afterward, you probably felt very good and quite relaxed, with a positive sense of well-being. You might have even said something like, "Boy, did I need that!" This feeling is thought to be a direct result of endorphins.

> ### *Knowledge Connection*
> Name some of the effects pain can have on one's daily life. What is meant by *gate control theory?* Describe the role of endorphins and their effects in pain perception and pain relief.

Classifications of Pain

There are many different classifications of pain. Pain that comes on suddenly and has a short duration (less than 6 months) is known as **acute pain**. Pain that lasts longer than 6 months is termed **chronic pain**. *Intermittent pain* is pain that comes and goes at intervals. **Intractable pain** refers to pain that cannot be relieved, is incurable, or is resistant to treatment. **Referred pain** is pain felt in an area other than where the pain was produced. An example of referred pain is the pain that is felt in the left arm, jaw, and shoulder that often occurs from the lack of oxygen to the heart muscle during a myocardial infarction. Figure 19-1 shows specific sites of referred pain. **Radiating pain** is pain that begins at a specific site and shoots out from or extends to a larger area beyond the site of origin.

Nociceptive Pain Versus Neuropathic Pain

Pain is derived in one of two ways:

1. From the stimulation of nerve pain receptors, called **nociceptors**
2. From damage to the nerves themselves

Nociceptors are randomly dispersed throughout the skin, subcutaneous tissue, and muscular tissue. These nerve pain receptors can be stimulated by temperature changes, tissue damage, and certain chemicals. Two of these chemicals that can stimulate the nerve pain receptors are substance P and prostaglandins, which are released during injury and damage to tissue. **Substance P** plays a role in eliciting localized tissue reactions similar to inflammation. **Prostaglandins** are hormones that act in the immediate area to initiate inflammation. Nonsteroidal anti-inflammatory drugs block the production of prostaglandins. The resulting pain is known as *nociceptive pain* and is generally localized within a specific area, from which the receptors send impulses to the central nervous system via afferent nerve pathways.

Neuropathic pain occurs due to injury or destruction of peripheral nerves or the central nervous system itself. This pain may extend beyond the local region to encompass a broadening area of discomfort that follows along the pathway of the damaged nerves.

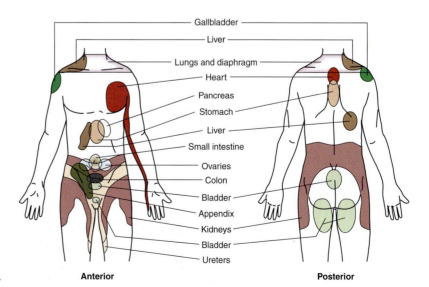

Figure 19-1 Sites of referred pain.

Anterior   **Posterior**

Nociceptive Pain

Nociceptive pain can be broken down into three different types:

1. **Cutaneous pain** is pain that is more superficial or pertaining to the skin's surface and underlying subcutaneous tissue. An example might be a paper cut or a mild burn.
2. **Visceral pain**, sometimes known as *soft tissue pain*, is the pain experienced from stimulation of deep internal pain receptors. Examples include pain that results from traumatic injury or surgery, or with metastatic invasion of the soft tissues such as the skin, muscles, and organs. It is generally described as an ache or a cramping-type pain, and can be intermittent or continuous.
3. **Deep somatic pain**, also known as *osteogenic pain*, is bone, ligament, tendon, and blood vessel pain. The pain may be diffuse and of longer duration than cutaneous pain. Bone cancer, fractures, and arthritic-type diseases are common sources of this type of pain. Your patient may describe it as pain with movement.

Neuropathic Pain

Neuropathic pain is the burning, stabbing or sometimes deep ache that your patient describes when there is nerve compression caused by pressure from tumors, lymphedema, or compression fractures of the spine. Nerve destruction can cause sharp, jagged, knife-like pain or even numbness. An example of this numbness is diabetic neuropathy. During the late stages of diabetes, a patient may develop total numbness of the feet that is extremely uncomfortable and dangerous for the patient.

One type of neuropathic pain is **phantom limb pain**, which feels as though it is coming from an extremity that has been *amputated,* meaning that is has been surgically or traumatically removed. A common example of phantom pain is the complaint of foot pain after the lower leg and foot have been surgically amputated.

Knowledge Connection

Differentiate between nociceptive pain and neuropathic pain. Describe three types of nociceptive pain.

Factors Affecting Pain

There are various factors that affect pain and its expression. They include the following:

- Ethnic and cultural beliefs
- Developmental stage
- Individual values
- Previous pain experiences
- Personal support system
- Emotions
- Fatigue

Ethnic and Cultural Beliefs

Certain cultures and ethnic groups view pain as something to be tolerated without overt expression. Individuals from northern Europe often feel that pain should be suffered in silence, as do some Native Americans and Asians. Older Irish individuals are known to be more tolerant of pain, while the younger generation finds it acceptable to complain of discomfort and to use medication for relief. The Saudi culture is similar to the Irish in the differences noted between older and newer generations; the older generation feels they must tolerate any discomfort so that they can fulfill their work duties. Jewish individuals are known to use facial expressions and gestures to express pain, but may not verbalize it. Most South Africans do not verbalize their pain. The women consider themselves stronger because they endure the pain of childbirth. Latino individuals may be comforted by moaning to express their pain or discomfort, though some feel that the men should endure pain without complaining, and that alleviating their pain would be demeaning. While it is important to consider the patient's cultural beliefs, you should never assume that a patient will react in the same manner as another patient of that particular ethnic group.

Developmental Stage

Infants and children experience the same levels of physiological pain, but are less able to express or articulate what they are feeling than adults. Infants usually respond with loud or shrill crying, changes in facial expression, waving their arms wildly, kicking their legs, and increases in pulse and respiratory rates. Older children may respond much like infants or may only whimper when experiencing pain. Their pain response may be affected by previous pain experiences. As children get older and have a better grasp of language, they are better able to verbalize pain or discomfort. Part of a child's expression of pain may directly relate to a lack of understanding of what is happening to him or her, anxiety, and fear.

Pain perception does not change with advancing age, nor is it natural for elderly individuals to have more pain simply because they are aging. When older adults suffer from multiple chronic and acute diseases, these individuals sometimes believe that they are expected to hurt more as they become more elderly. As a consequence, they may suffer in silence.

Individual Values and Previous Pain Experiences

Some individuals value stoicism. Some want to be independent and not rely on others to assist with their pain relief. Some individuals are simply very private regarding their personal feelings. Others may believe that being stoic about pain is illogical and unnecessary or may feel free to express their discomfort to anyone and everyone.

A patient may respond to pain based upon his or her previous pain experiences. No matter what your patient's values are, no matter what previous pain experiences there have been, it is your responsibility to educate the patient and ensure understanding regarding methods and availability of pain relief for that patient. To better understand your patient's pain, it is helpful to identify your own personal values regarding pain and to consider your previous pain experiences. How did you respond when in pain? What are your values regarding pain?

Personal Support System

Individuals who do not have a personal support system of family or friends may cope with pain differently than those who can depend upon the support and assistance of a spouse, loved ones, or close friends. This is especially true for children, who generally do better if a parent remains with the child at all times. Even though the patient has a personal support system, if those individuals are absent or are far away, the patient may experience more discomfort along with a sense of loneliness. Or the patient may simply find the pain experience to be more stressful without someone close by.

Emotions

All emotions affect the level and tolerance of pain and discomfort. Unpleasant emotions such as anxiety, stress, loneliness, and fear generally increase perception of pain, or decrease the patient's tolerance of pain. Conversely, positive emotions such as joy, happiness, and love, are more apt to decrease the perception of pain or render the patient more tolerant of the pain.

Fatigue

Patients who are not resting well or are fatigued will usually have an increased perception of pain as well as a lower capacity to cope with the pain. When patients experience continual pain, they relate that it worsens in the evening and night unless they rest or nap during the day.

Responses to Pain

The body responds to pain physiologically, psychologically, and behaviorally. Initially pain stimulates the sympathetic nervous system, which initiates the fight-or-flight response. A patient's pulse, respiratory rate, and blood pressure may rise. The pupils dilate, as do the cerebral blood vessels, delivering more blood to the brain to increase awareness. If the pain continues for days or weeks, the body begins to adapt to the pain, allowing the parasympathetic nervous system to reverse many of the sympathetic system responses, returning vital signs, pupils, and cerebral blood vessels back to normal. Thus, there are signs and symptoms that may be noted in acute pain that are not seen in chronic pain. Table 19-1 presents signs and symptoms of acute and chronic pain.

Knowledge Connection

Describe five factors and how they affect pain perception and pain relief. Compare the signs and symptoms of acute pain to those of chronic pain.

Management and Treatment of Pain

Before pain can be effectively treated, you must acquire as much information about the pain as possible, known as a pain assessment. It is important to know a number of things about the complaint of pain, including:

• **Level or extent of the pain:** Consistently use the same pain scale, such as a scale from 0 to 10, with 0 being none and 10 being the worst pain the patient can imagine.

Table 19-1 Signs and Symptoms of Pain

	Physiological Signs	Behavioral Signs	Psychological Signs
Acute	Recent onset Diminishes with healing **Fight/flight response:** 　Heart rate increases 　Respirations increase 　Systolic blood pressure 　increases 　Pupils dilate **As it worsens:** 　Diaphoresis 　Blood pressure drops 　Syncope 　Pupils constrict	Wincing or facial grimacing Moaning or crying Restlessness, such as nervous finger tapping or foot bouncing Rigid body posture Slow movement Holding or guarding the area Worsens during anxiety/fear Rocking or pacing	Reduced attention span Focused only on pain Anger Fear or anxiety Irritability
Chronic	Onset longer than 6 months ago Few or none Pupils may constrict Vital signs may not change	Lassitude Impaired mobility/activity Sleep disturbance Withdrawal from family and friends	Low self-esteem Depression Fatigue Anger Irritability

- **Site of pain:** Be specific—for example, not just the abdomen, but which quadrant. Not just the back, but whether it is right, left, or midline; and whether it is in the cervical, thoracic, lumbar, or sacral area of the back. Not just the leg, but whether it is right or left; in the foot, ankle, calf, thigh, or groin; and anterior, lateral, or posterior.
- **Characteristics of the pain:** Is it sharp, dull, intermittent, constant, burning, cramping, stinging, aching, or pressure-like? Does it feel like a vice grip, knife-like, pulling, tension or tightness, or spasmodic?
- **Whether the pain is acute or chronic:** When did it begin?
- **What elicits the pain:** Does eating, deep breathing, palpation, coughing, sneezing, repositioning, movement, or activity bring about the pain?
- **Patient's desires in relation to the pain:** This includes whether the patient wants medication or prefers nonpharmacological methods of pain relief.

The use of a pain scale for assessment of pain was covered in Chapter 17.

Acknowledgment and Acceptance

The first step in assisting your patient to obtain maximum pain relief is that of letting the patient know that you believe that he or she is in pain. Remember that the patient is the *expert* about whether or not he or she is suffering, not the health care provider. You should be the expert in relieving the pain, not interpreting whether or not the patient is really hurting. Listen to how the patient describes the discomfort and verbally acknowledge that you understand that he or she is hurting. After obtaining a complete description of the patient's pain, be quick to respond with relief measures. Explain to the patient your intent; let the patient know what you are going to do to effect pain relief for him or her. If it is too soon for medication, be certain to offer other methods of relief and distraction. Never tell the patient that it is too soon for more medication and leave needs unmet. There is always something that you can do to help reduce discomfort.

Nonpharmaceutical Methods

There are numerous ways to decrease pain or the perception of pain. The Agency for Healthcare Research and Quality (AHRQ) has printed guidelines encouraging health care providers to incorporate nonpharmaceutical methods of pain relief in situations that are appropriate, such as lower levels of discomfort in which the patient desires to avoid use of medication. When the pain is beyond mild levels, these nonpharmaceutical methods should serve as an adjuvant along with pharmacological therapies. **Adjuvant** means to assist or aid another treatment, therefore increasing the effectiveness.

Hot and Cold Packs

Both heat and cold therapy are especially good sources of relief for musculoskeletal pain and discomfort. More information regarding the use and effects of hot and cold packs is included in Chapter 18.

Massage and Effleurage

Cutaneous relief measures such as massage and effleurage are simple to provide, but can be extremely effective in some painful conditions. **Effleurage** is the repetitive gentle, gliding stroking of your fingertips over the surface of the skin. This technique is particularly effective during back massage to relax muscles or on the head to reduce tension headaches. You can use both hands to stroke two side-by-side circles over the abdomen of a woman in labor to decrease her discomfort from contractions. Firmer massage of muscles is often helpful to reduce limb, neck, and back pain. The method of relief is thought to stimulate the *closing of the gate* and production of endorphins that you read about earlier in this chapter.

Transcutaneous Electrical Nerve Stimulation

A TENS unit is a battery-powered device, about the size of a small pager, with lead wires and electrode pads, which you apply to the skin over the painful area (Fig. 19-2). The device delivers electrical stimulation to the large-diameter nerve fibers, which is thought to work similarly to massage, by closing the gate and stimulating the production of endorphins. The frequency and strength of impulse delivery is controlled by gradually increasing the dials on the TENS unit to a level at which the impulses are described as "gentle tapping" by the patient. The impulses should not be strong enough to feel like an irritant or produce discomfort. Skill 19-1 (page 403) provides instructions regarding application of a TENS unit.

Acupressure and Acupuncture

Acupressure involves applying fingertip pressure, and acupuncture is the insertion of ultrafine needles into specific body areas; both are thought to stimulate endorphin production. Further explanation is found in Chapter 11.

Relaxation

Helping a patient relax can be done in a number of ways, two of which we will explain here: progressive relaxation

Figure 19-2 A TENS unit.

and guided imagery. *Progressive relaxation* is a systematic process of using the mind to actually relax the patient's muscles from the top of the head to the toes. By focusing the patient's conscious mind on the tightening and relaxing of muscles, it interferes with perception of pain impulses, and the physiological reaction of muscle relaxation can directly relieve some types of pain. The patient lays in bed in the most comfortable position he or she can find with the eyes closed. You verbally direct the patient to focus on specific muscles, first tensing and then relaxing them, beginning at the head and progressing to the toes (Box 19-1). There are also many commercial tapes and compact disks that can be purchased and utilized for progressive relaxation.

Guided imagery is another method of using the mind to help control the body and guide the patient toward a more relaxed state. This process can help the patient feel more in control of emotions and thought processes, and provide relief of discomfort and induction of rest or sleep. Guided imagery can be done verbally or by use of tapes or compact disks. Using verbal suggestions, you direct the patient's thoughts to a place that is pictured as comfortable, calming, relaxing, and perfect. By asking the patient to use several of his or her senses, the body seems to respond as though what is imagined is real. A picturesque location, such as a beach, garden, mountaintop, or forest, is described in great detail as the patient lies quietly with the eyes closed. The patient is asked to visualize the specified place and to feel all the comforts of this place as you describe them in a soft, quiet, melodious voice (Box 19-2).

Distraction

Some patients will respond to distraction, others will not. If distraction works, it helps to take the mind off the pain and focus on something else. This simply decreases the conscious awareness of the pain. It should not be used as the sole method of pain relief, but is a good aid to **analgesics** (pain medications). Distraction is at work when a patient is talking and laughing with visitors, but asks for pain medication only a few minutes after the visitors leave. It can be accomplished through use of different senses as well as the cognitive mind, including:

- **Visual distraction:** watching television or reading a good book
- **Auditory distraction:** listening to music or someone reading aloud; an infant will often respond to soft whispering or singing close to his or her ear while being held or rocked
- **Tactile distraction:** receiving a back rub, having the hair brushed, rocking, receiving hugs, holding a pet, playing with a toy, taking a warm bath; an infant may respond to being patted or effleurage on the cheek or back of the neck, around the ear, or on the back
- **Intellectual distraction:** conversing with another individual; working; doing sudoku, crossword, or other types of puzzles; playing card games

Knowledge Connection

Who is the expert on the pain level the patient is experiencing? What characteristics should you assess during pain assessment? Discuss at least four methods of nonpharmacological pain relief.

Pharmaceutical Methods

There are various classifications of medications that are effective against pain, including nonsteroidal anti-inflammatory drugs (NSAIDs), non-opioids, opioid narcotics, and adjuvant drugs. These medications can be used alone or in conjunction with nonpharmaceutical methods of pain relief.

Non-Opioid Analgesics

Non-opioids are non-narcotic pain relievers used for mild to moderate pain. Acetaminophen is one of the most common, is available over the counter, and is used alone as well as in combination with other drugs such as codeine or hydrocodone for more severe pain. Besides having analgesic effects,

---

Box 19-1

Progressive Relaxation

Instruct the patient to find a comfortable position, dim the lights, close the door, and reduce as much noise and distraction as possible. Verbally guide the patient, using a quiet voice, in the following steps, beginning at the top of the head:

- Take a deep breath, breathing in slowly through your nose. Feel your chest and stomach rise until they can't rise any further. Exhale slowly through your mouth. Feel your chest and stomach relax. (Repeat the deep breath two or three times.)
- Focus on the top of your head. Feel the tightness of the skin and muscles. Contract those muscles. Feel how tight they are.
- Now, relax the top of your head. Feel all the tightness and tension drain away. Feel it leaving your body as you exhale. Let the top of your head just go limp. Feel it totally relaxed and limp. Feel any discomfort leave your body as you breathe out. Doesn't it feel good to relax?

Continue to use this same phrasing on the successive parts of the body as you progress to the toes. Include the following body parts:

Forehead	Tongue	Shoulders	Hips	Calves
Eyes	Chin	Chest & back	Pelvis	Ankles
Cheeks	Neck	Stomach	Thighs	Feet & toes

Most patients are either asleep or very relaxed by the time you reach the toes. This is particularly effective for anxious or stressed patients, those who cannot seem to fall asleep, and those who are in pain. It takes a few minutes of your time, but your patients will benefit from it, thus making it very rewarding for you.

Box 19-2
Guided Imagery

The following is an example of a scenario to use for guided imagery:

Close your eyes and take a deep, deep breath. As you exhale, feel all your stresses and discomforts leave your body. Picture in your mind a beautiful white sandy beach, close to the ocean, with lots of palm trees. You are lying comfortably in a hammock made of the softest silk fabric that you have ever felt. Feel its silkiness, its soothing caress on your skin. Feel how it supports your body. Let your body relax against the silk. Let it support you in complete and utter comfort. See the soft, puffy, white clouds as they drift lazily overhead. Watch their shapes as they change from one shape to another. Feel the warmth of the sun on your face, on your arms. It is just the perfect temperature, with the cool tropical breeze that blows gently across your skin. It's such a peaceful place. Breathe in the fresh tropical air and smell the ocean. Hear the waves as they lap onto shore and then trickle back to the sea. Listen as the birds echo their sweet calls, each a little different, soothing in their own ways. Hear the palm leaves rustle in the breeze. Smell the tropical flowers and see their vibrant colors. What a perfect place to be, a place where you can rest.

acetaminophen also has *antipyretic* (fever-reducing) effects. The maximum dosage allowed in adults is 4 grams, or 4,000 milligrams, every 24 hours. Even though it is an over-the-counter drug, acetaminophen can cause *hepatotoxicity* (damage to the liver) and death.

Real-World Connection

Over-the-Counter Pain Relief Carries Risks

A 19-year-old female was brought into the emergency room unresponsive and died a short time later from liver failure, secondary to acetaminophen overdose. She had been having recurring headaches for several weeks and taking acetaminophen around the clock in an effort to obtain relief. She thought that, since it was a common, over-the-counter drug, one that you could "even give to infants," it was harmless. She failed to follow the dose limits printed on the label and it ended tragically in the loss of her life.

Nonsteroidal Anti-inflammatory Drugs

NSAIDs are a medication class that helps to reduce inflammation and pain by preventing the release of inflammatory mediators, such as histamine, serotonin, prostaglandins, and leukotrienes, at the site of injury or inflammation. NSAIDs are useful in relieving cutaneous pain, visceral pain, and deep somatic pain. The most common over-the-counter drugs in this class are ibuprofen, naproxen, and aspirin, all of which have anti-inflammatory, analgesic, and antipyretic effects. Aspirin also has *antiplatelet* effects, which means that it decreases platelet clumping, which is the first step in clotting. Aspirin is commonly used for its antiplatelet effects to reduce risk of clotting in patients who might be prone to heart attacks or strokes, such as a patient with an elevated cholesterol level or hypertension. The dosage of aspirin is reduced from that used for analgesic, antipyretic, and anti-inflammatory purposes, which is 600 to 1,000 milligrams several times a day, to a mere 81 to 300 milligrams once daily. Because these drugs can cause severe gastric irritation and bleeding, they should be administered with food.

Opiate/Opioid Analgesics (Narcotics)

When non-opioid medications are ineffective in relieving moderate to severe pain, opiates or opioids may be needed. They are usually effective in relieving visceral pain and deep somatic pain. These analgesics work by binding with opiate receptors and stimulating the brain's production of enkephalin and beta-endorphin, compounds that decrease pain perception. They come from opium and its derivatives, known as opiates; and also in synthetic forms, known as opioids. They are **controlled substances** and therefore require a prescription to obtain them. All controlled, or *scheduled*, drugs have greater capacity for addiction and abuse and are regulated by federal law. Meperidine, codeine, dilaudid, morphine, and fentanyl are some of the more common drugs used in this class. Please note that meperidine use should be avoided in patients older than 65 years of age and in those patients with renal function impairment, due to production of normeperidine, a metabolite that can cause adverse side effects by irritating the cerebrum. Cerebral irritation can range from minor mood alterations to seizures in patients who do not have adequate kidney function to remove the products of drug breakdown.

Opiates and opioids can be administered by the oral, rectal, and transcutaneous routes, and they are also used extensively via the intramuscular (IM) and intravenous (IV) routes for intense pain. Along with pain relief, they may cause side effects of nausea, vomiting, constipation, itching, sedation, and even respiratory depression and pupil constriction in higher dosages. If a patient becomes only minimally responsive, administer the antagonist naloxone (Narcan) to counteract the opiate/opioid effects.

These drugs may be administered, within preset boundaries, by the patient, who controls the frequency and administration of his or her pain medication, a process known as **patient-controlled analgesia (PCA)**. It uses a computerized IV infusion device consisting of a pump, a large syringe containing the analgesic, IV tubing, and a push button the patient presses for delivery of analgesic (Fig. 19-3). The physician orders the maximum dosage and the intervals at which the drug may be administered, and the nurse or pharmacist calibrates the PCA pump accordingly. Initially, the nurse administers a larger dose known as the loading dose, or *bolus*, which provides an optimum blood level to get the pain under control. Then the patient pushes the hand-controlled button whenever he or she feels additional pain relief is needed. The preset dose limits and intervals (lockout times) prevent the patient from overdosing. The PCA offers the patient a sense of control over his or her own medication and provides more consistent pain relief with less medication. Box 19-3 lists additional advantages of PCA.

Figure 19-3 A woman pushes the button on her PCA pump to deliver pain medication.

Box 19-3

Advantages of Patient-Controlled Analgesia

There are numerous advantages of using patient-controlled analgesia, and it is helpful to explain these benefits to the patient and patient's family. Proper explanation will generally improve compliance as well as understanding, which are both necessary to achieve optimal benefits of this type of pain control.

- Provides patient with control over pain relief
- Reduces waiting for nurse response
- Avoids repeated injections
- Provides rapid relief via IV route
- Reduces anxiety and fear that pain will get out of control
- Allows for more frequent and evenly controlled pain relief
- Allows for smaller dosing, ultimately resulting in use of less medication
- Enables patient to achieve more comfortable ambulation over a continuum of time, therefore reducing complications of immobility

Adjuvant Analgesics
Adjuvant analgesics are classes of medication that produce pain relief either through a mechanism different than traditional analgesics or by potentiating or increasing the effects of opiates, opioids, and non-opioid drugs. Two examples are anticonvulsants and antidepressants. A blood level of anticonvulsants and antidepressants must be reached and maintained before pain relief will be noticed, generally taking 2 to 3 weeks. Anticonvulsants such as gabapentin and carbamazepine, and antidepressants such as amitriptyline, are used to treat nerve pain, a complication found in diabetics.

Skeletal muscle relaxants, benzodiazepines, and caffeine are helpful in relieving pain due to muscle spasms. Antispasmodics or anticholinergics are used to treat pain from intestinal colic.

Knowledge Connection

Compare the different ways NSAIDs, non-opioids, and narcotic opiates/opioids work to effect pain relief. List three categories of adjuvant medications that are sometimes used in pain relief. Explain what *controlled* or *scheduled drug* means. What are the benefits of using PCA?

Rest and Restorative Sleep

Rest and restorative sleep are not only necessary for pain relief and comfort, but are imperative for good physiological, psychological, and emotional health. **Restorative sleep** is that which allows an individual to awaken feeling rested, refreshed, rejuvenated, and energized, ready to meet new challenges. *Resting* may or may not involve sleep. It is any time that an individual feels relaxed and free from anxiety, such as when visiting with a loved one he or she has not seen in a long time, laughing during a funny movie, reading a good book, or napping. When napping, one is disturbed by external noises and awakens easily, but during restorative sleep the individual experiences a partial loss of consciousness and is more difficult to arouse. During restorative sleep, external noises may be incorporated into dreams that will not cause the individual to awaken.

What Happens During Restorative Sleep?

It is impossible to maintain good health without adequate restorative sleep, for this is when the brain works to repair the small injuries to the body, mind, and emotions that occur as part of the natural wear and tear of daily living, including such things as cellular repair and synthesis of protein. Of course, during illness and trauma there is much more damage that must heal before the body can be restored to optimum health. Without adequate rest and restorative sleep:

- Healing is slow and incomplete
- Immunity decreases
- Pain tolerance decreases
- Fragile emotions and impatience affect relationships
- Cognitive functions are impaired, making concentration difficult, resulting in poor decision making
- Work performance suffers
- Accidents increase dramatically

The brain also uses sleep time to *sort out* all the data that were received by the senses while awake, determining which information is important to keep and which is unimportant and can be purged. The trivial things such as hearing a car horn honk or smelling the aroma of dinner as you cooked are probably forgotten. If the brain identifies new information as useful, it will then not only process and store the new data, but will also associate it with previously acquired and stored knowledge. This allows the individual to learn more and better apply the new data in different ways. This explains a mind and body mechanism that you have probably experienced: worrying about a problem but finding yourself unable to decide what to do about it. So, rather than continue to fight with yourself over the matter, you decide to go to bed and worry about it tomorrow. The next morning when you awaken, the solution to the problem just comes to you. This occurs because the central nervous system (CNS) was sorting and processing all the data perceived yesterday while you slept.

Sleep Cycle

The body has a 24-hour cyclical pattern known as the **circadian rhythm**, during which body metabolism and functions increase and decrease in rhythmic patterns. For example, body temperature is usually lowest in the predawn hours and highest in the late evening hours, which is why children tend to spike fevers more in the evening and early nighttime hours, after the physician's office has closed.

Sleep is cyclical and alternates with longer periods of wakefulness. Two sleep cycles have been identified: *non–rapid eye movement sleep*, known as NREM sleep, and *rapid eye movement sleep*, known as REM sleep. NREM sleep involves four stages and is considered the deepest and most restful sleep cycle (Table 19-2). It makes up approximately 60% of an infant's sleep time and 80% of an adult's.

These sleep cycles are repeated several times a night, depending upon the length of time spent in sleep. Antianxiety and sleep-promoting medications can interfere with REM sleep, preventing the individual from feeling "rested" even after having slept several hours.

Knowledge Connection

Compare rest with restorative sleep. What are the CNS functions that occur during sleep? Differentiate between REM and NREM sleep.

Amount of Sleep Required

The body requires different amounts of sleep, dependent upon age, health, and fatigue level. The average number of hours of sleep required in healthy individuals is:

- **Newborns:** 16 to 18 hours per day
- **Infants up to 2 years:** 12 to 14 hours per day, including naps
- **Children 3 to 6 years:** 12 hours per day, including naps
- **Children 7 to 12:** 10 hours per night
- **Adolescents:** 8.5 to 9.5 hours per night
- **Young adults:** 7.5 to 8 hours per night
- **Older adults:** gradually decreases to 5.5 or 6 hours per night, may begin to nap

Societal pressures to earn more money and participate in extracurricular activities tend to lead us to think we must

Table 19-2   Stages of REM and NREM Sleep

NREM Sleep	
Stage I	Relaxation begins during this stage, as metabolism and vital signs begin to slow. The lightest sleep occurs, lasting only a few minutes. The individual is easily aroused and, if awakened, feels as if he or she has been daydreaming.
Stage II	Relaxation deepens as metabolism continues to slow. The individual begins to experience sound sleep, but arousal is still relatively easy. This stage lasts 10 to 20 minutes.
Stage III	Stage III lasts 15 to 30 minutes. Deep sleep begins as muscles are now completely relaxed. The parasympathetic nervous system slows vital signs further and the body becomes immobile. Arousal is more difficult.
Stage IV	It becomes very difficult to arouse the person during this deepest sleep that lasts 15 to 30 minutes. If he or she is sleep deprived, more time will be spent here. The body rests and is restored during this deep sleep. Even though the eyes are still, dreaming may occur during this stage.

REM Sleep
REM sleep occurs at end of each NREM cycle. The first cycle occurs about 90 minutes after sleep begins. Rapid eye movement begins and vital signs fluctuate. The brain is very active, and engaged in vivid dreaming that may be remembered after awakening occurs. The duration increases with each cycle, averaging 20 minutes. REM sleep is not as restful as NREM sleep.

work longer hours and be doing something all the time, interfering with sleep and rest requirements of children and adults alike. Studies show that most Americans do not get enough sleep and complain that they feel sleepy during the day. These studies also show that automobile accidents and on-the-job injuries increase dramatically in sleep-deprived people. Statistics indicate that nursing errors increase during the last 4 hours of 12-hour shifts. Because of this, it behooves you to evaluate your sleep and work habits. How much sleep is optimum for you? Do you get adequate sleep so that you do not feel sleepy the next day?

Knowledge Connection

How much sleep does a newborn require? A school-age child? A young adult?

Patient Teaching Connection

We Need to Educate Parents About Sleep

It is important that you educate parents regarding sleep requirements of infants and children in an effort to promote better health and increase learning abilities of school-age children. Teach parents to establish a time for going to bed and to be consistent in its enforcement. This sometimes requires limiting a child's participation in extracurricular activities to only one or two per week. Explain that certain bedtime rituals are helpful in gaining cooperation from the child; these rituals may include:

• Giving a warm bath at a set time
• Brushing the child's hair or applying lotion to the child's skin
• Giving each family member good-night kisses
• Allowing the child to select a stuffed animal or doll to sleep with
• Reading a bedtime story or Bible verse to the child
• Saying a bedtime prayer

Use of such rituals helps establish more regular sleep habits for children. Teach parents that use of night-lights may be helpful to allay fears of the dark.

Factors Affecting Rest and Restorative Sleep

There are many factors that affect the body's ability to rest and obtain the restorative sleep that it needs. The factors may be physiological, emotional, or environmental. Chronic sleep deprivation can result in fatigue, irritability, slow response time, blurred vision, headaches, forgetfulness, and confusion.

Lifestyle

Components of a lifestyle that many view as normal may have detrimental effects on rest and sleep. Caffeine, nicotine, alcohol, and sleep-inducing medications all can impair the body's ability to get adequate sleep. Caffeine and nicotine interfere with initiation of sleep, whereas alcohol causes awakening during the night. Individuals who work the night shift often have difficulty getting enough sleep during the day. Exercise is conducive to sleep when performed early in

the day, but if performed within 1 to 2 hours of bedtime, inhibits sleep in most people. Individuals who work in high-stress jobs often complain of continual problems sleeping.

Stress and Anxiety

All humans experience stress and anxiety and often take those stresses and worries to bed with them at night. Stress can prevent one from falling asleep and cause one to awaken during the night.

Environmental

Environmental temperatures that are too warm or cold, hospital noises and bright lights, waking the patient for nursing care, and other hospital routines interfere with a patient's ability to sleep. An uncomfortable hospital bed can also play havoc with a patient's comfort and sleep. Patients in intensive care units commonly complain of interruption of sleep due to noise produced by hospital staff, other patients, and equipment, such as bright lights, beeping sounds, alarms, telephones, and pagers.

Illness and Health Problems

Individuals who have health problems, illnesses, or injuries may suffer symptoms that interfere with their sleep, including:

• Pain or discomfort
• Shortness of breath or dyspnea
• Itching
• Reflux of gastric contents into throat
• Sinus drainage, congestion, or coughing
• Fever or diaphoresis
• Frequent elimination

Sleep Disorders

Various sleep disorders also interfere with the body's ability to obtain adequate restorative sleep (Table 19-3). The effects of these disorders range from annoying to life threatening.

Interventions to Promote Restorative Sleep

Promotion of sleep is an important nursing function that is sometimes overlooked. Most interventions are easy and simple to perform and produce increased comfort, cleanliness, and relaxation. They can also assist normal body functions and make the environment more conducive to sleep.

Prepare the Environment

Prepare the patient's room by modifying the room temperature to the patient's preference. Some individuals prefer a slightly cooler temperature for sleeping; others may have difficulty staying warm at night and want the temperature set a bit warmer. Provide blankets and pillows as desired by the patient. Clear the pathway from the door to the bed and from the bed to the bathroom. Turn on a night-light or provide dim lighting, enough for safety and orientation in the unfamiliar environment, but not enough to disturb sleep. Close the room door to increase noise reduction.

Table 19-3   **Sleep Disorders**

Disorder	Description
Bruxism	Grinding of teeth during sleep.
Insomnia	Chronic inability to fall asleep or stay asleep.
Narcolepsy	Condition causing uncontrollable, recurrent daytime episodes of sleepiness; can hinder driving and operating dangerous equipment.
Night terrors	Nightmares in children that cause awakening and fear.
Restless legs syndrome	An intolerable crawling sensation in the legs that results in an irresistible urge to move the legs.
Sleep apnea	Inability to maintain breathing while sleeping. The patient usually snores, accompanied by periods of apnea lasting from 10 seconds to 2 minutes. Can be life threatening.
Somnambulism	Sleepwalking; has the potential for serious consequences.
Sundowning	Confusion and disorientation in elderly patients that occurs in the evening hours. The patient is at higher risk for injury.

Comfort

To provide comfort at bedtime, begin by washing the patient's face and hands, detangling and brushing the hair, brushing the teeth, and moistening the lips with petroleum jelly, if needed. Offer a snack if hungry, and offer fresh water or cold or warm milk if preferred. Assist the patient with toileting as needed. Assess to determine if the patient has any pain or discomforts that require medication. Straighten and remove wrinkles in gown and bed linens, reposition the patient, and provide support with pillows.

Relaxation

One of the easiest ways to help a patient relax is by administering a back massage. Another intervention that helps to relax the patient is providing range-of-motion exercises, which stretch the muscles and stimulate the circulation. Playing soft, relaxing music is a good source of relaxation for some patients, while other individuals prefer meditation to initiate the relaxation process. Ask about the patient's concerns. Sometimes a patient needs validation of his or her feelings or needs to vent frustration or worries. Learn to be an active listener. Often 5 minutes spent listening and expressing empathy is all it takes to help a patient begin to relax.

Pain Relief

Pain must also be relieved in order for a patient to sleep soundly and deeply. If analgesics are required, they should be administered. There is a common myth perpetuated by some nurses: "The patient could not be hurting too badly. He complained of pain but was asleep when I got there with his pain medication. So I didn't give it to him." It is totally possible for some patients to sleep even though they are in pain. Sleep is sometimes exactly what the body needs to heal. Remember that much repair and healing takes place during sleep. The residual effects of general anesthesia can affect the level of consciousness of a patient for 24 to 48 hours. If a patient is drowsy or falls asleep after requesting pain medication, do not ignore his or her request for pain relief. Treat the pain.

Sleep Medications

Some patients just cannot sleep when hospitalized, no matter what interventions you try. Most physicians will order sleep medication that may be used on an as-needed basis. They are effective for short-term use, but interfere with sleep with chronic use. It is always better for the patient if you can promote sleep without medications that can interfere with REM sleep.

Supervision/Delegation Connection

Delegation of Tasks Does Not Relieve You of Your Responsibilities

Delegation of most of the nonpharmaceutical interventions to CNAs and UAPs is common and acceptable. However, it is important that you perform assessments as needed to determine the patient's usual sleep habits and to identify what problems may be preventing the patient from sleeping. It is also your responsibility to work with the patient and other staff members to determine which nonpharmaceutical interventions would be most appropriate.

Skill 19-1 Application of TENS Unit

Assessment Steps

1. Review the physician's order for site of application, settings for the TENS unit, and length of treatment. *This reduces the risk of administering incorrect treatment.*

2. Assess the patient's knowledge level regarding a TENS unit. *This determines patient learning needs.*

Planning Steps

1. Gather needed equipment and supplies: TENS unit, battery, lead wires, electrodes, conduction gel if the electrodes are not precoated, tape if the electrodes are not self-adhesive. *Preparation saves time and effort.*

2. Assess the patient's level of pain or discomfort using a scale of 0 to 10. *Using the same pain scale each time allows for more consistent pain measurement.*

Implementation Steps

1. Follow the Initial Implementation Steps located on the inside front cover.

2. Insert battery and lead wires into the TENS unit, making certain the unit is turned off *to avoid premature delivery of electrical impulses.*

3. Safety: *Apply conductive gel to electrodes if not precoated, to assure conduction and avoid shocks due to noncontinuous conduction.*

4. Secure the electrodes to their designated sites. If necessary, use tape to hold the electrodes in place.

5. Turn on the TENS unit. Instruct the patient to inform you as soon as he or she can feel the tingling sensation.

6. Gradually increase the amplitude according to the patient's response. Inform the patient that he should tell you when it feels like a gentle tapping. The electrical impulses should be well within the patient's comfort range. Caution the patient to avoid trying

to "tolerate it at higher, more uncomfortable amplitudes." *Discomfort prevents complete relaxation and tightens muscles, which increases pain.*

7. Assess the patient's comfort level every 15 minutes during the first hour of use. If the physician's order states to leave the TENS unit on longer than 1 hour, continue to assess comfort level every 1 to 2 hours. *This helps to assess the effectiveness of the treatment.*

8. At the designated time, turn the unit off before removing the electrodes. *Removing them while the unit is still on can result in shocks from current, which are uncomfortable.*

9. Remove adhesive electrodes and wipe the patient's skin to remove gel.

10. Follow the Ending Implementation Steps located on the inside back cover.

Evaluation Steps

1. Assess how the patient tolerated the treatment, along with the level of discomfort according to the 0 to 10 scale.

Sample Documentation

4/22/09   3:30 p.m.   States Rt. & Lt. lumbar area is tight and hurting, a 6 on a scale of 0 to 10. TENS unit applied to left and right lumbar area, pulse mode, and amplitude. ——————
———————————————————— Nurse's signature and credentials

4:30 p.m.   TENS unit removed. States lumbar pain is now 2 on 0-to-10 scale. ——————— Nurse's signature and credentials

---

 Post Conference

Other students were aware that your patient was angry and that his wife left in tears. They ask if the patient was difficult for you. You explain that your patient was experiencing phantom pain that he would not describe because he thought it was impossible to feel pain in his amputated foot. Your evaluation of your clinical day is very positive. It felt good to relieve his fears by explaining phantom pain to him. Several interventions helped him relax, especially the back massage. After medicating him with an ordered opiate for pain, he slept soundly for 3 hours and woke up refreshed. He was much more pleasant and wanted to call his wife to apologize.

KEY POINTS

- Pain is a warning sign that something is wrong or that tissue damage has occurred or is about to occur.
- Pain is always what the patient says it is. The patient is the expert on his or her pain.
- Pain can affect numerous aspects of a patient's life, including activities of daily living, sleep, nutrition, activity level, family relationships, job performance, social life, cognitive abilities, and spiritual beliefs.
- Pain is classified as either nociceptive or neuropathic pain.
- Factors that affect pain are ethnic and cultural beliefs, developmental stage, individual values, previous pain experiences, personal support system, emotions, and fatigue.
- The body responds to pain physiologically, psychologically, and behaviorally.
- Management and treatment of pain may include acknowledgment and acceptance, hot and cold packs, massage, TENS unit, acupressure and acupuncture, relaxation, distraction, non-opioid analgesics, NSAIDs, opiate/opioid analgesics, and adjuvant analgesics.
- Rest and restorative sleep are necessary for pain relief, comfort, and physiological, psychological, and emotional health.
- Sleep cycles include both REM and NREM sleep.
- The average adult requires 7.5 to 8 hours of sleep per night.
- Factors that affect rest and restorative sleep include lifestyle, stress level, environmental factors, illness, and sleep disorders.
- Interventions that promote sleep include preparing the environment, providing comfort, relaxation, active listening to patient concerns, and medications as needed.

REVIEW QUESTIONS

Select the answer that is most appropriate for each of the following questions. Some questions may have more than one correct answer. Check all that apply.

1. Pain can indicate which of the following?

   a. Damage has occurred to tissue.

   b. Edema is increasing and placing pressure on nerve endings.

   c. The wound is healing normally.

   d. Circulation to the site is adequate.

   e. There is a potential for damage to the tissues.

2. Which of the following individuals is the expert regarding the amount of pain Brad Monett is experiencing?

   a. The nurse

   b. The physician

   c. Brad

   d. The pain clinic representative

   e. All of the above

3. Christy Leigh is complaining of burning, searing pain along the lateral aspect of her left foot. When you assess Christy's foot, you see no wounds or abnormalities. She tells you that she has not injured the foot but has been having this pain intermittently for approximately 1 month. Upon reviewing her chart, you read that Christy has severe diabetes. Which type pain do you think Christy is having?

   a. Neuropathic pain

   b. Cutaneous pain

   c. Visceral pain

   d. Nociceptive pain

4. Alex Ganner has pancreatic cancer in the advanced stages and has been at home. He has been attempting to get relief of severe abdominal pain with prescription opioids for 6 days, but the pain is not responding. He finally agrees to be admitted for treatment of pain. Which type pain is Mr. Ganner experiencing?

   a. Cutaneous pain

   b. Neuropathic pain

   c. Chronic pain

   d. Intractable pain

   e. Referred pain

FILL-IN-THE-BLANK QUESTIONS

5. Captain Julius James, a veteran of the Vietnam War, lost his right foot in combat. He is hospitalized with pneumonia and you are assigned to admit and care for him during your shift. While interviewing Captain James, he tells you that he has right foot pain a lot in the evenings. You would document this as _____ pain in the admission assessment.

6. You are administering medications to Ruth Smith, who has severe arthritis in most of the joints of her hands and lower extremities, causing her significant joint and muscle pain. Her medication administration record shows that she is to receive 800 milligrams of ibuprofen three times per day for this pain. You know that ibuprofen is not a narcotic and is classified as a(n) _____ _____ due to its anti-inflammatory effects.

SHORT ANSWER QUESTIONS

7. List at least five factors that affect an individual's pain perception.

8. Explain the functions of the brain during restorative sleep.

9. Compare NREM and REM sleep cycles.

CRITICAL THINKING EXERCISE

10. It is 1:00 a.m. and one of the elderly patients on your unit is unable to sleep tonight. He tells you that he is worried about his cat at home. He knows his neighbor is feeding the cat each day, but he is concerned that the cat is lonesome without him. You know that the patient needs restorative sleep to help him recover from a urinary tract infection. What interventions might you try to help him get some rest?

ADDITIONAL RESOURCES

For additional Resources, Questions, and Activities, please see:

 Student Resource Disk

 http://davisplus.fadavis.com

 Student Study Guide

REFERENCES

D'Arcy Y. Are opioids safe for your patient? *Nursing2009.* 2009;39(4):40-44.

D'Arcy Y. Controlling Pain: Pain management by the numbers: using rating scales effectively. *Nursing2007.* 2007;37(11):14-15.

D'Arcy Y. Managing the Pain: Assessing pain with pain-rating scales. *LPN2007.* 2007;3(6):13-18.

D'Arcy Y. Managing the Pain: Getting a grip on neuropathic pain. *LPN2008.* 2008;4(2):14-19.

Dillon PM. *Nursing Health Assessment—A Critical Thinking Case Studies Approach.* Philadelphia: FA Davis; 2007.

Flaherty E. How to try this: using pain-rating scales with older adults. *Am J Nurs.* 2008;108(6):40-47.

Horgas A, Miller L. Pain assessment in people with dementia. *Am J Nurs.* 2008;108(7):62-70.

Managing the Pain: Assessing and managing pain in the pediatric patient. *LPN2009.* 2009;5(1):9-13.

Menefee LA, Monti DA. Nonpharmacologic and complementary approaches to cancer pain management. *J Am Osteopath Assoc.* 2005;105(Suppl): S15-S20.

Pack AI, Maislin G, Staley B, Pack FM, Rogers WC, George CF, et al. Impaired performance in commercial drivers: role of sleep apnea and short sleep duration. *Am J Respir Crit Care Med.* 2006;174:446-454.

Spira AP, Blackwell T, Stone KL, Redline S, Cauley JA, Ancoli-Israel S, et al. Sleep-disordered breathing and cognition in older women. *J Am Geriatr Soc.* 2008;56:45-50.

The Joint Commission. *2009 National Patient Safety Goals.* Available at: http://www.jointcommission.org/patientsafety/nationalpatientsafetygoals/. Accessed September 2, 2009.

University of Texas Southwestern Medical Center. Physicians seek strategies to improve the quality of sleep in icu, researchers report. December 10, 2007. Available at: http://www.utsouthwestern.edu/ utsw/cda/dept353744/files/430175.html. Accessed September 2, 2009.

Wilkinson JM, Van Leuven K. *Fundamentals of Nursing: Theory, Concepts & Applications.* Philadelphia: FA Davis; 2007.

Williams LS, Hopper PD. *Understanding Medical-Surgical Nursing.* 3rd ed. Philadelphia: FA Davis; 2007.

Admission, Transfer, and Discharge

Key Terms

Admission process

Discharge instruction form

Discharge planning

Discharge process

Leaving AMA

Separation anxiety

Terminal cleaning

Transfer summary form

Objectives

1. Identify four common patient reactions to admission.
2. Describe nursing interventions for common reactions to admission.
3. Explain the importance of making the patient feel welcome during the admission process.
4. Relate specific ways you can enhance communication in a culturally diverse patient population.
5. List the nurse's responsibilities during patient admission.
6. Name two populations who are prone to separation anxiety.
7. Discuss the importance of completing an admission orientation checklist.
8. Describe the information that should be included in a discharge summary.
9. Outline the nursing responsibilities during the patient discharge process.
10. Compare the transfer of a patient to another facility to a transfer within the same facility.

Clinical Connection

Your Assignment: You will be caring for a 67-year-old male who fell on the ice and shattered his right femur. He had surgery to repair it, using plates, screws, and wire. He cannot bear any weight on his right leg for a minimum of 8 weeks. He is married, but his wife is in poor physical health and is unable to care for him. As soon as you arrive on the floor, you learn that he is to be discharged today because his insurance will no longer pay for hospitalization. No decisions have yet been made about where he will go upon discharge.

Your Actions: Although you will not be responsible for making placement decisions, you will be involved in preparing the patient for discharge. He may be distressed about the abrupt change in his care and apprehensive over where he will go next. The social worker at the hospital is working on getting him placed in either a rehabilitation facility or a nursing home with physical therapists. You will need to reconcile his medications, ensuring that an accurate and complete list of all medicines he is to take is provided to the next caregiver. You will also assist with the discharge, ensuring that all of his belongings are gathered, including any valuables in the safe. You will be responsible for assisting with his discharge instructions and encouraging him in his rehabilitation plan.

Many individuals have never been admitted to a hospital as a patient nor even had a loved one hospitalized. Maybe you have not been through this traumatic experience or have not thought about hospitalization being traumatic. Maybe it does not seem like it is a big deal to become hospitalized. However, those who either have been a patient or have attended a close friend or relative while he or she was hospitalized know differently.

In this chapter, you will learn some possible patient reactions and how you can respond to them to decrease the trauma for your patients and their loved ones. You will also learn the guidelines and processes of admitting, transferring, and discharging patients. At the end of this chapter, you will be better prepared to meet your patients' needs during these periods of transition.

Admission

As the nurse, you have the opportunity, ability, and responsibility to make admission less stressful for your patients. It is during the **admission process** that you will make your first impression on the patient, one that can either help improve your patient's stay or make it a negative experience. This is the time to begin establishing rapport and a trusting relationship with the patient.

It is so important for you to begin the process of admission with the most positive approach possible. Walk into the room with a smile on your face. Make it a requirement for yourself! Make a conscious effort to avoid letting unpleasantries, such as being short-handed or behind schedule, show in your speech, facial expression, or body language. It

is amazing how easily expressions can sometimes be read or interpreted. Speak kindly and respectfully to the new patient. Introduce yourself and include your credentials so the patient will know whether you are a registered nurse, licensed practical/vocational nurse, student nurse, or someone from another department such as the business office or laboratory. Shake the patient's hand (Fig. 20-1).

Make brief eye contact and speak at a rate that does not sound hurried. Address the patient by his or her surname, such as Mr. or Mrs. Stephens. Avoid use of first names unless the patient specifically asks you to address him or her by first name. Avoid using terms of endearment such as "honey" and "sweetie." Use of these terms may be considered condescending or patronizing.

Figure 20-1 Making a good first impression helps the process of establishing rapport and trust with the patient.

Reactions to Admission

When admitting a patient, make certain that he or she is made to feel welcome. It is very difficult to establish rapport and a trusting relationship with a patient who feels that he or she is viewed by staff as a burden and not welcome. Box 20-1 presents some of the possible reactions your patients may experience during admission and hospitalization.

Fear

Fear of the unknown falls under *safety and security* in Maslow's hierarchy of human needs and can result in insecurity if the unknowns are not revealed in a timely manner. It is something most individuals have experienced at different points in their lives. With hospitalization, it is probably one of the most common responses due to the many unknowns. Some of the questions plaguing a patient during admission may include:

- What is wrong with me? What is my unknown diagnosis? What does it mean?
- What tests, procedures, treatments, or surgeries will I undergo?
- Will there be discomfort or pain?
- Who are all these people who keep coming into my room, one after another?
- How long will I have to be here?

It is helpful if you tell the patient what you are about to do, explain what he or she can expect, and ask if there are any questions you might answer. Reducing the number of

unknowns for your patient will lower his or her fear and stress levels and gain better compliance.

If the patient is a child, it is often helpful to allow the child to hold and become familiar with supplies or equipment that will be used in his or her care. For example, allow the child to take a teddy bear's tympanic temperature or listen to mommy's heart with your stethoscope (Fig. 20-2). Never tell the child that a procedure will not hurt unless it is the truth. It is important to be honest and admit that it "will hurt a little bit." You can then follow up with the child by describing what can be done to decrease the discomfort. If you tell the child that something will not hurt and it does, you instill distrust rather than trust and damage your credibility with the child.

Anxiety

Anxiety is another *safety and security* concern in Maslow's hierarchy. The physician and nurses may view the patient's diagnosis as a common occurrence that is easily treated, with the expectation the patient will recover quickly and return to normal routines. However, the patient will most likely not have the knowledge that his or her caregivers possess, and the diagnosis probably will not feel common or simple. Fear of the diagnosis can result in high levels of anxiety, especially if it is something as serious or frightening as cancer.

Anxiety can also develop due to separation from familiar surroundings and significant others; this is known as **separation anxiety**. Most individuals prefer to recover from illness or injury at home, where they are most comfortable and where care can be provided by family or loved ones rather than strangers.

A patient may worry about responsibilities as well, such as who will care for his or her children or other

Box 20-1

Common Patient Reactions to Admission

Becoming a patient in a hospital or outpatient clinic is stressful, at best. Even when it may bring relief, comfort, or even a cure, it is still not the most relaxing situation in which to find oneself. So many things are unfamiliar: the environment, the diagnosis or illness, the diagnostic testing and treatment it requires, the staff with whom the patient does not have an established relationship, the facility routines that will be imposed upon the patient, and the extent of the ensuing financial cost it will bring. The list of unknowns for the patient is endless, and each unknown has the potential to invoke unexpected or unusual reactions from the patient. Some of the more common reactions include:

- Fear of the unknown, which could be caused by a new diagnosis, tests or procedures, pain or discomfort, or even health care providers who are strangers
- Anxiety, which could be caused by problems with child care during hospitalization, effects of hospitalization on job, cost and expenses of hospitalization, and separation from familiar surrounds and significant others
- Loss of control over such things as attire, modesty, privacy, daily schedule of activities, and diet
- Loss of identity, because the patient may feel he or she is just one of many patients, a patient number, or a diagnosis

Figure 20-2   Attempt to familiarize the child with the stethoscope, penlight, or other equipment to reduce the child's anxiety.

dependent loved ones, such as an elderly parent. Individuals may not have strong support systems or families who live nearby.

A common cause of anxiety is financial concern. The patient may worry about the cost of hospitalization if there is no insurance coverage, the added expense of missing work, or the expense of hiring someone to care for his or her dependents. It is important to identify these problems and involve appropriate hospital resources as soon as possible. Social workers can generally assist the patient with these types of problems.

To help decrease anxieties, encourage the patient to ask questions and look for signs of understanding as you answer them. Provide a brief but factual explanation of the patient's diagnosis. Avoid the use of medical terminology unless it is clear the patient understands it; otherwise, use layperson's terms. Reassure the patient whenever possible without giving false reassurance. Encourage a child's parent or guardian to stay with the child if at all possible to reduce separation anxiety. Ask the parent to bring a couple toys or a favorite blanket from home to help familiarize the room for the child. The patient who is elderly may also be comforted by allowing a family member to stay.

Loss of Control

Another response common to hospitalization is loss of control, and it, too, comes under Maslow's *safety and security* needs. There is generally a steady stream of individuals at the patient's bedside. Visitors can come from the laboratory, radiology department, and business offices; they can be interns and residents, and they can be nurse assistants, primary care nurses, or a registered nurse case manager. And this is only a partial list of hospital staff who can visit the patient at the bedside. They all ask numerous questions, many of them repeated by several individuals, leading patients to complain of repetition. Effective communication by health care providers can prevent some of the question duplication. Pay attention to what has already been documented by others.

Many of the questions are of a private nature, some being very personal, to the point of discomfort for the patient, and the patient may feel the answers to some of the questions are not the business of health care providers. If your patient feels this way, explain why some of the more personal questions are asked and how they may be applicable to his or her care. Also, make certain the door to the patient's room is closed when interviewing the new patient. Avoid asking questions out in the hall, at the nurse's station, or at any site where other individuals could overhear.

Other aspects of hospitalization that may make a patient feel a loss of control include:

- Sleeping in a different bed
- Using a different toilet
- Eating whatever food is provided regardless of how it was prepared
- Being awakened during the night for provision of nursing care

Attire and Modesty

Other areas where loss of control may be felt include attire, modesty, and privacy. For example, when a patient is admitted for certain tests, surgeries, or procedures, the nurse may request that the patient wear a hospital gown rather than the patient's personal pajamas. It may seem a small issue to you, but to the patient it may represent a loss of control. Whenever possible, allow the patient to wear his or her own pajamas or gown if the patient has a preference.

Take care to protect the patient's modesty while assisting the patient to dress or undress as well as during examinations, tests, and treatments. Failure to do so can result in substantial patient embarrassment. It is important to remember that your patient may view exposure of his or her own body differently than would a health care provider. It is not an everyday occurrence for patients to view and handle other people's bodies as it is for you. Demonstrate sensitivity and respect by preserving your patient's modesty at all times. If it is necessary for the patient to wear a typical hospital gown, be vigilant in keeping the gown edges together and overlapping in the back, tying the strings to keep the gown closed as much as possible. Use drapes to prevent unnecessary exposure during delivery of nursing care.

Always knock before entering the patient's room. If the curtain is pulled, ask for permission to enter. While providing personal care, protect the patient's modesty by closing the door and pulling the privacy curtain around the bed. Avoid exposing more of the patient's body than is necessary; use a sheet or bath blanket for coverage, if needed. Allow the patient to do as much changing of his or her own clothes as possible. Encourage independence unless there are restrictions in activity. Let the patient wear his or her own pajamas if possible, and allow underwear to remain in place unless contraindicated. If the patient must wear a hospital gown, use a second gown put on backward to serve as a robe for added modesty.

An older adult may be mortified when the gender of the nurse differs from his or her gender. In certain cultures, it is even prohibited for a female to provide nursing care for a male, and vice versa. It is pertinent to make efforts to accommodate patients who feel strongly about this issue, especially for personal body functions such as bathing and toileting. When you must provide care to a patient of different gender than yourself, be vigilant to demonstrate respect and provide for privacy as much as possible while delivering nursing care. This will help to establish rapport in a situation that may be uncomfortable for the patient of a different gender.

Patient Rooms

Although private rooms are now more commonly available to patients, there is still the possibility in some hospital settings that the patient will have to share a room with a stranger. Generally, the two patients not only share a room, but they also share bathroom facilities and are able to overhear each other's conversations with health care providers and families. These situations can cause undue stress and feelings of loss of control for the patient.

If caring for a patient who is sharing a room, strive to keep the volume of your voice low when discussing sensitive issues. At times, it may be prudent to take the patient to a private examination room before divulging devastating or sensitive test results. It may also be possible to arrange for the roommate to be taken for a walk or a ride in a wheelchair to allow more privacy for personal interaction with the patient.

Decision Making

Allow the patient to make decisions when possible, even seemingly small ones such as:

• "Do you prefer ice water or tap water in your pitcher?"
• "Do you prefer your drinks with or without a straw?"
• "Would you like to leave your socks on?"

Provide choices and let the patient feel that he or she maintains some control over the situation as much as possible.

Loss of Identity

Some patients feel a loss of identity when they are hospitalized. It is easy to see how it develops: The patient now has a room number, a patient number, and a call light that he or she must use to obtain assistance. He or she is one patient of many patients, one who is often forced to wait for what he or she might consider to be routine services, such as:

• Performance of a test or procedure
• Delivery of pain medication
• Delivery of lunch tray
• Call light being answered
• Visit from the physician

Explain to the patient why you are placing an identification band on his or her wrist. Make it a priority to learn the new patient's name quickly and call him or her by Mr., Miss, Ms., or Mrs. with the last name. As stated before, avoid calling patients by first name unless requested to do so. This is especially important to show respect to patients who are older than you and grew up as part of a different generation. Never refer to patients by a room number or a disease or condition. Calling the patient by his or her name helps maintain identity and eases the patient's feeling of being "just another number."

Knowledge Connection

What age groups of patients are most prone to suffer separation anxiety? How can you help to relieve this anxiety?

Cultural Considerations

Patients will come from many different cultures and may have values, attitudes, beliefs, traditions, and customs that deviate from yours. They may not view the place of religion in daily life in the same way that you do, or see the medical world as you see it. These cultural differences can magnify the problems of fear, anxiety, loss of control, and loss of identity. Fear and anxiety can increase if the patient feels that he or she will not be treated in a culturally acceptable manner. When someone of a different culture provides the patient's care, the patient may be concerned that cultural rituals surrounding religion, hygiene, manner of dress, nutrition, and even food preparation may not be possible. This can increase the feelings of loss of control and loss of identity. Cultural differences can also cause additional problems by hindering verbal and nonverbal communication with the patient (Box 20-2). It is extremely important not only that you are aware of these differences, but that you display sensitivity and respect for patients' beliefs, whether you agree with them or not. Acceptance is necessary to establish a trust-based rapport with your patients.

Admitting Procedure

The patient's chart is initiated during the admitting process and includes various admission forms specific to each facility's policies and procedures. Admitting office staff obtain demographic data, such as the patient's:

• Full name
• Social security number
• Age
• Date of birth
• Residential address
• Telephone number
• Next of kin name and contact information
• Religious preference
• Place of employment
• Insurance and billing data
• Physician's name
• Reason for admission

Box 20-2
Culturally Savvy Communication

Communication between nurses and those with whom we share some of the same ethnic and cultural backgrounds, and maybe even similar religious beliefs, is not always easy or as clear as we think it is. It is of particular importance when there are cultural differences between two individuals, and especially if there are language barriers that exacerbate the problem. Work hard to become a culturally savvy communicator; it will bring unforeseen rapport, respect, trust, and rewards.

- Always address your patient by Mr., Mrs., Miss, or Ms. and his or her last name. Never use first names to address a patient unless the patient requests it.
- Avoid use of slang.
- Use simple, common, proper English.
- If there is a language barrier, provide an interpreter. Only use the patient's relatives to interpret if requested by the patient or there is no one else available.
- Do not attempt to use ethnic dialects unless you are fluent in the language.
- Use eye contact judiciously. Some cultures consider it disrespectful or a challenge to authority to look someone in the eye. A few of these cultures are Hispanics, some Native Americans, and various Eastern Asians.
- Position yourself so the patient can see your face and read your lips if necessary.
- Pay attention to the patient's facial expressions and other nonverbal communication. This may help you determine when the patient does not understand your communication.
- Exhibit respect for the patient's beliefs regarding health care, family, traditions, and religion.
- Clarify information when you do not understand what the patient has said.

Figure 20-3 Hospital identification bands: the white band is the identification band, the blue band indicates the patient's fall risk level, and the red band lists the patient's allergies.

Nursing Responsibilities During Patient Admission

Once the patient is brought to his or her room, you have numerous tasks to perform as part of the admission process. If the patient's condition warrants direct admission from the physician's office or the emergency room without going to the admitting office, send a family member to the admitting office to complete paperwork.

Introduction

When greeting the patient and family, remember to smile genuinely and introduce yourself, including your credentials. If the identification band has already been applied, check the band for confirmation of identity. If a band has not yet been applied, do so at this time. If there is a roommate, introduce the patients to each other. It is important to be courteous and respectful in your interactions with the new patient. The impression you make may be the lasting impression that goes home with the patient.

Orient the patient and family to the room, showing them how to obtain assistance and operate various room furnishings; also show them the availability and location of amenities (Box 20-3).

Admission Kit

Most hospitals have a basic admission kit that consists of a water pitcher or carafe, drinking glass, wash basin, emesis basin, soap dish, and box of tissues (Fig. 20-4). Make certain the admission kit is present at the bedside table; if it is missing, retrieve one from the supply room. Also provide a bedpan and urinal as appropriate. If the physician's orders indicate the patient may have oral fluids, fill the pitcher with water and ice according to the patient's preference.

Provide the patient assistance as needed with undressing and donning either a hospital gown or his or her personal pajamas, ensuring privacy by closing the room door and pulling the privacy curtain. If the patient is able to perform this task without your assistance, allow her or him to do so. This reduces some of the initial embarrassment the patient may feel.

Authority to Treat

Each facility has a form that must be completed and signed, granting permission for treatment. If the patient is a minor, the authorization for treatment must be signed by a parent or legal guardian. The age at which an individual is no longer considered a minor differs from state to state. In most states, the patient may provide authority to treat at age 18.

Identification Bands

Either the nurse or the admission office personnel apply an identification wristband containing patient name, room number, hospital identification number, age, birth date, and physician's name. The identification wristband stays on the patient throughout the entire hospitalization. *Safety: This band is one of the methods used to identify the patient prior to any procedure or administration of medications. If the patient is allergic to any medications, herbs, or foods, an allergy identification band is also applied.* An allergy band is normally red so that it is more easily noticed (Fig. 20-3).

Box 20-3
Admission Orientation Checklist

Each patient should be oriented upon admission to reduce anxiety and promote patient compliance. By providing the patient with a proper orientation, you allow the patient to maintain a better sense of control over the hospital experience, which is conducive to healing and a sense of well-being. Orientation of the patient to his or her room and hospital routines should include the following information:

- Location of the nurse's station in relation to the patient's room
- How to use the call light, intercom system, and emergency call light. *This is a good time to inform the patient of the physician's orders regarding whether or not the patient is allowed to get out of bed.*
- Location of the bathroom
- How to use the telephone
- How to operate the bed. *Safety: Explain that the bed should be kept in its lowest position.*
- How to adjust lighting
- How to operate the television and radio
- Location of personal care items; closet and drawer space for patient's belongings

- Times meals are served and any dietary restrictions ordered by the physician
- Location of cafeteria and snack machines
- Hours that you will be his or her nurse and how often your visits are to be expected
- Any policies that apply to the patient or family, such as visitation times, cell phone usage, or tobacco use policy
- When the physician normally makes visits

Safety: Make certain the patient is wearing an identification band and any necessary allergy alert band. Explain to the patient that each individual who provides care for the patient should check the name on the ID band as well as use a second identifier prior to delivery of all care. This will help to reduce the patient's irritation at being asked to state his or her name repeatedly. Plus, should a staff member fail to read the ID band as required, it provides the patient with the additional control of "offering the ID band for verification" to ensure that the staff member does indeed have the correct patient before beginning a treatment or administering medication.

Complete an inventory of clothing and personal items, such as eyeglasses, dentures, and hearing aids, brought to the hospital. These items may be kept at the bedside. Instruct the patient to send all valuables, such as money, credit cards, or jewelry, home with family members. If there is no family member available or the patient desires to keep valuables at the hospital, review with the patient the hospital's policy for storing valuables. Inventory the valuables and list them using only general descriptions. You cannot, with certainty, tell by simply observing a piece of jewelry whether it is real gold, silver, platinum, diamond, or zirconium. Whatever you list on the inventory is what the hospital is responsible for returning to the patient. It does not matter what subjective information the patient may tell you; you must document only objective data, that which you can see with your own eyes and state factually. For example, rather than

writing "24-carat yellow gold ring with 1-carat diamond," write "gold-colored ring with clear stone." Then document whether the patient kept the valuables at the bedside or placed them in a valuables envelope in the hospital safe. In order to provide extra protection against patient claims for "lost valuables," some facility policies require a second nurse's signature as witness of the valuables placed in the envelope. A copy of the inventoried items kept at the bedside should be given to the patient and another copy should be placed in the patient's chart.

Data Collection

An initial assessment database includes both objective and subjective data and is completed by interviewing the patient and performing physical assessment of all body systems. Objective data are those that you can perceive or measure, such as something you can hear, see, touch, or smell. Subjective data are those that only the patient can perceive and tell you about, such as pain, family history, or the patient's feelings. During the interview, it is important to obtain a thorough patient medical and surgical history, as well as a social history, including:

- Diseases, injuries, and surgeries experienced by the patient
- Family medical history
- Food, drug, seasonal, or environmental allergies
- Current prescription and over-the-counter medications, herbs, nutritional supplements, and illicit drugs
- Pertinent health habits practiced by the patient, such as a special diet, use of sleep aids, smoking, alcohol use, dependency upon laxatives for regular bowel movements, or use of assistive devices

Figure 20-4 Typical items that might be found in a hospital admission kit.

- List of the patient's complaints, such as discomfort, nausea, weakness, congestion, shortness of breath, or itching
- Living arrangements—for example, whether the patient lives alone, with a spouse, in an assisted living facility, with children
- Employment and type of work performed

The initial physical assessment should include:

- Vital signs, including blood pressure, temperature, pulse, respirations, oxygen saturation level, and pain level, location, and characteristics
- Level of consciousness
- Orientation to person, place, time, and situation
- Auscultation of heart, breath, and bowel sounds
- Assessment of bowel and bladder status and habits
- Examination of pupils, mucous membranes, and skin
- Peripheral pulses, capillary refill, color, temperature, range of motion, and strength of all extremities
- Weight and height

This assessment provides a baseline against which changes in patient condition, both improvement and deterioration, can be measured. For further information regarding physical assessment, see Chapter 21.

Supervision/Delegation Connection

Admission Assessments
The Joint Commission, an accrediting agency for health care facilities, requires each patient to be assessed by an RN upon admission, although portions of the assessment may be delegated to the LPN/LVN. A few assessments may be delegated to the CNA, such as assessment of vital signs, weight, and height.

Inquire about and answer any questions or concerns the patient or family may have. If you do not know the answer to a particular question, be honest and say you do not know. Then find out the answer and report back to the patient as soon as possible. Work to convey confidence as well as competence in order to help establish the trust and rapport that is so important.

Analyze Data
You will then compile and analyze the collected data to identify the actual problems the patient has, as well as any potential problems the patient is at risk for developing. These identified problems are used in development of the plan of care.

Though it may sound strange, **discharge planning** should be initiated during the admission process. You should collect data regarding the patient's living arrangements, physical limitations, and ability to perform activities of daily living, such as bathing, dressing, toileting, and meal preparation. This provides you with a better picture of the patient's current needs as well as needs that must be addressed in planning for discharge.

The patient's chart is compiled and physician's orders are noted and carried out according to protocol. You should explain any diagnostic tests and treatments that are ordered, assist the patient in collection of specimens such as urine or sputum, and arrange for transportation to laboratory or radiology departments. After explaining a test or procedure to the patient, observe for objective and subjective signs of understanding or confusion. This is part of the nursing process known as evaluation.

Knowledge Connection
Describe the objective and subjective components of an initial assessment database.

Discharge

The primary goal when a patient is hospitalized is to keep the patient's stay in the hospital as short as possible without endangering the patient's health. Discharge planning that has been ongoing since admission helps to make the discharge process go smoothly. The typical **discharge process** involves:

- Obtaining a physician's order
- Notifying the business office of impending discharge
- Reconciling the patient's medications
- Providing discharge instructions, prescriptions, and appropriate patient teaching
- Assisting the patient to gather his or her personal belongings and valuables
- Documenting the patient's condition, including vital signs
- Assisting the patient to the car
- Documenting the time of discharge and method of transportation
- Notifying housekeeping so that the room can be cleaned

Some facilities require the discharging nurse to schedule the patient's follow-up appointment with the physician as a patient courtesy.

Discharge Planning

Discharge planning should begin during or shortly after admission to the hospital and continue until the patient is discharged from the hospital. You and the patient work together and systematically plan how to best meet the patient's needs after hospitalization. Discharge planning may involve:

- Teaching about the patient's illness and how it may impact the patient's life
- Teaching dietary alterations to meet patient's needs
- Teaching safe and effective use of medications
- Teaching how to perform treatments, such as assessment of finger stick blood sugar level, colostomy irrigation, or dressing changes

- Teaching methods of adaptation for daily living
- Recommending various support groups, such as the Mastectomy Support Group or Alcoholics Anonymous
- Providing the patient with a list of available community resources, such as Meals on Wheels or Women, Infants, and Children Services (WIC)
- Making referrals to appropriate agencies such as home health care or hospice
- Assisting the family to find a long-term care or assisted living facility that will meet their needs

Knowledge Connection

When should you begin discharge planning for each patient?

Physician's Discharge Order

When the physician feels the patient is well enough to be discharged, a discharge order is written. If a patient becomes unhappy with his or her care, decides against treatment, or for any other reason simply decides to leave the hospital before the physician authorizes a discharge, this is known as "leaving against medical advice" or **leaving AMA**.

If the patient decides to leave AMA, your responsibility is to attempt to reason with him or her and to explain why it is not in his or her best interest to leave without authorization of the physician. If that fails to convince the patient to stay, you will ask the patient to sign a Leaving AMA form, which releases the hospital and physician from responsibility for the patient's health status after leaving. If the patient refuses to sign the Leaving AMA form, document in the nurse's notes that the form was offered but the patient refused to sign it. Most facilities require you to notify the attending physician regarding the situation.

Reconcile Medications

One of the most important discharge responsibilities of the nurse is medication reconciliation. The medication list must be reconciled with prescription and over-the-counter medications the patient was taking at home and with the physicians' orders while the individual was a patient in the facility. Patients often have more than one physician providing care and writing medication orders. This can result in physicians writing orders for similar drugs or for drugs that are contraindicated, meaning they are not supposed to be administered together. The nurse compares the medications that the patient was taking at home to the medications the patient is to take after discharge, to ensure the following:

- There are no duplications in ordered medications.
- Dosages are correct and any differences or changes in dosage were intended.
- All previous home medications have either been continued or discontinued, not overlooked.
- Prescriptions have been provided for new medications.
- A written list of medications is provided to the patient.

This safety measure was adopted in an effort to decrease medication omissions and duplications and potential drug interactions.

Discharge Instructions

When the physician writes a discharge order for a patient, the nurse completes a **discharge instruction form**, which includes:

- When to return to the physician's office for follow-up
- A list of medications and how to take them, and what side effects to watch for
- Required modifications or restrictions of diet or activity level
- Signs and symptoms of worsening condition that warrant physician notification
- Care or treatment that the patient is to continue at home

Figure 20-5 presents an example of a discharge instruction form.

After reviewing the discharge instructions verbally, ask the patient for questions and verify understanding of information. Once the patient acknowledges understanding, have the patient sign the discharge instruction form. Give one copy to the patient and place one copy in the patient chart. In the nurse's notes, you should document that instructions were reviewed verbally and given in writing, noting the patient's response to the instructions.

Patient Teaching Connection

Discharge Teaching

You are in the process of preparing a patient for discharge from the hospital in 2 days. The patient has been started on a new medication, nitroglycerin, for heart-related chest pain, known as angina. It is your responsibility to teach the patient what he needs to know so that he can safely and correctly take the new medication. You must teach him to protect the nitroglycerin from light and moisture to maintain its *efficacy*—its ability to achieve its desired effect. Explain that the drug is not to be taken after the expiration date on the bottle. Teach the patient to always take the medication with him when he leaves home. Explain that the drug is taken *sublingually,* which means that it is placed underneath the tongue to dissolve, and should never be swallowed. Tell him to place one tablet under his tongue as soon as he begins to have chest pain. If chest pain is not relieved, tell him that he is to repeat the tablet every 5 minutes for a maximum of three tablets. If the chest pain has not resolved after three tablets, he is to contact the physician or go immediately to the emergency room. Discuss the safety of having another individual drive the patient to the physician's office or emergency room to prevent risk should the patient lose consciousness while driving himself. Explain to the patient that the nitroglycerin may cause a headache as a side effect.

This information generally needs to be given verbally and written down for later reference. Ask for clarification that the patient understands.

TAKE THIS SHEET WITH YOU WHEN YOU RETURN TO YOUR DOCTOR

DISCHARGE INSTRUCTIONS

Name _____ Age _____ Doctor _____ Pharmacy _____

Discharge Date/Time _____ Diagnosis _____

MEDICATIONS   ALLERGIES _____   DIET _____

WOUND CARE
   Keep Clean and Dry
   May Shower
   Watch for signs of Infection
      (redness, pain, swelling, temperature, drainage)

ACTIVITY INSTRUCTIONS:
   (driving, sex, lifting, walking, exercise, etc.)
_____
_____
_____

RETURN TO CLINIC: _____

SPECIAL INSTRUCTIONS:
_____
_____
_____
_____

Call for Appointment:
Dr. S. Arthurs   375–3752
Dr. T. Stough   263–7263
Dr. J. Gerber   263–7263
Dr. R. Matson   375–3433
Dr. B. Krablin   375–7935

Nurse's Signature _____

Meds sent with patient Yes _____ No _____

Patient/Guardian Signature _____

Discharged by: w/c _____ amb. _____ carrier _____

DISCHARGE ASSESSMENT   Discharged to: _____ home   _____ N.H.

BEHAVIOR
___ alert
___ anxious
___ confused
___ oriented
___ lethargic
CIRCULATORY
___ no difficulty
___ edema
___ numbness
___ dizziness
___ palpitations
___ angina
___ anemia
___ bruising
URINARY
___ no difficulty
___ incontinence
___ hematuria
___ UTI
___ urostomy

ELIMINATION
___ no difficulty
___ constipation
___ diarrhea
___ uncontinence
___ ostomy
___ bleeding
___ laxative
MOBILITY
___ self
___ with help
___ cane/walker
___ bedfast
VISION
___ no difficulty
___ glasses
___ blurring
HEARING
___ no difficulty
___ limited
SPEECH
___ no difficulty
___ aphasic

NEUROLOGICAL
___ no difficulty
___ incoordination
___ parathesis
___ weakness
MUSCULOSKELETAL
___ no difficulty
___ pain/stiffness
___ contractures
___ arthritis
___ prosthesis
RESPIRATORY
___ no difficulty
___ dyspnea
___ cough
___ sputum
___ asthma
___ breath sounds
   ___ R
   ___ L
P ___ R ___
T ___ BP ___

GASTROINTESTINAL
___ no difficulty
___ dysphagia
___ nausea
___ vomitting
___ pain
___ bleeding
SKIN
___ warm
___ cold
___ dry
___ clammy
___ diaphoretic
___ pale
___ color pink
___ flushed
___ cyanosis
Turgor

COMMENTS:
_____
_____
_____
(RN's Signature)

Figure 20-5 An example of a discharge instruction form.

Notification of Business Office

As soon as you are aware of an impending discharge, you should notify the business office so that records can be assessed for completeness. If the patient has health insurance, a form authorizing the release of information to the insurance company will be checked for the patient's signature. If the patient does not have health insurance, it is important to make payment arrangements with the patient. Notifying the business office as soon as possible allows time to complete the necessary paperwork before the patient is ready to leave.

Gathering of Belongings and Valuables

In preparation for discharge, assist the patient to gather personal belongings together. Make certain any assistive devices such as eyeglasses, hearing aids, and dentures are safely placed with the personal belongings. Check to see if the patient has valuables locked in the hospital safe. Remember to have the patient sign the form for the receipt of the valuables and then sign it yourself. If necessary, obtain a cart on which to place the patient's belongings, as well as any gifts and flowers, to take them to the car.

Final Nursing Responsibilities

Discontinue any equipment and tubes that are to be removed prior to discharge and assess the patient's vital signs if they have not been assessed within the last hour. Document the patient's condition and vital signs in the nurse's notes, along with the time the patient actually leaves and the method of transportation. Most facility insurance carriers require that patients be taken to the car in a wheelchair to reduce risk of falls or injury.

Also make sure to notify housekeeping so the room can be given **terminal cleaning**. This includes disinfecting the bed, furniture, bathroom, sink, and floor. The bed must be made with fresh linens and the room prepared for admission of the next patient.

Knowledge Connection
Summarize the steps of the discharge process. What subjects should be included in discharge teaching? List the information that should be included in the nurse's discharge note.

Patient Transfer

An improvement or deterioration in the patient's condition may necessitate transferring the patient from one unit to another within the same facility or from the hospital to another facility, such as a long-term care facility or specialty hospital. A transfer from the hospital to another facility includes discharge as well as transfer papers be completed.

Transfer Within the Facility

The simplest transfer is to transfer a patient from one unit to another unit within the same facility. To complete this type of transfer you will need to:

- Obtain the physician's order for transfer.
- Explain the reason for the transfer to the patient and family.
- *Safety: reconcile the patient's list of medications, both prescription and over-the-counter, with home medications and new physician's orders to assure that nothing has been duplicated or omitted.* The list is then reviewed with the nurse receiving the patient at transfer. (This is another safety requirement of The Joint Commission's 2009 National Patient Safety Goals. The Joint Commission is in the process of revising the manner in which the medication reconciliation goal is to be achieved for the 2010 National Patient Safety Goals.)
- Gather the patient's personal belongings, medications, nursing supplies, and complete chart.
- Complete a **transfer summary form**, used to document the patient's condition and the reason for transfer, and a comprehensive list of the patient's medications.
- Phone a full report of the patient's condition and plan of care to the receiving nurse on the new unit.
- Document the time of transfer in the nurse's notes.
- Transfer the patient with all his or her belongings and chart to the new unit.

Discharge planning may involve multiple disciplines. Though generally the nurse or a specified discharge planner coordinates this process, it typically involves some of the following health care team members to effectively develop a plan that meets all the patient's needs after discharge:

- Physical therapist
- Occupational therapist
- Speech therapist
- Dietitian
- Social worker
- Home health nurse
- Ostomy nurse

Transfer to Another Facility

The process of transferring a patient to another facility is more complex. After obtaining the physician's transfer order, notify the business office of impending transfer. Assist the patient in arranging for transportation, such as calling for an ambulance or notifying a family member if the patient can go via private automobile. Some facilities require both a transfer summary form and a discharge summary to be sent to the receiving facility. You are responsible for knowing the facility's policies and procedures. If you are uncertain what the policy is, refer to the facility policy and procedure book.

A transfer summary form is prepared that contains information about the patient's condition and vital signs at time of discharge; discharge instructions that include a list of the patient's discharge medications, diet, activity restrictions, patient teaching that has been done, and follow-up appointments; time of transfer; and method of transportation. This form is usually completed by the transferring nurse and a copy is sent with the patient to the receiving facility. Another document commonly sent with the patient transferring to another facility is a document called a discharge summary. The physician completes this document, which summarizes the patient's condition, diseases, pertinent diagnostic results, medications and treatments, as well as where the patient is to go after discharge and follow-up treatment plans.

Any valuables in the hospital safe should be sent with the patient and notation made in the hospital chart and the transfer record. Make certain the patient has signed consent to release medical information to third parties to comply with the Health Insurance Portability and Accountability Act. All patient records that are sent with the patient should be sealed in a large manila envelope to protect confidentiality. Some facilities prefer to send the data via fax machine. It is important to phone the receiving facility informing them of the impending transmission. This helps ensure that the proper personnel receive the medical records.

Knowledge Connection

List the different health care providers who may contribute to the discharge planning of a patient. Describe the information that should be included in a transfer summary.

Post Conference

At your post conference, you have many thoughts to share. Several students were frustrated to learn that your patient was discharged, not based on the physician's determination, but based on the insurance company's rules. As you evaluate your clinical performance, you question if you did all you could for this gentleman. Did you:
- Explain what was happening to the patient?
- Gather all his belongings, including his valuables from the safe?
- Listen to his discharge instructions when presented by the staff nurse?
- Ensure that he had all his discharge instructions, list of all current medications, and prescriptions with him when he left?
- Relay any questions or concerns about discharge to the appropriate staff person?
- Act in a calm, reassuring manner even if you were rushed?
- Encourage him in the rehabilitation program he is about to begin?

If you strongly feel the patient is not ready for discharge, it is your responsibility as patient advocate to discuss your concerns and possible options with the physician. Sometimes there does not seem to be a resolution to the problem. If this is the case, it is difficult to see your patient discharged before he seems ready to go, but you will have done all you can do to help the patient transition from the hospital to his next destination.

KEY POINTS

- The first impression you make on your patient is during admission and can either help improve your patient's stay or make it a negative experience.
- Four common reactions to admission are fear, anxiety, loss of control, and loss of identity.
- Separation anxiety is common in children and older adults.
- Ways to improve the admission process for your patient include using effective communication,

introducing yourself and other direct health care providers, orienting the patient to the hospital room and typical hospital routines, providing as much information as possible regarding the patient's stay in the facility, encouraging the patient and family to ask questions and taking the time to stay and listen, avoiding the appearance of being "too busy" or "unconcerned," explaining procedures before performing them, protecting the patient's modesty and privacy, encouraging independence wherever possible, addressing the patient using title and surname, and displaying sensitivity and respect for and acceptance of the patient's beliefs.

- The admission process includes obtaining authority to treat; application of identification bands; assisting the patient to change into gown or pajamas; orienting the patient and family to the environment; inventory of clothing, personal items, and valuables; provision of a basic admission kit and carafe of water if allowed; completion of the initial assessment database; and compilation of the patient chart.
- Discharge planning begins at or shortly after admission.
- The discharge process includes obtaining a physician's order; notifying the business office; assisting the patient to gather personal belongings and valuables; discharge teaching; documentation of the patient's condition along with time of discharge and method of transportation; and notification of housekeeping.

REVIEW QUESTIONS

Select the answer that is most appropriate for each of the following questions. Some questions may have more than one correct answer. Check all that apply.

1. The first impression you make on the patient:

   a. will not affect the outcome of the hospitalization.

   b. can be a negative one.

   c. is not important.

   d. can lead to improving the patient's stay.

   e. can be the first step in establishing rapport with the patient.

   f. is partially determined by your facial expression.

   g. is partially determined by the time you take to explain things to the patient during the admission process.

2. Which of the following data should be included in a discharge summary?

   a. List of discharge medications

   b. Activity restrictions

   c. Patient's condition

   d. Follow-up appointment

   e. Diet

   f. Discharge teaching that has been done

3. Children and older adults are more prone to:

   a. feeling loss of identity.

   b. experiencing separation anxiety.

   c. feeling loss of control.

   d. adapting more readily to admission to a health care facility.

4. You can help prevent loss of identity for your patients by:

   a. calling them "honey," "sweetie," or other endearments.

   b. addressing them by title and surname.

   c. referring to them as a room number to protect privacy.

   d. referring to them by their diagnosis.

   e. addressing all patients with their first name to provide a sense of familiarity.

5. Which of the following should be included on an admission orientation checklist?

   a. How to use the call light

   b. Times meals will be served

   c. Location of the nurses' supply room

   d. How to raise the height of the bed

   e. How busy it is on the unit and that you may not be available as much as you would like to be

   f. Location of the bathroom

   g. Two methods staff will use to check the patient's identity before each procedure or medication administration

6. Which of the following will enhance communication with a patient from a different culture?

   a. Make jokes about the patient's beliefs and traditions to put the patient at ease.

   b. Clarify information when you do not understand what the patient has said.

   c. Use simple, common, and proper English.

   d. Avoid use of slang.

   e. Make eye contact at all times while conversing with the patient.

   f. Demonstrate respect for and acceptance of the patient's cultural and religious differences.

   g. Attempt to emulate the dialect and accent of the different culture.

SHORT ANSWER QUESTIONS

7. What accrediting agency requires that each patient be assessed by an RN upon admission?

8. At what point before discharge should discharge planning begin?

9. What information should be found on a patient identification band?

10. What should you always do before entering a patient's room?

11. You are preparing to transfer a patient to another facility and the physician asks you to fax the discharge summary to the receiving facility. Prior to faxing patient records to the receiving facility, what should you do to help ensure privacy is maintained?

12. You are admitting a small child to your unit at the hospital. What things could you do that might decrease fear and anxiety for the child?

CRITICAL THINKING EXERCISE

13. You are completing a valuables inventory for a new patient. The patient tells you that the ring is platinum with a 1.5-carat diamond and six emeralds totaling 1.2 carats total weight. How can you objectively describe the ring on the inventory? Why would it be a problem to describe it as it is written in this question?

ADDITIONAL RESOURCES

For additional Resources, Questions, and Activities, please see:

 Student Resource Disk

 DavisPlus http://davisplus.fadavis.com

 Student Study Guide

REFERENCES

Bergstrom J, Fraser L, Quinn M, Wheeler H. Doing it better: all roads lead to scheduled discharges. *Nursing2008*. 2008;38(12):61-63.

Emergency Nurses Association. Care of the critically ill or injured patient during interfacility transfer. 2005. Available at: http://www.ena.org/SiteCollectionDocuments/Position%20Statements/Interfacility_Transfer_ENA_White_Paper.pdf. Accessed September 9, 2009.

Institute for Healthcare Improvement. Schedule the discharge. Available at: http://www.ihi.org/IHI/Topics/Flow/PatientFlow/Changes/ScheduletheDischarge.htm. Accessed September 9, 2009.

Kravet SJ, Levine RB, Rubin HR, Wright SM. Discharging patients earlier in the day: a concept worth evaluating. *Health Care Manager*. 2007;26:142-146.

Lane BS, Jackson J, Odom SE, Cannella KAS, Hinshaw L. Nurse satisfaction and creation of an admission, discharge, and teaching nurse position. *J Nurs Care Quality*. 2009;24:148-152.

Lewis M, Tampara CD. *Medical Law Ethics & Bioethics for the Health Professions*. 6th ed. Philadelphia: FA Davis; 2007.

Merriman M. Pre-hospital discharge planning empowering elderly patients through choice. *Crit Care Nurs Q*. 2008;31:52-58.

Neeb K. *Mental Health Nursing*. 3rd ed. Philadelphia: FA Davis; 2006.

Nsameluh K, Holland DE, Gaspar P. Patient functional status changes during hospitalization: impact on early discharge planning. *Clin Nurse Specialist*. 2007;21:214-219.

Sudden Cardiac Arrest Prevention Medical Advisory Team. Heart failure admission to discharge checklist. April 2007. Available at: http://www.americanheart.org/presenter.jhtml?identifier=3065872. Accessed September 9, 2009.

The Joint Commission. *2009 National Patient Safety Goals: Hospital Program*. October 31, 2008. Available at: http://www.jointcommission.org/PatientSafety/NationalPatientSafetyGoals/09_hap_npsgs.htm. Accessed September 9, 2009.

Walker C, Hogstel MO, Curry LC. Hospital discharge of older adults: how nurses can ease the transition. *Am J Nurs*. 2007;107(6):60-70.

Wilkinson JM, Van Leuven K. *Fundamentals of Nursing: Theory, Concepts & Applications*. Philadelphia: FA Davis; 2007.

Williams L, Hopper P. *Understanding Medical-Surgical Nursing*. 3rd ed. Philadelphia: FA Davis; 2007.

Key Terms

Accommodation response

Adventitious breath sounds

Aphasia

Auscultation

Consensual reflex

Dysphasia

Excursion

Guarding

Halitosis

Jaundice

Lethargy

Orthopnea

Palpation

Paresthesia

Percussion

PERLA

Ptosis

Retractions

Signs

Sordes

Symptoms

Objectives

1. Define key terms associated with physical assessment.
2. Describe three purposes of physical assessment.
3. Differentiate between a comprehensive health assessment, a focused assessment, and an initial head-to-toe shift assessment.
4. Summarize the six techniques used for physical assessment.
5. Distinguish the different components to be examined during an initial head-to-toe shift assessment.
6. Relate each component of assessment to its associated body system(s).
7. Explain the significance of abnormal assessment findings.
8. Describe adaptations in assessment techniques that are necessary due to the age of the patient.
9. Perform an initial head-to-toe shift assessment.
10. Document the results of an initial head-to-toe assessment.

Skills

21-1 Measuring a Patient's Height

21-2 Measuring a Patient's Weight

21-3 Measuring an Infant's Weight and Length

21-4 Performing an Initial Head-to-Toe Shift Assessment

21-5 Performing a Basic Neurological Examination

21-6 Auscultating Breath Sounds

21-7 Auscultating Heart Sounds

Clinical Connection

Your Assignment: You are assigned to care for a 62-year-old male patient with congestive heart failure and emphysema. The staff nurse came in to do a shift assessment. She checked the oxygen flowmeter and the IV pump and site, listened to his heart, listened to the anterior lung fields, and checked his ankles for edema. She tells the patient, "Everything looks good," and leaves the room. As you care for him, you notice that he becomes short of breath when turning or moving in the bed. When you listen to his posterior lung sounds, you hear crackles throughout. You also notice edema over his low back area when he is turned. When you check his vital signs, his blood pressure has elevated some in the past 4 hours, and is now 158/88.

Your Actions: You think that the staff nurse may have missed some important information, but then doubt yourself because you are a student. The patient seems to be worsening and becoming more short of breath. You wonder if there are other things you should be checking to give a clearer picture of what might be going on with this patient.

As a nurse, your goal for all nursing care will be to provide care that is coherent, or logically connected to the patient's actual condition. What does this really mean? If nursing care is to be of any benefit to your patient, the care must be relevant to that specific patient and his or her needs and problems. It is important to remember that not all patients, even those with the same diagnosis, will have the same needs. That is the beauty of the human body: Even though we are technically similar to each other, we each have highly individualized differences. For example, you could line up 20 healthy individuals who all have "normal breath sounds," yet all 20 individuals' breath sounds will sound slightly different when you listen with your stethoscope. Regardless of this fact, it will be necessary for you to identify the presence of any abnormal breath sounds in all 20 of these patients.

How can you meet the individual needs of a patient if you are unaware of how that patient is different from another? The full value of each and every task, procedure, and skill you perform as a nurse is dependent upon whether or not you can accurately assess the patient's condition prior to, during, and after completion of the task, procedure, or skill. In this chapter, you will learn how to perform physical assessment in a thorough manner, and critically evaluate the assessment findings, and determine the significance of abnormal findings.

What Is Physical Assessment?

As you learned in Chapter 4, assessment is the first step of the nursing process and is ongoing throughout the nurse-patient relationship. It is the process you use to collect physical data that are relevant to the patient's health. To collect physical data about the patient's current condition, you will perform a physical examination of the patient, using four of your senses: sight, smell, hearing, and touch.

Purpose of Physical Assessment

Assessments are performed for several purposes:

- To establish the patient's current condition, a baseline against which future changes may be measured
- To identify problems the patient may have or have the potential to develop
- To evaluate the effectiveness of nursing interventions
- To monitor for changes in body function
- To detect specific body systems that need further assessment or testing

Three Levels of Physical Assessment

A *comprehensive health assessment* involves an in-depth assessment of the whole person, including the physical, mental, emotional, cultural, and spiritual aspects of the patient's health. The data, or information about the patient, are collected through physical examination and interview that may take as long as 2 hours to complete. This assessment is generally performed when a patient is admitted. The depth of assessment and the specific data to collect vary from facility to facility.

A *focused assessment* is less encompassing and involves an examination and an interview regarding a specific body system, such as examining solely the integumentary system or the respiratory system. It provides a cluster of data about just the one body system being assessed, which is usually the system involved in the illness or injury. Focused assessments are performed when time constraints allow you to check only the system or systems related to the patient's disease process, or when performing reassessment of a system in which abnormal findings were obtained earlier.

An *initial head-to-toe shift assessment* provides you with a quick overall assessment of the patient's condition to establish a baseline against which you can compare later assessments. This baseline is necessary for you to be able to identify changes in the patient's condition, whether it be improvement or deterioration. An initial head-to-toe shift assessment consists of performing a focused assessment of the following systems, conducted in a sequence beginning at the head and moving down to the toes:

- Neurological
- Cardiovascular
- Respiratory
- Integumentary
- Gastrointestinal
- Genitourinary
- Muscular
- Skeletal

An initial head-to-toe shift assessment also includes specific assessment of the patient's:

- Vital signs, including pain and oxygen saturation (SpO_2)
- Appearance
- Speech
- Safety risk factors
- Tubes and equipment
- Comfort or complaints
- Needs

Although the immune system is not assessed in depth, it should be mentioned because the vital signs, along with the focused assessments of the eight systems included in an initial shift assessment, will provide you with a meager amount of information that also relates to the patient's immune system.

Knowledge Connection

Explain the differences between a comprehensive health assessment, a focused assessment, and an initial head-to-toe shift assessment. List the eight systems and seven specific items to assess during an initial head-to-toe shift assessment.

When Is Physical Assessment Performed?

Assessment is an ongoing process that the nurse performs every time he or she encounters a patient, even when passing the patient walking down the hall. The nurse should always be looking and observing for changes in any aspect of the patient's condition. This continual assessment may not be recorded unless the nurse encounters what he or she determines to be a change from previous assessments. For the most part, though, the physical assessments we are talking about in this chapter are performed at typical times, including:

- On admission: comprehensive, in depth
- At the beginning of each shift: shorter, more focused
- When patient condition changes
- When evaluating the effectiveness of nursing care
- Anytime things do not *feel right*

When assessment findings are outside the normal range for the specific patient, they are considered to be abnormal. Abnormal findings should be reassessed within at least a 4-hour window, and sooner depending on the severity of the finding. Some abnormal assessment findings are minor or maybe even expected, while others are totally unexpected or represent potentially serious conditions. For example, if a patient admitted with an upper respiratory illness is noted to have developed an occasional dry cough, you might request that he or she let you know if it gets worse. Then you would reassess the cough within 4 hours to determine if it has worsened, improved, or remains the same. But if you assess a fever of 103°F, you must not only take immediate action to treat the fever, but also reassess the temperature within an hour to see if further intervention is required.

Knowledge Connection

Which of the three types of assessment are done on admission? At the beginning of each shift? How often should you reassess abnormal findings?

Assessment Techniques

You will begin your assessment with a method that produces subjective data: interviewing or asking questions of the patient. You will continue to make inquiries of the patient throughout the assessment, even as you begin to collect objective data.

Five techniques are used to collect objective data in the performance of physical assessment. They include inspection or observation, palpation, percussion, auscultation, and olfaction. They are performed in this order, except when you are conducting an abdominal assessment; when conducting an abdominal assessment, auscultation comes before palpation and percussion so that bowel sounds are not altered.

Although you may use additional tools to assist you in assessment, the most important tools you will need are your eyes, ears, hands, nose, and critical thinking ability. When use of the four senses produces evidence of illness or injury, the findings are objective, measurable, and classified as **signs**. When evidence of illness or injury is verbalized by the patient, the findings are subjective, not directly measurable, and classified as **symptoms**. In other words, signs of disease are those that can be detected by the nurse, while symptoms of disease are apparent only to the patient, so they must be verbally communicated by the patient to the nurse.

Interviewing

An inordinate amount of data are obtainable solely by interviewing or asking questions of the patient. You will ask questions to determine the patient's:

- Personal identity and demographics
- Details regarding current condition, including complaints, problems, concerns, and the specific reason the patient is seeking medical care at this time
- Medical history

• Social history
• Food and drug allergies
• Height and normal weight
• Expectations for hospitalization

As you learned in Chapter 6, rapport and trust are influential during the interviewing process. It is difficult to convince a patient who does not trust you to impart personal feelings or information. Box 21-1 lists ways to foster rapport and communication. Unless it is culturally contraindicated, make frequent eye contact with the patient while conversing. Remember to observe nonverbal behavior as well as verbal. If you see nonverbal evidence that does not correlate with what the patient says, assess further to clarify. For instance, a patient may deny pain but winces when you palpate the epigastric area. Inquire if the area is tender or hurts: "Does it feel uncomfortable when I press here?" Some patients interpret pain as something different and more severe than discomfort or tenderness. Ask if the patient has experienced "indigestion," "nausea," "reflux," or "heartburn," or use any other terminology that could elicit further information that might relate to the observed nonverbal behavior.

Therapeutic Communication

Remember to utilize the therapeutic communication techniques you learned in Chapter 6, as they will help you in establishing and maintaining rapport and interpersonal relationships. Avoid communication blocks that might discourage interaction and feedback. If there is a language barrier, make all efforts to obtain the assistance of an interpreter to avoid miscommunication and omission of important data.

Inspection

Inspection is the visual observation of anything about the body that you can see with the naked eye or with the assistance of other equipment such as a penlight, otoscope, or ophthalmoscope (Fig. 21-1). A penlight is used for assessment of pupil constriction of the eyes and examination of the oral and nasal mucous membranes. An otoscope is used to inspect the lining of the nose, tympanic membranes, and ear canals. An ophthalmoscope is used to assess the internal structures of the eyes. Without using any other equipment, you can use your powers of observation to inspect the patient's:

• General appearance
• Affect
• General body shape and size
• Posture
• Pupil size
• Color and condition of skin, sclera, and mucous membranes
• Respiratory efforts
• Skin for beads of perspiration
• Muscle movements and coordination
• Size and shape of abdomen
• Extremities for edema
• Equipment and tubes

Weight and Height

Although you may obtain a patient's verbal estimation of body weight and height, there are times that you will need to verify the data by weighing and measuring the patient. The weight may be assessed using bed scales or stand-alone scales, on which the height can also be measured. Some facilities require that all patients be weighed and have their height measured during admission. Other times that assessment of weight and height may be ordered include:

• For a newborn infant
• For assessment of nutritional or growth status

Box 21-1

Ways to Foster Rapport and Communication

When meeting and talking with a patient, it is important to establish a trusting, professional relationship. The following techniques can be used to foster rapport and communication with your patient:
• Smile.
• Greet the patient using his or her surname.
• Provide for privacy.
• Introduce yourself and explain your intent.
• Exhibit an open and relaxed posture.
• Be professional.
• Demonstrate active listening.
• Be attentive to the patient's responses and needs.
• Be aware of cultural influences and restrictions.
• Be sincere.
• Be nonjudgmental.
• Use touch purposefully and judiciously.

Figure 21-1 Front row: penlight. Second row: otoscope for assessing the tympanic membrane of the ear. Third row, left to right: ophthalmic head to convert otoscope to ophthalmoscope for assessing the internal eye and retina; nasal speculum for assessing the nasal passageway; two sizes of otic speculum for assessing the ear.

- For assessment of dehydration or fluid excess
- To determine the effectiveness of diuretic medications
- For calculation of certain medication dosages

Information on measuring a patient's height and weight can be found in Skill 21-1 (page 447) and Skill 21-2 (page 448), and Skill 21-3 (page 448) presents the procedure for obtaining the length and weight of an infant.

Palpation

Palpation is the application of your hands to the external surfaces of the body to detect abnormalities of the skin or tissues lying below the skin; to examine by touch or feel. By application of the fingertips, you can detect such things as:

- Skin turgor
- Growths on or below the skin
- Edema
- Size and location of body parts
- Distention of the bladder or abdomen
- Firmness versus softness of tissue, such as muscle rigidity
- Location and strength of pulses
- Temperature, texture, and moisture of the skin
- Pain

The dorsal or back surface of the hand provides for more sensitive assessment of temperature changes in the lower extremities (Fig. 21-2).

Palpation is classified according to depth of tissue compression. For example:

- Light palpation only depresses the tissue between 1 and 2 cm.
- Moderate compression depresses the tissue between 2 and 3 cm.
- Deep palpation depresses the tissue between 4 and 5 cm.

Figure 21-2 Use the dorsal aspect of the hand, which is more sensitive, to detect subtle differences in skin temperature.

Using the palmar surface of the hands, you can palpate for masses below the skin surface and accumulation of fluid in the peritoneal cavity called *ascites;* you can also determine if palpation elicits pain anywhere on the body. When palpating the abdomen, observe the patient's face for grimacing and feel for tensing of the abdominal muscles, both of which may indicate discomfort. When an area of discomfort is detected in the abdomen, you may want to assess further for what is known as rebound tenderness. This is done by applying moderately deep pressure and holding it for a couple of seconds. Then quickly release the pressure from the abdomen. Reflexive tensing of abdominal muscles or verbalization of *increased pain* with the *release* of pressure is termed *rebound tenderness,* which is common in appendicitis.

People and Places Connection

Cultural Beliefs in Assessment

It is important to consider cultural beliefs regarding the use of physical touch and modesty. Some cultures maintain differing views regarding exposure of and touching of the body, and your sensitivity to these views is critical. Some Mormons believe that underwear can only be removed in emergency situations. Muslims prefer health care providers of the same gender. The women are strictly modest and their bodies must be kept covered. Some Hispanic Americans may request a same-gender health care provider also. They may exhibit extreme modesty, and some women may even refuse to allow a male to provide nursing care to them. Individuals from China, India, and some Middle Eastern countries restrict male health care providers from touching the women and may request females. African Americans may not like to be touched until permission has been obtained; some tend to be distrustful and cautious with nurses and physicians until they know them better. Native Americans may frown on public displays of affection and touching. They, too, prefer permission be obtained before being touched. Hindus are extremely modest and private.

Percussion

Percussion is the technique used least for assessment. **Percussion** involves striking body parts with the tips of the fingers to:

- Elicit sounds that can help locate and determine the size of structures beneath the surface
- Identify whether the structure is solid or hollow
- Detect areas containing air or fluid

For example, percussion is used to detect the size of the liver and to identify lungs that are chronically hyperinflated due to disease. It may also be used to detect urinary bladder distention and peritoneal ascites. Blunt percussion uses the fist rather than the finger to tap or *percuss* and is useful to detect tenderness of the kidneys.

The fingers of the nondominant hand are placed flat on the surface to be percussed, generally either the abdomen or the chest. Then, using the dominant hand, the middle finger-tip taps lightly and quickly on the middle finger of the non-dominant hand two to three times (Fig. 21-3). It is best to avoid moving the entire forearm of the dominant tapping hand. Flexing the wrist in dart-throwing movements produces quick, sequential taps.

A medium-loud, resonant, hollow sound is heard on the chest surface over a healthy lung. Percussion of the chest of a patient with chronic obstructive pulmonary disease (COPD) may produce a louder, long, low-pitched hyperresonant sound, indicating a hyperinflated lung. When you percuss over a bowel or stomach containing a lot of air, you will detect a high-pitched tympanic or drum-like sound. A thud-like or soft dull sound is generally heard over solid organs such as the liver and spleen, as well as over fluid-filled compartments such as peritoneal ascites. If ascites is suspected, you may further assess for it using the *fluid wave test.* The patient assists you by placing the lateral aspect of his or her hand vertically in the middle of his or her abdomen, with the wrist pointing toward the patient's head and the fingertips pointing toward the feet (Fig. 21-4). Place your hands on each side of the abdomen. Use your fingers to tap on one side of the abdomen while the other hand

Figure 21-3   To perform percussion of the abdomen or chest, strike the stationary middle finger with the tip of the opposite hand's curved middle finger, allowing the moving hand to flex freely at the wrist. This allows the finger to strike in a hammer-like manner that produces the best sound.

Figure 21-4   Fluid wave test.

palpates the opposite side. The tapping will cause a fluid wave felt by the palpating hand if ascites is present.

To be skilled in abdominal assessment by palpation requires practice. Do not allow yourself to become frustrated as you are learning this important assessment technique. *Note: It is important that you keep your fingernails short to use this technique.*

Percussion is also used to assess for distention of the urinary bladder. The bladder does not normally rise superiorly, or above, the symphysis pubis. Begin percussion immediately above the symphysis pubis and percuss toward the umbilicus, noting any *dullness,* which may indicate a full bladder.

To assess the kidneys for tenderness, you will use *blunt percussion,* also known as *fist percussion.* Lay your nondominant hand palmar side down over the *costovertebral angle (CVA),* which is where the bottom of the posterior rib cage meets the vertebral column to form a 45-degree angle. Make a fist with your dominant hand and tap or strike the dorsal side of the hand laying over the CVA. Do this on both the right and left sides. Any pain or tenderness resulting is considered to be from the kidneys.

Auscultation

Auscultation is listening to the sounds produced by the body. Some sounds may be heard with the naked ear, such as belching, also known as *eructation;* passing of *flatus* or rectal gas; loud wheezing or gurgling; and loud bowel sounds. A stethoscope is used to assess the typically quieter sounds made by the heart, lungs, intestinal tract, and arteries of the neck. The bell side of the stethoscope (the cupped smaller piece) is used to assess lower pitched sounds such as abnormal heart valve sounds, known as *murmurs;* and the rushing of blood through a vessel such as the carotid artery, known as a *bruit.*

The bell is held lightly against the skin. Avoid pressing firmly or you will not be able to detect the sounds. The larger flat piece, or diaphragm side of the stethoscope, is used to assess higher pitched sounds, such as the normal heart sounds (S_1 and S_2), breath sounds, and bowel sounds. The diaphragm should be pressed firmly against the skin. To help you remember which side of the chest piece to use for different sounds, remember that the *little side is for lower* sounds and the *larger side for higher* sounds. Box 21-2 presents further stethoscope usage hints.

Olfaction

Olfaction, or the sense of smell, is used to detect odors characteristic of different health problems. For example, the smell of a patient's breath can often be revealing. A patient with bad breath, known as **halitosis,** may have poor oral hygiene, a sinus infection, or gastric upset. Individuals with high stress levels often have sour-smelling breath. A patient with kidney failure and uremia may have the smell of ammonia or urine on the breath. A smoker usually has a characteristic smoker's breath, just as one who has drunk alcohol may reek of alcohol. A patient with liver disease may have breath that has either a musty or sweet odor. When the

Box 21-2

Tips for Stethoscope Use

When using a stethoscope, it is important to use it correctly or the results you get from your assessment may not be accurate. Keep the following tips in mind:

- Point the earpieces forward toward your face.
- Clean the chest piece with alcohol between patients.
- Clean the earpieces between staff usage.
- The chest piece must be rotated to the bell or the diaphragm side to hear.
- Apply light pressure to the bell.
- Apply firm pressure to the diaphragm.
- Apply the chest piece directly to skin, not clothing.

To improve sound transmission:

- Use a stethoscope with dual tubing rather than single tubing.
- If the tubing is 28 inches or longer, remove the chest piece and trim the tubing to a length between 22 and 27 inches.
- Avoid tubing contact with clothing/rails.

breath smells like acetone or has a fruity smell, it may be an indicator of diabetes that is out of control.

Infectious drainage generally has a foul odor. The stools of a patient with cystic fibrosis usually are extremely foul smelling. Stools containing old blood have a very characteristic odor to them. *Cerumen,* or earwax, even has its own characteristic odors with some diseases. Cerumen that smells mousy may be indicative of a *Proteus* infection, while cerumen that has a putrid smell is due to a *Pseudomonas* infection. Cancer often has its own characteristic odor, sometimes detectable in an advanced stage that has yet to be diagnosed. Researchers are doing studies regarding the use of dogs and their acute sense of smell for detection of cancer in patients.

The sense of smell is stronger in some individuals than others. Some individuals have such an acute sense of smell that they can detect the odor of normal menstrual flow, even in women with scrupulous hygiene. Some health care providers are even able to differentiate the odor of strep throat from other throat infections. However, not all individuals have a sensitive sense of smell. For instance, someone with severe nasal allergies may have a more difficult time detecting odors than someone who does not have these allergies.

Knowledge Connection

What is the difference between a sign and a symptom? Explain the techniques used in assessment. Why are patient rapport and trust important?

Assessment Components Related to Each Body System

There are numerous components to be assessed to evaluate each body system. Table 21-1 presents a breakdown of assessments by body system.

Table 21-1 Assessment Components Related to Body Systems

System	Components Assessed
Neurological	Vital signs and level of consciousness Orientation Facial symmetry Pupillary size and reaction Ability to follow simple commands Speech Hand grip Feet flexion
Cardiovascular	Blood pressure and pulse Skin color, moisture, and temperature Color of mucous membranes Jugular vein distention Heart sounds Peripheral pulses Capillary refill of extremities Edema Color and temperature of extremities Clubbing of fingertips Activity tolerance Results of laboratory tests, such as blood counts, cardiac enzymes, and bleeding and clotting studies Results of radiological tests, such as chest x-ray Results of other tests, such as electrocardiogram

(table continues on page 428)

Table 21-1 Assessment Components Related to Body Systems (continued)

System	Components Assessed
Respiratory	Respiratory rate and characteristics Respiratory effort Respiratory pattern Symmetry of excursion SpO_2 Breath sounds Use of accessory respiratory muscles Shape of chest Retractions Cough and sputum Skin color Color of nailbeds Tolerance for activity Laboratory test results, such as arterial blood gases Radiological test results, such as chest x-ray
Integumentary	Skin color, texture, moisture, and temperature Turgor Skin integrity, including pressure points and lesions Surgical incisions
Gastrointestinal	Anorexia Nausea or vomiting Shape or distention of abdomen Consistency of abdomen Bowel sounds Bowel elimination Incontinence Flatus
Genitourinary	Last voiding Distention of bladder Frequency, burning, or urgency Color and clarity of urine Incontinence
Musculoskeletal	Range of motion in joints Presence of contractures Strength of hand grip Strength of foot flexion Ability to sit up or turn to side

Performing an Initial Head-to-Toe Shift Assessment

Gather the necessary equipment to perform the assessment, including a stethoscope, sphygmomanometer, thermometer, pulse oximeter, and penlight. Upon entering the patient's room, ask any visitors to step out into the hallway or waiting room. Close the door, provide privacy, and explain what you are about to do. Give the patient time to empty the bowel or bladder if needed. If you require urine or stool specimens, now is a good time to collect them. Be careful to protect the patient's modesty by keeping the patient covered with a sheet, except for the body part that is being assessed. Make certain the room temperature is comfortable for the patient. Maintain a professional demeanor at all times. Speak in a relaxed tone of voice and exhibit a relaxed facial expression. These preparatory steps serve to gain the patient's cooperation and decrease his or her anxiety. Skill 21-4 (page 449) provides the steps of initial head-to-toe shift assessment.

General Appearance

Note the patient's general appearance upon entering the room. In what position do you find the patient? Does the patient appear to be comfortable? Are there any signs of respiratory distress? Is there an indication of fear in the patient's face, such as wide eyes? What is the patient's skin color? Does the patient respond to the stimulus of your voice? Is the patient fidgeting? Is he or she unkempt? Visiting with guests? What indicators of mood or emotional tone are noted? Is the patient smiling or frowning? Research has related increased stress levels to a decrease in an individual's immunity. Is the patient making eye contact as is appropriate to his or her culture? Is the patient *mouth-breathing,* or breathing through the mouth rather than through the nose?

Vital Signs

Begin each head-to-toe shift assessment by assessing the patient's six vital signs: blood pressure, temperature, pulse, respirations, SpO_2, and pain level. Because the vital signs serve as important indicators of numerous processes occurring throughout the body, their assessment serves to establish a basic foundation of the patient's condition, possibly alerting you to problems or areas of concern that you may want to assess in more depth. All six vital signs can also serve as possible indicators of infection, and all but the SpO_2 and pain may relate to function of the immune system.

Blood Pressure

Blood pressure provides data associated with the cardiovascular system. As we age, *atherosclerosis* (hardening of the arteries) increases, contributing to the widening of the pulse pressure, or the difference between the systolic and diastolic readings. Blood pressure also relates information regarding the kidneys, which excrete renin, a major component in the control of blood pressure. Blood pressure also provides us with data relating to the level of hydration or fluid volume within the cardiovascular system. A pulse pressure of 20 mm Hg or less may be indicative of severe dehydration. In a patient who has fluid overload, blood pressure will be increased.

Temperature

An elevated temperature can direct your attention to infection or injury to the hypothalamus, the portion of the central nervous system that helps regulate body temperature. If the immune system is working correctly, it raises the body temperature whenever there are signs of microorganism invasion of the body. Hypothermia might indicate exposure to an environment that was too cold or a disorder of the body's temperature-regulating mechanisms. In a newborn, hypothermia may identify that the infant is not yet able to regulate body temperature. It can also be a sign of sepsis or severe hypothyroidism, or be a result of trauma.

Pulse

Pulse assessment may reveal hypovolemia, due to either dehydration or blood loss. An elevated pulse rate can possibly indicate pain, anxiety, fear, stress, physical exertion, low blood pressure, infection, effects of medication, and many other conditions.

Respirations

Assessment of respirations provides detail about the patient's respiratory system as well as the acid-base balance of the blood. The rate and depth of respirations may provide insight into the patient's pain intensity and level, anxiety or fear, or recent exertion.

SpO$_2$

The patient's SpO_2 level provides further insight as to the state of oxygenation.

Pain

Pain assessment includes the site of pain, characteristics of the pain, and strength of the pain, which can affect assessment of the other vital signs. Include any body language that may be exhibited supporting the idea that the patient is in pain, such as facial grimacing; rubbing, holding, or guarding any particular part of the body such as the abdomen or head; or any additional verbal sounds such as moaning. Pain can also direct you to problems in any of the body systems. The intensity and characteristics of pain can relate the severity of illness or injury and also detail the effectiveness of pain medication.

Neurological Examination

The vital signs also play a major role in a neurological assessment because they relate to function of the central nervous system, as all are controlled by the brain except the SpO_2. The medulla and the pons control the respiratory rate portion of oxygenation. The hypothalamus controls the body temperature and the autonomic nervous system, which controls the blood pressure and pulse. The medulla oblongata extends some control over the blood pressure and pulse.

Additional aspects of a basic neurological assessment will be performed throughout the head-to-toe process. However, when the components of the neurological assessment are performed together as a single assessment, this is commonly known as a *"neuro exam."* Box 21-3 lists all the components of a basic neurological examination. Skill 21-5 (page 450) details the steps of performing a basic neurological examination.

Head and Neck

As you begin the actual physical assessment, begin assessing at the head and work in a sequential order toward the toes. Begin by assessing the skin color, which provides data about the circulatory and respiratory systems. Pallor indicates poor circulation or anemia, while cyanosis indicates hypoxia.

Level of Consciousness

One of the first steps is to identify the patient's level of consciousness (LOC), a function of the neurological system. The LOC can be anywhere on a continuum from alert

Box 21-3

Components of a Basic Neurological Examination

The following are components of a *basic* neurological examination only. More advanced neurological evaluation can include various other assessments.
- Vital signs
- Level of consciousness
- Orientation to four spheres
- Pupil size, equality, and reaction to light
- Facial symmetry
- Speech clarity and appropriateness
- Response to simple commands
- Movement and strength of four extremities

to comatose. Note if the patient is awake or asleep. Is the patient alert or lethargic? **Lethargy** means drowsiness or mental sluggishness.

How do you determine if a patient is truly alert or if he or she is simply awake? A patient who is wide awake and responds to questions spontaneously is classified as alert. If the patient does not respond to verbal stimulus, the next level of stronger stimulus to use is tactile, or touch. If the patient still does not respond to the tactile stimulus, then you will use the third and strongest level of stimulus, which is pain. Slight pressure on the sternum or on a nailbed will produce discomfort. Careful use of one of the painful stimuli will determine if the patient is responsive or not. A patient who is heavily sedated may not respond, but otherwise, if the patient does not respond to a painful stimulus, the patient is considered to be *comatose*, or in a state of unconsciousness from which he or she cannot be aroused. The Glasgow Coma Scale, a scale used to assess LOC, is shown in Table 21-2.

If the patient is responsive to stimuli, you will then assess the patient's orientation level. There are four spheres of orientation to assess: person, place, time, and situation. To gather these data, ask the patient questions that will demonstrate the patient's knowledge regarding all four spheres. The easiest and most basic questions include questions similar to the following:

- **Person:** "What is your name?" or "Who is the President of the United States?"
- **Place:** "Can you tell me where you are?"
- **Time:** "What is today's date?" or "What day is it?"
- **Situation:** "What problem brought you to the hospital?" or "Do you know why you are here?"

Table 21-2 Glasgow Coma Scale

Function Assessed	Patient's Response	Score
Eye response	Opens spontaneously	4
	Opens to verbal command	3
	Opens to pain stimulus	2
	No response	1
Motor response	Reacts to verbal command	6
	Reacts to localized pain	5
	Flexes and withdraws from pain	4
	*Positions to decorticate posturing	3
	**Positions to decerebrate posturing	2
	No response	1
Verbal Response	Oriented, converses	5
	Disoriented, converses	4
	Uses inappropriate words	3
	Makes incomprehensible sounds	2
	No response	1

*Arms flexed to chest, hands clenched into fists and rotated internally, feet extended: Indicates problem is at or above the brainstem. Also known as *flexor posturing*.

**Arms extended, hands clenched into fists, wrists flexed, and forearms severely pronated (internally rotated): Indicates the problem is at the level of the midbrain or pons and is the more ominous of the two postures. Also known as *extension posturing*.

The total points possible ranges from 3 to 15. The highest possible score is 15, indicating the patient has full level of consciousness (LOC); is awake, alert, oriented, and follows simple commands. The lower the score, the higher the degree of neurological impairment.

Reprinted from Teasdale G, Jennett B. Assessment of coma and impaired consciousness: a practical scale. *Lancet.* 1974;304:81-84, with permission from Elsevier.

With practice and experience, you will learn to garner the same information from the conversation you have with the patient without having to ask the same questions each time you want to assess orientation. For example, the patient says, "The night nurse told me that Dr. Smith was going to discharge me either Tuesday or Wednesday." If this is accurate information, it is clear that the patient is oriented to person, place, time, and situation.

Documentation of LOC might appear as: *"awake, alert, oriented to person and time, disoriented to place and situation."* Using acceptable abbreviations to chart the same information would look something like this: *"AAO to person and time, disoriented to place and situation."* Documentation for a patient who is awake, alert, and oriented to all four spheres would look like this: *"AAOX4."*

Eyes

Next, assess the eyes. The sclera should be smooth, white, and glistening. In dark-skinned patients, the sclera may have a normal, slightly darker cast around the outside edges. Abnormalities might include redness or a bloodshot appearance, which can be a sign of inflammation, lack of sleep, or allergies. Yellowish-orange color of the sclera is normally an indication of elevated bilirubin, known as **jaundice**. Gently pull down the lower eyelids to observe the conjunctival sacs, which are normally pink and moist. Tissue redness, or *erythema,* may indicate inflammation and possibly infection. If the conjunctiva is receiving less oxygen than it requires, the naturally pink conjunctival sac may appear to be *cyanotic,* or blue. The cornea and lens should be clear and smooth. Older adults may have an opaque white ring around the outer edge of the cornea, known as *arcus senilis* (Fig. 21-5). Abnormalities include cloudiness, which is a sign of infection

or vitamin A deficiency, and opaqueness of the lens, which is usually a cataract. Young adults may have cataracts, but they occur more frequently in older adults.

Pupils

Normally pupils are black, round, between 3 and 7 mm diameter, and equal in size and reaction (Fig. 21-6). If the pupils are different sizes, it is called *anisocoria.* Unless it was a congenital abnormality that the patient was born with, anisocoria is indicative of neurological impairment. Observe the eyelids for drooping, or **ptosis**, of one side. This is most commonly associated with paralysis from a stroke.

After assessing the pupils for size and shape, you will use a penlight to assess equality of direct response to light, consensual response to light, and accommodation. To assess direct pupil response to light, dim the room lights, allowing the pupils to dilate slightly so they are easier to detect. Then briefly shine the penlight in one eye and observe the response of the pupil in that eye. Remove the light, allowing the pupil to dilate back to normal size. Then shine the light into the same eye a second time while observing the pupil in the opposite eye. It should constrict at the same rate and to the same size as the first pupil. Because the optic nerve divides or *bifurcates* at the distal end, stimulation of the nerve by shining a light in either eye should cause both pupils to rapidly constrict simultaneously and equally, known as the **consensual reflex** or *consensual response.* Repeat the process for the opposite eye.

Next, you will assess for the **accommodation response**. Hold your finger in front of the patient's face and ask the patient to focus on your finger as it moves. Slowly increase the distance between the patient's face and your finger to approximately 1.5 to 2 feet. The pupils should both dilate to allow in more light to see better at a distance. Then slowly move your finger closer to the patient's face until your finger nearly touches the patient's nose. The pupils should both constrict because they will not require entrance of as much light to see something up close. A difference in the rate of constriction or size of the pupils, failure to constrict simultaneously, or failure to accommodate are indications of neurological impairment. Document that the pupils are bilaterally brisk and equally reactive to light and accommodation as *"pupils equal* and *reactive* to *light* and *accommodation"* or **PERLA**.

Oral Mucous Membranes

Use a penlight to examine the oral mucous membranes for color, integrity, moisture, and odor. Normally the mouth, tongue, and gums should be intact, pink, and moist. A dry mouth is an indication of inadequate hydration, but it may also be a side effect of certain medications. Erythema is an

Figure 21-5a   Normal lens.

Figure 21-5b   Arcus senilis.

Figure 21-6   Pupil size in millimeters.

indicator of inflammation, and pallor is a sign of poor circulation or anemia. If the mucosa is erythematous and tender with white patches, it may be due to *Candida albicans,* a fungus commonly known as yeast. Cyanosis indicates either hypoxia or severe vasoconstriction.

Observe for ulcerations, lesions, coating of the tongue, bleeding of gums, and poor oral hygiene. Halitosis may be due to poor oral hygiene, stomach problems, or a sinus or oral infection. Small, painful ulcerations may be due to a virus, stress, or trauma. Painless ulcerations can be a sign of syphilis. White lesions and erythema of the tonsils are due to infection. Severe ulcerations or growths on the oral mucosa may be cancerous. An ulceration that has perforated the hard palate or roof of the mouth may be indicative of cocaine use (Fig. 21-7). Reddish-purple or hemorrhagic-appearing gums may be a sign of leukemia. Receding gums can be a sign of peridontal problems. A black, hairy appearance on the tongue indicates a fungal infection (Fig. 21-8), while a red, beefy-looking tongue is a sign of pernicious anemia (Fig. 21-9). A smooth, painful tongue is termed *glossitis* and can be due to inflammation or a side effect of medication.

Lips

Observe for *cheilitis,* or inflammation of the lips, as well as excessive dryness and cracking, all of which may be due to wind chapping, braces, dentures, dehydration, or seasonal allergies. A patient who repeatedly licks his or her lips or a patient who excessively applies lip balm may show the same

Figure 21-7 Perforation of hard palate as a result of cocaine use.

Figure 21-8 Black, hairy tongue caused by fungal infection.

Figure 21-9 Red, beefy tongue due to pernicious anemia.

signs of dryness or cracking. Sun exposure without sunscreen lip protection can also cause excessively dry and peeling lips. Fissures or cracking at the corners of the mouth are known as *cheilosis* and are usually related to vitamin B deficiencies.

If the lips are grossly swollen, especially if the edema occurred rapidly, the patient may have angioedema (Fig. 21-10), which is associated with serious allergic reactions such as anaphylaxis, a life-threatening allergic response. Allergic angioedema of the lips is usually seen along with other facial swelling and hives. It requires immediate medical treatment.

Lip color is also informative. Cherry-red lips may be a sign of carbon monoxide poisoning and acidosis. Pale lips are associated with anemia, but when the pallor is *circumoral,* meaning that it encircles the mouth area, it may indicate scarlet fever.

Dried mucus or food caked on the lips and teeth is termed **sordes** and can be easily treated with good oral hygiene. The objective data gathered in assessment of the lips provides you with information regarding the patient's nutritional status and hydration level.

Teeth

Does the patient have dentures? Is the patient without teeth, or *edentulous?* Inspect for excessive dental cavities, or *caries.* Are the teeth and mouth clean? Research has related poor oral hygiene to health care facility–acquired pneumonia

Figure 21-10 Angioedema caused by an allergic response.

as well as an increased risk of developing heart disease. Inquire if the patient has any difficulties chewing or eating. An elderly individual with dentures may not wear the dentures anymore because of poor fit. He or she may complain that the dentures rub sores when worn. Problems of this type may indicate special dietary needs.

Speech

Is the patient's speech appropriate, clear, and easy to understand? Or is it rambling, incoherent, inappropriate, or slurred? Some patients who have had strokes or other types of brain damage may be able to understand spoken and written words. The patient may even know what he or she wants to say, but cannot say the words. This is known as **aphasia** and is usually frustrating to the patient.

An individual who has difficulty coordinating and organizing the words correctly in a sentence may be suffering from an impairment known as **dysphasia**. Patients with dementia may have difficulty finding the right words to express themselves, often resulting in frustration and further confusion. Impairment of speech often is related to impairment of the central nervous system.

Neck

Are the jugular veins *distended,* or full enough that you can see them? If they are distended, this is indicative of fluid overload of the cardiovascular system, as in congestive heart failure (CHF). When you detect distended jugular veins, it necessitates further assessment, including auscultating breath sounds, weighing the patient, and reviewing the fluid intake and urine output for balance. Make note if the patient has a tracheostomy, as tracheostomies require special assessments and nursing care.

Dressings and Equipment on the Head and Neck

The patient may have dressings, incisions, supplemental oxygen, nasogastric tubes, tracheostomy tubes, or artificial airways in place on the head or neck. Assess their status and make certain all equipment is operating correctly.

Knowledge Connection

What findings can be noted by just observing as you enter the patient's room? Which vital signs provide information about each of the eight body systems mentioned? Which portion of the head and neck assessment pertains to the neurological system? The level of hydration? Circulation? What does PERLA stand for? Explain how to assess the consensual reflex and what it means. How is accommodation assessed?

Chest and Abdomen

Chest

As you move down to the chest area, observe the chest during respiration, noting the characteristics and pattern of respirations. Do they appear effortless? Or does the patient appear to have shortness of breath or difficulty breathing,

known as *dyspnea?* Does difficulty breathing in the supine position, known as **orthopnea**, force the patient to sit upright to ease the breathing? Even if you do not observe these problems, inquire if the patient has had any shortness of breath. Also ask the patient if he or she has a cough. If so, is it frequent or occasional? Is it a dry cough, known as a *nonproductive cough,* or does it produce sputum, known as a *productive cough?* If it is a productive cough, what amount of sputum is produced? Is it yellow, green, white, or clear, or is it blood-tinged? Is the sputum frothy or pink-tinged? Both of these are indicative of pulmonary edema as a result of worsening congestive heart failure. Blood-tinged sputum may be due to tuberculosis, and rust-colored sputum is common with pneumonia. Does the patient produce sputum each and every time he or she coughs? Or is it only a few times a day? Does the cough occur mostly at night? This is known as a *nocturnal* cough and may be a sign of pulmonary edema and congestive heart failure. Does the patient have to sleep sitting up due to orthopnea? This is often seen in patients with chronic obstructive pulmonary disease.

Also observe the respiratory rhythm and pattern. Is the breathing within normal parameters? If so, the term for this is *eupnea.* Or do you observe a pattern of respirations such as Biot's, Cheyne-Stokes, or Kussmaul's respirations? Table 21-3 lists different patterns of respirations and their meanings. Observe for equal chest expansion, or **excursion**, of both sides as the patient inhales. A more exact way to determine if the excursion of both sides of the chest is equal is to place both of your hands vertically on the patient's back with both thumbs on the spine at the level of the 9th or 10th ribs. Have the patient take a deep breath while observing the increasing distance that develops between your thumbs, noting whether both hands raise the same distance or not. Lack of or decreased excursion on one side of the chest can be caused by severe pneumonia or lung collapse, known as *atelectasis.* If one side does not expand, it might be documented as *"excursion absent on the [designated either left or right] side."* If the right side does expand, but not as well as the left side, you might document it as *"decreased excursion of right side"* or *"right side excursion less than left side."*

Note whether the patient uses the normal respiratory muscles (the diaphragm, chest, and abdominal muscles) or the accessory respiratory muscles (the sternocleidomastoid, scalene, trapezius, intercostal, and rhomboid muscles). Patients with chronic respiratory diseases such as emphysema often require use of these accessory respiratory muscles to breathe and develop a barrel-shaped chest. The shoulders should be the same height. Notice the shape of the anterior, lateral, and posterior aspects of the thorax. When viewing the thorax from the lateral view, there should be a slight convex curve of the midthoracic area and mild concave curve noted at the lumbar area. If the lumbar concavity is increased, it is known as *lordosis.* When the convexity of the midthorax is increased, it is called *kyphosis.* The older adult may develop severe kyphosis and a stooped posture, which must be taken into consideration when auscultating breath

Table 21-3 Respiratory Patterns

Pattern	Characteristics	When Seen?	Illustration
Eupnea	Normal rate and pattern: regular, equal-depth respirations.	Normal conditions	
Tachypnea	Increased respiratory rate.	Fever, stress, fear, anxiety, pain, exercise, hypoxia	
Bradypnea	Abnormally slow respiratory rate.	Opioid medications, sedatives, brain damage, metabolic alkalosis	
Kussmaul's	Abnormally deep and rapid respirations, rhythm regular, blows off excess CO_2.	Compensatory breathing mechanism seen during periods of metabolic acidosis	
Cheyne-Stokes	Cyclic breathing. Depth of respirations begin as very shallow, then each respiration gradually increases in depth until reaching a peak, at which time the depth begins to decrease with each breath until the depth is barely discernible. Then there is a period of apnea, from 5 to 20 seconds in length, after which the cycle begins again.	Increased intracranial pressure, brain damage, impending death	
Biot's	A sequence of several breaths of equal depth that alternate with periods of apnea.	Brain damage	
Apnea	Temporary or periodic absence of breathing.	Cheyne-Stokes respirations, sleep apnea, sudden infant death syndrome	

sounds and heart sounds. When viewing the spine from posterior, the vertebrae should be midline and straight. Curvature to either the left or right is called *scoliosis*.

Make note whether the patient's chest wall appears depressed, or sunken in, between the ribs or under the xiphoid process when the patient inhales. These abnormal movements are called **retractions** and indicate acute respiratory problems that need attention.

Landmarks for Auscultation
To accurately place the stethoscope for auscultation of breath and heart sounds, it is necessary to be familiar with the landmark terms and to know their locations (Fig. 21-11). Anteriorly, there are three vertical lines of reference: the

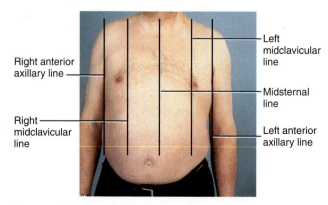

Figure 21-11a Vertical lines drawn to indicate anterior chest landmarks.

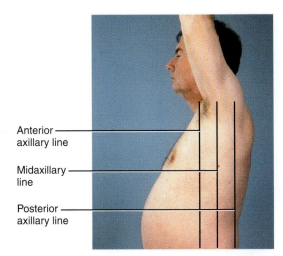

Figure 21-11b Vertical lines indicating lateral chest landmarks.

Figure 21-11c Vertical lines indicating posterior chest landmarks.

midsternal line and the left and right midclavicular lines. Laterally, there are also three vertical lines of reference: the anterior axillary line, midaxillary line, and posterior axillary line. Posteriorly, the three vertical lines include the midspinal line and the left and right scapular lines.

Auscultation of Breath Sounds

To help you hear the breath sounds, assist the patient to sit on the side of the bed or in the high Fowler's position. If the patient cannot sit up, try to place the patient in at least a semi-Fowler's position if tolerated. Otherwise, place the patient in the supine or lateral position for lung auscultation.

Warm the diaphragm or flat surface of the stethoscope with your hands. Place the diaphragm directly against the skin and listen from the top or apex of each lung to the base, alternating sides. Avoid listening through the gown or clothing; you will be able to hear more clearly and better detect abnormalities when the diaphragm is placed directly on the skin. Auscultate the breath sounds anteriorly, laterally, and posteriorly using the flat diaphragm side of your stethoscope. To perform this assessment correctly, you must know where the five lobes of the lungs are located.

Anatomy and Physiology Connection

The Lungs

Anteriorly, the superior, cone-shaped portion of each lung is known as the *apex* and extends approximately 1 inch above the medial aspect of the clavicle. The bottom, or base, of each lung is located at the sixth intercostal space in the midclavicular line. The bases extend down to the eighth intercostal space on the lateral aspect of the chest (Figs. 21-12 and 21-13). On the posterior aspect of the thorax, the apexes of the lungs begin at the first intercostal space, just below the first thoracic vertebrae. The bases of the lungs are located at approximately the tenth intercostal space, just below the tenth thoracic vertebrae, but extend down to the twelfth intercostal space upon deep inspiration. There are two lobes in the left lung and three lobes in the right lung, but only the upper and lower lobes can be auscultated posteriorly. The right middle lobe is positioned where it can *only* be accessed from the anterior and lateral aspects. The acronyms used to designate the five lobes are as follows: *LUL* is used for the left upper lobe, *LLL* for the left lower lobe, *RUL* for the right upper lobe, *RML* for the right middle lobe, and *RLL* for the right lower lobe.

When you auscultate breath sounds, listen for a complete respiration, both the inspiratory and expiratory phases, at each site. You should hear the air moving into the lungs and out of the lungs and there should be equality of breath sounds comparing the left to the right. As you move the stethoscope over different areas of the chest, listen to the pitch and duration of the sounds and the length of the inspiratory phase compared to the expiratory phase. Sounds heard over different portions of the chest will vary in these three characteristics.

The sounds heard over the bronchi, located under the manubrium, will have a shorter inspiratory and longer expiratory phase, and will sound louder and slightly harsher than other breath sounds. These are the bronchial breath sounds.

Over the middle chest and sternum, you will hear the bronchovesicular sounds, which have equal inspiration and expiration phases. They are quieter than the bronchial sounds and less harsh sounding.

The vesicular sounds can be heard over the periphery of the lungs. They have a longer inspiratory phase than expiratory, and are softer rustling sounds.

Abnormal and Adventitious Breath Sounds

If there are fewer breath sounds on one side, this is known as decreased breath sounds. When secretions and exudate from pneumonia solidify in lung tissues, this is known as

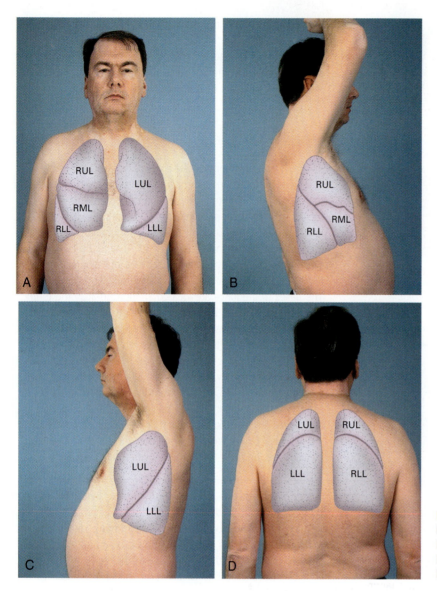

Figure 21-12 (A) Anterior view of both lungs' lobes. (B) Lateral view of right lung lobes. (C) Lateral view of left lung lobes. (D) Posterior view of both lungs' lobes.

consolidation, and may result in absence of breath sounds in that lobe. If there are no breath sounds, you will note them as absent. **Adventitious breath sounds** are those extra sounds superimposed over the normal breath sounds. They include crackles, rhonchi, wheezes, pleural friction rub, and stridor.

Crackles, also called *rales,* are discontinuous, usually heard during inspiration, and may be either fine or coarse. These adventitious breath sounds may be caused by the movement of air over secretions in the lung or the sudden opening of alveoli that have been closed. Crackles cannot be cleared by coughing. To learn to distinguish the sound of fine crackles, try rubbing several hairs together between your fingers just in front of your ear, and listen.

Rhonchi include sounds described as snoring, rattling, gurgling, squeaking, and low-pitched wheezes, caused by either secretions or partial occlusion of the airways. They are deeper and more rumbling sounds than crackles and are usually heard during expiration. Rhonchi are intermittent and may clear by having the patient cough. They can be caused by secretions in the airway, tumors, and partial airway obstruction.

Wheezes are continuous melodious, musical, or whistling sounds. They are due to constriction of the airways, and can be inspiratory or expiratory.

A *pleural friction rub* is a grating, creaking sound that is due to inflamed, edematous pleural surfaces rubbing together during breathing. These sounds are often heard during the first couple of days of lung inflammation.

Stridor can usually be heard with or without use of a stethoscope and is a sign of a life-threatening upper airway obstruction caused by a foreign body, tumor, swelling, or

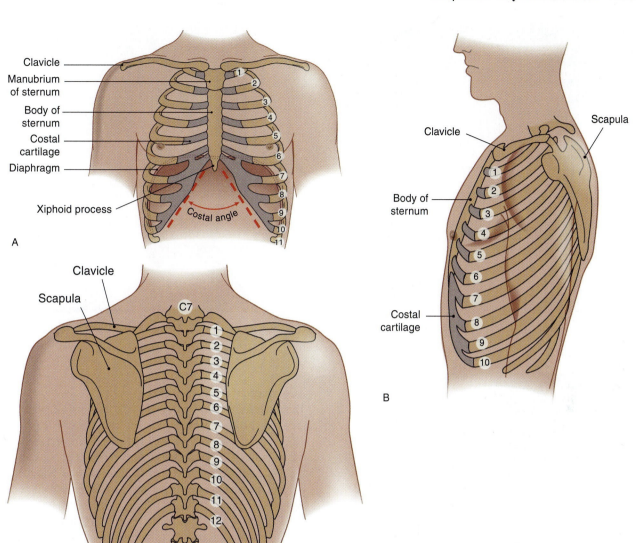

Figure 21-13 (A) Anterior view of chest with landmarks and ribs numbered. (B) Left lateral view of chest with landmarks and ribs numbered. (C) Posterior view of chest with landmarks and ribs numbered.

bronchial spasms. It is a shrill, high-pitched, harsh, crowing sound and requires immediate intervention. Small children who are prone to croup may present in the emergency room with stridor.

Placement of Stethoscope

Figure 21-14 illustrates the sequencing and positioning of stethoscope placement for auscultation of breath sounds. Anteriorly, listen to the apex of the left lung and then listen to the corresponding site on the right. The air movement should sound the same. If one side exhibits decreased or increased sounds compared to the other side, or exhibits adventitious sounds, make note. Then place the

stethoscope on the next lower intercostal space to listen, and then cross over to the corresponding space on the opposite side. You will be able to auscultate all five lobes on the anterior chest. Posteriorly, listen from the apexes of the lungs downward toward the bases, alternating from side to side.

The breath sounds provide objective data regarding the function of the respiratory system. To document that breath sounds were equal and clear to auscultation (CTA), meaning that no adventitious sounds or abnormalities were identified, chart something like *"breath sounds CTA in all 5 lobes."* Skill 21-6 (page 451) provides further details regarding auscultation of breath sounds.

Figure 21-14a Sequence of anterior auscultation sites.

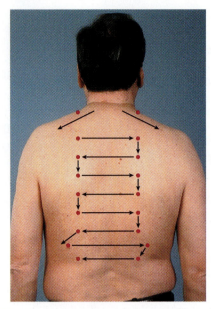

Figure 21-14c Sequence of posterior auscultation sites.

Figure 21-14b Sequence of lateral auscultation sites for both sides.

Knowledge Connection
What are the landmarks of the anterior, lateral, and posterior thorax? How many lobes are there in the lungs? Where can you access the sounds of each of these lobes: anteriorly, laterally, or posteriorly? What are the types of adventitious breath sounds? What does each mean? What intercostal space level indicates the bases of the lungs anteriorly? Posteriorly? How many sites of placement for the stethoscope are there for anterior assessment? Posterior assessment? What is the most life-threatening adventitious breath sound?

Auscultation of Heart Sounds

The preferred position to auscultate heart sounds is sitting, but they can also be heard using the left lateral or supine position. As you prepare to listen to the heart sounds, inspect the upper chest for an implanted pacemaker or central-line port. Either of these two devices when implanted under the skin will be visible as a firm, raised area in the shape of the implanted device. A port is a round device about 2 cm in diameter and provides continual IV access. A pacemaker is an approximately 3-cm by 4-cm rectangular-shaped box. It provides an automatic electrical impulse stimulus to initiate cardiac contraction when the patient's electrical conduction system is impaired.

Inspect and palpate the chest wall at the fifth intercostal space in the left midclavicular line for a pulsation. For most patients, this is the spot just inferior to the left nipple. It is easier to observe in thinner individuals. This location is known as the point of maximum impulse (PMI) because it is located over the apex of the left ventricle, which pumps the blood out of the heart to the rest of the body. This is the site where you can best hear the mitral valve, and where you will auscultate the apical pulse for rate, rhythm, and strength (Fig. 21-15). Three other sites are used to auscultate the heart sounds and hear the aortic, pulmonic, and tricuspid valves clearly:

- The aortic valve is best heard at the second intercostal space just to the right of the sternum and is known as the *right base heart sound.*
- The pulmonic valve can be auscultated at the second intercostal space just to the left of the sternum and is known as the *left base heart sound.*
- The tricuspid valve is best heard at the edge of the sternum, at the level of the fourth intercostal space just to the left of the sternum, and is known as the *left lateral sternal border (LLSB) heart sound.*

Figure 21-15 Cardiac auscultation sites.

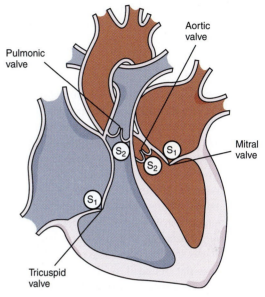

The first heart sound, known as the S_1 or *systolic sound,* is the louder, prolonged dull sound, usually of a lower frequency. Its source is ventricular contraction and the closure of the mitral and tricuspid valves. The S_1 is the "lubb" of the rhythmic *lubb-dupp* sound of the heartbeat.

After the S_1, there is a short pause before the second heart sound, the S_2. Also termed the *diastolic sound,* the S_2 is shorter and higher pitched than the S_1, and results from the closure of the aortic and pulmonary valves. The S_2 serves as the "dupp" of the *lubb-dupp* heart sound. Figure 21-16 illustrates where these sounds appear on an electrocardiogram.

Apical Pulse

The apical pulse (AP) is assessed for rate, rhythm, and strength. To assess the apical pulse, place the diaphragm of the stethoscope directly on the skin over the PMI and listen for both the S_1 and S_2 or "lubb-dupp." Remember, in identifying the S_1 and S_2, the S_1 will be the louder of the two sounds. The combination of the two sounds will equal one complete heartbeat. Some nurses find it helpful to close their eyes while auscultating heart sounds. This decreases sensory input and makes it easier to focus on the heart sounds.

Take the pulse for a full minute to provide a wider window of opportunity to detect abnormalities. Note the rate, and also compare the length of the intervals between the heartbeats. If they are all regularly or evenly spaced, the rhythm is said to be regular. If there is any variance in the length of time between beats, the rhythm is noted as irregular. The third assessment of the heart sounds is the strength of the beats. If both the S_1 and S_2 are clearly and distinctly heard, the strength may be documented as strong or distinct.

If you have a hard time hearing the apical pulse, have the patient lean forward and slightly to the left side, bringing the heart closer to the chest wall for better sound. If the sounds are still hard to hear or you can only hear one of the two sounds, document that the apical pulse strength is muffled or distant. A weak apical pulse may be a sign that the heart is not pumping adequately, as in congestive heart failure.

Figure 21-16 Occurrence of heart sounds shown on electrocardiogram. S_1 is heard at the beginning of systole. S_2 is heard at the beginning of diastole.

As you listen to the apical pulse, also feel the radial pulse (RP) to determine if they are the same rate. If the radial pulse is slower than the apical, it is documented as a *pulse deficit.* This is a common finding in patients with atrial fibrillation. If a pulse deficit is detected, seek another nurse to count the radial pulse at the same time you are counting the apical pulse to determine how many beats' difference there is between the two pulses. Once you are more experienced, you may become skilled enough to count both the apical rate and the number of skips at the radial site without the assistance of a second nurse, but it generally works best to utilize a second nurse to assist you. If there is a pulse deficit, be certain to also document it: for example, *"AP – 71, RP – 67, pulse deficit of 4."*

If you hear extra heart sounds, they may be due to a murmur. A *murmur* may present as a swishing, rumbling, or blowing sound and may be soft, loud, or booming. Some murmurs are normal, especially in children and young adults. Other murmurs are indicators of valvular problems. Murmurs may be heard during systole or diastole and are classified on a scale of 1 to 6. Murmurs are often difficult to auscultate, especially for the inexperienced nurse. As you progress in your clinicals and learn more about medical-surgical diseases, you will begin to increase your skills at murmur detection. As you begin clinicals, simply listen carefully and, if you think you are hearing extra heart sounds, solicit assistance from your instructor to clarify the sounds you hear. Skill 21-7 (page 452) presents further detail regarding auscultation of heart sounds.

Knowledge Connection

What is the PMI? Where do you assess the base heart sounds? The apical pulse? What are the names of the two heart sounds? How long do you listen to assess the apical rate? What is a pulse deficit?

Abdomen

As you progress down from the chest, you will next assess the abdomen. You will begin with inspection, move to auscultation of bowel sounds, and finally end with palpation and percussion if desired. This particular sequence of assessing the abdomen should always be followed. It is important that you auscultate the bowel sounds before you palpate the abdomen. If you deviate from the sequence and palpate the abdomen before auscultating the bowel sounds, you can stimulate bowel sounds that were not originally present, creating inaccuracy in your assessment findings.

First, inspect the shape and size of the abdomen, noting whether it is flat, rounded, or distended. Be certain to also gather subjective data by asking the patient if there is any problem with pain, indigestion, gas, nausea, vomiting, or *anorexia* (a lack of appetite). Anorexia, with its lack of nutritional intake, may contribute to decreased immunity. As people age, metabolism slows, activity decreases, and calorie requirements naturally decrease. Therefore, the appetite of older adults decreases over time. Be cautious and do not confuse a naturally lighter appetite of an older adult with anorexia. Also, a small child obviously will not require the amount of caloric intake needed by a teenager or adult.

Bowel Sounds

After visualization of the abdomen, auscultate the bowel sounds with the stethoscope, using the diaphragm. Mentally divide the abdomen in four equal quadrants, using the umbilicus as the midpoint (Fig. 21-17).

Begin listening in the right lower quadrant (RLQ), then the right upper quadrant (RUQ), then the left upper quadrant (LUQ), and lastly the left lower quadrant (LLQ). This pattern will track the ascending colon up to the transverse colon, and then to the descending colon and sigmoid. Place the stethoscope firmly against the skin and listen for clicks or gurgles. These are the sounds of *peristalsis,* the wave-like muscular contractions of the intestines that move intestinal contents through the alimentary canal, where absorption of nutrients and water takes place, toward the rectum for elimination.

There should be between 5 and 30 clicks or gurgles per minute in each of the four quadrants, and they should be somewhat high-pitched, which is known as *active* bowel sounds. Fewer than five clicks or gurgles per minute in any

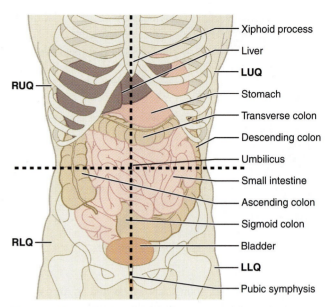

Figure 21-17 The four abdominal quadrants.

Labels: Xiphoid process; Liver; **LUQ**; RUQ; Stomach; Transverse colon; Descending colon; Umbilicus; Small intestine; Ascending colon; Sigmoid colon; RLQ; Bladder; **LLQ**; Pubic symphysis

quadrant is termed *hypoactive* bowel sounds, the result of slowed peristalsis, which can be caused by opioids, anesthesia, bedrest or decreased physical activity, infection in the peritoneal cavity, and bowel obstruction. The slower the peristalsis, the longer food remains in the intestines; this allows the large intestine to absorb more of the water from the food, making the remaining waste drier and harder. Therefore, a patient with hypoactive bowel sounds is more prone to constipation. More than 30 clicks or gurgles per minute is termed *hyperactive* bowel sounds and is the result of excessive peristalsis. Hyperactive bowel sounds may result from intestinal infection, irritable bowel disease, early bowel obstruction, and laxatives. This state of hyperactivity can cause cramping and rapid passage of food through the alimentary canal so that the colon does not have time to absorb the water from the digested food, leaving it in a liquid form to be expelled via the rectum, known as diarrhea. Some inflammatory diseases cause such excessive hyperactivity of the bowel that there is poor food absorption as a result of the severe diarrhea. If *gurgling* bowel sounds are loud enough to hear without a stethoscope, it is termed *borborygmus.*

A complete absence of bowel sounds may be due to late bowel obstruction, infection of the peritoneal cavity, or a paralytic ileus postoperatively. Therefore, it is important to be absolutely certain about a complete absence of bowel sounds. To be certain, listen for at least 3 to 5 minutes in each abdominal quadrant. This may seem like an excessively long time, but an absence of bowel sounds is significant and you must be certain before declaring that there are none.

Older adults may complain of not being able to control expulsion of flatus, because the rectal sphincter loses some of its elasticity, thereby decreasing voluntary control. Intestinal peristalsis also slows, increasing the risk of constipation.

Next, palpate the four quadrants of the abdomen to determine whether the abdomen is soft, firm, or hard. (Box 21-4 lists contraindications to palpation.) Observe for flinching, grimacing, or guarding while palpating. **Guarding** is the defense mechanism of tightening the abdominal muscles to prevent further compression of tender or inflamed areas. Ask the patient if the palpation elicits any pain or discomfort. Note any masses that may be felt.

Skin

Skin is assessed throughout the examination, as different areas of the body are exposed. The examination of the chest and abdomen is a particularly good time to further assess the skin. Assess for numbness or decreased sensation, known as **paresthesia**; if present, it indicates some type of nerve impairment, commonly seen as a complication of diabetes and as a result of a stroke.

Color

Skin color may vary from culture and ethnicity as well as from genetics. What color is the skin? Does it exhibit its normal pink, olive, tan, or brown tones? Or is it pale, lighter, or whiter than usual? As in the mucous membranes, pallor of the skin indicates decreased circulation or anemia. Individuals with dark skin usually have lips of a lighter color than the rest of the skin on the face. Though pallor can normally be detected on a dark-skinned person, the mucous membranes and nailbeds are the best indicator of circulation. Elderly patients often have numerous spots of yellowish-brown discoloration caused by years of sun exposure, known as *solar lentigines.* The older patient may refer to them as "liver spots." Box 21-5 lists skin color descriptors.

Temperature and Moisture

Skin is normally warm and dry. When assessing skin temperature, use the dorsal side of the hand because it is more sensitive. Is the skin warm or cool? Is it dry or moist? Moisture that can be felt on the skin surface may be due to fever, exertion, or even anxiety. If the patient is perspiring, he or she is considered *diaphoretic.* If the skin is hot, further assessment is needed. Is the room temperature comfortable? Has the patient had too many blankets as covering? Does the patient have a fever? If the skin is too cool or cold, further assessment is again needed. Is it due to environmental temperature or poor circulation?

Box 21-4

Contraindications to Abdominal Palpation

There are certain situations and conditions when it may be contraindicated to palpate a patient's abdomen. Never palpate the abdomen of a patient who:
- Has a known or suspected abdominal aortic aneurysm
- Has had an organ transplant
- Is known or suspected to have a Wilms' tumor (more common in children than in adults), as palpation may cause seeding or spreading of the tumor into the abdomen

Box 21-5

Skin Color Descriptors

Skin color provides you with data regarding multiple body system functions and is helpful in diagnosing certain conditions and disease processes. Skin color provides data related to the cardiovascular circulation as well as the efficiency of the respiratory system at providing adequate gas exchange of oxygen and carbon dioxide. It can serve as an indicator of liver disease and inflammation and infection. Below is a partial list of skin color descriptors and their possible *etiologies* (causes).
- **Pale:** a lighter color, more white than usual. If not the patient's normal "fair coloring," indicates poor circulation, anemia.
- **Erythematous:** redness of a designated site. Usually a sign of inflammation due to the increased circulation to the inflamed site.
- **Flushed:** widespread, diffuse red color of face; possibly includes the body. Usually caused by fever, embarrassment, exertion, or sunburn.
- **Jaundiced:** yellow or orange coloring of the skin and mucous membranes, easily detected in the sclera and palm of the hands. Jaundice is caused by liver impairment.
- **Cyanotic:** bluish-gray color of the skin and mucous membranes. Due to hypoxia and extreme vasoconstriction.
- **Ecchymotic:** Caused by bruising of the skin. Fresh bruises are bluish-purple; older bruises turn greenish-yellow as they begin to resolve.
- **Bronzing:** bronze pigmentation of the skin. Due to disorders of iron metabolism. Iron pigments are deposited in the body tissues.

Turgor

Evaluate the skin *turgor,* or elasticity, which is an indicator of hydration level in all ages of patients except elders. The skin of elderly patients loses its elasticity and is not a reliable assessment tool for hydration. Skin that has been exposed to the sun over the years is also considered not reliable because sunlight causes the skin to loose its elasticity. Gently pinch a fold of skin over the sternum or just below the clavicle between your index finger and thumb. Then release the skin; it should recoil immediately if the patient is well hydrated. If the skinfold remains *tented* for several seconds after release, it is considered to be nonelastic or to have slow recoil, a sign that may indicate a state of dehydration.

Integrity

Under normal conditions, the skin is intact without breaks or discontinuity. Assess whether the skin is intact, paying special attention to the pressure points as you continue to assess the rest of the body. Are there any areas of erythema and potential breakdown? Are there lesions or rashes? Older patients often have very thin and fragile skin, often so thin that it appears to be translucent and feels like tissue paper. Extra care must be taken during all aspects of nursing care for these individuals. It may take nothing more than a bump against a bed rail or wheelchair to cause a skin tear. Tape and bandage removal are frequent culprits causing skin tears in older adults. Care must be taken when removing tape; use of an adhesive remover is recommended. Any break in skin integrity, the first line of protection from microorganisms, will reduce the patient's ability to prevent infection.

Bowel and Bladder Status

Is the patient continent or incontinent of urine? When performing an initial shift assessment, it is important to determine when the patient last voided or urinated because the maximum time the patient should be allowed to go without voiding is 8 hours. If it has been close to 8 hours since the patient voided, palpate just above the symphysis pubis to determine if the bladder is distended, which would require intervention. If the patient has a Foley catheter, assess its patency, whether it is secured properly to the thigh, and the amount, color, and clarity of the urine. The kidneys should produce a minimum of 30 mL of urine per hour. Amounts less than 30 mL/hr indicate that the patient is severely dehydrated and needs fluids or that the patient's kidneys are not functioning properly, as in renal failure. Ask the patient if there is any problem with urination, such as burning, urgency, or frequency. These assessments provide you information regarding renal system function as well as information related to level of hydration.

When assessing young children, especially infants, an inadequate urinary output is even more significant because they normally have a higher body fluid ratio to maintain than do adults. This means that inadequate intake of fluids or smaller losses of fluid due to diarrhea or vomiting have a much higher and accelerated rate of dehydrating them to dangerous levels. Decreased urinary output may be severe enough to require IV fluids to prevent serious complications from dehydration. The older adult also dehydrates easier than the average adult and requires close observation of fluids taken in and urine output to maintain fluid and electrolyte balance.

Ask when the patient last had a bowel movement, and ask about the amount, color, and consistency of the stool. It is standard to make certain that each patient does not go longer than 3 days without having a bowel movement. The changes in dietary habits, source of drinking water, medications, and activity level that come with being hospitalized are enough to cause some patients to become constipated. Some elderly patients use laxatives on a daily basis and have become dependent upon them to have bowel movements, thus making it important to be aware of their laxative habits. These elimination problems can be avoided with regular assessment followed by appropriate nursing interventions.

If the patient has a colostomy or ileostomy, assess the stoma for erythema, edema, and excoriation, and assess for drainage bag intactness and content. You will learn more about stoma care in Chapter 30.

Unless the patient has a Foley catheter or some known problem of the perineal or anal area, these areas are normally not visualized until perineal care is provided or a bed bath is administered, or unless the patient is incontinent. If the patient is bedridden or incontinent, the perineum, coccyx, and buttocks should be assessed for cleanliness,

dryness, and integrity of the skin. Note any vaginal drainage, including color, amount, consistency, and odor.

Dressings and Equipment on the Chest or Abdomen

If the patient has telemetry electrodes, a chest tube, a surgical incision, a dressing, a drain, a binder, or any other piece of equipment attached to the chest or abdomen, assess it while you are in the vicinity for status or proper function.

Knowledge Connection

What is the order in which palpation, inspection, and auscultation should be performed on the abdomen? What are the four acronyms used to indicate the four sections of the abdomen? What is the longest period of time a patient should go without voiding? Without having a bowel movement?

Extremities

Assess the extremities for intact skin, erythema over pressure points, circulation, movement, coordination, strength, and joint flexibility.

Upper Extremities

Assess the peripheral pulses in both wrists for strength and equality. Are both radial pulses palpable? Do they both feel strong or weak, and is this strength equal on both the right and left side? Strength of peripheral pulses is documented using a scale of 0 to 3 and should include whether they are equal in strength (Box 21-6). This assessment provides you data about the circulatory system's function and fluid volume. A weak pulse may be a sign of decreased plasma volume as in hemorrhage or shock, or decreased pumping ability of the heart, or problems with the heart's electrical conduction system. An absent pulse indicates some type of blockage or lack of blood perfusion to the extremity due to inadequate pumping capacity of the heart. A bounding radial pulse can be related to hypertension or excess fluid volume.

After assessing the radial pulses, assess the patient's ability to freely move both arms and flex all joints. Note if

Box 21-6
Peripheral Pulse Scale

Peripheral pulses are assessed to determine not only their presence but also their strength. This provides you with data regarding the efficiency of the heart's pumping ability to deliver or *perfuse* blood to the farthest pulse sites from the heart. The following scale is commonly used to designate the strength of the peripheral pulses:

0	not able to palpate
1+	weak
2+	strong
3+	full, bounding

there is tightening and shortening of muscles that prevent full extension of joints, known as *contractures,* which provides data about the musculoskeletal system. Then hold out your hands with the index and middle finger extended on each hand, crossing your hands at the wrists. Ask the patient to squeeze your two fingers with each hand to test the grip strength. Note whether it is weak or strong and whether the grips are equal bilaterally. This assessment provides you with information regarding both the neurological and the musculoskeletal systems. It tells you whether the brain and the nerves are working together correctly to process your verbal instruction and deliver the impulse to the muscles, as well as the muscular strength of the hands.

Assess the color of the nailbeds. They should be pink if there is good circulation and if an ample supply of oxygen is being delivered to the tissues of the upper extremities. Cyanosis indicates hypoxia, and pallor signifies decreased blood flow to the extremity. This provides you with data regarding both the circulatory and the respiratory systems. Using the tip of your thumb, *gently* compress a nailbed on the patient's hand, emptying the capillaries of blood and causing the nailbed to turn white. Release the pressure and observe the length of time it takes the capillaries to refill with blood and turn the nailbed pink once again. Repeat the procedure on the other hand. The normal time for color return is 3 seconds or less in an adult and 5 seconds or less in elderly individuals. This assessment is known as the *capillary refill time* and serves as one indicator of adequate arterial circulation to the periphery. The elderly patient frequently has thickened and yellowed nails that make it difficult or impossible to blanch the nail bed, but there is another way to check capillary refill time in these patients. Simply press on the tip of one of the patient's fingers until it blanches. Release the pressure and count how many seconds before the color returns to pink. Also assess for clubbing of the fingertips; this may be indicative of chronic respiratory disease (Fig. 21-18).

Lower Extremities

Now move to the legs and feet and assess for the presence of edema. Recall that edema is the result of excess fluid shifting out of the cardiovascular space into the interstitial space between the individual cells. It may be due to a number of factors, such as hypertension, fluid volume retention or overload, inadequate blood level of albumin to maintain enough osmotic pull to hold fluid within the vascular system, inflammation of the lower extremities, or inadequate pumping of the heart, which would allow fluid to back up in the venous side of the vascular system. As fluid backs up in the vasculature, it increases hydrostatic pressure and forces excessive fluid through the capillary walls into the interstitial spaces. If edema is present, how much is there? Is it pitting edema (Fig. 21-19)? (Box 21-7 presents a pitting edema scale.) Where does the edema begin and end? Is it restricted to just the ankles, or does it extend from the toes to the midcalf or to the thigh?

Figure 21-18 Clubbing of fingertips.

Next assess the color of the legs and feet. Pallor of the legs and feet may be a sign of inadequate circulation to the lower extremities, which can be due to inadequate blood volume or vasoconstriction. A general erythema of the lower leg or foot may be indicative of inflammation or a blockage of the venous return, which can force an excessive volume of blood to remain in the lower extremity, making the extremity appear redder than normal. Cyanosis, or a bluish color, would be indicative of inadequate delivery of oxygen to the lower extremity. This could be the result of an arterial blockage, inadequate oxygen saturation of the blood's hemoglobin, inadequate blood volume due to hemorrhage or shock, or inadequate pumping of the heart, which fails to deliver sufficient oxygen-carrying blood to the feet. As you

Box 21-7

Pitting Edema

To assess for pitting edema, press the patient's skin over a bony prominence with your fingertip and hold for approximately 2 seconds, and then release the pressure. Pitting edema will leave a fingerprint even after removing your finger. The depth of the depression determines the amount of pitting edema present and can be measured using the following scale:

- **Trace pitting edema:** Minimal indention noted when pressure is applied; refills as soon as finger pressure is removed.
- **1+ pitting edema:** Slight indention depth of 2 mm; lasts no longer than 15 seconds after removing finger pressure.
- **2+ pitting edema:** Indention depth of 4 mm; lasts no longer than 15 seconds after removing finger pressure.
- **3+ pitting edema:** Indention depth of 6 mm; lasts a full minute after removing finger pressure.
- **4+ pitting edema:** Indention depth of 8 mm; lasts 2 minutes or longer after removing finger pressure.

Figure 21-19 Pitting edema of the foot.

can see, these assessments for color and edema provide a large volume of data relating to the circulatory system's function.

Assess for the other signs for which you assessed in the hands. Further assess circulation to the feet by feeling for the skin temperature of the lower extremities. Apply the dorsal surface of your hands to the lower legs and feet, noting whether they are warm or cool. If they are cooler than the legs or if one foot is cooler than the other, assess further. Were the patient's feet uncovered? Does the patient have peripheral vascular disease, a disease that impairs circulation to the extremities?

Assess both pedal pulses for strength and equality. They normally are strong and equal bilaterally. If you are unable to palpable the pedal pulse in either one of the feet, move up the extremity to palpate the posterior tibialis. If the posterior tibialis is not palpable, move up the leg to assess for the popliteal pulse. If it is not detected, assess for a femoral pulse. Once you have identified the most distal pulse that you can palpate, obtain a Doppler ultrasound machine and assess the pulse sites at which you were not able to palpate a pulse to ensure that there is adequate arterial circulation to the foot. It is imperative, in the absence of pulse detection by palpation, that you can identify which peripheral pulses can be obtained with Doppler ultrasound before notifying the physician.

Another assessment for circulation is the capillary refill time of the toenail beds. The normal refill time is the same as for the hands: In adults the capillaries should refill and turn pink again in 3 seconds or less, though in the elderly it may take up to 5 seconds. Any extremity with inadequate blood flow or oxygen delivery to the tissues has a reduced ability to prevent or fight infection.

To test neurological control and strength of the lower extremities, assess plantar flexion strength. Place the palms of your hands on the bottom or plantar side of the patient's feet. Ask the patient to press the soles of his or her feet against the palms of your hands. Note whether the movement is weak or strong or absent, and whether it is equal bilaterally. Now, lay the palms of your hands over the dorsal aspects of both feet and apply firm pressure. Then direct the patient to pull the toes of both feet toward his or her head while you provide resistance. Again, assess for the strength of this dorsiflexion and whether the strength is equal bilaterally. As with the upper extremities, this assessment provides you with information regarding both the neurological and the musculoskeletal systems. It tells you whether the brain and the nerves are working together correctly to process your verbal instruction and deliver the impulse to the muscles, as well as the muscular strength of the feet. An example of one cause of either a weaker or absent flexion on one side is a cerebrovascular accident (stroke).

Dressings and Equipment Applied to the Upper or Lower Extremities

Assess any dressings, IV access, dialysis shunts, antiembolism stockings, elbow or heel protectors, alternating compression devices, casts, splints, and any other equipment or supplies attached to any of the extremities to determine their condition or status, to ensure their proper function, and to monitor for signs and symptoms indicating possible adverse reactions or complications. Also make note if the patient is on any type of specialty bed, such as an eggcrate mattress overlay or an air-fluidized bed. These beds represent interventions for preventing skin breakdown and increasing comfort.

Knowledge Connection

What colors would be abnormal for the nailbeds? What would each abnormality signify? Compare the assessment of dorsiflexion to plantar flexion. Describe what to do if you are unable to palpate a pedal pulse. What supplies or equipment should also be assessed?

Needs and Comfort

A patient may have many and varied needs, and you will be responsible for meeting those needs. These needs are assessed as you perform the shift head-to-toe assessment (Box 21-8).

As you complete your assessment, give the patient one last opportunity to report any problems. Ask again if the patient is having any discomfort or pain. Inquire if the patient needs anything. If intake of fluid needs to be encouraged, ask the patient what fluids he or she likes. Provide one of the drinks of choice and remind the patient of the importance of adequate fluid intake. If the patient is on bedrest or requires assistance to get up, is on intake and output monitoring, or is NPO or on restricted oral fluids, remind the patient of these restrictions. Document any reinforcement or patient teaching that you provide along with the patient's

Box 21-8

Needs Assessment

Each individual will have various needs that will impact his or her health status and ability to heal. It will be your responsibility to assess for all possible needs of each patient, including those needs that may not be medical.

Oxygen and Circulatory Needs
- Respirations within normal ranges for rate, depth, effort, and pattern?
- SpO$_2$ adequate?
- Need for supplemental oxygen?
- Alert and oriented?
- Blood pressure within normal parameters?
- Pulse within normal parameters for rate, rhythm, and strength?
- Breath sounds clear to auscultation?
- Heart sounds distinct?
- Jugular vein distention?
- Peripheral pulses strong and equal bilaterally?
- Have a pacemaker or automatic defibrillator?
- Bruise easily?

Nutritional and Fluid Needs
- Today's weight? Weight gain or loss?
- Food preferences, including cultural considerations?
- Appetite?
- Dentures or edentulous?
- Food allergies?
- On a prescribed special diet? Patient compliant with diet?
- Presence of edema?
- Volume of fluid drunk in last 24 hours?
- Need input and output recorded?
- Nausea, vomiting, diarrhea, fluid losses?
- Special tubes such as nasogastric or gastrostomy tubes that affect fluid losses?

Safety and Security Needs
- Need for side rails to be up?
- Use of assistive devices?
- Prosthesis?
- Ability to communicate? Language barriers?
- Cultural barriers restricting care?
- Disorientation?
- Sensory deficits, such as deafness, aphasia, blindness, or paresthesia?

- Pain?
- Paralysis?
- Anxiety relating to hospitalization, child care, job security while hospitalized, cost of hospitalization, or disease prognosis?

Psychosocial and Cultural Needs
- Fears or anxieties?
- Depression?
- Pain?
- Coping strategies?
- Family or other support system?
- Social services needs?
- Cultural or religious differences needs?
- Need to contact spiritual advisor?
- Psychological consult required?
- Any concerns?
- Knowledge deficit?

Elimination Needs
- Amount and characteristics of urinary output?
- Amount, characteristics, and frequency of bowel movements?
- Any change in bowel habits?
- Able to perform act of elimination without assistance?
- Incontinent or continent?
- Foley catheter? Suprapubic catheter?
- Colostomy or urostomy?
- Use of diuretics or laxatives?

Rest and Activity Needs
- Tolerance for performance of activities of daily living, such as hygiene, toileting, feeding, and ambulation?
- Balance and equilibrium okay?
- Number of hours of sleep required?
- Sleeping aids utilized?

Grooming Needs
- Able to perform activities of daily living, such as bathing; oral, skin, nail, and hair care; shaving; toileting; feeding; and ambulation?
- Preferences for bathing, including time of day, type of bath?

response. *Safety: Return the bed to its lowest level and raise the bed rails. Position the patient's call light, water carafe, telephone, tissues, and any other items the patient might need within easy reach.* Inform the patient as to when you will return, and encourage the patient to push the call light if there is anything you can provide or do.

Documentation of Assessment Findings

All assessment findings must be documented as soon as possible. Some hospitals use computerized documentation, while others still use handwritten documentation. Each facility will have a specific policy and procedures to follow. Whether the documentation is computerized or not, there will be designated forms to complete for initial head-to-toe shift assessments. Some facilities will use a flow sheet or checklist format (Fig. 21-20). Other facilities may use a form that requires more narrative description (Fig. 21-21). An admission assessment form is normally 3 to 4 pages in length, with some checklists and some narrative sections. An example of this type of form may be found in the student workbook. For further assistance with documentation of assessments, see Chapter 5.

PATIENT FLOW SHEET (PT STAMP)

	Date: 9/16/11	0700	0800	0900	1000	1100	1200	1300	1400	1500	1600	1700	1800	1900	2000	2100	2200	2300	2400	0100	0200	0300	0400	0500	0600
Care Given	Doctor's Visit		✓																						
	Activity		CH	BB	AMB		CH		BR	AMB															
	Vital signs	✓			✓																				
	AM Care			✓																					
	Turn R-right L-left S-supine P-prone	R		S		L		S		R															
	Dressing Wound Care	n/a																							
	IV Therapy	n/a																							
	% of Diet		90				100																		
Skin	Skin Intact	✓																							
	Warm-Dry/ Color WNL	✓																							
	Comfort Measures	HP						HP																	
Neuro/Sensory	Alert & Oriented	✓																							
	Denies Pain	✓																							
	Denies Anxiety	✓																							
Respiratory	O₂ Therapy	n/a																							
	Breath Sounds Clear & Regular	✓																							
	TC & DB/IS	n/a																							
CV	Pulse Regular	P			P																				
	Heart Tones	CL																							
	Telemetry # ___	n/a																							
GI	Abdomen Soft	✓																							
	Bowel Sounds Present	✓					→																		
	BM								lg.																
Renal	Urine Clear	✓					→																		
	Foley Patent	✓					→																		
M/S	Moves All Extremities	✓																							
Safety	Side Rails Up	✓		✓		✓		✓	✓																
	Call Light in Reach	✓		✓		✓	✓	✓	✓																
	Bed in Low Position	✓		✓		✓		✓	✓																
Other	Braden Scale																								
	Nurse's Initials/ Signature	LL		*L. Ludwig, RN*																					
	Nurse's Initials/ Signature																	RN Assessment / Time							

CHARTING LEGEND
– = Within Normal Limits
X = problem, see NN
→ = no change
p = exception is normal for patient
n/a = not applicable

ACTIVITY KEY (x1 or x2 = NURSES ASSISTING)
BED = bedrest
DAN = dangle
CH = chair
AMB = ambulate
BR = bathroom
TUB = tub
ASL = asleep
BP = bedpan
B/B = bedbath
AST = assist
SHR = shower
BSC = bedside commode

O₂ KEY
NC = nasal cannula
M = mask
NRB = non-rebreather mask

HEART TONES KEY
CL = clear
DIM = diminished

COMFORT MEASURES
EM = eggcrate mattress
HP = heel protectors

WOUND DRESSING KEY
– = dry and intact
D = dressing ▲
SLC = suture line care
I = irrigation

IV KEY
IP = patent
D = dressing ▲
TU = tubing ▲
HL = hep lock
C = central line

Figure 21-20 Assessment flow sheet or checklist form.

Date:	Progress Note
8/24/10	0630 Lying supine with eyes closed. Snoring softly. Awakened to calling name.
	BP-116/68 T-99.6°F P-68 reg & strong R-15 reg & even. SpO₂ 97% on
	room air. Complains of aching in lumbar area of back, a 3 on a scale of 0-10.
	Denies need of pain med. Alert & oriented to 4 spheres. States slept well
	last night. Pearla. Sclera white & clear. Conjunctival sacs pink & moist. Oral
	mucosa is pink and moist, without lesions. No neck vein distention. Skin is
	pink, warm, dry, with elastic turgor. Respirations regular & even, with equal
	chest excursion. Breath sounds auscultated, all lobes CTA except fine rales
	in RLL. Heart sounds auscultated, AP 68, reg. & distinct. Denies cough since
	yesterday morning. Abdominal dressing clean, dry, & intact. Bowel sounds
	active in RLQ RUQ LUQ and hypoactive in LLQ. Abdomen flat & soft to
	palpation. Denies discomfort with palpation. Denies any further nausea
	since yesterday. States he is tolerating oral fluids without problems.
	Encouraged to drink at least 1200 mL on this shift. Acknowledged verbally
	he would. States his last BM was 2 days ago, but feels as if he will have one
	this morning. Foley catheter intact, patent, & draining clear, medium yellow
	urine to gravity. Denies discomfort. Catheter secured to thigh. IV in right
	wrist, 1000 mL D51/2NS infusing per pump at 80 ml/hr. Site is clean, dry,
	without edema, erythema, or tenderness. 4 ext. warm, pink, dry. No edema
	noted. Peripheral pulses strong & bilaterally equal in all 4 ext. Has full
	ROM x4 ext. Strong & equal hand-grips bilaterally. Strong & equal dorsal &
	plantar flexion bilaterally. Cap refill less than 3 seconds in all 4 ext. -------------
	---W. Weaver, LPN

Figure 21-21 Initial head-to-toe shift assessment documented in narrative format.

Skill 21-1 Measuring a Patient's Height

Assessment Steps

1. Assess whether the patient is able to stand unassisted.

Planning Steps

1. Obtain a platform scale or a wheelchair if the patient must be transported to the scale's location.

Implementation Steps

1. Follow the Initial Implementation Steps located on the inside front cover.
2. At the scale, remove the patient's shoes and have him or her step up on the scale with his or her back to the platform scale.

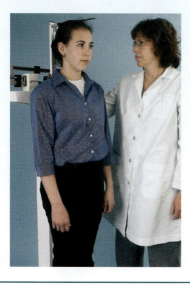

3. Raise the sliding ruler above the back of the patient's head and extend the height bar.
4. Carefully lower the height bar until it touches the highest point between the two parietal bones of the skull.
5. Have the patient step forward and off the scale without raising the height bar.
6. Read the height in feet and inches or centimeters according to facility policy.
 Note: The height will not be read at the top of the sliding ruler, but will be read at the point where the sliding ruler extends from its track.
7. Assist the patient back to bed as needed.
8. Follow the Ending Implementation Steps located on the inside back cover.

Evaluation Steps

1. Compare the patient's height to his or her weight, noting excessive or inqdequate weight for the height.

Sample Documentation

4/4/12   1000   Ht. 5 ft 9 in. ————————————
———————————— *Nurse's signature and credentials*

Skill 21-2 Measuring a Patient's Weight

Assessment Steps

1. Assess whether the patient's bed has built-in bed scales.
2. Assess the patient and the medical record *to ensure that the patient is allowed out of bed and is able to stand alone if platform scales are to be used.*
3. Review the medical record to assess the patient's previous weight *so that you can compare the current weight to determine whether there is a gain or loss.*

Planning Steps

1. Obtain a portable scale if necessary or a wheelchair if the patient must be transported to the scale's location.
2. If weight is to be assessed on a daily basis, plan to weigh the patient at the same time every day, such as before breakfast, *so that the weights will more accurately reflect gains or losses.*
3. Plan to consistently weigh the patient wearing the same amount of clothing, such as gown or pajamas, and without shoes, *so that the weights will more accurately reflect gains or losses.*
4. Make certain the scale is balanced before use.

Implementation Steps

1. Follow the Initial Implementation Steps located on the inside front cover.
2. Place clean paper towels on the platform scale *to keep the patient's feet clean.*

If Weighing an Adult or Child Who Can Stand Unassisted

3. Assist the patient as needed to get out of bed and stand, making certain that he or she is not experiencing dizziness. Assist in removal of shoes.

4. Have the patient step up on the scale. *Safety: Place your hand just a couple of inches behind the patient's back in case the patient begins to lose his or her balance.*
5. Read the weight while the patient is freestanding, without holding onto anything.
6. Assist the patient as needed to step off the scale and return to bed.
7. Follow the Ending Implementation Steps located on the inside back cover.

If Using a Built-in Bed Scale

3. The patient may be weighed lying in the bed.
4. Follow the steps as listed in the manufacturer's instructions.
5. Follow the Ending Implementation Steps located at the back of the book.

Evaluation Steps

1. Compare the new weight with the previous weight, noting whether there is an increase or decrease.

Sample Documentation

2-2-11   0800   *Weight 156 lbs, per bed scales, a loss of 3 lbs. since yesterday.* ————————
———————————— *Nurse's signature and credentials*

Skill 21-3 Measuring an Infant's Weight and Length

Assessment Steps

1. Review the patient's medical record to see the previous weight *so that you can compare the current weight to determine whether there is a gain or loss.*
2. Assess the room temperature where the scale is to be used, making certain that the environmental temperature is sufficiently warm *to prevent chilling the infant after removal of clothing.*

Planning Steps

1. Gather needed equipment and supplies: tabletop scale; separate tape measure if scale does not include length ruler; paper towels, lightweight cloth, or blanket.
2. Lay paper towels, cloth, or blanket in the scale cradle *to provide a barrier between the infant and the cold surface of the metal scale surface to prevent chilling the infant.*

3. Balance the scale with the paper or cloth barrier on the scale *to prevent inaccuracy.*

Implementation Steps

1. Follow the Initial Implementation Steps located on the inside front cover.
2. Remove all the infant's clothing or leave on the diaper, according to facility policy.
3. Lay the infant supine on the paper or cloth barrier in the scale cradle.
4. Gently extend the infant's leg at the thigh and knee. Use the scale's length marker or place a measuring tape along the posterior aspect of the infant's body. Measure the infant's length from the top of the head to the plantar surface of the infant's heel, reading the length in inches or centimeters.

Skill 21-3 (continued)

5. Next, weigh the infant. *Safety: Hold the palm of your hand 1 to 2 inches above the infant's abdomen to prevent the infant from falling. Even newborns can squirm and wiggle enough to present a fall risk. NEVER walk away and leave the infant unattended on the scale.*

6. Read the weight in pounds and ounces or kilograms and grams, dependent upon facility policy.
7. Remove infant from the scale and reapply clothing to prevent chilling.
8. Follow the Ending Implementation Steps located on the inside back cover.

Evaluation Steps

1. Compare the weight to the previously recorded weight, noting whether there is a gain or loss.

Sample Documentation

8/10/12	0930	Wt. 5 lbs. 2 oz. A loss of 1 oz since yesterday.
		———— Nurse's signature and credentials

Skill 21-4 Performing an Initial Head-to-Toe Shift Assessment

Assessment Steps

1. Assess the patient's chart to determine gender, age, and ethnicity *to assist you in planning size and type of sphygmomanometer and thermometer to use.*
2. Review the patient's chart to identify the patient's medical problems, including whether the patient can sit or stand. *This helps you to plan techniques for assessment.*

Planning Steps

1. Gather needed equipment and supplies: sphygmomanometer, stethoscope, thermometer, pulse oximeter, penlight, tongue depressor, examination gloves, scale if weight is needed. If body fluid samples are needed, include the appropriate specimen containers. Take pen and appropriate documentation form *for recording assessment findings.*
2. Have the patient empty the bladder before beginning assessment. Remember to collect urine if a specimen is required.
3. Turn off the radio and television *to provide a quiet environment in which to hear the heart, breath, and bowel sounds.*

Implementation Steps

1. Follow the Initial Implementation Steps located on the inside front cover.

2. Warm your hands before touching the patient *to avoid discomfort.* Limit use of examination gloves to portions of the examination that involve contact with body fluids, such as breaks in skin integrity or urine.
3. Assess the patient's vital signs first *to provide you with a baseline.* Be certain to include SpO_2 and pain assessment, *which can help to identify potential problem areas that may require extra assessment.*
4. Obtain weight if needed (see Skill 21-2).

Head and Neck

5. Assess level of consciousness, orientation to the four spheres, and speech. Inquire whether the patient has any pain, nausea, or other discomforts before you begin the assessment.
6. Assess the pupils and pupillary response to light and accommodation.
7. Assess both sclera and conjunctiva for color and moisture.
8. Inspect the face for symmetry and skin color. Note affect and eye contact.
9. Assess the lips and oral mucous membranes for color, integrity, moisture, and lesions.
10. Assess the teeth and gums for dentures, missing teeth, decay, gum recession, bleeding, sordes, and lesions.
11. Assess the neck veins for distention.

(skill continues on page 450)

Skill 21-4 (continued)

12. Assess any tubes, equipment, or dressings of the head or neck *to ensure patency and proper function.*

Chest and Abdomen

13. Inspect the chest for shape, symmetrical excursion, use of accessory respiratory muscles, and ease of breathing.
14. Assess skin turgor.
15. Auscultate the heart sounds for a full minute, noting the rate, rhythm, and strength. Compare the heart rate to the radial pulse to ensure there is not a pulse deficit.
16. Auscultate the breath sounds in all five lobes, listening anteriorly, posteriorly, and laterally. Note quality of sounds, adventitious sounds, and equality of left and right breath sounds.
17. Inquire about cough, sputum production, or shortness of breath upon exertion.
18. Inspect the abdomen for shape and size.
19. Auscultate for presence and activity level of bowel sounds in all four quadrants.
20. Palpate the abdomen for firmness and masses, noting if pain is elicited.
21. Inquire regarding nausea, vomiting, indigestion, and discomfort.
22. Inquire about the time of last voiding and bowel movement.
23. Inspect any tubes, equipment, or dressings of the chest and abdomen *to ensure patency and proper function.*

Extremities

24. Palpate the radial pulses for strength and equality of both sides.
25. Palpate the hands for edema and warmth.
26. Assess the nailbeds for color and capillary refill time.
27. Assess range of motion of the arms and hands.
28. Assess hand grip for bilateral equality of strength.
29. Inspect any tubes, equipment, or dressings of the arms *to ensure patency and proper function.*
30. Inspect the lower legs and feet for color.
31. Palpate the feet, ankles, and pretibial area for edema and skin temperature.
32. Palpate the pedal pulses for strength and equality.
33. Assess capillary refill time.
34. Assess for range of motion.
35. Assess for strength and equality of plantar flexion and dorsiflexion of both feet.
36. Inspect any tubes, equipment, or dressings of the legs *to ensure patency and proper function.*
37. Follow the Ending Implementation Steps located on the inside back cover.

Evaluation Steps

1. Evaluate the normal and abnormal findings and whether there are further actions you should take.
2. Determine if all aspects of assessment pertinent to the diseases and conditions of the patient have been addressed.
3. Determine that the patient has remained safe and warm during assessment.
4. Allow the patient to ask questions.
5. Inquire whether the patient is comfortable or has any needs.

Sample Documentation

An example of assessment documentation using a patient flow sheet is found in Figure 21-20. A sample using the narrative charting format can be found in Figure 21-21.

Skill 21-5 Performing a Basic Neurological Examination

Assessment Steps

1. Assess the patient's chart to determine gender, age, and ethnicity *to assist you in planning size and type of sphygmomanometer and thermometer to use.*
2. Review the patient's chart to identify the patient's medical problems, including the responses noted during the last neurological examination. *This helps you to plan techniques for assessment.*

Planning Steps

1. Gather needed equipment and supplies: sphygmomanometer, stethoscope, thermometer, pulse oximeter, penlight, tongue depressor. Take pen and appropriate documentation form *for recording neurological findings.*
2. Turn off the radio and television *to provide a quiet environment.*

Implementation Steps

1. Follow the Initial Implementation Steps located on the inside front cover.
2. Explain to the patient what you are about to do even if you believe the patient is comatose. *The hearing is thought to be the last sense to go.*
3. Try to arouse the patient by calling his or her name first in a normal tone of voice. If the patient does not respond, speak louder. If there still is no response, use tactile stimulus and gently touch the patient on the arm or hand. If there is no response, gently shake the patient. If no response, use an acceptable method of exerting mild pain, such as pressing moderately hard on a nailbed *to determine if the patient responds to painful stimulus.*
4. Assess vital signs, making note of elevated blood pressure and decreased pulse rate.

Skill 21-5 (continued)

5. If the patient is awake, ask the patient to identify his or her name and the place, time, and situation (the reason the patient is hospitalized) *to determine orientation to the four spheres.*

6. Ask the patient first to smile, then to clench the teeth, protrude the tongue and then move it side to side, furrow the brow, raise the eyebrows, and finally squeeze both eyes shut at the same time *so that you can observe for symmetry of muscle movement on both sides of the face.* The tongue should protrude at the midline of the mouth and move equally from left to right. Both eyebrows should rise equally. As both eyes are squeezed shut, both cheeks should rise and the wrinkling/bunching of tissue around the orbital areas should appear equal.

7. Ask the patient to squeeze your fingers with each of his or her hands *to test strength and equality of hand grip bilaterally.* Note if patient does not follow simple commands or if there is any difference in strength. If there is no response to your request, pick up the patient's arm. Raise it approximately 1 to 2 feet off the bed. Then release it and allow it to fall to the mattress. Note whether the arm falls flaccidly to the bed surface or if the patient offers any control of the muscles after releasing your hold on the arm.

8. Ask the patient to press the plantar side of the feet against the palms of your hands and then to pull the toes and feet toward his or her head as you provide resistance using the palms of your hands to pull against the dorsal surface of both the patient's feet. Note the strength and equality bilaterally. If there is

no response to your request, raise one leg off the bed as you did the arms, and release it. Allow it to fall to the bed surface. Note whether the leg falls limply or the patient offers some muscle control as it falls.

9. Follow the Ending Implementation Steps located on the inside back cover.

Evaluation Steps

1. Evaluate the normal and abnormal responses.

2. Compare to the previous neurological examination, noting any change in neurological response.

3. Determine whether further action is deemed necessary.

Sample Documentation

09/12/12   0745   BP – 128/68, T – 98.2, P – 73 reg & strong, R – 17. SpO₂ – 98%, denies any pain or discomfort. Does not respond to voice but awakens to tactile stimuli. Wife states he is hard of hearing. Alert and oriented to 4 spheres. PERLA. Follows simple commands. No facial drooping. Symmetrical raising of eyebrows, smiling, clenching teeth, and tongue movement. Speech is clear and appropriate. Hand grips are strong and equal bilaterally. Dorsal plantar flexion is strong and equal bilaterally. —————
————————— Nurse's signature and credentials

Skill 21-6 Auscultating Breath Sounds

Assessment Steps

1. Assess the patient's chart to determine gender and age *to assist you in planning techniques to use.*

2. Review the patient's chart *to identify the patient's medical problems, including whether the patient can sit up.*

Planning Steps

1. Obtain a stethoscope.

2. Turn off the radio and television *to provide a quiet environment in which to hear the breath sounds.*

Implementation Steps

1. Follow the Initial Implementation Steps located on the inside front cover.

2. Warm your hands and the diaphragm of the stethoscope before touching the patient *to avoid discomfort.*

3. Assist the patient into a sitting position or elevate the head of the bed between 45 and 90 degrees, if possible. If not, turn the patient to his or her left side.

4. Loosen the patient's gown and place the stethoscope diaphragm against the skin on the anterior chest wall and then the lateral aspects of the chest. Ask

the patient to breathe in and out through an open mouth. Listen for a full breath at each location, moving the stethoscope from the apexes to the bases, in a zigzag pattern from left to right (refer to Fig. 21-14).

5. Place the stethoscope on the back and listen to the posterior aspects of the lungs in the same manner.

6. Follow the Ending Implementation Steps located on the inside back cover.

Evaluation Steps

1. Evaluate the normal and abnormal breath sounds heard.

2. Evaluate whether further action is needed.

Sample Documentation

5/27/12   1815   Breath sounds auscultated, coarse crackles in RUL, RML, RLL; LUL & LLL clear to auscultation. —————
————————— Nurse's signature and credentials

Skill 21-7 Auscultating Heart Sounds

Assessment Steps

1. Assess the patient's chart to determine gender, age, and ethnicity *to assist you in planning techniques to use.*

2. Review the patient's chart *to identify the patient's medical problems, including whether the patient can sit up.*

Planning Steps

1. Obtain a stethoscope.

2. Turn off the radio and television *to provide a quiet environment in which to hear the heart sounds.*

Implementation Steps

1. Follow the Initial Implementation Steps located on the inside front cover.

2. Warm your hands and the diaphragm of the stethoscope before touching the patient *to avoid discomfort.*

3. Assist the patient into a sitting position or elevate the head of the bed between 45 and 90 degrees, if possible. If not, turn the patient to his or her left side.

4. Place the stethoscope diaphragm firmly against the patient's skin, not the gown, in the midclavicular line at the fifth intercostal space. Adjust the stethoscope slightly until you can best hear the heart sounds (refer to Fig. 21-15).

5. Listen for a few seconds while you identify the S_1 and S_2. *Remember that the heartbeat includes both the S_1 and the S_2.* Then count the number of heartbeats in 1 minute while observing the second hand of your watch. Assess for rate, rhythm, and strength. Make note of any extra sounds heard.

6. Move the stethoscope to the second intercostal space just to the right of the sternum *to listen to the right base heart sounds and the aortic valve.*

7. Move the stethoscope to the second intercostal space just to the left of the sternum *to listen to the left base heart sound and the pulmonic valve.*

8. Move the stethoscope to the edge of the sternum, at the level of the fourth intercostal space just to the left of the sternum, *to hear the left lateral sternal border heart sound and the tricuspid valve.*

9. Follow the Ending Implementation Steps located on the inside back cover.

Evaluation Steps

1. Evaluate the rate, rhythm, and strength of the heart sounds to determine normal and abnormal findings.

2. Determine that the patient has remained safe and warm during assessment.

Documentation Steps

5/26/12 2115 Heart sounds auscultated, S_1 & S_2 distinct and regular, rate equal to radial pulse. —————
——————————————— *Nurse's signature and credentials*

 Post Conference

At the end of the day, you feel good about the care you gave to this patient. After alerting your instructor to your patient's possibly worsening condition, you saw a thorough assessment in action. The staff nurse and your instructor showed you how to assess jugular vein distention, which was present in this patient. The patient's blood pressure continued to elevate as you monitored it every hour, eventually reaching 188/106. You learned the significance of sacral edema in a patient on bedrest. Your patient became more short of breath, even with increased oxygen. The staff nurse called the physician, and the patient was moved to the intensive care unit with severe congestive heart failure. Your instructor credited you with observing and reporting assessments necessary for detecting the worsening of his condition.

KEY POINTS

- Purposes of physical assessment include establishing a patient's current condition, establishing a baseline against which future changes may be measured, identifying problems the patient may have or have the potential to develop, evaluating the effectiveness of nursing interventions, monitoring for changes in body function, and detecting specific body systems that need further assessment or testing.

- Techniques of assessment include interviewing, inspection, palpation, percussion, auscultation, percussion, and olfaction.

- Assessment is performed in a head-to-toe sequence, beginning with the head and neck, progressing to the chest and abdomen, and then the four extremities.

- Components to be assessed during an initial shift assessment include the following systems: neurological, cardiovascular, respiratory, integumentary, gastrointestinal, genitourinary, and musculoskeletal. Also included in an initial shift assessment are vital signs, including pain and SpO$_2$; appearance; speech; safety risk factors; tubes and equipment; comfort or complaints; and a needs assessment.

- Various adaptations are necessary when assessing patients of different age groups.

REVIEW QUESTIONS

Select the answer that is most appropriate for each of the following questions. Some questions may have more than one correct answer. Check all that apply.

1. Which of the following assessments would be included in a focused cardiovascular assessment?

   a. Radial pulse

   b. Range of motion of extremities

   c. Vital signs

   d. Pupillary reaction to light

   e. Edema of extremities

   f. Neck vein distention

   g. Heart sounds

   h. Bowel sounds

   i. Use of accessory respiratory muscles

   j. Last bowel movement

   k. Color and warmth of lower extremities

2. During an assessment, you noted two new findings in a patient: unable to palpate peripheral pulse in lower extremities, and pupils that are not equal in size and rate of constriction. Which of these two findings provides you with information about the neurological system?

   a. Peripheral pulses

   b. Pupils

   c. Both findings

3. You have auscultated fine crackles in both the right and left lower lobes in a postoperative patient. What is the longest period of time you should allow to pass before you auscultate the breath sounds again?

   a. 1 hour

   b. 2 hours

   c. 3 hours

   d. 4 hours

   e. 5 hours

   f. 8 hours

4. While percussing over the upper quadrant where the liver is located, you know you are over the liver when you hear which of the following sounds?

   a. Drum-like sound

   b. Loud, hollow sound

   c. Soft, dull sound

   d. Low-pitched resonant sound

5. You would expect to hear which of the following sounds when percussing over a normal, healthy lung?

   a. Drum-like sound

   b. Loud, hollow sound

   c. Soft, dull sound

   d. Low-pitched resonant sound

6. Which of the following landmarks are used in anterior chest auscultation of the breath sounds?

   a. Right midscapular line

   b. Costovertebral angle

   c. Left midclavicular line

   d. Midsternal line

   e. Midspinal line

7. At which posterior intercostal space are the lung bases located during full inspiration?

   a. 1st

   b. 5th

   c. 8th

   d. 10th

   e. 12th

SHORT ANSWER QUESTIONS

8. Describe at least six assessments that you should perform when performing a focused assessment of the gastrointestinal system.

9. Describe the types of data that you can gather by simply observing a patient as you enter the room to perform a task.

10. Explain the difference between a sign and a symptom.

11. Which of the body systems are assessed in an initial head-to-toe shift assessment?

CRITICAL THINKING EXERCISE

12. How does the assessment of the cardiovascular system correlate with the assessment of the respiratory system?

ADDITIONAL RESOURCES

For additional Resources, Questions, and Activities, please see:

 Student Resource Disk

 http://davisplus.fadavis.com

 Student Study Guide

REFERENCES

Anderson J, Langemo D, Hanson D, Thompson P, Hunter S. Wound & skin care: What you can learn from a comprehensive skin assessment. *Nursing2007.* 2007;37(4):65-66.

Colleton LG. Peak technique: Beyond the stethoscope: respiratory assessment of the older adult. *Nursing Made Incredibly Easy.* 2008;6(5):11-14.

Core T, Hayes K. Acute abdominal pain: a systematic approach to adult assessment. *Nursing2009 Crit Care.* 2009;3(3):30-39.

D'Arcy Y. Managing the pain: Assessing pain with pain-rating scales. *LPN2007.* 2007;3(6):13-18.

Delville CL. Nutritional risk assessment: are your patients at nutritional risk? *Nurse Pract.* 2008;33(2):36-39.

Dillon PM. *Nursing Health Assessment: A Critical Thinking Case Studies Approach.* 2nd ed. Philadelphia: FA Davis; 2007.

Goolsby MJ. *Advanced Assessment—Interpreting Findings and Formulating Differential Diagnosis.* Philadelphia: FA Davis; 2005.

Gordon M. *Assess Notes: Assessment and Diagnostic Reasoning for Clinical Practice.* Philadelphia: FA Davis; 2008.

Halcomb SS. Acute abdomen: what a pain! *Nursing2008.* 2008;38(9):34-40.

Halcomb SS. What's causing your abdominal pain? Test your assessment skills. *Nursing2009.* 2009;39(4):57-58.

Hart A, Davidhizar R. What the nurse should know about the pulmonary system. *J Pract Nurs.* 2006-2007;56(4)-57(1):6-7, 11-13.

Hogstel MO. *Health Assessment Through the Life Span.* 4th ed. Philadelphia: FA Davis; 2005.

Holloway BW. *Nurse's Fast Facts—Your Quick Source for Core Clinical Content.* Philadelphia: FA Davis; 2004.

Huntley A. Chart smart: Documenting level of consciousness. *Nursing2008.* 2008;38(8):63-64.

Mullen-Fortino M, O'Brien N, Jones M. Critical care of a patient after CABG surgery. *Nursing2009 Crit Care.* 2009;4(4):46-53.

Pullen RL. Clinical do's & don'ts: Pulse oximetry. *Nursing2003.* 2003;33(9):30.

Rhoades J, Meeker BJ. *Davis's Guide to Clinical Nursing Skills.* Philadelphia: FA Davis; 2008.

Rushing J. Clinical do's & don'ts: Assessing a patient for lice infestation. *Nursing2008.* 2008;38(7):20.

Rushing J. Clinical do's & don'ts: Assessing for orthostatic hypotension. *Nursing2005.* 2005;35(1):30.

Scanlon V, Sanders T. *Essentials of Anatomy and Physiology.* 5th ed. Philadelphia: FA Davis; 2007.

Shindler DM. Practical cardiac auscultation. *Crit Care Nurs Q.* 2007;30:166-180.

Stanley M, Blair KA, Beare PG. *Gerontological Nursing—Promoting Successful Aging With Older Adults.* 3rd ed. Philadelphia: FA Davis; 2005.

The Joint Commission. *2009 National Patient Safety Goals.* Available at: http://www.jointcommission.org/patientsafety/nationalpatientsafetygoals/. Accessed September 10, 2009.

Venes D, ed. *Taber's Cyclopedic Medical Dictionary.* 20th ed. Philadelphia: FA Davis; 2005.

Wallace MA. How to try this: Assessment of sexual health in older adults. *Am J Nurs.* 2008;108(7):52-60.

Wilkinson JM, Van Leuven K. *Fundamentals of Nursing: Theory, Concepts & Applications.* Philadelphia: FA Davis; 2007.

Williams LS, Hopper PD. *Understanding Medical-Surgical Nursing.* 3rd ed. Philadelphia: FA Davis; 2007.

Surgical Asepsis

Key Terms

Autoclaving

Boiling

Chemical disinfection

Circulating nurse

Contamination

Disinfected

Gaseous disinfection

Ionizing radiation

Scrub nurse

Sterile conscience

Sterile field

Sterile technique

Sterilized

Surgical asepsis

Objectives

1. Define key terms associated with surgical asepsis.
2. Differentiate between medical asepsis and surgical asepsis.
3. Describe five methods of sterilization.
4. Explain how to tell if supplies are sterile.
5. Enumerate restricted settings in the hospital where aseptic surroundings are maintained.
6. Explain the necessity of developing a sterile conscience.
7. Identify guidelines for using sterile technique while opening sterile supplies, setting up and adding items to the sterile field, opening sterile packs, and working with a sterile field.
8. Determine when to use sterile technique.

Skills

22-1 Setting up a Sterile Field, Opening Sterile Packs, and Pouring Sterile Liquids

22-2 Donning Sterile Gloves—Open Method

22-3 Performing a Surgical Hand Scrub

22-4 Donning a Sterile Gown and Sterile Gloves—Closed Method

🌐 Clinical Connection

Your Assignment: During your clinical experience, you are asked to assist a physician while he inserts a *central line,* a special type of IV catheter that is inserted through the subclavian vein near the patient's neck. Using sterile technique, the physician makes a small incision, isolates the subclavian vein, and then inserts the *catheter,* a narrow tube. You have very little time to think about what you will need to do as an assistant in this bedside procedure.

Your Actions: You must consider the principles of sterile technique. You must decide how you will help without contaminating the sterile field or any of the supplies or equipment. You will need to obtain sterile supplies, check the expiration dates, and examine the packages for any tears or other open areas. You will need to obtain needed equipment and have it ready at the bedside, including the correct size of sterile gloves needed by the physician. While you will have help with this as a student, when you work as a nurse, this is a common scenario in which you will function independently.

The use of medical asepsis and clean technique was discussed in Chapter 14, and by now you are very familiar with the principles of using medical asepsis, as well as using standard precautions. But what about situations like the Clinical Connection above? What about the times when you are assigned for clinical experience in the operating room or other areas of the hospital where invasive procedures occur? You need to know more than simple clean technique in those areas. You will be using **surgical asepsis**, or **sterile technique**, which is the method used to prevent contamination during invasive procedures, or procedures that involve entering body cavities. Surgical asepsis requires the use of sterile supplies and equipment that have been treated to kill all pathogens and spores.

Disinfection and Sterilization

When you use surgical asepsis, you use supplies and equipment that have been **disinfected** by being cleaned with solutions to kill pathogens, or that have been **sterilized** using steam under pressure, gas, or radiation, to kill all pathogens and their spores. Some items, such as an IV pump, cannot be sterilized, so they must be disinfected with a solution to kill microorganisms and prevent the spread of pathogens from one patient to the next.

Before being sterilized, instruments and equipment are cleaned. This may be done by first rinsing with cold or warm water, then washing them in warm soapy water, followed by rinsing in clear water, or through the use of ultrasound to loosen organic material from tiny crevices in the equipment. All instruments that are hinged are left open to prevent damage to the hinges when they are being prepared for sterilization.

Types of Sterilization

Equipment and supplies may be treated in a variety of ways to kill pathogens. Some of the most common treatments include:

- **Autoclaving**: This method delivers steam under pressure, with heat ranging from 250°F to 270°F, to sterilize instruments that will not be harmed by heat and water under pressure.
- **Boiling**: This method of boiling instruments and supplies in water for 10 minutes kills non–spore-forming organisms but does not kill spores.
- **Ionizing radiation**: This method kills pathogens on sutures, some plastics, and biological materials that cannot be boiled or autoclaved.
- **Chemical disinfection**: This method is used to kill pathogens on equipment and supplies that cannot be heated. An example of such a chemical would be Cidex, which is used to sterilize rubber-based catheters used in urological procedures.
- **Gaseous disinfection**: This method kills pathogens on supplies and equipment that are heat sensitive or must remain dry.

Indications of Sterility

When you use supplies and equipment that have been disinfected or sterilized, you must ensure that they have not been contaminated in any way. Surgical instruments are often double-wrapped in a surgical towel and an outside wrapper, then sterilized in an autoclave. A piece of indicator tape is applied to the outer wrapper, across the final flap. Once the pack has been sterilized in an autoclave, the indicator tape shows black marks every half-inch (Fig. 22-1). The person who autoclaves the pack writes his or her initials, as well as the date and the expiration date, on the tape. Evidence that

Figure 22-1 These sterilized packs show exposed indicator tape with dark hash marks.

the wrapper has been wet appears as a discolored line at the level reached by the fluids. This is referred to as "strike-through." If you see strike-through, do not use the pack.

Single instruments or small items may be sterilized in individual peel-apart packs (Fig. 22-2). These packs are made of paper, with a clear cover so the contents can be visualized. If they are commercially prepared, they are stamped with an expiration date. Always check the expiration date, and examine the packaging to ensure that it remains intact. The item can no longer be considered sterile if the peel-apart pack is open anywhere or if the expiration date has passed.

Sterile Settings

Although it is impossible to truly sterilize an entire unit in a hospital, some areas are considered restricted to help maintain surgical asepsis. In these areas, staff remove street clothes and dress in hospital-laundered scrubs upon entering the unit. This prevents contamination of the unit with lint, pet hair, or other potential pathogens from outside the area. If you do not keep a pair of shoes at the hospital to wear in the unit, you may be required to place shoe covers over your shoes to protect against outside contaminants. Examples of

Figure 22-2 An example of a peel-apart pack being opened.

restricted areas in most hospitals include surgical suites, heart catheterization laboratories, delivery rooms, neonatal intensive care units, burn units, transplantation intensive care units, and oncology units.

To help maintain the aseptic surroundings in these types of units, you will be required to cover your scrubs with a lab coat or cloth isolation gown when you leave the restricted unit to go to other areas of the hospital. When you return, you will remove the outer coverings before entering the patient care area of the unit. This helps keep pathogens from hospital areas outside the unit from entering the restricted area.

Using Sterile Technique in Other Settings

You may be called on to assist a physician with a sterile procedure at the patient's bedside. Such a situation might include the insertion of chest tubes, insertion of an IV line into the subclavian vein, or performing a lumbar puncture. It is important that you know how to assist without contaminating the sterile field, are able to anticipate the physician's needs, and know how to provide supplies and equipment using sterile technique.

Nurses use sterile technique frequently during patient care activities. When they give injections, start peripheral IV lines, flush intermittent access devices, insert urinary catheters, and suction deep airways, they use sterile technique. All of these procedures require meticulous use of surgical asepsis to prevent infection.

During the insertion of these tubes or needles, the nurse is entering body tissues not normally exposed to pathogens. He or she is effectively bypassing some of the usual mechanisms for defending against invading pathogens.

> **Knowledge Connection**
> Describe five types of sterilization. How can you tell that a wrapped pack has been sterilized? Give four examples of restricted areas in the hospital. List four situations in patient care that require sterile technique.

Principles of Sterile Technique

When you perform skills requiring surgical asepsis, it is important to realize the consequences to the patient should contamination occur. **Contamination** refers to the potential presence of pathogens on a sterile field or sterile object, due to contact with an unsterile surface. A **sterile field** is an area that is free from all microorganisms where additional sterile items can be placed until they are ready for use. Because skin cannot be sterilized, sterile gloves are used to touch sterile items on the sterile field. Skill 22-1 (page 461) presents the steps involved in setting up a sterile field, and Skill 22-2 (page 463) presents the steps needed to don sterile gloves.

Even if an object or surface is considered clean, pathogens are still present. Therefore, if the clean object touches the sterile field or a sterile object, transfer of pathogens could take place. An example of this would be when a nurse is preparing a sterile dressing to apply to an open wound and accidentally drops the dressing onto the bedside table, contaminating it. In this case, the nurse would need to obtain another sterile dressing rather than risk introducing pathogens from the bedside table into the patient's open wound. In many situations, it is up to the nurse to admit the error and correct it. Often others do not observe the contamination.

Sterile Conscience

As you learn about and practice sterile technique, you will need to develop a **sterile conscience**. This means always being aware of potential or certain contamination of the sterile field or sterile objects, and taking appropriate steps to correct the situation, such as replacing the contaminated object or reassembling the sterile field with new supplies.

It is quite possible that no one other than you would be aware if contamination occurs. Therefore, you must be honest in admitting that such a thing did occur or could have occurred. *Safety: You must also put the patient's safety above your own convenience and correct the error, starting the procedure over if necessary.* When contamination occurs, you can no longer use the contaminated supplies. They must be replaced with new sterile supplies. Sometimes it is possible to have a second person open a sterile pack and add supplies to your sterile field, or open a sterile pack and allow you to use your sterile gloved fingers to lift the item from the pack without contamination. Box 22-1 provides additional information on opening sterile packs and adding sterile supplies.

Box 22-1

Opening Sterile Packs and Adding Sterile Supplies

There are several rules to follow when you open sterile packs and when you add sterile supplies to a sterile field.

- When a person not wearing sterile gloves opens a peel-apart pack for a person wearing sterile gloves, he or she peels the pack apart with the opening toward the sterile person. The nonsterile person peels the packaging so as to cover his or her bare hands. The sterile person then grasps the item, touching only the sterile item and possibly the inside of the sterile pack.
- Use the same procedure if you are not wearing sterile gloves and are unwrapping a sterile item to hand off to a sterile person. Open the flaps in such a way that you are holding the item through the wrapper with one hand and holding the flaps out of the way with your other hand. This allows the sterile person to grasp the sterile item without contamination (see Fig. 22-5).
- When opening sterile supplies to add to the sterile field, open the peel pack away from you. Allow the item to drop onto the sterile field without reaching across the field. Come in from the side to drop the item onto the field, being careful that it lands in the middle of the field and does not touch the outer 1 inch of drape that is considered contaminated.

Remember that you are responsible for your own sterile conscience and for the safety of your patients during sterile procedures, whether or not errors are observed by others.

Supervision/Delegation Connection

Sterile Technique and Assistive Personnel

In most situations, procedures requiring sterile technique are not delegated to assistive personnel, but are performed by the licensed nurse. In some states, UAPs are allowed to insert urinary catheters using sterile technique. No states allow CNAs to perform sterile procedures. Be sure you know your facility's policy and follow it carefully. If any task requiring sterile technique is permitted to be delegated, it is your responsibility to supervise and know that the UAP can correctly perform the task. It is also your responsibility to perform complicated procedures or perform skills requiring sterile technique if the patient is unstable. In these situations, the task should not be delegated to assistive personnel.

Guidelines for Using Sterile Technique

The principles of sterile technique are the same, regardless of the setting. Whether you are assisting in the operating room or the emergency room or performing a sterile procedure at the patient's bedside on a nursing unit, the guidelines are the same. One clear guiding principle to remember is:

Sterile + sterile = sterile
Sterile + unsterile = contaminated
Unsterile + unsterile = contaminated

This means that anything sterile remains sterile, as long as it only touches other sterile items. Anything sterile that touches anything unsterile must always be considered contaminated. Anything unsterile, no matter what it touches, is considered contaminated.

Opening Sterile Supplies

Before opening any sterile supplies, always be sure to do the following:

- Check the expiration date for sterility.
- Check the sterilization tape, if present, for color change—the hash marks should be dark.
- Check the packaging for any holes or tears, which would render the contents unsterile.

Setting Up the Sterile Field

When you are setting up a sterile field, keep the following guidelines in mind:

- The outer 1 inch of the sterile drape is considered contaminated because you must touch it as you set it up. Do not touch any other area of the sterile drape with your bare hands or any other nonsterile item (see Skill 22-1).
- Anything below the surface of the draped table is considered unsterile because you cannot see if it is touched by an unsterile surface.

- All parts of the sterile drape below the table surface are considered unsterile because they cannot be kept in your line of sight.
- Only sterile items can be placed on the sterile field.
- If the sterile field becomes damp or wet, it is no longer sterile because pathogens can be transmitted from the table through the drape when it is damp. The exception is a drape that is backed with moisture-proof material.

Adding Items to the Sterile Field

When you add items to an established sterile field, follow these guidelines to prevent contamination:

- Add sterile items to the field by opening peel-apart packs and dropping the item onto the field, staying away from the contaminated 1-inch outer border. As the sterile item drops from the package, do not allow the item to touch the edges of the package, as they are considered contaminated (see Skill 22-1).
- Add sterile liquids to a basin in a sterile field by holding the bottle so that the label is against the palm of your hand to prevent dripping onto the label, which could obscure the writing. Pour the liquid by holding the bottle approximately 4 to 6 inches above the basin. Pour slowly to avoid splashing, which could cause the sterile field to become wet. (See Skill 22-1, for more information on pouring sterile liquids.)
- Only after you have donned sterile gloves can you touch the sterile field and the items in the sterile field (see Skill 22-2).

Opening Sterile Packs

While certain sterile supplies, such as gauze 4×4s or a pair of scissors, may be packaged individually, there are various supplies that may be sterilized together in a pack. A pack contains all, or most of, the supplies needed to perform a particular procedure, such as a circumcision, vaginal examination, or laceration suturing. Some commercially wrapped packs have a single-layer paper top that peels off to reveal a plastic tray of sterile supplies. The tray itself can serve as a mini–sterile field if desired. Other commercially wrapped packs have an outer wrapper, somewhat like a plastic bag, that is removed to reveal an inner sterile wrapper that is used to set up the sterile field (Fig. 22-3).

If the sterile pack is sterilized by the facility, it will have both an outer and an inner wrapper. The outer wrapper

is opened without touching the inside of it and serves as an additional barrier between the table and the sterile supplies inside the pack. The inner wrap, when opened, will serve as the actual sterile field surface upon which all sterile supplies are placed and arranged for use (Fig. 22-4). If you are not wearing sterile gloves and must hand a facility-sterilized pack to another person who is wearing sterile gloves, you will use the method demonstrated in Figure 22-5 and explained in Box 22-1.

Figure 22-4 This nurse is opening an autoclaved, two-wrapper pack. The inner wrap remains sterile and rests on a sterile field created by the open outer wrapper.

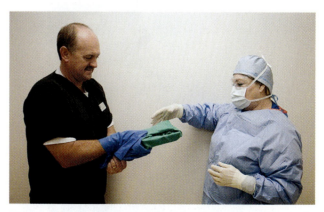

Figure 22-5 This unsterile nurse is handing off a sterile item by holding outer wrapper gathered back around her unsterile hand. The nurse in sterile garb wearing sterile gloves can then grasp it without contamination.

Figure 22-3 This nurse is removing the outer plastic bag wrap to access the inner sterile wrapper of a prepackaged kit.

When you open sterile packs to set up or add to a sterile field, it is important to follow these guidelines:

- Set the sterile pack on the clean surface positioned so that the first flap will open away from you.
- Open the flap that folds away from you first, and then open each of the side flaps. Open the flap that folds toward you last (Fig. 22-6). This prevents you from reaching across the sterile pack while you are opening it. If the pack is institutionally sterilized and has two wrappers, open each wrapper in the same manner, taking care to avoid touching the inner surface of the inner wrapper.

Working With a Sterile Field

Once the sterile field has been established, follow these rules:

- Do not reach across the sterile field unless you are wearing a sterile gown and gloves. Your arms and hands are not sterile, so you will contaminate the field by reaching across it.
- Keep the sterile field in view at all times to ensure that contamination does not occur.
- Never turn your back on the sterile field, as you cannot see if it becomes contaminated.
- Once you have applied your sterile gloves, keep your gloved hands in the *safety zone,* which is above waist level, below eye level, and in front of your body at all times. If they fall below the waist, above eye level, or outside your peripheral vision, they are out of your line of vision, so they could accidentally brush against an unsterile surface, causing contamination. Any time they are outside of the safety zone, they must be considered contaminated, requiring you to apply a new pair of sterile gloves before

Figure 22-6 This nurse is opening the last flap of a sterile pack toward himself as he sets up a sterile field.

continuing. For example, this means that you cannot reach behind you, nor can you reach below your waist to put anything in the trash can. You must learn to discard items by "dropping" the items from your hand and letting them fall to their intended target, while keeping your hand within the safety zone.

- When sterile objects are exposed to the air for a long period of time, they are no longer considered sterile. It is very important to wait to prepare the sterile field until just prior to its use.

Knowledge Connection
What should you do if a sterile supply becomes contaminated? What is meant by "developing a sterile conscience"? What portion of a sterile drape is always considered unsterile?

When to Use Sterile Technique

Physicians' orders do not usually include directions to use sterile technique. Part of developing nursing judgment involves knowing when to use sterile technique and when clean technique is adequate. Use sterile technique in the following circumstances:

- When entering a sterile body cavity with a tube or other invasive equipment. Examples would be inserting a catheter into the bladder, inserting an IV needle into the vein, and injecting medications into the muscles or subcutaneous tissue.
- When caring for patients whose skin is not intact, creating exposure to pathogens. Examples would be caring for patients with burns or open wounds.
- During procedures that expose body cavities or enter major blood vessels, such as surgery, heart catheterizations, and delivery of babies.
- When handling needles, syringes, and lancets. Box 22-2 presents tips on using sterile technique when handling these items.

Real-World Connection

The Importance of Sterile Supplies
A group of nurses working in a coronary care unit noticed that several patients had developed infections at their IV insertion sites. One patient's infection spread to his bloodstream, causing septicemia, and even spread to his heart. He became quite ill and had to have emergency surgery. The nurses pressed for an investigation into the situation. Eventually, the infections were traced back to a batch of IV catheters that apparently had not been sterilized correctly, leading to these patients' infections.

Preparation for Entering the Operating Room

When you enter restricted areas, including the operating room (OR), you will be expected to perform a surgical hand scrub. This type of handwashing is more extensive than the skill you learned in Chapter 14. It involves cleaning the

Box 22-2

Tips for Handling Needles, Syringes, and Lancets

When you handle needles, syringes, and lancets, you must follow sterile technique to prevent contamination and potential for infection for your patient.

- Keep needles and lancing devices sterile at all times.
- The shaft, bevel, and hub of the needle and tip of syringe (Fig. 22-7) should be kept sterile.
- Do not touch the sharp portion of the lancet.
- After use, immediately put a used needle or lancet into a puncture-proof sharps container. Do not recap a used needle as the risk of puncturing yourself is too great.

hands and arms up to the elbows to ensure that shedding skin cells and pathogens have been removed.

In the actual surgical area of the hospital, you will first change into hospital-laundered scrubs, then apply shoe covers, head cover, and mask before you begin the surgical hand scrub. Skill 22-3 (page 466) provides the steps needed to perform a surgical hand scrub.

You will then dry your hands with a sterile towel and proceed into the anteroom, where you will be assisted into a sterile gown by the circulating nurse. The **circulating nurse** is a registered nurse who assists in the OR by obtaining needed equipment and supplies. The circulating nurse is not "scrubbed in" on the case, so that he or she may leave the operating suite to obtain needed items. The **scrub nurse** assists the physician throughout the surgery by handing instruments, holding retractors, and performing other tasks that require sterile garb. This person, who may be a surgical technologist or a licensed practical nurse, does scrub in on the case. After donning your sterile gown with the assistance of the circulating nurse, you will don sterile gloves using the closed gloving method. Skill 22-4 (page 467) provides the steps involved in donning the sterile gown and performing closed gloving.

People and Places Connection

Sterile Technique and Different Practice Settings

Some procedures that require sterile technique in the hospital setting may not be performed using sterile technique in the home setting. For example, patients with nerve damage affecting their ability to empty their bladder must catheterize the bladder several times a day to drain it. In that situation, a sterile catheter is used, but clean technique is used for the insertion. The reason for this is that the number and type of pathogens found in the hospital have a much greater risk of causing severe infection than the pathogens in the patient's home.

In the long-term care setting, the variety and number of pathogens is a concern as it is in hospitals. Because it is a more residential setting, sterile procedures may be performed infrequently. However, it is not uncommon for residents to have indwelling catheters or wounds requiring sterile treatment. Nurses in long-term care settings administer injections of insulin and other medications frequently. It is important to use meticulous sterile technique to prevent possible infections.

Knowledge Connection

How will you know when to use sterile technique when you perform patient care procedures? What must you do before you enter the operating room? Which portions of the needle and syringe must always remain sterile?

Figure 22-7 Areas of the needle and syringe that should remain sterile.

Plunger   Barrel   Tip   Hub   Shaft   Bevel

Avoid touching   Measure dose here   Gauge number   **Keep sterile**

Skill 22-1 Setting up a Sterile Field, Opening Sterile Packs, and Pouring Sterile Liquids

Assessment Steps

1. Assess the room for a clean, dry, waist-high area to use for setting up the sterile field, *to ensure sterility when the field is established.*

2. Assess the patient for any needs prior to the procedure, such as toileting or pain medication, *to prevent interruptions during the sterile procedure.*

Planning Steps

1. Gather needed equipment and supplies: sterile gloves in the correct size, sterile supplies needed for the procedure.

2. Determine where to place the over-the-bed table or other surface selected for establishing the sterile field.

3. Determine where to place additional supplies so they will be convenient but do not require that you reach over the sterile field to obtain them. *Reaching over a sterile field causes contamination of the field.*

Implementation Steps

1. Follow the Initial Implementation Steps located on the inside front cover for procedures during which you will be working at the patient's bedside.

(skill continues on page 462)

Skill 22-1 (continued)

2. **If you are establishing a sterile field with a wrapper:**

   a. Place the sterile pack on the selected surface.

   b. Open the first flap of the wrapper away from you, then open the side flaps. Open the last flap toward you to avoid reaching across the sterile field.

   If you are establishing a sterile field with a drape from a commercial pack:

   a. Open the sterile container and remove the drape, touching only the outer 1-inch margin. Avoid touching any other items located in the pack, underneath the sterile drape.

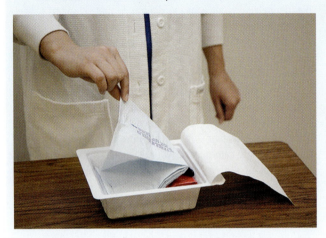

   b. Allow the drape to unfold and place it on the selected surface without contaminating the top working surface of the drape.

3. To add sterile items to the sterile field, open the peel-apart pack and drop the contents onto the drape, being careful not to touch the sterile items or the drape with your bare hands. The two inside surfaces of the peel-apart pack, which are sterile, should be the sides that are exposed to the sterile field as you drop the sterile item onto the field. Your non-sterile hands should be *behind* the sterile surface as the item is dropped. Avoid reaching over the sterile field *to prevent contamination.*

4. To add liquids to a sterile container such as a basin or bowl, follow these steps:

   a. Check the container for the expiration date. If the container has been previously opened, follow facility policy for how long it can be used, generally 24 to 48 hours. Solutions are no longer sterile if they have been opened for too long or are past their expiration date. *Safety: Write the date, time, and your initials on the label of the sterile solution when you open it for the first time.*

   b. Hold the container with the label in your palm. *This prevents any drips from the bottle from running onto the label and obscuring the printing on it.*

   c. Remove the lid from the solution bottle and place it with the edges up on a clean surface, but not on the sterile field. *The outside of the lid is not sterile, but the inside is and should not touch unsterile surfaces.*

   d. Pour a small amount of solution across the lip of the bottle into a cup or trash can *to remove dust or microorganisms that may be present to prevent them from being washed into the sterile basin.* This is referred to as "lipping" the bottle.

   e. Hold the bottle 4 to 6 inches above the sterile basin and pour in a gentle stream to avoid splashing. *If you splash fluid on a sterile drape, your field becomes contaminated, unless you have used a barrier-style drape that has a plastic, moisture-proof backing on it. Moisture cannot permeate the backing and therefore the drape would still be considered sterile.*

   f. Carefully replace the lid on the container, touching only the outer surface. The inner surface of the lid is considered sterile.

5. Don sterile gloves according to Skill 22-2. Then you can touch the items on your sterile field and continue with the procedure.

6. Follow the Initial Implementation Steps located on the inside front cover for procedures during which you are working at the patient's bedside.

Evaluation Steps

1. Evaluate whether the procedure was completed without contamination of the sterile field, sterile supplies, or sterile gloves.

Skill 22-2 Donning Sterile Gloves—Open Method

Assessment Steps

1. Determine the correct size of glove needed.

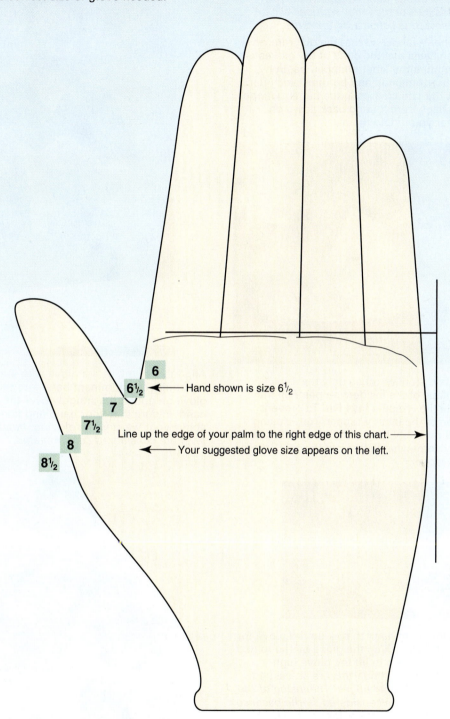

6
6½ ← Hand shown is size 6½
7
7½
8 Line up the edge of your palm to the right edge of this chart. →
8½ ← Your suggested glove size appears on the left.

2. Assess the glove packaging for the expiration date and any holes or tears. Check to be sure the packaging is dry. *Any open areas or wet areas would compromise sterility and the gloves could not be used.*

Planning Steps

1. Determine where you will open the wrapper containing the sterile gloves, thereby establishing a mini–sterile field. Remember to choose a clean, dry surface that is waist-high *to prevent potential contamination of the field.*

Implementation Steps

1. Follow the Initial Implementation Steps located on the inside front cover for procedures during which you will be working at the patient's bedside.

(skill continues on page 464)

Skill 22-2 (continued)

2. Open the outer wrapper and discard it. You may touch the outside of the inner wrapper with your bare hands. *This part of the inner wrapper will be against the table and is considered unsterile.*

3. Position the inner wrapper so that the diagram on the wrapper indicates that the cuffs of the gloves are toward you. To open the inner wrapper, begin by unfolding the horizontal top and bottom 1-inch flaps, smoothing flat the fold creases in the paper wrapper to prevent the flaps from folding back down on themselves after you unfold them.

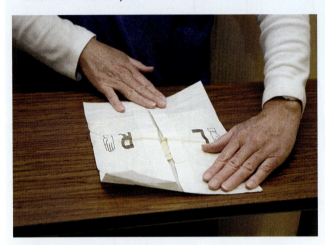

4. Then, to maintain sterility, touch only the 1-inch outer vertical flaps of the inside wrapper. Pull the flaps open until the wrapper lays flat. To prevent these two sides of the inner wrapper from closing again, you will probably have to gently pull the two flaps until they somewhat flatten out the fold creases in the paper wrapper.

6. Align the thumb of the glove with your thumb before inserting your dominant hand into the glove. Pull the glove on until it fits snuggly over the dominant hand. Ensure that your hand and fingers remain above your waist while gloving. *Items below waist level are considered contaminated.*

5. Use your nondominant hand to pick up the glove for your dominant hand. Pick up the glove by the folded cuff edge, making certain to lift the glove high enough so that the glove fingertips are at least 4 to 6 inches above the wrapper edges. *The inside of the cuff and glove will not be considered sterile because they will touch your bare hands.* Take a step back away from your package of sterile gloves. *This provides you with extra room to help prevent contamination by touching the package or surface upon which it lies, while you apply the glove.*

7. To pick up the second glove, slip your sterile gloved fingers underneath the cuff, between the cuff and the sterile palmar surface of the glove. *In this way, your sterile gloved hand touches only sterile surfaces of the glove for the nondominant hand.*

Skill 22-2 (continued)

Remember to lift the glove above the package and take a step backward *to allow yourself more room to prevent contamination*

8. Slide your nondominant hand into the glove, being sure the thumb of the glove aligns with your thumb. Pull the glove on until it fits snuggly over the nondominant hand.

   Note: While donning the second glove, keep the thumb of your dominant hand abducted away from your nondominant hand *to prevent possible contamination by accidental contact with bare skin.*

9. Now that gloves are on both hands, slip the gloved fingertips of your dominant hand underneath the cuff flap of the nondominant hand. Pull the cuff up using the gloved fingers only. Keep the dominant hand thumb abducted. *Using the gloved thumb will likely cause contamination as the cuff unfolds.* When the cuff has been pulled up most of the way on the forearm, remove your dominant hand fingers from underneath the cuff, allowing the cuff to recoil against the nonsterile surface of the forearm.

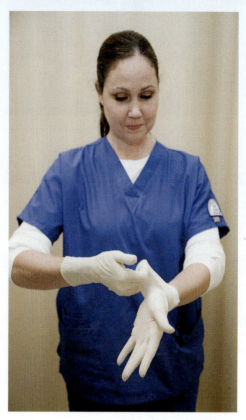

10. Slip the gloved fingertips of your nondominant hand underneath the cuff flap of the glove on your dominant hand, keeping your thumb abducted to prevent contamination. Using the gloved fingers only, pull the cuff up most of the way on the forearm, removing your nondominant hand fingers from underneath the cuff to allow the cuff to recoil against the nonsterile surface of the forearm.

11. Put your gloved hands together with your fingers interlaced to snug the fingers of the gloves against your fingertips so that no extra room remains at the fingertips.

(skill continues on page 466)

Skill 22-2 (continued)

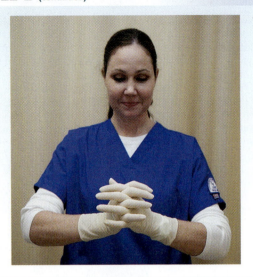

12. Follow the Initial Implementation Steps located on the inside front cover for procedures during which you are working at the patient's bedside.

Evaluation Steps

1. Determine that the procedure was completed without contaminating the sterile gloves or the sterile field.
2. Evaluate the fit of the gloves to determine if you have the correct size. They should fit closely without wrinkles, without excess material at the fingertips, and without bowing due to tightness.

Skill 22-3 Performing a Surgical Hand Scrub

Assessment Steps

1. Assess your readiness to perform the scrub:
   a. You are wearing hospital-laundered scrubs.
   b. You are wearing appropriate shoes or shoe covers.
   c. You have a hair cover and mask in place.

Planning Steps

1. Determine that sterile supplies you will need after completing the hand scrub are available, including sterile towels, a sterile gown, and sterile gloves in the correct size.
2. Determine that needed supplies are available for the hand scrub: knee- or foot-controlled water source, antiseptic soap, and an orangewood stick or other tool for cleaning nails.
3. Remove all jewelry from your hands and arms, such as rings and watches. Remove nail polish if it is chipped.

Implementation Steps

1. Turn on the water to a comfortable warm temperature. *Water that is too hot destroys natural oils and causes cracking of skin. Water that is too cold does not wash off soap or destroy bacteria, and causes chapping.*
2. Rinse each hand and arm from the fingertips to the elbows. Keep your fingertips above your elbows as you wash and rinse *to prevent water from your arms from running down over your clean hands.*
3. Obtain a palmful of antibacterial soap using a foot control. *This prevents your rinsed hands from touching a dirty soap dispenser.*
4. For the first handwash, lather your hands and up your arms to 2 inches above the elbow. *This removes some microorganisms before you begin the actual scrub.*
5. Under running water, use a clean orangewood stick or other tool to clean beneath your nails and around the cuticles.

6. Rinse your hands and arms again from fingertips to elbows, with the hands kept above the elbows. *Avoid touching the sink or dispensers with your hands as they are considered contaminated.*
7. Begin the hand scrub. **When scrubbing with an antimicrobial agent, follow these steps:**
   a. Dispense the antimicrobial soap into your hand according to facility policy.
   b. Apply to one hand and arm up to 2 inches above the elbow.
   c. Divide each finger, hand, and arm into four surfaces in your mind: ventral (palm side of hand), dorsal (back of hand), and two lateral (sides of hand) surfaces.
   d. Now divide your arm into the distal section, from the wrist to 4 inches up the forearm, and the proximal section, from 4 inches up the forearm to 2 inches above the elbow.

Skill 22-3 (continued)

e. Rub the lather for at least 10 strokes on each surface, for a total of 40 strokes on each finger, 40 strokes on the hand, and 40 strokes on the wrist and distal arm, and 40 strokes on the proximal arm and above the elbow. **Note:** The total scrub time is 3 to 5 minutes. Follow facility policy.

f. Repeat for the other hand and arm.

g. Repeat the scrub process if directed by facility policy.

h. Rinse from the fingertips to the elbows, keeping the hands above the elbows *so that contaminated water flows away from your hands.*

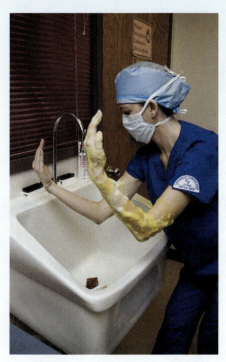

i. Dry your hands from the fingertips to the elbows using one sterile towel for each arm and hand. While drying, lean forward, bending from the waist, *to prevent the sterile towel with which you are drying from coming in contact with your scrubs.*

When using an alcohol-based surgical hand gel, follow these steps:

a. Dry hands thoroughly after the first handwash with a paper towel.

b. Obtain the recommended amount of surgical hand gel. Follow facility policy.

c. Apply the product to completely cover your hands and forearms, rubbing until it is dry.

d. Repeat the application of the product if that is what is recommended by the manufacturer. Again, follow facility policy.

8. Proceed to the anteroom of the operating room or other sterile area, keeping your cleansed hands raised above your elbows and positioned in front of you *so that they remain within the "safe zone,"* and don your sterile gown and gloves according to Skill 22-4.

Evaluation Steps

1. Determine if you completed the hand scrub according to facility policy, within the appropriate time frame and number of strokes recommended.

2. Evaluate whether you touched any contaminated surfaces during or after the surgical hand scrub. If this occurred, repeat the hand scrub.

Skill 22-4   Donning a Sterile Gown and Sterile Gloves—Closed Method

Assessment Steps

1. Assess your readiness to gown and glove to enter the sterile area:

a. Are you dressed in appropriate scrubs, shoe covers, hair cover, and mask?

b. Have you determined if needed supplies of sterile towels, gown, and gloves are available before beginning the surgical hand scrub?

c. Have you completed a surgical hand scrub? (See Skill 22-3).

Planning Steps

1. Arrange for a circulating nurse to assist you.

Implementation Steps

1. Pick up the sterile gown at the inner neckline and allow it to unfold, keeping the gown away from unsterile surfaces *to prevent contamination.*

2. Slip both of your arms into the arms of the gown and grasp the inside of the arms, leaving your hands within the cuffs of the gown.

(skill continues on page 468)

Skill 22-4 (continued)

3. Have the circulating nurse pull the neck area of the gown together, *touching only the inside to prevent contamination.* The circulating nurse will also tie the gown at the neck.

4. Do not push your hands through the gown sleeves. Keep them within the cuffs of the gown.

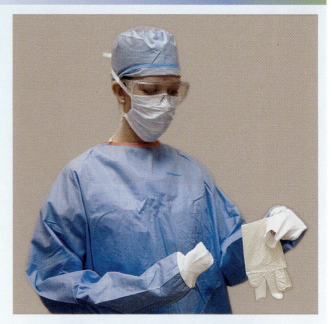

7. Place the glove on the forearm of your dominant hand, palm side down, with the glove fingers pointing toward your elbow and the glove thumb aligned with your thumb.

5. With your hands still inside the gown sleeves, open the sterile glove wrapper by grasping it through the gown material.
   Note: If the glove package is lying on a sterile field, the outer wrapper will already have been removed. If it is lying on a nonsterile field, the outer wrapper will have been opened, and the sterile inner wrapper will be lying on the sterile inside surface of the outer wrapper. As you open this sterile inner wrapper, do not allow your sterile gown cuffs to touch anything other than the sterile inner wrapper and gloves.

6. Pick up the glove for your dominant hand at the cuff with your nondominant hand, which is still inside the gown sleeve.

8. Grasp the inside of the cuff with the fingers of your dominant hand, which is still inside the gown sleeve.

9. Using your nondominant hand through the gown material, pull the dominant glove cuff over the gown cuff.

Skill 22-4 (continued)

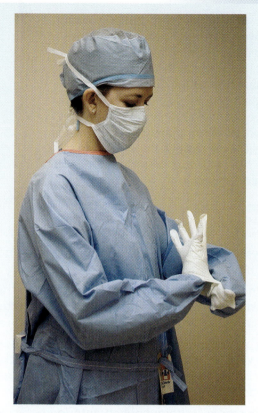

10. Slide your dominant hand into the glove as you pull up the glove cuff and gown cuff with your nondominant hand, which still remains within the gown sleeve.

11. Pick up the glove for your nondominant hand and place it on your forearm with the glove fingers pointing toward your elbow and the glove thumb aligned with your thumb.

12. Using your dominant gloved hand, pull the nondominant glove cuff over the gown cuff.

13. Slide your nondominant hand into the glove as you pull up the glove cuff and gown cuff with your gloved dominant hand.

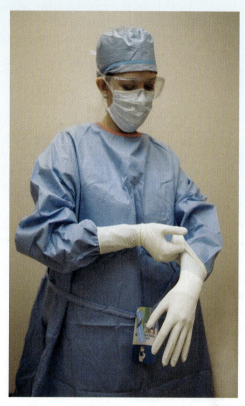

14. Adjust the fingers and smooth out any glove wrinkles. Ensure that the glove cuffs cover the gown cuffs so that no skin is exposed.
    Note: Although your skin has been scrubbed, it cannot actually be sterile and therefore may still harbor some pathogens.

15. Keep your hands together and above your waist. Enter the operating room by backing through the swinging doors, using care to avoid touching the front and sleeves of your sterile gown, as well as your gloves, against any unsterile surface.

Evaluation Steps

1. Evaluate whether you put on the sterile gown and sterile gloves with the closed method without contaminating them:

   a. Did your bare hands touch any part of the sterile gown other than the inside?

   b. Did your bare hands touch any part of the sterile gloves other than the inside?

   c. Once the sterile gloves were donned, did they remain covering the cuffs of the sterile gown so that no bare skin was exposed at any time?

Post Conference

Your instructor asks you to share your experience with the other students during Post Conference. You tell them that, although you were very nervous, you were able to set up everything needed for the procedure. The staff nurse reminded you to obtain masks and goggles for the physician, the nurse, and yourself. You remembered the principles of sterile technique while setting up the field and adding items to it. During the procedure, the physician asked for more gauze 4x4s, which you had not opened, but did have in the room. You remembered to peel apart the pack, with the opening toward the physician. You kept your bare hands away from the sterile gauze, allowing the physician to remove the 4x4s from the pack without contaminating his sterile gloves. The procedure went smoothly and safely for the patient with no breaches of sterile technique.

KEY POINTS

- Sterile technique is the method used for invasive procedures to prevent pathogens from entering the body by careful cleaning and sterilization of equipment and supplies, as well as the use of sterile gowns and gloves.

- Common types of sterilization include autoclaving, boiling, ionizing radiation, chemical disinfection, and gaseous disinfection.

- To check the sterility of an item, look at the expiration date, check for black hash marks on indicator tape, and examine the packaging for evidence that it has been wet (strike-through) or for holes or tears.

- Sterile technique is used in restricted areas of the hospital as well as at the patient's bedside for invasive procedures.

- Contamination occurs when a sterile field or sterile object may be exposed to pathogens due to potential or full contact with a nonsterile surface.

- A sterile conscience is the awareness of potential or certain contamination of a sterile field or items. It is up to you to admit that possible contamination occurred and start the procedure again with fresh sterile supplies, even if no one else observed the contamination.

- If anything unsterile touches a sterile field or item, it becomes unsterile. If in doubt, consider it unsterile.

- When setting up a sterile field, anything below the table surface is considered contaminated, as well as the outer 1 inch of the sterile drape. If it becomes damp or wet, it is no longer sterile.

- When adding items to the sterile field, follow specific guidelines to avoid contamination with sterile liquids and avoid contamination of items you wish to add.

- When opening sterile packs, always open the first flap away from you and the last flap toward you.

- Avoid reaching across a sterile field and keep it in view at all times, never turning your back to it. Set up the sterile field just before you are ready to use it.

- Use sterile technique when entering body cavities, veins, or arteries; when caring for patients with nonintact skin; and when handling needles, syringes, and lancets.

REVIEW QUESTIONS

Select the answer that is most appropriate for each of the following questions. Some questions may have more than one correct answer. Check all that apply.

1. Your patient has been discharged from the hospital. Remaining in the room are an IV pump and a *hemostat*, a metal-hinged instrument used to clamp off tubes or blood vessels. Which actions will you take?

   a. Clean the pump with disinfectant and rinse the hemostat in cool or warm water before sending it to be sterilized.

   b. Take both items to the central supply area to be cleaned and then sterilized.

   c. Return the IV pump to the storage area on the nursing unit and throw away the hemostat.

   d. Call the housekeeping staff and ask them to dispose of the equipment when they clean the room.

2. You are preparing to use a sterile pack. Which of these findings would concern you the most?

  a. The expiration date is 2 weeks in the future.

  b. It is difficult to read the initials of the person who sterilized the pack.

  c. The hash marks on the indicator tape are the same color as the tape.

  d. There are no holes or tears, and no evidence of strike-through.

3. As you prepare for a rotation in the heart catheterization laboratory, you will expect:

  a. to change into hospital-laundered scrubs.

  b. to wear street clothes covered by a lab coat in the patient care area.

  c. that it is a restricted area to maintain asepsis.

  d. to wear your regular scrubs covered by a gown, as well as wearing a mask and goggles.

4. The nurse will use sterile technique when performing which of the following procedures?

  a. Insertion of a urinary catheter

  b. Emptying a catheter drainage bag

  c. Starting an IV line

  d. Assessing the IV drip rate

  e. Performing a bed bath

  f. Suctioning the trachea

  g. Administering an insulin injection

5. A nurse is attempting to insert a sterile catheter into a patient's bladder. The nurse accidentally brushes the tip of the catheter against the side rail of the bed. The patient is unaware of this incident. Which action will the nurse take?

  a. Clean the tip of the catheter with an alcohol swab and continue with the procedure.

  b. Discard the contaminated catheter and begin the procedure over again.

  c. Say nothing and use the catheter anyway, since no one saw what happened.

  d. Stop the procedure, leave the room to get a fresh catheter, and resume the procedure.

6. A nurse wearing sterile gloves pushes up his glasses with his gloved hand. The nurse's next action is to:

  a. wash his hands while wearing his sterile gloves.

  b. remove the sterile gloves and wash his hands.

  c. obtain and don a second pair of sterile gloves.

  d. b and c.

CRITICAL THINKING EXERCISES

7. You are a student assigned to observe in the operating room. During the preparations for the surgery, you notice that the physician touches the sterile field before donning sterile gloves. What, if any, action will you take?

8. You are assigned to teach a patient with bladder problems how to perform self-catheterizations at home. The physician tells you to teach the patient to do this using medical asepsis rather than surgical asepsis. What is the rationale for such an order?

9. You are preparing to enter the operating room for clinical observation. List, in order, the steps you will take to make yourself as sterile as possible before entering the operating suite.

ADDITIONAL RESOURCES

For additional Resources, Questions, and Activities, please see:

 Student Resource Disk

 http://davisplus.fadavis.com

 Student Study Guide

REFERENCES

AORN Recommended Practices Committee. Recommended practices for surgical hand antisepsis/hand scrubs. *AORN J.* 2004;79:416-418, 421-426, 429-431.

Groves N. Decontamination of surgical instruments is no place to cut corners. *Ophthalmol Times.* 2008;September 15.

Gupta C, Czubatyj AM, Briski LE, Malani AK. Comparison of two alcohol-based surgical scrub solutions with an iodine-based scrub brush for presurgical antiseptic effectiveness in a community hospital. *J Hosp Infect.* 2007;65(1):65-71.

Johns Hopkins Medicine. Surgical scrub solution: It's good for patients, too. September 4, 2009. Available at: http://www.medicalnewstoday.com/articles/163005.php. Accessed September 5, 2009.

Johnson AW. Is sterile technique vital in the cath lab? *Cath Lab Digest.* 2008;16(6).

Kortgen A, Neiderprüm P, Bauer M. Implementation of an evidenced-based "standard operating procedure" and outcome in septic shock. *Crit Care Med.* 2006;34:943-949.

McLachlan E. Proper sterilization of instruments is essential to patient safety. Association for Professionals in Infection Control and Epidemiology Web site. Available at: http://www.apic.org. Accessed November 9, 2008.

Ogg M, Peterson C. Surgical hand antisepsis; hand lotions and creams; gel overlays as artificial nails; benchmarking. *AORN J.* 2007;85: 815-818.

Venes D, ed. *Taber's Cyclopedic Medical Dictionary.* 20th ed. Philadelphia: FA Davis; 2005.

Taurasi R. Maintain sterility in setting up procedure trays, and what is thermal equilibrium? *Healthcare Purchasing News.* 2004;October 4.

Wilkinson JM, Van Leuven K. *Fundamentals of Nursing: Theory, Concepts & Applications.* Philadelphia: FA Davis; 2007.

Clinical Skills and Care

Key Terms

Absorption

Antioxidants

Body mass index (BMI)

Catabolism

Complex carbohydrates

Dietary Reference Intakes (DRIs)

Digestion

Essential amino acids

Metabolism

Nitrogen balance

Nonessential amino acids

Nutrient interaction

Peristalsis

Satiety

Simple carbohydrates

Water balance

Objectives

1. Describe saturated, monounsaturated, polyunsaturated, and trans fats.
2. Define simple and complex carbohydrates.
3. List sources of complex carbohydrates.
4. Explain the difference between complete and incomplete proteins, including sources of each.
5. Contrast fat-soluble and water-soluble vitamins.
6. Describe general functions and sources of minerals.
7. Describe how to use food labels to make better food choices.
8. Explain how culture influences food choices.
9. Explain the importance of adequate fluid intake, including the recommended amounts for men, women, and pregnant women.

Clinical Connection

Your Assignment: You are caring for a 68-year-old male who is hospitalized for extreme constipation. He is having bowel movements now, but has had a poor diet that contributed to his constipation problems. His wife died 9 months ago. He eats mostly canned soups and processed lunch meats on white bread because he does not cook much. He sometimes gets fast food, such as hamburgers or fried chicken. He likes meat but does not eat vegetables or fruits. He tells you they go bad before he can eat them all, so they are a waste of money. He mostly drinks soft drinks throughout the day.

Your Actions: Not only do you need to monitor your patient's response to laxatives and stool softeners to be sure that his bowels are emptying properly, you also need to help your patient find ways to prevent re-hospitalization for constipation in the future. What nutritional concerns do you have for this patient? How can improving his diet help prevent constipation? What will you do to help him manage this problem?

The body requires adequate amounts of nutrients to maintain proper functioning. Even a relatively small nutrient imbalance can cause severe health problems. Proper nutrition is essential for a stronger immune system, less illness, and better health. To maintain life, nutrients must provide energy, build tissue, and regulate metabolic processes. Nutrients are essential to **metabolism**, the physical and chemical processes in the body that create and use energy. This chapter will show you the importance of nutrition and specific nutrients pertinent for optimal health. You will learn how nutritional needs differ through the life span, sources of nutrients, and how culture influences individual food preferences.

Nutrition

Nutrients are provided through natural (food) and artificial (supplements) sources. Nutrients include protein, carbohydrates, fats, vitamins, minerals, and water. The principle of **nutrient interaction** states that individual nutrients have primary and secondary functions and must work together to sustain the body's metabolic processes. Food provides energy, which is measured in kilocalories (kcal). Energy enables cells to perform all of their functions, including building proteins and other substances needed by the body. This energy can be used immediately or stored to be used later. Energy requirements vary throughout life. Typically, to maintain body weight, sedentary women, young children, and older adults need about 1,600 calories a day; older children, active adult women, and sedentary men need about 2,000 calories; and active adolescent boys and men need about 2,400 calories.

Nutrients are classified as either macronutrients or micronutrients. *Macronutrients* are required by the body on a daily basis in large amounts (grams) and include protein, carbohydrates, fats, water, and some minerals.

Micronutrients are also required daily, but in much smaller amounts (milligrams). Micronutrients include vitamins and trace minerals.

Knowledge Connection

How many calories does the average active adult male need per day? A sedentary woman? A young child? Which categories of individuals need around 2,400 calories per day?

FDA Guidelines and Food Labels

The Food and Drug Administration (FDA) first established standards for the minimum amount of nutrients necessary to protect most individuals from disease. These standard guidelines are known as **Dietary Reference Intakes (DRIs)** and contain recommendations for gender, age, pregnancy, and lactation. The DRIs are composed of four categories of nutrient recommendations:

1. **Recommended Dietary Allowance (RDA):** the amounts of selected nutrients considered adequate to meet the known nutrient needs of healthy people
2. **Estimated Average Requirement (EAR):** the intake level for a nutrient at which the needs of 50% of the population will be met.
3. **Adequate Intake (AI):** the amount of a nutrient that appears to maintain good health
4. **Tolerable Upper Intake Level (UL):** the maximum level of daily nutrient intake that is likely to pose no risk of adverse effects

The Nutrition Labeling and Education Act was passed in 1990 to ensure that food product labels include accurate information regarding nutritional content of foods. The U.S. Department of Agriculture (USDA) labeling laws ensure that meat and poultry products are safe, wholesome, and accurately labeled. Nutrition Facts food labels are found on all processed food products. Each label provides an ingredient list and nutritional descriptions (Fig. 23-1). These labels are meant to give consumers the facts they need to make informed decisions as they shop.

Each food label consists of six major components:

1. Food amount and energy content
2. Macronutrient content
3. Vitamin and mineral content
4. Daily Reference Value
5. Health claims
6. Labels for special needs

Dietary Guidelines for Americans

The *Dietary Guidelines for Americans* has been published jointly every 5 years since 1980 by the U.S. Department of Health and Human Services (DHHS) and the USDA. These guidelines provide authoritative advice for people 2 years and older about how good dietary habits can promote health and reduce risk for major chronic diseases. They serve as the basis for federal food and nutrition education programs. Key recommendations include:

• Consuming a variety of nutrient-dense foods and beverages within and among the basic food groups while choosing foods that limit the intake of saturated fats and trans-fatty acids (trans fats), cholesterol, added sugars, salt, and alcohol.
• Meeting recommended intakes within energy needs by adopting a balanced eating pattern.

Nutrition Facts	
Serving Size 1/2 cup (114g)	
Servings Per Container 4	

Amount Per Serving	
Calories 90	Calories from Fat 30

	% Daily Value *
Total Fat 3g	5%
Saturated Fat 0g	0%
Trans Fat 0g	0%
Cholesterol 0mg	0%
Sodium 300mg	13%
Total Carbohydrate 13g	4%
Dietary Fiber 3g	12%
Sugars 3g	
Protein 3g	

Vitamin A	80%	•	Vitamin C	60%
Calcium	4%	•	Iron	4%

* Percent Daily Values are based on a 2,000 calorie diet. Your daily values may be higher or lower depending on your calorie needs:

		Calories	2,000	2,500
Total Fat	Less than		65g	80g
Sat Fat	Less than		20g	25g
Cholesterol	Less than		300mg	300mg
Sodium	Less than		2,400mg	2,400mg
Total Carbohydrate			300g	375g
Dietary Fiber			25g	30g

Calories per gram:			
Fat 9	•	Carbohydrate 4	•	Protein 4

Figure 23-1 An example of a food label.

Key Dietary Recommendations for Specific Population Groups

As nutritional research advances, certain nutritional recommendations are made for specific population groups. Some important recommendations include the following:

• **People older than age 50 years:** Consume vitamin B_{12} in its crystalline form, such as in fortified foods or supplements.
• **Women of childbearing age who may become pregnant:** Eat foods high in heme-iron or consume iron-rich plant foods or iron-fortified foods with an enhancer of iron absorption, such as vitamin C–rich foods.
• **Women of childbearing age who may become pregnant and those in the first trimester of pregnancy:** Consume adequate synthetic folic acid daily (from fortified foods or supplements) in addition to food forms of folate from spinach, dried beans and peas, and citrus fruits.
• **Older adults, people with dark skin, and people exposed to insufficient ultraviolet-band radiation (sunlight):** Consume extra vitamin D from vitamin D–fortified foods or supplements.

Box 23-1 features key dietary recommendations for specific population groups.

Two examples of balanced eating patterns that exemplify the *Dietary Guidelines* are the Dietary Approaches to Stop Hypertension (DASH) Eating Plan and the USDA Food Guide, as shown in the MyPyramid food management system. These two similar eating patterns are designed to integrate dietary recommendations into a healthy way to eat and are used in the *Dietary Guidelines* to provide examples of how nutrient-focused recommendations can be expressed in terms of food choices. Table 23-1 provides a comparison of the USDA Food Guide and the DASH Eating Plan.

Both the USDA Food Guide and the DASH Eating Plan differ in important ways from common food consumption patterns in the United States. In general, they include:

• *More* dark green vegetables, orange vegetables, legumes, fruits, whole grains, and low-fat milk and milk products
• *Less* refined grains, total fats (especially cholesterol and saturated and trans fats), added sugars, and calories

Knowledge Connection

What dietary recommendation is made for people older than 50? Women who are pregnant? According to the consumption habits of the United States, relate at least one recommendation for healthier eating habits.

The DASH Eating Plan

The DASH diet is rich in vegetables and fruits; low in fat dairy products, saturated and total fat, and cholesterol; high in fiber, potassium, calcium, and magnesium; and moderately high in protein. The DASH eating plan follows

Table 23-1 Comparison of USDA Food Guide and DASH Eating Plan

Food Categories	DASH Eating Plan Recommendations	USDA Food Guide Recommendations
Fruits	2–2.5 cups per day	2 cups per day
Vegetables	2–2.5 cups per day	2.5 cups per day
Grains	7–8 servings per day	6 servings per day
Dairy	2–3 servings per day	6 ounces per day
Meats, Poultry, Fish,	6 ounces or less per day	5.5 ounces per day
Nuts, Seeds, Dry Beans	4–5 servings per week	Not considered a separate category; included in vegetable group
Oils	2–3 tsp. per day	6 tsp. per day
Added Sugar and Solid Fats	Limit to 2 tsp. per day	8 tsp. per day

Source: Adapted from U.S. Department of Health and Human Services. Dietary Guidelines for Americans. January 12, 2005. Available at: http://www.health.gov/dietaryguidelines/dga2005/document/default.htm.

heart-healthy guidelines to limit saturated fat and cholesterol. It focuses on increasing intake of foods rich in nutrients that are expected to lower blood pressure—mainly minerals such as potassium, calcium, and magnesium; protein; and fiber. It includes nutrient-rich foods so that it meets other nutrient requirements as recommended by the Institute of Medicine.

MyPyramid

The USDA's Center for Nutrition Policy and Promotion developed the MyPyramid food management system to establish recommendations for amount of food per group based on age, gender, and activity level. This food guidance system visually represents the five basic food groups: grains, vegetables, fruits, milk, and meat and beans (Fig. 23-2). The MyPyramid guide found at *www.MyPyramid.gov* is interactive and can be adapted to various groups according to cultural and religious preferences. MyPyramid can also be adapted to meet the nutritional needs of pregnant or lactating women.

American Heart Association Diet

The American Heart Association (AHA) is on a mission to build healthier lives that are free of heart disease and stroke. Proper nutrition is essential in prevention of disease. The AHA recommends tracking calories, getting regular exercise of at least 30 minutes a day, and eating a variety of nutritious foods from all food groups. Healthy choices include vegetables and fruits, whole grains, and fish. It is recommended that individuals eat less saturated fat, trans fat, and processed foods.

Anatomy and Physiology Connection

Digestion

Digestion is the process in which food is broken down in the gastrointestinal (GI) tract, releasing nutrients for the body to use. The process of digestion begins in the mouth, where a digestive enzyme called *salivary amylase* begins breaking down simple carbohydrates and fat. The mechanical motion of chewing breaks down starches into smaller products, with saliva moistening the foods. The esophagus transports foods from the mouth into the stomach through a process called *motility*. Muscles and nerves work together to spontaneously move food down the GI tract. No chemical or mechanical digestion occurs in the esophagus.

The gastric juices of the stomach are acidic in nature, which *hydrolyzes* (adds water to break down) carbohydrates into maltose and sucrose. Proteolytic and lypolytic enzymes mix with food and break down small amounts of proteins and fat. The stomach gently contracts and expands to further break down food particles. The gastrointestinal contractions known as **peristalsis** gently propel the food bolus into the small intestine.

Most digestion occurs in the first several feet of the small intestine through absorption. **Absorption** is the process in which nutrients are taken from the end products of digestion into the blood of the capillaries that are located in the villi that line the small intestine. Once food leaves the stomach, the digestion process in the small intestine is activated. Digestive enzymes are released from the liver, gallbladder, pancreas, and small intestine, resulting in the breakdown of starches

MyPyramid
STEPS TO A HEALTHIER YOU
MyPyramid.gov

GRAINS	VEGETABLES	FRUITS	MILK	MEAT & BEANS
Make half your grains whole	Vary your veggies	Focus on fruits	Get your calcium-rich foods	Go lean with protein
Eat at least 3 oz. of whole-grain cereals, breads, crackers, rice, or pasta every day 1 oz. is about 1 slice of bread, about 1 cup of breakfast cereal, or 1/2 cup of cooked rice, cereal, or pasta	Eat more dark-green veggies like broccoli, spinach, and other dark leafy greens Eat more orange vegetables like carrots and sweetpotatoes Eat more dry beans and peas like pinto beans, kidney beans, lentils	Eat a variety of fruit Choose fresh, frozen, canned, or dried fruit Go easy on fruit juices	Go low-fat or fat-free when you choose milk, yogurt, and other milk products If you don't or can't consume milk, choose lactose-free products or other calcium sources such as fortified foods and beverages	Choose low-fat or lean meats and poultry Bake it, broil it, or grill it Vary your protein routine – choose more fish, beans, peas, nuts, and seeds

For a 2,000-calorie diet, you need the amounts below from each food group. To find the amounts that are right for you, go to MyPyramid.gov.

Eat 6 oz. every day	Eat 2½ cups every day	Eat 2 cups every day	Get 3 cups every day; for kids aged 2 to 8, it's 2 cups	Eat 5½ oz. every day

Find your balance between food and physical activity

- Be sure to stay within your daily calorie needs.
- Be physically active for at least 30 minutes most days of the week.
- About 60 minutes a day of physical activity may be needed to prevent weight gain.
- For sustaining weight loss, at least 60 to 90 minutes a day of physical activity may be required.
- Children and teenagers should be physically active for 60 minutes every day, or most days.

Know the limits on fats, sugars, and salt (sodium)

- Make most of your fat sources from fish, nuts, and vegetable oils.
- Limit solid fats like butter, margarine, shortening, and lard, as well as foods that contain these.
- Check the Nutrition Facts label to keep saturated fats, *trans* fats, and sodium low.
- Choose food and beverages low in added sugars. Added sugars contribute calories with few, if any, nutrients.

U.S. Department of Agriculture
Center for Nutrition Policy and Promotion
April 2005
CNPP-14

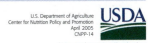

Figure 23-2   MyPyramid shows the number of recommended servings and food sources for the various food groups.

and proteins. Dietary fats are reduced to free fatty acids and monoglycerides. Almost all macronutrients, minerals, vitamins, and fluid are absorbed in the small intestine.

The colon and rectum absorb most of the fluid in digestion, along with small amounts of remaining nutrients and electrolytes. The colon plays an essential role in fermentation of starches, which produces short-chain fatty acids. These substances are important in maintaining normal mucosal functioning and assist in absorption of remaining water and sodium.

Nutrients absorbed from the GI tract travel through the portal vein to the liver, where they are either stored, transformed into other products, or released into circulation. Once released into circulation, nutrients are delivered via the bloodstream or lymphatic system to areas of need. Certain nutrients, such as fatty acids, that are not immediately used are stored in the body as adipose tissue.

Essential Nutrients and Their General Function

Water and all the essential nutrients must be ingested in a balanced ratio. Inadequate or excessive intake of any one nutrient or water can result in imbalances that are capable of impairing the body's ability for optimal functioning.

Water

Water is essential to life. The total body weight of an average adult is approximately 60% water. Water is found throughout the body and is the major component of blood and urine. Each body system depends on water for proper functioning all the way down to the cellular level. Some of the functions of water are to help maintain body temperature and blood pressure, flush out toxins from your system, carry nutrients to your cells, and provide lubrication for the ear, nose, and mouth. To maintain proper **water balance**, water intake should equal urine output and other water losses.

In general, the average adult needs a minimum of six to eight 8-ounce glasses, or 1,440 to 1,920 mL, of water per day. Some individuals need more, up to 3,100 mL/day. Most ingested fluids are generally counted as water or fluid intake. The actual amount of water required per individual will increase or decrease related to body needs. Certain factors affect water needs, including:

- **Exercise:** Increased perspiration related to exercise increases the body's need for water.
- **Environment:** Elevated temperatures in the summer, along with high humidity levels, increase the need for water.
- **Illness:** The body's need for water is increased in patients with fever, diarrhea, vomiting, or other hypermetabolic processes.
- **Pregnancy or breastfeeding:** Women who are expecting or breastfeeding need additional fluids to stay hydrated. Large amounts of fluid are used, especially when nursing.

The Institute of Medicine recommends that pregnant women drink 2.3 liters (approximately 10 cups or 2,290 mL) of fluids daily, and women who breastfeed should consume 3.1 liters (approximately 13 cups or 3,086 mL) of fluids a day.

Knowledge Connection
Explain at least four functions of water. What is the recommended volume of fluid intake per day? Which groups of people require more intake of water than the average person? How much water do you drink daily?

Protein

The body contains large amounts of protein. Protein, the main building block in the body, is the primary component of most cells and is essential for growth and development. For example, muscle, connective tissues, and skin are all built of protein. Protein is required for the following body functions:

- Producing energy and heat
- Building new tissue
- Manufacturing hormones and enzymes
- Forming antibodies
- Maintaining acid-base balance

The human body contains more than 100,000 different types of protein. Approximately 50% of this protein is found in skeletal muscle tissue. Body proteins are continuously broken down into amino acids through a process known as **catabolism**. These excess amino acids are then reorganized, or built, into tissue products through *anabolism*. The intake and use of dietary protein is measured by the amount of nitrogen intake in food protein and the amount of nitrogen excreted in the urine.

Nitrogen balance must be maintained for the body to remain in equilibrium. For every 1 gram of urinary nitrogen that is excreted, 6.25 grams of protein must be ingested. Positive nitrogen balance exists when the body takes in more nitrogen than it excretes, which allows the body to use the excess nitrogen to grow new tissue. This condition occurs normally during periods of rapid growth, such as childhood, and during pregnancy. Negative nitrogen balance occurs when excess nitrogen is excreted, with inadequate amounts of protein being consumed. Negative nitrogen balance occurs commonly in malnutrition. This condition can cause loss of muscle tone and growth retardation.

Proteins are composed of amino acids that are broken down into two categories: essential and nonessential. **Essential amino acids** cannot be made by the body and must be ingested through food. Examples of essential amino acids include lysine, histidine, and tryptophan. Essential amino acids can be found in:

- Milk
- Cheese
- Eggs
- Grains

Nonessential amino acids are made by the body through the breakdown of essential amino acids or through the normal breakdown of protein. Examples include alanine, glutamine, and tyrosine.

In a well-balanced diet, protein should provide between 10% and 35% of the total daily calories. Adults need to eat about 60 grams of protein per day. Proteins are grouped together as either complete or incomplete proteins. *Complete proteins* contain all nine essential amino acids. These are found in animal sources such as meat, fish, eggs, milk, and milk products. Soy is the only plant protein that is considered to be a complete protein. *Incomplete proteins* lack one or more of the essential amino acids. Foods containing incomplete proteins include:

- Nuts
- Corn
- Wheat
- Beans
- Seeds
- Brown rice

Eating combinations of incomplete proteins provides the body with all nine amino acids needed for complete protein synthesis. By consuming two or more of the incomplete protein sources, the vegetarian is still able to meet his or her protein requirements. Commonly used combinations include:

- Red beans and brown rice
- Peanut butter and whole wheat bread
- Brown beans and cornbread

Protein Digestion

Protein digestion begins in the stomach, where hydrochloric acid breaks down large proteins into amino acids. At the same time, the digestive enzyme pepsin works to digest these amino acids. As the food moves through the GI tract into the duodenum, the digestive enzymes trypsin and chymotrypsin further break down amino acids until they are small enough to be absorbed through the *villi*, or small vascular protrusions that line the small intestine. Once in the bloodstream, the amino acids are distributed by both red blood cells and plasma to tissues throughout the body, where they are used in the creation and repair of cell structures. The demand for protein is so great that the body maintains a constant balance of amino acids in the blood. Without adequate protein, the body cannot repair or heal tissues adequately or as quickly as is needed.

Knowledge Connection

What is the primary bodily function of protein? What does the body maintain in constant supply to ensure adequate protein availability? Explain the difference between complete and incomplete proteins. Which of the two requires consumption of two types of food in order to provide essential proteins?

Fats

Fats are another important source of energy for the body. Fat is the most concentrated source of energy in the diet, providing 9 kcal/g compared with 4 kcal/g from either carbohydrates or protein. Fat supplies essential fatty acids, is required for maintenance of healthy skin, and aids in the absorption of fat-soluble vitamins. The largest amount of fat is stored in the body's adipose or fat cells, but some fat is found in blood plasma and other body cells. These fat deposits not only store energy, but also are important in insulating the body and supporting and cushioning organs.

Dietary fat is broken down into several categories, including saturated, monounsaturated, polyunsaturated, and trans fats. *Saturated fats* are solid at room temperature and are implicated in cardiovascular disease because they raise blood cholesterol. Box 23-2 lists the main food sources of these fats.

Saturated fats are found primarily in animal sources, but are also found in plant oils such as coconut oil and palm oil. These oils are commonly added to packaged foods such as cookies, cakes, doughnuts, and pies. *Trans fats* are partially hydrogenated oils that are used to keep foods fresh. Historically, trans fats have been added to packaged foods, but most manufacturers have recently reduced the amount of trans fats used in their products due to the association of trans fats with elevated cholesterol.

Cholesterol is a naturally occurring fat that is found in the bloodstream. Cholesterol is vital in the production of cell membranes, in hormone production, and for the metabolism of fat-soluble vitamins. It is manufactured by the liver, which produces about 75% of total body cholesterol. The remaining 25% comes from food sources. Cholesterol is carried through the body by substances called *lipoproteins*. *Low-density lipoproteins (LDLs)* are known as *bad cholesterol*. LDLs carry cholesterol throughout the body, depositing excess cholesterol in the coronary arteries and brain.

Box 23-2

Fats That Elevate Total Cholesterol

Some fats are healthy and needed, while other fats are detrimental to health, making it very important to differentiate between the good fats and the bad ones. Educate your patients regarding the three types of fat that tend to elevate one's cholesterol level. Teach patients to avoid or at least limit consumption of the following three fats:

- **Trans fats:** Found in partially hydrogenated vegetable oils. Usually found in processed foods such as cookies and crackers, cakes and doughnuts, and french fries.
- **Dietary cholesterol:** From animal sources, such as beef and pork (especially liver and heart), fish, poultry, egg yolks, and dairy products.
- **Saturated fats:** From animal sources, and found in such foods as whole milk and whole-milk cheeses, ice cream, butter, lard, and most meats.

High levels of blood cholesterol are a major risk factor for coronary artery disease and stroke. Trans fats are implicated in raising LDL cholesterol, leading to increased rates of coronary artery disease and stroke. *High-density lipoproteins (HDLs)*, or *good cholesterol*, remove cholesterol from the arteries, transporting it back to the liver for excretion. Laboratory values for total cholesterol, LDLs, HDLs, and triglycerides are grouped into a *lipid profile* (Table 23-2). A trick for remembering which cholesterol is desired at higher ranges and which one at lower ranges is that the *L*DL (bad cholesterol) should be *l*ow and the *H*DL (good cholesterol) should be *h*igh.

Monounsaturated fats have one double-bonded (unsaturated) carbon in the molecule. Monounsaturated fats are liquid at room temperature but start to turn solid when chilled. Olive oil is an example of a type of oil that contains monounsaturated fats. These fats have been shown to decrease levels of LDL cholesterol, which have a positive impact on total blood cholesterol levels. Examples of foods high in monounsaturated fats include vegetable oils such as olive oil, canola oil, peanut oil, sunflower oil, and sesame oil. Other sources include avocados, peanut butter, and many nuts and seeds.

Polyunsaturated fats have more than one double-bonded (unsaturated) carbon in the molecule. Polyunsaturated fats are usually liquid at room temperature and when chilled. Polyunsaturated fats provide the essential fats that the body needs for normal cell development. Examples of polyunsaturated fats include omega-6 and omega-3 fatty acids; they can be found in fatty fish such as salmon, mackerel, herring, and trout.

Fat Digestion

The first step in digestion of fat is to dissolve it in the watery content of the intestine. The bile acids produced by the liver dissolve fat into tiny droplets and allow pancreatic and intestinal enzymes to break the large fat molecules into smaller ones. Bile acids then combine with the smaller fatty acids and cholesterol molecules and move them into the cells of the intestinal mucosa. Here, the smaller molecules are reformed into larger fat molecules and transported via the bloodstream for use in different areas of the body.

Knowledge Connection

How many calories does a gram of protein provide? A gram of fat? Which type of cholesterol is desired in higher ranges? Which of the types of fat are considered to contribute to cardiovascular disease? List several sources of trans fat, saturated fat, monounsaturated fat, and polyunsaturated fat. Which type of fat is known to decrease the bad cholesterol known as LDL? What are some food sources that a person might consume to help keep LDLs in the lower range?

Carbohydrates

Carbohydrates provide 4 kcal of energy per gram and are the main source of energy for the heart, brain, and skeletal muscles. They are widely available and are found in most food sources. Carbohydrates have been given a bad reputation recently due to their possible link to obesity. While overindulgence in carbohydrates can cause weight gain, these substances play a crucial role in metabolism and serve as the primary fuel for the body.

There are two types of carbohydrates: simple and complex. **Simple carbohydrates**, also known as *simple sugars*, are chemically made up of one or two sugar molecules and are absorbed very quickly. Sources of simple carbohydrates include:

- Fruit
- Milk
- Table sugar
- Syrup
- Candy
- Soda pop

Complex carbohydrates are starches and fiber, made up of long chains of three or more molecules of sugar, and take longer to digest than simple carbohydrates. Starch must be broken down before it can be used as a source of energy

Table 23-2 Lipid Profile Laboratory Value Ranges

Element	Optimal	Borderline	High Risk
LDL	<100 mg/dl	130–159 mg/dl	160+ mg/dl
HDL	>60 mg/dl	40–59 mg/dl	<40 mg/dl
Triglycerides	<150 mg/dl	150–199 mg/dl	>200 mg/dl
Total Cholesterol	<200 mg/dl	200–239 mg/dl	>240 mg/dl

Source: Adapted from National Heart, Lung and Blood Institute. How is high blood cholesterol diagnosed? Available at: http://www.nhlbi.nih.gov/health/dci/Diseases/Hbc/HBC_Diagnosis.html.

for the body. Sugars and starches occur naturally in many foods that also supply other nutrients. Food sources of complex carbohydrates include:

- Potatoes
- Rice
- Whole-grain bread
- Pasta
- Whole-grain cereals, such as oatmeal
- Broccoli
- Corn
- Beans
- Peas

Complex carbohydrates assist the body in maintaining a more stable blood glucose level, while simple carbohydrates quickly raise the blood glucose to higher levels, which stimulates increased insulin production that rapidly drops the glucose level. Most sources recommend that 45% to 65% of one's total calorie consumption come from complex carbohydrates. If the carbohydrate consumption is inadequate, there will be insufficient stores of glycogen. This forces the body to break down and utilize stores of protein and fats for use as energy, which prevents the protein from being available for tissue growth and repair. The minimum amount of carbohydrates needed to "spare" protein is between 50 and 100 g/day. Before fats can be burned as fuel for energy, they must be changed to ketones. If an inordinate level of ketones is produced, as in hyperglycemia or diabetes, the ketones cause the blood to become more acidic, which can lead to the acid-base imbalance known as ketoacidosis.

Diets rich in dietary fiber have been shown to have a number of beneficial effects, including decreased risk of coronary heart disease and improvement in bowel habits. Soluble fiber plays a more complex role in digestion than does insoluble fiber. The process of breaking down, or *fermenting,* soluble fiber produces gases such as methane, nitrogen, and carbon dioxide and short-chain fatty acids. The short chain fatty acids are responsible for many health benefits, including stabilization of blood glucose levels, decreasing LDL cholesterol, increased absorption of minerals, and promoting colon health and the immune system by lowering the pH of the large intestine. This lowered pH inhibits growth of pathogens and cancer cells. The soluble fiber also serves as a food source for the normal flora of the GI tract. Soluble or viscous fibers modestly reduce LDL cholesterol beyond levels achieved by a diet low in saturated and trans fats and cholesterol alone. Oats have the highest proportion of soluble fiber of any grain. Foods high in soluble fiber include oat bran, oatmeal, beans, peas, rice bran, barley, citrus fruits, strawberries, and apple pulp.

Insoluble fiber has been associated with decreased cardiovascular risk and slower progression of cardiovascular disease in high-risk individuals. Because insoluble dietary fiber does not break down as it passes through the GI tract, it attracts water and helps to provide bowel regularity. It is thought by some scientists to promote **satiety** (satisfaction

of hunger) by slowing gastric emptying, leading to an overall decrease in calorie intake. Foods high in insoluble fiber include whole wheat breads, wheat cereals, wheat bran, rye, rice, barley, most other grains, cabbage, beets, carrots, brussels sprouts, cauliflower, and apple peel.

Most Americans fail to consume adequate quantities of fiber on a regular basis. The average adult requires 25 to 35 grams of fiber per day for optimal health. Fruits, vegetables, whole-grain foods, high-fiber foods, beans, and legumes are good sources of both soluble and insoluble dietary fiber. While fiber has many health benefits, large and sudden increases of fiber intake may result in an increase of gastrointestinal flatus or gas. Therefore, when you teach patients of the need to increase their fiber intake, it is important to inform them that it should be gradually increased over 2 to 3 weeks to decrease the problem of flatus.

Carbohydrate Digestion

During digestion, all carbohydrates except fiber break down into sugars. Carbohydrate digestion begins in the mouth, where salivary amylase begins breaking down large complex carbohydrates into smaller molecules. This process continues to a small degree in the stomach. Once the carbohydrates reach the duodenum, the pancreatic enzymes break the carbohydrates down into simple sugars: maltose, lactose, and sucrose. These simple sugars are eventually broken down into glucose, which is then absorbed through the intestinal wall villi, transported by the bloodstream to the liver for storage as glycogen, or transported directly to the cells for immediate use.

Soluble fiber dissolves in water and ferments in the large intestine, producing short-chain fatty acids. Insoluble fiber does not break down as it passes through the GI tract.

Knowledge Connection

How many calories per gram are in carbohydrates compared to fats and protein? Explain the difference between simple carbohydrates and complex carbohydrates. List at least four food sources of fiber. What is the recommended daily intake of fiber?

Vitamins

Vitamins are naturally occurring substances that are found in plants and animals. They occur naturally in foods in small amounts and play a crucial role in many body functions, including blood clotting, bone formation, new tissue growth and repair, and nerve impulse conduction. The body is not able to synthesize adequate amounts of vitamins to meet physiological needs, so vitamins must be ingested through foods or supplements. Vitamins are classified as either water soluble or fat soluble.

Water-soluble vitamins are absorbed directly into the bloodstream from the GI tract. Because the body is unable to store these vitamins, they must be consumed daily. Water-soluble vitamins include the B vitamins—B_1 (thiamine),

B$_2$ (riboflavin), B$_3$ (niacin), B$_6$, and B$_{12}$—as well as vitamin C. These vitamins are found in a variety of foods, including cereal grains, meat, eggs, fish, and citrus fruits.

The B vitamins work to maintain healthy nerves, skin, and hair and serve as coenzymes in most areas of the body. Vitamin C is essential in immune system functioning and promotes the formation of collagen. In some cases, vitamins are used as drugs to treat specific disease conditions: Niacin is used to treat hyperlipidemia, and vitamin C aids wound healing.

Fat-soluble vitamins are absorbed from the small intestine into body fat and can be stored when intake exceeds need. Because of this, fat-soluble vitamins can become toxic when consumed in excess doses over a long period of time. Likewise, malabsorption of fat is associated with poor absorption of these vitamins. Fat-soluble vitamins include A, D, E, and K and are found in green leafy vegetables, dairy products, carrots, and liver.

Certain vitamins are known as **antioxidants**. These substances are thought to protect cells from the damage caused by unstable molecules known as *free radicals*. Free radical damage may lead to cancer. Antioxidants interact with and stabilize free radicals and may prevent some of the damage free radicals otherwise might cause. Examples of antioxidants include beta carotene, lycopene, vitamins C, E, and A, and other substances.

Knowledge Connection

Which vitamins are water soluble? Fat soluble? Which vitamins are toxic when consumed in excessive doses? Explain the function of antioxidants. Relate at least three functions of the B vitamins. Which vitamin is important for growing new tissue such as is required after surgery? What are free radicals?

Minerals

Minerals are inorganic elements that originate from the earth; they are found in all body tissues and fluids. Minerals cannot be digested and retain their original chemical identities in the body. They provide structure to the body, assist in fluid balance and acid-base balance, regulate nerve cell transmission and muscle contraction, and assist in the activation of vitamins, enzymes, and hormones. Minerals are classified into two groups: major and trace, both of which are essential for life.

Major minerals are those that are present in the body in amounts greater than 5 grams. These include calcium, phosphorus, sodium, potassium, and magnesium. Trace minerals are present in the body in amounts of 5 grams or less, but are equally important to body function as the major minerals. Trace minerals include iron, iodine, zinc, chromium, fluoride, copper, and selenium.

Calcium is the most abundant mineral in the body and has multiple functions, including muscle contraction, hormone and enzyme secretion, and nervous system performance. Up to 99% of calcium is stored in the bones, with the remaining 1% circulating in the bloodstream. Calcium is found in milk, yogurt, and cheese, as well as spinach, kale, and broccoli. Major functions and sources of calcium and other minerals are listed in Table 23-3.

Nutritional Deficiencies and Excesses

Too much of certain nutrients can be as problematic to the body's functioning as inadequate intake. You will need to understand these imbalances to better educate your patients.

Table 23-3 Functions and Sources of Minerals

Mineral	Function	Recommended Dietary Allowance	General Sources	Factors Affecting Absorption
Sodium	Regulates extracellular fluid levels, acid-base balance; controls nerve impulses and muscle contraction	1,000 mg	Salt, processed foods, cured meats	Excessive sweat losses
Potassium	Supports cardiac, skeletal, and smooth muscle contraction	3.5 grams	Fruits, vegetables, legumes	Excessive use of sodium, diarrhea, vomiting, use of diuretics
Magnesium	Supports muscle and nerve function, cardiac conduction, energy metabolism	320 mg for women 420 mg for men	Spinach, legumes, nuts and seeds	Alcoholism, poorly controlled diabetes, gastrointestinal disorders such as Crohn's disease, nausea, vomiting

Table 23-3 **Functions and Sources of Minerals** (continued)

Mineral	Function	Recommended Dietary Allowance	General Sources	Factors Affecting Absorption
Phosphorus	Acts as a structural component of bone and cell membranes	700 mg	Dairy products, meat, fish, soft drinks	High fructose intake, alcoholism, diabetic ketoacidosis
Iron	Acts as an essential component of protein that transports oxygen in the blood; cell growth and differentiation	8 mg for men 18 mg for women younger than age 50 years (premenopause) 27 mg for pregnant women	Red meats, fish, poultry, lentils, and beans	Type of dietary iron consumed, storage levels, tea and calcium consumption
Calcium	99% of calcium is used for maintenance of bone and teeth, 1% in serum is vital for electrical conduction of cardiac and muscular tissues	1,000 mg 1,500 mg for pregnant, lactating, and postmenopausal women, and men over 65 years	Dairy products, salmon, spinach, okra, broccoli, almonds, calcium-fortified foods such as cereal and juice	Vitamin D is essential for absorption, vitamin C helps absorption, high-fiber and high-fat diets can inhibit absorption, also controlled by parathyroid hormone and calcitonin and albumin levels
Zinc	Supports immune system, essential in wound healing, helps maintain sense of smell and taste	15 mg	Oysters, red meat, poultry, fortified breakfast cereal, beans, and nuts	Digestive diseases, alcoholism

Protein

Protein deficiencies are found throughout the world, but they are particularly prevalent in underdeveloped countries. Poverty and lack of resources such as livestock, seed, and farming equipment, or an insufficient knowledge base regarding foods containing protein, lead to disease conditions such as *kwashiorkor,* which is a type of malnutrition believed to be caused by insufficient protein intake. Signs of kwashiorkor include a swollen abdomen, ascites, dermatitis, and weight loss. The enlarged abdomen is related to *hepatomegaly,* or liver enlargement, and *ascites* is the collection of free fluid in the peritoneal cavity. Another sign of kwashiorkor is the flag sign, which is alternating bands of pale and dark hair.

Protein deficiencies in developed nations are related to poverty and lack of available protein sources, but they can also occur in people in higher socioeconomic groups who simply fail to eat adequate amounts of available complete proteins. Vegetarians typically do not develop protein deficiencies if they maintain adequate intake of dairy and soy products.

If more protein is consumed than is needed, the body does not build more protein or muscle. Instead, the body breaks the protein down and stores its components as fat, which can be broken down and used for energy later as needed.

Fats

Excessive dietary fat is one of the leading causes of overweight and obesity in the United States. As you learned in Chapter 7, one of the main objectives of Healthy People 2010 is to decrease morbidity related to obesity in the United States. Over the years of promotion of this ongoing U.S. Department of Health and Human Services program, this goal has fallen short, and it appears that Americans continue to gain weight, as the number of obese adults has risen from 15% in 1980 to 32.9% in 2004. Obesity is measured by many scales, most commonly through measurement of the **body mass index (BMI)**.

The BMI is a number calculated from a person's weight and height. It provides a reliable indicator of body fatness for most people and is used to screen for weight

Table 23-4 Body Mass Index Table

To use the table, find the appropriate height in the left-hand column labeled Height. Move across to a given weight (in pounds). The number at the top of the column is the BMI at that height and weight. Pounds have been rounded off.

BMI	19	20	21	22	23	24	25	26	27	28	29	30	31	32	33	34	35
Height/Inches							**Body Weight/Pounds**										
60	97	102	107	112	118	123	128	133	138	143	148	153	158	163	168	174	179
61	100	106	111	116	122	127	132	137	143	148	153	158	164	169	174	180	185
62	104	109	115	120	126	131	136	142	147	153	158	164	169	175	180	186	191
63	107	113	118	124	130	135	141	146	152	158	163	169	175	180	186	191	197
64	110	116	122	128	134	140	145	151	157	163	169	174	180	186	192	197	204
65	114	120	126	132	138	144	150	156	162	168	174	180	186	192	198	204	210
66	118	124	130	136	142	148	155	161	167	173	179	186	192	198	204	210	216
67	121	127	134	140	146	153	159	166	172	178	185	191	198	204	211	217	223
68	125	131	138	144	151	158	164	171	177	184	190	197	203	210	216	223	230
69	128	135	142	149	155	162	169	176	182	189	196	203	209	216	223	230	236
70	132	139	146	153	160	167	174	181	188	195	202	209	216	222	229	236	243
71	136	143	150	157	165	172	179	186	193	200	208	215	222	229	236	243	250
72	140	147	154	162	169	177	184	191	199	206	213	221	228	235	242	250	258
73	144	151	159	166	174	182	189	197	204	212	219	227	235	242	250	257	265
74	148	155	163	171	179	186	194	202	210	218	225	233	241	249	256	264	272

Source: National Heart, Lung and Blood Institute. Body mass index table. Available at: http://www.nhlbi.nih.gov/guidelines/obesity/bmi_tbl.htm.

categories that may lead to health problems. The BMI chart is simple to use (Table 23-4). Individuals whose BMI falls under 18.5 are generally considered to be underweight, and those with BMIs between 18.5 and 24.9 are within the normal weight range (Box 23-3). Those whose BMIs are between 25 and 29.9 are considered to be overweight, and a BMI greater than 30 is classified as obese.

However, certain factors should be taken into consideration when calculating the BMI of special groups of individuals, as some people may not be overweight even though they fall into the 25.0 to 29.9 range. For example, athletes may have higher BMIs due to increased muscle mass, and pregnant women have more weight than they do under normal conditions. BMI calculations would indicate a higher amount of body fat in people in these groups than they really have. The opposite might be true in groups such as the elderly or those with physically disabilities. Because they typically have less fat, BMI calculations would likely underestimate the amount of body fat. BMI measurements are also inaccurate for the morbidly obese. Even though there are categories for which the BMI is not accurate, it is still the best tool to use as an indicator of body fatness in the general population.

Knowledge Connection

In which groups of people might the BMI calculation be inaccurate? Calculate your BMI. Do you need to modify your eating habits and weight?

Carbohydrates

Weight gain and obesity are the most common conditions associated with eating excess carbohydrates. Eating carbohydrates raises insulin, which then lowers blood sugar. This causes a desire (or craving) for more food and, in some people, carbohydrates. As more food and calories are taken in, energy must be burned to prevent weight gain. Insulin release also triggers sugars to be converted into fat for storage.

Foods that are high in added sugar, such as soda, cookies, cake, candy, frozen desserts, and some fruit drinks, tend to also be high in calories and low in other valuable nutrients. Sugars and starches also contribute to dental caries by providing substrate for bacterial fermentation in the mouth.

Carbohydrate deficiency may result from carbohydrate intolerances related to enzyme deficiencies. Although not common, a deficiency in the enzymes needed to digest lactose, maltose, and sucrose is sometimes present at birth. Intestinal lactase enzymes usually decrease naturally with age, but this happens to varying degrees. Because of the uneven distribution of enzyme deficiency based on race and ethnic heritage, especially in lactose intolerance, genetics are believed to play a role in the cause of primary carbohydrate intolerance.

Digestive diseases such as celiac disease and tropical sprue, which affect absorption in the intestine, as well as intestinal infections and injuries, can reduce the amount of enzymes produced. In cancer patients, treatment with radiation therapy or chemotherapy may affect the cells in the intestine that normally secrete lactase, leading to intolerance.

Vitamins

Vitamin deficiencies are common in underdeveloped countries. Deficiencies in the United States are related to disease conditions, such as intestinal malabsorption disorders, including Crohn's disease. Other vitamin deficiencies, such as deficiencies of vitamin B_{12} or folic acid, are likely to occur in alcoholics. Signs and symptoms of vitamin deficiencies are numerous (Table 23-5).

Water-soluble vitamins were once thought to be relatively safe in large amounts. However, recent research shows that consumption of vitamin C in doses many times greater than the recommended daily allowance (RDA), known as *megadosing,* can cause gastric upset, and large doses of vitamin B_6 can lead to neurological abnormalities.

Minerals

Mineral deficiencies typically do not develop in adults who eat a well-balanced diet. However, people who follow restrictive diets may not consume enough of a particular mineral. For example, vegetarians, including those who eat eggs and dairy products, are at risk of iron deficiency.

Mineral toxicities are usually related to improper use of supplements, environmental exposure, or alterations in metabolism. Trace mineral imbalances can occur due to hereditary disorders such as Wilson's disease, in which copper is deposited into body tissues instead of being excreted.

Box 23-3

BMI Categories

The Body Mass Index Table establishes general ranges of BMI reflecting when an individual is underweight, within normal weight ranges, overweight, or obese.
- Underweight: less than 18.5
- Normal weight: 18.5–24.9
- Overweight: 25–29.9
- Obese: 30 or greater

Source: National Heart, Lung, and Blood Institute. Calculate your body mass index. Available at: http://www.nhlbisupport.com/bmi/.

Knowledge Connection

What does the body do with excess intake of protein? Vegetarians who fail to include adequate soy and dairy products in their diets are more prone to have what type of deficiency?

Table 23-5 Vitamin Deficiencies and Excesses

Vitamin	Source	Physiological Functions	Deficiency	Excess
Fat-Soluble Vitamins				
A	Liver, vitamin A–fortified milk and dairy products, butter, whole milk, cheese, egg yolk.	Helps to form skin and mucous membranes and keep them healthy, thus increasing resistance to infections. Essential for night vision. Promotes bone and tooth development. Beta carotene, the precursor of vitamin A, is an antioxidant and may protect against cancer.	*Mild:* night blindness, diarrhea, intestinal infections, impaired vision *Severe:* inflammation of eyes, keratinization of skin and eyes, blindness in children	*Mild:* nausea, irritability, blurred vision *Severe:* growth retardation, enlargement of liver and spleen, loss of hair, bone pain, increased pressure in skull, skin changes
D	Vitamin D–fortified dairy products, fortified margarine, fish oils, egg yolk. Synthesized by sunlight action on skin.	Promotes hardening of bones and teeth. Increases the absorption of calcium.	*Severe:* Rickets in children; osteomalacia in adults	*Mild:* nausea, weight loss, irritability *Severe:* mental and physical growth retardation, kidney damage, movement of calcium from bones into soft tissues
E	Vegetable oil, margarine, butter, shortening, green and leafy vegetables, wheat germ, whole-grain products, nuts, egg yolk, liver.	Protects vitamins A and C and fatty acids. Prevents damage to cell membranes, antioxidant.	Almost impossible to produce without starvation; possible anemia in low-birth-weight infants	Nontoxic under normal conditions *Severe:* nausea, digestive tract disorders
K	Dark green leafy vegetables, liver; made by intestinal bacteria.	Factor in blood clotting.	Excessive bleeding	No toxicity symptoms reported

Water-Soluble Vitamins

	Sources	Function	Deficiency	Toxicity
B₁ (thiamine)	Whole-grain and enriched breads, enriched cereals, dried peas and beans.	Coenzyme in energy metabolism. Promotes normal appetite and nervous system functioning.	*Beriberi:* mental confusion, fatigue, peripheral paralysis, edema, cardiomyopathy, sudden death	No toxicity symptoms reported
B₂ (riboflavin)	Milk and dairy products, enriched breads and cereals, green leafy vegetables.	Coenzyme in energy metabolism. Aids in red blood cell development. Assists in releasing energy from carbohydrates.	*Uncommon:* dermatitis, glossitis, photophobia, anemia	No toxicity symptoms reported
B₃ (niacin)	Meat, fish, milk, eggs, peanuts.	Essential in the breakdown of fats and protein. Role in maintaining muscle tone and nervous system functioning.	*Pellagra:* Four Ds • Dermatitis • Diarrhea • Dementia • Death	Flushing, liver damage, gastric ulcers, nausea and vomiting
B₆	Meat, fish, poultry, fruits, whole grains, dried peas and beans.	Essential in protein metabolism, nervous and immune system function.	Dermatitis, glossitis, depression, confusion	Neuropathy
B₁₂	Fish, meat, poultry, fortified breakfast cereals.	Helps maintain nervous system, red blood cell production, DNA production.	Macrocytic anemia, GI disturbances, neurological deficits	No toxicity symptoms reported
C	Citrus fruits, strawberries, green peppers, turnip greens.	Growth and repair of tissues, wound healing, antioxidant.	*Scurvy:* hemorrhage, skin changes, delayed wound healing, softening of bones, anemia	Diarrhea, abdominal cramping, nausea

If a Little Is Good, Is More Better?

A young RN who had only been out of nursing school for 3 years was very health conscious and physically active. She exercised 5 to 6 days a week, participated in various sports, drank lots of water, took time to have fun and play regularly, worked to eat a balanced diet, and took a daily multiple vitamin. After having several bouts of colds and allergies, she decided to boost her immunity by taking a vitamin C supplement, adding up to an additional 4,000 milligrams (mg) of vitamin C per day. After 7 months of taking the supplement, she tired of taking so many pills every day and discontinued the supplement. A week or so later, she noticed large areas of *petechiae,* pinpoint-size flat red spots due to capillary rupture, over much of her body. The rash continued to spread daily for 4 days. Though the rash did not itch, it was a source of concern to her and she decided to seek medical attention. Ultimately, it was determined that, even though she ate well and was in good nutritional condition, she was suffering from some of the symptoms of scurvy, a disease caused by inadequate intake of vitamin C. By ingesting such high levels of vitamin C supplements for several months and then stopping the supplements cold turkey rather than weaning herself off them slowly, she had subjected her body to a *faux* scurvy. Even though she was still getting adequate vitamin C in her diet, her body misinterpreted the sudden and dramatic drop in vitamin C intake to be a deficiency of vitamin C.

Differing Nutritional Needs Over the Life Span

Nutritional requirements constantly change throughout one's life span. Certain conditions such as pregnancy may also change an individual's nutritional needs.

Pregnancy

The pregnant woman has significantly increased nutritional needs. The old saying "eating for two" is not entirely correct, but the body does require increased nutrients for proper fetal development. The American College of Obstetricians and Gynecologists (ACOG) recommends an average weight gain of 25 to 30 pounds (11.4 to 13.6 kg) during pregnancy. On average, women are recommended to eat between 2,500 and 2,700 calories daily. Recent research shows that women who gain more than the recommended amount during pregnancy and who fail to lose this weight within 6 months after giving birth are at much higher risk of being obese nearly 10 years later.

No specific recommendations exist for the amount of carbohydrate or fat intake in pregnancy. Protein needs during the second and third trimesters of pregnancy are 300 kcal more than pre-pregnancy needs. Pregnant women should try to eat seven or more servings of fruits and vegetables combined (for example, three servings of fruit and four of vegetables) daily; six to nine servings of whole-grain or enriched breads or cereals; four or more servings of low-fat or nonfat milk, yogurt, cheese, or other dairy products; and 60 grams of protein every day.

Pregnant women require vitamin and mineral supplements to ensure proper development of the fetus and to limit strain on the mother's body. All women who are considering pregnancy should begin supplements of folic acid to prevent neural tube defects. Daily recommendations for folic acid are 0.4 mg. The Centers for Disease Control and Prevention (CDC) recommends that pregnant women start taking a low-dose iron supplement (around 30 mg/day), or a multivitamin with iron beginning at the time of their first prenatal visit.

The World Health Organization/UNICEF infant feeding guidelines support exclusive breastfeeding for the first 6 months of the infant's life and the continuation of breastfeeding, together with appropriate complementary feeding, up to 2 years of age or beyond. Both mothers and infants receive multiple benefits from breastfeeding. Breast milk contains multiple maternal antibodies that protect infants from bacterial and viral infections. It is also easy to digest, and some sources state that breastfed babies have fewer allergies later in life. Women who breastfeed have reduced rates of breast and ovarian cancer. A recent meta-analysis of breastfeeding effectiveness found that breastfeeding was associated with a reduction in the risk of acute otitis media, nonspecific gastroenteritis, severe lower respiratory tract infections, atopic dermatitis, asthma in young children, obesity, types 1 and 2 diabetes, childhood leukemia, sudden infant death syndrome (SIDS), and necrotizing enterocolitis.

Women who breastfeed require healthy diets similar to those for any adult. The La Leche League supports eating a varied diet that includes all food groups. Most women are advised to eat approximately 500 extra calories daily while breastfeeding. While breastfeeding mothers who eat a nutritionally balanced diet do not need vitamin or mineral supplements, the American Academy of Pediatrics advises daily drops of vitamin D for all breastfed babies.

Toddlers and Preschool Children

A wide variety of foods rich in essential nutrients is necessary for growing bodies, and forms the basis of most nutritional recommendations. Children age 2 years and older should be encouraged to eat at least five servings of fruits and vegetables daily, as well as a wide variety of other foods low in saturated fat and cholesterol. Following a diet such as this will help them maintain normal blood cholesterol levels and promote cardiovascular health.

In children younger than 2 years of age, dietary fats play a key role in the formation of vital nerve and brain tissues. Health professionals do not recommend feeding reduced-fat foods to children of this age. For example, use of whole milk rather than low-fat or fat-free milk is advised.

Although severe nutrient deficiencies are rare in the United States, calcium, iron, zinc, vitamin B_6, folic acid, and vitamin A are the nutrients most likely to be low in children as a result of poor dietary habits. The American Academy of Pediatrics does not support routine supplementation for normal, healthy children. Although there is no harm in giving children a standard children's supplement, megadoses should always be avoided, and caution should be used when supplementing the fat-soluble vitamins A, D, E, and K.

School-age Children

While undernutrition continues to be a major problem in many developing countries, the problem of overweight and obesity has reached epidemic proportions globally, and both developed and developing countries are seriously affected. Being overweight in childhood can lead to type 2 diabetes mellitus and cardiovascular disease. Also, overweight children often face social discrimination, which can lead to low self-esteem and depression.

Establishing good dietary habits during childhood decreases the possibility of inappropriate eating behavior later in life. Children should eat foods from all food groups, including lean meats, dairy products, whole-grain enriched cereal products, fruits, vegetables, and legumes. The primary emphasis of diets for children is on providing adequate calories and nutrients for normal physical activity, growth, and development.

Total fat intake should be between 30% and 35% of calories for children 2 to 3 years of age and between 25% and 35% of calories for children and adolescents 4 to 18 years of age, with most fats coming from sources of polyunsaturated and monounsaturated fatty acids, such as fish, nuts, and vegetable oils.

Several cross-sectional surveys on U.S. children and adolescents have found inadequate intake of dietary fiber, which could be improved by increasing consumption of whole fruits, vegetables, and whole-grain products.

Adolescents

Adolescents experience a period of rapid growth that requires increased nutrient needs. Adolescents' caloric needs vary depending on their growth rate, degree of physical maturation, body composition, and activity level. However, they do need extra nutrients to support the adolescent growth spurt, which, for girls, begins at age 10 or 11, reaches its peak at age 12, and is completed by about age 15. In boys, it begins at 12 or 13 years of age, peaks at age 14, and ends by about age 19. Males require greater amounts of calories and protein due to increased muscle mass, lean body tissue, and bone development.

Sufficient amounts of iron and calcium are particularly important as the adolescent body undergoes this intensive growth period. From ages 9 to 18 years, both males and females are encouraged to consume a calcium-rich diet, about 1,300 mg daily, in order to ensure adequate calcium deposits in the bones. The recommended calcium intake can be achieved by getting at least 3 cups of milk daily or the equivalent amount of yogurt or cheese. For those who do not wish to consume dairy products, a variety of other calcium sources are available, such as green, leafy vegetables; calcium-fortified soy products; and other calcium-fortified foods and beverages.

Adolescent females experience an increase in body fat. This can lead to obesity and eating disorders. According to the National Mental Health Information Center, as many as 10 million girls and women and 1 million boys and men are struggling with eating disorders such as *anorexia nervosa,* a disorder causing people to severely limit their food intake, or *bulimia,* a disorder in which people binge and purge by vomiting or using laxatives. A comprehensive nutritional regimen and psychotherapy and medical nutritional therapy that focuses attention on acceptable weight limits and establishment of good eating habits is needed in this population.

Adolescent females who experience teenage pregnancy have special nutrient needs. Similar to adult females who are pregnant, adolescents require supplements of folic acid, iron, zinc, and calcium. Pregnant teenagers should undergo a comprehensive nutritional assessment to determine any deficiencies and to promote adequate weight gain.

Patient Teaching Connection

Pregnancy: Weight Gain and Diet

You are working with a group of pregnant teenagers at a local clinic. Many of the teens express concern about weight gain during pregnancy. It is vital to teach these girls that weight gain during pregnancy is an important determinate of fetal growth, and that poor weight gain is directly associated with low calorie intake and lower intake of important nutrients. This makes it pertinent that the young mothers eat enough to prevent scrawny and unhealthy babies. Explain that weight gain is based on a person's pre-pregnancy BMI. Weight gain for a young adolescent should fall between 28 and 40 lbs. (12.7 to 18.2 kg). During the second and third trimesters, adolescents should gain approximately 1 lb. (2.2 kg) per week. The best way for a pregnant teenager to meet her dietary needs is to maintain a regular three-meal schedule with three nutritious snacks, keeping in mind that adequate servings from all the different food groups in the Food Guide Pyramid is important. A varied, balanced eating plan is the only way to provide enough nutrients and food energy during pregnancy and to "feed" an unborn baby.

Adulthood

Nutritional needs of adults are established from several guidelines, including MyPyramid and the Dietary Guidelines for Americans. Generally, nutritional requirements will vary due to age, weight, height, and physical activity. As adults age, overall energy and calorie needs typically decrease, but required amounts of selected nutrients may increase. Calcium needs increase for women due to decrease in calcium absorption and increase in bone loss. As women age and enter menopause, iron needs decrease.

Adults must balance caloric intake with energy expenditure to maintain weight and avoid fat storage. At the onset of adulthood, energy requirements usually reach a plateau that will last until one's mid-40s, after which they begin to decline, primarily because activity levels and lean muscle mass (amount of muscle versus body fat), which represents the basal metabolic rate or BMR, decrease. Weight gain in adulthood is associated with the development of cardiovascular disease and diabetes.

Poor food habits, such as eating fast foods, develop in early adulthood and are generally continued throughout life. Younger adults are more likely to eat fast foods several times a week, which can lead to cardiovascular disease related to increased intake of saturated fats. Younger adults consume a large amount of calories through beverages such as soft drinks and flavored waters. These beverages contain large amounts of simple carbohydrates, leading to excess intake of "empty" calories that have little nutritional benefit.

Older Adults

Many factors affect the nutritional status of older adults. Many are at risk for undernutrition and malnutrition, while others have special nutrient requirements due to the effects of aging on the GI tract, kidneys, and metabolism. As we age, basal metabolic rate decreases. As energy needs decrease, appetite decreases, which can lead to undernutrition. Older adults are at risk for vitamin B_{12} deficiency related to decreased absorption and conversion by the GI tract. Vitamin D deficiency is also common in older adults due to decreased ability of the kidneys to convert it to its active form.

As adults age, losses of lean muscle mass, body water, and bone mass increase. Fat stores increase, leading to fat deposits in the abdomen. This condition, known as *central obesity,* leads to release of fatty acids into the blood, leading to increased blood lipid levels and increased blood insulin levels. This process leads to the development of cardiovascular disease and diabetes.

Studies show that a good diet in later years helps both in reducing the risk of these diseases and in managing the diseases' signs and symptoms. This contributes to a higher quality of life, enabling older people to maintain their independence by continuing to perform basic daily activities, such as bathing, dressing and eating. Poor nutrition, on the other hand, can prolong recovery from illnesses, increase the costs and incidence of institutionalization, and lead to a poorer quality of life.

Lack of calcium in the diet can lead to osteoporosis. Sources of calcium include milk and dairy products, which can be expensive to purchase for some older adults. Calcium supplements are widely available, but can cause constipation.

Since constipation may affect up to 20% of people older than 65 years of age, older adults should choose to consume foods rich in natural calcium and dietary fiber.

Knowledge Connection
Describe at least two differences in nutritional needs for each age group through the life span.

Cultural Influences on Nutrition

A person's culture is a learned behavior that is passed down from previous generations, and each culture has values and beliefs that guide dietary habits. Food choices are determined by cultural laws and preferences. Food selection may depend on a cultural belief, such as whether the food is considered edible or taboo. Foods can take on symbolic meanings related to major life experiences such as birth and death. Traditional foods have strong meanings and bind families and communities in fellowship.

While many factors affect dietary choices, Hispanic people of the southwestern United States typically eat a diet rich in complex carbohydrates with an emphasis on corn and corn products, beans, rice, and bread. Common meats include pork, poultry, and goat. People of Puerto Rican heritage eat similar foods, with addition of tropical fruits such as plantain and bananas. The main cooking fat is usually lard.

The African American culture has developed much of what is known as "Southern cooking." While dietary patterns vary according to regional differences, in general African Americans tend to follow diet choices from the four basic food groups. Breads such as biscuits and cornbread are a common staple. Because many African Americans are prone to lactose intolerance, milk and dairy products are not highly consumed. Green leafy vegetables are frequently eaten and usually cooked with bacon or salted pork. Other common vegetables include corn, potatoes, okra, and tomatoes. Pork dishes, such as ribs, ham, and sausage, are commonly eaten. Other common meats include poultry, liver, and fish. Most meats are fried in lard, shortening, or vegetable oil.

Jewish cuisine is incredibly varied, and it is hard to single out a specific culinary tradition as particularly Jewish. In accordance with Jewish dietary law, Jewish cuisine does not include pork or shellfish. Many dishes in Jewish cuisine also have religious symbolism, especially breads and cakes. Challah, for example, is bread braided together to represent manna, or plaited like a ladder leading to heaven. Bread may also be baked into shapes such as doves and keys to represent various symbolic events in Jewish history, and sweet desserts are also considered symbolically important, as they imply wishes for good fortune.

Jewish American diets are well known for the cleaning process that determines if a food is kosher. *Kosher* food meets Jewish dietary laws, or *kashrut,* which comes from the Hebrew word for "fit" or "proper." Kosher food laws are rather extensive. Some are derived directly from the Bible and others through rabbinic interpretations over the years. According to the Torah, meats such as cloven-hoofed, cud-chewing mammals are kosher, as are chicken, duck, and turkey. Milk and meat cannot be served together. Poultry and meat must be slaughtered under strict guidelines called *shechita,* which means the animal must not suffer pain.

Asian American food patterns are varied and based on the particular cultural belief of the population. Asian Americans have emigrated from the Philippines, China, Hong Kong, Cambodia, Vietnam, Laos, Thailand, Korea, and Japan. Chinese Americans eat less meat and more fresh vegetables than Americans in general. Vegetables are served freshly cooked in a wok, or steamed to preserve crispness. Milk products are used sparingly. Eggs and soy products are main sources of protein. Rice is the staple grain and is eaten with most meals. Most meals are cooked using peanut oil. Studies have shown that the Chinese American diet contains far less saturated fat than the diets of African Americans, Hispanic Americans, or Caucasians.

Japanese American dietary patterns are similar to those of Chinese Americans, with both cultures using rice as the primary grain. This culture prefers seafood and fish as the main meat source. Vegetables are usually steamed, and fresh fruits are eaten at main meals. Japanese Americans are very concerned about the visual appeal of the food and the "separateness" of the foods and tastes. Garlic and hot pepper are not common ingredients.

Acculturation

Acculturation is the modification of the culture of a group or individual as a result of contact with a different culture. As Mexican immigrants become acculturated to the dietary habits of Americans, Mexican American children begin to eat foods with higher caloric intake and increased amounts of dietary fats. Foods that are recommended as part of a healthy diet and are accessible and affordable to families in Mexico may not be affordable to low-income families in the United States. Because of this, common feeding practices that are not associated with being overweight in Mexico, where the foods available are more nutritious, may put children at risk for obesity in America, where low-cost foods are generally energy dense and nutrient poor.

Because of the many health problems associated with overweight and obesity, immigrants should be encouraged to continue dietary traditions that include fresh fruits and vegetables, beans, and whole grains. Immigrants should be taught to avoid increased dietary fat.

 Post Conference

At Post Conference, you talk about your patient and his misunderstandings about diet and how it affects constipation. He told you that he cannot eat fiber because it gives him gas. After you asked a few questions, you learned that he had tried only one time to increase the fiber in his diet, increasing his fiber intake from 14 to 15 grams one day to 30 grams the next day, rather than gradually increasing fiber intake by a couple of grams per day. You know that such a large increase all at one time could cause flatus, and you were able to explain to him how to gradually increase fiber in his diet to prevent that from happening. You also helped him choose foods he likes and can easily prepare that have higher fiber content than what he has been eating. In addition, you were able to explain to him how drinking tea, coffee, or water would help increase the amount of fluid his body could use, while colas can cause the body to lose water.

KEY POINTS

- Nutrients are needed by the body to carry out essential metabolic functions.
- Carbohydrates are classified as simple or complex.
- The average adult needs between 50 and 65 grams of protein daily.
- Vitamins are classified as either water soluble or fat soluble.
- Excessive ingestion of fat-soluble vitamins can lead to toxicity.
- Low levels of folic acid in pregnant women are associated with neural tube defects in their infants.

- Water is the body's principal chemical component, making up 60% of body weight.
- The Recommended Dietary Allowance (RDA) is the level of nutrient intake that is sufficient to meet the needs of almost all healthy individuals of a given life stage and gender group.
- Absorption is the process by which substances pass through the intestinal mucosa into the blood or lymph so nutrients can be delivered to cells throughout the body.

REVIEW QUESTIONS

Select the answer that is most appropriate for each of the following questions. Some questions may have more than one correct answer. Check all that apply.

1. The primary function of carbohydrates as a food source is to:
   a. regulate metabolic processes.
   b. build body tissue.
   c. supply energy.
   d. provide bulk.

2. The primary function of protein in the body is to:
   a. supply energy.
   b. regulate metabolic processes.
   c. control muscle contractions.
   d. build tissue.

3. A characteristic of saturated fats is that they are:
   a. found primarily in animal products.
   b. liquid at room temperatures.
   c. composed of many double bonds.
   d. found primarily in vegetable products.

4. Rickets is caused by a deficiency of which vitamin?
   a. Vitamin A
   b. Cobalamin
   c. Niacin
   d. Vitamin D

5. Which foods are commonly fortified with vitamin D?
   a. Flour
   b. Cereal
   c. Milk
   d. Tuna
   e. Margarine

6. Which foods provide the most calcium per serving?
   a. Legumes
   b. Whole grains
   c. Dairy products
   d. Leafy vegetables

7. It is important that energy needs are met in pregnancy so that:
   a. maternal vitamins are spared.
   b. optimal fetal growth is ensured.
   c. adipose tissue stores are spared.
   d. adequate blood volume is provided.

8. The vitamin that may help prevent fetal neural tube defects when consumed before pregnancy and through the early weeks of pregnancy is:
   a. vitamin B_6.
   b. niacin.
   c. vitamin C.
   d. folate.

9. The largest source of sodium in the typical American diet is:
   a. processed foods.
   b. salt added at the table.
   c. salt added while cooking.
   d. foods naturally high in salt.

10. A patient with a BMI of 22 should be considered:
   a. overweight.
   b. at a healthy weight.
   c. underweight.
   d. obese.

Critical Thinking Exercises

11. Mr. Baze is a 71-year-old African American who is being seen in the clinic for hypertension. His primary care provider wants him to follow a low-sodium diet. He asks you about foods that he should avoid. What is your response?

12. Ms. Havner is concerned about her nutritional status. She has access to the Internet and has become confused about the many nutritional websites. What information can you give her to assess her current nutritional status?

Additional Resources

For additional Resources, Questions, and Activities, please see:

 Student Resource Disk

 http://davisplus.fadavis.com

 Student Study Guide

References

American Heart Association. Know your fats. 2008. Available at: http://www.americanheart.org/presenter.jhtml?identifier=532. Accessed September 21, 2009.

Anderson J, Young L. Fat-soluble vitamins. Available at: http://www.ext.colostate.edu/pubs/foodnut/09315.html. Accessed September 21, 2009.

Centers for Disease Control and Prevention. Overweight and obesity. Available at: http://www.cdc.gov/nccdphp/dnpa/obesity/index.htm. Accessed September 21, 2009.

Edelstein S, Sharlin J. *Life Cycle Nutrition: An Evidenced Based Approach.* Sudbury, MA: Jones and Bartlett; 2009.

Grodner M. *Foundations and Clinical Applications of Nutrition: A Nursing Approach.* 4th ed. St. Louis: Mosby Elsevier Health Science; 2007.

International Food Information Council. Child & adolescent nutrition, health & physical activity. Available at: http://www.ific.org/nutrition/kids. Accessed September 21, 2009.

Lutz C, Przytulski K. *NutriNotes.* Philadelphia: FA Davis; 2004.

Lutz C, Przytulski K. *Nutrition and Diet Therapy: Evidence-Based Applications.* 4th ed. Philadelphia: FA Davis; 2006.

Mahan LK, Escott-Stump S, eds. *Krause's Food, Nutrition & Diet Therapy.* 12th ed. Philadelphia: Saunders Elsevier; 2007.

Manzella, D. What's the difference between simple and complex carbohydrates? 2006. Available at: http://diabetes.about.com/od/carbohydratefaq/f/typesofcarbs.htm. Accessed September 21, 2009.

MedlinePlus. Carbohydrates. Available at: http://www.nlm.nih.gov/medlineplus/ency/article/002469.htm. Accessed September 21, 2009.

MedlinePlus. Drinking water. Available at: http://www.nlm.nih.gov/medlineplus/drinkingwater.html. Accessed September 21, 2009.

MedlinePlus. Nutrition. Available at: http://www.nlm.nih.gov/medlineplus/nutrition.html. Accessed September 21, 2009.

National Heart, Lung, and Blood Institute. Healthy eating. Available at: http://www.nhlbi.nih.gov/hbp/prevent/h_eating/h_eating.htm. Accessed September 21, 2009.

Wilkinson JM, Van Leuven K. *Fundamentals of Nursing: Theory, Concepts & Applications.* Philadelphia: FA Davis; 2007.

Williams LS, Hopper PD. *Understanding Medical-Surgical Nursing.* 3rd ed. Philadelphia: FA Davis; 2007.

Nutritional Care and Support

Key Terms

Anaphylaxis

Anorexia nervosa

Bolus feedings

Bulimia nervosa

Clear liquid diet

Dysphagia

Enteral nutrition

Food intolerance

Full liquid diet

Gastric decompression

Glycosolated hemoglobin

Jejunostomy tube (J-tube)

Mechanical soft diet

Nasogastric (NG) tube

NPO

Parenteral nutrition

Partial parenteral nutrition (PPN)

Percutaneous endoscopic gastrostomy (PEG) tube

Pureed diet

Total parenteral nutrition (TPN)

Objectives

1. Define key terms related to the nutritional care of patients.
2. Discuss methods to assist with meals and improve the patient eating experience in the hospital.
3. Describe how to monitor intake and output and why it is important.
4. Discuss the various types of therapeutic diets and modifications.
5. Describe the nurse's responsibilities associated with mealtimes and therapeutic diets.
6. Explain how the glycosylated hemoglobin test is useful in treating patients with diabetes.
7. List at least six guidelines to employ in teaching patients with diabetes.
8. Contrast anorexia nervosa and bulimia nervosa.
9. Discuss the various effects drugs may have on food intake.
10. Identify the indications for use of enteral and parenteral nutrition.
11. Compare the various nasogastric and nasointestinal tubes and their uses.
12. Explain what is meant by gastric decompression.
13. Identify risk factors for aspiration and interventions to prevent it.
14. Differentiate between partial and total parenteral nutrition.
15. Identify specific diagnostic tests and monitoring that are used to assess a patient's response to supplemental nutrition therapy.
16. Describe potential complications associated with tube feedings.
17. Review nursing responsibilities in the management of patients receiving therapeutic diets, enteral nutrition, and parenteral nutrition.

Skills

24-1 Assisting a Patient with Feeding

24-2 Recording Intake and Output

24-3 Inserting a Nasogastric Tube

24-4 Irrigating a Nasogastric Tube

24-5 Removing a Nasogastric Tube

24-6 Administering Intermittent Bolus Enteral Feedings

24-7 Using a Feeding Pump

Clinical Connection

Your Assignment: You are assigned to care for a 58-year-old male patient who has suffered a severe cerebrovascular accident (CVA). He is unable to swallow any food or fluids without choking and has been hydrated with IV fluids for the 2 days since the CVA occurred. The physician has decided that the best course of action is to place a nasogastric tube and provide tube feedings for the next few weeks. After that, the patient may be able to regain his ability to swallow and can begin to eat soft foods again.

Your Actions: Your instructor turns to you in report and says, "Good. It looks like you will get to place a nasogastric tube today." You are suddenly very insecure about performing this procedure. You think to yourself, "If I do not place the tube correctly, the feedings can go into the patient's lungs and cause aspiration, even death." Your hands start to sweat as you think about what could go wrong, and you wish some other student had this assignment.

As you provide care to patients, you will encounter those who require nutritional support in the form of modified diets, nutritional restrictions, supplementation, or mechanical assistance with nutrition. In this chapter, you will learn about the nutritional needs of patients and different types of therapeutic diets, including diets modified for disease states. You will learn to assess a patient's ability to eat or need for alternative means of nutrition, as well as how to assist a patient with eating and how to make mealtimes pleasant. You will also learn to care for patients receiving enteral and parenteral nutrition, patients with feeding tubes, the different types of feeding formulas, and the care and management of feeding tubes.

Supporting Nutritional Intake

Hospitalized patients may experience a variety of factors related to illness or medication that impede their nutritional intake, such as anxiety, pain, fatigue, lack of appetite (called *anorexia*) or nausea and vomiting. Your role as the nurse in the nutritional care of the patient is to be supportive and ensure that he or she has adequate nutrient intake. This is more than just ensuring that the patient's meal is ordered or that the meal tray is delivered to the correct patient. Food and mealtimes in our society are often associated with social events or cultural or ethnic traditions, and most people have their own preferred routine for meals. For those patients receiving care in an institutional setting, individual patient needs may become secondary to the needs of the organization. Patient meal choices are often limited and mealtimes are dictated by the needs of the various organizational services. Nursing intervention can improve the patient experience and optimize nutritional intake.

Assessment

When a patient is admitted to the hospital, it is important to assess his or her nutritional problems and needs. It is impossible to meet a patient's specific needs if you do not know what the patient's needs are. During the initial assessment, you should ask questions to identify specific allergies, special diets the patient may have been following at home, and dietary preferences the patient may have, including cultural or ethnic requirements or restrictions. You will also want to assess the patient's physical capabilities and identify any type of assistance with feeding that he or she may require, such as cutting up foods, assistance in opening containers, or feeding the patient who is blind or too weak to feed himself or herself.

Another assessment you will perform is to determine what medications the patient has been taking at home, because many medications can create side effects such as nausea, diminished appetite, or altered sense taste. It is often possible to assist the patient to overcome medication side effects with simple interventions such as helping the patient to select foods or to arrange meal and snack times that minimize nausea, thus helping to improve the patient's food intake.

Mealtime Preparation

It is important to provide patients with a pleasant environment that is free of clutter and odors to enhance mealtimes. Odors can adversely affect the patient's desire to eat or trigger nausea. Work to eliminate body excretion smells such as feces and infectious or bloody drainage. It is important for you to guard against breath odor (known as *halitosis*), body odor, and food odor on your hands, all of which can be a source of nausea, headache, or allergic reaction for the patient. Take care to eliminate these odors if present before mealtime.

Odors

Ill patients are often negatively affected by odors that normally would be pleasant or, at the very least, not offensive, such as perfume or aftershave, fragranced hair products, lotions, and strong fabric softeners. Avoid all personal care products that contain fragrance and laundry products that result in a strong residual fragrance on your clothing.

Environment

Plan to prepare the patient's room prior to the delivery of meal trays, so that the over-the-bed table upon which you will set the tray is ready. Make certain that it is free of offensive items such as an emesis basin containing sputum, a urinal with or without urine in it, a roll of toilet tissue, a hair brush, or soiled tissues or washcloths. Remove anything that you would not want on your dining room table during mealtime. Wipe the table surface with a damp cloth.

Toileting

Inquire whether or not the patient needs to go to the bathroom, and if so, assist the patient to the bathroom or with use of a bedpan. A patient who has a full bladder or needs to have a bowel movement will probably not eat as much as he or she would after toileting. If a patient has to interrupt a meal to attend to toileting, there is little likelihood that the patient will resume eating afterward.

Patient Comfort

Make certain the patient is comfortable because pain or discomfort can inhibit eating. Make certain that the patient has slippers or socks on to keep the feet warm, and either a robe

or a second gown worn backward, with the opening in front similar to a robe. The patient may also need a blanket placed across the lap if he or she feels cold. If the patient wears dentures or glasses, obtain them and make sure that they are clean. Then assist the patient as needed to insert the dentures or put on the glasses.

Patient Positioning

If the patient is able to sit on the side of the bed or get up to sit in a chair, assist the patient to do so. An upright position is more conducive to eating. If not, make certain that the patient is positioned properly in the bed with good body alignment and then elevate the head of the bed between 60 and 90 degrees, depending upon the patient's condition and preference. Position the over-the-bed table over the patient's lap so that it is directly in front of the patient (Fig. 24-1). Adjust the height of the table according to the patient's needs.

Patient Cleanliness

To reduce risk of bacterial contamination while eating, provide the patient with two warm wet washcloths, one with soap and one without for rinsing, to wash his or her face and hands before eating. If the patient is unable to perform this task independently, assist as needed.

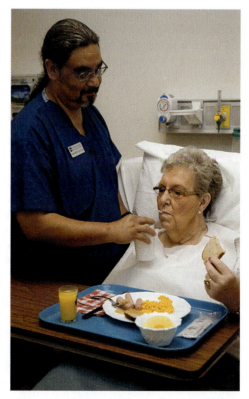

Figure 24-1   When feeding a patient, position the over-the-bed table in front of the patient, not off to the patient's side at the side of the bed.

Assistance With Eating

Your time spent assisting patients with meals can be used to learn more about your patients and to develop and enhance the nurse-patient relationship. Patients who require assistance often find themselves in a position that they are not used to, that of dependency on others to help them meet their needs. During mealtime, take time to talk with your patient and ask questions about his or her life situations and experiences. Probe to determine if the patient has anxiety, concerns, or questions that have not been answered, or gather insight into the dynamics of his or her life. Help to make mealtime more of a social event or at least a more pleasant interaction for the patient, unless the patient's culture views it differently. Mealtimes also offer an opportune time to educate patients regarding dietary changes they may need to make or the use of adaptive equipment. Box 24-1 offers tips on ways to assist patient with meal planning and eating. For more information regarding the steps of assisting a patient with feeding, see Skill 24-1 (page 527).

Assisting a patient with meals is a task that can be delegated to UAPs or CNAs. However, before delegating the task, make certain that the UAP understands the ethnic and cultural considerations related to different foods, nutrition, and mealtime. You may need to educate the UAP regarding ethnic and cultural beliefs and customs related to food and its consumption. It is also your responsibility to ensure that the UAP is knowledgeable about the patient's physiologic status as it relates to impaired swallowing, requiring the patient to be fed slowly. He or she must know what to do if the patient chokes or aspirates.

Monitoring Intake and Output

Because fluid and electrolyte balance is critical to optimal health and recovery from illness and injury, ensuring adequate fluid intake is even more important than ensuring consumption of food. This should be a primary focus in your care of each patient. When there are concerns regarding a patient's fluid and electrolyte balance, it will be your responsibility to monitor the patient's intake and output, commonly called I/O. This simply means to measure and record all fluids taken in and all fluid volumes that are lost.

Intake includes fluids taken by mouth, those administered IV, and fluids administered by enteral or parenteral feedings, which will be discussed later in this chapter. A clear plastic drinking cup marked in increments of ounces and milliliters can be used to measure the amount of fluid that is drunk. It is also used to measure the remaining volume after the patient drinks only part of a container with a specified volume in it. For example, if a can of carbonated cola contained 360 mL and the patient only drank part of the cola, you would measure the remainder and subtract that from the 360 mL to determine the amount ingested. The cup should be held at approximately eye level to accurately read the volume (Fig. 24-2). Most hospitals have standardized volumes listed for their commonly used containers, making it easier to calculate intake. Box 24-2 provides a list of common container volumes.

Box 24-1

Tips for Assisting Patients With Meal Planning and Eating

Because good nutrition is so important to the healing process, it must be monitored and evaluated for adequacy. The patient commonly does not feel like eating much, so it is your responsibility to make it a priority to do everything you can to ensure optimal nutritional intake. Below are a few tips to help you to do this.

- Spend time getting to know the patient. Be warm and compassionate, letting the patient know you understand that his or her pain, anxiety, or other psychosocial factors are affecting appetite.
- If the patient is nauseated or hurting, provide appropriate medication before mealtime.
- Supervise the assistive personnel and ensure that they assist the patient in preparing for mealtime by getting the patient comfortable in a bed or chair, providing a warm wet washcloth to wash the hands and face, and clearing the over-the-bed table of clutter and unpleasantries to provide ample room for the meal tray. Wipe the over-the-bed table off with disinfectant if a urinal or other contaminated items have lain on it. This preparation should be carried out prior to tray arrival as it is impossible to do these tasks with a tray of food in one's hands.
- Ensure that assistive personnel wash their hands prior to passing out meal trays.

- Teach assistive personnel to check each tray for the correct diet and appropriate temperature of food; to open containers on the tray; and how to safely assist those patients who require assistance.
- Help the patient identify factors that would improve the eating experience, such as selecting foods he or she likes, creating a comfortable environment, arranging for early or later trays if the patient's normal routine is quite different than the hospital routine, or allowing friends and family to bring in foods from home provided there are no dietary restrictions.
- If the patient's appetite is limited, provide five to six smaller feedings per day rather than three larger ones. The physician will generally write an order for this if you ask.
- Educate your patient as to the importance of nutritional intake and drinking adequate fluids in the healing process.
- Make rounds to your patients' rooms during mealtimes. Ask your patients if they have any needs or if they are satisfied with their meals; help facilitate a pleasant experience by being a problem-solver.

Figure 24-2   Use a graduated cup and hold up at eye level to accurately measure intake.

Box 24-2

Examples of Standard Container Volumes

Different facilities will use glasses, cups, and bowls of various sizes that will hold differing volumes of liquid. Each facility will have its own list of standard container volumes. Become familiar with the volumes where you work. Below is a list of common container volumes.

- **Popsicle:** 90 mL
- **Juice glass:** 120 mL
- **Individual ice cream cup:** 120 mL
- **Coffee cup:** 150 mL
- **Small gelatin cup:** 180 mL
- **Drinking glass:** 180 mL or 240 mL
- **Small soup bowl:** 180 mL
- **Large soup bowl:** 240 mL
- **Small carton of milk:** 240 mL

Output includes all bodily fluids that are lost, including urine, emesis, liquid stool, blood, suctioned gastric contents, and drainage from drainage devices such as a Hemovac or Jackson-Pratt drain, which you will read about in Chapter 26. You will measure urine and emesis in clear containers that are larger than the one used to measure oral intake. The units of measurement will be the same: ounces and milliliters. You may hear the containers referred to as graduated containers or receptacles. When you measure any form of output, you will write it on the I/O sheet at the bedside, indicating the type of output, such as Hemovac drainage or gastric suction. Each category is totaled separately and documented on the I/O sheet or flow sheet in the patient's chart at the end of each shift. Then the total of all intake is calculated and compared with the calculated total of all output. The average adult requires between 1,500 and 2,500 mL of fluid intake per 24 hours, depending upon size and health status. The total urinary output should closely balance with the total intake, usually within 200 to 300 mL of the intake. Skill 24-2 (page 528) provides additional information regarding intake and output recording.

Supporting Patients With Special Nutritional Needs

As you provide nursing care and nutritional support to patients, you will encounter patients who have special nutritional requirements. These patients may have an inability to tolerate certain nutrients or an actual eating disorder. Food allergies or intolerances present significant challenges. Food allergies are most commonly identified in infancy or early childhood. When identified in children, the patient and family have not had time to develop adaptive measures; they are frequently anxious and uncertain about their ability to effectively manage and meet their nutritional needs.

Food Allergies

A *food allergy* is a reaction by the patient's immune system to an allergen, which is a food protein that once ingested causes the immune system to develop antibodies. The most common food allergies are:

- Peanuts
- Wheat
- Dairy products
- Eggs

Typically, a patient with food allergy will experience such symptoms as skin, respiratory, and gastrointestinal reactions, which get increasingly worse with repeated exposures to the offending agent. It is important that the nurse gather assessment data on the history of the allergy, when it was first identified, symptoms experienced, and interventions used in the event of a reaction. Allergic reactions can present as a rash or hives, or can be severe and result in anaphylaxis. **Anaphylaxis** is a life-threatening emergency as it involves swelling of the upper respiratory tract and can result in occlusion of the airway. The patient, patient's family, and all persons involved with the care of the patient need to be aware of the signs and symptoms of anaphylaxis and the appropriate and immediate treatment of the reaction.

Food Intolerances

Food intolerance is not an allergic reaction; it is an adverse reaction to a food without activation of the immune response. The symptoms generated by the food intolerance can be triggered by distinct properties of the food, such as tyramine in aged cheese or wine, or by metabolic disorders, such as gluten intolerance. Food intolerance can stem from the body's lack of digestive enzymes or an inability to utilize these enzymes. The resultant symptoms of intolerance are usually of a gastrointestinal nature, such as bloating, flatulence, diarrhea, or nausea. Treatment of food intolerances requires identification of the offending agent; this can be accomplished by eliminating various foods from the diet over a period of time. Once the offending agent is identified, the patient will need to modify his or her diet to limit or eliminate the offending foods. Lactose intolerance, for example, would require that a patient limit milk intake. However, the patient would also have to evaluate other foods to determine if they contain lactose.

Knowledge Connection
Discuss the differences between food allergy and food intolerance. Describe common symptoms of each.

Therapeutic Diets

Many patients must follow a modified diet to help manage their illness or injury. Hospital food comes in a variety of regular and modified diets. Diets may be modified singularly, such as a 1,500-calorie diet, or may be modified in combinations, such as a 1,500-calorie, low-sodium, mechanical soft diet. Each facility will have a diet manual that contains details about each type of diet and the foods that are allowed. All patients must have a diet ordered by their primary care physician unless there is an order for the patient to remain NPO, which is explained below. Dietary modifications are made in collaboration with a hospital or institutional dietitian. The following represent the most commonly prescribed restrictions and modified diets.

NPO

NPO stands for "nothing per os," or mouth. It means the patient is restricted from oral intake of food or fluid, including water. This is frequently ordered before surgery, invasive procedures, and certain diagnostic studies to reduce the risk of aspiration. Common orders may be "NPO after midnight" or "NPO 8 hours prior to procedure." A patient who is vomiting may have an NPO order specified to be in effect until nausea and vomiting are no longer a problem.

Most patients who are nourished can tolerate brief periods without food or fluid; however, prolonged periods of NPO status, such as when a procedure or surgery is delayed for 24 hours, should be avoided. During prolonged periods of NPO status, IV fluids may be given to maintain hydration and a minimally supportive caloric intake.

Anytime a patient is NPO, the patient and family should be informed regarding the NPO status and the reason why it is ordered. This will help to increase compliance. An NPO sign should be placed on the door and on the wall over the patient's bed to serve as a reminder for staff and visitors. You should empty and remove the patient's water carafe and drinking glass from the bedside as a reminder that the patient is not to drink anything.

Regular Diet

A regular diet is appropriate for those patients without special nutritional needs. This diet provides approximately 2,000 calories per day and offers a balanced meal plan. The nutritional value of this diet can vary widely depending on the food choices of the patient. Hospital meals offer the patient the opportunity to have adequate caloric intake but are not necessarily designed to be low in sodium, fat, or cholesterol. You may need to educate your patient to make nutritionally sound choices. Regular diets are adapted to meet the age-specific needs of patients as the nutritional needs of a child differ from those of an elderly person and from those of a middle-aged adult.

For patients with specific cultural or ethnic needs, many facilities provide ethnic variances such as Asian, kosher, or vegetarian. If a facility does not provide these variations, you may want to encourage the patient's family or friends to bring ethnic foods from home that will allow or encourage the patient to eat more.

Even though patients typically order their daily meals from a selection of menu choices, you may encounter patients with complaints related to the taste or texture of hospital food. They may complain of it being "bland and tasteless." This may be true, because house diets must be prepared to meet the needs and tastes of a wide variety of patients. Usually foods available for selection on the hospital menu are limited to avoid unpopular food items such as turnips, or those that are fatty, fried, or gas producing.

Diets Modified by Consistency

Patients with acute illnesses and those undergoing surgery or bowel procedures may need a diet that is modified in consistency to assist in the management of their illness. The physician may order "Clear liquids, advance as tolerated." This means the patient is allowed to gradually progress from a diet of clear liquids to full liquids, then on to a soft diet and finally to a regular diet, as the patient is able to tolerate the increasing consistencies without nausea, vomiting, or distress.

For some elderly patients or those with chewing problems or difficulty swallowing, termed **dysphagia**, a long-term diet modification may be necessary. Common diets with consistency modifications include clear liquid, full liquid, mechanical soft, and pureed.

• A **clear liquid diet** is ordered to provide hydration and calories in the form of simple carbohydrates that help meet some of the body's energy needs. The defining characteristic that separates a clear liquid from a full liquid has to do with its clarity. Is the liquid, as is or diluted with water, clear enough that you can "read a newspaper" through it? For example, a dark carbonated cola that is diluted with water would become clear enough to see through it. If so, it may be considered a clear liquid. Examples of clear liquids include water, broth, and tea without milk. As clear liquid diets do not provide adequate calories, proteins, fats, vitamins, or minerals to meet the body's needs, a patient should be progressed as quickly as possible to a more nutritious diet.

Common examples of when a clear liquid diet might be appropriate include postoperatively or during recovery from gastrointestinal disease such as vomiting and diarrhea, when the gut must be introduced slowly to food. When the clear liquids are tolerated, the patient may be advanced to a full liquid diet. It will be your responsibility to determine when to advance the diet by assessing how the patient tolerates each new level of diet.

• A **full liquid diet** consists of all the liquids found in a clear liquid diet with the addition of all other opaque liquids and food items that become liquid at room temperature. Examples of full liquids might include milk, pudding, and ice cream. As is the case with the clear liquid diet, this diet also provides limited nutrients, so patients should remain on this plan for a limited period of time. Patients who need to remain on a liquid diet for an extended period of time should have the diet planned by a dietitian, who may recommend the addition of high-calorie, high-protein supplements.

• A **mechanical soft diet** is the diet of choice for patients with acute or chronic difficulties with chewing, such as those with jaw problems, missing teeth, poorly fitting dentures, or severe weakness or fatigue. This diet includes all of the items from the full liquid diet plus the addition of such foods as scrambled eggs and cottage cheese. Many items can be included in this diet by altering their texture through extensive cooking or use of a blender or food processor. Through the inclusion of a wide variety of foods, this diet is better able to meet a person's nutritional needs; however, it is quite low in fiber so patients may be at risk for constipation.

• A **pureed diet** is one that is processed in a blender/food processor. Any food item can be included, but its consistency must be changed. Food items are placed in a blender while liquid is added to moisten them, creating a texture that is somewhat thicker than full liquid but that can still be swallowed easily.

Table 24-1 provides examples of foods for each of the four diets listed above.

Knowledge Connection
What are the categories of diets modified by consistency? What are the key nutrients these provide, and which may need to be supplemented?

Diets Modified for Disease

Certain patient conditions may require that the patient's diet be modified to either increase or restrict the intake of certain nutrients. The following will identify the most common of these diets:

• **Diabetic:** Used to manage calorie and carbohydrate intake for patients with diabetes mellitus, primarily those who are insulin dependent.

• **Calorie-restricted:** Used for those patients who must lose weight.

• **Sodium-restricted:** Used for those patients with hypertension, congestive heart failure, or kidney or liver failure, and those who require help to prevent or correct fluid retention. The degree of restriction is commensurate with disease severity, severity of symptoms, and the medication regimen prescribed. Typically sodium restrictions range from

Table 24-1   Partial List of Foods by Consistency

Clear Liquid	Full Liquid	Mechanical Soft	Pureed
• Water	• All clear liquids	• All liquids and pureed foods	• All liquids
• Broth/bouillon	• Cream soups	• All soups	• Scrambled eggs
• Black coffee	• Milk	• Ground/finely diced meats	• Pureed meats
• Tea	• Cream	• Finely diced/flaked fish	• Pureed vegetables
• Carbonated drinks	• Ice cream	• Cottage cheese	• Pureed fruits
• Clear fruit juices:	• Yogurt	• Soft cheeses	• Mashed potatoes
• Apple	• Milkshakes	• Mashed or riced potatoes	• Gravy
• Grape	• Sherbet	• Rice	• Applesauce
• Cranberry	• Custards/puddings	• Oatmeal	• Baby foods
• Gelatin	• Vegetable juices	• Grits	
• Popsicles	• Pureed vegetables	• Pancakes	
• Clear sports drinks:	• All fruit juices	• Soft breads	
Gatorade	• Protein drinks	• Soda and graham crackers	
• Electrolyte drinks:	• Liquid supplements	• Cooked soft vegetables	
Pedialyte	• Refined cooked cereals:	• Cooked or canned fruits	
	• Cream of Wheat	• Bananas	
	• Malto-Meal	• Soft pastries	

2,000 to 3,000 mg/day. While many patients think that simply not adding salt to foods provides adequate sodium restriction, that is not the case. Most of the sodium people ingest comes from processed foods, making it necessary to read labels for sodium content if the patient is sent home on this diet.

- **Fat-restricted:** Used for patients who are experiencing problems with fat malabsorption, such as those with disorders affecting the gallbladder, liver, lymphatic system, pancreas, or intestines. It may also be used with those patients who have elevated triglyceride, lipid, or cholesterol levels, or for patients needing general weight loss.

- **Fiber-restricted:** Used during the acute phase of intestinal disorders when the presence of fiber may exacerbate intestinal pain, produce diarrhea, or cause an intestinal blockage. This diet is often used prior to intestinal surgery to minimize fecal volume or postsurgery to allow the gastrointestinal system to transition gradually to a regular diet.

- **Renal:** Used to manage or limit fluids and electrolytes for patients with renal insufficiency or disease. The renal diet is complex, and the patient's nutritional needs change over the course of the disease. A dietitian specializing in renal disorders may guide the nutritional therapy.

- **Protein-restricted:** Used to manage protein intake for those patients with liver or kidney disease.

- **High-calorie, high-protein:** Used to increase calorie and protein intake in those patients with increased need related to wound healing, growth promotion, and increasing or maintaining weight. High-fat foods may also be added to increase calories available for energy use.

- **Antigen-avoidance:** Used for patients allergic to or with an intolerance of certain foods, such as gluten-free diets for patients with celiac disease. These diets are often difficult to maintain once the patient is home, due to the rarity of commercial businesses that carry the special products made without these ingredients.

- **Five to six small, frequent feedings:** A physician may order any type of diet to be provided in several smaller feedings throughout the day rather than the traditional three meals per day. This is used with those patients who have difficulty tolerating larger meals or simply are unable to eat more than a few bites at a time, as well as those who need to have food gradually reintroduced. Often elderly patients are only able to eat small amounts at a time, thus making it difficult to obtain the needed nutrients in the traditional three meals a day. By increasing the number of meal or snack times from three to five or six per day, the patient has a better chance of receiving the needed nutrients.

Knowledge Connection

Give an example of an illness or condition that might necessitate a high-protein diet. Identify one type of diet that might be ordered to help decrease swelling of a patient's hands and legs. For what type conditions might the physician order a fat-restricted diet?

Nursing Responsibilities

You will be responsible for monitoring the diet type, percentage eaten, and whether or not the patient tolerated the meal. When the physician has ordered "clear liquids, advance as tolerated," such as might be appropriate postoperatively or during recovery from gastrointestinal illness, it will be your responsibility to determine when to advance the patient's diet. Utilizing the nursing process, you will assess how much the patient eats and record this as a percentage, record how the patient tolerates each meal, and evaluate whether he or she is ready to have the diet advanced to the next level of consistency. Factors indicating that the patient is not yet ready to advance the diet may include any of the following:

- Nausea
- Vomiting
- Abdominal distention
- Cramping
- Absent or hypoactive bowel sounds
- Complaints of indigestion
- Diarrhea

Once you evaluate how the patient is tolerating each level of increased consistency, you will notify the dietary service to advance the diet to the next level.

Laboratory and Diagnostic Connection

Diabetes

In order to effectively manage insulin-dependent diabetes, also known as type 1 diabetes, it is imperative to maintain *glycemic control,* which refers to the blood glucose level. This is done by thorough monitoring of blood glucose levels on a prescribed basis, such as once daily or before meals and at bedtime. Blood glucose should remain within a prescribed range established by the patient's physician. The 2008 American Diabetes Association guidelines state that a range of 90 to 130 mg/dL before meals is acceptable for existing diabetics. Glucose testing provides valuable immediate information allowing patients to adjust their food intake, medications, or activity level, and for preventing hypoglycemic events.

Glucose in the blood freely enters red blood cells and attaches to hemoglobin molecules, directly proportional to the amount of glucose present. Health care providers evaluate a patient's long-term glycemic control by measuring **glycosylated hemoglobin**, known as hemoglobin (Hb) A_{1c}. A red blood cell has an average life span of 120 days, so the Hb A_{1c} measures the amount of glucose present over a period of 2 to 3 months, giving a better overall picture of glycemic control. In nondiabetics, Hb A_{1c} is usually less than 6% of the hemoglobin. The goal of diabetes treatment is to maintain an Hb A_{1c} less than 7%. For diabetics without adequate control, it can range as high as 12% to 20%.

Diabetes

The diagnosis of diabetes can be overwhelming. It is a disease that requires new medications, developing an awareness of blood glucose levels, and modification of various aspects of the patient's lifestyle as well as nutritional habits. Eating a healthier diet is among the most significant modifications the patient with diabetes must make. It is important that the patient with diabetes understand his or her disease, how diet aids in symptom management, and the prevention of short- and long-term complications. Many patients with newly diagnosed diabetes erroneously believe that their disease is related to sugar intake and therefore should be alleviated by the diet.

Before discharge, you will need to teach the patient about effective meal planning and nutritional intake. Using the following patient instructions will help you emphasize the most important points about healthy eating:

- Eat a well-balanced diet, which includes carbohydrates, moderate protein, and fat in sparing amounts.
- Know the differences between simple and complex carbohydrates:
  - *Simple carbohydrates,* which are found primarily in fruits, fruit juices, processed baked goods, and sugar, are quickly converted to glucose and can be used to quickly raise the blood glucose. There is no need to totally eliminate them from the diet, but simple carbohydrates should be ingested in moderation and the carbohydrate intake should be consistent from day to day to maintain better balanced blood glucose.
  - *Complex carbohydrates,* which are found in whole grains, vegetables high in fiber, and legumes such as dried peas and beans, require the body to work harder to break them down to use for energy, helping to maintain a more consistent blood glucose level. The majority of ingested carbohydrates should be complex carbohydrates rather than simple carbohydrates.
- Eat three meals and an evening snack daily. Some physicians may prefer you to eat an additional snack in midmorning and midafternoon. Each of these should contain some protein.
- Do not skip meals.
- Increase your fiber intake.
- Reduce your fat intake by baking, broiling, or grilling foods.
- Lose weight if you are overweight. Studies show that even a loss of 10% of total body weight is significant to help lower blood glucose.

Eating Disorders

Eating disorders are evidenced by extreme disturbances in eating habits, to such a point that the patient's health can be severely affected or even result in death. The most common of these disorders are anorexia nervosa and bulimia nervosa, both of which involve the patient's relationship with food and eating and their body image. Women and girls are more at risk to develop an eating disorder than males. Most eating disorders occur during adolescence or early adulthood, but are not restricted to these phases of life. Eating disorders may result from either physical or psychological causes and result in both physical and psychological effects. These patients have an impaired perception of self and do not see their eating or lack of eating as problematic.

Anorexia Nervosa

Anorexia nervosa is characterized by an excessive leanness or wasting of the body, known as *emaciation.* There is relentless self-starvation in an effort to reduce the body weight below normal. These patients do not see themselves accurately and perceive that they are overweight, even when they are at the point of physical starvation. Given the freedom to choose their meals, patients who are anorexic will continue to restrict their intake. They will also exhibit obsessive thoughts related to their body shape and weight, and display an intense fear of obesity. Physical symptoms commonly seen in the severely underweight anorexic patient are:

- Brittle nails
- Dull, dry, brittle hair
- Amenorrhea
- Severe constipation
- Lethargy or fatigue
- Below-normal vital signs
- Muscle weakness
- Muscle wasting
- Anemia

Possible complications include electrolyte imbalances, such as abnormally low levels of calcium, magnesium, zinc, and phosphorus; and dehydration and metabolic acidosis or alkalosis from overuse of diuretics and laxatives. Patients with anorexia may struggle with the disease for a decade or longer, resulting in death if medical treatment is not sought before the damage is too severe to reverse.

Bulimia Nervosa

Bulimia nervosa is commonly referred to as *binge eating* and is frequently accompanied by some type of behavior that will help to get rid of some of the calories that were ingested while bingeing, such as self- or medication-induced vomiting (known as *purging),* excessive exercise, fasting, or overuse of laxatives. Some patients will also abuse diuretics to reduce water weight. Psychologically, the bulimic patient is also obsessed with body shape and weight; the binge-purge cycles are triggered by stressful events or may be influenced by peer pressure in adolescents. The acts of bingeing and purging are generally hidden from friends and family. These patients may horde junk food and hide it for later bingeing. Physical symptoms that may be observed in a patient with bulimia nervosa include:

- Chronic inflammation or soreness of throat due to retching and exposure to gastric acid during vomiting
- Diarrhea from laxative abuse
- Increasing dental decay from exposure to gastric acid when vomiting
- Indigestion
- Regurgitation of gastric fluids into the esophagus, known as *gastric reflux*
- Dehydration

Possible complications include renal damage, fluid and electrolyte imbalances, and gastroesophogeal reflux disease. Patients with bulimia may also suffer from anorexia, increasing the extent and severity of damage, as well as the risk of death.

Patients with eating disorders pose a significant challenge for the nurses working with them. They are most effectively managed by an interdisciplinary team with expert knowledge and skill in managing these disorders.

Knowledge Connection

Describe the common symptoms of the patient with anorexia nervosa and the patient with bulimia nervosa.

Food-Drug Interactions

Certain drugs and foods can interact and alter the effects of the medication. Some drug and food combinations result in less serious interactions and should simply be monitored, while others significantly change the drug's effect and can result in a serious adverse reaction, making it imperative to avoid the offending food while administration of the drug is necessary. Some of the general types of food-drug interactions include the following:

- Some medications can affect nutrient intake by inhibiting appetite, causing gastrointestinal (GI) discomfort, or causing some other reaction that inhibits food intake by making it unpleasant or painful. Other medications can stimulate appetite, increasing the quantity of food ingested.
- Certain medications can alter the absorption, metabolism, or excretion of nutrients; alternatively, some nutrients can alter the absorption, metabolism, or excretion of medications.
- Other food-drug interactions can create medication toxicity.

Prevention of these adverse events is avoidable with education. You have a primary responsibility to be aware of potential food-drug interactions and to educate your patients to be alert to these possibilities. There are numerous food-drug interactions, and as more medications are developed, the potential for new food-drug interactions increases. It would be impossible to memorize all of these adverse combinations, so you must faithfully research each new or unfamiliar drug in a drug book before you administer it. Many facilities have pharmacology software programs installed on their computers for the health care providers to use to look up medications. Another good resource is your pharmacist.

Drug Effects on Food Intake

The side effects of medication, such as nausea, vomiting, altered taste sensation, anorexia, decreased salivation, and sores or lesions in the mouth or the upper GI tract, can inhibit appetite or make food intake painful. Some medications can be very sedating or cause the patient to feel confused; this will in turn interfere with nutritional intake. These side effects may be monitored and managed when they occur on a short-term basis without causing significant weight loss. However, when the side effects are chronic, a plan of intervention must be developed to prevent weight loss and emaciation. For example, chemotherapy patients with severe nausea or vomiting would probably require the use of *antiemetics,* medications that help to prevent or reduce nausea and vomiting.

Many medications, such as corticosteroids, some antidepressants, and the atypical antipsychotics, can cause unintentional weight gain. For example, corticosteroids dramatically increase the appetite of some patients, resulting in increased consumption of food intake. These patients can gain large amounts of weight, often greater than 20 pounds, in a short period of time. It is important to teach patients about these potential problems and devise strategies to manage them before the weight is gained. For some patients, such as those with *cachexia* (malnutrition and wasting associated with cancer), weight gain is desirable. These patients may be prescribed medications to increase their appetite.

Drug Effects on Absorption

Dietary effects that reduce medication absorption typically occur through the influence of increased gastric motility, conditions within the GI tract that are either too acidic or too alkaline, or direct interaction of food with a medication. Most medications are absorbed in the small intestine and may be absorbed more quickly if the stomach is empty during drug administration. While it may be best that certain medications be given on an empty stomach to enhance absorption, there are others such as ibuprofen or aspirin that should be taken with food to decrease gastric irritation. Some medications are best absorbed in an acidic medium but others may be damaged by acidity. Those that are damaged by acidity are often available in an enteric-coated formulation that dissolves in the small intestine, thereby promoting better absorption. High-fiber foods and diets may decrease the absorption of certain medications.

Medications can also influence the absorption of nutrients. Drugs that damage the intestinal mucosa, such as nonsteroidal anti-inflammatory drugs or antineoplastics (cancer drugs), and certain antibiotics can cause malabsorption. Binding of drugs to nutrients will impair absorption of the drug and/or the nutrient. For example, some antibiotics bind to the calcium in foods or supplements, which reduces the absorption of both the antibiotic and the calcium. Certain medications, such as histamine$_2$ (H$_2$) blockers or proton pump inhibitors, can reduce stomach acidity and impede the absorption of vitamin B$_{12}$, iron, and folate. Finally, medications can directly impede nutrient absorption by interfering with intestinal metabolism.

Drug Effects on Metabolism

Metabolism of food and medications occurs through the use of enzyme systems in the small intestine and liver. Some medications can inhibit or induce the activities of these enzyme systems, impairing the metabolism of nutrients. For example, the anticonvulsant phenytoin induces the liver system that metabolizes folate, vitamin D, and vitamin K, resulting in patients on this anticonvulsant needing additional supplements of these vitamins.

Many other medications can impact metabolism by mimicking the body's natural hormones, such as corticosteroid drugs that mimic the body-produced hormone cortisol. The human body, when exposed to these medications, acts as if it is experiencing an additional release of hormone. In the case of long-term treatment with corticosteroids, the patient may experience weight gain, rounding of the face shape called *moon facies,* hyperglycemia, bone loss, and muscle wasting.

Foods or their components can affect the enzyme systems as well and interfere with medication metabolism. Grapefruit juice, for example, has been found to inactivate or inhibit enzymes necessary for the metabolism of a number of medications. The outcome of this can be that levels of the medication are greatly increased, yielding a much stronger physiologic effect. Another high-risk interaction occurs between many foods and herbs and the drug warfarin, an anticoagulant that is prescribed for patients with a history of blood clots. The patient taking warfarin should avoid eating foods containing moderate to high levels of vitamin K, as vitamin K can significantly weaken the anticoagulant effect of warfarin, increasing the risk of recurrent blood clots. In addition, the popular herbal supplements ginkgo, ginseng, St. John's wort, dong quai, and garlic, among others, contain compounds that enhance the effects of warfarin, which could possibly result in bleeding or hemorrhage. Patients who take warfarin should be educated to limit or avoid these foods and herbs. This education is your responsibility as well as that of the physician and the pharmacist. Table 24-2 presents a sampling of foods and drugs that should not be administered at the same time, and foods that should be completely avoided while taking a particular drug.

Drug Effects on Excretion

Excretion refers to the process of eliminating a medication or its metabolites or nutritional components from the body; this is usually performed by the kidneys. The length of time it takes to excrete a medication influences the extent of the medication's therapeutic effects. Slowed or inadequate excretion can raise the blood level of a medication and cause toxicity as successive scheduled doses are administered. Rapid or increased excretion can limit or greatly reduce the medication's therapeutic effect.

Certain medications can alter the kidney's excretion of nutrients such as minerals. Such diuretics as furosemide, for example, can cause increased excretion of important

Table 24-2 **Selected Food-Drug Interactions**

Food or Drink	Drug
Large amounts of potassium-rich foods: bananas, oranges, leafy green vegetables	Potassium-sparing diuretics: spironolactone, amiloride, triamterene
Foods high in vitamin K: broccoli, spinach, cauliflower, kale	Anticoagulant: warfarin
Grapefruit, grapefruit juice, alcohol	Statin drug for high cholesterol: Lipitor
Orange juice, large amounts of licorice	Beta blocker for angina and hypertension: Tenormin
Alcohol	Beta blocker for angina, hypertension, and migraine headaches: Inderal
Dairy products	Quinolone anti-infectives: Cipro, Levaquin Tetracycline anti-infectives: doxycycline Antifungals: Diflucan, Nizoral, Sporanox
Apple juice, orange juice, grapefruit juice	Antihistamine: Allegra

minerals such as potassium, sodium, chloride, calcium, and magnesium. Long-term use of furosemide requires regular monitoring of the patient's fluid and electrolyte status and usually requires potassium supplementation. Similarly, isoniazid (INH), a medication used to treat tuberculosis, can lead to increased excretion of vitamin B_6. Patients receiving INH therapy must be treated for more than 6 months, which can lead to vitamin B_6 deficiency. To prevent the deficiency, patients are started on B_6 as soon as INH is prescribed.

Many foods and nutrients can impact the excretion of medications. Lithium, a mood-stabilizing agent, is metabolized by the kidneys, where some of it is also reabsorbed and the remainder is excreted. This process is influenced by blood levels of sodium. Because lithium is similar in chemical structure to sodium, the kidneys often excrete lithium as if it were sodium. A person with a high level of sodium will excrete high levels of sodium and also lithium, which can lead to subtherapeutic levels of the medication. Conversely, those with low sodium levels will retain extra lithium, leading to increased levels. Lithium is a medication that must be maintained in a specific therapeutic range, and increased levels can lead to adverse effects or even toxicity. This makes it extremely important to monitor the sodium levels in a patient taking lithium.

Knowledge Connection
Identify a few high-risk problems associated with absorption and excretion in relation to food-drug interactions. Why is it important to educate patients about potential food-drug interactions?

Enteral Tubes

Enteral tubes come in various styles and lengths and are used for multiple purposes. They may be used to decompress the stomach postoperatively, following abdominal injury, or as treatment for intestinal obstruction. These tubes may also be inserted and used for nutritional support or medication administration, as well as for collecting a specimen of stomach contents for diagnostic assessment of the GI tract, such as analyzing the gastric contents for pH or testing for blood.

Knowledge Connection
Explain four purposes for insertion of enteric tubes.

Anatomy and Physiology Connection

Gastrointestinal Tract
A review of the anatomy of the gastrointestinal (GI) tract can help you to visualize the digestive organs and processes that occur as food moves through the body. The GI tract grows and changes through a person's life span, allowing greater digestion

of food particles as it matures. This is part of the reason solids are introduced to older infants, as the partially broken down food particles may contribute to a heightened allergic response.

The organs that comprise the GI tract include the mouth; pharynx; esophagus; stomach; small intestine, which is further divided into the duodenum, jejunum and ileum; and large intestine. The accessory organs include the liver and the gallbladder (Fig. 24-3). Digestion begins as food enters the mouth, where enzymes begin to break down the food, and continues as it travels through the GI tract. Along the way, peristalsis and the musculature of the GI tract guide the mechanical digestion; enzymes and secretions are added by various organs for chemical digestion. Nutrient absorption primarily occurs in the small intestine. Absorption is the process by which nutrients pass through the walls of the small intestine and enter into the bloodstream in the capillaries. Absorption occurs by varying mechanisms that include passive diffusion and osmosis, facilitated diffusion, and energy-dependent active transport. The process of *passive diffusion* occurs when the pressure on one side of the membrane is greater and the nutrients move from the area of greater pressure through the mucosa to the area of less pressure. At this point, the nutrients enter the circulatory system and are used for energy or stored for later use. While most nutrients are absorbed in the small intestine, most of the water absorption occurs within the large intestine, helping to maintain water and electrolyte balance and to solidify the remaining waste product into soft, formed feces to be expelled per the rectum.

Nasogastric and Nasointestinal Tubes

The **nasogastric (NG) tube** is shorter than the nasointestinal (NI) tube, and is inserted through the nose, down the esophagus, and into the stomach; the longer NI tube is also inserted through the nose and continues through the stomach, into the duodenum or even further into the jejunum. The terms *nasointestinal tube and nasoenteric (NE) tube* are often used interchangeably. The NI or NE tube is usually smaller in bore size and more flexible than an NG tube. Some of them are weighted on the tip to help pull the tube through the stomach into the duodenum or jejunum; one commonly used NI tube is the Dobhoff (Fig. 24-4). They are mostly used for enteral feedings in patients who are at increased risk for aspiration, such as those with absent or diminished gag reflex or severe gastroesophageal reflux disease (GERD).

Tube Size and Length
The outside diameter of the NG or NI tube is measured using the French (Fr) scale: the larger the number, the larger the outside diameter of the tube. The most common sizes of feeding tubes are those measuring 8 to 12 Fr and with a length of 36 to 43 inches (90 to 108 cm). Larger bore NG tubes such as 16 or 18 Fr are most commonly used for patients requiring gastric decompression or washing out the

Figure 24-3   Organs of the digestive tract.

stomach (termed *lavage),* obtaining gastric specimens, and instilling charcoal for poisoning or drug overdose.

Single-lumen Versus Double-lumen

One style of NG tube is the Salem sump tube, a double-lumen tube, meaning that it has two separate channels inside the tube. One lumen is an air vent and the other is for drainage of stomach contents, irrigation, instillation of medications, and obtaining gastric samples. The vent lumen extends like a "pigtail" from the side of the tube near the end that connects to the suction tubing. Some manufacturers make the pigtail blue to differentiate it as the *air vent.*

A second type of large-bore NG tube is Levin's tube, which has only one lumen. It can be used for the same

purposes as the Salem sump tube, but does not have the air vent lumen to allow equalization of vacuum pressure. Both the Salem sump and Levin's tube are intended for short-term use only. Leaving them in place for more than 10 to 14 days can result in necrosis of the nasal septum.

Gastric Decompression

Gastric decompression is the process of reducing the pressure within the stomach by emptying it of its contents, including ingested food and liquids, gastric juices, and gas. The stomach contents are removed by inserting a double-lumen NG tube through the nose into the stomach and

Figure 24-4 a. Nasogastric tube: the holes in the end of the tube allow contents to be suctioned from the stomach or fluid to be instilled into the stomach. b. Weighted nasointestinal tube: smaller and more flexible than nasogastric tube, usually preferred for feeding.

connecting the drainage lumen to a suction source. The gastric contents are drained into a graduated container where contents are assessed for volume, color, and consistency.

Several small holes are distributed over 3 to 6 inches of the end of the NG tube lumen that is inserted into the stomach (refer back to Fig. 24-4). Once the suction begins to pull a vacuum through these small openings, it can cause the end of the tube to adhere to the wall of the stomach, serving to irritate the mucosal lining. If it remains adhered to the same spot for an extended period of time, it can damage the mucosa. The smaller second lumen is usually blue to differentiate it from the primary lumen, and is designed to allow for atmospheric air to be drawn into the tube to equalize the vacuum pressure in the stomach caused by the suction, helping to prevent the tube from adhering to the gastric mucosa.

Knowledge Connection
What does it mean to decompress the stomach? Describe the purpose of a double-lumen nasogastric tube.

Insertion of NG Tube for Gastric Decompression

Placement of an NG tube requires a physician's order, normally stating the type and size of tube and the purpose for the tube. If the physician does not include this information, clarify all three pieces of information before inserting tube. After reviewing the order on the medical record, and clarifying if necessary, review the record for conditions that might contraindicate insertion of the tube.

Preparing the Patient
Inquire of the patient whether he or she has ever experienced an NG tube insertion. Then explain the process to the patient, being honest but choosing your words carefully and observing the patient's responses. This helps you to know when the patient does not understand something, when he or she has a question, and when the patient begins to exhibit fear or anxiety. Your words and approach can have a dramatic impact on the patient's response. You can help a patient to better understand what you are about to do, gain the patient's confidence and cooperation, and alleviate some of his or her anxiety. However if you fail to choose your words carefully, offer an incomplete explanation of what you are about to do, appear to be in a hurry, or display an apathetic or thoughtless attitude, you can raise his or her fear and anxiety level, resulting in lack of patient cooperation that can make the insertion process much more uncomfortable for the patient and more difficult for you.

Preparing Supplies for Use
Gather your supplies, wash your hands, verify the patient's identity, provide for privacy, raise the bed to working height, and lower the rails. (See Skill 24-3, page 530, for a list of supplies and equipment that you will need.) Talk to the patient while you are preparing your work area and during the actual insertion of the tube. This will help to reduce the patient's anxiety and keep the patient focused on what you are saying rather than stressing as he or she watches you.

Arrange your supplies so they are ready to use. Tear two pieces of 1-inch-wide silk tape, one piece approximately 1 inch and the second piece 3 inches in length. Beginning at one end of the 3-inch piece of tape, tear the tape lengthwise down the middle for approximately two-thirds of its length, leaving two 1/2-inch-wide tails that are about 2 inches long. The other end of the tape should still be 1 inch wide for about 1 inch of the tape's length. You will use the tape to secure the tube to the patient's nose; if the facility stocks them, you may obtain the adhesive securing device designed specifically for this purpose. Squeeze a small amount of water-soluble lubricant on a paper towel for lubricating the tip of the NG tube; place it within easy reach. Place your stethoscope on your neck so that it is ready for you to raise to your ears. Place a protective pad or towel over the patient's chest to prevent soiling his or her gown. Ask the patient to hold a finger against one side of his or her nose and exhale. Then have the patient repeat the action on the opposite side. Ask which side feels the most open. This will be the side you will want to use for inserting the NG tube.

Using the NG tube, measure the length from the tip of the patient's nose to the earlobe and then from the earlobe to the xiphoid process. Mark this spot on the tubing with a piece of tape, but do not wrap the tape around the tube so tightly that it is difficult to remove once the tube has been inserted. Obtain an irrigation syringe that will:

• Hold 50 or 60 mL
• Have a plunger that is used to fill and empty the syringe
• Have a catheter tip or slip-tip so that the tip will fit into the NG tube opening

Connect the irrigation syringe to the open end of the NG tube and pull the plunger about halfway back to allow room for gastric contents. Then lay the tube with attached syringe within easy reach. Connecting the irrigation syringe before insertion of the tube will prevent gastric juices from soiling the bed, requiring an extra linen change. Provide the patient with an emesis basin and tissue or washcloth to hold in the nondominant hand and a glass of ice water with a straw to hold in the dominant hand. Apply your clean examination gloves.

Inserting an NG Tube

Communicate to the patient some type of hand signal that he or she is to use if it becomes too uncomfortable or the patient would like you to pause. Tell the patient that you will tell him or her when to take a drink and swallow. Explain that, if he or she can do this each time you cue him or her, that it will make the tube go down much easier and faster.

Have the patient hyperextend the head just slightly. Gently insert the lubricated tip of the NG into the intended naris (Fig. 24-5). Remember that the nasal passageway begins to descend within a couple of centimeters. Avoid pushing the tip of the tube upward against the top side of the nasal passage as it is quite painful and can damage tissue. Never force the tube. You should feel the tube begin to curve downward toward the nasopharynx. If not, gently lift the portion of the tube in your hand so that it directs the tip of the tube downward in the back of the patient's nasal passage. As soon as you reach the point of stimulating the patient's gag reflex, stop advancing the tube and pull it back just a tiny distance, no more than 1/4 inch (0.6 cm), *just to the point that the gag reflex is not being stimulated,* and instruct the patient to take a deep breath and relax. After giving the patient a couple seconds to relax, instruct the patient to begin drinking from the straw. Then, as the patient swallows, advance the tube, cueing the patient to "swallow, ...

swallow." The advancement of the tube coordinated with swallowing allows normal peristalsis to help pull the NG tube along. Repeat this until the tube is inserted to the tape marking. If the patient begins to gag or cough or gives you the designated hand signal to stop, pause and allow the patient to relax and breathe. Coax the patient along in this manner until the insertion is completed. *Safety: If the patient gags or coughs continually and does not seem able to stop, the tube may be curled up in the back of the throat. Use a flashlight and tongue blade to view posterior pharynx to look for the tube. If the patient cannot speak, becomes cyanotic, or coughs incessantly, the tube is likely to be in the lungs. Immediately remove the tube.* (Refer to Box 24-3 for more on what to do when an NG tube enters the lungs.)

Securing the NG Tube

Once the tube is where you want it, remove the tape marker and apply the two pieces of tape you prepared to secure the tube to the patient's nose. There are various methods of taping the tube to the nose, and once you have managed several NG tubes, you will probably find that you prefer a particular method over the others. Here is one common way to apply the two pieces of tape. Apply the end of the 3-inch strip of silk tape (that you previously tore down the middle) to the patient's nose with the two tails hanging down toward the NG tube. Then wrap one of the tails around the tube, spiraling tape down the tube until the entire tail of tape is secured to the tube. Then wrap the second tail the opposite direction around the tube in the same manner. Finally, apply the other piece of tape that is 1 inch wide and 1 inch long directly across the end of the first piece of tape on the patient's nose. This helps to further secure the tape to reduce risk of the NG tube coming out unintentionally. *Safety: Never let go of the tube until it is secured. It can come out in the blink of an eye, especially if the patient coughs, gags, or moves.* The patient would be very upset if you allowed it to fall out and

Figure 24-5   Gently insert the tip of the nasogastric tube into the most patent naris. As the tube begins to advance through the oropharynx, encourage the patient to sip water and swallow. This produces peristalsis that helps to advance the tube into the stomach.

Box 24-3

Reacting When an NG Tube Enters the Lungs

When inserting a nasogastric (NG) tube, it is important to know the signs and symptoms of the tube entering the lungs and the interventions to take if you believe the tube has entered the lungs. Signs and symptoms of a tube entering the lungs include the patient:
• Becoming cyanotic
• Being unable to make a verbal sound
• Coughing spasmodically and uncontrollably
If any of these signs and symptoms are present during NG tube insertion, the tube has likely entered the lungs. If this occurs, immediately and completely withdraw the NG tube. Once removed, the patient will most likely resume normal breathing and regain his or her proper coloring. However, if the patient continues to show signs of distress, take appropriate steps to restore his or her airway and breathing.

put the patient through a repeat insertion. *Safety: Be certain to tape the tube so that it is centered in the naris opening and does not press against any portion of the naris. If the tube presses against the nose, it can cause a pressure ulcer.*

Verifying Placement of the NG Tube

Now verify tube placement by aspirating with the irrigation syringe to see if you get a return of gastric contents. If a patient has a large volume of gastric contents in the stomach, the contents may already be returning into the NG tube and attached syringe before you even have time to tape it to the patient's nose. Check the color to determine if it is green or yellowish-brown, common colors of gastric contents. Check the pH of the aspirated contents with litmus paper strips to verify that it is between 1 and 4. Using either a red or black indelible marker, mark the NG tube boldly at the point of insertion into the nose. This mark will be used as a point of reference for subsequent assessments of tube placement.

Once you have assessed the gastric contents for color and pH, it is still the gold standard of patient care to verify its placement by performing an x-ray. The tube has a radiopaque line that shows up on x-ray, confirming the location of the NG tube tip. *Safety: X-ray confirmation of NG tube location should always be performed immediately after the insertion of any type of enteral tub, whether it is placed for gastric decompression, gastric analysis, or administration of medications or feedings.*

Skill 24-3 provides step-by-step instructions regarding how to insert a nasogastric tube.

Attaching the NG Tube to Suction

Attach the primary lumen to a connecting tube that extends from the suction device. Set the suction on low continuous or intermittent suction according to physician's orders. High suction is typically used only with intermittent suction.

Maintaining Patency of an NG Tube

To prevent an NG tube from clogging, it is important to assess the tube for *patency,* or the condition of being wide open, every 2 hours. Observe for the continual fluctuation and movement of gastric contents through the NG tube and connecting tube into the drainage container indicating patency. The physician may write an "as needed" order for irrigation of the NG tube to maintain patency. Skill 24-4 (page 532) explains how to irrigate an NG tube.

Real-World Connection

Inserting an NG Tube

A patient presented to the emergency room around 2000 with complaints of severe pain, nausea, and vomiting for over 6 hours. After examining the patient and performing a couple of diagnostic procedures, it was determined the patient was suffering from an obstruction of the large intestine, which was causing the portion of the bowel proximal to the obstruction to distend as it filled up with gastric juices and gas. Normal peristalsis was attempting to move the intestinal contents from the stomach through the small and large intestines, but was unable to do so because of the obstruction, which explained why the patient was experiencing so much pain and nausea.

The patient was admitted and orders were written to place the patient on NPO status, start IV fluids, and insert an NG tube connected to low intermittent suction. While the nurse was preparing to insert the NG tube, the patient vomited several hundred milliliters of brown semiliquid fecal material. Once the tube was successfully inserted, the extreme abdominal distention, pain, nausea, and vomiting began to improve immediately. With the administration of an analgesic and antiemetic, the patient got almost total relief by the time she had been there 1 hour. Within that first hour, a total of 2,000 mL of gastric contents and brown, foul-smelling, semiliquid stool were suctioned from the patient's GI tract. That particular patient later told the nurse that the insertion of that NG tube was the best thing that had ever happened to her and she knew that it had saved her life.

Nursing Responsibilities for an NG Tube Connected to Suction

Your responsibilities when caring for an NG tube connected to suction include the following:

- Assess the tube every 2 to 4 hours to ensure patency.
- When necessary, irrigate a clogged tube according to the physician's orders and facility policy.
- Monitor vacuum source settings for correct high or low suction and intermittent or continuous suction every 2 to 4 hours.
- Assess tubing connections to prevent accidental disconnection.
- Assess the color, amount, and consistency of gastric drainage.
- Assess the tube positioning and method of securing the tube so that the tube does not put pressure on the naris, which can result in a pressure ulcer.
- Manually clamp off the NG tube and auscultate bowel sounds every 4 hours, noting hyperactive, hypoactive, and absent sounds.
- Assess the abdomen for abdominal distention and palpate the abdomen, noting firmness.
- Assess the patient for reports of nausea, vomiting, pain, cramping, abdominal fullness, and discomfort every 2 hours.
- Assess for passage of rectal flatus, which may indicate the return of the bowel function known as *peristalsis.*
- Provide mouth care and apply lip moisturizer every 2 hours to prevent drying of the mucous membranes.
- Provide ice chips if allowed to keep the mouth moist.
- Monitor I/O to prevent fluid volume deficit or overload.
- Monitor the serum potassium level, noting a level below normal, known as *hypokalemia.*

Removing an NG Tube

Once the physician has ordered the NG tube to be discontinued, it will be your job to remove it. This procedure is not complicated and takes only a few minutes to accomplish. Explain the process to the patient to alleviate any anxiety and gain the patient's cooperation. Provide the patient with a tissue to wipe mucus from the nose. Wear protective gloves and position a waterproof pad across the patient's chest to prevent soiling of the patient's gown. Instill 10 to 20 mL of air into the NG tube's main lumen to empty the tube of any gastric contents. This prevents fluid from dripping onto the epiglottis during removal. Remove the tape securing the tube to the patient's nose, pinch off the tube, and ask the patient to hold his or her breath to close off the epiglottis. Twist the tube gently to loosen any dried secretions that may be making the tube stick to the lining of the nasal passage or throat, and quickly withdraw the tube from the patient's nose. Wrap it up in the waterproof pad you positioned on the patient's chest and dispose of it in a biohazard bag. You will want to remove it from the patient's view because it may be covered with unsightly mucus and secretions. Assist the patient to wash the face and perform mouth care. Document the procedure and the patient's tolerance of it. Skill 24-5 (page 532) presents more information on removing an NG tube.

Enteral Nutrition

Patients you care for are often too weak or too ill to take in sufficient nutrients by eating. Certain illnesses can interfere with eating, swallowing, digestion, or absorption of food to the degree that the body is not receiving adequate nourishment. In these cases, nutritional support, in the form of liquid formulations of nutrients, can be administered to meet a person's energy needs. The two types of nutritional support are enteral nutrition and parenteral nutrition.

Enteral nutrition uses the GI tract as a delivery system and involves tube feedings that usually replace all oral intake, but may also be given as a supplement to oral ingestion of nutrients. Enteral nutrition is the preferred method for patients with high nutritional needs and an intact GI system, such as those with burns, trauma, severe malnutrition, or neurological problems that impair swallowing. Choosing an enteral feeding route depends on a number of factors. These include the patient's medical condition and stability, current nutritional status, and nutrient requirements for healing and recovery.

Feeding Tubes

As you read earlier, NG and NI tubes inserted for instillation of nutritional feedings are generally softer and smaller than those used for gastric decompression or lavage. They are inserted using basically the same method described previously; however, they tend to go down easier due to being smaller and softer.

Percutaneous Endoscopic Gastrostomy and Jejunostomy Tubes

Patients requiring long-term feedings have surgical endoscopic placement of a percutaneous feeding tube. *Percutaneous* means that an incision is made through the skin and abdominal wall, allowing the tube to extend from either the stomach or jejunum to the external surface of the abdomen. If the tube is placed in the stomach, it is known as a **percutaneous endoscopic gastrostomy (PEG) tube** (Fig. 24-6); if the tube is inserted into the jejunum, it is called a **jejunostomy tube** or **J-tube**. Figure 24-7 shows the insertion sites of different tubes. The tube is secured by the tight suturing of the incision around the tube. This also helps to prevent leakage of formula during feedings. For patients with newly inserted PEG or J-tubes, the nurse must provide care for the surgical incision until it is completely healed. Of all the feeding tubes, the PEG is the most comfortable for the patient. Originally it was used for those patients needing long-term nutritional support, though current trends in addressing patient comfort and improved technology have made this a good option for short-term therapy. The PEG or J-tube should also be marked at the point of insertion into the skin and measured from the point of insertion to the distal end of the tube. These two pieces of data should be recorded for use as a reference point when checking placement of the tube prior to instillations of feedings or medications.

Knowledge Connection

Discuss the various types of feeding tubes. When is enteral nutrition the preferred feeding method?

Tube Feeding Formulas

The selection of formula will be dependent on where the tube is placed and where formula will enter the GI tract. The patient's ability to digest and absorb nutrients will determine

Figure 24-6 A percutaneous endoscopic gastrostomy (PEG) tube.

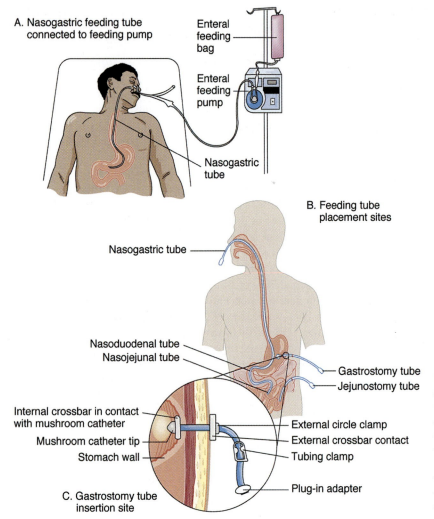

A. Nasogastric feeding tube connected to feeding pump

Enteral feeding bag

Enteral feeding pump

Nasogastric tube

B. Feeding tube placement sites

Nasogastric tube

Nasoduodenal tube
Nasojejunal tube

Gastrostomy tube
Jejunostomy tube

Internal crossbar in contact with mushroom catheter

Mushroom catheter tip

Stomach wall

External circle clamp
External crossbar contact
Tubing clamp

Plug-in adapter

C. Gastrostomy tube insertion site

Figure 24-7   Feeding tubes: a. Nasogastric tube connected to feeding pump. b. Feeding tube placement sites: gastrostomy, jejunostomy. c. View of gastrostomy tube insertion site showing the integument, subcutaneous, and muscle layers, as well as the stomach wall, that a percutaneous gastrostomy tube must go through before entering the stomach.

which type of formula is used. Table 24-3 describes the most common types of enteral feeding formulas.

Enteral Feeding Methods

The delivery method is chosen with consideration of a number of factors, such as the type and location of the feeding tube, the patient's medical condition and status of the digestive system, the type of formula being administered, and the length of time the patient has been on enteral feedings.

Feedings may be ordered for intermittent infusion and administered over 30 to 60 minutes or ordered continuously to be delivered over an 8- or even 24-hour period. The infusion rate will be regulated by either an infusion pump or gravity drip set according to the physician's order.

Intermittent Tube Feedings

Intermittent feedings are used in patients who are on long-term enteral feedings and no longer acutely ill. These patients may be in a long-term health care facility or at home. Intermittent feedings are administered in equal portions periodically throughout the day. The patient will usually receive 200 to 300 mL of formula every 4 to 6 hours.

The formula is delivered by gravity via a bolus or drip set, or with a feeding pump, and administered over a 30- to 60-minute period. The amount of formula delivered per feeding will depend on the total quantity of formula the patient needs to receive in a 24-hour period. Feedings are divided into equal portions and scheduled over the course of the day, or scheduled only during waking hours to provide patients with uninterrupted sleep time. This latter schedule is preferable for those patients on long-term feedings as this allows the patient a schedule that more closely resembles normal.

Intermittent feedings are generally well tolerated; maintaining the formula at room temperature decreases the potential for gastric discomfort. Because of the high risk of aspiration with enteral feedings, the head of the bed should be elevated at least 30 to 45 degrees during the entire feeding and for 1 hour after the feeding to help reduce the risk of reflux and aspiration.

Bolus Feedings

Bolus feedings are a type of intermittent feeding that is frequently used. To administer a bolus feeding, a large irrigating syringe (50 mL or greater) is attached to the feeding

Table 24-3   Types of Enteral Feeding Formulas

Type of Formula	Formula Description	Use for Patient Diagnoses
Standard formulas	Contain protein isolates from milk, soybeans, or a combination of purified proteins. They provide 1 kcal/mL of solution and are proportionally balanced, delivering 12%–20% of kcal as protein, 45%–60% of kcal as carbohydrates, and 30%–40% of kcal as fats. They also contain vitamins and minerals and meet the nutritional needs of most patients.	Patients who can digest and absorb nutrients without difficulty but are unable to eat or swallow sufficiently; or patients who need additional nutrition above their oral consumption.
Hydrolyzed formulas	Contain macronutrients that are *predigested,* or have been partially or fully broken down to components that require little digestion before absorption. These formulas are often low in fat and may be enriched with medium-chain triglycerides to ease digestion and absorption.	Patients who have compromised digestive or absorptive functions.
High-protein formulas	Contain normal nutrients with additional protein.	Burns Large open wounds Malnutrition
Diabetic formulas	Contain reduced levels of simple carbohydrates.	Diabetes mellitus type 1 Diabetes mellitus type 2
Renal formulas	Contain reduced levels of potassium, sodium, and nitrogen.	Renal insufficiency Renal failure
Pulmonary formulas	Provide 55% of the calories as fat so that less CO_2 is produced as oxygen is consumed.	Lung cancer Chronic emphysema Chronic asthma Pulmonary fibrosis
Fiber-containing formulas	Contain higher levels of fiber.	Diverticulosis Colon cancer Diabetes Heart disease Those in long-term care

tube. The size of the feeding tube will determine the size and type of syringe tip that can be used: a catheter-tipped 50- or 60-mL irrigation or piston syringe for larger tubes, or a 20- to 30-mL slip-tipped injection syringe for smaller tubes. If using the larger catheter-tipped irrigation syringe, remove the plunger from the syringe barrel and then insert the tip of the syringe into the open lumen of the feeding tube. Bend or crimp the tubing just below where it attaches to the syringe. This will prevent formula from flowing through the feeding tube before you are ready. Flush the tube by pouring 30 to 60 mL of water into the syringe. Release the bend or crimp in the tube so water can flow through the feeding tube and then re-crimp tube. Carefully begin to pour the formula into the syringe barrel until it is almost full. Then release the bend or crimp in the tubing, allowing formula to flow through the feeding tube until the syringe is almost empty (Fig. 24-8). At this time, you may stop the flow by bending the tubing again while you refill the syringe or, if you are steady enough, you may continue pouring formula into the syringe as it is instilling, until feeding is completed. Use whichever method works best for you, but *use caution to prevent air from entering the tube in between refilling the syringe.* Instilling air will increase gastric distress and should be avoided. This method should permit you to instill the feeding over a short period of time, generally 15 to 20 minutes, directly into the stomach or small intestine.

Feedings will be scheduled four to six times per day. Residuals should be checked before administering each feeding (see section on Checking Residual Gastric Volume below). Bolus feedings can be poorly tolerated, causing a number of problems such as cramping, gastric distention, diarrhea, and aspiration. For further information regarding administration of intermittent bolus enteral feedings, see Skill 24-6 (page 533).

Figure 24-8 Nurse administering intermittent bolus PEG feeding.

Continuous Infusion Feedings

Continuous feedings are best administered via an infusion pump at a constant rate over an 8- to 24-hour period. The continuous infusion method promotes better tolerance of feedings and nutrient absorption. The use of the pump provides greater control of the rate and amount of feeding delivered. This method is used with critically ill patients due to the decrease in hypermetabolic response to stress, risk for aspiration, and incidence of diarrhea. Continuous feedings should be interrupted every 4 hours to check placement and residual volume, to administer water for hydration if ordered, and to flush the tube to prevent clogging. These patients must have the head of the bed raised at least 30 degrees continually to reduce the risk of aspiration.

Tube feedings are typically initiated at full strength but at a slower rate to allow the intestinal tract time to adapt. You will monitor the patients for symptoms indicating poor tolerance, such as nausea, diarrhea, abdominal cramping, vomiting, or high gastric residuals. Once the patient exhibits tolerance of the feeding, the hourly rate can be increased every 8 to 12 hours until the desired rate of infusion is achieved. Feeding by the enteral route has been shown to improve nutritional status, strengthen immune response and reduce sepsis, minimize the hypermetabolic response to trauma, and maintain the function of the intestinal tract. Skill 24-7 (page 534) provides information on how to use a feeding pump.

Checking Placement of a Feeding Tube

You read earlier in the chapter that you must assess placement of any type of NG or NI tube prior to instillation of medication, irrigant, or feedings. It is so important that we want to emphasize it once more. *Safety: If the placement of a tube is not confirmed prior to administering a feeding or medication, there is a risk of instilling the formula or medication directly into the lungs via an NG tube or into the sterile peritoneal cavity via a PEG or J-tube.* Some patients have developed pneumonia, and other patients have actually died, from failure to confirm tube placement prior to instillations.

Checking Residual Gastric Volume

Before you can safely administer a tube feeding, not only must you check tube placement but you must also assess the *residual gastric volume,* or the amount of formula that still remains in the stomach from the previous feeding. If the previous feeding has not been absorbed and remains within the stomach and you proceed to instill another formula feeding, the additional formula can fill the stomach, which increases the risk of reflux via the cardiac sphincter into the esophagus. The esophagus lies in the immediate vicinity of the opening to the larynx at the superior end of the trachea, allowing refluxed formula to be aspirated into the lungs. Aspiration of fluids can initiate laryngeal spasms and/or result in pneumonia. *Safety: It is vital that you check the residual volume as well as tube placement before instilling each tube feeding.*

The process of checking residual volume is not complicated. It can be performed after the tube placement check, but it makes more sense to perform it at the same time. While you are aspirating for stomach contents to verify placement, simply aspirate contents until the stomach is empty. If residual amount is greater than the syringe can hold, measure the aspirate volume using a graduated container. Do not discard the residual aspirate, as it is rich in electrolytes and should be re-instilled into the stomach to prevent an electrolyte imbalance, unless physician's orders state otherwise. Determine whether the residual volume exceeds the physician's order for the amount at which to withhold the feeding. If the physician does not write specific orders for handling residuals, then follow the facility's policy and procedure. However, if the physician fails to provide specific instructions and the facility's policy and procedure manual does not specify a residual volume at which to withhold the feeding, then you must rely on what you learned as a student.

For intermittent feedings, check to see if the residual volume is more than half the volume of formula given at the previous feeding (maximum residual volume). If so, you should re-instill the aspirated residual unless it is *equal to or greater than* the total volume of formula previously administered. Withhold the scheduled feeding for 1 hour and then recheck the residual volume. If the residual volume is now less than half the volume an hour earlier, you may proceed to administer the feeding.

If the patient is receiving continuous tube feedings, the maximum residual volume is half of the volume instilled during the last hour. If the residual exceeds half the volume, discontinue the feeding or slow it to half the normal rate for 1 hour, then recheck the residual. If the residual is now less than half of 1 hour's volume, proceed with the scheduled feeding. If in doubt regarding whether or not to re-instill the aspirate, notify the physician for orders.

Nursing Care of the PEG or J-Tube Insertion Site

Inspect the insertion site each day, noting any redness, tenderness, irritation, or drainage that might indicate infection. New PEG or J-tube sites should be cleaned daily with gauze and sterile saline. Using a circular motion, cleanse from the inner aspects of the site to the outer aspects. Ensure that the site is thoroughly dry and then cover it with a split-gauze dressing, also known as a *drain gauze,* which fits around the tube. For existing mature sites, cleansing should occur daily with a clean washcloth, warm water, and soap. The inner aspects of the site should be cleaned with a cotton swab to remove any drainage or leakage. Allow the site to dry thoroughly and leave it uncovered.

Nursing Responsibilities for a Patient with a PEG or J-Tube

Your responsibilities for a PEG or J-tube include:

- Assessing tube placement by checking the tube markings to determine that the tube has not shifted or dislodged prior to each instillation
- Maintaining patency of the tube
- Performing daily assessment of skin integrity surrounding the tube
- Performing daily cleansing of the tube insertion site as appropriate
- Assessing bowel sounds daily, noting absent, hypoactive, or hyperactive sounds
- Assessing the abdomen, noting distention
- Assessing for gastric residual prior to instillation of medications or formula
- Elevating the head of the bed during feedings and for 30 to 60 minutes afterward
- Monitoring intake and output to ensure proper balance
- Monitoring weight, noting any loss
- Monitoring for diarrhea or constipation that might result from certain feeding formulas

Complications Associated With Tube Feedings

Tube feedings are an artificial means of feeding a patient, and complications can arise. Common complications such as nausea and diarrhea are related to the patient's inability to tolerate the type of formula. The problem can usually be resolved by changing to a different formula.

Clogged feeding tubes are a problem that can stem from the processes associated with the feedings. It is important to prevent clogging by flushing the tube before and after instillations. If the feeding tube does clog, obtain a physician's order to irrigate the tube to restore patency.

Patients receiving tube feedings may have impaired swallowing ability due to stroke or debilitation from chronic illness, or may be unconscious. *Aspiration* is an adverse event that places these patients at risk for additional serious illness. Aspirated material can include oropharyngeal bacteria, particulate matter, and acidified gastric contents. Aspiration of bacteria can cause aspiration pneumonia. Aspirated particulates can cause severe laryngospasm and bronchial constriction, wheezing, chest pain, and even respiratory failure. Aspiration of acidified gastric contents produces a chemical burn to the alveolar walls, causing a rapid movement of protein and fluids into the alveoli. This results in a decline in lung compliance with respiratory failure ensuing. The nurse can undertake a number of preventative measures to avoid aspiration (Box 24-4).

Metabolic problems are also potential complications: hyperglycemia, dehydration, fluid overload, or electrolyte imbalances can occur in patients receiving tube feedings. The proper choice of formula, a slow rate of infusion, and ensuring adequate hydration with water can help minimize and eliminate these complications.

Another serious complication associated with tube feedings is contamination of formula. Feeding formulas should be kept refrigerated until you are ready to use them. Contaminated formula can cause severe gastrointestinal problems, including cramping, vomiting and diarrhea, or food poisoning. Your patients receiving enteral feedings are already seriously medically compromised, and contaminated formula can lead to serious adverse consequences. Patients tolerate room-temperature formula better than cold,

Box 24-4
Techniques to Prevent Aspiration

Because aspiration may be life threatening, you are responsible for implementing interventions to reduce the risk of aspiration. This is a partial list of interventions that you should implement.

- Use the smallest diameter feeding tube possible.
- Confirm tube placement with x-ray immediately after insertion and prior to initiating tube feeding.
- Confirm tube placement prior to each instillation of medication, water, or formula.
- Make certain that active bowel sounds are present prior to instillations.
- Assess for abdominal distention before feedings.
- Elevate the head of the patient's bed to 30 to 45 degrees during intermittent feedings and at least 1 hour afterward; for continual feedings, the head of the bed must remain elevated at 30 to 45 degrees.
- Check gastric residual volumes prior to intermittent feedings and every 4 hours during continuous feedings.

so you will need to plan to take formula out of the refrigerator and allow it to warm to room temperature approximately 1 hour before administering it. Box 24-5 presents key points related to managing formula.

Knowledge Connection

When is enteral nutrition the preferred feeding method? Why cannot all medications be administered via an enteral tube?

Supervision/Delegation Connection

Tube Feedings

UAPs work under the supervision of the RN or LPN/LVN. Tasks that may be delegated include administration of enteral tube feedings via an NG, NI, PEG, or J-tube. The delegation of feeding can only occur after the verification of the feeding tube placement. You are responsible for this assessment and cannot delegate performance of tube placement verification. You are also responsible to supervise the UAP in preparing and positioning the patient to receive the tube feeding. The UAP can document the intake and output and report these data. Remember that the rules governing delegation are dictated by each state's Nurse Practice Act. It is your responsibility to know the role and scope of practice for both yourself and the UAPs whom you supervise, as well as delegating nursing care appropriately.

Box 24-5

Tips for Managing Tube Feeding Formulas

Tube feeding formulas should be carefully managed to prevent spoilage, just as you protect the food you serve to patients as well as your own family. Patients receiving tube feedings may have compromised immunity, making it an even higher priority to prevent bacterial contamination of the formula. Here are some basic tips to remember.

- Wash hands thoroughly before handling formula or the feeding system.
- Rinse and wipe the top of the can before opening.
- Label all opened formula with the patient's name, date, and time when opened; follow the label instructions regarding the length of time you may use the formula once opened.
- Make sure all open cans are covered and stored in the refrigerator when not in use.
- Do not use and discard all unlabeled formula and out-of-date formula.
- Rinse the feeding bag and tubing with clean water before adding new formula.
- Flush the tube with water before and after each use.
- Hang only the amount of formula that can be administered in 6 hours; discard formula that hangs for more than 6 hours.
- Never add new formula to old.
- Change the feeding bag and syringe every 24 hours.

Parenteral Nutrition

Parenteral nutrition is administered directly into the bloodstream via a central venous catheter, bypassing the GI tract. Aseptic technique is required, and the bag of solution must be changed every 24 hours. It is used for patients with one or more problems that are complicated by malnutrition and low protein levels. These patients generally do not have functioning GI tracts or are unable to absorb adequate nutrients through enteral feedings. Box 24-6 presents a partial list of conditions in which parenteral nutrition might be appropriate.

Depending on the patient's nutritional needs and the expected length of time parenteral feedings will be required, **partial parenteral nutrition (PPN)** may be administered through a peripherally inserted central catheter (PICC) inserted into a smaller peripheral vein, or **total parenteral nutrition (TPN)** may be administered through a central venous catheter (CVC) placed in a larger central vein. The core differences between TPN and PPN are the vessel selected to receive the nutrition and the concentration of solution infused. Only the "least hypertonic" solutions may be infused into the peripheral veins, whereas it is possible to deliver higher concentrations through the larger central veins.

Partial Parenteral Nutrition

PPN is used for those patients who are able to meet some of their nutritional needs orally but require additional calories or nutrients for a limited period of time due to their illness. PPN does not meet the patient's total nutritional needs without concurrent ingestion of food via the GI tract. Patients with short bowel syndrome or malabsorption syndromes often require PPN in addition to oral intake. Solutions infused into peripheral veins must be isotonic or only mildly hypertonic to prevent phlebitis and decrease the risk of

---

Box 24-6

Conditions That Might Require Parenteral Feeding

There are many medical conditions for which parenteral feeding may be required. Here is a partial list of conditions that may be treated with parenteral feeding.

- Burns or trauma, severe
- Cancer
- Chemotherapy
- Hepatic failure
- Intestinal obstruction
- Intractable vomiting or diarrhea
- Malabsorption disorders
- Necrotizing enterocolitis
- Paralytic ileus, unrelenting
- Renal failure
- Short bowel syndrome

thrombus. Parenteral nutrition solutions include a mixture of dextrose, amino acids, lipid emulsions, electrolytes, vitamins, and trace minerals in sterile water. The Infusion Nurses Society states that peripherally administered PPN solution cannot contain a concentration that exceeds 10% dextrose and 5% amino acids. Due to these restrictions, PPN will provide a limited amount of calories, necessitating oral supplementation for the patient to have adequate daily caloric intake.

Total Parenteral Nutrition

TPN is a hypertonic, nutritionally complete solution that is delivered via a large-diameter central vein. It provides calories, essential vitamins, minerals, and electrolytes and restores nitrogen balance, promoting tissue growth and wound healing, which makes it useful in patients who are nutritionally depleted. Infusion into a large vein allows for the TPN solution to be diluted quickly. TPN is used when a patient's nutritional requirements are high and it is anticipated that the need will be long term. Patients for whom it may be used are those being treated for extensive trauma, burns, or sepsis; those undergoing aggressive cancer treatment; or those with gastrointestinal illnesses that interfere with metabolism and absorption of nutrients.

The CVC that is used for TPN can have two, three, or four separate lumens, or channels (Fig. 24-9), and must be inserted surgically into one of the larger central veins, such as the subclavian vein or internal jugular vein, and advanced until the catheter tip is positioned in the superior vena cava (Fig. 24-10). The insertion site where the catheter perforates the cutaneous layer must be continually covered with a sterile dressing, usually a transparent occlusive dressing. Often the patient who is a candidate for insertion of a central line for TPN already has a suppressed or impaired immune system. Because this extremely invasive procedure places the patient at risk for infection, you should receive specific training before providing nursing care for a central line.

Figure 24-10 Central venous catheters are typically inserted into larger central veins such as the subclavian or jugular veins and threaded into the superior vena cava.

Some facilities limit care of central lines to RNs only, while others permit LPN/LVNs once they have been trained. It is your responsibility to know the facility policies and procedures where you are employed, as well as knowing what the Nurse Practice Act in your state allows.

Patients receiving TPN may receive their medications mixed into their solution or intravenously infused into the designated lumen or a port linked to the central line. They often receive insulin to help control serum glucose, as the TPN solution has a high glucose concentration. In general, due to the potential for incompatibilities, the addition of medications to TPN solution should be limited and compatibility must be ensured. TPN is expensive, administration requires that the patient be continually monitored, and it increases the risk for the development of infection or mechanical or metabolic problems. TPN therefore is discontinued as soon as the patient's nutritional needs have been met or the patient can tolerate enteral or oral feedings.

TPN Infusion

Initially, TPN is infused slowly to give the body time to adapt to the infusion of a highly concentrated glucose solution, increasing in increments of 25 mL/hr until the desired rate of infusion is achieved. It will be administered via a continuous drip infusion on a pump to ensure a controlled rate of infusion. It is essential that infusion be slow and controlled, as a rapid infusion of TPN solution can cause severe hyper- or hypoglycemia, with the potential for further complications such as coma or death. Initially, a patient will receive 1 liter of solution infused over 24 hours, with the rate being increased by 1 L/day until the desired volume delivery is reached.

When caring for a patient receiving parenteral nutrition, it is important that you monitor laboratory values closely to assess for fluid or electrolyte imbalance until the patient is fully stable on a parenteral formula. Before you can discontinue a patient's TPN, the patient must be

Slide clamp

Proximal lumen port (18-gauge lumen)

Distal lumen port (16-gauge lumen)

Medial lumen port (18-gauge lumen)

Figure 24-9 Triple-lumen central venous catheter (CVC) injection ports.

gradually weaned from TPN to either enteral or oral feedings in order to prevent metabolic complications.

Knowledge Connection

What is the difference between TPN and PPN? Why is TPN administered via a central line catheter?

Monitoring Nutritional Status

Patients receiving parenteral nutrition should be monitored closely for nutritional status. This includes monitoring daily weights until stable and certain laboratory results. Electrolyte levels should be monitored daily for 1 week before decreasing to twice a week. Prealbumin, albumin, and total protein should be monitored, but do not have to be monitored as frequently as the electrolytes. The glucose level should be monitored at least twice daily, usually four times, in order to determine how often the patient requires insulin, and how much, to maintain a stable blood glucose level.

Prealbumin is produced primarily by cells in the liver but is also produced by gastrointestinal mucosa and the pancreas. It is quite sensitive to changes in nutritional status, has a relatively short half-life, and is rapidly responsive to protein depletion. These characteristics make prealbumin a good indicator of acute changes, while albumin remains the standard for monitoring chronic malnutrition. Normal prealbumin levels are 15 to 35 mg/dL. Finger stick blood sugars should be assessed every hour during the initial TPN infusion and then every 4 to 6 hours thereafter to provide a reference for insulin administration.

People and Places Connection

Home Health and Nutritional Support

Patients receiving enteral or parenteral therapy may be on these feedings for long periods of time. Many patients will not require lengthy hospital stays and will be discharged home on feedings. The home health nurse's role in management of the patient requiring nutritional support is one of patient/family advocate, coordinator, and educator. A key factor in the success of enteral or parenteral nutrition will be family or caregiver involvement. This should begin early in the process, ideally as soon as parenteral nutrition is implemented in the hospital setting. Caregivers should be involved in discussions regarding site selection, nutrient delivery method, and formula selection, with consideration given to their ability to manage the care and the affordability of the feeding formula. The nurse will educate the patient and caregiver regarding care of the feeding tube, tube placement site, flushing the tube, administering feedings, safety issues, and managing complications that may arise, such as a clogged tube. Safety in the administration of enteral and parenteral feedings is important; caregivers must be taught how to verify the tube placement, how to minimize risk for aspiration, and how to manage air in the PPN or TPN line. The nurse will also teach the caregiver how to safely store formula and minimize the risk of contamination. Signs and symptoms of problems for which the patient should be monitored must be taught and made available in printed format for later referral.

The home health nurse will follow the patient to assist with management of feedings as the patient transitions to home; however, the nurse will gradually assume a more supportive role as he or she teaches the caregiver to assume responsibility for the feedings and care and management of the tube. Once the caregiver has assumed full responsibility, the nurse will remain involved and continue to follow the patient, assessing for adequate nutrition as evidenced by maintenance of weight and normal laboratory values, including glucose and albumin levels. The nurse will also perform physical assessments regularly, monitoring skin integrity by looking for areas of pressure ulceration or risk for breakdown, checking for signs of muscle wasting, monitoring the lungs to look for signs indicating aspiration of particulates and evolving pneumonia, and monitoring for signs of difficulty tolerating tube feedings, such as increased abdominal discomfort, bloating, or diarrhea. The nurse will serve as the primary communicator with the physician and assist to coordinate care as the patient's condition changes.

Nursing Care Plan for a Patient Post-CVA With a PEG Tube

You have been assigned to provide care for Mr. Ayala, who was transferred from a distant hospital to your facility because he lives nearby. He was admitted a few hours ago and is 5 days post–cerebrovascular accident (CVA), more commonly called a "stroke." You know that he also has insulin-dependent diabetes mellitus and being fed through a PEG tube. What do you need to know before you may begin to plan his nursing care? What questions might you want to ask yourself as you collect data? What are the areas in which the patient might have problems or be at high risk for developing problems? For Mr. Ayala, you would probably seek to answer the following questions:

- What is the status of his neurological and cardiovascular systems?
- How old is he?
- What residual deficits from the stroke does he have?

Nursing Care Plan for a Patient Post-CVA With a PEG Tube (continued)

- How is he coping with those deficits?
- Does he have impaired mobility?
- Is he at risk for injury?
- Is he at risk for aspiration?
- Is his diabetes stable or are his glucose levels elevated?
- Is he continent of bowel and bladder?
- Is he able to communicate?
- Does he have a strong system of support locally?

Assessment

Now that you have an idea of what data you need to collect, your initial step will be to review the current medical record. Specifically, you need to review the patient's medical history, noting medical conditions that alter the patient's nutritional needs and influence the type of feeding formula selected. You will also want to know why the patient is receiving enteral nutrition and approximately how long it is anticipated to continue. While reviewing the patient's chart, observe for data that indicate possible complications or may influence such things as the timing of administration or formula selection, such as:

- Height and weight
- Aspiration risk
- Diarrhea or constipation
- Fluid or electrolyte imbalance
- Hyperglycemia
- Nausea and vomiting
- Skin breakdown

Your next step will be to review the patient's laboratory result for the following tests if they have been ordered:

- Hemoglobin and hematocrit levels
- Blood glucose levels
- Protein level
- Fluid and electrolyte status

Review of the patient's graphic sheet shows his current vital signs tend to be stable: blood pressure – 136/82; temperature – 99°F; pulse – 70; respirations – 16. You also note his intake on the previous day was 2,000 mL of IV dextrose 5% in water (D5W) with a urine output of 1,400 mL. This morning his fasting glucose was 125 mg/dL, his serum albumin was 34 g/L, and his electrolyte panel indicated normal results. Part of his blood count, the hematocrit (Hct) and hemoglobin (Hgb), were within normal range, indicating no anemia, but there was not an order to check his protein level.

The chart shows that a continuous enteral feeding was initiated this morning, infusing at 20 mL/hr via feeding pump. You noted in the chart that he is unable to speak, known as *dysphasia,* but is able to answer questions by blinking: once for "yes" and twice for "no."

Next you will need to review the patient's medication record, checking listed medications for incompatibility with feeding formulas; those that may in some way affect the GI tract functions, such as increasing or decreasing peristalsis; or those that cause *diuresis,* the increase in removal of water by increasing urine output.

You enter Mr. Ayala's room to perform your morning assessment. It is early, but you note that, even though he is still in bed, he is awake and alert and makes eye contact as you introduce yourself. He also attempts to smile; however, only the left side of his face moves. He reaches out with his right hand to shake your hand. You are glad to learn that his hemiparesis is on his nondominant side. He moves about easily in bed without assistance and writes on a tablet that he still needs help to take a pan bath and dress, but that he is slowly learning. He can use the urinal but still requires assistance to get up to the bedside commode. You find that he has difficulty swallowing since the stroke, termed *dysphagia,* and a PEG tube was surgically placed yesterday. You proceed with your assessment, taking care to observe his response to questions. He shakes his head when you inquire if he is experiencing any pain or discomfort, and writes that he would like to be bathed and get up in a chair as soon as someone can help him. You explain that part of your nursing care will be to check his PEG tube and site to ensure that healing has begun, assess the security of the PEG tube, and check for signs of infection. You check the site and note an approximately ¼-inch ring of mild erythema but no signs of purulent drainage or leakage of gastric contents. The tube is secured to the patient's abdomen with tape and the feeding system is connected, infusing formula at 20 mL/hr. He shakes his head to indicate that he has had no nausea, vomiting, diarrhea, or other GI complaints since the feeding was started and that he has been passing rectal flatus. You auscultate active bowel sounds in all four quadrants.

You previously noted physician orders to advance the feeding to 30 mL/hr by 3 p.m. You end the assessment with an evaluation of his skin,

(care plan continues on page 522)

Nursing Care Plan for a Patient Post-CVA With a PEG Tube (continued)

noting a slight reddening of intact skin over the coccyx. The rest of the initial shift assessment findings were within normal limits.

Prior to leaving the room, you say good-bye to Mr. Ayala, explaining that you will send a nursing assistant to give him a bath and assist him to the chair. You also lower the bed to its lowest position, raise the head of the bed to 30 degrees, confirm that its wheels are locked and side rails are up, and position his call light and tissues where he can easily reach them.

What have you learned from your assessment and data collection? From your review of the patient and chart, you have determined that he is a 56-year-old Hispanic male, alert and oriented to all four spheres, and is experiencing no pain or discomfort. He makes good eye contact and smiles during your assessment and interaction with him. He has right-sided hemiparesis, putting him at high risk for falls and limb injury. He is unable to speak but can write messages with his right hand, is able to respond to questions by eye-blinking, and can use the call bell to summon assistance; however, he could not call out for help if his call light was out of reach. He does not exhibit any evidence of poor self-esteem, depression, or powerlessness as you might expect to see in some post-stroke patients with residual deficits. According to his laboratory results, he has no fluid or electrolyte imbalance and no anemia. His glucose level is only slightly elevated. You do not know about his protein level because it was not ordered. His vital signs indicate stable cardiovascular and respiratory status without fever. His dysphagia required insertion of a PEG tube yesterday. The new PEG insertion site, located on the left upper quadrant of his abdomen, exhibits no signs of infection or bleeding. His PEG tube is intact and patent, with a continuous infusion of formula at 20 mL/hr that needs to be increased to 30 mL/hr over the next 6 hours. He is continent of both bowel and bladder. He has a 2-cm reddened area on the coccyx that blanches and returns to normal color after repositioning. The data tell you that your patient is status post-CVA with stable cardiovascular status, vital signs, and glucose level. Thus far, he is tolerating his enteral feedings, he has had adequate I/O, and his fluid and electrolyte panels indicate adequate hydration and nutritional status.

It is now time to use the data to identify problems the patient is experiencing. You will establish the nursing diagnoses and prioritize them. It is important to remember that a nursing diagnosis is the same thing as a patient problem; it simply represents a specific need the patient has at this time. As you learn the nursing process, remember that it is the same problem-solving process that you use every day to make decisions in your own life.

Nursing Diagnoses

After analyzing the data, you determine that Mr. Ayala has a few high-risk and problem areas. Your first priority is his safety, as he has right-sided hemiparesis and has difficulty swallowing. The appropriate nursing diagnoses for these problems include:

• Impaired swallowing
• Impaired physical mobility

The patient has two actual problems that place him at risk to develop additional problems. When there is evidence that a problem could develop, that is known as a *potential* problem. For example, the impaired swallowing places the patient in danger of aspirating, resulting in the additional nursing diagnosis "Risk for aspiration." Because the patient actually suffers impaired physical mobility, this problem places him at risk for developing additional problems, resulting in the following nursing diagnoses:

• Risk for falls
• Risk for constipation
• Risk for impaired skin integrity

Assessment of the coccyx found the skin reddened, further data reinforcing his risk for impaired skin integrity in the form of a pressure ulcer. This potential problem requires that action be taken to prevent its occurrence. He already has one site of impaired skin integrity: the new incision made to insert his PEG tube. The skin is the first line of defense against invading microorganisms and infection. By incising through this first line of defense, there is now potential for bacteria to enter the body and cause an infection. The following nursing diagnosis also applies to this patient: "Impaired skin integrity."

Because the 56-year-old patient, sole provider for his family, is unable to speak and suffers the above deficits, you know that he has impaired verbal communication and also has the nursing diagnosis "Risk for situational low self-esteem."

Now it is time to develop a plan of care for a few of these problems.

Nursing Care Plan for a Patient Post-CVA With a PEG Tube (continued)

Planning

Your nursing care plan will include your role and that of the UAPs, CNAs, and other health care providers working with you. Your plan of care will be tailored to meet Mr. Ayala's needs; therefore, the interventions will be specific to him. Your first priority will be his safety, then his nutrition, and next his activities of daily living (ADLs). You must remain aware of his psychosocial needs as he is experiencing role change, isolation, and impaired verbal communication. You need to provide care that will help him adapt to his body changes while preventing problems that are directly related to mobility impairments.

Because the top priority is impaired swallowing, your plan must ensure that the patient is identified as high risk for aspiration. Interventions to prevent aspiration might include the following:

- Note in the care plan and on the Kardex that the patient is NPO and may have only ice chips.
- Post an NPO sign above the patient's bed.
- Reinforce this with the patient and family members.
- Keep the head of the bed elevated a minimum of 30 degrees at all times.
- Ensure that suction equipment at the bedside is ready for use at all times.
- Keep the call light within reach at all times.
- Assist the patient with mouth care every 2 hours to prevent dryness. Apply moisturizer to the lips PRN.
- Provide ice chips PRN.
- Infuse the designated formula via PEG tube at a controlled rate of 30 mL/hr. If tolerated for 24 hours without GI distress, increase the rate to 50 mL/hr. If tolerated for 24 hours, increase the rate to 75 mL/hr.
- Check tube placement and residual volume every 4 hours. If volume is greater than half the previous hour's infused volume, re-instill the aspirate, stop the infusion for 1 hour, and restart at the previous rate.
- Monitor I/O closely for 2 weeks, reporting variances.
- Record daily weights each a.m. at 0800.

The patient has impaired mobility, and because of this he is at risk for falls and at risk for constipation. Interventions include the following:

- Assist the patient up into a chair at least three times per day and to a bedside commode as needed.

- Cue the patient to reposition every 2 hours, and teach him the importance of activity.
- Encourage and assist the patient as needed to perform active/passive range of motion (ROM) to all extremities twice a day.
- Assess pressure points for erythema and apply lotion to his back and all pressure points three times per day.
- Keep a hand roll positioned in the left hand.
- Keep the bed in its lowest position with the wheels locked.
- Raise both bed rails continually.
- Assess bowel sounds with each tube placement check, noting hyper- or hypoactivity.
- Monitor and document bowel movements (BMs) for frequency, consistency, color, and amount.
- Administer a laxative of choice if there is no BM after 2 days.

The patient has impaired skin integrity related to the newly inserted PEG tube and is at risk for infection at the site. Interventions include the following:

- Assess the PEG insertion site each shift, noting erythema, edema, increased warmth, or drainage.
- Clean the insertion site with soap and water and pat it dry each day during a.m. and p.m. care.
- Keep the PEG tube securely taped to the abdomen at least until the site is well healed.
- Monitor for fever once each shift.

The patient is bound to eventually exhibit some evidence of low self-esteem or depression, so make certain that he knows what resources are available to him. Interventions include the following:

- Take 10 minutes a couple of times a day to go in and visit with him. Sit down and show him that you are willing to listen. You may not do anything but sit with him for this time, but it will evidence your availability.
- Offer the services of the social worker and a counselor should he feel he might benefit from their help.
- Explain to and educate the patient and family regarding different ways to increase his independence.
- Make certain the physician orders occupational therapy (OT), physical therapy (PT), and speech therapy (ST) evaluation and treatment.

(care plan continues on page 524)

Nursing Care Plan for a Patient Post-CVA With a PEG Tube (continued)

Implementation

Now that you have developed a plan, you need to put it into action. Explain to the patient why he is NPO and discuss his plan of care with him. Retrieve the NPO sign and send it with an unlicensed staff member to hang above his bed (Table 24-4). Direct the UAP or CNA to bathe him and provide a.m. care, perform ROM, assess pressure points and apply lotion, and ensure repositioning every 2 hours. After the bath, call the lift team to assist the patient from bed to chair, requesting to be notified once he is up so that you can assess his comfort and pain, observe how well he sits and maintains balance in the chair, and take appropriate action. You will take responsibility for checking tube placement and residual volume every 4 hours. Once you are sure he is tolerating the formula, you will gradually increase the rate by 5 mL/hr; 4 hours later you will increase it again by 5 mL/hr, reaching today's desired rate by 3 p.m. Remind the physician to order the OC, PT, and ST.

Evaluation

Now that you have enacted the patient's care plan, you will want to evaluate its effectiveness and your patient's progress toward health. You have already evaluated his laboratory results and know that his fluid and electrolytes are balanced at this time, but this will be an ongoing assessment to be evaluated each time you care for him. You will continue to monitor his fluid intake and output, observing for indications of fluid retention. You will compare the intake to the output and determine if they are both adequate and that the output is within 300 to 500 mL of his intake. You will evaluate his blood glucose levels to determine whether or not you need to administer the sliding-scale insulin. You will also monitor for trends in the glucose level, reporting if it consistently climbs or shows a pattern of dropping a little lower each day. You know that his skin integrity is good at this time and that there are no signs or symptoms of infection at the insertion site, but will continue to monitor for changes each day.

Mr. Ayala tolerated being up in the chair for 2 hours, was able to maintain his balance without dropping his blood pressure, and experienced no discomfort (see Table 24-4). He remembered to use his dominant hand to lift his left arm and leg to prevent them from dragging or banging against the bed and chair. He was able to summon staff when he felt fatigued and was ready to go back to bed. You were able to successfully increase the rate of his tube feeding, and he tolerated the formula well. He asked you several questions regarding rehabilitation and how it might help him to regain some functions. It appears that this plan of care provided for the patient's safety, comfort, and progress toward improved health status thus far. You will wait and see how tomorrow goes.

Table 24-4 Care Plan for a Patient Post-CVA With a PEG Tube

Nursing Diagnosis: Impaired swallowing
Expected Outcomes: Will maintain patent airway. No aspiration.

Interventions	Evaluations
Note in the care plan and on the Kardex that patient is NPO with only occasional ice chips. Post NPO sign on the door and above the bed.	8/2/12: Eats ice chips sparingly. Remains NPO. 8/4/12: No change.
Keep the head of the bed elevated a minimum of 30 degrees at all times.	8/1/12: HOB maintained at 30 degrees. No signs of aspiration. 8/5/12: No aspiration.
Reinforce NPO status, elevation of bed, and risk of providing oral fluids with the patient and family members.	8/1/12: Verbally instructed patient, wife, grown daughter regarding importance of NPO status and risk of aspiration. Family verbally acknowledged understanding. Patient nodded agreement. 8/2/12: Following instructions.

Nursing Care Plan for a Patient Post-CVA With a PEG Tube (continued)

Table 24-4 Care Plan for a Patient Post-CVA With a PEG Tube (continued)

Nursing Diagnosis: Impaired swallowing
Expected Outcomes: Will maintain patent airway. No aspiration.

Interventions	Evaluations
Assist the patient with mouth care to prevent dryness four times per day. Apply lip moisturizer to lips prn.	8/2/12: Mucous membranes pink, moist, and intact. Able to apply lip balm unassisted. 8/5/12: Mucous membranes remain pink, intact, and moist.
Keep suction equipment at the bedside ready for use at all times. *Discontinued 8/14*	8/1/12: Suction not needed. 8/2/12: No choking or aspiration. 8/3/12: Working to relearn swallowing technique with therapists. 8/6/12: Makes effort to swallow melted ice chips without problems. No suction needed. 8/14/12: Suction removed from room.
Keep the call light within reach at all times.	8/1/12: Uses call light when assistance is needed. 8/5/12: Calls staff as needed.
Infuse Jevity per PEG tube with pump at 30 mL/hr. If tolerated for 24 hours without GI distress, increase to 50 mL/hr. If tolerated for 24 hours, increase to 75 mL/hr.	8/1/12: Tolerated 30 mL/hr without nausea or distention; bowel sounds active in all quads except RLQ, which was hyperactive. 8/2/12: Tolerated 50 mL/hr. No distention, nausea, or diarrhea. 8/3/12: Rate increased to 75 mL/hr. 8/4/12: Active bowel sounds throughout; no reports of gastric distress.
Check PEG tube placement and residual volume every 4 hours. If volume is greater than half the previous hour's infused volume, re-instill aspirate, stop infusion for 1 hour, and then restart at previous rate.	8/1/12: Placement confirmed; residuals 30 mL and less. 8/2/12: Placement confirmed; residuals 40 mL, 50 mL, 35 mL. 8/4/12: Residuals less than 50 mL consistently. 8/6/12: Residuals and placement checks unchanged.
Monitor I&O closely for 2 weeks; report variances.	8/1/12: In – 880 mL; Out – 630 mL. 8/3/12: In – 1,925 mL; Out – 1,475 mL. 8/9/12: I&O balanced. 8/14/12: I&O remains balanced.
Record daily weights at 0800 a.m.; report losses. *Discontinued 8/14/12*	8/1/12: Admission: 179 lbs. 8/2/12: 177 lbs. 8/4/12: 177 lbs. 8/8/12: 177.5 lbs. 8/14/12: 179 lbs.; stable; daily weights discontinued.

(table continues on page 526)

Nursing Care Plan for a Patient Post-CVA With a PEG Tube (continued)

Table 24-4   Care Plan for a Patient Post-CVA With a PEG Tube (continued)

Nursing Diagnosis: Impaired physical mobility
Expected Outcomes: During hospitalization: (1) Skin integrity will remain intact. (2) No development of contractures. (3) Will remain injury-free. (4) No development of constipation. Maintain bowel elimination with a BM at least every 3 days.

Interventions	Evaluations
Assist the patient to get up into a chair a minimum of three times per day and to a bedside commode as needed.	8/1/12: Requires 2 assists to stand and pivot to chair; reported fatigue afterward. 8/4/12: Assists with right arm; can bear weight on unaffected leg with 2 assists to balance. 8/7/12: Still unable to move left leg voluntarily; no longer reports fatigue after up. 8/14/12: Able to transfer to bedside commode with retractable arms, unassisted, using short slide board.
Cue the patient to reposition every 2 hours; teach him the importance of activity. *Discontinued 8/13*	8/1/12: Cued every 2 hr. Requires 2 assists to turn to either side. 8/3/12: Continues to require 2 assists to turn to right side, but can turn to left side unassisted; needs help to position support pillows. 8/5/12: Continues to help reposition self and do a little more each day. 8/13/12: Moves about unassisted in bed; no longer requires staff to cue or assist.
Encourage and assist the patient as needed to perform active/passive ROM to all extremities twice a day.	8/1/12: Active ROM exercises performed; 5 sets of each movement. 8/3/12: Active-passive ROM today; able to move unaffected joints and use right hand to move left arm and hand; states he feels so much better after exercises. 8/5/12: Reported sleeping better at night; believes it is due to ROM; working hard to move left leg; some left shoulder lift performed independently. 8/10/12: Increasing strength; slight movement of left arm.
Assess pressure points for erythema and apply lotion to back and all pressure points three times per day. Day 9: Modified to twice per day, during bath and p.m. care.	8/1/12: Skin over pressure points intact; mild redness over coccyx, 2-inch circle, resolves 15 min after repositioning. 8/4/12: No redness noted on pressure points except pale pink area on right elbow where patient leans on elbow to sit up; gel-filled elbow pads applied. 8/6/12: No further redness of elbows or other pressure points. 8/8/12: Able to sit up without leaning on elbow; removed elbow pads; skin intact; no redness.
Keep a hand roll positioned in the left hand.	8/1/12: States the hand roll keeps the left hand from sweating so badly. 8/3/12: Left fingers still flaccid; hand roll replaced daily. 8/7/12: No signs of contractures in left hand. 8/8/12: Exercises his left hand 8 to 10 times/day, even while watching TV and visiting; only places hand roll during sleep hours.
Keep the bed in its lowest position with the wheels locked.	8/1/12: Bed kept in low position and brakes locked; does not attempt to get up unassisted. 8/5/12: Calls for assistance when he needs to get up.

Nursing Care Plan for a Patient Post-CVA With a PEG Tube (continued)

Table 24-4   Care Plan for a Patient Post-CVA With a PEG Tube (continued)

Nursing Diagnosis: Impaired physical mobility
Expected Outcomes: During hospitalization: (1) Skin integrity will remain intact. (2) No development of contractures. (3) Will remain injury-free. (4) No development of constipation. Maintain bowel elimination with a BM at least every 3 days.

Interventions	Evaluations
Raise both bed rails continually.	8/1/12: 2 rails up; doesn't try to get out of bed alone. 8/4/12: Pulls on bed rail with right hand to help turn him.
Assess bowel sounds with each tube placement check, noting hyper- or hypoactivity.	8/1/12: Active bowel sounds in RLQ, RUQ, LUQ and hyperactive in LLQ. 8/5/12: Active times 4 quadrants. 8/8/12: Hypoactive.
Monitor and document bowel movements for frequency, consistency, color, and amount.	8/1/12: Chart shows last BM 2 days prior. 8/2/12: Continent of small, brown, soft BM. 8/3/12: None. 8/4/12: Large, soft dark brown BM. 8/5/12: 3 semi-soft BMs. 8/7/12: None in 2 days. 8/8/12: Moderate amount soft brown BM. 8/10/12: None for 2 days; milk of magnesia 30 mL given.
Administer a laxative of choice, if there is no BM after 2 days.	8/5/12: Having BMs without difficulty. 8/10/12: Laxative requested and given.

Skill 24-1 Assisting a Patient with Feeding

Assessment Steps

1. Review the patient's medical record *to determine diet orders.* Review the chart for problems that might impair the patient's ability to self-feed.
2. Assess the patient for risk of aspiration. *Patients at high risk are those with dysphagia, decreased gag or cough reflex, or decreased level of consciousness, and those with difficulty managing saliva. If the patient is at high risk, ensure that suction is available at the bedside.*
3. Assess the patient's intake and output, weights, and laboratory values. *This helps to evaluate nutritional status.*

Planning Steps

1. Gather needed equipment and supplies: a protective barrier to protect the patient's gown, assistive devices. *Being prepared saves you time and effort and increases efficiency.*
2. Provide the patient an opportunity to use the bathroom. *This helps to reduce mealtime interruptions.*
3. Clean the over-the-bed table of clutter and unpleasantries such as a urinal, toilet tissue, or emesis basin containing sputum. *A clean and neat table is more conducive to eating.*

Implementation Steps

1. Follow the Initial Implementation Steps located on the inside front cover.
2. Assist the patient to a chair or elevate the head of bed to the high Fowler's position. *This positions the patient for eating and decreases risk of aspiration.*
3. Provide a warm, wet washcloth to wash the face and hands *to reduce microorganisms.*
4. Place a protective barrier beneath the patient's chin so that it covers the patient's gown, *to prevent the gown from soiling.*
5. Provide as much assistance as the patient needs, while encouraging optimal independent feeding. *It is important to encourage optimal independence for the patient's self-esteem, but still ensure that adequate assistance is provided to optimize nutritional intake.*
6. Position the over-the-bed table directly in front of the patient so food is in front of the patient, as it is at one's own dining room table. *This helps to make it more like mealtimes at home and is more conducive to eating. Avoid placing the table along the side of the bed, which puts the "dining table" at the patient's side rather than in front of the patient. This requires you to turn to pick up each bite of food and*

(skill continues on page 528)

Skill 24-1 (continued)

then carry each spoonful the distance from the side of the bed across the patient to his or her mouth.

7. If the patient is able to feed himself or herself, assist with tray setup as needed: open containers, cut up meat, butter bread, and open condiments and apply them if the patient desires. If the patient is unable to feed himself or herself, proceed with feeding the patient. *It is important to do everything possible to encourage nutritional intake.*

8. If possible, sit down while feeding the patient. *This shows the patient that you are not in a hurry, encouraging the patient to eat more.*

If the patient is blind:

a. First identify whether the sight impairment is long-standing or a new loss. If the patient is not used to being blind, you will probably need to feed the patient or assist the patient in feeding himself or herself. If the patient has been blind for a long time, you will need to ask the patient if you can help feed him or her.

b. Be certain to approach the subject judiciously and compassionately, as the patient may be very sensitive about the inability to do certain things, and the loss of independence.

If a blind patient is able to self-feed:

a. Open containers and cellophane-wrapped flatware or condiments, cut meat, butter bread, and season food if the patient desires.

b. Verbally inform the patient where each food item is located on the plate using the numbers on the face of a clock and the relationship of plates, bowls, glasses, and flatware for identifiers. For example: "Your meatloaf is at 12:00, mashed potatoes are at 3:00, green beans are at 6:00, a glass of iced tea is on the right above your fork and spoon, a bowl of peaches is on the left above your knife, and apple cobbler is to the far left of the bowl of peaches. Here is your napkin."

c. It is helpful to gently guide the patient's hands to feel the sides of the dinner plate as you begin to tell where the food contained on the plate is located. Also guide the patient's hand to feel the glass, flatware, and extra bowls. *These things will encourage more intake.*

9. Allow the patient to determine the order in which he or she will eat foods *to allow the patient more control.*

10. Encourage the patient to handle easy-to-eat foods such as bread or small pieces of fruit *to promote independence.*

11. Keep food bits small and allow the patient adequate time to chew and swallow food *to reduce the risk of choking.*

12. Make mealtime a pleasant social occasion, engaging in conversation while feeding and encourage the patient to talk about his or her life, children, or favorite hobbies. Smile during the meal. *This makes mealtime more conducive to eating.*

13. Follow the Ending Implementation Steps located on the inside back cover.

Evaluation Steps

1. Observe the level of independence and amount of assistance required *to determine if additional assistance is needed.*

2. Observe for signs of difficulty swallowing, such as gagging, choking, or significant coughing, during oral intake *to prevent aspiration.*

3. Measure the amount of oral fluid intake each meal. Estimate the percentage of the solid foods eaten. Measure liquids in milliliters (mL). Document this in the appropriate location in the chart.

4. Observe the patient's ability to tolerate his or her diet, monitoring for signs such as abdominal distention and complaints of cramping, nausea or vomiting, or indigestion, and document in the chart. *This helps to determine if the diet should be changed or not.*

Sample Documentation

5/25/12   1230   Required total assistance with soft diet. Consumed 50% of potatoes, green beans, & chicken without swallowing problems. No complaints of GI distress. ————————
———————————— Nurse's signature and credentials

Skill 24-2 Recording Intake and Output

Assessment Steps

1. Review the patient's medical record for previous intake and output to see if there are imbalances. *This helps you to know if you need to encourage fluids or not.*

2. Introduce yourself to the patient and explain the procedure. Review the rationale for the monitoring of intake and output so that the patient and family understand the importance of measuring. *This results in better compliance.*

Planning Steps

1. Gather needed equipment and supplies: paper and pen, specimen pan, urinal, graduated receptacle, drinking glass with increments marked in milliliters. *Being prepared saves you time and effort and increases efficiency.*

2. Instruct the unlicensed personnel who will be assisting in the patient's care. *It is your responsibility to communicate the needs of the patient to the unlicensed personnel.*

Skill 24-2 (continued)

3. Place paper and pen at the bedside for recording the intake and output *to increase compliance.*

Implementation Steps

1. Follow the Initial Implementation Steps located on the inside front cover.

2. Measure, do not estimate, the volume of liquid consumed, except when the exact volume of an empty container is known, such as a milk carton that holds 240 mL. If only part of it was consumed, measure what is left and record the difference *to increase accuracy.*

3. Document on the intake and output sheet in the room; at the end of the shift, transcribe the total to the flow sheet. *Documenting at the bedside increases accuracy.*

4. If intake volumes are less than desired, encourage the patient to drink more. Find out the patient's likes and dislikes and provide the preferred items, as long as they are not contraindicated by his or her diet order. If necessary, offer a few ounces every hour to get adequate fluid in the patient. *Don't wait until the end of the shift to become concerned about inadequate intake. Be proactive. This helps to more accurately determine fluid balance.*

5. Measure the amount of urine and other sources of output, such as the amount emptied from drainage devices, stomach aspirate, emesis, or diarrhea excreted by the patient, and document on the flow sheet in the chart. *This helps to more accurately determine fluid balance.*

6. Document all output in the room immediately after measurement. Avoid trying to remember totals until the end of the shift. At the end of the shift, transcribe the totals to the flow sheet in the chart *to increase accuracy.*

7. Follow the Ending Implementation Steps located on the inside back cover.

Evaluation Steps

1. Compare the intake and output amounts, noting any significant imbalance. *The output total should be within 300 to 500 mL of the intake, allowing the difference for the insensible losses.*

Sample Documentation

At the bedside:

Date _Jan 1_	Shift _3/11_	
	Output	
Intake	**Urine**	**Emesis**
240 mL	255 ml	130 mL
70 mL	155 mL	
240 mL	530 mL	
85 mL	940 mL	
90 mL		
725 mL		

Then, the end-of-shift totals are transcribed to the intake and output sheet in the chart as follows:

Date		INTAKE				OUTPUT				
	Shift	**Oral**	**IV**	**Irrig**	**Total Shift intake**	**Urine**	**Emesis**	**NG**	**Drains**	**Total Shift Output**
10/1	7/3	1,050 mL	240 mL		1,290 mL	1,115 mL	275 mL			1,390 mL
	3/11	725 mL	240 mL		965 mL	940 mL	130 mL			1,070 mL
	11/7									
	24-hour Total									

Skill 24-3 Inserting a Nasogastric Tube

Assessment Steps

1. Review the medical record for medical history, current diagnoses and problems, and conditions that might limit the patient's ability to cooperate during the procedure or that contraindicate insertion of an NG tube.

Planning Steps

1. Gather needed equipment and supplies: correct type and size of NG tube, catheter-tipped irrigation syringe or a 50-mL syringe with a smaller slip-tip if required to fit the feeding tube, container of water, litmus paper to measure pH, emesis basin, wash cloth, towel or waterproof pad, examination gloves, lubricating jelly, tape or device to secure tubing to nose, glass of ice water and straw, stethoscope, adapter (to connect NG tube to suction connector tube or feeding tubing or plug for end of NG tube), flashlight, tongue blade, suction setup with a long connector tube or feeding setup, indelible marker, tape measure. *Being prepared saves time and effort and increases efficiency.*

2. Explain the procedure to the patient, discussing it fully and instructing the patient in ways in which he or she can assist to make the procedure go smoothly. *This reduces anxiety and increases patient compliance during the procedure.*

3. **If the NG tube is to be connected to suction:** Set up the suction apparatus, including a canister and connector tube that connects to the NG tube adaptor.

4. Measure the length of the NG tube by measuring from the tip of the patient's nose to the earlobe and then to the xiphoid process. Mark this length on the tube with a small piece of tape, but do not wrap the tape so tightly around the tube that it is difficult to remove once the tube has been inserted. *This determines the approximate length to insert the NG tube.*

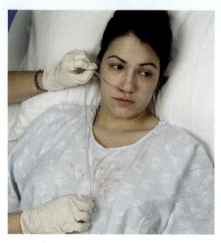

5. Determine the patency of the patient's nares before selecting an acceptable naris.

Implementation Steps

1. Follow the Initial Implementation Steps located on the inside front cover.

2. Wearing clean examination gloves *to protect yourself from potential contact with body fluids,* pull the plunger back on the irrigation syringe *to make room for gastric contents to drain into the syringe.* Snugly insert the tip of the irrigation syringe into the open end of the NG tube. *This will prevent soiling the bed with gastric contents as the NG tube reaches the stomach, which saves you from having to change linens.*

3. Lubricate 3 to 4 inches of the tip of the NG tube with a small amount of water-soluble lubricant. *This reduces friction and increases ease of passage of the tube. Safety: Avoid using petroleum-based lubricants, as they increase the risk of pneumonia due to inhaling petrolatum products.*

4. Repeat the instructions for the patient and ask if he or she has further questions. *This procedure frightens many patients, and repeating the instructions is sometimes helpful to alleviate anxiety.*

5. Have the patient hyperextend the neck. Insert the tube through the patient's naris, slowly advancing the tube downward into the nasopharynx. You may feel slight resistance as the tube enters the nasopharynx; gentle rotation of the tube typically overcomes this. *Safety: Never force the tube if there is more than the slightest resistance. Forcing the tube can result in serious damage to the nasal mucosa. If you meet resistance, remove the tube, relubricate the end of the tube, and attempt insertion in the opposite naris.* It is typical for the patient's eyes to water during tube insertion.

Skill 24-3 (continued)

6. When the patient begins to gag, you know that the tube is in the posterior nasopharynx; stop advancing the tube and withdraw it a very short distance (about ⅛ inch), *just enough to stop the gagging.* Encourage the patient to take a couple of deep breaths and relax. Then instruct the patient to flex his or her head forward, drink a sip of water, and swallow. *This position aids passage of the tube through the posterior pharynx and esophagus rather than the larynx.*

   a. Continue to cue the patient to "swallow... swallow... swallow...". Continue to gently guide the tube each time the patient swallows. If the patient continues to gag and cough, use a penlight and tongue blade *to make certain the tube has not curled up in the back of the patient's throat.* *Safety: If the patient exhibits symptoms of respiratory distress or cyanosis, stop the procedure and withdraw the tube immediately.*

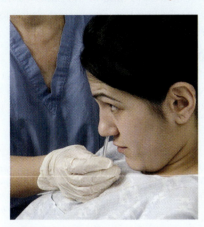

   b. Once the tube is in place, secure the end by taping it to the patient's nose. As you tape the tube, make certain to avoid positioning the tube where it is pressing against the naris *to prevent accidental dislodgment of the tube.*

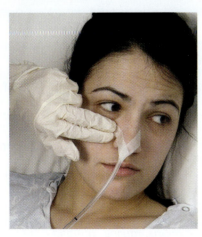

   c. Using an indelible marker, boldly mark the tube at the point of insertion and measure the length of tube extending from the body. Record this measurement *for comparison at future placement checks.*

7. Check placement of the tube by aspirating gastric contents with the irrigation syringe. Note the color and check the pH of the fluid with litmus paper. The pH should be acidic, between 1 and 4. *This ensures proper placement.*

8. Apply a tubing clamp or insert a plug. *Safety: Until placement has been verified by x-ray, nothing can be instilled into the NG tube, including a normal saline flush, water, medications, and formula.*

9. Notify radiology and transport the patient to the radiology department for an x-ray. After tube placement has been verified, return the patient to his or her room and connect the NG tube to suction or feeding as ordered.

10. Follow the Ending Implementation Steps located on the inside back cover.

11. Document the procedure, time it was performed, patient's tolerance of the procedure, length of tube extending from insertion site, method used to determine correct placement and findings, characteristics of any drainage, and patient's current respiratory status.

Evaluation Steps

1. Confirm tube placement by x-ray *to ensure proper placement.*

2. Assess the patient's level of comfort *to enable you to provide optimal comfort.*

3. Assess the characteristics of any aspirate or drainage: color, consistency, and amount.

Sample Documentation

5/31/12   1015   Explained procedure. States she has had an NG tube previously and understands the process. Inserted 18 Fr Salem sump NG tube into Rt. naris without resistance or difficulty, per physician's order. 17.5-inch NG tube extending from insertion site. Obtained 450 mL thick, dark green gastric contents within a few minutes. Checked contents with litmus paper — pH 2.5. Denies discomfort. ————————— Nurse's signature and credentials

5/31/12   1035   To x-ray per W/C accompanied by UAP. Tube placement confirmed in the stomach. Returned to room per W/C. NG tube attached to low intermittent suction per physician's order.
———————————— Nurse's signature and credentials

Skill 24-4 Irrigating a Nasogastric Tube

Assessment Steps

1. Check the patient's medical record for orders and a radiographic report verifying correct placement of the NG tube. *This helps to prevent instilling irrigant into a displaced tube.*

2. Observe the NG tube and assess for secure placement, *to prevent accidental dislodgment of the tube.*

Planning Steps

1. Gather needed equipment and supplies: catheter-tipped irrigating syringe or a 50-mL syringe with a smaller slip-tip if required to fit the feeding tube, normal saline (NS), litmus paper to measure pH, tape measure, emesis basin, towel or waterproof pad, examination gloves, lubricating jelly, tape or device to secure tubing to nose. *Being prepared saves time and effort and increases efficiency.*

Implementation Steps

1. Follow the Initial Implementation Steps located on the inside front cover.

2. Place the patient in a sitting or high Fowler's position *to help reduce reflux and aspiration.*

3. Position waterproof pad under the end of the NG tube and unclamp the end of the NG tube if clamped. Otherwise, disconnect the tube from suction or the feeding setup. *This protects linens from soiling and allows access to the tube.*

4. To verify placement, assess whether the insertion mark is still positioned at the point of entry and measure the length of tube extending from the insertion site, comparing it with the recorded length. Then use a syringe to withdraw 5 to 10 mL of gastric residuals, observe the color of the contents, and measure the pH.

Patients who have been fasting at least 4 hours have a pH of 1 to 4; those on continuous feedings will have a slightly higher pH. *This ensures that the irrigant enters the stomach.*

5. Re-instill aspirated gastric contents *to prevent electrolyte imbalance,* and disconnect the syringe from the NG tube.

6. Draw up the ordered volume of normal saline (usually 30 to 60 mL) into the syringe and reconnect the syringe to the NG tube.

7. Gently instill the normal saline into the tube. *Excessive force increases risk of reflux and aspiration.*

8. Gently aspirate the irrigant back into the syringe. *Excessive suction can damage the gastric mucosa.*

9. Remove the syringe from the tube; clamp or plug the proximal end of the tube or reconnect it to suction. Secure the tube to the patient's gown.

10. Follow the Ending Implementation Steps located on the inside back cover.

Evaluation Steps

1. Assess the patient's tolerance of the procedure.

2. If the NG tube was connected to a suction source, observe for fluid movement through tube *to verify patency.*

Sample Documentation

6/4/12 0920 NG tube irrigated with 30 mL NS according to physician's orders. Irrigated without difficulty. NG tube patent. Reconnected to low intermittent suction. No C/O discomfort during irrigation. ——————— Nurse's signature and credentials

---

Skill 24-5 Removing a Nasogastric Tube

Assessment Steps

1. Review the patient's intake and output *to determine fluid imbalances.*

Planning Steps

1. Gather needed equipment and supplies: towel or protective pad; washcloth; tissues; examination gloves; irrigation syringe; patient's toothbrush, toothpaste, and mouthwash. *Being prepared saves time and effort and increases efficiency.*

Implementation Steps

1. Follow the Initial Implementation Steps located on the inside front cover.

2. Place the patient in the high Fowler's position and hand the patient some tissues.

3. Clear the tube of any secretions by using an irrigation syringe to inject 10 mL of air through the main lumen. *This reduces the risk of fluid dripping into the airway as the tube is withdrawn.*

4. Remove all tape from the patient's nose and the NG tube *so the tube can be removed.*

5. Have the patient hold his or her breath and gently but quickly withdraw the tube, immediately wrapping it in the disposable protective pad to remove it from the patient's line of vision. *This reduces the risk of aspiration during removal of the tube.*

6. Discard all contaminated supplies in the appropriate biohazard waste receptacle.

7. Provide the patient with a warm, wet washcloth to wash the face.

8. Assist the patient as needed to brush the teeth and rinse the mouth with mouthwash *to rid the mouth of debris, mucus, and bad taste from the tube removal.*

9. Offer a glass of cold water to drink, if the patient is not NPO, *to soothe a dry throat.*

10. Follow the Ending Implementation Steps located on the inside back cover.

Skill 24-5 (continued)

Evaluation Steps

1. Determine if the patient is experiencing any discomfort or pain related to the procedure and medicate accordingly. *This provides for patient comfort.*
2. Assess for active bowel sounds and repeat in 4 hours, while observing for abdominal distention, nausea, or vomiting. *This helps to determine GI tract tolerance of tube removal.*

Sample Documentation

> 11/21/12 0930 NG tube removed without difficulty per Dr's orders. Abdomen flat and soft; no complaints of nausea. Bowel sounds active in all 4 quadrants. Instructed to eat no more than one teaspoon of ice every 30 minutes and to report any nausea or bloating to staff. ————— Nurse's signature and credentials

Skill 24-6 Administering Intermittent Bolus Enteral Feedings

Assessment Steps

1. Review the patient's medical record and physician's order to determine the rate, route, and type of formula to be administered and *to reduce the risk of error.*
2. Evaluate the patient's current nutritional status. Review the laboratory data and other available diagnostic data, such as finger stick blood sugar readings. Assess for fluid volume excess or deficit, and metabolic or electrolyte imbalances. *This helps to determine patient's nutritional needs.*
3. Assess whether the patient has impaired swallowing, or has had facial trauma or surgeries of the alimentary canal, head, or neck. *These conditions indicate the patient's need for enteral tube feedings.*
4. Obtain a baseline weight to determine increases or decreases after initiation of feedings. *This provides for later comparisons to help evaluate the effectiveness of feedings.*
5. Assess for active bowel sounds; if absent, withhold feeding until you check with the physician.

Planning Steps

1. Gather needed equipment and supplies: clean gloves; pH litmus strips; prescribed enteral formula; an irrigation syringe or a 30-mL or larger syringe with a smaller slip-tip catheter tip if required for a snug fit into the NG, NI, or PEG tube; tape measure; cup of water. *Being prepared saves time and effort and increases efficiency.*

Implementation Steps

1. Follow the Initial Implementation Steps located on the inside front cover.
2. Raise the head of the bed 30 to 45 degrees *to reduce the risk of reflux and aspiration.*
3. Have the tube feeding formula at room temperature *to reduce intestinal cramping.*
4. Check the expiration date of the formula and the integrity of its container *to determine the safety of the formula.*
5. Arrange supplies on the over-the-bed table within easy reach.
6. Check for correct tube placement and gastric content residual volume by assessing whether the insertion mark is still located at the insertion point, measuring the length of the tube from the point of insertion to the distal end and comparing with the recorded measurement, and using the irrigation syringe to aspirate all stomach contents. *Safety: If the tube is a Salem sump tube, do not insert the syringe tip into the blue air vent.* Measure the amount of residual aspirate and check the pH with litmus paper. Be sure the pH is acidic, between 1 and 4. *This prevents instillation of fluids into a displaced tube.* Re-instill aspirate *unless* the amount is equal to or greater than half the last feeding, in which case you will:
   a. First, follow the physician's orders if indicated.
   b. If there is no physician's order regarding residual volume, then follow the facility policy.
   c. If neither addresses the issue, re-instill the aspirate and wait an hour. Then repeat assessment of residual gastric volume.

   This helps to prevent electrolyte imbalance.

   With a J-Tube: Proceed as above; however, you will aspirate intestinal secretions. Intestinal residuals tend to be small in amount and more alkaline. Residuals of more than 10 mL with an acidic pH may indicate that the tube has dislodged and is displaced to the stomach.
7. Shake the feeding formula *to ensure that it is mixed well.*
8. Remove the plunger or rubber bulb from the irrigation syringe barrel and attach the tip to the feeding tube.
9. Bend or crimp the feeding tube just below the connection to the tip of the irrigation syringe *to prevent the flow of formula as you fill the syringe.*
10. Carefully pour the formula into the syringe barrel.
11. Release the bent or crimped tube, allowing formula *to begin to flow.* Do not raise the syringe more than 15 to 18 inches above the tube insertion site, which can cause discomfort due to excessive pressure and too rapid instillation. Recrimp the tube before the syringe runs completely dry *to prevent air from filling the line and infusing, as added formula pushes the air in front of it.*
12. Keep refilling the syringe in the same manner until the infusion is competed. Monitor the patient throughout the feeding, *observing for any signs of respiratory distress.*
13. Flush the tube with 30 to 60 mL of water to clear formula from the line and ensure that the tube is patent. *This will reduce clogging and bacterial growth.*

(skill continues on page 534)

Skill 24-6 (continued)

14. Administer water via the feeding tube between feedings or as ordered.

15. Maintain the patient in a semi-Fowler's position or with the head of bed elevated at least 30 degrees for 1 hour *to promote gastric emptying and prevent vomiting or aspiration.*

16. Follow the Ending Implementation Steps located on the inside back cover.

Evaluation Steps

1. Observe and assess the patient's respiratory status postfeeding, as changes such as increased rate, wheezing, increased coughing, or sudden decrease in O_2 saturation *can indicate aspiration.*

2. Auscultate breath sounds at least once every 8 hours *to detect adventitious sounds that may indicate aspiration.*

3. Measure aspirate every 4 hours *to evaluate the patient's tolerance of feedings.*

4. Monitor laboratory values, including albumin, prealbumin, and transferrin. Notify the physician of significant changes. *This provides information to determine if the nutritional status is stable, improving, or worsening.*

5. Monitor intake and output every shift and calculate 24-hour totals, *noting if there is an imbalance.*

6. Weigh the patient daily, at the same time of day and with the same scale to maintain consistency, until the tube feeding maximum rate has been reached, then weigh three times per week or per the physician's order, noting if weight begins to decline. *Evaluate the effectiveness of feedings.*

7. For patients with tubes placed through the abdominal wall, inspect the insertion site for erythema, edema, increased warmth, and drainage *to detect signs and symptoms of infection.*

Sample Documentation

6/2/11   0645   *Awake and alert, lying supine. NG tube placement checked by aspirating residual gastric contents, obtained 75 mL of yellowish-brown gastric contents, pH = 3. Insertion mark remains at point of entry. C/O of mild discomfort in left nostril, no erythema noted, skin intact. Replaced tape securing NG tube to nose. States it feels better. Head of bed elevated 45 degrees. Tube flushed with 30 mL of water, and 250 mL of Jevity instilled per gravity. Tube flushed with 30 mL water. No signs of gastric or respiratory distress noted. ————————*
———————————— *Nurse's signature and credentials*

Skill 24-7 Using a Feeding Pump

Assessment Steps

1. Review the patient's medical record and physician's order to determine the rate, route, and type of formula to be administered *to reduce the risk of error.*

2. Evaluate the patient's current nutritional status. Review the laboratory data and other available diagnostic data, such as finger stick blood sugar readings. Assess for fluid volume excess or deficit, and metabolic or electrolyte imbalances.

3. Assess whether the patient has impaired swallowing, or has had facial trauma or surgeries of the alimentary canal, head, or neck. *These conditions indicate the patient's need for enteral tube feedings.*

4. Obtain a baseline weight to determine increases or decreases after initiation of feedings. *This provides for later comparisons to help evaluate effectiveness of feedings.*

5. For PEG or J-tubes, inspect the skin around the tube for irritation, signs of skin breakdown, infection, or drainage.

6. Auscultate bowel sounds before feeding. If no bowel sounds are heard, consult the physician before initiating feeding.

Planning Steps

1. Gather needed equipment and supplies: clean gloves, stethoscope, pH litmus strips, tape measure, prescribed enteral formula, disposable feeding bag and tubing or ready-to-hang system, 30-mL or larger irrigation syringe, feeding pump. *Being prepared saves time and effort and increases efficiency.*

Safety: Note that a feeding pump is not the same as an IV pump.

Implementation Steps

1. Follow the Initial Implementation Steps located on the inside front cover.

2. Have the tube feeding formula at room temperature *to reduce intestinal cramping.*

3. Check the expiration date of the formula and the integrity of its container *to prevent using outdated or spoiled formula.*

4. Prepare a ready-to-hang system or pour formula into a disposable feeding bag with clamped tubing. Hang the formula bag on the IV pole.

5. Place the patient in the high Fowler's position or elevate the head of the bed 30 to 45 degrees *to reduce the risk of reflux and aspiration.*

6. Prime the tubing from the formula bag by opening the clamp and allowing formula to flow until all air in the tubing is displaced with formula. *Instillation of air can cause discomfort, belching, and reflux.*

7. Position a waterproof pad under the distal end of the NG, PEG, or J-tube *to protect the bed from soiling.*

8. Put on clean gloves and proceed to verify tube placement. Assess the location of the insertion mark to determine that it is still at the point of entry. Measure the length of the tube extending from the insertion site to the distal end of the tube. Use an irrigation syringe to aspirate residual gastric contents. Observe appearance of aspirate and check the pH

Skill 24-7 (continued)

to make certain the acidity is between 1 and 4. *This reduces the risk of installation into a displaced tube.*

9. Return the entire aspirate to the stomach unless the amount is equal to or greater than half the volume of formula that infused in the last hour or half the volume of the last intermittent feeding, *to prevent electrolyte imbalance.* If this is the case, withhold the feeding and reassess the residual in 1 hour. Once the residual volume is within acceptable parameters, you may proceed with the feeding process.

10. Flush the tube with 30 mL of water *to ensure that the tube is clear and patent.*

11. Connect the feeding setup tubing to the patient's feeding tube, thread it through the feeding pump, set the volume and rate, and initiate the feeding.

12. Maintain the patient in the semi-Fowler's position or with the head of the bed elevated continuously *to promote gastric emptying and prevent vomiting or aspiration.*

13. Follow the Ending Implementation Steps located on the inside back cover.

Evaluation Steps

1. Measure aspirate every 4 hours *to evaluate the patient's tolerance of feedings.*

2. Monitor all laboratory values regularly; albumin, prealbumin, and transferrin indicate stable, improving, or worsening nutritional status. Notify the physician of significant changes. *This evaluates nutritional status and effectiveness of feedings.*

3. Observe and assess the patient's respiratory status postfeeding, as changes such as increased rate, wheezing, increased coughing, or sudden decrease in O_2 saturation *can indicate aspiration.*

4. Monitor intake and output every shift and calculate 24-hour totals, *noting imbalance.*

5. Weigh the patient daily, at the same time of day and with same scale to maintain consistency, for the first 2 weeks of continuous feeding, noting any decrease. Then weigh three times per week or per the physician's order, noting if weight begins to decline. *This evaluates the effectiveness of feedings.*

Sample Documentation

3/24/12   1130   NG tube placement verified by x-ray. Jevity 500 mL tube feeding initiated per feeding pump 50 mL/hr. Hob elevated 45 degrees. ———— *Nurse's signature and credentials*

Post Conference

After caring for your patient for 2 days, you feel much more comfortable around nasogastric tubes. You inserted his tube on the first day and placement was verified by aspirating greenish stomach contents, which had a pH of 3, and also by x-ray before instilling anything into the tube. You were still nervous, though, when you first attached the feeding pump and started the feedings. You kept watching the patient and checking for any signs of aspiration. On the second day, the patient pulled out his tube, and you had to insert a new one. This time it went even more smoothly and you began to feel confidence about this skill. Now you are glad that you were the lucky student assigned to this patient.

KEY POINTS

- Oral diets may be modified in consistency or in nutrient concentration depending on the needs and disease state of the individual patient. Combination diets such as mechanical soft, low sodium may be ordered.

- Nutritional supplements are often ordered for patients with decreased appetites, increased nutritional requirements, and digestion or absorption problems.

- Patients with difficulties tolerating oral intake may receive enteral feedings. Tube feedings can be nasogastric or nasointestinal or via the lower gastrointestinal tract via PEG or J-tube.

- The choice of tube feeding method will depend on the patient's digestive and absorptive abilities, the size of the feeding tube, infusion site, nutritional requirements, current and past medical history, and tolerance.

- Verification of NG/NI tube placement by radiography is the most accurate method. It is done following the initial placement of the tube; thereafter, the insertion mark made on the tube at the point of insertion is assessed to ensure that the tube has not migrated, along with measuring the length of the tube extending from the insertion site to its distal end and comparing it with the recorded measurement. Aspiration of gastric contents and assessment of the pH is used to verify continued presence of the tube in the proper location of the GI tract.

- Standard tube feeding formulas require normal digestion and contain intact molecules of protein, carbohydrates, and fat.

- Tube feedings can be continuous or intermittent bolus. Continuous feedings should be administered with a feeding pump.

- Gastric residuals should be checked prior to each feeding or every 4 hours during continuous feedings.

- The tube should be flushed with water before and after feedings or administration of medications.

- Complications can arise with enteral tube feeding, such as clogged tubes, aspiration, electrolyte imbalance, hyperglycemia, and severe diarrhea.

- Enteral nutrition is the preferred method of providing supplemental nutrition to patients. It is administered via the gastrointestinal tract and supports GI functioning.

- Nursing care of the patient with a percutaneous tube includes care of the tube insertion site.

- Parenteral nutrition is the administration of nutrition intravenously for patients who are unable to adequately ingest enough nutrients through the GI tract to meet their nutritional requirements.

- There are two types of parenteral nutrition: partial parenteral nutrition (PPN) and total parenteral nutrition (TPN). PPN solutions contain a lower concentration of dextrose than TPN. PPN can frequently be given via a large peripheral vein, while TPN is given via a central venous line.

- When administering any type of parenteral nutrition, the nurse must adhere strictly to sterile technique; contamination can lead to serious infection and septicemia.

- Patients receiving parenteral nutrition should have their laboratory values monitored frequently to assess for electrolyte imbalances, hyper- or hypoglycemia, and malnutrition.

- Prealbumin is the standard measure for monitoring acute changes in patients' nutritional status.

- Patients may receive enteral or parenteral nutrition in the hospital or at home.

REVIEW QUESTIONS

Select the answer that is most appropriate for each of the following questions. Some questions may have more than one correct answer. Check all that apply.

1. You are caring for an 80-year-old female who has poorly fitting dentures and significant difficulty chewing food. Which diet would be most appropriate for her?

   a. Full liquid diet

   b. Regular diet

   c. Pureed, low-residue diet

   d. Mechanical soft diet

   e. Clear liquid diet

2. You are caring for a patient receiving intermittent bolus feedings and it is time for the next feeding. Which of these interventions will you perform first?

   a. Total the intake and output for the shift.

   b. Have the patient move from the chair to the bed to lie down.

   c. Aspirate the residual gastric contents, test the pH, and measure it.

   d. Flush the tube with 30 mL of water.

   e. Measure the length of the tube extending from the insertion site.

3. A patient is receiving total parenteral nutrition (TPN) via central venous catheter. The patient's wife is concerned about his care and wants to know why the TPN bag is not changed as often as a regular IV bag of solution would be. You respond by telling her the standard for changing the TPN bag is every:

   a. 6 hours

   b. 8 hours

   c. 12 hours

   d. 24 hours

4. You are caring for a patient who is scheduled for surgery. Your teaching will include information about nutrition and healing. You will tell the patient which of the following macronutrients is required for tissue repair?

   a. Carbohydrates

   b. Fat

   c. Vitamin E

   d. Protein

   e. Vitamin K

5. As a home health nurse, you will be caring for the patients noted below. Which patient is at greatest risk for experiencing inadequate nutrition?

   a. A 60-year-old white male recently diagnosed with type 2 diabetes.

   b. A 72-year-old widow who had a mild cerebrovascular accident (CVA) 3 days ago.

   c. A 25-year-old mother with two preschoolers, who is recovering from a tonsillectomy.

   d. A 55-year-old black male recovering at home following coronary artery bypass surgery.

6. Critically ill tube-fed patients should have the head of the bed raised to _____ during the feeding and for up to 1 hour after feeding.

   a. 5 to 10 degrees

   b. 15 to 25 degrees

   c. 30 to 45 degrees

   d. 50 to 60 degrees

   e. 90 degrees

7. What intervention(s) should you prepare for when caring for a patient who is 6 hours postburn with 30% second-degree burns and has absent bowel sounds?

   a. Withholding oral intake.

   b. Insertion of a nasogastric tube to low intermittent suction.

   c. Starting a diet of clear liquids only.

   d. Inserting a feeding tube for nutrition.

   e. Feeding the patient a soft diet.

8. Which actions are taken to verify the correct placement of a small-bore NG tube immediately after insertion? (Select all that apply and rank in correct order.)

   a. Aspirate the gastric contents, check the pH of contents, and observe the color.

   b. Confirm the size of the feeding tube after taping.

   c. Place the distal end of the tube in a glass of water and observe for bubbles indicating air exchange.

   d. Take an x-ray.

   e. Flush the tube with 15 to 30 mL of water to ensure its correct placement.

Short Answer Question

9. You are working in a pediatric clinic when the mother of a 15-year-old female patient calls about her daughter. She is concerned because her daughter is constantly worried about her weight, talks about various foods and their nutritional quality, and exercises 2 to 3 hours daily. She states that the daughter constantly complains of a sore throat and indigestion. What disorder would you suspect? How would you explain the daughter's complaints?

Critical Thinking Exercises

10. You are working on a cardiovascular unit and are assigned to care for a 68-year-old black female who is being admitted. She has advanced multiple sclerosis and has virtually no motor function from the neck down, and suffers from significant dysphagia. What are your nursing priorities for this patient? Develop a plan of care to assist her in meeting her nutritional needs.

11. A 75-year-old white male has been ill with nausea, vomiting, and diarrhea for the last 4 days. He transferred from his long-term care (LTC) facility to your hospital. His weight 1 week ago at the LTC was 165 lbs. (75 kg); today it is 156 lbs. (70.9 kg). Your assessment reveals hyperactive bowel sounds, a soft and slightly tender abdomen in all four quadrants, and continued nausea and diarrhea but no vomiting in the last 8 hours. He is afebrile with normal electrolyte values. What type of diet order would be the best choice for him? What nursing interventions should you perform during your 7-to-3 shift?

12. You are caring for a patient receiving 250 mL of formula via intermittent enteral feedings. You withdraw 50 mL of residual gastric content when you check his nasogastric tube's placement, patency, and residual. Should you return the gastric aspirate to the patient's stomach or discard it? Provide a rationale for your response.

ADDITIONAL RESOURCES

For additional Resources, Questions, and Activities, please see:

 Student Resource Disk

 http://davisplus.fadavis.com

 Student Study Guide

REFERENCES

American Association of Critical-Care Nurses. *Practice Alert: Verification of Feeding Tube Placement.* Aliso Viejo, CA: American Association of Critical-Care Nurses; 2005.

American Diabetes Association. Standards of medical care in diabetes. *Diabetes Care.* 2008;31(Suppl 1):512-544.

Davidson J. Strategies for improving glycemic control: effective use of glucose monitoring. *Am J Med.* 2005;118:27-32.

Gregory KE, Mainous RO. Research abstracts: the influence of enteral feeding regimens on necrotizing enterocolitis in preterm infants. *Adv Neonatal Care.* 2009;9(2):86.

Lourenco R. Enteral feeding: drug-nutrient interaction. *Clin Nutr.* 2001;20:187-193.

Magnuson BL, Clifford TM, Hoskins LA, Bernard AC. Enteral nutrition and drug administration, interaction, and complications. *Nutr Clin Pract.* 2005;20:618-624.

Metheny NA. Preventing respiratory complications of tube feedings: evidence based practice. *Am J Crit Care.* 2006;15:360.

Metheny NA, Schallom L, Oliver DA, Clouse RE. Gastric residual volume and aspiration in critically ill patients receiving gastric feedings. *Am J Crit Care.* 2008;17:512-519.

Mitchell JF. Oral dosage forms that should not be crushed. Institute for Safe Medication Practices Web site. 2008. Available at: http://www.ismp.org/tools/donotcrush.pdf. Accessed September 23, 2009.

National Institutes of Health. Eating disorders. 2007. Available at: http://www.nimh.nih.gov/health/publications/eating-disorders/nimheatingdisorders.pdf. Accessed September 23, 2009.

Palmer JL, Metheny NA. Preventing aspiration in older adults with dysphagia. *Am J Nurs.* 2008;108(2):40-48.

Rhoades J, Meeker BJ. *Davis's Guide to Clinical Nursing Skills.* Philadelphia: FA Davis; 2008.

Rolfes S, Pinna K, Whitney E. *Understanding Normal and Clinical Nutrition.* 7th ed. Belmont, CA: Wadsworth and Thomson Learning; 2006.

Scanlon V, Sanders T. *Essentials of Anatomy and Physiology.* Philadelphia: FA Davis; 2007.

Siow E. Enteral versus parenteral nutrition for acute pancreatitis. *Crit Care Nurse.* 2008;28(4):19-25, 27-31.

Smeltzer S, Bare R. *Brunner & Suddarth's Textbook of Medical-Surgical Nursing.* 11th ed. Philadelphia: Lippincott Williams & Wilkins; 2008.

Society of Gastroenterology Nurses and Associates. *Gastroenterology Nursing: A Core Curriculum.* 4th ed. Chicago: Society of Gastroenterology Nurses and Associates; 2008.

Society of Gastroenterology Nurses and Associates. Position Statement: The role of the nurses and associates in placement of percutaneous endoscopic gastrostomy (PEG) tube. 2008. Available at: http://www.sgna.org/Resources/PEGplacementFINAL_308.pdf. Accessed September 23, 2009.

The Joint Commission. 2009 National Patient Safety Goals. Available at: http://www.jointcommission.org/patientsafety/nationalpatientsafetygoals/. Accessed September 23, 2009.

Wilkinson JM, Van Leuven K. *Fundamentals of Nursing: Theory, Concepts & Applications.* Philadelphia: FA Davis; 2007.

Williams LS, Hopper PD. *Understanding Medical-Surgical Nursing.* 3rd ed. Philadelphia: FA Davis; 2007.

Williams NT. Medication administration through enteral feeding tubes. *Am J Health Syst Pharm.* 2008;65:2347-2357.

Diagnostic Tests

Key Terms

Arteriography

Barium enema

Bone marrow aspiration

Chest x-ray (CXR)

Colonoscopy

Complete blood cell count (CBC)

Complete metabolic panel

Computed tomography (CT)

Differential

Electrocardiography (EKG)

Electroencephalography (EEG)

Esophagogastroduodenoscopy (EGD)

Glomerular filtration rate (GFR)

Intravenous pyelogram

Left shift

Lumbar puncture

Magnetic resonance imaging (MRI)

Oral glucose tolerance test

Paracentesis

Right shift

Ultrasonography

Objectives

1. Correctly use key terms associated with diagnostic tests.
2. Explain the nurse's role and responsibilities in relation to diagnostic tests.
3. Explain all the components of a complete blood cell count, including a white count differential.
4. Contrast the functions of the five types of white blood cells.
5. Relate the normal adult ranges of complete blood cell count components.
6. Identify the normal findings of a urinalysis.
7. Discuss aspects of diagnostic tests and procedures that the nurse should teach the patient.
8. Name at least two tests that evaluate renal function.
9. Identify three diagnostic tests that would provide you information relating to nutrition.
10. Name three diagnostic tests that would be useful in evaluating liver function.
11. Identify allergies for which the nurse should assess prior to procedures and tests requiring use of contrast medium.
12. Differentiate between esophagogastroduodenoscopy, barium enema, and colonoscopy, and between magnetic resonance imaging and computed tomography, including purposes and preparations for each.
13. Explain the purpose of a lumbar puncture and how to position a patient for the procedure.
14. Prioritize the postprocedure nursing actions to be performed after a femoral arteriogram.
15. Relate the purposes of a glucose tolerance test, intravenous pyelogram, and bone marrow aspiration.

Skills

25-1 Assisting with Aspiration Procedures: Bone Marrow, Lumbar Puncture, and Paracentesis

25-2 Performing a 12-Lead Electrocardiogram (EKG)

 Clinical Connection

Your Assignment: You are caring for a 37-year-old female hospitalized with abdominal pain, nausea, and vomiting of unknown origin. The physician has ordered an esophagogastroduodenoscopy (EGD), ultrasound of the gallbladder and pancreas, and blood work to include a blood chemistry, electrolyte panel, alkaline phosphatase (ALP), glomerular filtration rate (GFR), and creatinine. Your patient tells you that she hopes they do it all quickly because she hates needles and has no idea what the other tests are like.

Your Actions: You will need to prepare your patient for each test, explain the tests to her, and assess her after some of the tests. It is important that you know the purpose of each test and the normal findings, so you can notify the physician of abnormal results.

Diagnostic tests are those tests and examinations that help to make a medical diagnosis by ruling out possible diagnoses or by specifically pinpointing the disease process or injury afflicting the patient. This chapter will assist you to identify your role as a nurse in relation to diagnostic tests and to familiarize you with some of the more commonly used examinations.

Please note that this chapter does not provide a comprehensive review of diagnostic testing, as it concentrates its focus on routine tests that you will likely see on a daily basis. As you will find out through the course of your schooling and even as you start your career, the number of diagnostic tests available to health care professionals cannot be covered in a single chapter. The authors encourage you to utilize books dedicated solely to this specialized subject to further your knowledge.

Nursing's Role in Diagnostic Testing

As the nurse, you will not be performing many of the tests discussed in this chapter, but you will have numerous responsibilities relating to physician-ordered diagnostic tests and procedures. Depending on the test, your responsibilities may include:

- Noting the physician's order
- Occasionally scheduling the test or procedure
- Educating the patient regarding the process
- *Safety: Determining that the patient is not allergic to any dyes or preparations that may be used for the test,*
includes allergies to iodine, shellfish, and contrast medium
- Making certain written consent is obtained, if the procedure requires it
- Knowing when to withhold food and fluids (Box 25-1)
- Preparing the patient
- Obtaining specimens or delivering specimens to the laboratory

Box 25-1

When to Withhold Food and Fluids

Withholding food and fluids, or permitting "nothing by mouth," is known as keeping the patient NPO. Many tests require that the patient be kept NPO prior to the test, but there are no hard and fast rules for which tests require this. Each facility will have its own policies for diagnostic tests and whether or not preparation includes being kept NPO. Which blood chemistry tests include being kept NPO varies widely from site to site. Some of the tests more commonly requiring the patient to be kept NPO for 6 to 8 hours include:
- Any type of endoscopy, such as barium enema and colonoscopy
- Cardiac catheterization
- Any computed tomography with contrast medium or dye
- Any scope procedures that require conscious sedation or general anesthesia
- Any test reflecting glucose levels, such as glucose tolerance test, fasting blood glucose, and hemoglobin A_{1c}
- Lung and brain scans if contrast medium is used
- Cholesterol and lipid tests

- Reassuring or supporting the patient as needed
- Assisting the examiner with performance of the test or procedure
- Notifying the physician of significant abnormal results
- Monitoring for complications
- Providing necessary postprocedure nursing care
- Being able to relate the significance of the test findings to the patient's condition
- Administering laxatives or enemas to remove fecal material from the intestinal tract, which allows for better visualization of the intestine for various imaging tests

Some tests will even require administration of a *radiopaque substance,* which is a substance impenetrable to x-rays and other forms of radiation, or a *radionuclide,* which is an atom that emits electromagnetic rays as it disintegrates.

With all of these responsibilities, you can easily see that understanding the purposes, preparation for, and processes of commonly administered diagnostic tests is paramount to your role as a nurse. Table 25-1 details the preparation and post-test nursing care for selected tests.

Patient Teaching Connection

Diagnostic Tests
Prepare the patient for upcoming tests or procedures to alleviate the patient's anxiety and increase compliance. Using terminology that the patient will understand, explain the purpose of the test or procedure, as well as the test's benefits and dangers. The patient has a legal right to know the risks involved. Describe what will occur, including any preparatory steps that must be performed prior to the test. If a specimen such as urine or sputum is required, explain how to correctly obtain the specimen. Avoid using acronyms for the name of the test or procedure; instead, use the complete name. For example, use "white blood cell count" rather than "WDC." Remember that the average patient is not a health care provider. However, this does not mean that you should talk down to the patient as if he or she is ignorant.

It is generally helpful to provide the patient with a written pamphlet or brochure about the procedure. Some patients prefer to read about it before you verbally explain it, while others would rather discuss it with you first and then relax and read the pamphlet to reinforce your teaching. If written consent must be obtained to perform the procedure, be certain that all patient teaching is completed before the consent is signed.

Knowledge Connection
Discuss at least eight responsibilities you will have regarding diagnostic testing. What types of preparations are common prior to diagnostic procedures?

Categories of Diagnostic Tests

There are five general categories of diagnostic tests that we will discuss in this chapter:

1. Laboratory tests
2. Radiology and imaging tests and procedures
3. Ultrasonography
4. Endoscopic examinations
5. Graphic recording tests

Laboratory Tests

Laboratory test is a broad classification for numerous types of examinations performed on some type of body fluid, such as whole blood or the serum portion of the blood, spinal fluid, sputum, urine, gastric contents, feces, and bone marrow.

Anatomy and Physiology Connection

Blood
Let's briefly review the production of blood cells. In adults, red blood cells (RBCs) are produced by the bone marrow within the sternum, vertebrae, ribs, and pelvis. The kidneys release a protein known as erythropoietin, which acts on stem cells in the bone marrow to produce more RBCs. The RBC has a relatively short life span of approximately 120 days, after which it is destroyed by the reticuloendothelial system. White blood cells (WBCs) are mostly produced in the bone marrow, with limited production in the lymphoid tissues. Platelets are produced from large bone marrow cells known as *megakaryocytes.*

Hematology
Hematology is the study of blood cells and the blood-forming tissues (the bone marrow). The most common test ordered is the **complete blood cell count (CBC)**, which measures the number of leukocytes, or WBCs; erythrocytes, or RBCs; and thrombocytes, or platelets (PLTs). It also differentiates the percentages of the five types of WBCs (lymphocytes, neutrophils, eosinophils, basophils, and monocytes); measures the hemoglobin (Hgb), or iron pigment; and measures the hematocrit (Hct), which is the measurement of the percentage of packed RBCs compared to the whole blood volume. Each of these tests may be ordered as a stand-alone test as well as components of a CBC. *Even as a new nursing student attending clinical experiences, it is important to comprehend the different components of a CBC because it is performed on every patient upon admission to a hospital.* Table 25-2 lists the normal CBC values.

When the WBC count is elevated above normal, it is termed *leukocytosis;* when it is below normal, it is called *leukopenia.* WBCs, especially the neutrophils, function

Table 25-1 **Preparation and Post-Test Nursing Care for Selected Tests**

Test	Description	Purpose	Preparation	Post-Test Nursing Care
Barium enema	Rectal instillation of barium (a contrast medium) to provide for radiographic visualization of the large intestine, to see its shape and any abnormalities that might be present.	To detect cancerous tumors, obstructions, polyps, inflammatory disease, or diverticula in the colon.	Explain procedure. Offer assurance and support. The day before, perform bowel prep of laxatives and enemas according to facility or physician orders. Clear liquid diet. NPO after midnight.	Administer milk of magnesia or laxative of choice to remove barium before it hardens. Monitor for constipation. Explain that stools will be white until barium is eliminated. Provide fluids and physician-ordered diet.
Bone marrow aspiration (See Skill 25-1, page 551, for more information on assisting with bone marrow aspiration.)	Under local anesthetic, a sample of marrow is removed from the sternum, tibia, or iliac crest by needle aspiration for evaluation of blood cell production.	To diagnose some serious anemias, thrombocytopenia, and cancerous tumors, and to stage Hodgkin's disease.	Describe procedure and explain that it only takes 10–20 minutes to perform. Assess for allergy to local anesthetic to be used. Explain there will be a feeling of pressure and a brief period of discomfort when the marrow is actually aspirated. Offer reassurance and support. Make certain written consent has been obtained. Administer sedative or analgesic 60–90 minutes prior to test. Assess vital signs for baseline.	Hold pressure to puncture site and observe for bleeding at site. Apply dressing. Monitor vital signs for shock: ↓ BP, ↑ P Monitor for signs of infection: ↑ T, ↑ P
Intravenous pyelogram (also known as excretory urogram)	An iodine-based contrast dye is injected intravenously. X-rays are taken for visualization of the kidney parenchyma, pelvis, calyces, ureters, and bladder.	Evaluation of renal structure and function; aids in detection of kidney stones, obstruction, tumors, urinary tract disease, and trauma.	Explain procedure. Assess for allergy to iodine, shellfish, contrast medium dyes. Keep patient NPO for 8 hours prior to test. Make certain a consent form has been signed.	Observe for hematoma at the injection site. Observe for delayed reaction to the contrast dye. Assess for adequate urination. Encourage PO fluids to rehydrate patient and flush dye from body. Provide physician-ordered diet.

Test	Description	Purpose	Preparation	Post-Test Nursing Care
Lumbar puncture (See Skill 25-1, for more information on assisting with lumbar puncture.)	Insertion of a spinal needle between vertebral spinous processes into the lumbar section of the arachnoid space to obtain cerebrospinal fluid (CSF) sample to culture for organisms and measure the CSF pressure.	To diagnose meningitis, subarachnoid hemorrhage, tumors, and other infections of the central nervous system.	Explain procedure and that it takes 10–15 minutes. Make certain written consent is obtained. Assess allergy to iodine prep and local anesthetic. When ready for procedure, position patient on his or her side at the edge of the bed. Have patient draw knees up to abdomen and tuck chin down to chest to flex the spine for ease of needle insertion (Fig. 25-1). Help to hold patient in this position for duration of test.	Keep patient flat in bed for 8 hours. May turn from side to side, but may not raise head. Encourage plenty of PO fluids to reduce risk of spinal headache. Provide a flexible straw for drinking. Monitor needle insertion site for bleeding or drainage of CSF hourly for 4 hours and then every 4 hours for a period of 24 hours. Perform neurological status checks as ordered by physician. Assess for numbness and tingling of extremities, fever, neck rigidity, change in level of consciousness, BP changes, widening pulse pressure, ↓ P, or irregular respirations for the first 24 hours.
Oral glucose tolerance test	Patient drinks concentrated glucose syrup to stimulate pancreatic production of insulin. Blood and urine samples are collected at five to six intervals over a 3- to 6-hour span to evaluate glucose levels.	To diagnose diabetes mellitus or hypoglycemia.	Explain procedure. Keep patient NPO for 12 hours, except for water, which must be drunk for production of urine samples.	Provide physician-ordered diet and fluids. Observe for hypoglycemia and hyperglycemia.
Paracentesis (See Skill 25-1, for more information on assisting with paracentesis.)	Under local anesthetic, a needle is inserted through the abdominal wall into the peritoneal cavity to remove free fluid from within the cavity (ascites) (Fig. 25-2).	To relieve discomfort of the pressure of ascites, common in abdominal organ cancers and liver disease.	Explain procedure. Assess for allergy to local anesthetic to be used. Offer assurance and support. Make certain written consent has been obtained. Weigh patient. Measure abdominal girth. Have patient empty bladder. Assess baseline vital signs.	Document amount of fluid removed. Monitor vital signs. Assess for *syncope* (fainting). Encourage rest for several hours. Observe needle insertion site for hematoma. Weigh patient and compare to pretest weight. Measure abdominal girth and compare to pretest girth.

Figure 25-1 For a lumbar puncture, the patient is positioned on his or her side close to the edge of the bed, with thighs and head flexed as much as possible toward the abdomen. The needle is inserted into the subarachnoid space.

Figure 25-2 An abdominal paracentesis is performed to drain the accumulation of fluid in the abdominal cavity, called *ascites*.

Table 25-2   Complete Blood Count Normal Values

Blood Component	Normal Range
WBC, total	4,300–10,800/mm^3
WBC, differential	
Total neutrophils	55%–70% of total WBC
(Bands)*	(0%–5%)
(Segmented)	(54%–65%)
Lymphocytes†	20%–40% of total WBC
Monocytes	2%–8% of total WBC
Eosinophils	1%–4% of total WBC
Basophils	0%–1% of total WBC
Red blood cells	Males: 4.6–6.2 million/mm^3
	Females: 4.2–5.4 million/mm^3
Hemoglobin	Males: 13–18 g/dL
	Females: 12–16 g/dL
	Children: 11.2–16.5 g/dL
	Newborns: 16.5–19.5 g/dL
Hematocrit	Males: 40–54 mL/dL
	Females: 37–47 mL/dL
	Children: 34–49 mL/dL
	Newborns: 49–54 mL/dL
Platelets	150,000–400,000/mm^3

*When bands elevate to higher percentage levels, called a *left shift,* this indicates bacterial infection.

†When lymphocytes elevate to higher percentage levels, called a *right shift,* this indicates viral infection.

primarily to protect the body from infection. Once a bacterial infection begins, the bone marrow increases the production of WBCs, specifically the neutrophils, monocytes, and a few lymphocytes. The lymph tissue produces the majority of lymphocytes. A **differential** is the breakdown of the total WBC into percentages of the five types of white cells, each of which elevates in response to different situations:

- *Neutrophils elevate* with infection. Slightly immature neutrophils are called *bands;* when their level is elevated, as opposed to the more mature segmented neutrophils, it is known as a **left shift**, which generally indicates bacterial infection.
- *Eosinophils* elevate in response to allergic reactions and parasites.
- *Basophils* contain large amounts of histamine and elevate in hypersensitivity reactions, such as stings, iodine, or medications. These reactions, known as *anaphylactic reactions,* are life-threatening allergic reactions.
- *Monocyte* levels rise as a second line of defense against bacterial infections.

- *Lymphocytes* increase with viral infections and allergic conditions; when their level is elevated, it is known as a **right shift**, a typical indicator of viral infection.

As shown above, a differential can help to discern whether there is a bacterial or viral infection, an allergic or hypersensitivity reaction, a parasitic invasion, or a disease of the blood-forming organs.

An RBC count provides the number of RBCs in a cubic millimeter (mm^3) of whole blood, whose function is to carry the Hgb, which binds with oxygen to be delivered to cells throughout the body. When the RBC count is lower than normal, it is known as *erythropenia or erythrocytopenia*. A lower-than-normal level of RBCs can help to diagnose hemorrhage beyond 24 hours, fluid overload, or anemia. *Anemia* is a condition in which there is a reduction in the delivery of oxygen to the tissues; it is usually indicated by depressed RBC and Hgb levels. *Polycythemia* describes an elevated RBC count.

Closely related to the RBC count—and part of a CBC—is the Hgb test. This test helps to determine the presence and severity of the different types of anemia. When Hgb is decreased, the body's oxygen-carrying capacity is reduced, which interferes with the ability of different body tissues and systems to function at optimal level.

The RBC, Hgb, and Hct levels are closely related and are useful in diagnosing dehydration, anemia, and polycythemia. As well as being ordered as a stand-alone Hct or as part of a CBC, the Hgb and Hct are often ordered as an *H&H.*

PLTs are the blood cells that aid in the blood-clotting process to prevent hemorrhage and help to protect vascular surfaces. If a patient has too many PLTs, the patient has *thrombocytosis,* which can result in abnormal clotting. If a patient has too few PLTs, *thrombocytopenia* develops, which hinders the body's hemostatic ability, or ability to stop bleeding.

Knowledge Connection

Differentiate between the five types of WBCs, including possible etiologies of their elevations. What are the medical terms for the different types of blood cells, including RBCs, WBCs, and PLTs? Describe the components of a complete WBC count. List three ways a Hgb level may be ordered. Describe what is meant by a *left shift.*

Blood Chemistry Tests

Blood chemistry tests may be performed on whole blood, plasma, or serum. They are generally performed to detect changes in the biological chemical reactions in the body. They may be used to rule out certain conditions as well as to diagnose a disease or syndrome. Some of the more common chemistry tests include:

- **Blood glucose:** The glucose level in the blood is helpful in diagnosis and treatment of diabetes mellitus.

- **Electrolyte levels:** Potassium (K^+), chloride (Cl^-), sodium (Na^+), magnesium (Mg^{2+}), calcium (Ca^{2+}), and phosphate (PO_4^-) levels are obtained to evaluate fluid and electrolyte balance and acid-base balance, which you will learn more about in Chapter 29.

- **Enzymes and isoenzymes:** These substances are released into the blood from specific tissue cells when those cells are injured; the enzymes and isoenzymes present help identify damage to specific organs. Cardiac cells release troponin, creatine kinase-MB (CK-MB), and lactate dehydrogenase types 1 and 2 (LD_1, LD_2). Damaged liver cells release aspartate aminotransferase (AST), alanine aminotransferase (ALT), and alkaline phosphatase (ALP).

- **Blood urea nitrogen (BUN):** Nitrogen is an end product of protein metabolism, excreted by the kidneys into the urine. Elevated blood levels occur with dehydration. In the past the BUN was used as an indicator of renal function impairment; however, recently it has been determined that it does not accurately measure renal function. At this time, the BUN is still being ordered by some physicians, but many other physicians do not use the test.

- **Serum creatinine:** Creatinine is a product of metabolism, removed from blood by the kidneys. Elevated levels indicate impairment of kidney function.

- **Total protein:** Total protein is used to evaluate many conditions, such as malnutrition, dehydration, severe burns, gastrointestinal disease, renal disease, liver disease, and diabetes mellitus. It measures serum levels of albumin and globulins, which are vital to numerous body functions. These proteins:
  - Serve as a buffer in acid-base balance
  - Help to maintain osmolarity of body fluids
  - Act as carrier transporters of iron, copper, and other ions
  - Perform as enzymes and antibodies
  - Help to bind and detoxify medications
  - Serve as a resource for tissue nutrition

- **Total bilirubin:** Total bilirubin measures the blood level of *bilirubin,* which is an orange pigment that is released during the destruction or breakdown of hemoglobin. Once an RBC's normal life span is over, the RBC is destroyed, releasing the hemoglobin and, eventually, the bilirubin. Normally, Kupffer cells in the liver transform the bilirubin into bile, which aids in digestion and is excreted in the feces. Certain disease processes can interfere with this process, resulting in excessive blood levels of bilirubin that stain the skin and tissues a yellowish-orange color, a condition known as *jaundice.* The bilirubin test is performed to evaluate liver function and to help in the diagnosis of certain anemias and biliary obstruction.

Most facilities have designated names for specific clusters or groups of blood chemistry tests. For example, some facilities use terms such as *basic metabolic panel* or **complete metabolic panel**, each representing a specific grouping of tests in which 8 or 14 respective tests are to be done. Box 25-2 provides a list of the tests included in a complete metabolic panel.

Box 25-2

Complete Metabolic Panel

A complete, or comprehensive, metabolic panel (CMP) is the name for a group of 14 separate tests that provide an overview of some of the functions of the liver, kidneys, and pancreas. Tests included in a CMP are:

- **Albumin:** a protein produced by the liver
- **Alkaline phosphatase (ALP):** an enzyme produced by the liver
- **Alanine aminotransferase (ALT),** also known as **SGPT:** an enzyme produced by the liver
- **Aspartate aminotransferase (AST),** also known as **SGOT:** an enzyme produced by the liver
- **Bilirubin:** a waste product remaining after the liver destroys old red blood cells
- **Blood urea nitrogen:** a waste product filtered from the blood by the kidneys*
- **Calcium:** an electrolyte; excess levels are removed from the blood by the kidneys

- **Chloride:** an electrolyte; excess levels are removed from the blood by the kidneys
- **Creatinine:** a waste product filtered from the blood by the kidneys
- **Glucose:** a simple sugar fuel source for cellular energy; needs insulin (from the pancreas) to transport glucose into the cells
- **Potassium:** an electrolyte; excess levels are removed from the blood by the kidneys
- **Sodium:** an electrolyte; excess levels are removed from the blood by the kidneys
- **Total protein:** measures all serum proteins, including albumin and globulins
- **Total serum CO_2:** measures serum level of bicarbonate (HCO_3^-), which provides data about serum CO_2 level because 95% of serum CO_2 is carried as part of HCO_3^-

*The BUN has recently lost credibility as a measure of kidney function. Most physicians are now using a test called the glomerular filtration rate (GFR) as a more accurate gauge of kidney function.

Nursing Care for Blood Chemistry Tests

The patient should be informed that a blood sample will have to be drawn for any of the tests mentioned above. Most laboratories do not place restrictions on food or fluid for the tests we have listed. However, many other tests do require the patient to be kept NPO. Please refer to a laboratory diagnostic text book as you learn more about other diagnostic tests during your nurse's training and actual patient care. It will be your responsibility to know when to keep a patient NPO.

Knowledge Connection

Describe at least four common laboratory tests and their purposes. Name two tests that evaluate renal function. Identify three diagnostic tests that would provide you information relating to nutrition. Name three diagnostic tests that would be useful in evaluating liver function.

Urine Tests

Urine tests may be performed on voided or catheterized urine specimens, or urine may also be collected over 24 hours for examination (see Chapter 31). Analysis of the urine and its contents provides you with much useful information.

Urinalysis

Routine urinalysis tests are ordered frequently in medical clinics and are routinely ordered upon admission to hospitals. Normal findings in a routine urinalysis include:

- **Color:** straw to dark yellow
- **Odor:** slightly aromatic
- **Appearance:** clear
- **Specific gravity:** 1.005 to 1.035
- **pH:** 4.5 to 8.0

- **Glucose:** none
- **Protein:** none
- **Ketones:** none
- **Bilirubin:** none
- **RBCs:** 0 to 2 per high-power field
- **WBCs:** 0 to 5 per high-power field
- **Epithelial cells:** 0 to 5 per high-power field
- **Casts:** none
- **Bacteria:** none
- **Yeast:** none

A basic urinalysis is simple to perform but can provide you with valuable information about the patient's health status, not just about the renal system. For example, the urine of a dehydrated patient may be a darker color, even amber. Color changes and abnormal pH values can be due to different diseases, medications, or dietary habits. The appearance may be cloudy due to the presence of bacteria or WBCs, often indicating infection of the urinary system. The specific gravity, which is the weight of the urine, will increase as dehydration increases the urine's ratio of solutes to water and may also cause the odor to become stronger, even to the point that it smells like ammonia. Other systemic diseases and conditions can also affect the specific gravity, such as diabetes insipidus, congestive heart failure, and shock. Protein in the urine, known as *proteinuria,* is usually related to some type of renal disease. The presence of ketones in the urine, known as *ketonuria,* is generally related to diabetes mellitus, indicating that adequate blood glucose is not being delivered to individual cells throughout the body. Therefore, it is to your benefit, as well as important to your patients' well-being, to become familiar with the components normally present in the urine and the significance of elevated or decreased amounts. It is also important to know the significance of abnormal components present in the urine.

Glomerular Filtration Rate

Now considered the most accurate test for evaluating kidney function, the **glomerular filtration rate (GFR)** measures the volume of urine, in milliliters, that is filtered by the kidney within 1 minute. The test involves a 24-hour collection of urine and determination of a creatinine level, but more commonly an *estimated glomerular filtration rate (eGFR)* is performed. Using a formula and the creatinine results, the eGFR is calculated without waiting to collect a 24-hour urine sample. Anything below 60 mL/min is considered to be significant renal impairment (Table 25-3).

Radiology and Imaging Tests

Radiography or x-ray provides an image of the bones without any preparation and is the most common test performed on the skeletal system. It is useful in detecting bone fractures and displacement of bone structures.

Chest X-ray

Chest x-ray (CXR) not only will allow you to see the bony structures of the thorax, but also allow you to visualize:

- The heart's position and size
- The lungs and whether they are fully expanded or have collapsed lobes (known as *atelectasis),* and whether they are clear or congested
- Densities that may indicate malignant tumors or tuberculosis

Nursing Care for Chest X-ray
There is little nursing care necessary for a CXR. Explain that painless x-ray pictures will be taken, requiring removal of jewelry, bras, and shirts or blouses with buttons, zippers, or snaps. A hospital gown will be used to protect modesty.

Magnetic Resonance Imaging

Magnetic resonance imaging (MRI) is a form of radiology that uses a magnetic scanner to detect the magnetic properties of atoms, usually hydrogen, while radiofrequency energy produces images of body tissues. It produces slices of the site, similar to computed tomography scans, allowing the examiner to view organs and tissues at all depths. MRI is useful in evaluation of the brain, spinal cord, bone, organs, and vessels in motion, as well as other fluid-filled soft tissues. It aids in diagnosing hemorrhagic and embolic cerebrovascular accidents (CVAs), more commonly known as strokes; tumors; multiple sclerosis; spinal cord aberrations; and other fluid-filled soft tissue disorders. MRI can be done with or without contrast medium or dye.

The patient is placed in a tunnel opening within the scanner, which is not very large. Some patients become claustrophobic and require sedation, while others are unable to tolerate the procedure. These patients usually are better able to tolerate the procedure if performed in an open-style MRI machine.

Nursing Care for Magnetic Resonance Imaging
When an MRI is ordered, you will need to verify if contrast is to be used for enhanced visualization. The patient may need to be kept NPO, depending upon the organs to be scanned, whether or not contrast dye will be used, and the facility's policy. The contrast dye used in MRI is not iodine-based as with computed tomography.

It is important to educate the patient regarding an impending MRI, making certain to inquire if the patient has claustrophobia. You should inform the patient of the limited space inside the scanner tunnel and that there will be loud knocking and clicking sounds emitted from the scanner throughout the test. Ear plugs, music, and sound-reducing headphones are routinely used to muffle the noise. Inform the patient that, even though the MRI is painless, the noise can be annoying, and it generally takes from 30 to 90 minutes to complete the scan. For patients in whom claustrophobia is severe, a mild sedative or antianxiety medication may be ordered preprocedure. Most facilities require that a consent form be signed. *Safety: Ask the patient if he or she has any metal implants, aneurysm clips, residual buckshot from*

Table 25-3   Glomerular Filtration Rate

Glomerular Filtration Rate (mL/min)	Level of Kidney Impairment	Description
100–120	None	Normal function
90–99	1	Slight kidney impairment with adequate GFR
60–89	2	Mild kidney impairment
30–59	3	Moderate kidney impairment
15–29	4	Severe kidney impairment
Less than 15	5	Complete kidney failure

gunshot wounds, or a pacemaker. MRI is contraindicated for patients with any type of internal ferrous metal, due to the strong magnetic pull of the scanner.

Computed Tomography

Computed tomography (CT), also known as computed axial tomography or *CAT,* scanning, is an x-ray procedure that takes many x-ray images of body parts from different angles. It then uses a computer to combine all the images to generate cross-sectional pictures and three-dimensional images of the internal organs and structures of the body. In other words, a CT scan helps to visualize slices of the organ or structure being imaged or scanned. This form of imaging can be used to detect normal and abnormal structures in the body, such as tumors. A contrast medium or dye may be ingested or injected prior to the procedure to better differentiate certain structures.

Nursing Care for Computed Tomography

As with an MRI, it is pertinent to assess whether or not the patient has claustrophobia and explain the types of things that may be used to combat or decrease these feelings. *Safety: Be certain to ask the patient if he or she is allergic to iodine, shellfish, radiopaque dye, or any contrast medium.* Allergic reactions to iodine-based products may be more serious than just a "typical rash," often resulting in systemic anaphylaxis, which is a life-threatening reaction causing bronchospasm, laryngeal edema, and peripheral vasodilation, which drops the blood pressure.

If contrast medium is to be administered, assess the patient's kidney function tests to confirm adequate kidney function to handle the contrast medium if it is to be used. This would include the creatinine, BUN, and GFR. An elevated creatinine or BUN should be reported to the physician before proceeding with contrast medium administration. Poorly functioning kidneys are indicated by a lower GFR and should also be reported to the physician. If the patient is currently taking metformin, it should be withheld the day of the CT scan and for an additional 2 days to prevent lactic acidosis problems. To assist with the elimination of contrast dye after the procedure, encourage fluids.

Arteriography and Venography

Arteriography, also known as *angiography,* and *venography* are forms of radiology that require a contrast medium be instilled into designated arteries, in the case of arteriography, or veins, in the case of venography. This allows examination of the vessel to assess for abnormalities such as *thrombosis* (blood clots), tumors, constrictions, occlusions, and *aneurysms,* which are weakenings or dilations in a vessel wall that is at risk of rupturing. These studies are commonly used to examine vessels in the heart, brain, lungs, and lower extremities.

Nursing Care for Arteriography and Venography

Nursing care is dependent upon the vessels accessed during the procedure. For example, when arterial access is performed, such as on the femoral artery, written consent must be obtained and allergy to the dye must be assessed. You must assess whether the patient has been on anticoagulants and monitor bleeding and coagulation test results prior to the test and make certain they are within normal ranges. Vital signs are monitored prior to, during, and after the procedure. After completion of the femoral arteriogram, pressure must be maintained on the needle insertion site. The patient must be kept on bedrest for 6 to 8 hours, keeping the involved leg straight. Distal pulses, capillary refill, color, and temperature of the lower extremity must be assessed hourly.

Knowledge Connection

Name three purposes for performing a CXR. Why would femoral arteriography require so much assessment postprocedure? What safety concern must you address with a patient prior to an MRI?

Ultrasonography

In **ultrasonography**, ultrasound waves are used to produce images of organs and tissues that can be recorded and printed. It is painless and easy to use. Some of the areas in which ultrasound has been found beneficial include determining the size and position of the fetus or placenta, determining function of cardiac valves, identifying arterial blockages, detecting abscesses and cancerous tumors, and visualizing female reproductive organs. Generally, there is no preparation for ultrasound except for obstetrics, when the patient may be required to drink several glasses of water to provide a full urinary bladder for the test. However, it is important to educate the patient regarding the ease of the test to decrease anxiety and increase patient compliance.

Endoscopic Examinations

Endoscopic examinations use a flexible scope with optical capability that allows visualization of body cavities and hollow organs, such as the colon or urinary bladder. Most endoscopies are performed using light sedation to alleviate discomfort during the procedure. Some of the more common endoscopies include esophagogastroduodenoscopy and colonoscopy.

Esophagogastroduodenoscopy

In **esophagogastroduodenoscopy (EGD)**, after spraying the mouth and throat with a local anesthetic or administering mild sedation, a flexible scope is inserted through the mouth, down the esophagus, through the stomach, and into the upper duodenum, allowing visualization of the lining of each. It is useful in detection and biopsy of polyps, ulcers, tumors, and constrictions, as well as evaluation of chemical burns after ingestion of poisons.

Nursing Care for Esophagogastroduodenoscopy

The only preparation for EGD is to place the patient on NPO status for 8 to 12 hours prior to the test. The patient needs to be educated regarding the procedure and that there is minimal or no discomfort. Assess vital signs prior to the procedure for a baseline, during the procedure, and every 15 minutes for 1 hour and every hour for 4 hours after the procedure. Cardiac, neurological, respiratory, and gastrointestinal assessments should be performed upon arrival back to the floor to make certain the patient is stable. Observe the patient for possible perforation. Signs of perforation might include severe pain or difficulty swallowing; epigastric, abdominal, shoulder or back pain that increases with torso movement; and dyspnea or cyanosis.

Colonoscopy

In **colonoscopy**, once the patient is sedated, a flexible endoscope is inserted via the rectum into the colon and terminal ileum, allowing the physician to visualize the lining for abnormalities such as polyps, ulcerations, and tumors and to biopsy tissue as needed. The patient usually feels no discomfort during the examination and is unable to remember anything about the procedure after awakening. This examination should be performed at least every 5 to 10 years after the age of 50, more often is there is a familial history of colon cancer.

Nursing Care for Colonoscopy

The preparation for a colonoscopy requires limiting the patient's intake to clear liquids for 24 hours before the examination, with avoidance of ingestion of anything "red" such as red jello, popsicles, or soda. Laxatives of the physician's choice are administered, usually beginning about 2 p.m. the day before the examination. This may or may not be followed with one to three enemas the evening prior to the test to completely clean out the bowel. The rest of the nursing care required is the same as for the EGD. Remember to reassure the patient that sedation will be administered, causing him or her to sleep during the procedure.

Knowledge Connection

Why would it be pertinent to have the large intestine clean and free of feces prior to a colonoscopy? What preparation is required for an EGD? What type of problems might be detected during an EGD? Name one major risk of EGD and colonoscopy. What type of problems could be discerned during a colonoscopy? What signs and symptoms would you observe for after an EGD?

Graphic Recording Tests

Numerous graphic recording tests are performed to detect abnormalities in the electrical activity of the heart, skeletal muscles, and brain. Two of the more common ones are electrocardiography and electroencephalography.

Electrocardiography

Electrocardiography, or **EKG** (also seen as ECG), uses six electrodes applied to specific locations on the chest wall and four electrodes applied to the four extremities to graphically record the electrical activity through the heart's electrical conduction pathway. It analyzes the heart's electrical activity from 12 different angles or views, detecting any abnormalities. The printout indicates how long it takes for the electrical impulse to travel from the sinoatrial (SA) node through the intra-atrial pathways to the atrioventricular (AV) node, then through the bundle of His and the Purkinje fibers. This time span is demonstrated by deflections of the baseline known as P waves, QRS complexes, and T waves as well as the P-R interval and the S-T interval (Fig. 25-3). Aberrations from normal time spans and complexes that are altered in shape indicate injury or malfunction of the heart. Skill 25-2 (page 552) provides more information on performing a 12-lead EKG.

Though an EKG can be beneficial in diagnosing heart attacks and *myocardial ischemia,* which is a lack of adequate blood flow and oxygen to the heart muscle itself, a normal EKG does not always rule out a heart problem. If you work in a cardiac unit, clinic, or hospital setting where you perform or view EKGs regularly, you will acquire a better working knowledge of how to interpret EKG waveforms.

Nursing Care for Electrocardiography

Inform the patient that an EKG helps to assess cardiac function and takes about 10 to 15 minutes. Describe the procedure and inform the patient that there should be no discomfort related to the EKG. Obtain a list of medications that the patient is currently taking, as well as a history of the patient's cardiovascular system symptoms if they have not already been documented in the medical record. Ask the patient to remove any jewelry that may interfere with electrode placement. Preserve the patient's modesty as much as possible while attaching the chest electrodes and during the procedure. Ask the patient to lie as still as possible during the actual EKG.

Real-World Connection

EKG Imperfection

A 44-year-old female had not been feeling well for 3 to 4 weeks and had visited her family practitioner on several occasions. Her complaints were vague and hard to describe. She was tired and said that she "just did not feel right." Various blood tests were run, producing normal results. After discussing her case with her physician during one of her visits, they mutually decided she should start taking a good multiple vitamin, pay more attention to her eating habits, drink plenty of water, and get plenty of rest and regular exercise.

The physician ran a routine EKG, just to be on the safe side, before she increased her exercise level above what she had been doing prior to their discussion. The EKG was the first one she had ever had, and the results appeared normal with no areas of concern. A couple days later, she was at work in her office, when she suddenly stood up and grabbed her chest. Before she could utter a word, she fell to the floor, unresponsive and without pulse or respiration. One of her employees called 911 and an ambulance was dispatched. She was pronounced dead-on-arrival at the local hospital emergency room. Autopsy results indicated that she had died of a massive myocardial infarction (MI) and that she had experienced numerous MIs previously that had gone undetected.

This real-life example demonstrates the fact that EKGs *cannot* rule out heart disease or a past or current MI. Though an EKG *may* be helpful and sometimes does detect *cardiac ischemia,* which is a lack of blood to the heart muscle, and an active MI, it is not 100% assured that a patient is not having heart problems—especially in women, whose cardiac signs and symptoms present differently than they do in men.

Telemetry Monitoring

A telemetry monitor is a portable heart monitor. The battery pack is about the size of a pager. Wires (also called leads) attached to the battery pack connect to electrodes placed on the patient's chest. The electrodes are disposable foam circles with a connection in the middle that transmit the electrical activity of the heart as a waveform. The patient can then get up and move around without being hardwired to a bedside monitor, while his or her heart rhythm is being continuously monitored. At a remote monitoring station, monitor technicians will watch the continuous waveform on a screen.

Any abnormalities in the heart's activity are detected by the computerized equipment and printed out as an EKG strip. The monitor technician will notify the nurse caring for the patient of any abnormal rhythms.

You may get a call to check the telemetry unit on a patient if the monitor technician is not able to clearly see the waveform. Go to the patient's room promptly, then check each wire to be sure it is firmly inserted in the battery pack and firmly attached to the electrode. Check each electrode to be sure it is firmly stuck to the chest wall. If you need to change the battery, open the sliding cover at the bottom of the battery pack, replace the old battery with a fresh one, and close the cover. Telephone the monitor station from the patient's room to verify that a clearer picture has been obtained.

Safety: When you remove a telemetry unit for any reason, such as to give a bath or shower, you MUST first call the monitor station and tell the technician that you are going to remove the unit. The monitor technician will flag the patient's display with the reason the telemetry unit is off. Replace the unit immediately after completing the bath or shower; then telephone the monitor station from the patient's room to be sure the display is clear. It is also important to call the monitor technician prior to removing the unit when the health care provider has discontinued the order for it.

Figure 25-3 The electrical impulse initiating contraction of the heart muscle (heartbeat) begins in the sinoatrial node and is conveyed through the rest of the electrical conduction pathway. The P wave represents the depolarization of the atria, the result of which is contraction of the atria. The QRS complex represents the depolarization of the ventricles, resulting in contraction of the ventricles. The T wave represents the repolarization of the ventricles, during which the ventricles relax in preparation for the next depolarization. Each of the boxes on the EKG strip represents the length of time that it takes the impulse to travel through the designated sections of the conduction pathway.

The disposable electrodes are usually changed after the bath or when they no longer stick to the chest well. Replace the electrodes according to your facility's policy. Return the battery pack to the gown pocket or pouch. Be sure the pouch is clean and comfortable for the patient.

The electrodes and wires may be placed on the chest in a variety of patterns to transmit the heart's electrical activity. The right and left upper chest near the shoulders are used for the arm lead placements. The lower limb leads are usually placed on the lower ribs toward the patient's sides. A ground wire may be placed on the center of the chest when five wires are used. The wires are color-coded for placement. For example, the white wire is placed on the right upper chest to represent the right arm. Follow your facility's policy for electrode placement.

One way to remember electrode placement is to follow this guide:

- **White to the right:** White goes on right upper chest
- **Clouds over grass:** White on right upper chest, green on right lower chest
- **Smoke over fire:** Black on left upper chest, red on left lower chest
- **Brown is ground:** Brown goes in the middle of the chest

Holter Monitors

A Holter monitor is an even more portable electrocardiograph than the telemetry unit. This type of monitoring device can be worn by the patient at home. It is usually ordered for a 24- to 48-hour period. It weighs about 2 pounds and is placed in a harness that the patient wears on his or her back. Again, electrodes are placed on the patient's chest with lead wires attached. The Holter monitor records the patient's EKG for the entire period that it is worn. The patient is asked to keep a diary of his or her activities during the 24- to 48-hour period. If the patient feels symptoms, such as chest discomfort, pain, or palpitations, he or she will push the "event" button, which marks the EKG recording for later analysis by the physician. This type of monitoring works well for patients who have cardiac symptoms that occur with activity or at widely spaced intervals.

Electroencephalography

In **electroencephalography (EEG)**, electrodes are placed strategically on the scalp and record the electrical activity of the brain, known as *brain waves*. This study is beneficial in detecting epilepsy, diseases of the central nervous system, and tumors, and to confirm brain death.

Nursing Care for Electroencephalography

Explain the procedure to the patient and family, being careful to include that it is painless. Wash the patient's hair to remove all hair spray and styling products. After the patient returns to his or her room, it may be necessary to shampoo the hair to remove the electrode paste. If the EEG confirmed brain death, be prepared to support the family in this difficult time. It may be helpful to offer to telephone a minister or member of the clergy for the family.

Knowledge Connection
What is the purpose of an EKG? Does a normal EKG always prove that the patient does not have heart problems? Give three purposes for which an EEG might be performed.

Skill 25-1 Assisting with Aspiration Procedures: Bone Marrow, Lumbar Puncture, and Paracentesis

Assessment Steps

1. Verify the patient's understanding of preprocedure teaching.
2. Verify that written consent has been obtained for the procedure.
3. *Safety: Assess for patient allergies to local anesthetic, as well as iodine and shellfish if an iodine-based cleanser is to be used for the preparation.*

Planning Steps

1. Gather needed equipment and supplies:
   a. **Bone marrow aspiration:** bone marrow aspiration tray, sterile gloves, local anesthetic, prep cleansing solution, labels for laboratory specimens, dressing supplies (sterile gauze and tape or bandage).
   b. **Lumbar puncture:** lumbar puncture tray, extra spinal needle, sterile gloves, local anesthetic, prep cleansing solution, labels for laboratory specimens, vital sign equipment, dressing supplies (sterile gauze and tape, bandage, or small occlusive pressure dressing).
   c. **Paracentesis:** paracentesis tray, sterile gloves, large calibrated container, local anesthetic, prep cleansing solution, labels for laboratory specimens, vital sign equipment, dressing supplies (sterile gauze and tape or bandage).

Implementation Steps

1. Follow the Initial Implementation Steps located on the inside front cover.
2. Set up the sterile field *to prevent contamination.*
3. Position the patient for the procedure:
   a. **Bone marrow aspiration:** Supine for tibial or sternal aspiration, side-lying for iliac crest aspiration.
   b. **Lumbar puncture:** Side-lying with knees flexed onto abdomen and chin tucked against chest, close to the edge of the bed.
   c. **Paracentesis:** Semi-Fowler's position.
4. Assist the physician as needed with cleansing prep of injection site and drawing up of local anesthetic.

(skill continues on page 552)

Skill 25-1 (continued)

5. Reassure the patient and assist him or her to remain in the proper position throughout the procedure.

6. After completion of the procedure, hold pressure on the puncture site for at least 5 minutes *to prevent bleeding*. Once you are certain that bleeding has stopped, apply a bandage, small dressing, or occlusive pressure dressing as appropriate.

7. Apply labels to specimens before sending them to the laboratory.

8. Follow the Ending Implementation Steps located on the inside back cover.

9. Document the procedure and the patient's tolerance of it.

Evaluation Steps

1. Assess vital signs, noting any signs of hypotension or shock.

2. Assess the puncture site for bleeding or drainage.

3. Position the patient for comfort.

4. Send laboratory specimens to the laboratory.

Sample Documentation

12/1/10   0900   Placed in supine position. Baseline VS:
BP – 132/68, T – 98.6, P – 68 reg & strong, R – 14 reg & even.
Abdomen cleansing prep performed using Betadine. 1% lidocaine
injected at intended puncture site just above the umbilicus.
Paracentesis performed by Dr. Holsted with 750 mL cloudy, yellow
fluid returned. Pressure held on injection site for 5 minutes.
No signs of bleeding noted. No problems noted during procedure.
No complaints of discomfort. ———————————————
————————————— Nurse's signature and credentials
0925   VS: BP – 138/74, P – 74 reg & strong, R – 17 reg
& even. ————————— Nurse's signature and credentials.

Skill 25-2 Performing a 12-Lead Electrocardiogram (EKG)

Assessment Steps

1. Review the EKG machine manual for specifics of operating that particular model.

Planning Steps

1. Gather needed equipment and supplies: EKG machine with 10 lead wires, 10 new pre-gelled electrodes or 10 non-gelled electrodes with a bottle of conduction gel, alcohol sponges, razor, washcloth.

Implementation Steps

1. Follow the Initial Implementation Steps located on the inside front cover.

2. Position the patient in the semi-Fowler's or supine position, making him or her as comfortable as possible. Remove the patient's shirt or blouse and bra. Cover with a patient gown that opens in the front *to help preserve modesty*. Remove necklaces, bracelets, and watches *to prevent interference with the electrical tracing*.

3. If necessary, shave small areas on the chest at the sites for application of electrodes. If shaving is not necessary, remove body oil at the sites using alcohol sponges *so that electrodes will make good contact with the skin*.

4. Enter appropriate data into the EKG machine *to allow for proper identification and interpretation of results on the EKG printout*.

5. Apply 10 electrodes. The electrodes will either be pre-gelled or you may have to apply a small amount of conduction gel *to ensure adequate conduction of electrical impulses*. Apply four electrodes to the medial or inner aspects of both wrists and ankles,

ensuring good contact with skin. Then apply six electrodes to the chest:
- V_1 at the right sternal border in the fourth intercostal space
- V_2 at the left sternal border in the fourth intercostal space
- V_4 in the fifth intercostal space in the midclavicular line
- V_3 halfway between V_2 and V_4
- V_5 to the left of the V_4 electrode in the anterior axillary line
- V_6 to the left of the V_5 electrode in the midaxillary line.

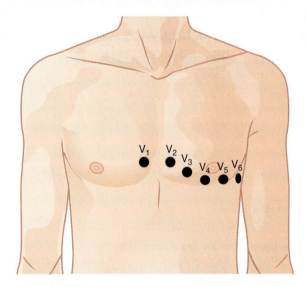

Ensure good contact with skin. *If the electrodes are not placed correctly, the tracing will not be reliable.*

Skill 25-2 (continued)

6. Attach the lead wires to the electrodes. The six chest lead wires will be marked V_1, V_2, V_3, V_4, V_5, and V_6. Attach the lead wires to the electrodes at the corresponding sites on the patient's chest.

7. Request that the patient hold completely still *to avoid interference during the EKG.*

8. Following the manual instructions, press the run button.

9. After reviewing the EKG printout for correct appearance, turn off the machine.

10. Remove the electrodes and clean the skin with alcohol wipes or a damp cloth *to remove any residue from the conduction gel.* Assist the patient to dress if necessary.

11. Follow the Ending Implementation Steps located on the inside back cover.

Evaluation Steps

1. Review the EKG printout and notify the physician of pertinent findings.

Sample Documentation

3/12/10   1415   12-lead EKG performed without difficulty. Results phoned to Dr. Heart. ————————
———————————— Nurse's signature and credentials

Post Conference

When you enter the conference room for Post Conference, another student says, "I bet you had an easy day. Your patient was just having tests, right?" You respond by saying, "She had quite a time of it. She was terrified of having her blood drawn, vomited while she was in the radiology department, and had abdominal pains during the ultrasound." Your patient benefited from your teaching and was relieved to know that, although four vials of blood were drawn, the technician only had to stick her once with the needle, not once for each test. She knew what to expect when she was sedated for the EGD, and was glad you were there when she had the ultrasound, which turned out to be painful because of her extreme abdominal tenderness. By the end of your shift, the physician was feeling confident about a diagnosis of pancreatitis. And you would never have the attitude that a patient was "just having tests," having seen firsthand what was involved in her care.

KEY POINTS

- CBC components include the WBC, RBC, PLTs, Hgb, and Hct.

- A differential assesses the level of the five types of leukocytes: lymphocytes, neutrophils, basophils, monocytes, and eosinophils. A left shift indicates bacterial infection and a right shift indicates viral infection.

- The nurse's role includes explanation of the test, verifying that written consent has been obtained, knowing when to keep the patient NPO, physically preparing the patient for the test, obtaining specimens, supporting the patient, assisting the examiner, monitoring for complications, providing post-test nursing care, and understanding the significance of the test results.

- Some of the most common diagnostic tests include the CBC, urinalysis, CXR, and EKG.

- CT scans and MRI are methods of producing and recording images of organs and tissues, done in sequential slices so the tissue can be examined at every depth.

- The nurse must assess for allergies to iodine, shellfish, radiopaque dye, and contrast media prior to any procedure that requires a contrast medium to be used.

- Common tests to evaluate renal function include the GFR and creatinine.

- Common tests to evaluate liver function include the AST, ALT, ALK, and bilirubin.

- Common tests to evaluate cardiac function include the EKG, troponin, CK-MB, and LD_1 and LD_2.

- Common tests to evaluate the gastrointestinal tract include the EGD, colonoscopy, and barium enema.

- Common tests to evaluate blood flow include arteriograms and venograms.

REVIEW QUESTIONS

Select the answer that is most important for each of the following questions. Some questions may have more than one correct answer. Check all that apply.

1. Which of the following urinalysis findings would you need to report to the physician?

   a. Protein: 2 +

   b. Bacteria: 0

   c. White blood cells: 3 to 4 per high-power field

   d. pH: 4.1

   e. Specific gravity: 1.025

   f. Red blood cells: 10 per high-power field

2. Which of the following preparatory steps would you be likely to perform prior to a barium enema?

   a. Start an IV line the day prior to the test.

   b. Keep the patient NPO 48 hours prior to the test.

   c. Administer a laxative the day before the test.

   d. Place the patient on a clear liquid diet for 24 hours prior to the test.

   e. Administer an enema the evening before the test.

3. Which of the following tests would be helpful evaluating the large intestine?

   a. Colonoscopy

   b. Esophagogastroduodenoscopy

   c. Barium enema

   d. Electrocardiography

   e. Intravenous pyelogram

   f. Hemoglobin and hematocrit

4. Which of the following findings indicate a left shift and bacterial infection in an adult?

   a. WBC: 13,900/mm³; total neutrophils: 82% (bands: 40%, segmented: 42%); eosinophils: 2%; basophils: 1%; lymphocytes: 15%

   b. WBC: 4,600/mm³; total neutrophils: 65% (bands: 5%, segmented: 60%); eosinophils: 4%; basophils: 1%; lymphocytes: 30%

   c. WBC: 11,350/mm³; total neutrophils: 55% (bands: 3%, segmented: 52%); eosinophils: 12%; basophils: 2%; lymphocytes: 31%

   d. WBC: 10,450/mm³; total neutrophils: 70% (bands: 5%, segmented: 65%); eosinophils: 2%; basophils: 0%; lymphocytes: 28%

5. Which of the following tests or procedures is (are) beneficial in evaluation of the kidneys?

   a. Intravenous pyelogram

   b. 24-hour urine

   c. Oral glucose tolerance test

   d. Urinalysis

   e. Glomerular filtration rate

   f. Creatinine

6. You are to provide nursing care for a patient who just had a femoral arteriogram. Which of the following actions would take priority?

   a. Assessment of vital signs

   b. Assessment of puncture site for bleeding

   c. Assessment of temperature of lower extremity on the affected side

   d. Keeping the affected leg straight

   e. Assessment of ability to void

   f. Providing PO fluids

7. You should measure the abdominal girth and weight of a patient who is about to undergo:

   a. glucose tolerance test.

   b. CT scan of the cerebrum.

   c. alkaline phosphatase test.

   d. paracentesis.

   e. lumbar puncture.

8. When performing a 12-lead EKG, you know that you will apply:

   a. 12 lead wires.

   b. 10 lead wires.

   c. 6 lead wires.

   d. 4 lead wires.

CRITICAL THINKING EXERCISES

9. You are assigned to provide nursing care for a patient who is scheduled for a colonoscopy tomorrow morning. In report, you are told that she is extremely nervous and frightened regarding the procedure. What can you to do help this patient?

10. Why is it so important that you provide thorough patient teaching regarding any upcoming tests or procedures?

ADDITIONAL RESOURCES

For additional Resources, Questions, and Activities, please see:

 Student Resource Disk

  http://davisplus.fadavis.com

Student Study Guide

REFERENCES

Dillon PM. *Nursing Health Assessment: A Critical Thinking Case Studies Approach.* 2nd ed. Philadelphia: FA Davis; 2007.

Fischer RA. Device safety: Danger: beware of unretrieved device fragments. *Nursing2007.* 2007;37(11):17.

Hopkins T. *Lab Notes: Guide to Lab & Diagnostic Tests.* 2nd ed. Philadelphia: FA Davis; 2009.

Lawrence BL, Taylor D. Eye on diagnostics: Esophageal pH monitoring goes wireless. *Nursing2007.* 2007;37(10):26-27.

Rhoads J, Meeker BJ. *Davis's Guide to Clinical Nursing Skills.* Philadelphia: FA Davis; 2007.

Scanlon V, Sanders T. *Essentials of Anatomy and Physiology.* 5th ed. Philadelphia: FA Davis; 2007.

Schoch L, Whiteman K. Eye on diagnostics: Monitoring liver function. *Nursing2007.* 2007;37(11):22-23.

Smeltzer SC, Bare BG, Hinkle JL, Cheever KH. *Brunner & Suddarth's Textbook of Medical-Surgical Nursing.* 11th ed. Philadelphia: Lippincott Williams & Wilkins; 2008.

Starkey C. *Therapeutic Modalities.* 3rd ed. Philadelphia: FA Davis; 2004.

The Joint Commission. *2010 National Patient Safety Goals.* Available at: http://www.jointcommission.org/PatientSafety/ NationalPatientSafetyGoals/. Accessed October 19, 2009.

Venes D, ed. *Taber's Cyclopedic Medical Dictionary.* 21st ed. Philadelphia: FA Davis; 2009.

Wilkinson JM, Van Leuven K. *Fundamentals of Nursing: Theory, Concepts & Applications.* Philadelphia: FA Davis; 2007.

Williams LS, Hopper PD. *Understanding Medical-Surgical Nursing.* 3rd ed. Philadelphia: FA Davis; 2007.

Key Terms

Abrasion

Débridement

Dehiscence

Edema

Erythema

Eschar

Evisceration

Granulation tissue

Hemorrhage

Ischemia

Laceration

Methicillin-resistant *Staphylococcus aureus* (MRSA)

Necrotic

Pressure ulcer

Purulent

Sanguineous

Serosanguineous

Serous

Sinus tract

Objectives

1. Define key terms related to wound care.
2. Contrast contusion, abrasion, puncture, penetrating, and laceration wounds.
3. Differentiate between clean, clean-contaminated, contaminated, infected, colonized, open, and closed wounds.
4. Identify risk factors for pressure ulcers.
5. Correctly stage pressure ulcers.
6. Outline nursing interventions to prevent pressure ulcers.
7. Describe other types of wounds: stasis ulcers, sinus tracts, and surgical incisions.
8. Explain the three phases of healing.
9. Compare first, second, and third intention wound closures.
10. Explain how different factors affect wound healing.
11. Describe possible complications of wound healing and appropriate nursing care for each.
12. Discuss wound treatments and the nursing responsibilities for oaoh.
13. Accurately assess a wound and wound drainage.
14. Describe types of dressings and their uses.
15. Relate low serum protein levels to wound healing
16. Identify information to document concerning wounds.
17. Develop a care plan for a patient with a pressure ulcer.

Skills

26-1 Removing Sutures and Staples

26-2 Caring for Drainage Devices

26-3 Irrigating a Wound

26-4 Obtaining a Wound Culture

26-5 Changing Sterile Dressings and Wet-to-Damp Dressings

26-6 Applying Transparent and Hydrocolloid Dressings

As you care for patients, you will encounter a variety of wounds requiring various treatments. In this chapter, you will learn about different types of wounds, ulcers, drains, drainage, and dressings. You will be able to determine the likelihood of infection by assessing a wound. You will learn to measure and describe a wound, and to evaluate healing in a wound. You will be prepared and confident that you will not miss anything.

Types of Wounds

Wounds are categorized as either open or closed. A wound in which the skin remains intact is considered a *closed wound*. A wound in which the skin integrity has been breached is an *open wound*. In addition to being categorized as open or closed, wounds may also be classified as contusions, abrasions, puncture wounds, penetrating wounds, lacerations, or pressure ulcers.

Contusions

A contusion is a closed discolored wound caused by blunt trauma, better known as a *bruise*. Though the skin is intact, there is injury to the tissues underneath the epidermis, which may swell as blood leaks from broken blood vessels into the *interstitial spaces* (the spaces between cells). This extra fluid in the interstitial space causes pressure on the nerve endings, resulting in pain or tenderness. The leakage of blood causes the skin to be discolored, generally a bright red or purple color that fades over a period of days to blue, bluish-green, and finally to yellow as the contusion heals (Fig. 26-1).

Abrasions

An **abrasion** is a superficial open wound; abrasions include scrapes, scratches, or rub-type wounds where the skin is broken, such as a carpet burn or a skinned knee. These wounds are generally superficial and heal well if kept clean (see Fig. 26-1).

Puncture Wounds

A puncture wound is an open wound that results when a sharp item, such as a needle, nail, or piece of wire, pierces the skin. The resulting wound is a round hole in the skin that extends down into the deeper tissues, according to the diameter and length of the offending sharp item (see Fig. 26-1).

Penetrating Wounds

A penetrating wound is similar to a puncture wound, with the difference being that the offending object remains embedded in the tissue. The degree of damage depends upon the size of the object and the tissues or organs affected by the penetration (see Fig. 26-1).

Lacerations

A **laceration** is an open wound made by the accidental cutting or tearing of tissue. Common sources of lacerations include knives and pieces of glass and metal. Unlike a surgical incision, it has jagged edges, often making closure of the wound more difficult and less aesthetically pleasing (see Fig. 26-1).

Pressure Ulcers

A **pressure ulcer** is a wound resulting from pressure and friction. The skin may be intact and *erythemic* (reddened), or the skin may be broken. If the skin is broken, the ulcer may be superficial or very deep.

Contamination of Wounds

Wounds fall into one of the following categories:

- **Clean:** A wound that is not infected.
- **Clean-contaminated:** A wound that was surgically made, is not infected, but has direct contact with the normal flora

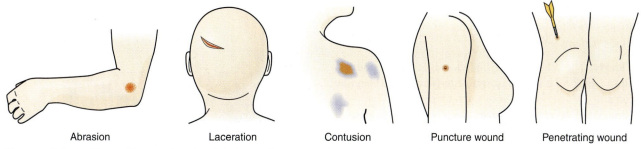

Figure 26-1   Types of wounds: abrasion, laceration, contusion, puncture, and penetrating.

| Abrasion | Laceration | Contusion | Puncture wound | Penetrating wound |

in either the respiratory tract, urinary tract, or gastrointestinal tract. It has more potential to become infected.

- **Contaminated:** This can be a surgical wound or a wound caused by trauma that has been grossly contaminated by breaking asepsis.
- **Infected:** An infected wound is one in which the infectious process is already established, evidenced by high numbers of microorganisms and either **purulent** (containing pus) drainage or **necrotic** (dead) tissue. The classic signs of infection include **erythema** (redness), increased warmth, **edema** (swelling), pain, odor, and drainage.
- **Colonized:** A colonized wound differs from an infected wound in that it has a high number of microorganisms present but is without signs of infection.

Knowledge Connection
Which type of wounds are considered *open?* Which type of wounds are considered *closed?* List the classic signs and symptoms of an infected wound.

Pressure Ulcers

A pressure ulcer, also known as a *decubitus ulcer or bedsore,* occurs when external pressure is exerted on soft tissues, especially over bony prominences, for a prolonged period of time. Tissues and capillaries are compressed, resulting in reduced blood flow to the area, known as **ischemia**. Under normal conditions, blood delivers the vital oxygen and nutrients required for cells to stay alive. Ischemia deprives the involved tissues of adequate oxygen and nutrients and, if this state persists, the cells will eventually *necrose* (die).

Pressure ulcers can also develop as a direct result of friction or shearing force. Shearing force occurs when the patient's skin and another item, such as bed linens or the surface of a chair, move in opposite directions while being pressed together by the weight of the body. This movement results in friction that can pull the tissue apart, or shear it from the body. If a patient is pulled or dragged across the bed rather than lifted, shearing force to the patient's skin can result in destruction of the epidermis and dermis.

The most common sites for development of pressure ulcers are over the bony prominences such as the sacrum, buttocks, greater trochanters, elbows, heels, ankles, occiput

(back of the head), and scapulae (Fig. 26-2). The longer the pressure is maintained on the area, the worse the extent of necrosis that occurs.

Knowledge Connection
What is the main cause of pressure ulcers? Where are the most common sites for them to develop?

Figure 26-2   Pressure points in the Fowler's, lateral, and supine positions.

Risk Factors for Pressure Ulcers

Patients who are prone to development of pressure ulcers include patients who are:

- **Elderly:** The skin of elderly individuals is thinner and less elastic, making it more susceptible to friction and shearing force.
- **Emaciated or malnourished:** *Emaciation* is the state of being very lean or having very little muscle.
- **Incontinent of bowel or bladder:** With incontinence of bowel or bladder, the skin of the perineal area tends to be wet much of the time, leading it to become *macerated,* or softened.
- **Immobile:** This includes patients who are paralyzed, or have casts or splints, as well as those restricted to a bed or chair.
- **Impaired circulation or chronic metabolic conditions:** Chronic metabolic conditions such as diabetes result in impairment of circulation, which can increase the risk of ischemic tissue.

Staging Pressure Ulcers

Pressure ulcers can range in appearance from a reddened area to deep craters that involve muscle and even bone. They are *staged,* or classified, according to the extent and depth of damage for a total of six classifications. This staging scale is utilized solely for pressure ulcers (Fig. 26-3).

Deep Tissue Injury

A deep tissue injury (DTI) usually begins with an area over a bony prominence that differs from the surrounding tissue, in either temperature, texture, firmness, or discomfort level. It may form a blood-filled blister or a thin blister that overlies a dark wound bed. The blister may break and reveal a thin layer of eschar underneath. However, a DTI may not include a blister at all. The area may simply turn a dark burgundy, purple, or maroon color, like a bruise. Any of these presentations represent injury to the underlying soft tissue.

Stage I

A stage I pressure ulcer is indicated by erythema, generally over a bony prominence, that remains for at least 15 to 30 minutes after relieving the pressure—and it will not *blanch,* or turn white, when you gently touch it with your fingertip. In a darker skinned individual, the skin may appear darkened rather than red. The area may feel warm and firm, soft, or boggy. Avoid massaging the erythematous area as this may cause further tissue damage. The patient may complain of burning or tingling at the site. Further damage and progression of the pressure ulcer can be prevented at this stage if appropriate measures are taken.

Stage II

A stage II pressure ulcer occurs when there is a partial-thickness loss of dermis. This would include intact serum-filled

Figure 26-3 The stages of pressure ulcers: a. Stage I pressure ulcer. b. Stage II pressure ulcer. c. Stage III pressure ulcer. d. Stage IV pressure ulcer. e. Unstageable pressure ulcer due to presence of eschar.

blisters and broken blisters that reveal a shallow, pink or red ulceration that can be either shiny or dry. Generally there is erythema surrounding the skin break. The erythematous area may feel warmer than the surrounding skin due to the increased blood flow.

A stage II ulcer is harder to heal than a stage I ulcer and may allow microorganisms to enter and multiply so that an infection is possible.

Stage III

The stage III pressure ulcer is a full-thickness loss involving damage to the epidermis, dermis, and subcutaneous tissue, but not involving muscle or bone. Undermining and tunneling may be seen in this stage. The depth of tissue loss is discernable even if slough is present. These wounds tend to be infected, may produce drainage, and take longer to heal than a stage I or II pressure ulcer, because a great deal of granulation tissue must be produced to fill the wound and repair the damage.

Stage IV

The stage IV pressure ulcer is also a full-thickness tissue loss, only it involves deep tissue necrosis of muscle, fascia, tendon, joint capsule, and sometimes bone. As in a stage III ulcer, there may be tunneling and undermining. Infection in a stage IV ulcer can involve deeper tissues such as the bone, a condition known as *osteomyelitis*. Due to the massive tissue destruction, this ulcer may be extremely slow to completely heal, depending upon the patient's health status.

Unstageable

These pressure ulcers also involve full-thickness tissue loss but are impossible to accurately stage due to the wound bed being completely obscured by eschar or excessive slough. **Eschar** is hard, dry, dead tissue that has a leathery appearance. It can be black, brown, or tan. The ulcer cannot be staged until there is at least a portion of the wound bed exposed to detect the depth of the ulcer. If eschar remains intact and stable, completely covering a site such as the heel, it should not be removed. It should be left alone to cover and protect the damaged tissue underneath it.

Knowledge Connection

Describe the differences between the six classifications of pressure ulcers. How do you explain the fact that eschar must be removed before an ulcer can be accurately staged?

Real-World Connection

How Deep Can a Pressure Ulcer Be?

In a skilled nursing facility, a 29-year-old male patient was admitted from a distant hospital. The patient was a paraplegic and had no feeling from the waist down, with bilateral above-the-knee amputations and severe uncontrolled diabetes. It was noted in the records that the patient had a pressure ulcer on the sacral-coccyx area and a Foley catheter to drain his bladder of urine. While admitting the patient and making him comfortable in the bed, the nursing staff noted that the linens under his hips were wet with urine, thought to be from a leaking catheter. As the assessment continued, the nursing staff

rolled the patient to one side to assess the pressure ulcer. When the dressing was removed, the nurses discovered that the inflated Foley catheter balloon was visible deep in the base of the ulcer. The ulcer was so large and deep that it extended through the subcutaneous layers, fascia, and muscular layers all the way through the posterior wall of his bladder. Most of the urine was leaking directly from the bladder onto the dressing and bed.

This is why it is important to take appropriate measures to prevent the development of pressure ulcers before they begin and to treat even mild stage I pressure ulcers as soon as they are identified. Otherwise, they can progress to unbelievable extents very quickly.

Prevention of Pressure Ulcers

The majority of pressure ulcers can be prevented with good nursing care, which starts with thorough assessment of the skin and pressure points. Many facilities use standardized scales of assessment, such as the Braden scale (Fig. 26-4).

Skin assessment should be done on a daily basis. If the patient is restricted in mobility to any degree, assess the skin every 8 hours at a minimum. If the patient is bedfast, assess the pressure points every 2 hours. In an individual with multiple risk factors for skin breakdown, it is possible for pressure ulcers to occur in 2 to 3 hours. Look for excessively dry skin as evidenced by flaking or peeling. Look for areas where the skin is broken, excoriated, or blistered. Assess the color of the skin, noting any:

- **Pallor:** related to impaired circulation, which is a major risk factor for skin breakdown
- **Erythema:** indicates the increased capillary blood flow associated with inflammation
- **Jaundice:** also known as yellowing of the skin, jaundice is a sign of an abnormally high serum level of bilirubin, which can make skin itch and be more susceptible to loss of integrity
- **Bruising:** discolored areas; make notations of any such areas that are found, so it is easy to determine if new breakdown occurs

Determine if skin turgor is elastic or nonelastic. This helps you determine whether the patient's hydration is adequate, another important factor for healthy skin. A patient who is dehydrated or edematous from overhydration will have increased risk for skin breakdown.

After establishing the skin's condition, reposition the patient at least every 2 hours to avoid pressure and compromise of circulation to the area. Keep the skin clean and dry. Assess an incontinent patient's incontinence pads or linens every hour. Keep linens free of wrinkles, which can cause further areas of increased pressure. Skin care for the immobile patient may include application of lotion to dry skin and assessment of pressure points for erythema every 1 to 2 hours. Immobile patients should be lifted with a draw sheet or mechanical lift rather than dragged across the bed or

BRADEN SCALE FOR PREDICTING PRESSURE SORE RISK

Patient's Name _____ Evaluator's Name _____ Date of Assessment _____

	1	2	3	4				
SENSORY PERCEPTION ability to respond meaningfully to pressure-related discomfort	**1. Completely Limited** Unresponsive (does not moan, flinch, or grasp) to painful stimuli, due to diminished level of consciousness or sedation. OR limited ability to feel pain over most of body.	**2. Very Limited** Responds only to painful stimuli. Cannot communicate discomfort except by moaning or restlessness OR has a sensory impairment which limits the ability to feel pain or discomfort over 1/2 of body.	**3. Slightly Limited** Responds to verbal commands, but cannot always communicate discomfort or the need to be turned. OR has some sensory impairment which limits ability to feel pain or discomfort in 1 or 2 extremities.	**4. No Impairment** Responds to verbal commands. Has no sensory deficit which would limit ability to feel or voice pain or discomfort.				
MOISTURE degree to which skin is exposed to moisture	**1. Constantly Moist** Skin is kept moist almost constantly by perspiration, urine, etc. Dampness is detected every time patient is moved or turned.	**2. Very Moist** Skin is often, but not always moist. Linen must be changed at least once a shift.	**3. Occasionally Moist:** Skin is occasionally moist, requiring an extra linen change approximately once a day.	**4. Rarely Moist** Skin is usually dry, linen only requires changing at routine intervals.				
ACTIVITY degree of physical activity	**1. Bedfast** Confined to bed.	**2. Chairfast** Ability to walk severely limited or non-existent. Cannot bear own weight and/or must be assisted into chair or wheelchair.	**3. Walks Occasionally** Walks occasionally during day, but for very short distances, with or without assistance. Spends majority of each shift in bed or chair.	**4. Walks Frequently** Walks outside room at least twice a day and inside room at least once every two hours during waking hours.				
MOBILITY ability to change and control body position	**1. Completely Immobile** Does not make even slight changes in body or extremity position without assistance.	**2. Very Limited** Makes occasional slight changes in body or extremity position but unable to make frequent or significant changes independently.	**3. Slightly Limited** Makes frequent though slight changes in body or extremity position independently.	**4. No Limitation** Makes major and frequent changes in position without assistance.				
NUTRITION usual food intake pattern	**1. Very Poor** Never eats a complete meal. Rarely eats more than 1/2 of any food offered. Eats 2 servings or less of protein (meat or dairy products) per day. Takes fluids poorly. Does not take a liquid dietary supplement OR is NPO and/or maintained on clear liquids or IVs for more than 5 days.	**2. Probably Inadequate** Rarely eats a complete meal and generally eats only about 1/2 of any food offered. Protein intake includes only 3 servings of meat or dairy products per day. Occasionally will take a dietary supplement. OR receives less than optimum amount of liquid diet or tube feeding.	**3. Adequate** Eats over half of most meals. Eats a total of 4 servings of protein (meat, dairy products) per day. Occasionally will refuse a meal, but will usually take a supplement when offered OR is on a tube feeding or TPN regimen which probably meets most of nutritional needs.	**4. Excellent** Eats most of every meal. Never refuses a meal. Usually eats a total of 4 or more servings of meat and dairy products. Occasionally eats between meals. Does not require supplementation.				
FRICTION & SHEAR	**1. Problem** Requires moderate to maximum assistance in moving. Complete lifting without sliding against sheets is impossible. Frequently slides down in bed or chair, requiring frequent repositioning with maximum assistance. Spasticity, contractures or agitation leads to almost constant friction.	**2. Potential Problem** Moves feebly or requires minimum assistance. During a move skin probably slides to some extent against sheets, chair, restraints or other devices. Maintains relatively good position in chair or bed most of the time but occasionally slides down.	**3. No Apparent Problem** Moves in bed and in chair independently and has sufficient muscle strength to lift up completely during move. Maintains good position in bed or chair.					

Total Score _____

Figure 26-4   Braden Scale for Predicting Pressure Sore Risk.

chair. To remove linens from underneath a patient, the patient should be rolled to one side and the linens folded to the center of the bed. Then the patient is rolled to the other side and linens are removed. This prevents the shearing that occurs when linens are simply pulled out from under the patient. It is also important to make certain the patient receives adequate fluids and nutrition. Protein, mineral, and vitamin drink supplements may be given when patients fail to consume adequate meats, fruits, and vegetables at mealtimes.

Numerous specialty beds and devices are available that help to decrease the risk of pressure ulcers. Pressure-relieving devices include sheepskin pads, foam eggcrate mattresses, gel-filled pads and mattresses, air-filled mattresses and overlays, and beds that pump air through mattresses filled with tiny beads, known as air-fluidized beds. (These devices are discussed in Chapter 16.) For extremities, there are foam and sheepskin protectors made to fit elbows and heels (Fig. 26-5).

Other Wounds Found in Hospitalized Patients

Pressure ulcers are only one kind of wound found in hospitalized patients. Other wounds include stasis ulcers, draining sinus tracts, and surgical incisions.

Stasis Ulcers

Stasis ulcers develop when the venous blood flow is sluggish, generally in the lower extremities, allowing deoxygenated blood to pool in the veins. These ulcers develop from chronic valve problems, blood clots, and other conditions that interrupt venous blood flow, such as chronic venous insufficiency. The resulting edema damages surrounding tissues and causes ulcers to develop. This chronic condition is very difficult to heal.

Draining Sinus Tracts

A **sinus tract** is a channel or tunnel that develops between two cavities or between an infected cavity and the surface of the skin, sometimes known as a *fistula* (Fig. 26-6). A sinus tract that forms due to infection usually produces purulent drainage that is thick and yellow or green. If the sinus tract opens onto the skin's surface, it usually has to be irrigated and packed with strips of tiny gauze-like material to absorb the drainage until the infection clears and the tract can be allowed to heal.

Surgical Incisions

Surgical incisions, intentionally made with sharp instruments, are linear with more sharply defined edges than most wounds. The two edges of an incision should have good *approximation,* meaning they should be close together. (See Figure 26-7 for an illustration of an incision with areas of poor approximation.) An incision may be closed with sutures, staples, Steri-Strips, or skin adhesive.

Wound Healing

To accurately assess a wound, you must know how a wound heals. Whether the wound is a surgical incision, a pressure ulcer, or due to trauma, the steps in the healing process are the same and occur in three phases.

Phases of the Healing Process

Inflammatory Phase

This phase occurs when the wound is fresh and includes both hemostasis and phagocytosis. During *hemostasis,* the body stops the bleeding associated with the fresh wound. The damaged blood vessels constrict and retract to decrease blood

Figure 26-5 Heel protectors are lined with soft material and strapped onto the foot. Elbow protectors slip over the patient's arms to prevent pressure on the bony prominences of the elbows.

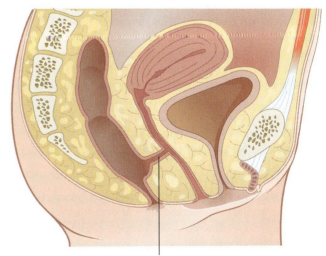

Fistula between rectum and vagina (enterovaginal)

Figure 26-6 A fistula or sinus tract can connect two body cavities, or can tunnel from a body cavity or wound to the skin. This fistula connects the vagina and the rectum.

Figure 26-7 The wound edges of this surgical incision are not well approximated. The *arrows* point to areas where the skin edges do not meet.

flow. A clot begins to form as fibrin is deposited in the wound. Eventually, a scab forms over the wound, protecting it from contamination. During *phagocytosis,* specialized white blood cells (macrophages) engulf and digest invading microorganisms and the remaining fragments of damaged cells.

Signs of inflammation include warmth, redness, pain, and edema. These are due to increased blood supply to the wound so that hemostasis and phagocytosis can occur. It is not always a wise choice to medicate with drugs that block inflammation, such as anti-inflammatories and steroids, because they interfere with the body's natural processes and therefore delay healing.

Reconstruction Phase

This phase occurs when the wound begins to heal, lasting for about 21 days after the injury. It is also referred to as the *proliferation phase.* The process of initiating healing begins with the presence of fibroblasts in the wound. These fibroblasts produce collagen, which is a tough protein material that forms scar tissue and helps strengthen the wound. The capillaries produce new networks so that the wound is supplied with oxygenated blood and nutrients. As new tissue begins to grow and fill in the wound, it looks red and semi-transparent. This new tissue, called **granulation tissue**, is extremely fragile. If it is irritated or abraded, it bleeds easily. When you measure a wound and find that it is getting smaller, filling with deep pink to red tissue, you know that the wound is healing, or "granulating."

Maturation Phase

This phase, also known as the *remodeling phase,* occurs when the wound contracts and the scar strengthens. Initially, a healing ridge develops just beneath the incision and approximately 1 cm on either side. Depending on the size of the wound and other factors, this phase can last 1 to 2 years. The macrophages continue to produce refined collagen to give the scar strength. As the scar thins and lightens in color, it also becomes firm and less elastic than the skin around it. This gives the area extra support to prevent reopening of the

wound. Overproduction of collagen results in a thick, raised scar called a *keloid.* Keloids can form on any type of skin, but are most common on darkly pigmented skin.

Types of Wound Closures for Healing

When a wound must be closed to promote healing, one of three methods will be employed: first, second, or third intention closure (Fig. 26-8).

First Intention

When the wound is clean with little tissue loss, such as a surgical incision, the edges are approximated and the wound is sutured closed. This helps prevent pathogens from entering the wound and allows healing to occur quickly. Box 26-1 describes the typical progression of healing in a healthy individual with a new surgical incision.

Second Intention

When there is greater tissue loss and the wound edges are irregular, the edges cannot be brought together. Examples of this would be a pressure ulcer or traumatic wound. In these situations, the wound must be left open to gradually heal by filling in with granulation tissue, which will leave a wide scar. Open wounds must be packed with moist gauze to absorb drainage and allow tissue to grow. They are covered with additional dressings to help prevent microorganisms from entering the wound. Strict sterile technique must be employed when applying dressings to open wounds in order to prevent infection.

Third Intention

When third intention healing is employed, the wound is left open for a time to allow granulation tissue to form; it is then sutured closed. An example of this would be a draining wound, which is left open until the drainage ceases and then is sutured closed.

Factors Affecting Wound Healing

For optimum wound healing, conditions must be favorable for new tissue growth. A number of factors can delay the healing process, including the age and lifestyle of the patient, additional illness and wounds, nutritional status, oxygenation, medications, and tension on the edges of the wound (Table 26-1).

Anatomy and Physiology Connection

The Inflammatory Process

The skin, consisting of the *epidermis* (outermost layer) and the *dermis* (innermost layer or true skin), serves as the first line of defense against microorganisms and foreign bodies. Whenever this first barrier is broken, the inflammatory process is initiated. The damaged cells release histamine and other chemicals, which cause the capillaries to *dilate,* or widen, and increase

(a) Primary intention

Clean wound

Sutured early

Results in hairline scar

(b) Secondary intention

Wound gaping and irregular

Granulation occurring

Epithelium fills in scar

(c) Tertiary intention

Figure 26-8 The three different types of closure: a. Primary intention healing with a clean wound sutured closed and well healed. b. Secondary intention healing with an irregular wound, unsutured for granulation to occur, and scar formation. c. Third intention healing with an unsutured wound, partially filled with granulation tissue, then closed with suture.

Wound not sutured

Granulation partially fills in wound

Granulating tissue sutured together

permeability of the capillary walls. The dilation allows increased blood flow to the site, causing erythema and increased warmth. More leukocytes are delivered to the site to help guard against infection. The increased permeability allows leukocytes to leave the vascular space and enter into the interstitial space and attack microorganisms directly, while red blood cells deliver more oxygen and nutrients to aid the healing process. This increase of fluid in the interstitial space results in edema. The edema causes pressure on nerve endings, producing discomfort and pain.

Complications of Wound Healing

Several types of complications can occur as a wound heals. It will be your responsibility to differentiate between normal healing and the presence of complications. You will be expected to assess your patients' wounds for signs and symptoms of these complications, and to know what to do if they occur. Some are considered medical emergencies, and your fast action can mean the difference between a good outcome and a poor one.

Box 26-1

Typical Healing of Surgical Incisions

Surgical incisions typically heal in the following manner:
- Within 48 hours after surgery, the incision begins to bind together.
- Due to the normal inflammatory reaction, you will observe slight swelling around staples or sutures and mild erythema of the incision in the first day or two.
- Most incisions have scant or no drainage at all, but some have a scant to moderate amount of sanguineous or serosanguineous drainage. It will change from sanguineous to serosanguineous to serous, and decrease in amount, over the first 5 postoperative days.
- By the fifth day postoperatively, you will be able to feel a ridge of granulation tissue directly below the incision. This ridge may extend to both sides of the incision for about a centimeter. Some patients become alarmed if they discover this ridge, but it is part of the normal healing process.

Table 26-1 **Factors Affecting Wound Healing**

Factor	Effect on Wound Healing	Example
Age	Wounds contract more slowly. Strength of scarred area is decreased. Skin is less elastic as people age. Collagen replacement is impaired.	An elderly patient with skin tears may heal slowly due to lack of collagen and elasticity.
Chronic illness	Illnesses affecting major body systems, such as heart, lung, and kidney disease, as well as neurological deficits affect optimal functioning of those systems. In turn, healing of wounds is negatively affected by impairment of other body systems.	A patient with chronic lung disease and congestive heart failure experiences very slow healing of an operative wound.
Diabetes mellitus	Causes decreased circulation due to narrowed peripheral blood vessels. Increased blood glucose interferes with the healing process.	A patient with diabetes whose blood glucose levels are poorly controlled could be expected to have slow wound healing.
Hypoxemia	Decreased oxygen delivered to the wound by the bloodstream causes impaired healing; oxygen is necessary for wounds to heal properly.	A patient with anemia or chronic lung disease may have hypoxemia, leading to impaired wound healing.
Lifestyle choices	Smoking decreases the oxygen content of the blood and constricts blood vessels, impeding circulation to wounds. Excessive alcohol intake can lead to poor nutrition, which affects wound healing. Obesity puts patients at risk for wound complications such as infection and dehiscence.	An obese patient who smokes and consumes alcohol in large amounts is at high risk for impaired wound healing and wound complications.
Lymphedema	When the area around a wound is edematous, circulation to and from the wound is impaired. Lack of efficient circulation decreases wound healing.	A patient with stasis ulcers on his or her leg experiences swelling in the area. Without compression applied by using leg wraps or support hose, the patient will be at risk for impaired healing of the leg ulcers.
Medications	Certain prescription medications delay the healing process and can mask symptoms of inflammation and infection.	A patient taking steroids or cytotoxic medications, such as chemotherapy, will be at risk for delayed or impaired wound healing.
Multiple wounds	Each wound competes for the available protein and substrates needed for tissue repair, resulting in delayed wound healing for all the wounds.	A patient injured in a motorcycle accident has multiple wounds and abrasions. It can be expected that all of them will be slow to heal.
Nutrition and hydration	Lack of calories and adequate protein impairs tissue growth. Deficiency in intake of vitamins A and C and zinc in the diet interferes with wound repair. Inadequate fluid intake causes the wound to be dry, restricting granulation of tissue.	A patient who is tube fed often receives a nominal amount of calories and protein, which delays wound healing.
Radiation exposure	Cancer treatments involving radiation can cause breakdown of underlying connective tissue, affecting repair capabilities.	A patient receiving radiation treatments for lung cancer after surgery on the lung is at risk for impaired wound healing of the surgical site or reopening of the surgical site.

Table 26-1 **Factors Affecting Wound Healing** (continued)

Factor	Effect on Wound Healing	Example
Wound tension	Extra tension placed on the wound edges can lead to *ischemia* (lack of blood supply to the area) and *necrosis* (death of tissue due to lack of blood supply). Tension on wound edges may be due to activities such as coughing, sneezing, lifting, and vomiting.	A patient who is vomiting repeatedly causes increased tension on the sutures of an abdominal wound, pulling the edges apart and infering with normal healing.

Infection

One of the most common wound complications is infection. A patient who has just undergone a surgical procedure or who has an open wound will have impaired defenses against infection. The most common microbial pathogen associated with wound infections is *Staphylococcus aureus*. This bacterium is present on the skin of all people, so it easily enters wounds unless special precautions are followed. In the operating room, strict sterile technique must be enforced. Surgical instruments, equipment, and personnel are all potential sources of infection.

Laboratory and Diagnostic Connection

Testing to Determine if a Wound Is Infected

In order to effectively treat an infected wound, you must identify the microorganism that is causing the infection and determine which antibiotics will be effective against the microorganism and kill it. This test is known as a wound *culture and sensitivity* (C&S). Some microorganisms have mutated so that they are no longer sensitive to certain antibiotics. These strains are labeled as resistant to the specific antibiotics. After the offending microorganism is identified, tiny disks, each saturated with a different antibiotic, are placed on the agar plate to observe whether or not the antibiotic kills the microorganism. If the antibiotic successfully kills the microorganism, the microorganism is sensitive to that specific drug. If it does not kill the microorganism, the microorganism is considered resistant to that antibiotic.

Another laboratory test valuable in treatment of wounds is the white blood cell (WBC) count and differential (WBC & Diff). A white blood cell count is a microscopic examination of the total number of WBCs that are present in the patient's blood. The normal range is 4,500 to 10,000/mm³, while infection may cause an increased level of WBCs. A differential shows the percentage of each of the five types of WBCs: neutrophils, lymphocytes, basophils, eosinophils, and monocytes. An increase in percentage of lymphocytes may be seen with chronic bacterial infections. An increased percentage of neutrophils may be seen with acute infections and a decreased percentage in widespread bacterial infections.

Methicillin-resistant Staphylococcus aureus

A resistant strain of *Staphylococcus aureus*, identified as **methicillin-resistant** *Staphylococcus aureus* **(MRSA)**, is an extremely serious issue. Like other staph microorganisms, this resistant form can live on the skin of healthy people without causing illness. However, when a wound becomes infected with MRSA, the physician has little choice in effective antibiotics for treatment. Although vancomycin is the current antibiotic of choice to treat MRSA, an even more resistant strain is now making an appearance. This strain, vancomycin-intermediate *Staphylococcus aureus* (VISA), is developing resistance even to vancomycin.

Escherichia coli

Another common infective pathogen appears in wounds after surgery on the gastrointestinal system. Bacteria normally found in the bowel are referred to as enterococci. One specific bacterium from this group, *Escherichia coli or E. coli*, helps to break down food for digestion. When the intestines are opened during surgery, the bacteria from the bowel, including *E. coli*, can easily infect the surgical wound. Special preparation before bowel surgery helps decrease the chances of such an infection. When emergency surgery is performed on the gastrointestinal tract, especially when perforation or rupture has occurred, infection is quite likely.

Clostridia

When a wound is infected with bacteria called *clostridia*, the result is a condition known as *gas gangrene*. This pathogen grows only in the absence of oxygen and is called an *anaerobe*. As the bacteria multiply in the wound, poisonous toxins and gases are emitted.

Gangrene most often occurs due to poor circulation to a body part, especially a digit or limb, or as a complication of an untreated infection in a wound. Essentially, a portion of the body dies while still attached to living tissue in the body. The area may become black due to tissue death and produce a characteristic foul odor associated with decaying tissue. When the affected area is pressed, a crackling sensation will be felt due to the gas produced by the bacteria.

This infection is treated with antibiotics and surgical removal of the dead tissue, a process known as **débridement**. If the condition is due to impaired circulation, the patient will be evaluated for revascularization surgery.

Infected wounds are débrided and may be treated in *a hyperbaric chamber*. Such a chamber delivers oxygen under high pressure to help kill anaerobic bacteria and promote wound healing. Aggressive antibiotic therapy is necessary to prevent the spread of toxins into the bloodstream. If other treatment fails, the affected limb may have to be amputated.

Stat Nursing Response to Wound Infection

You are responsible for assessing surgical and open wounds for any signs of infection. Be sure to differentiate normal wound healing from the early onset of infection. Inspect and assess surgical incisions and other wounds at least every 8 hours. When you assess an infected wound, you will see pronounced erythema around the staples or sutures and on the edges of the incision. Drainage may increase in amount with each successive day rather than decrease. The drainage may be purulent and *malodorous* (bad-smelling). The byproducts of the bacteria infecting the wound emit a strong odor. The incision itself may begin to open between sutures or staples. The patient's vital signs usually reflect infection: Elevated temperature and heart rate may be noted. Laboratory results often show an elevated WBC. The patient often complains of increasing incisional pain, rather than decreasing pain, with each postoperative day.

When you observe possible signs of infection in a wound, notify the physician of your findings immediately. Before calling, be sure to have all appropriate information at hand:

- Vital sign readings
- Laboratory results
- Amount and type of drainage
- Description of the wound, including observed signs of infection
- Patient's rating of incisional pain

If the patient is already on an oral or IV antibiotic, have the name and dosage of the medication available when you call the physician. Be prepared to obtain a specimen of wound drainage for culture and sensitivity.

Wound Dehiscence and Evisceration

Wound **dehiscence** is not a common complication of wound healing, but it is an extremely serious one. It occurs when there is a partial or complete separation of the outer layers of a wound (Fig. 26-9). Dehiscence occurs in about 3% of abdominal surgery patients, with a mortality rate between 14% and 50%. This condition occurs most often between the 5th and 12th postoperative day.

Several reasons for wound separation exist, and many occur in surgery. If sutures or staples are placed too far apart or too close to the edges of the incision, the edges do not meet together for optimum healing. Anything that can lead to necrosis of the wound edges, such as wound infection, extremely tight sutures, or impaired blood supply, can end in wound dehiscence. If the wound edges are separating between sutures, or if sutures are removed too soon, the wound may reopen (see Fig. 26-7). It is best not to remove sutures until the ridge of granulation tissue can be felt. Be sure to help your patient splint his or her incision with a pillow before coughing or sneezing to help prevent extra stress on wound edges. Provide patients with medications as ordered for nausea and stool softeners to prevent tension on the wound from vomiting or straining to have a bowel movement.

As you might imagine, if an abdominal wound reopens, the abdominal contents may protrude through the opening (Fig. 26-10). This condition is referred to as **evisceration** and is a life-threatening situation. The exposure of abdominal contents can lead to necrosis of the intestines or overwhelming sepsis. If a patient tells you, "I feel like something just split open," be ready to act quickly.

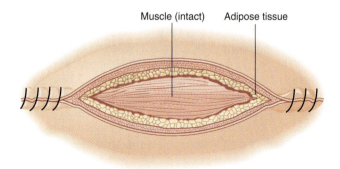

Muscle (intact)   Adipose tissue

Figure 26-9 This wound has separated and the muscle layer is visible beneath; it is an example of wound dehiscence.

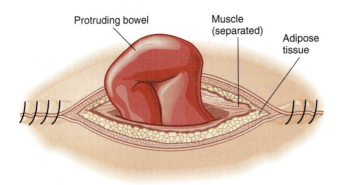

Figure 26-10   This wound and the muscle layer beneath have separated, allowing the intestine to protrude outward through the wound; it is an example of wound evisceration.

Stat Nursing Response to Wound Dehiscence and Evisceration

This situation usually occurs suddenly, often with the only warning being a pronounced increase in serosanguineous drainage from the wound. Should dehiscence occur, reassure your patient and assist him or her to a supine position. Stay with your patient and notify the physician immediately. Request that sterile supplies be brought to the room, including a basin, normal saline, abdominal dressings, 60-mL syringe, masks, gowns, gloves, and drapes. A suture removal kit may be necessary. Sterile adhesive strips should also be on hand.

If the wound is completely separated or a large portion of it has reopened, be prepared to send the patient to the operating room as soon as possible. If only a small portion of the wound has reopened, the physician may use sterile adhesive strip closures.

If evisceration has occurred as well, you must act immediately. *Safety: Do not attempt to replace the organs into the abdominal cavity.* Cover the exposed organs with sterile dressings soaked in normal saline. Keep the dressings moist by adding sterile saline using the sterile syringe. When you moisten the dressings, assess the exposed organs for signs of necrosis, such as a color change to blue, purple, or black. Position the patient in the low Fowler's position with the knees flexed to reduce strain on the abdominal wound. Do not give your patient anything by mouth (keep the patient NPO), as surgery will have to be performed. Be sure that you have a patent IV line, and administer fluids and medications as ordered through it. Monitor vital signs at least every 15 minutes to detect signs of shock. Be calm and continue to reassure your patient.

Knowledge Connection
What is the difference between wound dehiscence and evisceration? How are they treated similarly? How are they treated differently?

Hemorrhage

Rarely, a surgical wound may **hemorrhage**, or bleed profusely. This is also a medical emergency. When you check for bleeding postoperatively, always look and feel beneath the patient for blood that might pool there rather than be absorbed into the dressing. Hemorrhage may be due to a slipped suture, displaced blood clot, or trauma to the incision. A large amount of bright red blood indicates bleeding from an artery. Patients taking anticoagulant medications (blood thinners) and those with clotting disorders are at risk for hemorrhage postoperatively.

Hemorrhage may also occur internally. No discharge of blood is present, but symptoms of blood loss are the same. As blood gathers in the abdominal cavity, the abdomen becomes distended and taut. This is a cardinal sign of potential postoperative hemorrhage, and the patient should be evaluated immediately for that complication. Pale mucous membranes, rapid and thready pulse, hypotension, diaphoresis, and cool, clammy skin are later signs of hemorrhage. This condition can lead to death if not detected and treated without delay.

Stat Nursing Response to Hemorrhage

External or internal hemorrhage is a medical emergency. Notify the physician immediately. Position the patient in the low Fowler's position with the knees flexed. If you can see the source of the bleeding, put on gloves and apply firm pressure over the area. Administer oxygen via mask or nasal cannula. Monitor vital signs at least every 15 minutes and be prepared for the patient to return to the operating room as soon as possible. Ensure a patent IV line and administer fluids as ordered to help prevent circulatory collapse.

Knowledge Connection
What are possible causes of wound hemorrhage?

Wound Treatment

You will provide wound care as ordered by the physician. Treatments will differ for each wound, depending upon the type and extent of the wound, whether it is an open or closed wound, the level of contamination, and the physician's personal preference.

Closure

Surgical wounds and traumatic wounds with intact tissue are generally closed using some type of closure material. Most common are sutures, staples, surgical adhesive, and sterile adhesive strips, sometimes referred to by the brand name, Steri-Strips. A surgical wound is closed from the inner layers to the outer layers of tissue. Absorbable sutures are used in the inner tissue layers. The outer skin layers are approximated and held in place using one of several closure methods. Nonabsorbable sutures or staples are used on the outer layers of tissue and are removed after 7 to 14 days.

Surgical adhesive can only be used on the outer skin layers and "glues" the wound together. No removal is necessary, and the edges of the wound remain approximated during the healing process. Sterile adhesive strips are used to close small wounds, or wounds that are healing. For example, you may apply sterile adhesive strips to an incision after you remove the sutures or staples, to give it support as it continues to heal. Sterile adhesive strips are narrow reinforced tape strips and will eventually peel free of the skin.

Nursing Responsibilities for Suture/Staple Care

Your responsibilities include assessment of the suture line each time you inspect an incision. This may be when you perform a dressing change, or when you assess your patient at the beginning of your shift. Notice any sign of loosening sutures, gaps in the incision, or redness around the staples or sutures that indicates infection. Assess incisions every 8 hours to detect changes that may occur. You may also be responsible for removing sutures and staples when the wound has healed. Skill 26-1 (see page 578) shows how to remove sutures and staples.

Drains and Drainage

After traumatic injury or surgery, wounds generally produce drainage. At first, this drainage looks like blood (**sanguineous**), then it looks pink (**serosanguineous**), and finally, as the wound heals, the drainage becomes clearer to slightly yellow fluid (**serous**). This is a predictable pattern as a wound heals; deviations from this pattern indicate some type of wound complication. Box 26-2 describes types of wound drainage.

When a wound is expected to produce significant drainage, the surgeon will place a drain in the wound before closure. A tube then extends through the skin and to the outside of the body, ending in some type of collection receptacle. If drainage is allowed to remain in the tissues, it will prevent granulation from occurring and impede wound healing.

Closed drains attach to a device that, when compressed, causes gentle suction, allowing fluid to be drawn from the wound into the collection container. A Hemovac and a Jackson-Pratt, also called J-P, are both active drains that operate on the suction principle (Fig. 26-11). A T-tube is a passive drain. It is placed in the common bile duct after gallbladder surgery to drain excess bile from the area via gravity. It connects to a small collection bag but does not cause suction within the wound.

A Penrose drain is an open drain (see Fig. 26-11). A flat tube is inserted in the wound during surgery, then brought out through a "stab wound" or slit in the skin. A sterile safety pin is fastened through the flat tube to keep it from sliding into the wound. Drainage from the wound exits through the Penrose drain and is absorbed by the dressing. Several sterile gauze 4×4s are layered over and under the end of the drain to absorb the exudate. Open drains are used less frequently than in the past because they provide a pathway for pathogens to reach the wound. Closed drains are seen most frequently.

Nursing Responsibilities for Drain Care

You will be responsible for any drains that your patients may have. Empty drains every 8 hours or when they become one-half to two-thirds full. If the bulb on the Jackson-Pratt drain or the round receptacle on the Hemovac drain is no longer compressed, the container is full and must be emptied. When compression is absent, no suction is present. Skill 26-2 (see page 579) shows the steps required to care for and empty drainage devices.

Measure drainage in a calibrated container and record the amount on the intake and output record. Note the type of drainage. Report a significant increase in the amount of drainage and the presence of purulent drainage to the physician immediately, since these could indicate impaired healing and infection.

Box 26-2

Types of Wound Drainage

It is important to describe wound drainage accurately so that other health care workers can compare your findings with theirs.
- **Sanguineous:** Comes from the Latin word for "bloody" and means "containing blood"; it refers to red, bloody drainage.
- **Serous:** Comes from the Latin word for "serum," the clear liquid portion of the blood; it refers to clear to pale yellow drainage that looks like serum.
- **Purulent:** Comes from the Latin word meaning "full of pus," and means "containing pus"; it is thick yellow or green drainage and is a sign of infection.
- **Bilious:** Comes from the word "bile," which is made by the body to help break down fats for digestion. It is a dark greenish color and is often present in wound drainage after gallbladder surgery.

Sometimes more than one type of drainage is present. These words are then combined to indicate the two types of drainage from the wound:
- **Serosanguineous:** Both blood and clear drainage are present. Combined, they turn dressing materials a pink color.
- **Seropurulent:** Both clear drainage and drainage with pus are present.

Figure 26-11 These are different types of wound drains: Penrose on the left, Jackson-Pratt in the center, and Hemovac on the right.

If a Penrose drain is in use, change the dressings around the drain carefully to prevent dislodging the tube. The physician may order the drain to be shortened a specified length, for example, 2 inches. This involves removing the safety pin and pulling the specified length of tubing out of the wound, cutting off the excess tubing, and reattaching the safety pin. This procedure may not be in the entry-level nurse's scope of practice, so be sure to check facility policy before performing it.

Knowledge Connection

What are four ways wounds are closed? What is the purpose of a wound drain? When should wound drains be emptied?

Measurement of Wounds and Observation of Drainage

Assessing a wound is the only way to determine whether the wound is healing or if there are complications such as infection. So it is pertinent that you are skilled in wound assessment (Box 26-3). One of the first things you will note is the amount of drainage on the old dressing, which is generally referred to as a scant, small, moderate, or large amount. You must also describe the color of the drainage.

In some situations, the physician may not want the dressing to be changed for 24 or 48 hours, even though it contains drainage. If that is the case, nurses mark the drainage on the dressing to show increases over time. For example, a patient who has just returned from surgery has an abdominal dressing with a quarter-sized amount of drainage visible on the outside dressing. Draw around the drainage with a pen, then write the date, time, and your initials next to it. When the nurse on the next shift cares for this patient, he or she will be able to tell if the drainage has increased since that time.

If large amounts of drainage occur and the dressing is not to be changed for 24 hours, reinforce the dressing with additional abdominal dressings to absorb additional drainage. Notify the physician of the excessive drainage, because it is not normally expected after most surgeries.

Box 26-3

Wound Assessment Summary

When you assess a wound, be sure to include all of the following aspects of the wound.
- **Site:** anatomical location
- **Wound type:** open or closed
- **Wound closure:** sutures, staples, Steri-Strips, approximation
- **Size:** width, length, depth
- **Condition of wound bed:** color, texture, eschar, sloughing, presence of granulation tissue, undermining, or sinus tracts
- **Condition of skin surrounding wound:** color, texture, maceration
- **Pain:** rate discomfort/tenderness using pain scale
- **Drainage:** amount, type/color, odor

You will need to assess the size of a wound—its length, width, and depth. Use a ruler or a disposable paper wound measurement ruler. Without touching the paper or ruler to the skin, measure the width of the wound at its widest point. Do the same for the length of the wound. If the wound is completely round, you can measure the width and consider it the diameter of the wound. To measure depth, use a sterile cotton-tipped swab. Carefully insert the swab at the deepest area of the wound and mark skin level with your gloved finger against the handle portion of the swab. Then carefully hold the swab near the ruler or paper ruler to determine depth. It is common to measure wounds in centimeters or millimeters, rather than inches. If the wound has a sinus tract connected with it, the swab can be used to determine the length of the tract as well. Insert the swab as far as it will go, mark the handle portion with your finger, then measure the length of the tract.

If the wound is open, assess the base or bed of the wound for color of tissue, texture of tissue, granulation tissue, eschar, sinus tracts, and undermining. If the wound has been surgically closed, assess the number of staples, sutures, or Steri-Strips that are intact. To help you describe the appearance of different areas of the wound, visualize a clock face. Make notes using the clock face as a reference. For example, there may be eschar at 12 o'clock and granulation tissue at 6 o'clock. Once you have completed your wound and drainage assessment, you are ready to clean the wound.

Cleaning Wounds

Some wounds contain dissolved necrotic tissue and pus; others may hold tissue fluid and blood (*exudate*). In these situations, you will anticipate physician's orders to clean the wound with dressing changes. Cleaning of wounds may be accomplished in the physical therapy department of some hospitals, especially if vigorous cleansing in a whirlpool bath is ordered to remove dead tissue or wound contaminants. Irrigation is the more gentle method of wound cleansing and is ordered when fragile granulation tissue is present. Wounds can also be cleaned with soft gauze moistened with sterile saline, using a light patting movement. Use care to prevent damaging healthy tissue.

To clean around a drain exiting from a wound, use a sterile antiseptic swab or forceps and cotton balls soaked in antiseptic. Clean in a circular motion on the skin, starting as close as possible to the drain. Move outward in enlarging circles, overlapping slightly to be sure no gaps are left and all skin is cleansed. Make one circle with a swab or cotton ball, then dispose of it. Make the next slightly larger circle with a new swab or cotton ball.

To clean a long incision that is sutured or stapled closed with approximated edges, again use sterile antiseptic swabs or forceps and cotton balls soaked in antiseptic. Clean from the superior end of the incision to the inferior end. The superior portion of the wound is considered less contaminated than the inferior portion, because drainage usually flows downward. Do not go back over an area that has already been cleansed. If you do so, you can contaminate the cleansed area with pathogens from an unclean area. If the incision itself is contaminated, clean from the superior to the inferior end of the wound with one swab or cotton ball, then dispose of it. Continue cleaning using long strokes from superior to inferior along the incision, using a new swab or cotton ball for each stroke. Alternate cleaning one side of the incision, then cleaning the opposite side until an area of several inches on either side has been cleansed. Dispose of each swab or cotton ball after every stroke.

Nursing Responsibilities for Cleaning Wounds

When wound irrigation is ordered, the purpose is to remove surface debris without injuring granulation tissue. This is best accomplished by using mild pressure of 8 pounds per square inch. To deliver the correct amount of pressure, you will use a 35-mL syringe with a 19-gauge Angiocath attached. As you spray normal saline through the Angiocath, it will gently remove surface debris without causing damage to the wound. Hold a basin below the inferior margin of the wound to catch the irrigant. Skill 26-3 (page 580) presents the steps for performing a wound irrigation.

The most common irrigant is sterile normal saline because it is isotonic to the body. If a different fluid is to be used, the physician will order it. Be sure to assess the amount, color, and consistency of debris removed by the irrigation, and document this in the patient's chart.

Obtaining a Wound Culture

The physician may order a specimen of the wound drainage to be tested for culture and sensitivity to see which pathogens might be growing in the wound and determine the appropriate antibiotics for treatment. You will obtain the wound culture during the dressing change. If a wound irrigation is ordered, perform the irrigation first, then obtain the specimen of wound drainage for culture. Skill 26-4 (page 582) lists the steps for obtaining a wound culture specimen.

Dressings

Dressings serve several purposes. In the case of a surgical incision, dressings protect the incision and absorb drainage as the wound heals. In the case of chronic wounds, such as pressure ulcers and vascular ulcers, the dressings also protect from further injury, provide the moist environment required for healing, and fill the open space within the wound. Since healing of these ulcers must occur from the inside out, open spaces need to be packed until they fill with granulation tissue. Without packing, the pooling debris and exudate would cause the wound to become larger.

Wounds cannot heal without the appropriate amount of moisture. When a wound is covered and moisture is maintained within it, the epidermal cells can move freely through the moisture to promote healing. When wounds are dry, the

cells must first tunnel below the surface to a moist area where they secrete enzymes. The enzymes help dissolve the scab so the epidermal cells can begin healing. The purpose of many dressings is to preserve a moist wound environment so healing can occur.

Many different types of dressings exist. Some are designed simply to cover the wound. Others are intended to be packed into the wound. Still others have been developed specifically to maintain a moist wound bed. The physician will order the type of dressing to be used for each patient. However, you will be expected to know the appropriate use of each type of dressing and to assess wound healing response. Table 26-2 shows a comparison of common dressings and their uses.

Wet-to-Damp and Wet-to-Dry Dressings

Wet-to-damp wound dressings are ordered to maintain a moist wound bed and to wick out drainage from the wound. They are changed frequently to prevent the gauze in the wound from drying out completely. A wet-to-dry dressing may be ordered for the purpose of helping to débride the wound. The necrotic tissue in the wound sticks to the dry gauze so that, when the gauze is removed, the necrotic tissue is also removed. However, it is easy to damage granulation tissue with this method. Currently, wet-to-damp dressings are favored for wound healing over the wet-to-dry débridement method, because they preserve fragile granulating tissue. Skill 26-5 (page 582) gives the steps required to change a sterile dressing and a wet-to-damp dressing.

You may also apply other dressings, such as those listed in Table 26-2. Two of the most common dressings you will apply are transparent film dressings and hydrocolloid dressings. Skill 26-6 (page 585) provides directions for applying transparent and hydrocolloid dressings.

Knowledge Connection
When would you expect to see wound irrigation ordered for your patient? Why is moisture necessary for wounds to heal?

Securing Dressings

Once dressings are in place, they must be secured well enough to keep the outer dressing fixed, and to keep any additional dressings beneath it from becoming dislodged. Tape is one option for holding dressings in place. Several types of tapes are available, including foam tape, silk tape, and paper tape. Foam tape is thicker than the other types and anchors well. Paper tape is a good choice for those with thin, fragile skin, such as elderly individuals as well as patients who are allergic to other types of tape.

In addition to tape, dressings may be held in place with Montgomery straps or abdominal binders. Montgomery straps attach to the skin with adhesive on either side of the wound. The slotted flaps lay over the dressing and lace up with narrow gauze strips, much like you would lace up a shoe and tie

Table 26-2   **Types and Purposes of Dressings**

Type	Purpose	Composition	Examples
Alginate	Loosely packed or layered in wounds and sinus tracts; used for wounds with moderate to large amounts of drainage; also comes in "ropes" that are cut to fit in the wound; wound is covered with absorbent dressing.	Derived from seaweed; when it absorbs drainage, it turns into a soft gel that does not adhere to the wound; absorbs up to 20 times its own weight.	Algisite Curasorb Kaltogel Sorbsan Tegagel
Gauze	Used to loosely pack large wounds in wet-to-damp dressings for débridement; then covered with a thicker dressing to absorb drainage. May require irrigation with dressing change to remove all fibers from wound.	Cotton, polyester, or rayon fibers, loosely or tightly woven; filled dressings include absorbent material; unfilled are composed of woven threads only; Telfa pads are coated to prevent sticking.	ABD (abdominal dressing) Curity gauze sponge Gauze 4×4s Kerlix gauze fluff Telfa
Hydrocolloid	Used on wounds with minimal wound drainage and on dry, clean wounds. Not recommended for infected wounds.	Made of water-attracting gelling agents such as pectin or gelatin; absorbs excess fluid from the wound while still holding in moisture.	Combiderm Comfeel Duoderm
Hydrofiber	Used on wounds with excessive drainage or deep wounds that require packing. Cover dressing is required. Stays in place up to 7 days. One type (Aquacel-Ag) contains antimicrobial agents effective against MRSA and vancomycin-resistant enterococci.	Dressing in pad or ribbon form made from absorbent fibers (the same material as in hydrocolloid dressings).	Aquacel Aquacel-Ag Versiva
Negative pressure wound therapy (NPWT)	Used in deep open wounds and covered with transparent polyvinyl dressing. Uses gentle negative pressure to remove drainage and contaminants. Allows new growth of blood vessels and increased circulation to promote healing; maintains a moist environment.	Sterile foam dressing that is packed loosely into the wound or ulcer. An adhesive drape is applied over it to form an airtight seal; a vacuum source attaches to the motor unit and causes negative pressure.	Wound VAC
Polyvinyl	Used on clean wounds without drainage. Can be used to hold other dressings or IVs in place.	Transparent adhesive that is semipermeable; keeps oxygen and moisture in but bacteria out.	Bioclusive Opsite Skintact Tegaderm

it. They are used when frequent dressing changes are necessary, so tape does not have to be removed frequently from the skin. Figure 26-12 shows Montgomery straps in use.

Abdominal binders can also be used to hold abdominal dressings in place. Because they are made of elastic and held in place with Velcro, they tend to apply some pressure to the incision, which may be uncomfortable for the patient. They are often used when the incision needs extra support.

Taping Dressings

When taping a dressing to a joint, place the tape parallel to the bend of the joint, allowing movement without dislodging the dressing. When taping dressings to other areas, place the tape at the top and bottom edges, catching both dressing and skin, then add one or two pieces of tape across the middle. Use enough tape to overlap the dressing by 1½ to 2 inches on either side. Avoid allowing the edges of the dressing to

Figure 26-12 Montgomery straps may be used to hold an abdominal dressing in place to prevent the need to remove tape with each dressing change.

curl down over the tape at the top or bottom, since that can then contaminate the wound (Fig. 26-13).

Knowledge Connection

When would you consider using Montgomery straps? How would you tape a dressing to a patient's elbow area?

Nursing Responsibilities for Applying Dressings

Applying dressings to an open wound is considered a sterile procedure in most situations. Gloves should always be worn, and a gown, goggles, and mask are worn when there is danger of splashing. You must keep a good "sterile conscience," that is, you must admit any breaks in technique and start over to protect your patient from possible infection.

You are also responsible for assessing the wound during a dressing change. Measure the length, width, and depth of the wound. Inspect the wound for dark pink or red granulation tissue, as well as yellow or black tissue. Note the location and length of sinus tracts connected with the wound. Assess the type of drainage on the old dressing for color and amount. Remove your gloves and wash your hands before applying a new dressing. Follow orders for irrigation or cleansing of the wound. Apply the new dressing carefully, following orders for the type of dressing. Write the date, time, and your initials on the new dressing.

Figure 26-13 Incorrect placement of tape to secure a dressing.

People and Places Connection

Wound Care of Elderly Patients

Elderly patients with wounds can be a challenge. Because of physiological factors, wounds in elders heal more slowly. In addition, elders may not see well enough to observe changes in wounds, so infection may occur without the patient realizing it. It may be difficult for elderly patients to change their own dressings with good technique. The cost of supplies for wound care may deter them from getting care they need. Decreased circulation to extremities may prevent elderly patients from experiencing the degree of pain normally associated with a stasis ulcer or extremity wound, therefore leading to a delay in seeking treatment.

Wound Care in Home Health Care

Often nurses make visits in the home health care setting to perform dressing changes. The case manager generally opens the case, formulates the care plan, and manages the care. Field nurses make daily visits to change the dressing and observe the wound. In home health care, different nurses may make visits on different days. A "weekend nurse" may make the Saturday and Sunday visits. So, it is very important that each nurse document thoroughly his or her observations about the size, shape, and color of the wound, as well as the nature of the wound drainage. The nurses' description of the wound and how it is healing is the only information used to determine Medicare reimbursement, so it is important to show progress in wound healing or a change in the plan of care if the wound is not healing.

Supervision/Delegation Connection

Wound Care and Unlicensed Assistive Personnel

In some states the RN or LPN/LVN can delegate certain tasks to UAPs, including applying a simple dressing, such as a bandage or gauze and tape. Under no circumstances should the packing or assessment of a wound be delegated. In some states, UAPs may be allowed to obtain a wound specimen or empty a wound drainage container. Be sure you know the laws and rules in your state. When in doubt, do not delegate.

Documenting Wound Care

Accurate documentation of wound care is extremely important. Describe the amount and color of drainage on the old dressing. Document the length, width or diameter, and depth of the wound. Refer to a clock face to describe the interior of the wound, including sinus tracts and their length. Describe the color of the wound and appearance of the surrounding skin. Document the type of dressing applied. It is helpful to say how many gauze 4×4s you used, for example, in a wet-to-damp dressing, so the next nurse knows exactly what to prepare.

Review documentation to be sure that the wound is getting smaller, not larger. This is essential for third-party payers to continue to pay for care. If the wound is not getting smaller over several days or a week, notify the physician. Different orders may be necessary to promote healing.

Nursing Care Plan for a Patient With an Infected Stage II Pressure Ulcer

Assessment

Your first step in planning care for a patient with a pressure ulcer is to gather all the available data. An assessment of the ulcer must be made so it can be staged, including the location, size, depth, color, condition of the surrounding skin, drainage, odor, and discomfort level.

- **Location:** Where is the ulcer located? Is it over a bony prominence? Will pressure be exerted on it while sitting or lying in the supine, prone, or lateral position?
- **Size:** What is the width? Length? Measure both.
- **Depth:** How deep is the ulcer? Which layers of tissue are involved? If it goes beyond a shallow crater, you may use a long-handled sterile cotton-tipped swab to mark the depth. Insert it into the deepest part of the crater and mark the height of the skin surface with your thumb. Then hold the swab next to a measuring device to determine the actual measurement. Is there undermining? Are there any sinus tracts?
- **Color:** What color is the skin around the ulcer? What color is the base of the ulcer? Is there granulation tissue (grains of soft, fragile pinkish-red tissue)? Eschar (firm, brown or black)? Remember, if it has eschar, the ulcer cannot be staged until it has been débrided. Is there sloughing?
- **Condition of surrounding skin:** Is the skin around the ulcer sloughing? Intact? Macerated?
- **Drainage:** Is there drainage? Is it serous, serosanguineous, sanguineous, or purulent? How much drainage is there?
- **Odor:** Does the wound or drainage have a foul odor?
- **Discomfort level:** Is there tenderness or pain? What number on a pain scale of 0 to 10?

It is also important to note if the patient's white blood count is elevated.

You must assess nutritional factors relating to development and treatment of a pressure ulcer:

- Has the patient been eating a nutritious diet?
- Is the patient well hydrated?
- Is the patient's serum protein low?
- Is the patient's hemoglobin low?

Assess the patient's risk factors:

- Is the patient elderly?
- Is the patient emaciated?
- Is the patient incontinent of bowel or bladder?
- Does the patient suffer from impaired mobility? Is his or her circulation impaired?

- Is the patient diabetic?
- Are there circulatory problems?

The data you collect tells you the patient is an 81-year-old female with no circulatory diseases. She has a stage II pressure ulcer on her left heel that measures 1.5 × 2.5 cm with a depth of 0.5 cm. The skin around the ulcer is erythemic and slightly warmer than the surrounding skin. The ulcer bed is bright red with tiny red bumpy tissue across most of the ulcer. There is a moderate amount of yellow purulent drainage on the dressing. It has no odor, and the patient denies any discomfort. The patient can no longer walk, but she is able to sit in a chair with assistance. She tells you that she likes to be up most of the day, but at the nursing home where she resides, she only gets out of bed once or twice a day. Her records show that she is on a soft diet and eats at least 70% of most meals. She tells you she cannot chew meat very well with her dentures. Her hemoglobin and serum protein are both a little low. Her white blood cell count is within normal limits. She has lost 6 pounds in the last 2 weeks since she has been dealing with the pressure ulcer. The patient is continent of both bowel and bladder. Her capillary refill in her feet is less than 4 seconds, which is within normal limits for her age.

Nursing Diagnoses

After collecting all the data, you have to analyze this information and determine what kind of problems this patient might have or be at risk for developing. In other words, what are her nursing diagnoses? In order to determine this, you must review what you have learned about this particular patient.

She has no metabolic disease that would impair the circulation to her extremities. Her feet are warm and pink with brisk capillary refill and strong pedal pulses. There is no history of injury to the heel and yet there is an ulcer there. She is no longer able to walk, and is restricted to her bed and a chair, most frequently the bed. Without any evidence to indicate another cause, it is probably safe to assume the ulcer is a pressure ulcer. The granulation tissue indicates there is some healing taking place. The skin surrounding the

(care plan continues on page 576)

Nursing Care Plan for a Patient With an Infected Stage II Pressure Ulcer (continued)

ulcer is erythemic and warmer than the skin on the rest of her foot, and there is purulent drainage. This lets us know that the wound is infected. Because protein is necessary for growth of new tissue, her low *hemoglobin* (iron protein carried by the red blood cells) and serum protein are not conducive to rapid healing. If her dentures do not allow her to chew meat well, that will further decrease her source of protein. The loss of 6 pounds supports the need for more protein and calories as well.

By grouping the information this way, you can identify that this patient has a problem with skin integrity that seems to be related to direct pressure on the heel. You identify that the ulcer is not healing well and the problem may be a direct result of poor nutrition and continued pressure on the heel. After reviewing your NANDA-I list of nursing diagnoses, you are able to determine that she has at least two nursing diagnoses:

• Impaired skin integrity (a stage II pressure ulcer that is infected)
• Inadequate nutrition (less than her body demands)

Now you can begin planning how to care for these problems (see nursing diagnoses in Table 26-3).

Planning

For this patient, appropriate interventions begin with reducing pressure on the patient's left heel while she is in bed and up in a chair.

There are a number of pressure-relieving devices that can be used with the patient's bed, so it is important to evaluate which one will work best for this particular patient's situation. The ulcer is already present, so heel protectors will not work. A gel pad is a possibility, but the patient has other pressure points that have to be protected from developing further pressure ulcers. An eggcrate mattress might work, but probably not as well as a gel-filled mattress overlay. Also, the patient said that she prefers to be up several times a day, so the plan should be to get her into a chair at least three times daily.

Basic interventions may also be useful, including repositioning her at least every 2 hours and keeping pillows between her knees and ankles to avoid increased pressure on these areas while in bed. These interventions will help to prevent further skin breakdown, but relieving all pressure on the heels has to be a priority so the left heel can repair itself. Pillows can be used to elevate the lower legs and allow the patient's heels to overhang the pillows. When the patient is in a chair, a combination of a stool and pillows to prop her left leg so the heel does not rest on the stool would be an appropriate intervention.

With stage II pressure ulcers, it is important to watch the infection and monitor whether the wound is healing. This can best be accomplished by assessing the wound, drainage, and surrounding skin on a daily basis. Wounds heal better if they are kept slightly moist, so ask the physician if he or she would order some type of hydrocolloidal product to help maintain the wound's moisture.

The physician feels that the patient needs more protein and calories for healing and has ordered a high-protein, high-calorie supplement and a high-protein diet. List some high-protein foods for the patient and ask if she likes any of them, and then report her likes to the dietary service and nursing staff because she will eat more if she is eating food that she likes. If she has difficulty chewing meat, ask the dietary service to grind it for her.

To determine if these interventions are working, plan to monitor the patient's laboratory results to see if her hemoglobin and serum protein levels begin to rise after the dietary changes. Also plan to weigh the patient every day while hospitalized, to make certain she stops losing weight.

Implementation

At this stage of the nursing process, you can now implement the interventions that you have planned (see interventions in Table 26-3).

Evaluation

The last step in the nursing process is to evaluate whether the interventions you have been implementing are helping the ulcer to heal and preventing development of new pressure ulcers (see evaluations in Table 26-3). It appears that the ulcer is indeed healing, and the patient's blood levels of protein are slowly coming up toward normal. The patient still needs some further healing, but it looks like you are on the right track with your plan of care.

Nursing Care Plan for a Patient With an Infected Stage II Pressure Ulcer (continued)

Table 26-3   Care Plan for Infected Stage II Pressure Ulcer

Nursing Diagnosis: Impaired skin integrity, related to infected pressure ulcer on left heel, as evidenced by tissue destruction of stage II pressure ulcer
Expected Outcomes: Patient will have no evidence of infection at discharge: normal WBC, no fever, wound bed pink and moist. Patient will show no evidence of new skin breakdown nor extension of current wound dimensions at discharge.

Interventions	Evaluations
Keep a gel-filled overlay pad on top of the mattress.	Day 3: No new skin breakdown. States she sleeps better on the gel overlay. Day 7: No new skin breakdown. Day 12: No new skin breakdown.
Reposition the patient every 2 hours when in bed.	Day 3: Requires no assist to reposition, but has to be cued. Cap. refill brisk × 4 extremities. Day 6: Now turns self without cueing except while sleeping. Turning schedule maintained by staff at night. Cap. refill brisk bilaterally × 4 extremities.
Elevate both lower legs on a small pillow to keep the heels off the bed.	Day 2: Prefers to let heels overhang the end of the bed to avoid contact with bed. Skin around wound intact, pink, dry. Day 7: Skin on Rt. heel intact Day 12: Rt. heel without erythema.
Keep pillows between the knees and ankles when the patient is lying in the lateral position.	Day 3: Body alignment maintained. States the support feels better than letting bony places rub together. Day 7: No erythema on knees or ankles. Day 12: Skin on knees and ankles intact.
Assist the patient out of bed to sit in a chair for 1–2 hours at meal-times and at least one other time during the day that patient would like to be out of bed.	Day 3: States enjoys being up more. Often sits up most of evening. Day 7: Sits up most of evening and 2–2.5 hr in a.m. Day 12: Continues to voice enjoyment of time out of bed.
When the patient is up in a chair, elevate the feet on a footstool using a pillow to keep the left heel off the surface of the stool.	Day 3: Compliant, keeps feet elevated and heels off stool. Slight edema of Lt. heel. Day 7: Edema decreased, nearly gone. Day 10: No edema.
Assess ulcer and drainage, documenting in the nurse's notes daily.	Day 3: Continues w/ sm. amt. serous drainage. No change in size. Day 7: Scant serous drainage. Beginning to granulate. Day 12: Ulcer improving, granulating well, pink & moist. Measures 0.5 cm × 1.5 cm, depth 3–4 mm. No drainage for past 7 days.
Apply dressing and medication to the left heel ulcer daily as ordered by the physician: Using sterile technique, cleanse the ulcer daily with sterile normal saline and apply a light dusting of Brand X Hydrogel Powder over the surface of the ulcer. Cover with a sterile dressing.	Day 1: WBC 11,350/mm^3. Day 5: WBC 7,900/mm^3. Day 12: Healing well. See above assessment. Continue to use sterile technique. No fever. WBC 7,500/mm^3 (within normal limits).

(table continues on page 578)

Nursing Care Plan for a Patient With an Infected Stage II Pressure Ulcer (continued)

Table 26-3   Care Plan for Infected Stage II Pressure Ulcer (continued)

Nursing Diagnosis: Imbalanced nutrition, less than body requirements, related to inability to chew meat as evidenced by recent loss of 6 pounds (2.72 kg)
Expected Outcome: Patient will increase high-protein foods in diet, including protein supplements, and will increase weight by 5 pounds (2.27 kg) within 10 days.

Interventions	Evaluations
Provide Brand Z High-Calorie, High-Protein drink between meals and at bedtime.	Day 3: Consumes 100% of supplement consistently. Likes chocolate better than vanilla. Day 10: Consumes 100% of supplement most days.
Provide a high-protein diet. The patient likes peanut butter, beans, cheese, and eggs. Grind meat for ease of chewing.	Day 3: Eats 80%–100% of meals consistently. Frequently requests & eats peanut butter & crackers. Eats eggs for breakfast daily. Eating ground meat without problems. Day 10: Eats > 80% of meals & snacks.

Monitor laboratory results—hemoglobin, serum protein—noting drops or failure to increase	Serum protein @ admission: 5.8 g/dL (below normal).
	    7 days: 6.2 g/dL (WNL).
	    10 days: 6.4 g/dL.
	Hgb @ admission: 11.9 g/dL (little low).
	    10 days: 12.1 g/dL (low normal).

Record daily weights, noting losses.	Admit: 129 lbs. 3 days: 129.5 lbs. 7 days: 131 lbs. 10 days: 132 lbs.

Skill 26-1   Removing Sutures and Staples

Assessment Steps

1. Review the physician's order for specific instructions, such as orders to remove alternating staples rather than all staples. In orthopedic surgeries, orders are often written to remove alternating staples one day and remaining staples the next day.
2. Assess the patient's pain level and medicate if needed. Discomfort associated with suture or staple removal is usually mild and brief. However, *if the patient is already experiencing significant pain, removal of closures may exacerbate it.*

Planning Steps

1. Gather needed equipment and supplies: clean gloves; suture removal kit or staple removal kit; reinforced adhesive strips, such as Steri-Strips.

Intervention Steps

1. Follow the Initial Implementation Steps located on the inside front cover.
2. Open the peel pack containing the suture removal set or staple remover.

Removing Sutures

3. Using the forceps in the removal kit, grasp the knot of the suture with your nondominant hand, and lift the suture away from the skin.
4. Using the notched scissors for the removal kit in your dominant hand, slide the notched blade under the suture. Cut the suture next to the skin, adjacent to the knot.
5. As soon as the suture is clipped, pull smoothly and firmly with your nondominant hand. The suture will slide out, and *the contaminated portion of the suture will not be pulled through the skin.*
6. Remove every other suture and observe the wound edges for any signs of separation. *This helps prevent the possibility of dehiscence when all sutures are removed.*
7. Remove the remaining sutures, unless otherwise ordered.

Removing Staples

3. Hold the staple remover in your dominant hand.
4. Slide the lower hooked jaw under the middle of the staple.

Skill 26-1 (continued)

5. Gently squeeze the handles together. The staple ends will slide upward out of the skin.

6. Remove alternating staples while continually assessing wound edges for evidence of separation. *Safety: If there is any indication that edges might be separating, stop and do not remove any more staples. Apply Steri-Strips and notify the physician.*

7. If wound edges remain approximated, continue to remove the rest of the staples as ordered.

Cleaning and Dressing the Wound

8. Gently wipe the area with an alcohol pad *to remove debris and dried blood, which could become a medium for bacteria growth.*

9. Place Steri-Strips across the incision area. *This provides extra support to wound edges as healing continues.*

10. If desired by the patient, cover the incision with a gauze 4×4 *to protect the wound from irritation by clothing.*

11. Follow the Ending Implementation Steps located on the inside back cover.

12. Document the procedure and appearance of the wound.

Evaluation Steps

1. Check the incision line after a few hours *to be sure the incision edges remain approximated after patient activity.*

Sample Documentation

5-31-12   1120   *Rt. hip incision well approximated, without erythema, edema, or drainage. Every other staple (6 staples) removed and Steri-Strips applied (7 staples remaining). Incision integrity remains intact. Denies incisional discomfort.* ————
———————————————— *Nurse's signature and credentials*

Skill 26-2   Caring for Drainage Devices

Assessment Steps

1. Review the order for frequency to empty drainage device. It should be emptied at the end of the shift or when one-half to two-thirds full unless otherwise indicated in the physician's orders.

2. Assess the amount and characteristics of the drainage in the drain container.

Planning Steps

1. Gather needed equipment and supplies: water-repellant drape, graduated container, clean gloves, two alcohol sponges, goggles if splashing is possible.

Implementation Steps

1. Follow the Initial Implementation Steps located on the inside front cover.

2. Don clean gloves and apply goggles if needed *to follow standard precautions when handling the drainage device.*

3. Place the water-repellant drape under the drainage device *to prevent soiling linens.*

4. Assess the drain insertion site for erythema, edema, and drainage *to detect any signs of infection.*

5. Wipe the drain spout with an alcohol sponge *to prevent introducing microorganisms into the drain.* Avoid raising the drainage device above the insertion site. *This prevents reflux of contents into the wound bed, which decreases the risk of infection.*

6. Pointing the spout away from your face, open the spout and pour the contents into the graduated container so it can be measured, taking care to avoid splashing.

(skill continues on page 580)

Skill 26-2 (continued)

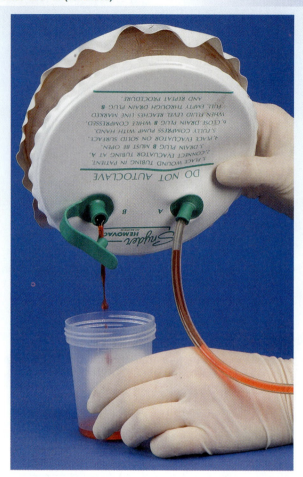

7. Clean around the drain spout with a new alcohol sponge.

8. Compress the drainage device *to establish suction* (known as *reactivating* the drain) and close the spout without contaminating it.

9. Note the amount, color, and other characteristics of the drainage before pouring contents down the toilet.

10. Follow the Ending Implementation Steps located on the inside back cover.

11. Document the volume and characteristics of the drainage emptied as well as the assessment of the drain insertion site.

Evaluation Steps

1. Compare the amount and appearance of the drainage with previous descriptions for evidence of decreasing drainage production.

2. Make certain the drainage system is draining and remains below wound height.

Sample Documentation

10-8-12   1100   JP drain emptied of 110 mL serosanguineous drainage. Drain insertion site in RUQ abdomen without erythema, drainage, or edema. JP reactivated and secured to gown below level of wound site. ———— Nurse's signature and credentials

Skill 26-3 Irrigating a Wound

Assessment Steps

1. Review the physician's orders *to determine the type of solution and frequency of irrigation.*

2. Assess the patient's pain level and medicate if needed. *Irrigation is usually part of a dressing change, which may be uncomfortable for the patient.*

Planning Steps

1. Gather needed equipment and supplies: emesis basin, sterile saline or other ordered solution, sterile irrigation kit or basin, 35-mL syringe and #19 Angiocath for correct pressure, bed protector, clean gloves.
   • Some nurses find it helpful to obtain a sterile towel or drape to use to prepare a small sterile field upon which to place sterile items.
   • Some irrigation kits will have a sterile tray that may also be used as a mini–sterile field.

2. Prepare for dressing change as well with biohazard bag, sterile dressings, and sterile gloves *because irrigation is usually performed during a dressing change.*

3. Enlist assistance if needed *to keep the patient in the correct position during the procedure.*

Intervention Steps

1. Follow the Initial Implementation Steps located on the inside front cover.

2. Set up the sterile field for your supplies. Remember to include any dressing supplies that you may need to redress the wound.

3. Pour sterile saline into a sterile basin or irrigation kit.

4. Open the Angiocath and the syringe packages without contaminating the sterile items and drop them onto the sterile field.

5. Position the patient in a manner that will best allow the irrigation solution to drain from the wound into the emesis basin that will be positioned at the wound's edge.

6. Don clean gloves.

7. Remove old dressing and place in the biohazard bag.

8. Place the bed protector on the bed *to prevent irrigant from soaking the bed.*

9. Position the emesis basin underneath the bottom edge of the wound and prop it with a towel or washcloth *to catch the irrigant as it flows from the wound.* If the patient is able to assist you, he or she may be able to hold it in place.

Skill 26-3 (continued)

10. Remove contaminated gloves.

11. Don sterile gloves.

12. Carefully remove the Angiocath sheath from the needle, laying the needle back on the sterile field. Touch the hub of the Angiocath only. Do not touch the sheath. Attach the hub of the 19-gauge Angiocath sheath to the 35-mL syringe. *These sizes ensure the ideal amount of pressure to remove debris without damaging any granulation tissue that may be present.*
    Safety: Leave the needle on the sterile field until you are done with the procedure so that you can open the lid to the wall-mounted sharps container without contaminating your sterile gloves.

13. Draw up 25 to 30 mL of irrigating solution into the syringe.

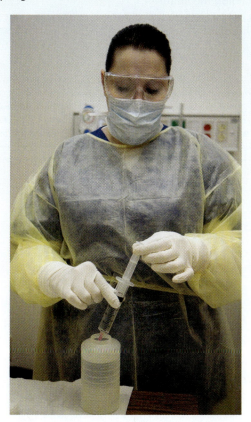

14. Hold the syringe so that the Angiocath is approximately 2 inches from the wound surface, at the superior edge of the wound. Depress the syringe plunger to cause a steady spray of fluid into the wound *to wash away debris.* Spray using a back-and-forth motion, moving from one side of the wound to the opposite side, and gradually working your way from the top of the wound to the bottom wound edge. *This prevents rinsing debris back into previously cleansed areas.*

15. Continue filling the syringe and irrigating the wound until the fluid leaving the wound is clear. *This ensures that all debris has been removed.*

16. Using a sterile gauze 4×4 with the four corners bunched up between your fingers, dry the skin around the outside perimeter of the wound. Avoid touching the interior of the wound *to prevent cross-contamination.*

17. Inspect the wound and note the size, depth, and color. Note the amount and color of any necrotic tissue.

18. Apply a new dressing following the steps in Skill 26-5.

19. Follow the Ending Implementation Steps located on the inside back cover.

20. Document the procedure, including the type and amount of solution used, the appearance of the return fluid, an assessment of the wound, and the type of dressing applied.

Evaluation Steps

1. Determine the effectiveness of wound cleansing using irrigation. Note whether loose, necrotic tissue is mostly removed after irrigation. Notify the physician if irrigation is not effective.

Sample Documentation

1-25-12   0930   *States no wound discomfort and does not desire pain med before irrigation. 4×4 dressing removed with 2-cm spot of dried serous drainage. Puncture wound edges mildly pink. Wound measures ½ cm across and 4 cm deep. Irrigated with sterile NS 100 mL using 19-g Angiocath and 35-mL syringe, using sterile technique. Wound covered with five sterile 4×4s. No c/o discomfort at any time.* ——— *Nurse's signature and credentials*

Skill 26-4 Obtaining a Wound Culture

Assessment Steps

1. Review the physician's order for an aerobic or anaerobic culture.
2. Assess the wound and the type of dressing, if there is one, *to determine supplies you will need to replace the dressing.*

Planning Steps

1. If the patient already has a dressing change scheduled, *performing the culture at the same time as the dressing change will save time.*
2. Gather needed equipment and supplies for the dressing change and supplies for the wound culture: clean gloves, sterile culturette tube with cotton-tipped swab.

Implementation Steps

1. Follow the Initial Implementation Steps located on the inside front cover.
2. Irrigate or cleanse the wound first *to remove exudate. Surface pathogens are not necessarily the cause of the wound infection.*
3. Don clean gloves and remove the old dressing if present.
4. Holding the culturette container in your nondominant hand, loosen the cap and remove the culturette swab from container with your dominant hand. *Use caution to avoid contaminating the distal cotton-tipped end of the swab.*
5. Holding only the proximal tip of the culturette swab, swirl the distal cotton-tipped end only on the granulation tissue in the wound bed. Avoid touching the cotton tip to the outer edges of the wound, *because normal flora (microorganisms that live on the patient's skin) can contaminate the culture.*

6. Quickly place the distal cotton-tipped end of the swab back into the culturette container, *using care to prevent touching it to the outside edges of the container.* Push the cap tightly onto the container.
7. If a dressing was present, replace it using sterile technique.
8. Label the container with the patient's name, room number, and ID number, the physician's name, the date and time, and the name of the test to be performed.
9. Follow the Ending Implementation Steps located on the inside back cover.

Evaluation Steps

1. Evaluate the patient's pain level during and after obtaining the culture.
2. Assess laboratory results of the culture after 48 and 72 hours.

Sample Documentation

8-13-12   0730 *Surgical incision on RLQ abdomen with poor approximation on lateral aspect, 1.5-cm open area, 0.5-cm deep, oozing moderate amount thick yellow purulent drainage. Wound irrigated per order. Wound culture obtained and sent to lab. C/o incisional tenderness using scale of 0 to 10, a 1 before performing culture, a 2 during, and a 1 afterward.* ———————————
———————————————— *Nurse's signature and credentials*

Skill 26-5 Changing Sterile Dressings and Wet-to-Damp Dressings

Assessment Steps

1. Review the physician's order and previous nurses' notes on the dressing change. *This will help you know how many dressings and what type you will need.*

2. Assess the patient's pain level. Medicate at least 30 minutes prior to performing the dressing change. *This will help keep the patient comfortable during a potentially uncomfortable procedure.*

Skill 26-5 (continued)

Planning Steps

1. Gather needed equipment and supplies: dressings (sterile gauze 4×4s and abdominal dressings), tape, clean gloves, biohazard discard bag, sterile cotton-tipped swabs, paper wound ruler, sterile gloves. *For the wet-to-damp dressing change,* you will also need a sterile basin or a dressing change kit and a pour-top bottle of sterile normal saline (NS).

2. Enlist assistance, if needed, to keep the patient positioned off of the wound during the dressing change *to prevent possible contamination of the wound during the procedure.*

Implementation Steps

1. Follow the Initial Implementation Steps located on the inside front cover.

2. Wash hands and follow standard precautions *to prevent transmission of blood-borne pathogens.*

3. Set up a sterile field, adding all additional sterile supplies that you will need. **Note:** *If you will be pouring sterile liquids, drape a sterile barrier with a moisture-proof backing over the clean over-the-bed table. This will keep your field sterile even if you splash sterile solution onto it.*

   If Applying a Wet-to-Damp Dressing: Additional supplies must be prepared as part of the sterile field:

   a. Check the label on the bottle of sterile NS three times *to make certain you have the right solution.* Check the manufacturer's date of expiration *to ensure it is still in date.* If the bottle has been previously opened, also check the date and time the nurse has written on the label. *If bottle has been open for longer than 24 hours, it can no longer be considered sterile. Dispose of it and obtain a new bottle of sterile NS.*

   b. If the bottle has never been opened, write the date, time, and your initials on the label. *This tells the next nurse to change the dressing when the NS was opened.*

   c. Remove the cap from the bottle and place it on the table next to the sterile field drape with the open rim pointing upward.

   d. *Note: If the bottle has been previously opened and is still within the 24-hour window, hold the bottle over the trash can and pour out a small amount of NS. The liquid pouring over the lip of the bottle helps to wash away any microorganisms that might be present. This process is known as "lipping" the bottle.*

   e. Pour saline into the sterile basin or the well of the dressing change kit to use to prepare the wet-to-damp dressings. **Alternative:** If bulk sterile gauze 4×4s are supplied in a separate plastic tub or tray, you can pour the saline directly over the 4×4s without taking them out of the sterile tray. It can serve as a mini–sterile field.

4. Open and position the biohazard bag *to receive contaminated waste.*

Remove Old Dressing

5. Don clean gloves *to follow standard precautions when handling the old dressing.*

6. Loosen the tape on the old dressing by gently pulling it from each side toward the wound. *This prevents tension on wound edges.*

7. Remove the old dressing and inspect the color and amount of the drainage present.

Assess the Wound

8. Inspect the wound and assess the color, odor, and presence of sinus tracts. Also assess for the presence of granulation tissue.

9. Measure the length, width, and depth of the wound *to determine degree of healing.* To measure the wound length and width, either a paper wound ruler or a transparent cellophane wound-sizing device may be used. Hold the measuring device above the wound without touching the wound surface. **Hint:** *Use a sterile cotton-tipped swab to measure the depth of the wound and of any sinus tracts.*
   • Information obtained in Steps 7, 8, and 9 is important for accurate documentation and may indicate complications to wound healing.

10. If there is a drain present, assess the drain insertion site for erythema and edema.

Cleanse the Wound

11. Remove contaminated gloves.

12. Apply sterile gloves, taking care to maintain sterility of gloves and sterile field.

13. Clean wound as ordered *to remove exudates and to promote granulation.* **Alternative:** If wound irrigation has been ordered, it should be done at this time (see Skill 26-3).

14. If there is a drain present, clean around it as well.

(skill continues on page 584)

Skill 26-5 (continued)

Apply a Sterile Dressing

15. Apply a new sterile dressing to the wound.
    For a Wet-to-Damp Dressing:
    a. Unfold the sterile gauze 4×4s completely and place them in the sterile saline you poured into the basin or well of the kit. **Alternative:** If the bulk 4×4s came in a sterile plastic tub or tray, you can pour saline directly on the 4×4s in their tray.

b. Press the excess saline out of a 4×4 until it is moist but not dripping. *Excessive moisture in the wound may cause maceration (softening) of the skin.*
c. Fluff the 4×4 *to increase the surface area of the gauze for contact with the wound.*

d. Carefully hold the moist 4×4 in your hand, and using sterile forceps from the kit or a sterile swab, gently pack the fluffed 4×4 into the wound. *Safety: Avoid pressing gauze tightly under any overhanging edges of the wound, as this will interfere with granulation tissue formation.*

e. Do not allow the gauze to touch the skin surface outside the wound. *This would cause contamination of the wound with surface microbes.*
f. Completely fill the wound with fluffed, saline-moistened gauze 4×4s *to keep all surfaces of the wound moist and promote healing.*

g. Cover the filled wound with damp, unfluffed 4×4s *to help maintain moisture.*
h. Cover the unfluffed 4×4s with an abdominal dressing pad, with the stripe on the pad facing outward so that it is visible after the dressing is in place. *This will hold moisture in the wound, protect it from contaminants, and absorb drainage.*

For a Dry Dressing:
a. Cover the wound with enough sterile gauze 4×4s for adequate absorption of drainage. If there is a wound drain, place a split 4×4 around it to prevent maceration of the skin.
b. Cover the 4×4s with an abdominal dressing pad. The stripe on the abdominal dressing should be facing outward so that it is visible after the dressing is in place. Use the correct size of abdominal dressing so that it completely covers the 4×4s and drain.

Skill 26-5 (continued)

Secure Dressing

16. Tape the superior and inferior edges of the dressing to the skin, taping from one lateral side to the opposite lateral side of the dressing. Then place another piece or two of tape across the middle of the dressing. Make strips of tape long enough to extend beyond dressing edges by 1½ to 2 inches.

Less length will not adequately secure the dressing. More will result in unnecessary discomfort upon removal.

— Too short
— Too long, narrow
— Too wide

Complete the Dressing Change

17. Remove gloves and wash hands.
18. Write the date, time, and your initials on the edge of the dressing.

19. Dispose of the biohazard bag and used supplies according to facility policy.
20. Follow the Ending Implementation Steps located on the inside back cover.
21. Document the date; time; wound appearance, including size, depth, color, and presence of granulation tissue; amount and type of drainage; dressing change procedure; signature; and credentials.

Evaluation Steps

1. Compare measurements and appearance of the wound with previous descriptions for evidence of healing.
2. Determine the patient's comfort level during the dressing change *to ensure adequate pain control with prescribed medications.*
3. Review any laboratory reports, such as wound culture and sensitivity results or white blood cell counts, for evidence of improving infection indicators.

Sample Documentation

> 7-19-11   0920   States pain med has reduced pain level from a 6 to a 1 on 0–10 scale. Removed 5½ in. × 9 in. ABD dressing from suprapubic incision. Removed damp packing with moderate amount green purulent drainage. Incision open end-to-end. 15 cm × 2 cm × 2.5 cm deep. Wound bed bright red and some pallor noted on medial aspect. Moderate amount granulation tissue on lateral aspect of wound bed. No erythema or edema of surrounding skin. Wound irrigated with 250 mL St. NS using 19-g Angiocath and 35-mL syringe, using sterile technique. Repacked wound with sterile moist gauze packing. Covered with ABD dressing. C/o pain @ 3 during irrigation and @ 1 on completion of dressing change.
> ———————————— *Nurse's signature and credentials*

Skill 26-6   Applying Transparent and Hydrocolloid Dressings

Assessment Steps

1. Review the physician's order for dressing change.
2. Determine the need for change of dressing: Has the barrier been in place 3 to 5 days? Is the barrier loosening, leaking, or developing an odor?

Planning Steps

1. Obtain needed equipment and supplies: clean gloves, scissors, biohazard bag, sterile saline and gauze 4×4s if the wound is to be cleansed, transparent or hydrocolloid dressing as ordered, tape, disposable paper ruler, alcohol swabs.
2. Ensure that the size of the dressing is appropriate. Transparent dressings should overlap the wound onto the skin for a 1-inch margin around the wound. For a hydrocolloid dressing, the overlap should be a 1¼- to 1½-inch margin around the wound. *This helps the dressing adhere to the skin and remain in place.*

Implementation Steps

1. Follow the Initial Implementation Steps located on the inside front cover.
2. Wash hands and don clean gloves *to follow standard precautions.*

Remove Old Dressing

3. Gently loosen the edges of the dressing and pull it toward the wound *to prevent tension on the wound edges.*
4. Dispose of the dressing in the biohazard bag *because it is contaminated with blood and body fluids.*
5. Inspect the wound for amount and type of drainage, odor, and color.
6. Measure the size of the wound using a disposable paper ruler, being careful not to touch the wound. *This information is needed for documentation.*
7. Remove gloves and wash hands.

(skill continues on page 586)

Skill 26-6 (continued)

Apply New Dressing

8. Apply clean gloves.

9. Clean the wound if ordered. Use sterile saline and sterile gauze 4×4s to gently clean the area. Gather the four corners of a 4×4 together and hold them with your fingers, forming a puff-ball with the central portion of the 4×4. Take care to avoid touching the central portion of the 4×4's sterile surface that is used to clean the wound. Pour a small amount of sterile NS over the central portion of the 4×4. Cleanse the wound from the center to the outer edges. Repeat the process using additional 4×4s as needed.

10. Use a final 4×4 to dry the surrounding skin thoroughly.

    Transparent Dressings:

    a. You may need to clean the skin around the wound with an alcohol pad to remove skin oils, *so the dressing will adhere better.*

    b. Apply the transparent dressing to one side of the wound. Remove the paper backing from the adhesive side of the dressing, pulling carefully away, while holding the dressing against the wound. *Safety: Do not stretch the transparent dressing tightly against the wound or it will impair movement and comfort.*

    c. Remove the surface film from the top of the transparent dressing, if present.

    d. Remove the edge pieces of the paper backing that remain on the adhesive side of the dressing.

    e. Write the date, time, and your initials on the edge of the transparent dressing.

    Hydrocolloid Dressings:

    a. Peel the paper backing from the hydrocolloid dressing.

    b. Place the dressing over the wound and smooth gently.

    c. Remove the surface paper from the hydrocolloid dressing, if present. *Hint: Hold your hand on the applied dressing for a few seconds. The warmth of your hand will help mold it to the skin and promote better adherence.*

    d. Write the date, time, and your initials on the edge of the hydrocolloid dressing.

Complete the Dressing Change

11. Inspect the dressing for any wrinkles and smooth them out *to prevent access to the wound by contaminants.*

12. Follow the Ending Implementation Steps located on the inside back cover.

13. Document the date, time, appearance of wound, size of wound, and type and amount of drainage.

Evaluation Steps

1. Apply tape to the edges of the dressings if they start to lift or roll up.

2. Inspect the wound through the transparent dressing daily. Inspect the hydrocolloid dressing daily for drainage escaping under the dressing, wrinkling, or excessive exudate absorption.

3. Evaluate appropriate use of the barrier dressing. These dressings are not indicated if excessive drainage occurs or if the wound is infected. Notify the physician if either of these situations occurs.

Sample Documentation

6-4-12   1415   States no wound pain. Denies need for pain med prior to dressing change. Hydrocolloid dressing removed from sacrum. 3 cm × 3.5 cm erythema, skin intact. No blistering. Cleansed with sterile NS using clean technique. New 5 cm × 8 cm hydrocolloid dressing applied. No c/o discomfort during or after dressing change. ———————— Nurse's signature and credentials

🌐 Post Conference

After your clinical experience, you have an opportunity to evaluate the care you gave. As you discussed your day with your classmates, you realized how much you had learned and accomplished during these two clinical days. You were able to maintain contact precautions as you cared for your patient with MRSA. You observed your patient for any reactions to the vancomycin he was taking to treat the MRSA. You changed the dressing very carefully, removing the old dressing and measuring the wound. You were able to identify granulation tissue and the location of infected tissue. Although it took some practice, you were able to fluff the wet gauze 4×4s and place them inside the wound without contaminating it; then you covered the wound with damp 4×4s, and covered the entire area with an abdominal dressing pad that you taped in place. Your instructor was very pleased with your accurate and detailed documentation of the procedure.

KEY POINTS

- The classic signs of infection include edema, erythema, drainage, and increased warmth.

- Pressure ulcers result when pressure is maintained on tissue until it becomes ischemic and begins to necrose.

- Friction and shear force damage tissue even more quickly than constant pressure does.

- The highest priority nursing intervention for preventing and treating pressure ulcers is to reposition the patient at least every 2 hours.

- The most common sites for development of pressure ulcers include the occiput, scapula, elbow, sacrum, coccyx, buttock, greater trochanter, ankle, and heel.

- Risk factors for pressure ulcers include emaciation, malnourishment, dehydration, overhydration, maceration, fragile skin as in the elderly or young children, incontinence, immobility, and metabolic conditions that impair circulation.

- There are four stages of pressure ulcers.

- A pressure ulcer covered with eschar cannot be staged until the eschar is débrided.

- Healing has three phases: the inflammatory phase, reconstruction phase, and maturation phase.

- All wounds heal by first, second, or third intention.

- Wound assessment should include width, length, depth, approximation of edges, color of wound bed and surrounding skin, texture, presence of granulation tissue, and drainage (amount, color, consistency, and odor).

- Wound evisceration is an emergency and requires stat nursing actions.

- When removing staples or sutures, remove every other one and replace it with a Steri-Strip to ensure wound integrity.

- Types of wound drainage include serous, serosanguineous, sanguineous, purulent, seropurulent, and bilious.

- The most common microorganism causing wound infections is *Staphylococcus aureus.*

- Tests that are valuable in the treatment of wounds are wound cultures, WBC, hemoglobin, and total protein level.

- The new tissue that indicates healing is occurring is fragile, translucent to pinkish-red, and grainy in appearance, and is known as granulation tissue.

- Hemovac and Jackson Pratt drains are active drainage devices. A T-tube drain is passive, draining via gravity.

- Wet-to-damp dressings are used to keep the wound bed slightly moist so it can heal.

- Débridement is removal of necrotic tissue from a wound.

- Appropriate personal protective equipment should be worn when providing wound care. Gloves should always be worn. A gown, goggles, and mask are worn when there is danger of splashing.

REVIEW QUESTIONS

Select the answer that is most appropriate for each of the following questions. Some questions may have more than one correct answer. Check all that apply.

1. A patient's J-P drain should be emptied:

   a. every 2 hours.

   b. every 8 hours.

   c. when one-half to two-thirds full.

   d. only when it needs to be reactivated.

   e. when the container is full.

2. Which one of the following assessment findings makes it impossible to stage a pressure ulcer?

   a. Purulent drainage

   b. Eschar

   c. Sloughing tissue

   d. Erythema

   e. Drainage

   f. Signs of infection

   g. Undermining

3. The phase of healing during which granulation tissue forms in a wound is the:

   a. inflammatory phase.

   b. reconstruction phase.

   c. maturation phase.

   d. remodeling phase.

4. You observe pink drainage from a patient's wound. You would describe this as:

   a. sanguineous.

   b. serous.

   c. purulent.

   d. seropurulent.

   e. serosanguineous.

5. Your patient has a large abdominal wound with copious drainage and many layers of gauze 4×4s in the dressing. The patient develops a skin reaction to the tape due to frequent dressing changes. What might you recommend for this patient?

   a. Change to surgical adhesive instead of tape to hold dressings in place.

   b. Call the doctor and ask for an order to decrease dressing change frequency.

   c. Ask the charge nurse about using Montgomery straps or an abdominal binder instead of tape.

   d. Wrap gauze around the patient's trunk to hold the dressings in place.

6. A patient returns from surgery with a left shoulder dressing. A 3-inch diameter spot of red drainage is visible on the anterior portion of the dressing. The physician does not want the dressing disturbed for 24 hours. What will you do?

   a. Call the physician to report the drainage and request a change in orders.

   b. Reinforce the dressing by adding several gauze 4×4s over the area.

   c. Draw a line on the dressing outlining the drainage, with the date, time, and your initials.

   d. Document the drainage in the chart and observe for further drainage over the next several hours.

7. A patient has signs of infection in his left shoulder incision—erythema, warmth, and a small amount of purulent drainage. You prepare to report this to the physician. Which information will you have ready when you call?

   a. Vital signs

   b. Name and dosage of pain medication currently ordered

   c. Appropriate laboratory results

   d. Patient's rating of incisional pain

   e. Description of the wound and drainage

   f. Names of all staff who have changed his dressing since surgery

   g. Signs of infection you observe

   h. Name and dosage of antibiotics currently ordered, if any

8. You are caring for a 67-year-old male who had a cerebrovascular accident 3 weeks ago. In addition, he has developed a pressure ulcer on his right hip. Which of the following data that you collected will be useful in developing a care plan that will address his pressure ulcer?

   a. Last week he weighed 165.5 lbs. and today he weighs 161.8 lbs.

   b. The pressure ulcer is a stage III.

   c. He has 250 mL clear yellow urine in his Foley catheter.

   d. He is not able to sit up in a chair for longer than 15 minutes at a time.

   e. He dislikes cheese, beans, chicken, and fish, but loves steak, eggs, all kinds of nuts, and peanut butter.

   f. His affect is flat.

   g. He has been on an eggcrate mattress while in the hospital.

9. Which one of the following interventions would you rate as the *most* important for care of his pressure ulcer?

   a. Change the wet-to-damp dressing on his right hip wound qid using sterile technique.

   b. Tell dietary service about his food likes and dislikes.

   c. Reposition the patient every 2 hours around the clock, avoiding the Rt. lateral position.

   d. Assess the condition of the pressure ulcer once daily.

   e. Provide Foley care every shift.

   f. Work to increase the length of time the patient can tolerate sitting in a chair.

CRITICAL THINKING EXERCISES

10. Create and describe a scenario of a patient with a wound in whom there are *at least four indicators* that a wound culture would be beneficial.

11. Describe a scenario when it would not be wise to remove all the staples in a surgical incision.

ADDITIONAL RESOURCES

For additional Resources, Questions, and Activities, please see:

 Student Resource Disk

 http://davisplus.fadavis.com

 Student Study Guide

REFERENCES

Ayello EA. New evidence for an enduring wound-healing concept: moisture control. *J Wound Ostomy Continence Nurs.* 2006; 33(6 Suppl):S1-S2.

Ayello EA, Baranoski S, Salati DS. Wound care survey report. *Nursing2005.* 2005;35(6):36-45.

Baldwin KM. Damage control: Preventing and treating pressure ulcers. *Nurs Made Incredibly Easy.* 2006;4(1):12-26.

Baugh N, Zuelzer H, Meador J, Blankenship J. Wounds in surgical patients who are obese. *Am J Nurs.* 2007;107(6):40-50.

Beatie S. Bedside emergency: wound dehiscence. *RN* [serial online]. 2007;June 1. Available at: http://www.modernmedicine.com/modernmedicine/CE+Library/Bedside-emergency-Wound-dehiscence/ArticleStandard/Article/detail/433110.

Black J, Baharestani M, Cuddigan J, Dorner B, Edsberg L, Langemo D, et al. From the NPUAP: National Pressure Ulcer Advisory Panel's updated pressure ulcer staging system. *Adv Skin Wound Care.* 2007;20:269-274.

Calianno C, Jakubek P. Wound wise: The need to debride. *Nurs Made Incredibly Easy.* Mar/Apr 2007;5(2):7-10.

Clinical Rounds: Staph super-bug on the move. *Nursing2007.* 2007;37(9):34-35.

Galli S, Constantinides M. Wound closure techniques. 2006. Available at: http://emedicine.medscape.com/article/884764-overview. Accessed October 8, 2009.

George EL, Panos A. Does a high WBC count signal infection? *Nursing2005.* 2005;35(1):20-21.

Greenfield R, Shaikh S. Gangrene. 2007. Available at: http://www.emedicinehealth.com/gangrene/article_em.htm. Accessed October 8, 2009.

Medline Plus. Blood differential. 2009. Available at: http://www.nlm.nih.gov/medlineplus/ency/article/003657.htm. Accessed October 8, 2009.

Medline Plus. Gangrene. 2008. Available at: http://www.nlm.nih.gov/medlineplus/ency/article/007218.htm. Accessed October 8, 2009.

Medline Plus. WBC count. 2009. Available at: http://www.nlm.nih.gov/medlineplus/ency/article/003643.htm. Accessed October 8, 2009.

Pittman J. Effect of aging on wound healing: current concepts. *J Wound Ostomy Continence Nurs.* July/Aug 2007;34:412-417.

Ratliff C, Taler G. National Pressure Ulcer Advisory Panel's updated pressure ulcer staging system. *Urol Nurs.* 2007;27:144-150.

Rhoads J, Meeker BJ. *Davis's Guide to Clinical Nursing Skills.* Philadelphia: FA Davis; 2007.

Scanlon VC, Sanders T. *Essentials of Anatomy and Physiology.* 5th ed. Philadelphia: FA Davis; 2007.

Schweon S. MRSA extends its reach. *RN* [serial online]. 2006;February 1. Available at: http://rn.modernmedicine.com/RNweb/CE+Library/MRSA-extends-its-reach/ArticleStandard/Article/detail/301785?ref25.

Sieggreen MY. Getting a leg up on managing venous ulcers. *Nurs Made Incredibly Easy.* 2006;4(6):52-60.

Singhal H, Kaur K, Zammit C. Wound infection. September 15, 2009. Available at: http://emedicine.medscape.com/article/188988-overview. Accessed October 8, 2009.

Stillman RM. Wound care. 2009. Available at: http://www.emedicine.com/med/topic2754.htm. Accessed October 8, 2009.

Wilkinson JM, Van Leuven K. *Fundamentals of Nursing: Theory, Concepts, and Applications.* Philadelphia: FA Davis; 2007.

Williams L, Hopper P. *Understanding Medical-Surgical Nursing.* 3rd ed. Philadelphia: FA Davis; 2007.

Wound, Ostomy, and Continence Nurses Society. Guidance on OASIS Skin and Wound Status M0 Items. 2006. Available at: http://www.wocn.org/pdfs/WOCN_Library/OASIS_Guidance_rev_07_24_2006.pdf. Accessed October 8, 2009.

Musculoskeletal Care

Key Terms

Amputate

Continuous passive motion (CPM) machine

External fixators

Fracture

Joint replacement

Osteoarthritis

Physical therapist

Prosthesis

Skeletal traction

Skin traction

Spica

Sprain

Stump

Objectives

1. Define key terms associated with musculoskeletal care.
2. Describe common musculoskeletal conditions that result in limited mobility.
3. Discuss the role of the physical therapist in the health care team.
4. Differentiate between indications for use of x-rays, CT scans, and MRIs to diagnose musculoskeletal conditions.
5. Enumerate six types of immobilizing devices used for musculoskeletal disorders.
6. Describe nursing care of patients with musculoskeletal conditions, including casts, traction, joint replacement, and amputation.
7. Discuss guidelines for patients using assistive devices for ambulation.
8. Describe the steps necessary to develop a plan of care for a patient with impaired mobility related to a musculoskeletal condition.

Skills

27-1 Performing Neurovascular Checks
27-2 Setting Up a Continuous Passive Motion Machine
27-3 Applying Elastic Bandages

Clinical Connection

Your Assignment: You have been assigned to care for a patient who is having a right total knee replacement due to osteoarthritis. She is scheduled to go to the operating room at 0730. You will be assisting with her preoperative care and performing postoperative care when she returns to her room on the patient unit.

Your Actions: You know very little about a total knee replacement or how to care for someone immediately following this surgery. It sounds painful and somewhat frightening to you when you get the assignment. You must find out about any special concerns during preoperative care, although you have sent several patients to surgery in earlier clinicals. You know about taking routine postoperative vital signs and managing pain after surgery, but your instructor mentioned a CPM and you have no idea what it is or what to do with it. You also wonder how soon this patient will be able to get up in a chair and what special care the replaced joint will require.

When you care for patients who have musculoskeletal disorders, they often will have at least some degree of restricted mobility. As you recall from Chapter 16, immobility can place patients at risk for a number of complications, in addition to potential complications from surgery or other procedures. You will study more details about different types of musculoskeletal disorders, their treatment, and their prognoses when you study medical-surgical nursing. The purpose of this chapter is to prepare you to care for patients with limited mobility related to musculoskeletal conditions.

Musculoskeletal Conditions Resulting in Limited Mobility

A variety of musculoskeletal conditions can result in immobilization of a joint, a limb, or the entire body. Some of the most common conditions are fractures, joint replacements, and lower limb amputation.

Common Musculoskeletal Conditions

A **sprain** is an injury to a joint that results in damage to muscles and ligaments. Severe sprains may cause ligaments to be completely torn. Mild sprains often cause only minor muscle and ligament damage. The ankle is the joint that is most often sprained, but a sprain can occur in other joints as well. The sprained joint must be supported and rested in order to heal. The acronym RICE is used to help you remember treatment for a sprain:

- **R**est: The joint must be rested and should not bear weight until it can do so without pain.
- **I**ce: Apply ice to the joint during the first 48 hours after the injury occurs to help decrease swelling and pain.
- **C**ompression: Apply an elastic bandage to compress the joint and prevent further swelling.
- **E**levation: Keep the joint elevated above the heart, again to help decrease swelling and pain.

Fractures are breaks in the bone. They may range from a narrow crack, called a *hairline fracture,* to a bone that is broken into many small pieces, called a *comminuted fracture.* To promote healing of a fracture, the broken ends of the bones must be supported in close proximity to one another for 4 to 8 weeks or longer to allow the bone to grow together. This may require the insertion of pins, wires, or screws to hold the bone pieces together. Generally, a cast or immobilizer is placed on a limb to accomplish this. If the fractured bones are in the trunk of the body, support may be provided in other ways, such as wires inserted into the bones to hold them together.

A **joint replacement** is a surgery to remove damaged articular bone surfaces and replace them with metal and plastic surfaces. It is performed when a joint has severe degenerative changes, usually due to advanced **osteoarthritis**, which causes degeneration and inflammation of joints over time. The most commonly replaced joints are the knees and the hips. Because these joints bear the body's weight, they may become stressed over time. If the joint has been injured in the past, osteoarthritis is more likely to develop in later life.

When a limb is so damaged by trauma that it cannot be saved, it will be **amputated**, or surgically removed. Other reasons for amputation include severely decreased blood flow to the limb and *gangrene* (death of tissue) in a limb. The remaining portion of a limb after amputation is referred to as a **stump**. While the stump is not immobilized after surgery, it requires specialized nursing care, discussed later in this chapter. When a lower limb is amputated, the patient will be dealing with mobility issues as well.

The result of immobilization is that the patient will need assistance to regain muscle strength and ambulation ability. **Physical therapists** are the health care team members responsible for assessing musculoskeletal deficiencies and developing the plan of care to strengthen muscles and restore mobility. The physician and physical therapist may order that the patient be ambulated a specific number of times per day, or a specific distance at each walk. It is your nursing responsibility to be sure that such orders are carried out, so the patient can gain strength and be prepared for discharge. Sometimes nurses may feel that they are too busy to get the patient up and assist with ambulation, but these activity orders are very important and must be carried out.

Knowledge Connection

List four musculoskeletal conditions that result in limited mobility. What is the role of the physical therapist in the health care team?

Laboratory and Diagnostic Connection

Testing for Musculoskeletal Conditions

Different types of diagnostic tests are used to diagnose different types of musculoskeletal conditions. X-rays are typically ordered for suspected fractures or significant trauma. Computed tomography (CT) scans are most helpful to further identify fractures that may be difficult to see on x-rays, as well to view congenital abnormalities of the musculoskeletal system. They can be used when magnetic resonance imaging (MRI) would be contraindicated because of metal implants, pacemakers, or claustrophobia. MRI is used when pathological fractures occur because these fractures are usually associated with bone

tumors. MRI is also used to examine congenital problems of the spine. MRIs are generally ordered to view soft tissue conditions such as injuries to joints, and ligament, tendon, or muscle tears. Bone scans are ordered when there is suspected widespread disease of the bones, as in a metabolic condition or cancer.

Types of Immobilization

When a bone or joint has to be immobilized, the physician chooses the appropriate device for the situation. The devices used for immobilization are varied, depending on the condition and the time needed for healing. Sometimes when students think about musculoskeletal conditions and immobilization, they think only of fractures and casts. However, you will see that there are many such conditions and devices. Table 27-1 contains descriptions of various types of immobilization devices used to treat musculoskeletal disorders.

External fixators are the wires, pins, tongs, and rods that may be used in skeletal traction. These devices are found on the outside of the limb, but are also fixed to the bone of the limb (Fig. 27-1). They may help hold the bone in place while healing occurs or may be used for attaching weight to move bones in traction.

Table 27-1   Immobilization Devices

Device	Description and Use
Abductor pillow	Wedge-shaped foam pillow, often with Velcro straps, placed between the legs of patients who have had total hip replacement surgery; keeps hips abducted while patient in bed; straps keep the pillow in place and prevent shifting.
Cast	Hard plaster or fiberglass encasement for a limb; used to immobilize joints, usually to stabilize fractures until they heal; sometimes used to immobilize severely sprained joints until healing can occur; often used after musculoskeletal surgeries to stabilize the joint and surgical sites.
Elastic bandages	Woven bandage containing elastic to stretch as it is wrapped around an injured area; elastic helps compress the area to decrease edema.
Immobilizer	Soft fabric with firm internal stays; opens and closes with Velcro fasteners; used to protect an injured limb and to keep its joints from flexing; often a "boot" for foot and ankle injuries.
Splint	Firm plastic molded form used to keep a joint or joints from flexing; may be applied to a limb and wrapped in place with gauze or an elastic bandage; sometimes "air splints" are used when transporting injured patients; can be slipped beneath the injured limb, wrapped around it, then inflated to immobilize the joint.
Traction	*Skin traction* involves use of ropes, pulleys, and weights to align bone ends after a fracture; weights are attached to a frame held in place with elastic bandages or other wrap on the skin; may be used to prevent severe muscle spasm due to displaced bones until surgery can be performed. *Skeletal traction* uses wires, rods, or tongs that penetrate the skin and subcutaneous tissue and are inserted into the bone; these then attach to a frame with weights or only to a frame to hold the bone in place or move the bone with the weights.

Figure 27-1   This patient has an external fixator in place on the lower leg.

An additional type of external fixator is the *Ilizarov frame,* named for the Russian doctor who developed it. This frame is composed of metal rings on the outside of the limb, with rods and wires that attach to those rings. The rods and wires also penetrate the skin and insert into the bone. This fixator is used to stabilize small bone pieces, such as in a comminuted fracture, keeping the fragments aligned while bone growth occurs. It is also used in situations in which one leg has been left shorter than the other after trauma. By turning screws in the frame, the rings separate slightly; over time, the bone grows to fill in the gap. This allows for a very gradual increase in bone length to help the legs become more even.

Knowledge Connection
What are the purposes of traction? When might an Ilizarov frame be used?

Caring for Patients With Musculoskeletal Immobilization

As a nurse, you will be expected to know how to care for patients with musculoskeletal immobilization devices. You will be responsible for delivering appropriate care to the patient regardless of the type of device being used. Cast care and traction care will be discussed here as fundamental nursing skills. If you care for a patient with a different type of device, be sure you look up information about the device in a medical-surgical textbook or are instructed in the appropriate care by nursing staff.

Caring for a Patient in a Cast

Casts may be made of plaster of Paris, fiberglass, or other types of polymers. Plaster casts are often preferred for lower limbs because they can support the body's weight better than fiberglass without breaking down easily. A **spica** cast encases the hips and one or both legs. There is an open area for the perineum, and an abductor bar keeps the legs and hips a specific distance apart. These casts are often used to correct hip dysplasia in young children. It is very important that you move the patient in a spica cast carefully, and do not use the abductor bar to lift the patient. It is not designed for that purpose, and doing so can damage the spica cast.

When a plaster cast is applied, it takes many hours for it to dry. If you are caring for a patient in a plaster cast that is not yet dry, follow these guidelines:

• Support the limb on pillows in such a way that air circulates all around the cast for even drying.
• Avoid touching the wet or damp cast with your fingers, because they can leave dents in the cast that will remain after it dries, causing pressure points on the skin beneath the cast.
• If it is necessary to touch the cast, use only the palms of your hands.

Fiberglass casts are more lightweight and dry very quickly compared to plaster casts. A special light may be used to promote drying of the fiberglass cast.

When you care for patients with dry casts, whether plaster or fiberglass, follow these guidelines:

• Teach the patient to avoid putting anything between the cast and the skin beneath it, especially for the purpose of scratching. Skin sheds outer epidermal cells, but when the cast is in place, the cells that have been shed tend to pile up rather than flake off, causing intense itching at times. If the patient uses an implement such as an ink pen or straightened coat hanger to scratch beneath the cast, it can abrade the skin. The warm, dark, moist area beneath the cast is a perfect medium for bacteria growth, leading to severe infection. One alternative is to use a portable hair dryer to blow cool air down the cast to relieve the itching.
• Observe for any drainage staining the cast or any malodorous discharge, which would indicate infection beneath the cast. Report such observations to the physician.
• Assess circulation to the casted limb. If swelling occurs, the cast may cause restricted circulation, which can lead to tissue necrosis or nerve damage. To assess circulation, perform neurovascular checks every 2 hours for the first 24 hours after the cast is applied or surgery is performed. The neurovascular checks then may be decreased to every 4 hours or according to facility policy (see Skill 27-1, page 605).
• Place tape "petals" over the edges of the cast if they begin to crack or crumble over time. To reinforce the edges of the

cast with tape, also called "petaling" a cast, cut 3- to 4-inch strips of tape. On one end of each strip, cut the tape in a point. Place the square end of the tape against the cast between the patient's skin and the cast. Fold the pointed edge of the tape over to the outside of the cast. This technique can also be used to cover rough edges of the cast that may irritate the skin and cause breakdown.

Caring for a Patient in Traction

Two types of traction may be employed: skin traction and skeletal traction. When **skin traction** is used, the limb is wrapped with an elastic bandage or fitted with a Velcro wrap to which a frame is attached. One or more ropes are attached to the frame; on the other end of each rope, a weight is attached. An overhead frame is affixed to the bed, with a *trapeze bar,* or triangular piece, attached for the patient to use as a hand grip when moving in bed. Figure 27-2 shows a patient in skin traction with the overhead frame and trapeze bar in place.

When **skeletal traction** is used, pins, screws, or tongs are surgically inserted into the bone. These devices, referred to as *external fixators,* require meticulous nursing care. Because these fixators penetrate the skin and enter the bone, they provide a pathway for pathogens to enter the body. Infections of the bone are very serious and sometimes quite difficult to treat. It is the nurse's responsibility to prevent such infections by performing pin-site care as ordered. Generally, orders for this care include cleansing the skin insertion sites using sterile gauze saturated with normal saline or hydrogen peroxide. In addition, you need to assess the pin sites for signs of infection. Small amounts of serous or serosanguineous drainage at the insertion site is a normal finding. Immediately report any purulent drainage to the physician as this is indicative of infection. Also report increasing redness of the skin around the insertion site. Most physicians do not order ointment at pin sites because the moisture can promote bacteria growth.

Tongs are used on the skull to provide cervical traction after surgery or fracture to the cervical vertebrae. The tong insertion sites are located on either side of the skull. The hair in the area has usually been shaved to decrease the chances of infection. Again, you will clean the insertion sites according to orders and make the same assessments as for pin sites.

In addition to pin-site care, nurses are responsible for monitoring traction to ensure that no complications occur:

- Ensure that the weights hang freely and do not rest on the floor.
- Ensure that the ropes pull in a straight line without crossing one another.
- Assess for skin breakdown beneath the external traction devices.
- When turning a patient in traction, have another person lift up on the weights, causing slack in the ropes while the patient is turned. After the patient is supported and aligned, the second person then gently and slowly releases the weights to hang freely.
- Ensure that the patient's body is in proper alignment so that the traction pulls correctly.

Knowledge Connection

Why does itching occur beneath a cast? How can it be safely relieved? What is the difference between skin traction and skeletal traction? When might tongs be used for traction? What do you need to do when turning a patient in traction?

Caring for a Patient After Joint Replacement

When a joint is replaced, specialized nursing care is needed to avoid postoperative dislocation or other complications. It is very important that you know the appropriate nursing care for joint replacements, during both your practice as a student and your practice as a nurse.

Total Hip Replacement

It is necessary to review the normal anatomy of the hip joint to understand how a total hip replacement is performed.

Figure 27-2   This patient is in traction, but can use the trapeze bar attached to the over-the-bed frame to assist with movement. Note that the weight is hanging freely off of the end of the bed.

Anatomy and Physiology Connection

The Hip Joint

The normal hip joint consists of the head of the femur, which fits into the acetabulum of the pelvis, forming a ball-and-socket joint (Fig. 27-3). The acetabulum is lined with smooth cartilage, and the rounded head of the femur rotates freely and smoothly in the socket. A small amount of fluid, called *synovial fluid*, is also found in the joint to lubricate that movement.

When a hip joint is replaced, the head and neck of the femur are removed and replaced with a titanium implant that is bonded into the top of the femur. It is in the shape of the head and neck of the femur. The acetabulum is revised and a titanium acetabular cup lined with smooth plastic is cemented into the pelvic bone. Now the new femur head fits exactly into the new acetabular cup and moves smoothly and easily. However, the muscles that had attached to the head of the femur do not attach to the artificial femur immediately, so muscular support for the joint is absent. Eventually, the muscles repair and support the new joint, but that takes several months.

Immediately after surgery and for several more months, the patient must avoid adducting the operative leg to the midpoint of the body or beyond. In addition, the patient must not flex the hip joint more than 90 degrees. Both of these actions could cause the new femur head to pop out of the acetabular cup, which would require treatment for a joint dislocation, often involving a return to surgery.

A wedge-shaped abductor pillow is used to keep the patient from accidentally moving the affected leg to or beyond the midline (Fig. 27-4). When you turn the patient to the unaffected side or the back, the abductor pillow must be kept in place. Generally, you will have orders not to turn the patient on the operative side during the immediate postoperative period.

When you assist the patient to get out of bed, to sit in a chair, or to use the bedside commode, you must be very careful that the patient does not lean forward at any time, as that would flex the hip beyond 90 degrees and possibly cause hip dislocation. Figure 27-5 illustrates the angle that occurs when a patient leans forward. After discharge,

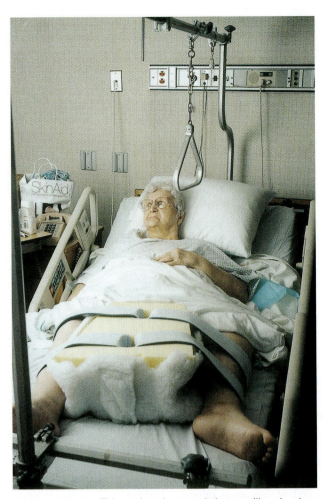

Figure 27-4 This patient has an abductor pillow in place to prevent adduction of the prosthetic right hip joint, causing possible dislocation.

patients are encouraged to use an extension gripper to pick up any dropped items, so that they do not flex the hip too far. Box 27-1 contains guidelines to follow when caring for patients who have had total hip replacements.

Real-World Connection

Researching the Right Condition

A nursing student was assigned to care for a patient who was 1 day postoperative with a total hip replacement. The student researched how to care for a patient with a fractured hip repaired with open reduction and internal fixation, rather than researching care for a patient who had a total hip replacement. During clinicals, the student turned the patient onto her operative side (contraindicated in either situation) and flexed the unaffected leg at the knee, bringing it over the operated leg. No abductor pillow was in use. This had the effect of adducting the operated leg beyond the midpoint of the body. The patient began to cry out in pain because the hip replacement had dislocated. It required a return trip to surgery to relocate the replaced joint.

Ball and socket
Acetabulum of
hip bone

Head of
femur

Figure 27-3 The hip joint includes the acetabulum and the head of the femur.

Correct hip flexion   Incorrect hip flexion

≤90°   >90°

Figure 27-5   If the patient with a total hip replacement leans forward, the hip angle is greater than 90 degrees, which can cause dislocation of the head of the femur.

Box 27-1

Mobility Guidelines for Patients With Total Hip Replacements

To prevent dislocation of a new total hip replacement, the patient and nursing staff must be careful to avoid hip flexion beyond 90 degrees. The following guidelines will help you keep the patient's hip prosthesis in place:

- Keep the abductor pillow in place while the patient is in bed.
- Avoid turning the patient on the operative side, according to physician's orders.
- Assist the patient out of bed carefully to prevent flexion of the hip more than 90 degrees.
- Ensure that the patient calls for help if any items are dropped, and that the patient does not lean forward, which would flex the hip beyond 90 degrees.
- Assist the patient to get up from the chair or bedside commode without leaning forward.

Total Knee Replacement

Another commonly replaced joint is the knee. In this surgery, the top of the tibia and lower end of the femur are replaced with titanium or other metal implants. The femoral component sits on the tibial component, which is topped with a durable plastic surface. The metal of the tibial component articulates against the plastic surface to allow smooth movement of the two surfaces. The patella may be completely replaced with a rounded piece of polyethylene or durable plastic. Sometimes plastic is affixed to the back of the existing patella to provide a smooth articular surface when the knee is flexed.

Some nursing concerns after a total knee replacement are different than those after a total hip replacement. Very soon after surgery, flexion of the new knee joint begins. To accomplish this, a **continuous passive motion (CPM) machine** is used. This machine is designed to gently flex the patient's knee according to the number of degrees of flexion on the setting, and then gently extend the knee. The leg is supported on a platform that gently bends and straightens the knee as it moves. The patient will require effective pain management in order to tolerate the passive exercise.

The CPM machine sits on the patient's bed and is connected to a power source. The platform where the patient's leg rests is lined with sheepskin to prevent skin breakdown. It is important that you line up the machine so that the break in the platform is centered beneath the patient's knee. It is also important to ensure that the CPM machine is positioned so that the supported leg is maintained in correct body alignment with the hips and rest of the body. The only way to verify this positioning is to stand at the foot of the bed and inspect the visual alignment of the CPM machine with the hips and torso. Place the machine so that the patient's leg rests comfortably on the platform, set the dial to the degrees of flexion and speed of flexion ordered by the physician, and turn on the machine. Remain with the patient for 10 to 20 repetitions to ensure that he or she is tolerating the passive exercise. The physician will order the length of time the CPM is to be on during a 24-hour period, as well as when to increase the degrees of flexion to improve joint function. Skill 27-2 (page 605) presents more information on setting up a CPM machine.

During the first 24 hours postoperatively, even with adequate pain medication, the patient may experience much discomfort when the machine first begins to flex the knee. The more the patient tenses the affected leg muscles, the more pain he or she will experience. This is a good time to teach and assist your patient to use relaxation breathing. Box 27-2 contains guidelines to follow when caring for patients with total knee replacements.

Knowledge Connection

Why must a patient with a new total hip replacement refrain from adducting the leg or flexing the hip more than 90 degrees? What is the function of a CPM machine after a total knee replacement?

Caring for a Patient After Amputation

Amputation of a body part is an emotionally traumatic event. Not only does the patient need physical care, but he or she requires emotional support as well. Physical care of the patient with an amputation is focused on rehabilitation,

Box 27-2

Guidelines for Caring for Patients With Total Knee Replacements

When a patient has had a total knee replacement, it is important that the CPM therapy be performed correctly to prevent limited range of motion in the prosthetic knee joint. These guidelines will be useful when caring for a patient with a total knee replacement:

- Ensure that the patient's pain is managed so that he or she can tolerate passive exercise.
- Set the degrees of flexion on the CPM machine according to the physician's orders.
- Follow orders exactly regarding the length of time the CPM machine is to be in use and advancing the degrees of flexion.
- Assist the patient in and out of bed using a walker or other assistive device.
- Follow the physician's orders regarding the amount of weight bearing allowed on the operative knee.

even immediately after surgery. It is important that the limb stump heal well and be shaped correctly to fit into a **prosthesis**, or artificial limb, such as an arm or leg.

Initially, observe the sutures or staples in the stump to ensure that all edges of the wound are approximated and growing together well. If the incision does not heal well, it may break open or the skin may break down with the pressure of a prosthesis. If left to heal on its own, the stump will have a squared-off shape. However, in order to fit into the socket of a prosthetic limb, the stump must have a smooth, rounded shape. That is the reason for wrapping the stump with an elastic bandage in the postoperative healing phase, so it will heal in the correct shape to fit into the prosthesis. Skill 27-3 (page 606) provides information about wrapping extremities with elastic bandages. In some situations, a compression sock is used to shape the stump, rather than elastic bandage.

In addition, the patient with an amputation is dealing with a disturbed body image and all the possible life changes that accompany it. It is important for you to be accepting of the patient and not communicate rejection of the altered body imagine, even nonverbally. You need to listen when the patient wants to talk about his or her feelings and lifestyle changes as a result of the amputation. It is not unusual for the patient to be angry and perhaps direct that anger at you. These patients are mourning a loss and often go through some or all of the stages of grieving discussed in Chapter 10.

Knowledge Connection

What is the purpose of wrapping a stump? How can you help a patient with an amputation adjust to body image changes?

Assistive Devices for Ambulation

Various types of assistive devices are available for people who are unable to ambulate independently. In most acute care settings, a physical therapist will fit the assistive device

to the patient and instruct him or her on its proper use. You may be responsible for reinforcing the therapist's teaching. The following information will help you do so.

Crutches

Crutches are used when a patient is unable to bear full weight on a lower limb. The patient may be restricted to no weight bearing or partial weight bearing. Crutches fit correctly when there are three fingerbreadths of space between the axillary pad and the patient's axilla, as the patient is standing with the crutch tips 4 to 6 inches (10 to 15 cm) to the side of the heel.

Guidelines for assisting patients using crutches include:

- Ensuring that the patient is bearing weight on the hands and wrists, not on the axillary pads. *Safety: Bearing weight on the axilla can cause compression of nerves and can lead to nerve damage affecting the arm and hand*.
- Instructing the patient that, when he or she is walking upstairs on crutches, the patient should place the unaffected leg on the step, then move up the crutches and the affected leg.
- Instructing the patient that, when he or she is walking downstairs on crutches, the patient should place the crutches and affected leg on the downward step, then bring down the unaffected leg.
- Assisting the patient, if needed, to use the appropriate crutch-walking gait. (Table 27-2 describes common gaits.)
- Reminding the patient to keep the affected foot slightly forward, rather than bending the knee and holding the foot behind the crutches. *Safety: If the knee is flexed and the foot held behind the crutches, it can affect the patient's balance, causing him or her to fall backward*.

Canes

A cane is used when a patient can bear weight on the affected leg but needs extra support while ambulating. Several styles of canes exist, but they generally fall into two categories: single-pronged or multipronged canes.

A single-pronged cane has one tip and may have a variety of handles (Fig. 27-6). A multipronged cane generally has three or four tips. A three-pronged tip may be called a tripod cane, and a four-pronged tip may be called a quad cane. In many situations, the multipronged cane is preferred because there is less chance that the cane could slide or slip as the patient leans on it. A cane is the correct height when the top of it is even with the patient's hip joint as the tip is positioned 4 inches (10 cm) away from the side of the foot.

Guidelines for assisting patients using a cane include:

- Ensuring that the patient holds the cane on the unaffected side.
- Reminding the patient to remain erect, rather than leaning over the cane.
- Ensuring that the patient moves the unaffected leg and the cane forward together, then moves the affected leg forward.

Table 27-2 **Common Crutch-walking Gaits**

Type	Description
Two-point gait	For patients who are able to bear partial weight on the affected limb; patient moves one foot and the opposite crutch forward at the same time, then moves remaining foot and crutch forward.
Three-point gait	For patients who are unable to bear weight on the affected limb; patient moves both crutches and the nonaffected foot forward at the same time, and then brings the affected foot forward without touching down or placing weight on it.
Four-point gait	For patients able to bear weight on the affected limb; patient moves the first crutch forward, then the opposite foot forward, patient then moves remaining crutch forward, then remaining affected foot forward.
Swing-to gait	For patients able to bear weight on the affected limb; patient is standing on both feet and moves both crutches forward at the same time; patient then swings both feet forward to the level of the crutches.
Swing-through gait	This is the same as the swing-to gait except that the patient swings both feet forward beyond the level of the crutches.

Walkers

Walkers are used by patients who can bear full weight on both legs but need assistance to maintain balance. Several styles of walkers are available. The most common style is a metal frame with four legs and one open side, so that the patient moves behind the walker and steps into the frame. Other styles include the type with two legs and two wheels. The wheels are located on the front of the walker, allowing the patient to push the walker rather than having to pick up the whole frame to advance it forward. A walker style popular for home use has four wheels with hand brakes and a seat where the person can sit to rest when the brakes are secured (Fig. 27-7). A walker that is the correct fit will come up to the patient's hip joint. When the patient grips the handles, his or her elbows should be bent at a 30-degree angle.

Guidelines for assisting patients using walkers include:

- Ensuring that the patient stands between the back legs of the walker. *Safety: Standing too far behind the walker can affect balance and lead to falls.*
- If the walker is the type that the patient must pick up and move forward, ensuring that the patient sets the walker

Figure 27-6 Two styles of single-tipped canes and a quad cane.

(a)   **(b)**

Figure 27-7 A standard walker (**a**) that the patient must lift and advance, and a rolling walker (**b**) with brakes and a seat.

down and steps forward into it, rather than simply carrying it.

- If the walker is the rolling style with hand brakes, ensuring that the brakes are set (handles pulled downward) before the patient attempts to sit on the walker seat.
- If one leg is weak, instructing the patient to move the affected leg forward with the walker, then move the unaffected leg forward.

Knowledge Connection

How should a patient using crutches bear his or her body weight? What is a quad cane? How do you instruct a patient to ambulate with a walker if he or she is weak on the left side?

People and Places Connection

Promoting Mobility in Home Health Care and Long-Term Care
When you care for patients in their homes, be sure that you evaluate the need for physical therapy if it is not already being given. Many times patients are weak from hospital stays and are unable to ambulate safely in the home as they did before their illness. If you see the need for physical therapy, let your nursing supervisor know, so that orders can be obtained from the physician.

Promoting Mobility in Long-Term Care
In the long-term care setting, it is so important that residents remain mobile for as long as possible. Be sure that you follow activity orders, such as assisting with ambulation and increasing time in sitting up in a chair, to help preserve the residents' mobility.

Nursing Care Plan for a Patient With Total Left Knee Replacement

When you plan care for a patient with impaired mobility, protection from injury and restoring mobility are two prominent concerns. If you were going to develop a care plan for the patient that you were assigned in the Clinical Connection of this chapter, you would need a little more information. Here is what you find from reading the chart:

> The patient is a 66-year-old female with a history of severe osteoarthritis in her left knee. She is overweight, weighing 240 pounds (109 kg), and is 64 inches (162.5 cm) tall. Her right knee is arthritic as well, but the left knee is worse, so the decision was made to replace the left knee first. She is a widow and lives alone. Her daughter is here from out of state and can stay with her for 2 weeks.

When your patient returns to her room after surgery, she has been medicated for pain and is very sleepy. Once she is moved from the stretcher to the bed, she becomes your responsibility. Figure 27-8 presents a concept map care plan for a patient with a total left knee replacement. Begin with your immediate postoperative assessment.

Assessment

One of the first assessments you will make is that of vital signs. Watch for changes that could indicate shock, such as decreasing blood pressure and increasing pulse, or changes that could indicate increasing pain, such as elevated blood pressure and pulse.

Next, assess the incision. It will most likely have a dressing in place. Look for drainage on the dressing. If any is present, draw a line around it and write the time, date, and your initials. This way, you can tell if and when the drainage increases. Check beneath the patient's knee for pooling blood or drainage.

Assess the patient's pain level. Although the patient was medicated in the recovery room, movement and transfer to the bed may exacerbate knee pain. Evaluate the pain using a 0-to-10 scale and assess the pain level frequently. Chapter 19 contains more information about managing pain and promoting rest and sleep.

Assess any tubes attached to the patient. This includes IV lines and pumps, drains, and catheters. In this case, the patient has only one IV line connected to a pump. Note the quantity and solution of the IV fluids, and note the setting on the pump, which is usually the number of milliliters per hour at which the fluid is infusing.

Assess the patient's circulation distal to the surgery site. It is important to detect any compromise as quickly as possible. Assess post-tibial and pedal pulses bilaterally. When you compare the operative side with the unaffected side, the pulses should be equal in strength. Check the foot for warmth, color, and capillary refill. (See Skill 27-1, for more detail on neurovascular checks.)

Follow the additional assessment guidelines in Chapter 21.

Nursing Diagnoses

Now it is time to determine the nursing diagnoses appropriate for this patient. One concern will be her postoperative pain and pain management. Another will be the incision and its healing.

Nursing Care Plan for a Patient With Total Left Knee Replacement (continued)

Another will be her limited mobility after surgery, and her weight, as well as limited function in the right knee, all of which may complicate her recovery. In addition, she needs to be mobile enough to perform self-care by the time her daughter leaves. The diagnoses that express these concerns include:

• Acute pain related to physical injury as evidenced by restlessness and verbal reports of pain
• Impaired skin integrity related to knee surgery as evidenced by incision into body structures
• Impaired physical mobility related to the loss of integrity of bone structures as evidenced by limited range of motion
• Risk for injury related to altered mobility
• Imbalanced nutrition, more than body requirements related to excessive intake in relationship to metabolic need

If you found other diagnoses that could be used as well, then you have done a great job. Some additional diagnoses could be:

• Chronic pain related to joint degeneration in the right knee
• Impaired transfer ability related to minimal weight bearing on left knee
• Impaired walking related to minimal weight bearing on left knee

As you can see, there are a number of possible nursing diagnoses for this patient. In this chapter, we will focus on the first six identified above.

Planning

When you plan care, you are not only planning what you need to do for the patient, you are also planning what outcomes or goals you want your patient to meet. In this case, planning involves deciding what interventions will be needed to help her manage her acute pain after surgery. You will want to look back at Chapter 19 for reminders on ways to manage pain in addition to administering pain medications as ordered. Then you can decide to use distraction, gate control theory, or other techniques to help her with her pain. Your obvious goal is to keep her comfortable, and when planning a goal for that, we often say that we want to keep the pain at a 4 or

below, as it may be impossible for her to be totally pain free in the first few days after surgery.

You must also plan to assess her left knee incision and to provide care as ordered by the physician. First, you plan how to assess drainage and hemorrhage while the dressing is in place. Then, when the dressing is removed, generally about the second day postoperatively, you will assess the incision itself. What will you be looking for? Signs of infection or wound dehiscence are certainly concerns. Review Chapter 26 for more details about assessing and dressing a wound. Your goal for her incision is that it will heal without infection or other problems.

Your patient will definitely need help to get out of bed, to use the bedside commode or bedpan, and to obtain items that are not within reach. When she is allowed to be up, she will probably not be able to bear weight on her operative leg at first and will use a walker for balance and ambulation. What nursing interventions will you need to provide to help her with these mobility issues? Your goal for her mobility is that she will be safe using the walker when she is up and that she will call for help when she needs to get out of bed.

The fact that your patient is significantly overweight will be of concern to you as well. You will need to plan ways to help her make good food choices and to learn appropriate serving sizes. You will also need to reinforce teaching done by the dietitian regarding weight loss. Your goal for her is to lose weight and make healthy food choices.

Implementation

You are now at the stage of the nursing process to implement, or actually perform, the interventions that you have planned. Refer to the interventions listed in Table 27-3.

Evaluation

Once the interventions, or nursing actions, have been performed, you will want to evaluate whether they were effective or not. Did they accomplish what you intended? Did they help the patient's problems? Refer to the evaluations listed in Table 27-3.

(care plan continues on page 602)

Nursing Care Plan for a Patient With Total Left Knee Replacement (continued)

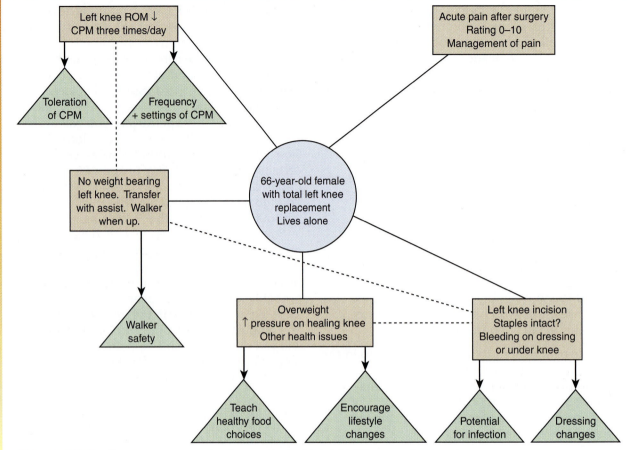

Figure 27-8 Concept map care plan for a patient with total left knee replacement.

Table 27-3 Care Plan for a Patient With a Total Left Knee Replacement

Nursing Diagnosis: Acute pain related to physical injury as evidenced by restlessness and verbal reports of pain
Expected Outcome: Patient will report that pain is consistently rated 4 or below before discharge from hospital.

Interventions	Evaluations
Use a pain scale of 1–10 to assess for pain and discomfort several times per shift.	Day 1: Initial c/o pain @ 8. Day 2: C/o pain @ 6. Day 3: C/o pain @ 4.
Encourage the patient to ask for pain medication before pain becomes severe.	Day 1: Waited until pain was 7 before asking for meds, reminded to call earlier to try to keep pain below 5. Day 3: Called for meds at level 5 pain.
Provide distraction and other nonpharmacological interventions for pain (see Chapter 19).	Day 2: Distracted from pain and CPM machine while visitors were present and while watching a movie on TV. Day 3: Laughing with family and able to wait longer between pain medication requests when family present.
Medicate for pain before starting the CPM machine.	Day 1: Medicated every 4 hours for pain. CPM on 1 hr ×3. Day 2: Medicated every 4–6 hours for pain, always within 1 hr of using CPM. Day 3: Able to tolerate CPM with lower strength pain med.

Table 27-3 Care Plan for a Patient With a Total Left Knee Replacement (continued)

Nursing Diagnosis: Impaired skin integrity related to knee surgery as evidenced by incision into body structures
Expected Outcome: Patient will display healing incision with edges approximated and without signs of infection by discharge from hospital. Patient will verbalize signs of infection and criteria for contacting the physician prior to discharge.

Interventions	Evaluations
Assess dressing for drainage and beneath the knee for bleeding postoperatively, every 4 hours for the first 24 hours; reinforce dressing as needed.	Day 1: Quarter-size drainage on dressing during first 8 hr after surgery. 8 hr later had increased to 4 inches in diameter. Day 2: Dressing removed by physician.
Change the left knee dressing every shift using 2 gauze 4×4s to protect the incision.	Day 1: Dressing changed every shift, quarter-sized amount serosanguinous drainage on old dressing. Day 2: Dressing changed each shift; quarter-sized amount serous drainage on old dressing. Day 3: Dressing changed each shift; dime-sized amount serous drainage on old dressing.
Assess the incision for approximated edges, signs of infection, and bleeding.	Day 1: Edges approximated, redness around all staples, no drainage or bleeding. Day 2: Less redness present, edges remain approximated, no drainage or bleeding. Day 3: Sl. redness around staples, 1-cm open area between staple #2 and #3 with sm. amount serous drainage present.
Teach the patient signs of infection (redness, heat, increasing pain, purulent drainage, elevated temperature) and wound dehiscence to report to the physician prior to discharge.	Day 1: Able to verbalize two signs of infection. Day 2: Able to verbalize signs of wound dehiscence, including gaping of wound or small deep openings with or without drainage. Day 3: Able to verbalize four signs of infection and signs of wound dehiscence.

Nursing Diagnosis: Impaired physical mobility related to loss of integrity of bone structures as evidenced by limited range of motion
Expected Outcome: Patient will demonstrate increased range of motion in knee to 80 degrees by discharge from the hospital. Patient will be able to participate in ADLs and desired activities using touch-down weight bearing within 5 days of surgery.

Interventions	Evaluations
Follow the physician's orders for the CPM machine: 1–2 hours tid; settings of 40 degrees of flexion at 10 degrees per minute to start and advance to 80 degrees of flexion at 30 degrees per minute as tolerated.	Day 1: CPM machine set at lowest setting tid. Day 2: CPM advanced to 50° of flexion at 20° per minute tid; tolerated with minor c/o discomfort. Day 3: CPM advanced to 60° of flexion at 30° per minute tid; pt. complained of increased discomfort on second session; decreased flexion by 5° for third session and tolerated without complaints.
Assist the patient when out of bed; instruct the patient not to get out of bed without assistance.	Day 1: Assisted to BSC ×3; pivoted well on right leg. Day 2: Assisted to BR with walker ×4 on 7–3 shift with toe touch-down only. Day 3: Ambulated with walker in room and hallway with minimal weight bearing on left leg.

(table continues on page 604)

Table 27-3 **Care Plan for a Patient With a Total Left Knee Replacement** (continued)

Nursing Diagnosis: Impaired physical mobility related to loss of integrity of bone structures as evidenced by limited range of motion
Expected Outcome: Patient will demonstrate increased range of motion in knee to 80 degrees by discharge from the hospital. Patient will be able participation in ADLs and desired activities using touch-down weight bearing within 5 days of surgery.

Interventions	Evaluations
Reinforce the teaching by the physical therapist.	Day 1: Reminded to pivot on right leg only and not to bear weight on left leg; instructed in active ROM for other joints. Day 2: Instructed to amb to BR; touch-down with foot only when using walker. Day 3: Instructed in minimal weight-bearing techniques while amb with walker in hallway.

Nursing Diagnosis: Risk for injury related to altered mobility
Expected Outcome: Patient will use walker safely and call for assistance to get out of bed during hospital stay. Patient will verbalize and demonstrate safe use of walker prior to discharge.

Interventions	Evaluations
Ensure that the patient knows where the call light is located and how to use it. Instruct the patient not to get out of bed without assistance.	Used call light all 3 days, which was answered promptly by nursing staff. Day 3: Attempted to get up to BR without assistance and experienced difficulty obtaining walker; sat down on side of bed and called for help.
Keep the pathway to the bathroom clear of equipment and supplies.	Day 2: Used walker to go to BR; it became entangled in IV pump power cord. Equipment rearranged to prevent further problem; nursing staff present and assisted; no injury occurred.

Nursing Diagnosis: Imbalanced nutrition, more than body requirements related to excessive intake in relationship to metabolic need as evidenced by weight 20% above ideal for height and frame
Expected Outcome: Patient will verbalize understanding of changes in lifestyle and behaviors needed for weight loss prior to discharge. Patient will demonstrate ability to choose healthy foods and identify activities to pursue to deal with food cravings by discharge.

Interventions	Evaluations
Reinforce the teaching of the dietitian regarding reduced calorie intake.	Day 2: Assisted with menu choices and discussed how they differed from food choices at home.
Help the patient identify "trigger foods" to avoid and praise the patient for making positive food choices.	Day 2: Stated that simple carbs made her want to eat more and more carbs. Listed trigger foods as chips, crackers, and ice cream. Day 3: States she is going to stop buying simple carbs; discussed alternate food choices. States she likes carrots and cauliflower with reduced-calorie dip and will buy these instead of chips and crackers.
Determine alternate activities during times of food cravings.	Day 3: Discussed what to do when food cravings hit; likes to dance with a DVD teaching dance steps and is not hungry after dancing. Encouraged her to do that when physician agrees knee is healed adequately.

Skill 27-1 Performing Neurovascular Checks

Assessment Steps

1. Determine the area of the limb distal to the surgical site or cast that is to be evaluated.

Planning Steps

1. Obtain a neurovascular check flow sheet.
2. Determine when the last neurovascular check was done. Perform checks every 2 hours for the first 24 hours after surgery or application of a cast unless otherwise ordered.

Implementation Steps

1. Follow the Initial Implementation Steps located on the inside front cover.
2. Ask the patient if he or she is experiencing numbness, burning, or tingling in the affected limb. Test sensation of the affected and unaffected limbs by touching each with a paper clip and asking the patient to tell you when he or she feels the sensation of the paper clip touching the limb. *A decreased sensation in the affected limb may indicate impairment of sensory nerve function.*
3. Assess for edema at the surgical site and distal to the site or cast. Compare the size of the distal aspect of the extremity to the unaffected extremity. *Edema indicates impairment of circulation and should be monitored closely to determine if it increases.*
4. Touch the patient's skin distal to the surgical site or cast with the back of your hand. Assess for warmth and compare to the warmth of the same area on the unaffected limb. *Cooler temperature of the affected limb may indicate impairment of circulation.*
5. Assess the color of the skin and nailbeds in the distal portion of the affected limb. These should be the same as in the unaffected limb; nailbeds should be pink. *Pallor or cyanosis indicates impairment of circulation.*

6. Test capillary refill in the nailbeds of the fingers or toes distal to the surgical site or cast. Compare it to that in the unaffected limb. *Slower refill time in the affected limb or refill longer than 5 seconds indicates that circulation is impaired.*
7. Ask the patient to move the fingers or toes of the affected extremity. *Movement should be free of discomfort if motor nerves are unimpaired.*
8. Palpate distal pulses if possible and compare with the pulses on the unaffected limb. *Each should be present and equal if no circulatory impairment is present.*
9. Ask the patient to describe his or her pain in the affected limb, including the type of pain and intensity. Ask him or her to rate it on a 0-to-10 scale. *Pain should gradually decrease in intensity as healing occurs. A sudden increase in pain could indicate infection or compression.*
10. Follow the Ending Implementation Steps located on the inside back cover.

Evaluation Steps

1. Determine deviations from normal during neurovascular checks and report them to the health care provider.
2. Evaluate the patient's pain level and report complaints of increasing pain, which could indicate impaired circulation.

Sample Documentation

1-22-12   0900   *Casted Lt. arm elevated on 2 pillows. Lt. fingers exhibit moderate edema with no increase from 0700, pink, warm, good motion & sensation, cap. refill less than 3 seconds. No C/O pain. ———————— Nurse's signature and credentials*

Skill 27-2 Setting Up a Continuous Passive Motion Machine

Assessment Steps

1. Review the physician's order. Note the degrees of flexion and the speed ordered, as well as the length of time the machine is to be in use.
2. Assess the patient's pain level. Determine the need for and administer pain medication before beginning CPM treatment.
3. Determine patient comfort needs before starting CPM treatment: assist to the bathroom or bedside commode if needed; place desired items within reach.

Planning Steps

1. Obtain needed equipment: CPM machine, sheepskin for platform. Follow the facility policy for charging out the equipment.

Implementation Steps

1. Follow the Initial Implementation Steps located on the inside front cover.
2. Place the CPM machine on the bed and connect it to the power source.
3. Place the sheepskin on the platform where the patient's leg will rest, especially at the end near the gluteal fold *to prevent pressure on the patient's skin, which could lead to a pressure ulcer.*
4. Position the CPM machine so that the break in the platform is centered beneath the patient's knee. Align the machine and the patient's leg with the hips and torso of the patient's body *to prevent injury or muscle spasms.*
5. Carefully assist the patient to place the affected leg on the CPM platform.

(skill continues on page 606)

Skill 27-2 (continued)

6. Set the degrees of flexion and speed as ordered by the physician.
7. Turn on the CPM machine.
8. Observe the machine as it flexes and extends the patient's knee and ensure that the passive exercise is being well tolerated by the patient. *Gentle passive exercise should not cause pain.*

9. Follow the Ending Implementation Steps located on the inside back cover.

Evaluation Steps

1. Evaluate the movement of the patient's knee for appropriate degrees of flexion and extension.
2. Evaluate the patient's pain level while using the CPM machine.
3. Ensure that the CPM therapy is in use for the length of time ordered.

Sample Documentation

> 8-12-11 1430 CPM machine in place and on. Set at 90° flexion at speed of 30° per minute per physician's order. States knee feels stiff but passive motion is not painful. ————
> ———————————————— Nurse's signature and credentials
> 8-12-11 1530 CPM off per physician's order. No edema noted. States pain is at a 4 after treatment. ————
> ———————————————— Nurse's signature and credentials

Skill 27-3 Applying Elastic Bandages

Assessment Steps

1. Check the physician's order for placement and purpose of the elastic bandage.
2. Assess the patient's limb or stump for skin breakdown or wounds.
3. Assess for edema in the limb or stump.

Planning Steps

1. Obtain the correct width of elastic bandage. *Use wider widths to cover larger areas, such as for stump wrapping.*
2. Obtain metal closures, safety pins, or tape *to hold wrap in place.*

Implementation Steps

1. Follow the Initial Implementation Steps located on the inside front cover.

For Figure-of-Eight Wrap on the Ankle
2. Wrap two turns around the instep of the foot to secure the end of the wrap.
3. Bring the bandage around the inner ankle and behind the lower leg.
4. Bring the bandage around the outer ankle, across the top of the foot, and back to the instep.
5. Bring the bandage under the foot, then across the top of the foot to the inner ankle.
6. Bring the bandage around the inner ankle and behind the lower leg.

7. Repeat the above steps until bandaging is complete. Each additional wrap should be approximately ¼ to ½ inch (0.51 to 1.3 cm) more proximal than the previous wrap, making an evenly distributed criss-cross pattern across the dorsal surface of the foot and ankle.
8. Secure the bandage end with tape, safety pins, or metal clasps.
9. Follow the Ending Implementation Steps located on the inside back cover.

Skill 27-3 (continued)

For Spiral Turn on the Forearm or Leg

2. Start at the narrower area of the lower leg or wrist area of the forearm.
3. Wrap two turns to anchor the wrap.
4. Wrap the bandage around the arm or leg, progressing up the limb with each turn at a 30-degree angle, overlapping the elastic bandage with each turn.

5. Repeat the above steps until bandaging is complete.
6. Secure the bandage end with tape, safety pins, or metal clasps.
7. Follow the Ending Implementation Steps located on the inside back cover.

To Wrap a Below-the-Knee Amputation

2. Wrap the elastic bandage two times above the knee joint.
3. Fold the bandage at an angle on itself and hold in place with your thumb.
4. Bring the bandage down the front of the stump, over the end of the stump, and up the back of the stump, holding it in place.

5. Fold the bandage back on itself and keep holding both turns in place while you wrap the back length of the stump, the end of the stump, and up the front length of the stump.
6. Repeat Steps 4 and 5 two more times, covering the stump entirely. Most stumps will require two elastic bandages in order to have adequate length to complete the recurrent turn wrap.
7. Anchor these folded layers of bandage by wrapping the bandage around the circumference of the leg, catching all the folds of the bandage.
8. Wrap the remaining bandage in a figure-of-eight style from the stump to below the knee joint, covering the sides of the stump.

9. Secure the bandage end with tape, safety pins, or metal clasps.

10. Follow the Ending Implementation Steps located on the inside back cover.

Evaluation Steps

1. Make certain the wrap is not too tight by ensuring that you can slip two fingers underneath the bandage at its proximal end. Ask the patient if it is painful or causing numbness or tingling in the limb. If so, remove and rewrap more loosely.
2. For all wraps except on a stump. Assess fingers and toes for edema, warmth, capillary refill, sensation, movement, and color. If circulation is impaired, remove and rewrap more loosely.
3. Determine if wrap is too loose, so that it sags or comes loose as the patient moves. If so, remove and rewrap more tightly.

Sample Documentation

8-18-11 1207 Elastic bandage applied to left ankle using figure-of-eight. States it is comfortable. Left toes pink, warm, with cap. refill less than 3 seconds, and without edema or numbness. Able to wiggle toes. Left ankle elevated on pillow. ————
———————— Nurse's signature and credentials

🌐 **Post Conference**

You followed this patient from her return from the recovery room to her third postoperative day and you found it amazing how mobile she was by that last day. She went from being nearly immobile to ambulating the length of the hall using a walker. She insisted that the surgical pain was less uncomfortable than the previous arthritic pain she experienced with every step. You learned how effective the CPM was at keeping the knee mobile and flexing it without the patient having to intentionally do so. She slept through the CPM use, even as it flexed her knee up to 60 degrees, more than she has been able to flex it in 20 years.

KEY POINTS

- Sprains, fractures, joint replacements, and amputations are common musculoskeletal conditions that limit mobility.

- Physical therapists are members of the health care team responsible for assessing deficiencies in musculoskeletal function and developing a plan of care. It is very important to follow the orders of the physician and recommendations of the physical therapist regarding patient activity and mobility.

- A variety of immobilization devices are used to promote healing of musculoskeletal disorders. These include casts, traction, splints, immobilizers, and abductor pillows.

- External fixators are used in skeletal traction to hold bone fragments in place or to attach weights to move bones. A specific type of such a fixator is the Ilizarov frame, which is used to stabilize small bone pieces while growth occurs and also may be used to help lengthen bone in a leg or arm shortened by trauma.

- When caring for a patient in a spica cast, do not move or lift the patient using the adduction bar.

- When a plaster cast is drying, handle it only with the palms of your hands since using your fingers may cause dents in the cast that can lead to pressure ulcers under the cast.

- When caring for patients with dry casts, observe carefully for drainage or discharge on or under the cast. Teach patients how to relieve itching under the cast without causing skin abrasions.

- Perform neurovascular checks every 2 hours in the first 24 hours after a cast is applied or surgery is performed on a limb, then every 4 hours or according to facility policy.

- When caring for a patient in traction, keep all ropes straight without kinks, aligned in pulleys, with weights hanging freely. Assess for skin breakdown beneath the traction boot or elastic bandage.

- When caring for a patient in skeletal traction, clean the pin sites using sterile technique with the solution ordered. Observe them carefully for signs of infection as any infection at the pin site can easily invade the bone.

- When caring for a patient with a total hip replacement, keep the abductor pillow in place while the patient is in bed. When the patient transfers from the bed to a chair, and while sitting in the chair, prevent him or her from flexing the hip more than 90 degrees. Adduction of the leg or flexion of the hip can cause dislocation of the hip prosthesis.

- When caring for a patient with a total knee replacement, a CPM machine will be ordered. This passively exercises the knee with flexion and extension and must be set at the speed and degree of flexion ordered by the physician.

- When caring for a patient with an amputated limb, it is important to give emotional as well as physical support. It is also important to constantly plan toward rehabilitation and the use of a prosthetic limb. Assess the incision for healing, and wrap the stump with an elastic bandage to form the proper shape for fitting into the socket of the prosthesis.

- Assistive devices for ambulation include crutches, canes, and walkers. It is important to ensure the correct fit of each device and then reinforce the teaching of the physical therapist on the use of each.

- When planning care for patients with impaired mobility, it is important to address pain before expecting the patient to exercise the affected limb or to ambulate. Plan for preventing injuries and keeping the patient safe when out of bed. Assess circulation and incisions after surgery to detect signs of infection or impaired circulation or neurological function.

REVIEW QUESTIONS

Select the answer that is most appropriate for each of the following questions. Some questions may have more than one correct answer. Check all that apply.

1. A coworker twisted her ankle going down the stairs. It is swollen and is painful when she bears weight on it. Which intervention would be the least helpful for healing this sprain?

   a. Avoiding bearing weight on her ankle.

   b. Wrapping her ankle with an elastic bandage.

   c. Applying heat to her ankle for 20 minutes at a time.

   d. Elevating her ankle on a pillow while she is lying down.

2. The purpose of which of the following devices is to prevent flexion of an affected joint?

   a. Cast

   b. Immobilizer

   c. Splint

   d. Elastic bandages

   e. Traction

   f. Abductor pillow

   g. Ilizarov frame

3. A patient comes into the clinic with his arm in a cast. You notice a small amount of thick, light yellow drainage coming from under the cast, and it has an unpleasant odor. There is no drainage staining the cast, and no open areas of skin are visible at the edge of the cast. Which question is most appropriate to ask this patient?

   a. "Have you inserted anything under the cast to scratch your arm?"

   b. "Have you had an upper respiratory infection recently?"

   c. "Do you have a skin rash anywhere on your body?"

   d. "Is the edge of the cast irritating your skin?"

4. A patient is in skeletal traction for a comminuted fracture of the tibia. While giving pin care, you notice a small amount of serous drainage around each pin site. Which observation is most accurate?

   a. The drainage is a symptom of skin infection.

   b. This finding is normal for skeletal traction.

   c. This is an indication of pin dislocation.

   d. The drainage is an indication of a bone infection.

5. Which surfaces are replaced when a patient has a total hip replacement?

   a. The articular surfaces of the femur and the tibia.

   b. The posterior surface of the patella and the tibia.

   c. The acetabular cup and head of the tibia and fibula.

   d. The head and neck of the femur and the acetabular cup.

6. You are caring for a patient with a fresh total hip replacement. Which statement would indicate that your patient needs more teaching?

   a. "I will sleep with the abductor pillow between my legs every night for several months."

   b. "I can cross my legs when I am sitting in a chair, as long as my feet are elevated on a footstool."

   c. "I need to use an extension gripper to pick up anything I drop."

   d. "I will sit in the recliner with the back slightly reclined when I am out of bed."

7. The purpose of the CPM machine is to provide:

   a. active abduction and adduction.

   b. active range of motion to all joints.

   c. passive flexion and extension.

   d. passive internal and external rotation.

SHORT ANSWER QUESTION

8. A patient has had his hand and part of his forearm amputated due to a traumatic injury. What would be the result if he refused to have his stump wrapped continuously with an elastic bandage?

CRITICAL THINKING EXERCISES

9. Why does a dislocated hip prosthesis cause pain to a patient, since the socket is not made of the patient's bones?

10. A patient with a left fractured ankle was put in an immobilizing boot and told to use crutches 2 days ago. She fell this morning and is complaining of left arm pain when she arrives at the clinic where you work. What would you ask her about her use of crutches?

ADDITIONAL RESOURCES

For additional Resources, Questions, and Activities, please see:

 Student Resource Disk

 http://davisplus.fadavis.com

 Student Study Guide

REFERENCES

American Academy of Orthopaedic Surgeons. Knee implants. 2007. Available at: http://orthoinfo.aaos.org/topic.cfm?topic=A00221. Accessed October 13, 2009.

American Academy of Orthopaedic Surgeons. Total hip replacement. 2009. Available at: http://orthoinfo.aaos.org/topic.cfm?topic=A00377. Accessed October 13, 2009.

Braddock EJ, Greenlee J, Hammer RE, Johnson SF, Martello MJ, O'Connell MR, et al. Manual Medicine Guidelines for Musculoskeletal Injuries. Lodi, CA: Academy for Chiropractic Education; April 1, 2007. AHRQ National Guidelines Clearinghouse Web site. Available at: http://www.guideline.gov/summary/summary. aspx?ss=15&doc_id=10798&nbr=5626. Accessed October 13, 2009.

Getting patients back on their feet. *LPN2005.* Sept/Oct 2005;1(5): 15-16.

Howell B. Joint surgery: paving the way to a smooth recovery. *RN* [serial online]. 2007;January 1. Available at: http://rn.modernmedicine.com/ RNweb/article/articleDetail.jsp?id=394867.

Lethaby A, Temple J, Santy J. Pin site care for preventing infections associated with external bone fixators and pins. *Cochrane Database Syst Rev.* 2008;(4):CD004551.

Scanlon V, Sanders T. *Essentials of Anatomy and Physiology.* 5th ed. Philadephia: FA Davis; 2007.

Tomić S, Bumbasirević M, Lesić A, Mitković M, Atkinson HD. Ilizarov frame fixation without bone graft for atrophic humeral shaft nonunion: 28 patients with a minimum 2-year follow-up. *J Orthop Trauma.* 2007;21:549-556.

Venes D, ed. *Taber's Cyclopedic Medical Dictionary.* 21st ed. Philadelphia: FA Davis; 2009.

Wilkinson JM, Van Leuven K. *Fundamentals of Nursing: Theory, Concepts, and Applications.* Philadelphia: FA Davis; 2007.

Williams LS, Hopper PD. *Understanding Medical-Surgical Nursing.* 3rd ed. Philadelphia: FA Davis; 2007.

Respiratory Care

Key Terms

Atelectasis

Crepitus

Cyanosis

Dyspnea

Endotracheal tube

Exhalation

Hemothorax

Hypoxemia

Hypoxia

Incentive spirometer

Inhalation

Nebulizer

Parietal pleura

Pleural effusion

Pneumothorax

Sputum

Tension pneumothorax

Tracheostomy

Visceral pleura

Objectives

1. Define key terms associated with respiratory care.
2. Explain the mechanics of inhalation and exhalation.
3. Describe chemical and nervous regulation of respirations.
4. Explain the changes in physiological regulation of respiration in patients with chronic lung disease.
5. Differentiate between internal and external respiration.
6. Describe the role of the pleural membrane in respiration.
7. Contrast hypoxia and hypoxemia.
8. Identify causes of impaired oxygenation.
9. List inspection points in the assessment of a patient with impaired oxygenation.
10. Describe palpation, auscultation, and other assessment findings that could indicate impaired oxygenation.
11. Discuss the significance of selected diagnostic tests when caring for patients with impaired oxygenation.
12. Explain nursing interventions to use for patients with impaired oxygenation.
13. Discuss safety measures to enforce when the patient is receiving supplemental oxygen.
14. Identify types of oxygen sources and delivery devices used for supplemental oxygen.
15. List tips for conservation of energy for patients with chronic lung disease.
16. Describe various artificial airways and how to suction the patient with the airway in place.
17. Describe a tracheostomy tube and the nursing care needed to keep it patent.
18. Illustrate chest tube placement and how the chest drainage system works.
19. Discuss nursing care of patients with chest tubes.
20. Plan care for a patient with a respiratory disorder.

Skills

28-1 Obtaining a Sputum Specimen

28-2 Obtaining a Throat Culture Specimen

28-3 Assisting With Incentive Spirometry

28-4 Administering a Nebulizer Treatment

28-5 Administering Supplemental Oxygen

28-6 Performing Nasopharyngeal and Oropharyngeal Suctioning

28-7 Performing Endotracheal and Tracheostomy Suctioning

28-8 Performing Tracheostomy Care

28-9 Maintaining Chest Tubes

🌐 Clinical Connection

Your Assignment: You are assigned to care for a hospitalized patient tomorrow in clinical who has a tracheostomy. He was injured in a car accident and was on a ventilator for several weeks. He is breathing on his own now, but still has the tracheostomy in place. In addition, he has recently developed pneumonia in his right lung. He has a large amount of secretions and requires suctioning every 2 to 3 hours. The tracheostomy will have to be cleaned on your shift and a new inner cannula put in place. He has humidified oxygen at 4 L/min via a tracheostomy collar.

Your Actions: You are not exactly sure what a tracheostomy is for or how it works, much less how to suction it or clean it. You know about oxygen delivery by nasal cannula and by mask, but you have no idea what a tracheostomy collar is. You know you have a whole lot of research to do before clinical in the morning.

It can be alarming to see a patient struggle to breathe or to have to assist a patient who must be suctioned to be able to breathe. As the patient becomes more anxious, it is easy for your anxiety to increase as well. This chapter will help you prepare to care for patients who have respiratory problems, assisting them to improve oxygenation and breathe more easily.

Normal Oxygenation

The term *airway* refers to the path that air takes as it enters and exits the lungs. The normal pathway is through the nostrils into the pharynx, into the trachea, and then either to the right or the left bronchus, which branches into the bronchioles that terminate into the alveoli. When this pathway is unblocked and air is moving freely, it is referred to as a patent airway.

The Mechanics of Breathing

When the airway is patent, air is inhaled and follows the pathway to the alveoli, where oxygen is absorbed into the blood and carbon dioxide leaves the blood to be exhaled.

Oxygen and carbon dioxide move across the alveolar cell membranes and the cell membranes of the capillaries surrounding the alveoli by the process of *diffusion*.

This process occurs involuntarily, meaning that there is no conscious thought given to it. It is important to understand the mechanics of how breathing occurs so that you can grasp the treatments for respiratory disorders affecting those mechanics, such as chest tubes, endotracheal tubes, and mechanical ventilation.

The diaphragm and the intercostals are the muscles required for breathing to occur. When the diaphragm contracts in response to stimulus from the phrenic nerves, it moves downward, which increases the size of the chest cavity. Intercostal muscles then contract, moving the ribs up and out, which also enlarges the chest cavity from side to side and from front to back. When the chest cavity size increases, it causes the lungs to expand. Then the pressure within the lungs drops below atmospheric pressure, or becomes negative pressure. This causes a sort of vacuum, and air is pulled into the lungs until the pressure in the lungs equals the pressure outside of the body. The term used to describe this is **inhalation**, also known as *inspiration*.

As these muscles relax, again in response to nerve stimulus, the size of the chest cavity decreases. The ribs come inward, the diaphragm rises upward, and the lungs are then compressed, forcing the air to go out. This is referred to as **exhalation**, also known as *expiration*.

Regulation of Respiration

Nerves and a chemical control mechanism both contribute to the regulation of respirations. The respiratory center is in the medulla, located in the brainstem. This brain function automatically controls inhalation by sending impulses to the phrenic nerve, which causes contraction of the diaphragm and intercostal muscles.

Chemical regulation of respirations is influenced by chemoreceptors located in the carotid and aortic bodies and in the medulla of the brain. When these chemoreceptors detect a decrease in the oxygen level of the blood or a change in blood pH, they send a message to the medulla, which in turn causes an increase in the rate and depth of respirations. When carbon dioxide increases above normal amounts, it causes the blood to become more acidic. The chemoreceptors respond by sending the message to the medulla, which in turn causes the respiratory rate to increase to "blow off" or remove excess carbon dioxide, returning the blood pH to normal levels. (See Chapter 29 for more information about acid-base balance and the role of the lungs in maintaining blood pH.)

Rising carbon dioxide levels that in turn cause the blood to become more acidic provide the brain's stimulus to breathe. That is why you cannot hold your breath for long periods of time—not because your oxygen level is falling, but because you are trapping carbon dioxide in your blood, causing a buildup of carbonic acid, which in turn prompts the medulla to make you breathe.

Regulation of Respiration in Chronic Lung Disease

People who have severe chronic lung disease gradually develop a different stimulus to breathe. Unlike those with healthy lung tissue, air is trapped in their alveoli for long periods of time because oxygen and carbon dioxide are unable to diffuse freely across the stiff, nonelastic alveolar membrane. This raises the blood's level of carbon dioxide and lowers the oxygen level. The body gradually acclimates to the higher carbon dioxide level because it cannot continue to increase the respiratory rate higher and higher to blow it off. Thus, the high carbon dioxide level no longer stimulates respiration and the body begins to respond to the lower level of oxygen, which now becomes its stimulus to breathe. Then, if the oxygen level is raised too high, it can impair the message from the medulla that instructs the body to breathe. It will be important to remember this later in the chapter when we discuss oxygen flow rates for patients with chronic lung disease.

Internal and External Respiration

External respiration occurs between the alveoli and the capillaries. The alveoli are air sacs encircled by tiny capillaries. Oxygen moves via diffusion from an area of higher concentration to an area of lower concentration. When you inhale, the inspired air contains more oxygen, so it passes from the alveoli into the capillaries.

Internal respiration occurs between the bloodstream and the body cells. When fresh oxygen enters the bloodstream, it is carried by the hemoglobin on the red blood cells through the arteries and arterioles to the capillaries. In the tiny capillaries, where the walls are just one cell thick, the oxygen diffuses to the tissue cells where the concentration is lower. At the same time, carbon dioxide and other waste products diffuse into the blood from the tissue cells for the same reason. The blood then returns to the heart and lungs through the venules and veins. Once it is pumped back to the lungs by the right side of the heart, the carbon dioxide and waste products leave the blood and enter the alveoli to leave the body with exhalation.

Anatomy and Physiology Connection

The Pleura

The chest cavity is lined with a thin membrane that also covers each lung, similar to a sac within a sac. This membrane is called the *pleura*. The portion of the pleura that lines the chest cavity is called the **parietal pleura**. This continuous membrane then covers the lungs, and that portion is called the **visceral pleura**. There is a very narrow space between the two layers, referred to as the *pleural space,* in which a negative pressure, or vacuum, must be maintained so that expansion of the chest wall will cause the lung to expand as the chest wall expands. If this vacuum is lost and air or fluid enters into the pleural space, the lung will collapse rather than expand. This space contains a small amount of fluid that helps hold the two layers together, but also allows them to glide smoothly against one another with each inhalation and exhalation. A similar situation occurs when you add a drop of water to a microscope slide, then place the coverslip over it. The water forms a film that holds the coverslip on the slide, but allows it to glide against the slide for correct placement.

Knowledge Connection

What role do muscles, nerves, and chemicals play in respiration? What are the similarities and differences between internal and external respiration?

Impaired Oxygenation

If a blockage occurs in the airway, or oxygen cannot pass into the blood in the alveolar capillaries, the patient is unable to obtain needed oxygen from room air. If oxygen cannot cross into the tissue cells in the peripheral capillaries, the patient is unable to provide oxygen to body cells. Each of these situations can lead to impaired oxygenation.

It is very important to recognize the signs and symptoms of decreased oxygen in the blood and tissues because oxygen is necessary for brain and organ function. Often the symptoms do not become noticeable until the oxygen level has dropped considerably.

When oxygen levels in the blood drop below normal range, it is referred to as **hypoxemia**. In the event of hypoxemia, the blood cannot take adequate amounts of oxygen to the tissues during internal respiration, causing **hypoxia**. Without enough oxygen in the tissues, you will see changes in mental function, in color of the skin and mucous membranes, and in respiratory rate and rhythm. Box 28-1 lists signs and symptoms of hypoxia.

Real-World Connection

Effects of Hypoxia on Thinking
Hypoxia to the brain can cause changes in mental function, including affecting judgment. A home health nurse went to visit a patient with chronic lung disease who had recently been hospitalized with respiratory failure. When the nurse arrived, she found that the patient had recently discharged his gun in his home. He had seen his reflection in a mirror and his hypoxic brain had misinterpreted the face as that of a stranger; he thought that someone was looking in the window of his home. After discharging the gun, he realized that he had shot at his own reflection. His oxygen saturation was very low at 66%, and he was readmitted to the hospital.

Box 28-1
Signs and Symptoms of Hypoxia

When patients become hypoxic, the early symptoms may be missed if you are not aware of them. By the time the later symptoms are evident, the patient is severely hypoxic. It is important to assess your patients for the early subtle signs as well as the more apparent ones.

Early
- Agitation
- Anxiety
- Changes in level of consciousness
- Disorientation
- Headache
- Irritability
- Restlessness
- Tachypnea

Late
- Bradycardia
- Cardiac dysrhythmias
- Cyanosis
- Decreased respiratory rate (bradypnea)
- Retractions

Causes of Impaired Oxygenation

A variety of situations can contribute to impaired oxygen exchange. It may be due to some type of obstruction in the pharynx, trachea, or bronchi causing a decrease in inspired air. If the nose is blocked due to mucus congestion, the body utilizes an alternate path and mouth breathing occurs. If the trachea is blocked by secretions, coughing clears them. If the trachea becomes blocked by a foreign body, such as a piece of food, and coughing is either impossible or not sufficient to remove the blockage, the Heimlich maneuver can be performed to clear the airway. If the bronchi or bronchioles are blocked by thick mucus or secretions, deep coughs and possibly mucus-thinning agents are required to clear it.

Another cause of impaired oxygenation may be secretions in the alveoli or damage to the alveoli caused by chronic lung disease. When the alveoli are not fully functional, less oxygen can cross into the blood and less carbon dioxide is able to leave the blood. Low oxygen in the blood may also be due to a situation in which the patient is unable to fully expand the lungs due to fluid or pus in the chest cavity, or a blood clot in the lung preventing circulation to the alveoli. Patients who have had surgery or chest trauma may have hypoxemia due to pain that prevents them from taking a deep breath.

Chronic lung disease is also a cause of hypoxemia. Over time, the alveoli and airways are damaged, making them unable to expand and move air in and out, so oxygen does not cross into the alveolar capillaries to be taken to the body tissues.

Damage or trauma to the lung itself can also cause hypoxemia. If a lung collapses, called **atelectasis**, expansion does not occur, so air is not pulled into the lungs. This may be the result of trauma such as a bullet or knife wound to the chest. It may also be due to blockage of the airway to the lung, preventing expansion of the lung. For example, if a large tumor is blocking the air path in the right main bronchus, inhaled air is unable to fill the lung.

Be aware that a patient can have a normal pulse oximetry reading and still suffer from hypoxia. If the blood is carrying adequate amounts of oxygen, the pulse oximetry reading will be normal. However, the oxygen may not be crossing the capillary wall and entering the tissue cells. Box 28-2 summarizes the causes of hypoxia and hypoxemia.

Caring for Patients With Impaired Oxygenation

You will care for many patients with impaired oxygenation. Generally, these patients are anxious and frightened; being unable to get your breath is a terrifying experience. As the patient's nurse, it is very important for you to remain calm. Speak in a normal tone of voice, without sounding excited or upset. Tell the patient what you need him or her to do. Help him or her slow down breathing by repeating "Breath in, breath out" at the tempo at which you want the patient to breathe. It is important that you reassure the patient that help is present. Do not leave the patient in acute respiratory distress alone, even if you think that the patient is "just anxious."

Causes of Hypoxia and Hypoxemia

A variety of conditions can lead to hypoxia and hypoxemia. These may be due to a mechanical problem that interferes with air entering the body, blood conditions interfering with the blood's ability to transport oxygen, side effects of medications, or environmental situations. Causes include:

- Airway obstruction due to tumor, choking on a foreign body, thick mucus, or swollen airways
- Anemia
- Atelectasis (collapsed lung)
- Decreased cardiac output
- High altitude
- Hypoventilation due to anesthetics, sedatives, or coma
- Poor peripheral circulation
- Pulmonary embolus

Assessing Respiratory Status

As you perform a respiratory assessment, you will inspect, palpate, and auscultate the patient. As you enter the room and interact with the patient, note the following:

- Color of skin and mucous membranes
- Respiratory effort
- Cough
- Chest appearance
- Oxygenation status
- Oxygen saturation

Color of Skin and Mucous Membranes

When oxygen levels in the tissues decrease, the lips take on a bluish color, called **cyanosis**. This color change may also be observed on the tip of the nose, on tops of the ears, and in the nailbeds. When the patient has dark skin, the color may appear more ashen than cyanotic and you will depend more upon the color of the mucous membranes. Check the palms of the hands and soles of the feet for color changes as well. *Safety: Cyanosis is a late sign of hypoxia. Take action immediately and notify the health care provider stat.*

Respiratory Effort

When the patient is having difficulty moving air in and out of the lungs, it is referred to as **dyspnea**. Notice if the patient is having difficulty breathing while at rest, and also if he or she becomes short of breath when ambulating a short distance, such as to the bathroom and back. If the patient has to stop to rest or catch his or her breath when ambulating a brief distance, then the patient is short of breath, known as *exertional dyspnea.* Patients with impaired oxygenation often assume a position of sitting upright and leaning slightly forward with arms and head over a table. This is the *orthopneic* position. It increases the intrathoracic area, allowing the patient to inhale more air. Watch for gasping respirations, or "air hunger," and expressions of grimacing or fear on the patient's face.

Cough

If the patient is bringing up **sputum**, or mucus from the lungs, when coughing, it is referred to as a *productive cough.* If the cough is dry, it is referred to as a *nonproductive cough.* It is important to notice the color, consistency, and amount of any sputum the patient produces. Sputum that is clear or white may indicate a viral infection; if it is yellow or green, it may be indicative of a bacterial infection. Rust-colored sputum indicates the presence of blood and may be seen in some pneumonia infections and tuberculosis. When sputum is gray or black, it usually indicates that the patient has inhaled smoke or soot. Pink and frothy, or bubbly, sputum is indicative of fluid and blood mixed together and is seen in a life-threatening condition called *pulmonary edema.*

In addition to the color of sputum, the consistency is also an important observation. Thick, tenacious, sticky mucus is difficult to cough out. It tends to remain in the lungs and provides a good medium for bacteria growth. If you observe this in your patient, encourage him or her to drink more fluids to help thin the mucus and make it easier to cough out.

Chest Assessment

Inspection

Look for muscular retractions between the ribs, substernally, and around the neck, evidenced by muscles and skin pulling inward as the patient inhales. *Safety: This is also a late sign of hypoxia and hypoxemia. Notify the health care provider immediately.* Observe the patient for the use of the accessory muscles in the neck and shoulders while breathing, indicating excessive muscular effort to breathe (Fig. 28-1).

Palpation

To begin palpating the chest, place your hands on either side of the chest. As the patient inhales and exhales, determine if each side of the chest is moving equally, called *excursion.*

Figure 28-1 This patient shows evidence of retractions in the neck and shoulders as he inhales.

Differences in chest wall movement, along with shortness of breath, can indicate a serious problem such as airway obstruction, pneumothorax, or **pleural effusion** (fluid in the chest cavity). A **pneumothorax** occurs when a hole allows air to enter the pleural space, also termed the *pleural cavity,* where there is supposed to be negative pressure. A life-threatening type of pneumothorax is a **tension pneumothorax**. When this occurs, air is trapped in the pleural cavity surrounding the lungs, which not only compresses and collapses the lungs but also causes pressure on the heart and major blood vessels and causes them to shift within the thorax. *Safety: Tension pneumothorax is a medical emergency. Notify the health care provider immediately.*

Feel for **crepitus**, or air in the subcutaneous tissues, in the chest wall, face, and neck. When you gently press your fingertips on the patient's skin, you will feel a crackling sensation, much like the feeling of crispy rice cereal being crushed beneath the patient's skin. Crepitus is usually felt beneath an area of edema. *Safety: Air in the subcutaneous tissues, also called subcutaneous emphysema, indicates that air that should be in the lungs is in the tissues. Notify the physician immediately.*

Auscultation

Now use your stethoscope to auscultate the lungs, as you learned in Chapter 21. As you listen to respirations, both with and without the stethoscope, observe the rate, character, and quality of respirations. Note if the rate is outside of the normal range of 12 to 20 breaths per minute. As you assess quality, determine if the respirations are shallow or deep, or if the patient is struggling to breathe. Determine the pattern of respirations. (Refer to Table 21-3 in Chapter 21 to refresh yourself on patterns of respirations, including tachypnea, bradypnea, eupnea, Kussmaul's, Cheyne-Stokes, Biot's, and apnea.) As you listen with the stethoscope to both the anterior and posterior chest, assess for adventitious breath sounds. If the patient has fluid in the lungs or airways, the sound is described as *crackles.* It is similar to the sound a soft drink makes after you pour it into a glass, because it is the sound of air moving through fluid. Refer to Chapter 21 for a review of adventitious lung sounds. To listen to adventitious lung sounds, use your student CD that accompanies this text.

Oxygenation Status

When beginning to assess the patient's oxygenation status, determine the patient's orientation to time, place, and person. Note restlessness and unusual irritability or confusion. Even minor changes can indicate hypoxia. *Safety: Remember that changes in level of consciousness can indicate decreased oxygen reaching the brain.*

Oxygen Saturation

Determine oxygen saturation using a pulse oximeter. (Refer to Chapter 17 for the procedure for using pulse oximetry). The pulse oximeter is used to measure the oxygen saturation of capillary blood (SaO_2). The normal range for the SaO_2 is 95% to 100%. In healthy people, a saturation of 94% or below is cause for concern. *Safety: Remember that nail polish, especially a dark color, and artificial nails will cause inaccurate pulse oximetry results.* Remove nail polish or use an alternative site such as the earlobe or forehead. You can check a patient's oxygen saturation without a physician's order. Be alert to subtle signs and symptoms of hypoxemia and check the oxygen saturation when indicated.

Knowledge Connection

What areas will you inspect when assessing a patient with impaired oxygenation? When you palpate, what two evaluations are you making? How can you tell if the patient is becoming hypoxic or hypoxemic?

Diagnostic Tests

In addition to your assessment, certain diagnostic tests help clearly explain the patient's oxygenation status. Table 28-1 shows types of diagnostic tests and the significance of abnormal results. Obtain sputum specimens and throat culture specimens when ordered by the health care provider to help diagnose respiratory conditions.

Sputum Specimens

When you obtain a sputum specimen, keep in mind that the best time to do this is first thing in the morning. Patients may have mucus that has pooled during the night, making it easier to obtain a specimen. There are two ways to obtain a sputum specimen:

1. The patient coughs and brings up mucus from the lungs and expectorates it into a sterile specimen container.
2. You suction the throat or trachea and trap the mucus in a specimen container attached to the suctioning tubing.

The results of sputum testing help diagnose infection, tuberculosis, bleeding, and fluids in the lungs. Skill 28-1 (page 631) gives the steps needed to obtain a sputum specimen.

Throat Culture Specimens

Specimens from the throat for culture and sensitivity are frequently obtained by nurses in physician's offices and clinics, but sometimes may be ordered in home health care and hospitals as well. Generally a throat culture is ordered to detect a *Streptococcus* infection in the throat, commonly referred to as *strep throat,* so that it may be treated promptly. If such an infection is present and is not treated, it can lead to other illnesses including rheumatic fever and rheumatic heart disease. Skill 28-2 (page 632) gives the steps in obtaining a throat culture specimen.

Laboratory and Diagnostic Connection

Arterial Blood Gases

Arterial blood gases (ABGs) are drawn from an artery rather than a vein as are other blood tests. The most commonly used arteries are the radial, femoral, and brachial. A glass or plastic syringe is used; the syringe has had a small amount of heparin added, which is an anticoagulant to prevent the blood from clotting.

After testing for collateral circulation, the health care professional inserts the needle into the artery at a 90-degree angle. Unlike other blood samples, no vacuum tube is used for ABGs. Instead, the pressure of the blood in the artery causes the plunger of the syringe to rise as blood enters the syringe.

After the needle is withdrawn from the artery, the health care professional inserts it into a cork to prevent additional air from entering the syringe. The syringe is then transported to the laboratory in a bag or cup containing ice to keep it cold.

ABGs measure the pH, the partial pressures of oxygen (PaO_2) and carbon dioxide ($PaCO_2$), the bicarbonate level (HCO_3^-), and the oxygen saturation (SaO_2) of arterial blood. Information from ABGs will help you know your patient's pH status. If the pH is above 7.45, the patient is in alkalosis. If the pH is below 7.35, the patient is in acidosis. Both of these conditions require immediate action by the health care provider to correct.

Blood gases also show if the cause of the acidosis or alkalosis is due to a respiratory problem, which would cause the $PaCO_2$ to be increased or decreased, or a metabolic problem as a result of kidney regulation of bicarbonate. In that case, the patient's HCO_3^- levels would be above or below normal. Normal ranges for ABGs, along with the significance of findings above and below normal, can be found in Table 28-2.

ABGs are usually drawn by respiratory therapists or specially trained nurses or laboratory technicians. Registered nurses also may take a sample of arterial blood for ABGs from an arterial line in a critical care setting.

Nursing Interventions for Patients With Impaired Oxygenation

There are a variety of nursing interventions you will use to help prevent decreased oxygenation in your patients who have had surgery or who must remain in bed. In addition, there are a number of actions to take to improve oxygenation in your patients with lung disorders.

Turn, Cough, and Deep Breathe

Patients who have had surgery or are on bedrest must be turned every 2 hours to prevent respiratory complications due to immobility. (See Chapter 16 for a review of complications of immobility.) In addition to assisting patients to turn from side to side, you must encourage patients to take three deep breaths and then cough to remove secretions from the lungs and airways. *Safety: You need to assist the patient to turn, cough, and deep breathe every 2 hours to help prevent hypostatic pneumonia.* If the patient has an incision or is weak, he or she may find this difficult to perform. If the patient has an abdominal or chest incision, encourage him or her to hold a pillow against the incision while taking deep breaths and coughing. The pillow will splint the incision, making it less uncomfortable for the patient to comply with coughing and deep breathing.

Incentive Spirometry

One way to encourage patients to take frequent deep breaths is through the use of an **incentive spirometer**, which is a device with one or more chambers and a mouthpiece. As the

Table 28-1   **Respiratory Diagnostic Tests and Their Purposes**

Diagnostic Test	Purpose	Significance of Abnormal Results
Pulmonary function tests	To determine lung capacity, volume, and flow rates.	Used to diagnose obstructive or restrictive lung diseases such as COPD and asthma.
Peak flow	Measures the amount of air that can be exhaled with force using a peak flowmeter.	Used to determine dosage and frequency of some respiratory medications. Can be used by patient to monitor the effectiveness of medications.
Chest x-ray	Used to visualize lung fields; air appears dark so it can be determined if all lobes are filling with air. Fluid, dense tissue, and infiltrate appear white.	Used to determine lung filling and size of cardiac silhouette, and to identify tumors, pneumonia, infiltrate, and effusions.
Tuberculin skin test	To determine reaction to presence of tuberculin bacillus in skin layers.	If skin over and around injection site elevates and *indurates* (gets hard) with or without redness, the result is positive. This indicates past exposure to the disease or current disease. Must be followed up with chest x-ray for confirmation. False positives are caused by the malaria vaccine given in many African countries.

Table 28-2 **Normal Ranges for ABGs and the Significance of Abnormal Levels**

Blood Gas Component	Normal Range	Significance of Levels Above Normal	Significance of Levels Below Normal
pH	7.35–7.45	Alkalosis	Acidosis
PaO_2	75–100 mm Hg	Hyperventilation	Hypoxemia
$PaCO_2$	35–45 mm Hg	Converts to carbonic acid and causes acidosis	Lack of carbonic acid causes alkalosis
HCO_3^-	22–26	Excess of alkalinity causes alkalosis	Lack of alkalinity leads to acidosis
SaO_2	95%–100%	Hyperventilation or excess supplemental oxygen	Hypoxemia and hypoxia

patient inhales, a set of balls or a piston with a platform top rises, showing the patient the volume of the inhalation. The patient continues to try to improve the volume of inhalations to raise the balls or piston higher, which helps to expand the lungs fully and prevent atelectasis. Instruct the patient to use the incentive spirometer every hour and to repeat the inhalations 10 times. Skill 28-3 (page 632) provides more information on assisting with incentive spirometry.

Patient Teaching Connection

Incentive Spirometry

When you instruct the patient to use an incentive spirometer, it is important to give clear directions. Often, patients think they should blow into the device using a forceful exhalation, which could cause lung injury. Explain that the purpose of the incentive spirometer is to increase the amount of air inhaled, which expands the air sacs in the lungs. This decreases the patient's risk for developing pneumonia and atelectasis, or a collapsed lung.

Instruct the patient to breathe in slowly and deeply, trying to raise the platform above the piston to the preset slide pointer. Alternately, if you are using a three-chamber device, the patient tries to inhale slowly and deeply enough to raise all three balls in the chambers.

Instruct the patient to use the incentive spirometer 10 times each hour to expand the lungs fully. However, your responsibility does not end with those instructions. Follow up with your patient several times during your shift to ensure that he or she is using the incentive spirometer. Ask the patient to demonstrate using it for you so you can be sure that he or she is performing the procedure correctly and you can see the volume of air the patient is inhaling. Enlist the assistance of family or friends if necessary to help remind the patient to use the incentive spirometer.

Nebulizer Treatments

A **nebulizer** is a medication delivery system containing an air compressor and a mask or handheld mouthpiece. Liquid medication, usually a bronchodilator, is ordered by the physician and is placed in a small cup that attaches to the air compressor via tubing. The medication may be ordered to be mixed with saline. *Safety: Follow orders carefully as failing to mix the medication as ordered could lead to an overdose.* Saline without medication may also be used to provide moisture to the airways to thin tenacious mucus. The compressed air travels through the liquid medication or saline, converting it into a fine mist that the patient inhales directly into the airways and lungs. A physician's order is required for all nebulizer treatments.

Once you add the liquid medication, medication with saline, or saline alone to the cup, you will assemble the remaining apparatus for medication delivery. When the compressor is turned on, you will see vapor in the mask or from the spacer on the back side of the handheld mouthpiece. The patient then breathes the vapor in, slowly and deeply. If the patient is using the mouthpiece, he or she must close the lips around it and breathe in through the mouth and out through the nose. If the patient is unable to breathe in this manner during the nebulizer treatment, you will want to use the mask apparatus rather than the mouthpiece. The patient can then breathe in and out through the nose or mouth and still inhale the medication effectively. Skill 28-4 (page 633) gives the steps for preparing a nebulizer and administering a nebulizer treatment.

Supplemental Oxygen

When a patient is hypoxemic, the health care provider orders supplemental oxygen. It is important to understand the purpose of this; remember that room air contains 21% oxygen, so it is always available as we breathe. However, in the presence of lung disease or other conditions that interfere with external respiration, supplemental oxygen increases the amount of available oxygen with each inhalation.

Oxygen is not without its risks, however. *Safety: Oxygen supports combustion, meaning that its presence will cause any fire to burn faster and hotter.* Anytime oxygen is in use, you must ensure that safety precautions are followed:

- Ensure that "No Smoking" signs are on the doors and above the bed. In hospitals, smoking is no longer allowed anywhere. However, in home health care and some long-term care or assisted living facilities, smoking could still be an issue. In those settings, be sure the signs are in place and the restrictions on smoking are enforced.
- Ensure that no open flames are in the same room as an oxygen source. In home health care, this refers to open-flame heaters, candles, and fireplaces. The oxygen source must be in another room away from any flame.
- Check electrical devices such as electric razors to ensure that there are no frayed wires that could cause sparks, which could lead to a fire.
- Eliminate the possibility of static electricity, which could also spark a fire. Use cotton gowns and linens, not synthetics.
- Avoid using petroleum-based products such as petroleum jelly on the lips of patients using supplemental oxygen. Use a water-soluble or non–petroleum-based product instead.

Oxygen can cause toxicity in some situations. If a person breathes a high concentration of oxygen for long periods, it can cause central nervous system damage. If a high liter flow of oxygen is given to patients with chronic lung disease, it can cause severe respiratory problems. Remember that their stimulus to breathe is low oxygen in the blood rather than higher than normal carbon dioxide levels. During a severe exacerbation, such as an acute worsening of chronic lung disease, higher levels of oxygen may be used *short-term only* to help get the patient through the crisis. If the patient receives supplemental oxygen at a liter flow above 2 to 3 L/min beyond the acute crisis, it can cause respiratory depression and even death. *Safety: Always keep routine supplemental oxygen liter flow for patients with chronic obstructive lung disease below 3 L/min.*

Oxygen Delivery

Supplemental oxygen can be delivered in a variety of ways. The health care provider will order the specific device. However, it is important for you to evaluate the effectiveness of such orders and suggest a change if it is appropriate. It is also important for you to understand how oxygen is delivered by each device. For example, if a patient who is using a nasal cannula, which delivers oxygen via nasal prongs, is breathing mostly through his or her mouth, a mask may be more appropriate for oxygen delivery.

Oxygen may be derived from different types of sources. For example, in the hospital setting, oxygen is piped in through the walls and accessed by inserting a flowmeter into a valve. The oxygen then flows through tubing to the patient (Fig. 28-2). When the patient leaves the hospital room, a portable oxygen tank, called an E-cylinder, is used to provide continuous oxygen. This is a small portable tank on a wheeled cart (Fig. 28-3). You will need to know how to switch the patient from one type of source to another when

Figure 28-2 An oxygen flowmeter connected to piped-in oxygen.

you ambulate a patient in the hallway of the hospital. Patients at home may use liquid oxygen. When they leave home or move about the house, they can use a portable container called a stroller, which is light enough to be carried by the patient (Fig. 28-4). Table 28-3 lists the types of oxygen sources with a description of each.

There are a variety of ways that oxygen is supplied from the source to the patient. The nasal cannula, which has short curved prongs designed to fit inside the nostrils, interferes the least with eating and talking. It works best for patients who breathe through the nose. Masks of various types are used for different needs. Table 28-4 describes the different oxygen delivery devices, their liter flows, and the purposes of each. Skill 28-5 (page 634) gives the steps in administering supplemental oxygen.

Conservation of Energy

Patients with chronic lung disease often must use the accessory muscles in the neck and shoulders to move air in and out of their lungs. When this is the case, the patient cannot

Figure 28-3 This is an example of an E-cylinder.

Figure 28-4 This patient is using a liquid oxygen stroller.

terrycloth robe. During the shower, the patient can sit while applying soap and rinsing the body. After the shower, the patient can slip on the robe and sit and rest outside of the shower. The robe will absorb water and the patient will not have to use the shoulder and neck muscles to dry off with a towel. Often just the activity of taking a shower is exhausting for the patient with chronic lung disease.

• For nutritional assistance, encourage the patient to use PulmoCare or a similar meal supplement to increase protein and calories without high carbohydrate intake. Metabolism of carbohydrates produces carbonic acid, which in turn can contribute to acidosis in the patient with chronic lung disease.

Encourage the patient to eat frequent, small meals several times per day, rather than three larger meals. This will help him or her get in more calories before tiring. The patient may become weary after eating only a few bites of a meal because of the use of accessory muscles to eat instead of breathe.

• For other activities of daily living, encourage the patient to take frequent rest periods during these activities. When you care for a patient with chronic lung disease in the hospital setting, plan to take a longer time than usual for bathing, dressing, grooming, and oral care. The patient will require frequent breaks to rest and breathe with those accessory muscles rather than using them for daily care.

Be patient and kind. Rushing the patient causes more stress for both of you. The patient cannot go any faster and needs your understanding and patience regarding the pace required to complete activities.

Knowledge Connection

How often should patients be turned and asked to deep breathe and cough? What is the purpose of delivering a medication via a nebulizer? Why is conservation of energy important for patients with chronic lung disease? What safety issues are of concern to home health care patients with supplemental oxygen?

use the same muscles to perform tasks such as bathing and eating. The patient must then make a choice between bathing and breathing or eating and breathing. That is why you often see patients with chronic lung disease who are very thin and have poor nutritional status.

You can help these patients conserve their energy so that they can use those accessory muscles to breathe, but still be able to obtain nourishment and perform some activities of daily living. Some tips for assisting them include:

• For bathing assistance, encourage the patient to place a nonrusting chair or bench in the shower and to get a

Table 28-3   Types of Oxygen Sources

Type	Description
Piped-in oxygen	Found in health care facilities with a wall outlet above the bed. The flowmeter is inserted into the wall to access oxygen within the pipe (see Fig. 28-2). When the patient ambulates in the hall or is taken to other departments in the hospital, an E-cylinder is used.
Oxygen tank	Large, green, heavy tanks that hold oxygen gas and must be exchanged for a full tank when empty. They are usually delivered by an oxygen supply or medical equipment company. The patient is connected to the tank with extension tubing, allowing for a limited area for ambulation.
Oxygen E-cylinder	Small green tank that holds oxygen gas and sits on a wheeled holder, allowing patient mobility (see Fig. 28-3). It can be used when the patient leaves the hospital room, home, or a facility and is wheeled alongside as he or she walks. When empty, it must be exchanged for a full one.
Oxygen concentrator	Removes some oxygen from room air and concentrates it for oxygen delivery of up to 4 L/min. Requires electricity to work and may increase the cost of the patient's electric bill. Looks similar to a piece of furniture. If the patient leaves home or a facility, he or she must use an E-cylinder.
Liquid oxygen	Oxygen that is kept cold so that it is a liquid rather than a gas. A larger barrel-shaped tank contains the oxygen supply. A smaller stroller is filled from the large tank (see Fig. 28-4). It is lightweight and easy to carry with a shoulder strap. The contents of the stroller last up to 10 hours set on 2 L/min. Can be refilled from the main tank by the patient.

Table 28-4   Oxygen Delivery Devices

Delivery Device	Liter Flow	Description	Tips for Use
Nasal cannula 	1–6 L/min	Delivers oxygen into the nares; patient can more easily eat and talk with it in place; patient must breathe mostly through the nose for full benefit.	Apply correctly. Nasal prongs curve inward when inserted into the nares, and tubing slips over the ears. The slider fits under the chin.
Simple face mask 	5–10 L/min	Delivers oxygen directly to the nose and mouth; patient may breathe through nose or mouth; flow rate less than 5 L/min will cause carbon dioxide to accumulate in the mask.	May cause patient to feel claustrophobic and hot; elastic straps hold mask in place and may irritate skin above the ears, causing pressure. Pad with gauze 4×4s if needed.

(table continues on page 622)

Table 28-4 Oxygen Delivery Devices (continued)

Delivery Device	Liter Flow	Description	Tips for Use
Partial rebreathing mask	6–15 L/min	Mask with bag attached that traps carbon dioxide for rebreathing to lower pH levels; ports on the side of the mask allow most exhaled air to discharge.	When used correctly, rebreathing bag will not collapse during inhalation; if collapse occurs, increase flow rate according to prescriber's orders.
Non-rebreathing mask	6–15 L/min	Prevents the patient from rebreathing any exhaled air; it escapes through a one-way valve that does not allow room air to enter. The bag traps oxygen as a reservoir for inhalation; only delivery device that can provide 100% oxygen when set at 15 L/min.	When used correctly, rebreathing bag will not collapse during inhalation; it should remain at least half full. If it does not, increase the oxygen flow rate according to prescriber's orders.
Venturi mask	24%–80%	Contains a plastic valve between the tubing from the oxygen source and the mask, which allows a precise mix of room air and oxygen to equal a specific percentage of oxygen. The dial on the valve (or interchangeable adapter) indicates the liter flow to use to equal a specific percentage of oxygen. This gives more exact control of inspired oxygen, especially for patients with COPD.	The physician orders percentage of oxygen, not liter flow. You must check the dial or adapter to determine the liter flow necessary to equal the oxygen percentage and set the flowmeter accordingly.
Face tent	8–12 L/min	Used for patients who feel claustrophobic with other masks because the top is open; allows for high amounts of humidity to be used due to open top.	Oxygen delivery is not as precise, so it is important to assess oxygen saturation and signs and symptoms of hypoxia in your patient using this device.

Table 28-4   **Oxygen Delivery Devices** (continued)

Delivery Device	Liter Flow	Description	Tips for Use
Tracheostomy collar	4–10 L/min	Delivers highly humidified oxygen through large tubing; rests over the tracheostomy with an elastic band that goes around the neck and can be tightened at the sides.	Due to high humidity, condensation builds up in the large tubing. Be cautious when turning or moving the patient so that pooled water does not migrate into the tracheostomy and cause choking.
T-piece	4–10 L/min	Attaches to the flange of the tracheostomy; oxygen flows from one side of the T-piece to the trachea. During exhalation, air exits through the open end of the T-piece.	Keep the connection to the tracheostomy intact, being careful not to allow tension on it to pull out the inner cannula.

Nursing Interventions for Patients Needing Airway Assistance

In some situations, the patient cannot maintain his or her own open airway due to decreased level of consciousness, recent surgery, or other situations. An *artificial airway* is used to assist in maintaining a patent airway. It is usually made of hard plastic or soft rubber and may be placed in the oropharynx, in the nasopharynx, or within the trachea. An endotracheal airway may be inserted through the nose or mouth.

Pharyngeal Airways

An *oropharyngeal airway* is made of hard plastic in a slightly curved shape and is designed to hold the tongue in place so that it cannot obstruct the airway of an unconscious patient (Fig. 28-5). They come in a variety of sizes, from infant through adult. This type of airway is not used for conscious patients since it can cause gagging or vomiting.

A *nasopharyngeal airway* is made of pliable rubber and is designed to be inserted through the nose into the pharynx. This type of airway is also referred to as a nasal trumpet due to its shape (see Fig. 28-5).

Suctioning With Pharyngeal Airways in Place

The patient may be unable to clear the airway for a variety of reasons, including a weak cough, decreased level of consciousness, or postoperative pain. It is important to be aware of signs that the patient needs to be suctioned, such as rattling sounds in the throat, shortness of breath, ineffective cough, and crackles on auscultating the lungs.

You will use a *suction catheter,* a thin pliable tube with holes in the end, to remove secretions from the patient's nose, throat, and mouth. If an oropharyngeal airway is in place, you will pass the suction catheter along the grooves in the sides of the airway. If a nasopharyngeal airway is in place, you can pass the suction catheter through the airway to the throat. If no airway is in place, you can use the pliable suction catheter to suction through the nose and down the

Figure 28-5   A variety of airway sizes and types.

throat. Skill 28-6 (page 635) gives the steps in performing nasopharyngeal and oropharyngeal suctioning. Then you can switch to a hard plastic tube with a larger diameter to suction the mouth. This type of suction device is referred to as a Yankauer suction catheter or tonsil tip suction tube (Fig. 28-6). If the patient reacts to the presence of the tube in his or her mouth by biting down, it will not damage the tonsil tip and you will still be able to suction. If that occurs with the softer type of suction catheter, it will impede suction and damage the catheter. Skill 28-6 also discusses the steps of using a tonsil-tip suction device.

Endotracheal Airways

Some airways are designed to enter the trachea, not the pharynx. These airways are used when the patient is unable to breathe independently due to airway obstruction or respiratory arrest. An **endotracheal tube** is a firm but flexible plastic tube that may be inserted through the nose or the mouth. The tube is usually inserted by a physician or specially trained respiratory therapist. These tubes are often placed in the surgery suite to support ventilation during surgery. Their purpose is to connect the patient to the ventilator so oxygen and air is delivered directly to the lungs. The positive pressure of the ventilator causes the air to go into the lungs.

To ensure that air does not exit through the trachea around the tube, the endotracheal tube contains an inflatable cuff located near the distal end. When the cuff is inflated, air cannot leak around the tube, but goes completely into the lungs for full ventilation (Fig. 28-7).

Suctioning an Endotracheal Tube

Patients with endotracheal tubes are cared for in critical care settings. It is considered a sterile procedure to suction the tube because it goes deep into the trachea, and poor technique could introduce pathogens into the lungs. The sterile suction catheter is inserted using sterile technique through the endotracheal tube, and suction is applied as the catheter is pulled outward. Some suction catheters are inside a sleeve of clear plastic, keeping the catheter itself sterile, but allowing you to touch the outside of the sleeve without putting on sterile gloves. Skill 28-7 (page 637) gives the steps in performing endotracheal suctioning using a sleeved catheter.

Figure 28-6   A Yankauer or tonsil-tip suction tube.

Figure 28-7   An endotracheal tube placed through the mouth and into the trachea with the cuff inflated to prevent air leaks.

Tracheostomy

A **tracheostomy**, an incision into the trachea that is held open with a tube to promote breathing, may be performed for several reasons. If a patient has had an endotracheal tube for 7 to 10 days and will require longer term ventilator support, a tracheostomy is usually performed. A tracheostomy is also performed when the airway is obstructed, either temporarily or permanently. In many cases, the obstruction is due to cancerous tumors in the laryngeal area.

Because the endotracheal tube can erode the trachea after being in place longer than 2 weeks, the tracheostomy is necessary. First, an incision is made into the trachea, called a *tracheotomy*. Then the shorter tracheostomy tube is inserted directly into the trachea and anchored in place. The ventilator is then attached to the tracheostomy tube.

A tracheostomy tube has three parts (Fig. 28-8):

1. The *outer cannula,* with or without a cuff. The cuff is inflated to prevent air leakage when the patient is on a ventilator, just as it is on the endotracheal tube. The cuff on the tracheostomy tube should remain inflated while the patient eats to prevent aspiration of food or fluids. Most hospitals have a policy for deflating the cuff periodically to prevent erosion of the trachea due to pressure. You can tell if the cuff is inflated or deflated by checking the "pillow" on the tracheostomy. If it is inflated, the cuff is inflated.

2. The *obturator,* which fits inside the outer cannula and forms a smooth end for inserting the tracheostomy tube into the tracheotomy. The obturator is removed once the tube is in place and kept at the bedside in case the tube comes out and must be reinserted. The blunt edge of the open tube could not easily be inserted into the trachea. The obturator fills the blunt edge with a smooth, rounded end for ease of insertion.

3. The *inner cannula* is inserted after the obturator is removed. It may be a disposable tube or it may be designed to be cleaned and replaced every 8 hours. Mucus collects in the inner cannula and can block the patient's airway if it is not suctioned frequently and cleaned or replaced regularly.

Figure 28-8   A tracheostomy tube with inflatable cuff and "pillow," inner cannula, and obturator.

Labels: Outer tube with cuff and inflating tube; Cuff; Inner cannula; Obturator.

Suctioning and Cleaning a Tracheostomy

To clear a tracheostomy tube, you will use aseptic technique to insert a suction catheter into the inner cannula and apply suction as you withdraw it. When you are applying suction, you are also removing oxygen as you remove mucus. Therefore, this procedure should be done quickly and effectively. The suction catheter may be sheathed or unsheathed. As with the sheathed catheter for suctioning an endotracheal tube, you do not have to wear sterile gloves to touch the sheath because the sterile catheter remains protected inside it. Skill 28-7 explains the process of suctioning a tracheostomy.

When you clean a tracheostomy, you will remove the inner cannula and clean it in hydrogen peroxide mixed half-strength with saline, then rinse it in saline, dry it, and reinsert it. This is done every 8 hours using aseptic technique to prevent introducing pathogens into the trachea and lungs. If the inner cannula is disposable, you will remove it and reinsert a new one rather than cleaning and reinserting.

Tracheostomy ties are generally changed at this time. *Safety: If possible, have an assistant hold the tracheostomy tube in place while you change the ties or holders. If you are performing this procedure alone, do NOT remove the old ties until the new ties are in place and secured. The patient can easily cough the tube completely out of the trachea if it does not remain secured in place.* You may use foam tracheostomy tube holders that are held in place by Velcro, or twill ties that you thread through the slots on the tracheostomy tube and tie. Skill 28-8 (page 639) gives the steps for cleaning a tracheostomy tube and changing tracheostomy ties.

Knowledge Connection

What is the difference between an oropharyngeal airway and a nasopharyngeal airway? What is the purpose of an endotracheal tube? What is an obturator and how is it used?

Chest Tubes

If the negative pressure in the pleural cavity is disrupted, the lungs can no longer fully expand. This causes dyspnea, chest pain, hypoxia, and respiratory distress. It may be due to secretions obstructing the airways or traumatic injuries that penetrate the chest wall—for example, gunshot or stab wounds. This disruption also occurs after surgery that involves opening the chest, such as surgery on the lungs or heart. To re-establish the negative pressure within the pleural space, also known as the *pleural cavity,* the physician will insert chest tubes.

Placement of Chest Tubes

When air enters the pleural space, it rises to the top of the cavity. As you learned earlier, this is referred to as a *pneumothorax.* A chest tube is inserted into the pleural space through an incision in the anterior superior surface of the chest in the second to fourth intercostal space to release this air. When blood and drainage are present in the pleural space, they pool in the lower portion of the cavity; this is called a **hemothorax.** The chest tube to drain this fluid is inserted in the anterior inferior area of the chest, between the eighth and ninth intercostal space, and enters the pleural space. In situations in which both air and blood are in the pleural cavity, two tubes are placed, one higher and one lower, joined by a Y-connector, then attached to tubing leading to a drainage system.

Chest tubes may be inserted at the bedside or in the emergency department. They may also be placed in surgery during a thoracic procedure. When chest tubes are placed outside of surgery, a nurse must immediately connect them to the drainage system and tape all connections thoroughly to prevent leaks.

Chest Drainage System

The drainage system for chest tubes is most commonly a single molded plastic unit containing three chambers (Fig. 28-9).

Chamber One

The chamber on the left (chamber one) is for wet suction. This is used when drainage needs to be gently pulled out of the pleural space. While the drainage unit may be connected to wall suction, the amount of suction is actually controlled by the amount of water in this chamber. Follow the physician's order for the amount of water to add. You will generally fill the chamber to the –20 cm line with sterile water. When the suction source is attached, bubbles will be present in this chamber, which you will be able to see and hear. Set the suction so that gentle bubbling occurs. Rapid bubbling will just cause the water to evaporate faster; it will not change the amount of suction.

In systems with dry suction, a dial on the drainage unit is set to the suction ordered by the physician, then the unit is connected to wall suction. The same amount of suction, –20 cm, is operating, but there is no continuous bubbling and no fluid that can evaporate. *Safety: Be sure you*

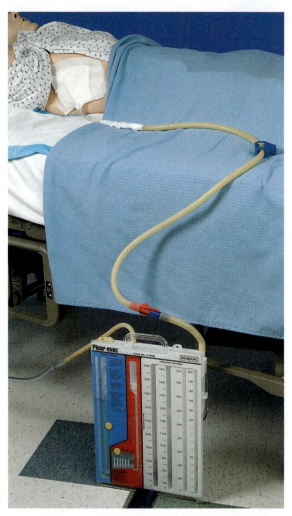

Figure 28-9 A chest drainage system with the tubes in the correct position for gravity drainage. Note the taped connections and the three sections of the drainage system. The blue area is the suction chamber, the red area is the water-seal chamber, and the white area is the collection chamber.

know how to use and evaluate the chest drainage system used in your facility.

Chamber Two

The middle chamber (chamber two) is for the water seal. This is required to re-establish negative pressure in the pleural space and prevent air from entering the cavity through the chest tube. It is standard to establish a 2-cm water seal, which means that you will add sterile water up to the 2-cm mark on the middle chamber.

Observe this chamber closely. It is not unusual to see the water level rise as the patient inhales and fall as the patient exhales. This motion is referred to as *tidaling* and will stop when the lung has reinflated.

Another observation to make about this chamber is that, when the patient has a pneumothorax, you will see the air leave the chest cavity and make bubbles in this chamber. Some types of drainage systems have a scale from 1 to 7

measuring the amount of escaping air. This allows you to document the resolution of the pneumothorax.

Once the air is removed and the pneumothorax resolved, you should not see bubbles in the water-seal chamber; if you do see bubbles in the water-seal chamber, there is an air leak in the system. *Safety: At the first sign of bubbles in the water-seal chamber of a patient with a resolved pneumothorax, check all tubing connections and the dressings at the insertion site for possible air leaks.*

Chamber Three

The remaining chamber (chamber three) on the right is the collection chamber. This is where blood and other fluids from the pleural cavity are trapped and measured. Because this is a closed system that re-establishes negative pressure within the pleural space, the drainage is never emptied. Rather, you will mark the level of drainage on the writable surface adjacent to the collection chamber. You will also write the date and time, along with your initials, next to the amount of drainage. Then you will determine the amount of output for an 8-hour period. Take the following scenario as an example:

When you come on shift, you find the collection chamber contains 325 mL of output counted by the previous shift. Eight hours later, the collection chamber contains 440 mL. To determine the amount of output for your shift, subtract 325 from 440 and record 115 mL as the chest tube output.

You should expect the amount of drainage to gradually decrease each day until the pleural space has been drained and the physician removes the chest tube. It is important for you to assess the color and amount of chest tube drainage several times during your shift. *Safety: If a sudden increase in total output or a sudden increase in bright red output occurs in the chest tube drainage unit, notify the physician immediately since this could indicate hemorrhage.*

Nursing Interventions for Patients With Chest Tubes

Patients with chest tubes may be in critical care units, but they may also be on regular nursing units, which is why it is important for you to know how to care for them. Your responsibilities include assessing the patient's respiratory status every 2 hours to ensure that no complications occur. The patient should have audible breath sounds in all lung fields as the pneumothorax and/or hemothorax resolve. It is possible that you will hear a friction rub due to the presence of the chest tube in the pleural space.

It is important for you to assess for clots that might occlude the tubing, preventing the suction from maintaining the "vacuum" necessary to restore the negative pressure within the pleural space. An increase of positive pressure can build up within the pleural space and, if it is not resolved, can cause a tension pneumothorax. This condition can eventually shift the entire mediastinal area, which includes the heart, bronchial trees, and major blood vessels, from the center to one side, causing compression of the heart. This shift can prevent the previously unaffected lung from optimally exchanging gases, further adding to the problem. If clots are noted, follow your facility's policy and your physician's orders. The previous practice of "stripping" the tubes that lead to the drainage unit (pinching the tubing closed and sliding your fingers down the tubing to pull clots toward the drainage unit) is no longer recommended because it increases positive pressure within the pleural space. However, a clot that occludes the tubing can have the same result. "Milking" chest tubes refers to pinching the tube above the clot briefly and repeating this action to work the clot gently toward the drainage unit. *Safety: Know your facility's policy for intervening when clots are present in the tubing from the chest tube to the drainage unit.* In many situations, the response to a blood clot in chest tubing lies with the physician's preference.

It is also important to know what to do if a chest tube comes out. A special dressing impregnated with petroleum jelly makes an occlusive barrier to cover the opening and prevent air from entering. It is the policy at some hospitals to keep such a dressing at the bedside of the patient with chest tubes. However, if the patient has an unresolved pneumothorax, placing petroleum gauze over the opening could cause a tension pneumothorax due to air trapped in the chest. In that case, some researchers recommend placing regular gauze over the opening and preparing for reinsertion. *Safety: Notify the physician immediately if a chest tube comes out. Follow facility policy regarding the use of petroleum gauze.*

If the chest tube becomes disconnected from the drainage unit, place the end of the tube in a bottle of sterile saline or sterile water so that it is 2 cm below the surface of the fluid to re-establish the water seal. You can then connect the tube to a new drainage system. It is no longer recommended that chest tubes be clamped with padded hemostats except for very short periods in specific circumstances, such as to change the drainage unit or to test the patient's ability to tolerate the removal of the chest tube.

If the drainage unit is a wet suction setup, it must be kept upright at all times. Inspect tubing to be sure that there are no kinks and that the fluids are draining to gravity. Eliminate any loops that would require drainage to run up-hill. Always check for leaks. Keep all connections securely taped. Keep all dressings around the insertion site intact. These are petroleum gauze dressings covered with regular gauze. Check the patient for *subcutaneous emphysema,* the feeling of crepitus under the skin, to detect any air leaks into the tissue. Skill 28-9 (page 640) gives the steps for maintaining chest tubes.

Knowledge Connection

Why is the chest tube for a pneumothorax placed in the upper area of the chest? List the three chambers of a standard chest tube drainage system. What might indicate hemorrhage in a patient with chest tubes?

Nursing Care Plan for a Patient With COPD and Pneumonia

You are planning care for a 60-year-old male patient with a diagnosis of bilateral pneumonia and chronic obstructive pulmonary disease (COPD). He lives with his wife, who is also having health problems, but she is his primary caregiver. He has had pneumonia several times in the past 2 years, but this is the most severe case. The following are questions you might ask yourself as you assess him and collect data:

• What are his lung sounds like?
• Is he hypoxemic?
• Does he have a productive cough?
• What is the amount, color, and consistency of the sputum?

Figure 28-10 presents a concept map care plan for a patient with COPD and pneumonia.

Assessment
When you research his chart and perform your assessment, you discover that your patient is 5 feet, 10 inches (177.6 cm) tall and weighs

135 pounds (61.2 kg). His skin color is pale with a bluish tinge to his lips and nailbeds. His temperature is elevated at 102.2°F (39°C), his pulse is 108, respirations 26, and blood pressure 144/86. His SaO₂ using a pulse oximeter is 89%. He is short of breath with any movement and has oxygen on at 2 L/min per nasal cannula (2L/NC).

He has a history of smoking 2 packs per day for 20 years. He has a weak cough that is often non-productive. When he does expectorate sputum, it is a small amount of rust-colored sputum. He appears anxious and is sitting in the high Fowler's position in bed. His activity orders are for bedrest with bathroom privileges. When you assist him to the bathroom, he is extremely short of breath with exertion. When you auscultate his lungs, you hear coarse crackles in the lower lobes bilaterally that do not clear with coughing.

He has a poor nutritional intake. His wife says he eats a few bites of a meal and then becomes short of breath and must rest. The physician has ordered a sputum specimen for culture and sensitivity.

(care plan continues on page 628)

Nursing Care Plan for a Patient with COPD and Pneumonia (continued)

Nursing Diagnoses

Now you must identify the appropriate nursing diagnoses for this patient based upon your assessment findings. Several diagnoses are appropriate. In addition, you have identified nutritional concerns for this patient and an inability to tolerate activity. You determine the highest priority nursing diagnoses for him are:

- Ineffective airway clearance related to secretions in the airways as evidenced by ineffective cough and adventitious breath sounds
- Impaired gas exchange related to chronic lung changes as evidenced by dyspnea and decreased oxygen saturation.
- Activity intolerance related to imbalance between oxygen supply and demand as evidenced by dyspnea with exertion
- Nutrition: less than body requirements related to poor endurance during eating as evidenced by low body weight

Planning

You will now plan your interventions and the outcomes for this patient. You decide that the outcomes for him will be that he will cough more effectively to remove secretions before discharge, that his gas exchange will then improve when the secretions are removed, and therefore his oxygen saturation will also improve. You determine that his activity tolerance can be increased when his oxygenation improves, and that he can increase his body weight by changing some eating habits to accommodate his poor endurance. You begin to think of a number of nursing interventions to help him accomplish these outcomes, including ways to help him conserve his energy, ways to help him expectorate sputum and keep his lungs expanded, and ways to help improve his nutritional status.

Implementation

Now that you have developed a care plan, it is time to put it into action. One of the first actions you take is to place him in high Fowler's position to help him expand his lungs more effectively. You find out which fluids he likes to drink and offer them frequently to help thin his mucus. You suction him as needed to clear the airway and encourage him to cough and deep breath every 2 hours. You continue to assess him for signs of improving or worsening hypoxia and hypoxemia. You assist him with activities and teach him ways to conserve his energy so he can breathe with less effort. You also include his wife in this instruction, as well as teaching them both about ways to improve his nutritional status. Table 28-5 contains your interventions for each of the nursing diagnoses you identified for this patient.

Evaluation

Once you have put the care plan into action, you need to evaluate its effectiveness in resolving the patient's nursing diagnoses and reaching the desired outcomes. His breath sounds are clearer and he is now able to do huff coughing to remove secretions from the airways. His oxygen remains on at 2L/NC as ordered and his oxygen saturations are improving. You continue to assess his oxygen saturation every 4 hours, as well as his color and appearance. He is now able to ambulate to the bathroom with assistance for personal care at the sink. He is using energy conservation techniques during exertion and plans to use your ideas at home to help him be able to do more personal care without getting so short of breath. His nutritional status is improving some, and he is learning which foods are easiest for him to eat. He is using the PulmoCare supplement to provide calories and nutrition without increasing carbonic acid production. Table 28-5 shows daily evaluations of the nursing interventions for this patient.

Nursing Care Plan for a Patient with COPD and Pneumonia (continued)

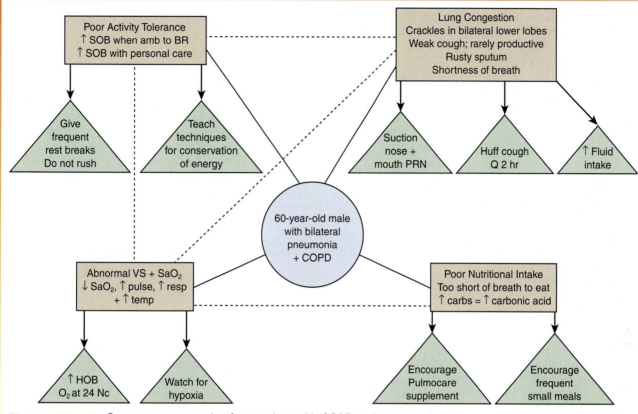

Figure 28-10 Concept map care plan for a patient with COPD and pneumonia.

Table 28-5 Care Plan for a Patient With COPD and Pneumonia

Nursing Diagnosis: Ineffective airway clearance related to secretions in the airways as evidenced by ineffective cough and adventitious breath sounds

Expected Outcomes: Patient will demonstrate effective huff coughing prior to discharge. Patient will verbalize the importance of drinking 8 ounces of fluid every 2 hours while awake to thin mucus by discharge.

Interventions	Evaluation
Encourage fluid intake to help thin mucus, making it easier to cough up and expectorate. Find out what liquids the patient prefers to drink and offer 8 ounces every 2 hours.	Day 1: Likes to drink apple juice and iced tea. Taking fluids every 2 hours. Day 2: Coughing better, able to bring up some sputum that is now a greenish-yellow color. Continues to take fluids well. Day 3: Breath sounds clearer, fewer coarse crackles in the bases of the lungs.
Obtain an order to perform oropharyngeal and nasopharyngeal suctioning as needed until the patient can cough more effectively. Use Yankauer catheter for oral suctioning. Teach the patient how to huff cough and encourage him to do so every 2 hours.	Day 1: Suctioned and obtained thick rust-colored secretions from the nasopharynx. Instructed on huff coughing, but effort still weak. Day 2: Doing better with huff coughing. Day 3: Huff coughing well, without being prompted.

(table continues on page 630)

Table 28-5 **Care Plan for a Patient With COPD and Pneumonia** (continued)

Nursing Diagnosis: Impaired gas exchange related to chronic lung changes as evidenced by dyspnea and decreased oxygen saturation
Expected Outcome: Patient will be able to ambulate to bathroom without dyspnea before discharge. Patient will maintain oxygen saturation of 92% or above before discharge.

Interventions	Evaluation
Maintain supplemental oxygen as ordered at 2 liters per nasal cannula. Assess pulse oximetry every 4 hours to determine effective oxygenation. Assess the patient for signs and symptoms of hypoxia, including confusion, restlessness, and irritability. Assess color and circulation by evaluating the nailbeds, lips, and mucous membranes every 2 hours.	Day 1: Oxygen maintained as ordered. SaO_2 still low at 90%. Mild restlessness, but no other signs of hypoxia. Lips and mucous membranes dusky. Day 2: Lung sounds improving. SaO_2 now at 91%. No signs or symptoms of hypoxia. Nailbeds less dusky. Day 3: Oxygen continued as ordered. SaO_2 at 92%, which is very good for his situation. Cough more effective and lung sounds clearer. Nailbeds and mucous membranes remain slightly dusky.

Nursing Diagnosis: Activity intolerance related to imbalance between oxygen supply and demand as evidenced by dyspnea with exertion
Expected Outcome: Patient will be able to participate in ADLs with minimal dyspnea by discharge. Patient will verbalize ways to conserve energy when performing ADLs at home prior to discharge.

Interventions	Evaluation
Assist the patient with conservation-of-energy techniques: • Decrease activities that require use of accessory muscles. Use a bench or chair in the shower; use a terrycloth robe instead of drying after a shower when home. • Take frequent rest breaks during activities. Do not rush the patient; plan for extra time when assisting with ADLs.	Day 1: Refused bed bath due to shortness of breath. Allowed nurse to sponge off perineal area and armpits only. Day 2: Able to tolerate full bed bath with assistance. Became short of breath after washing arms and face. Took a 10-minute break, then able to assist by washing own perineal area. Day 3: Able to ambulate to bathroom. Had to rest on chair once at the sink. Waited for him to regain energy, then assisted with sponge bath at sink. Verbalizes plans to try chair in shower at home and using a terrycloth robe instead of drying after shower.

Nursing Diagnosis: Nutrition: less than body requirements related to poor endurance during eating as evidenced by low body weight
Expected Outcomes: Patient will verbalize food choices that do not increase carbonic acid buildup or require excessive chewing prior to discharge. Patient will supplement oral intake with meal replacement formulas appropriate for pulmonary disorders before discharge. Patient will gain 2 lbs. within 5 days.

Interventions	Evaluation
Explain that increased carbohydrate intake can lead to excess carbonic acid buildup. Encourage the patient to drink PulmoCare or a similar product for meal replacement if he is too exhausted to eat. Encourage the patient to eat frequent small meals to decrease energy demands while eating. Encourage foods that do not require a great deal of chewing, which uses accessory muscles. Recommend foods such as soups, stews, tender meats, puddings, and applesauce.	Day 1: Ate very little all day. Stated "just too tired to eat." Day 2: Ate small amount of eggs and bacon at breakfast, then agreed to a can of PulmoCare midmorning. Able to drink about half of it. Ate about ⅓ of lunch and ⅓ of dinner before becoming too short of breath to continue. Took another half can of PulmoCare before bed. Day 3: Ate about ⅓ of breakfast with PulmoCare midmorning. Ate more at lunch than yesterday, nearly ½ of meal, then ate a snack of hard-boiled eggs brought in by wife midafternoon. Ate about ½ of supper and drank more PulmoCare before bed. Weight up slightly at 135.8 lbs.

Skill 28-1 Obtaining a Sputum Specimen

Assessment Steps

1. Verify the health care provider's order for the sputum specimen.
2. Determine the frequency and type of cough the patient is experiencing. If it is frequent and productive, you may be able to get the specimen at any time. If not, plan to obtain the specimen in the early morning *when the most sputum is available for expectoration.*
3. Determine the patient's pain level and medicate if necessary. *The patient may be unable to give good cough effort if he or she is in pain.*

Planning Steps

1. Gather needed equipment and supplies: sputum specimen container, clean gloves. If obtaining a suctioned specimen, you will need a sputum trap that attaches to the suction tubing.

Implementation Steps

1. Follow the Initial Implementation Steps located on the inside front cover.

For Obtaining a Sputum Specimen by Coughing and Expectoration

2. Assist the patient to sit upright *to facilitate lung expansion.*
3. Splint the abdominal or chest incisions with a pillow *to help prevent incisional pain.*
4. Instruct the patient to inhale deeply two times, then take a third deep breath and cough while exhaling. *This expands the lungs and opens the airways to allow mucus production with cough.*
5. Instruct the patient to expectorate the mucus into a sterile specimen container. Ask the patient to avoid touching the inside of the container with his or her mouth or tongue, and avoid touching the inside with your hands, *to prevent cross-contamination.*
6. Repeat Steps 4 and 5 until approximately 30 mL of sputum has been obtained. *This is the minimum amount needed for laboratory testing.*
7. Follow the Ending Implementation Steps located on the inside back cover.

For Obtaining a Sputum Specimen by Suction

2. Follow the steps for suctioning the nasopharynx in Skill 28-6 except that, when you assemble the suction tubing and suction catheter, you will attach a sputum trap between them. When you suction the nasopharynx, you will go deep into the trachea and obtain sputum that will be suctioned into the sputum trap for testing.

3. After obtaining the specimen, remove the suction tubing from the connection and attach the rubber tubing on the specimen trap to the port where the suction tubing was attached.
4. Follow the Ending Implementation Steps located on the inside back cover.

Evaluation Steps

1. Ensure that you have at least 30 mL of sputum in the container.
2. Determine the patient's response to the procedure.
3. Ensure that the specimen is labeled and placed in the appropriate biohazard specimen bag with the requisition.
4. Ensure that the specimen is taken to the laboratory promptly or refrigerated until it can be transported.

Sample Documentation

10/10/12   1330   Sputum spec of 30 mL of thick yellow mucus obtained. C/o fatigue after coughing effort. Resp increased to 26/min. Assisted to Fowler's position to rest. Sputum spec labeled and delivered to lab. ———— Nurse's signature and credentials

Skill 28-2 Obtaining a Throat Culture Specimen

Assessment Steps

1. Verify the physician's order for throat culture.

Planning Steps

1. Gather needed equipment and supplies: throat culture swab, tongue blade, clean gloves, examination light if needed.

Implementation Steps

1. Follow the Initial Implementation Steps located on the inside front cover.

2. Assist the patient to an upright position in the bed or chair *to allow better visualization of the throat.* If the room is dark, use an examination light *to make it easier to visualize the throat.*

3. Ask the patient to open his or her mouth widely and say "Ah" *to allow access to the back of the throat.* Place the tongue blade on the tongue *to hold it down during the procedure.* Tell the patient to breathe through the mouth. *This helps prevent gagging.*

4. Remove the swab from the tube without touching any part of the swab itself. Hold onto the cap into which the swab handle is inserted. *Touching any part of the swab, even while wearing clean gloves, can contaminate the specimen.*

5. Insert the swab into the patient's mouth without touching the teeth, cheeks, lips, or gums, *which would cause contamination of the specimen.*

6. Using one side of the swab, slide it against the back of the throat and tonsils to the right of the uvula. Target reddened areas or patches of white or yellow exudate *to ensure that pathogens are obtained.*

7. Using the other side of the swab, slide it against the back of the throat and tonsils to the left of the uvula, targeting the same type of areas. *This allows collection of specimens from different areas of the throat to more easily identify pathogens.*

8. Carefully replace the swab into the sterile tube. *Contamination of the swab or tube can lead to misdiagnosis and inappropriate treatment for the patient.*

9. Crush the capsule in the end of the tube *to provide a moist environment for the pathogens until the culture is done.*

10. Label the tube according to facility policy.

11. Follow the Ending Implementation Steps located on the inside back cover.

Evaluation Steps

1. Ensure that an adequate specimen has been taken *so the culture will grow any pathogens present in the patient's throat.*

2. Evaluate the patient's tolerance of the procedure. Did it cause gagging or throat discomfort?

3. Ensure that the throat culture tube is placed in the appropriate biohazard specimen bag with the requisition and taken to the laboratory.

Sample Documentation

10/10/12   1330   Throat culture obtained per order and delivered to the lab. Pharynx red with yellowish-white patches noted on tonsils bilaterally. Culture taken from these areas. C/o sore throat before and after procedure. ———— Nurse's signature and credentials

Skill 28-3 Assisting With Incentive Spirometry

Assessment Steps

1. Verify the physician's order for incentive spirometry. **Note:** Some hospitals do not require a physician's order for this because it is considered a nursing or respiratory therapy order. Always follow your facility's policy.

2. Determine the patient's pain level, availability, and willingness to perform the procedure. It may be necessary to medicate the patient for pain before beginning the procedure.

Planning Steps

1. Obtain an incentive spirometer.

2. Plan for appropriate time for incentive spirometry; avoid mealtimes.

Implementation Steps

1. Follow the Initial Implementation Steps located on the inside front cover.

2. Assist the patient to an upright position in the bed or chair *to enlarge the rib cage and allow for maximum lung expansion.*

3. Splint abdominal or chest incisions with a pillow *to prevent pain during deep inhalation and exhalation.*

4. Place the mouthpiece of the incentive spirometer between the patient's lips *to prevent air from escaping around it during inhalation.*

5. Instruct the patient to take a deep breath through the mouth, then exhale through the nose. *This helps the patient understand that the focus is on deep inhalation, not exhalation.*

Skill 28-3 (continued)

6. Show the patient how far the platform or balls moved. Identify the goal for the patient to work toward. Set the slide pointer to the goal volume on the spirometer.

7. Instruct the patient to repeat the inhalations 10 times every hour while awake *to prevent respiratory complications of immobility such as pneumonia and atelectasis.*

8. Follow the Ending Implementation Steps located on the inside back cover.

Evaluation Steps

1. Ask the patient to demonstrate the use of the incentive spirometer without verbal cues *to ensure that he or she understands how to correctly use it.*

2. Check back frequently *to be sure the patient is using the incentive spirometer as ordered.*

Sample Documentation

10/10/12   1100   *Assisted with incentive spirometry. Able to raise 2 out of 3 balls in unit. Instructed to repeat 10 times each hour.* ———————— *Nurse's signature and credentials*

Skill 28-4 Administering a Nebulizer Treatment

Assessment Steps

1. Verify the physician's order for nebulizer treatment and medication. Determine if the medication is to be diluted with saline or administered full strength.

2. Research the medication if you are unfamiliar with it. Know the expected effects, side effects, and contraindications before administering any medication. (See Chapter 35 for more information on researching medications.)

3. Assess the patient's lungs for adventitious breath sounds and the patient for dyspnea.

Planning Steps

1. Obtain a nebulizer if one is not already in place at the bedside. Obtain ordered respiratory medications according to facility policy.

2. Determine if the patient can use a handheld mouthpiece or needs a mask for treatment. *Use a mask if the patient is unable to hold the mouthpiece or to breathe in through the mouth and out through the nose during the treatment.*

3. Pour the ordered medication and saline into the medication cup, checking the medication three times (see Chapter 35).

4. Assemble the mouthpiece parts or mask parts and attach the compressor tubing to the medication cup.

Implementation Steps

1. Follow the Initial Implementation Steps located on the inside front cover.

2. Assist the patient to an upright position in the bed or chair *to enlarge the rib cage and allow for maximum lung expansion.*

3. Check the patient's pulse. *Safety: Bronchodilators, if ordered, will increase the pulse rate. If the pulse is above 100, you may want to consult with the physician before administering a bronchodilator.*

4. Place the mouthpiece between the patient's teeth and have him or her close the lips about it *to prevent escape of medication around the mouthpiece.* If using a mask, place it over the nose and mouth and tighten the elastic straps *to keep it in place.*

5. Turn on the air compressor. *This causes the medication to be converted to a fine mist for inhalation.*

6. Instruct the patient to breathe slowly and deeply *to inhale the medication into the small airways and lungs.*

7. Instruct the patient to continue the treatment until the vapor is no longer visible from the spacer on the mouthpiece or in the mask. *This indicates that the medication has been completely inhaled.*

8. Remain with the patient if necessary *to ensure that the treatment is completed correctly.*

9. Turn off the air compressor when the vapor is gone and the medication cup is empty.

10. Check the patient's pulse again *to determine the effect of the medication.* Expect an increase of approximately 20 beats per minute. *Safety: If the pulse rate is significantly higher than expected, notify the physician.*

11. Disassemble the parts of the mouthpiece or mask and rinse them in warm water *to remove any remnants of medication or saline that could crust in openings and affect function.*

12. Allow the parts to drain on a clean paper towel and air dry *to be ready for the patient's next treatment.*

(skill continues on page 634)

Skill 28-4 (continued)

13. Follow the Ending Implementation Steps located on the inside back cover.

Evaluation Steps

1. Determine the effectiveness of the treatment. Auscultate the lungs to evaluate for decreased adventitious sounds.

2. Determine how the patient tolerated the treatment: Did it cause exhaustion? Was the patient able to follow directions? Did the patient inhale all the medication? Does the patient feel relief of dyspnea after treatment?

Sample Documentation

10/10/12   1340   C/o tightness in chest with inhalation. Lungs auscultated. Bilateral wheezes and coarse crackles noted bilaterally throughout lung fields. —————————
————————— *Nurse's signature and credentials*
10/10/12   1400   Nebulizer treatment with 2 mL DuoNeb administered per order. Able to use mouthpiece with deep inhalations. Tolerated without c/o discomfort or fatigue. States "breathing easier" afterward. Lungs auscultated. Scattered coarse crackles heard in bilateral lower lobes. ————— *Nurse's signature and credentials*

Skill 28-5 Administering Supplemental Oxygen

Assessment Steps

1. Verify the physician's order for oxygen. Be certain of liter flow and type of delivery device ordered *as some types are contraindicated in certain lung diseases.*

2. Assess the patient's respiratory status, including pulse oximetry *to document improved SaO₂ with oxygen.*

Planning Steps

1. Gather needed equipment and supplies: oxygen flowmeter, humidifier bottle, ordered delivery device.

2. Obtain appropriate safety signs regarding smoking and open flames and post them.

Implementation Steps

1. Follow the Initial Implementation Steps located on the inside front cover.

2. Connect the oxygen flowmeter to the oxygen source. For piped-in oxygen, follow facility guidelines. The flowmeter may have to be positioned in a certain way to enter the valve, or a release button may have to be pressed for the flowmeter to enter.

3. Fill the oxygen humidifier with distilled water so the level is between the minimum and maximum lines. *Safety: Oxygen at low flow rates (below 3 L/min) does not have to be humidified. Any flow rate of about 3 L/min or higher must be humidified to prevent excessive drying of the mucous membranes.*

4. Attach the humidifier to the flowmeter by screwing it onto the connector completely.

5. Attach the tubing from the oxygen device to the humidifier.

6. Place the oxygen delivery device on the patient:
   • **Nasal cannula:** Place the prongs so the curve is toward the nares and loop the tubing over the ears. Push the slider up under the patient's chin *to hold it securely in place.*

• **Simple, rebreathing, and non-rebreathing masks:** Place the mask over the patient's nose and mouth and the elastic strip around the head, above the ears. Pull the strap at the sides of the mask to tighten *so the mask fits snugly over the face.* Bend the metal nosepiece *to conform to the bridge of the nose.*

Skill 28-5 (continued)

- **Venturi mask:** Ensure that the dial or interchangeable valve between the mask and the oxygen source is correct *to deliver the ordered percentage of oxygen.* Apply the mask the same as the other masks.

- Adjustable nose clip
- Oxygen regulator
- Venturi barrel

- **Face tent:** Fit the tent under the patient's chin with the elastic strap around the head. Tighten at sides as needed *for a snug chin fit.*

- **Tracheostomy collar:** Place the collar loosely over the tracheostomy tube with the elastic strap around the patient's neck. Tighten at the sides as needed *to keep the collar in place.*
- **T-Piece:** Attach to the tracheostomy tube and ensure that it is arranged in such a way that any condensation within the tubing drains away from the patient.

7. Set the ordered liter flow. Turn the dial on the flowmeter so that the silver ball rises to the ordered liters per minute. The line of the selected liter number should cross the middle of the silver ball for correct flow.

8. Follow the Ending Implementation Steps located on the inside back cover.

Evaluation Steps

1. Ensure that oxygen is flowing through the delivery device. There should be bubbles in the humidifier, *indicating the flow of oxygen through it.* To check low liter flow through an unhumidified cannula, place the cannula in a cup of water. *If you see bubbles, the oxygen is flowing.*

2. Measure pulse oximetry after 30 minutes *to evaluate improvement of* SaO_2 *due to supplemental oxygen.*

3. Evaluate the patient's comfort with oxygen. Does he or she complain of feeling claustrophobic? Is he or she mouth-breathing? It may be necessary to consider a change of delivery device with the health care provider's approval.

Sample Documentation

10/10/12	1440	SaO_2 on room air was 90%. O_2 started per order at 2L/NC. ———— Nurse's signature and credentials
10/10/12	1520	SaO_2 94%. Tolerating cannula without c/o discomfort. States, "easier to breathe now." ———— ———— Nurse's signature and credentials

Skill 28-6 Performing Nasopharyngeal and Oropharyngeal Suctioning

Assessment Steps

1. Verify the physician's order for nasopharyngeal or oropharyngeal suctioning. **Note:** In some hospital settings, a physician's order may not be required for suctioning. Follow facility policy.

2. Assess the patient and the need for suctioning. Auscultate the lungs and listen for rattling or moist sounds in the airways as the patient breathes.

Planning Steps

1. Gather needed equipment and supplies: sterile suction catheter and glove kit, saline, sterile basin or cup to hold saline, goggles and mask or mask and face

shield. For oropharyngeal suctioning, obtain a Yankauer or tonsil-tip suction device and clean gloves.

Intervention Steps

1. Follow the Initial Implementation Steps located on the inside front cover.

For Nasopharyngeal Suctioning

2. Ensure that the connection tubing is attached to the suction catheter on the wall and set the regulator at 80 to 120 mm Hg. Test the suction by placing your thumb over the tubing *to determine that it is working correctly.*

(skill continues on page 636)

Skill 28-6 (continued)

3. Open the sterile saline and mark it with the date and time if it is a multiuse container *to ensure that it is not used beyond 24 hours or hospital policy.*

4. Pour some saline into the sterile basin or cup. *This will be used to moisten and rinse the suction catheter between suctioning.*

5. Put a clean glove on your nondominant hand for controlling the suction.

6. Open the sterile catheter and glove kit. Put the sterile glove in the kit on your dominant hand *as this is the hand that will hold and manipulate the suction catheter.* If two gloves come in the kit, put them both on, but consider your nondominant hand as not sterile.

7. Hold the sterile suction catheter in your sterilely gloved dominant hand, being careful to keep the tip within your grasp *to prevent it from becoming contaminated.*

8. Hold the nonsterile connection tubing connected to the suction canister in your nondominant hand.

9. Hold the proximal end of the sterile suction catheter in your dominant hand and connect it to the nonsterile connection tubing without contaminating your dominant hand.

10. Place the thumb-valve portion of the sterile suction catheter in your nondominant hand.

11. Lubricate the first 3 to 4 inches of the suction catheter with the saline by placing it in the cup or basin and placing your thumb over the valve, suctioning in the liquid.

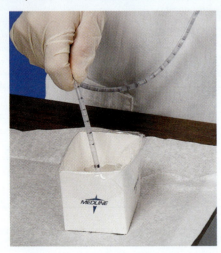

12. Insert the sterile catheter into the right nostril. *Safety: Do not apply your thumb while entering the nose and throat to prevent causing hypoxia.*

13. Continue inserting the catheter through the nose to the back of the throat.

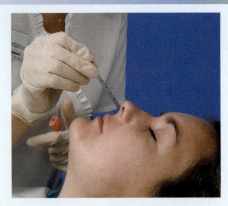

14. Apply your thumb to the valve as you gently but quickly pull the catheter out of the throat and nose. *Safety: Use intermittent suction by lifting your thumb periodically. Suction for no longer than 10 seconds at a time to prevent hypoxia.*

15. Insert the catheter into the basin or cup of saline and apply your thumb to the valve *to rinse the inside and outside of the catheter.*

16. Repeat Steps 11 through 14 going through the left nostril.

17. The suction catheter can now be used to suction the patient's mouth, which has a higher number of bacteria and pathogens present, so it is suctioned last. However, some patients may find this objectionable. Also, the patient may bite down on the suction catheter if it is inserted into the mouth. It is appropriate to change to a Yankauer, or tonsil-tip, suction device at this time.

For Oropharyngeal Suctioning

18. Disconnect the suction catheter from the suction tubing. Hold the catheter in the palm of your dominant hand and remove the glove over the catheter. *This contains the catheter for disposal and prevents contamination of the hands.*

19. Remove the glove from your nondominant hand and wash or sanitize your hands *to prevent cross-contamination.*

20. Put on clean gloves *because oral suctioning is not a sterile procedure.*

21. Attach the Yankauer, or tonsil-tip, suction device to the suction tubing.

22. Insert the tonsil tip into the patient's mouth to the back of the throat, then cover the opening with your thumb or finger *to create suction.*

Skill 28-6 (continued)

23. Suction each side of the throat, in the cheek pouches, and around the tongue *to remove mucus.*

24. Insert the tonsil tip into the saline in the basin or cup and place your thumb or finger over the valve *to rinse the inside and outside of the tonsil tip.* Repeat as necessary during suctioning of the mouth.

25. Disconnect the rinsed tonsil tip and replace it in the wrapper for reuse. Follow facility policy for the length of time it can be used.

26. Follow the Ending Implementation Steps located on the inside back cover.

Evaluation Steps

1. Auscultate the patient's lungs and listen to the patient breathe to determine that the airways are clearer after suctioning.

2. Evaluate the patient's response to the procedure: Did he or she complain of shortness of breath? Pain or discomfort? Fatigue?

Sample Documentation

10/11/12	1730	*Respirations moist sounding, with rattling in throat. Coarse crackles heard in bilateral upper lobes.* ———————————————————— *Nurse's signature and credentials*
10/11/12	1745	*Nasopharyngeal suctioning performed. Lrg amt of thick white mucus obtained. Suctioned orally for sm amt of yellow mucus. Lung sounds clear bilaterally. Resp quiet and even at 20/min.* ———————— *Nurse's signature and credentials*

Skill 28-7 Performing Endotracheal and Tracheostomy Suctioning

Assessment Steps

1. Verify the physician's order for endotracheal or tracheostomy suctioning.

2. Assess the patient for the need for suctioning. Auscultate the lungs and listen for moist respirations through the tracheostomy. If the patient is on a ventilator, you may hear the pressure alarm go off, indicating the need for suctioning.

Planning Steps

1. Gather needed equipment and supplies: sterile suction catheter kit (contains gloves, catheter, and cup for saline), sterile saline, goggles and mask or mask and face shield, gown if indicated, Ambu bag for tracheostomy suctioning.

Intervention Steps

1. Follow the Initial Implementation Steps located on the inside front cover.

Suctioning an Endotracheal Tube When Patient Is Connected to a Ventilator

2. Turn the suction on between 80 and 120 mm Hg.

3. Put on the sterile gloves and prepare the sterile suction catheter and saline as you did in Skill 28-6, keeping in mind that your nondominant hand is not sterile.

4. Lubricate the suction catheter in the sterile saline as in Skill 28-6.

5. Push the button on the ventilator to give 100% oxygen. *This gives 100% oxygen to the patient for 2 minutes while you perform suctioning to help prevent hypoxia.*

6. Insert the catheter into the endotracheal tube until you meet resistance, which is the carina of the trachea. *Safety: Do not apply suction while inserting the catheter to prevent hypoxia.*

7. Apply suction with your thumb as you withdraw the catheter. Use a circular motion and rotate the catheter between your thumb and first finger as you withdraw it *to ensure that you suction all areas inside the endotracheal tube.*

8. Perform suctioning quickly. *Safety: Suctioning for longer than 10 seconds at a time can cause hypoxia.*

9. Rinse the suction catheter by placing it in the cup of sterile saline and using your thumb on the valve to create suction.

10. Repeat Steps 8 to 12 as needed to clear the endotracheal tube of secretions.

11. Disconnect the suction catheter from the suction tubing. Hold the catheter in the palm of your dominant hand and remove the glove over the catheter. *This contains the catheter for disposal and prevents contamination of the hands.*

12. Remove the glove from your nondominant hand and wash or sanitize your hands *to prevent cross-contamination.*

13. Follow the Ending Implementation Steps located on the inside back cover.

For In-Line Suction of an Endotracheal Tube

2. Turn the suction on between 80 and 120 mm Hg.

3. It is unnecessary to use sterile gloves for in-line suction because the suction catheter is contained inside a sterile sleeve, which is connected to the endotracheal tube.

4. Push the button on the ventilator to give 100% oxygen. *This gives 100% oxygen to the patient for 2 minutes while you perform suctioning to help prevent hypoxia.*

Skill 28-7 (continued)

5. Wearing clean gloves, gently insert the suction catheter into the endotracheal tube until you meet resistance.

6. Apply suction by pressing the button over the suction port as you withdraw the catheter. Again, apply suction for no longer than 10 seconds at a time. Repeat suctioning as needed to clear the endotracheal tube of secretions.

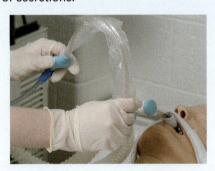

7. Rather than placing the suction catheter in saline to clear it, squeeze a 10-mL plastic container of saline into the port located on the in-line setup. As you insert the saline, apply suction so it will clear the suction catheter.

8. Follow the Ending Implementation Steps located on the inside back cover.

For Suctioning a Tracheostomy When Patient Is Not Connected to a Ventilator

2. Turn the suction on between 80 and 120 mm Hg.

3. Attach the Ambu bag to 100% oxygen from the piped-in oxygen.

4. Enlist the assistance of another health care worker. *Safety: It is very difficult to attach the Ambu bag to the tracheostomy and squeeze the bag to hyperoxygenate the patient using only one hand since your other hand will be sterile.*

5. Put on the sterile gloves and prepare the sterile suction catheter and saline as you did in Skill 28-6, keeping in mind that your nondominant hand is not sterile.

6. Lubricate the suction catheter in the sterile saline as in Skill 28-6.

7. Have your assistant attach the Ambu bag to the tracheostomy tubing and give the patient three to five breaths, then disconnect it from the tracheostomy tube. If you have no assistant, you must do this while keeping your dominant hand sterile and holding the sterile suction catheter.

8. Insert the catheter into the tracheostomy tube until you meet resistance, which is at the carina of the trachea. *Safety: Do not apply suction while inserting the catheter to prevent hypoxia.*

9. Apply suction with your thumb as you withdraw the catheter. Use a circular motion and rotate the catheter between your thumb and first finger as you withdraw it *to ensure that you suction all areas inside the tracheostomy tube.*

10. Lift your thumb off of the valve after a few seconds and then return it to the valve. *This helps prevent the suction catheter from sticking against tracheal tissue and causing trauma to it.*

11. Perform suctioning quickly. *Safety: Suctioning for longer than 10 seconds at a time can cause hypoxia.*

12. Rinse the suction catheter by placing it in the cup of sterile saline and using your thumb on the valve to create suction.

13. Repeat Steps 9 to 12 as needed to clear the tracheostomy tube of secretions. Wait at least 30 seconds between suctionings *to allow the patient to breathe easily.* Reoxygenate with Ambu bag between suctionings. Avoid suctioning for more than a total of 5 minutes *to prevent fatigue, trauma, and hypoxia. Safety: It is a good idea to hold your breath while you are suctioning a patient with a tracheostomy, since this will remind you that the patient cannot breathe while the suction catheter is in the tracheostomy.*

14. Disconnect the suction catheter from the suction tubing. Hold the catheter in the palm of your dominant hand and remove the glove over the catheter. *This contains the catheter for disposal and prevents contamination of the hands.*

15. Remove the glove from your nondominant hand and wash or sanitize your hands *to prevent cross-contamination.*

16. Follow the Ending Implementation Steps located on the inside back cover.

Evaluation Steps

1. Evaluate the patient's ease of respirations after suctioning. Is the ventilator working properly without pressure alarms? Can the patient with a tracheostomy breathe without mucus bubbling or rattling?

2. Determine how the patient tolerated the procedure. Was he or she frightened? Anxious? Did he or she complain of fatigue or discomfort afterward?

Sample Documentation

10/11/12   2010   Respirations moist with rattling noted in trach. Suctioned for mod amt of light yellow mucus. Coughed repeatedly during procedure and do fatigue after suctioning complete. Resp quiet and even at 22/min. ————————————————— Nurse's signature and credentials

Skill 28-8 Performing Tracheostomy Care

Assessment Steps

1. Verify the physician's order for tracheostomy care. Standard orders are to perform the care every 8 hours.
2. Assess the type of tracheostomy the patient has. If the inner cannula is disposable, you will need to obtain a new replacement cannula. If it is reuseable, you will need to obtain a kit for cleaning the inner cannula.

Planning Steps

1. Gather needed equipment and supplies: replacement cannula or tracheostomy care kit, hydrogen peroxide, sterile saline, sterile gloves, clean gloves, goggles and mask or mask and face shield. You will need a tracheostomy holder if the patient does not use ties. You will also need a suction catheter and glove kit.

Intervention Steps

1. Follow the Initial Implementation Steps located on the inside front cover.
2. Suction the tracheostomy following the steps in Skill 28-7. *This removes secretions and helps keep the tracheostomy patent during the cleaning of the inner cannula.*
3. Don clean gloves. *This will allow you to touch the inner cannula to remove it without contaminating your sterile gloves or exposing yourself to blood or body fluids.*

Cannula Care
To Replace a Disposable Inner Cannula

4. Open the package containing the new inner cannula, keeping the cannula on the sterile inner surface of the package.
5. Remove the inner cannula by unlocking it, either by turning it slightly to the side or by pinching the connecting flanges *so it will easily slide out.*
6. Dispose of the inner cannula in the biohazard trash.
7. Insert the new inner cannula by turning it so the end you are holding is at about the 9 o'clock position. Then, as you insert it into the outer cannula, turn it gently to the 6 o'clock position. *Safety: Once the new inner cannula is inserted, ensure that it clicks into place or is tightened to stay in place.*

To Clean and Replace a Reusable Cannula

4. Open the tracheostomy care kit and set up your sterile field. Dump the contents of the kit onto the sterile field. *This allows you to use the basin for your liquids.*
5. Open and pour hydrogen peroxide into the larger compartment in the basin to a depth of ½ inch. Add saline to a depth of another ½ inch to dilute the hydrogen peroxide. *Safety: Full-strength hydrogen peroxide can be irritating to the tissues.*
6. Pour sterile saline in the other two compartments in the basin *to be prepared to clean and rinse the inner cannula.*

7. Remove the inner cannula from the tracheostomy. Remember to unlock it by turning it slightly to the side or pinching the connecting flanges so it will easily slide out.
8. Drop the inner cannula into the basin compartment containing the peroxide and saline *to allow the cannula to soak.*
9. Remove your clean gloves and sanitize your hands *to prevent cross-contamination.*
10. Put on sterile gloves and arrange your supplies on your sterile field *so that you can easily obtain what you need as you complete the procedure.*
11. Use the sterile small bottle brush to clean the inside and outside of the inner cannula with the peroxide/saline solution.
12. Place the inner cannula in a basin compartment containing only sterile saline and agitate it *to rinse off the peroxide.*
13. Remove the inner cannula from the saline and use a sterile gauze 4×4 to dry the outside. Use both pipe cleaners together to dry the inside of the cannula by pulling them through it. *Safety: It is important to dry the inside and outside of the cannula to prevent introducing saline into the trachea and causing choking. Be alert to any threads from the 4×4 that could cling to the cannula. It should be dry and debris free.*
14. Insert the cleaned inner cannula by turning it so the end you are holding is at about the 9 o'clock position. Then, as you insert it into the outer cannula, turn it gently to the 6 o'clock position. *Safety: Once the cleaned inner cannula is inserted, ensure that it clicks into place or is tightened to stay in place.*

To Clean Faceplate

15. Dip a cotton-tipped applicator from your sterile field into the unused basin compartment containing sterile saline. Use the moistened applicator to clean around the stoma *to loosen dried or crusted mucus.* Get a new moistened swab for each swipe *to prevent cross-contamination.*

16. Dampen a sterile gauze 4×4 in the saline and clean the faceplate of the tracheostomy. Dry the faceplate with another gauze 4×4.

To Change the Tracheostomy Ties or Tracheostomy Holder
For Twill Ties

4. Insert one end of the tie into the slit at the side of the faceplate.
5. Bring the other end behind the patient's neck and pull it through the slit on the other side of the faceplate.

(skill continues on page 640)

Skill 28-8 (continued)

6. Tie the two ends together at the side of the patient's neck *so that he or she does not lay on a knot that could cause skin breakdown.*

For Velcro Holders

4. Insert the Velcro ends through the slits in the faceplate from back to front.

5. Ensure that the foam holder is laying smoothly behind the patient's neck.

6. Pull the Velcro through the slits and press it down against the foam, leaving about a one-finger space between the patient's neck and the holder. *Safety: Do NOT remove the old ties until the new ties are in place and secured. The patient will cough as you work with the tracheostomy and can cough it out if it is not secured.*

Completion of Tracheostomy Care

7. Remove the old tracheostomy dressing from beneath the faceplate and replace it with a clean tracheostomy dressing. This is placed so that the open ends point toward the patient's chin and are brought together above the tracheostomy. The dressing absorbs drainage and mucus from around the stoma.

8. Ensure that the tracheostomy collar is in place over the tracheostomy if ordered and that oxygen is being delivered per order.

9. Follow the Ending Implementation Steps located on the inside back cover.

Evaluation Steps

1. Determine the effectiveness of the procedure. Is the tracheostomy clean and patent?

2. Evaluate the patient's response to the procedure. Did he or she complain of pain, discomfort, fatigue, or shortness of breath?

Sample Documentation

10/11/12   2100   *Trach care performed. Suctioned for mod amt of thick white mucus. Inner cannula partially obstructed with sm amt thick white mucus. Tolerated without c/o discomfort or fatigue. Writes "can breath better" after procedure completed.* ———
—————————— *Nurse's signature and credentials*

Skill 28-9 Maintaining Chest Tubes

Assessment Steps

1. Verify the physician's order for level of suction in the chest drainage system.

2. Assess for an emergency situation if chest tubes are being inserted at the bedside. Enlist the help of other staff members *to help you gather and assemble all equipment as quickly as possible.*

Planning Steps

1. Gather needed equipment and supplies: chest tube with insertion tray, drainage system, sterile water, connectors, petroleum jelly (Vaseline) gauze dressings, split drain sponges, abdominal dressing pad, padded Kelly clamps; sterile gloves, masks, gowns, and goggles as needed.

2. Organize your equipment. Set up the suction and water seal per order *to have the drainage system ready when the tube is attached.*

Intervention Steps

1. Follow the Initial Implementation Steps located on the inside front cover.

2. Assist the physician as required by opening packages, handing items, and pouring solutions. Reassure the patient during the procedure.

3. Once the tube is in place, attach it to the drainage system and remove the padded Kelly clamp.

4. Apply Vaseline gauze dressing around the chest tube site, sealing any area where an air leak could occur. Cover the Vaseline gauze with drain sponges and abdominal dressing pads (ABDs). Tape the dressing area completely *to help prevent air from entering the chest cavity.*

5. Tape all connections thoroughly, taping away from the patient first, then back toward the patient. Attach the chest tube to the patient with a loop of tape *to prevent tension on the insertion site as you tape the connections.*

6. Turn on suction as ordered until gentle bubbling is noted, if it is a wet suction system.

7. Place drainage system securely on the floor and arrange the tubing so that there are no kinks or downward loops *so drainage can flow by gravity to the collection chamber.*

8. Maintain the drainage system in an upright position below the level of the chest at all times *to prevent the water seal or suction fluids from being disturbed.*

9. Frequently assess the tubes for kinks or loops, and the drainage in the tubing for clots, *which could cause increased negative pressure in the chest cavity. Safety: If clots are blocking the tubing, follow facility policy and physician's orders. Do NOT milk or strip the tubes unless you are specifically ordered to do so.*

Skill 28-9 (continued)

10. Ensure that Vaseline gauze and 4×4s are at the bedside in case of air leakage or other emergency. Follow facility policy for appropriate action to take if the chest tube is dislodged.

11. Assess output in the collection chamber. Be aware of the color and amount draining each hour.
    Safety: Notify the physician immediately if the drainage changes to a bright red color or is greater than 100 mL/hr.

12. Assess for air leaks in the drainage system. Remember that wet suction will bubble gently in the suction chamber. If the patient has a pneumothorax, expect to see air in the water-seal chamber as well as tidaling in the chamber. As the pneumothorax resolves and the lung reinflates, the air in the water-seal chamber and the tidaling in the chamber will cease.

13. Mark output for your shift on the writable surface of the collection chamber. Mark the level of the output, then write the date, time, and your initials. Calculate drainage output for your shift by subtracting the amount in the drainage chamber when you started your shift from the amount in the chamber at the end of your shift.

14. Assist the patient to a comfortable position and reassure him or her regarding the chest tubes. Encourage the patient to change position, cough, and deep breathe every 2 hours *to help re-expand the lung and remove drainage from the chest cavity.*

15. Follow the Ending Implementation Steps located on the inside back cover.

Evaluation Steps

1. Evaluate the effectiveness of the chest tubes. Is the patient breathing with less difficulty? Is the suction set correctly? Is the water seal at 2 cm of water? Are there signs of escaping pneumothorax? Are there any signs of additional air leaks?

2. Evaluate the patient's response to the procedure. Is the patient resting comfortably? Is pain medication needed for the incision site? Is the patient complaining of any other problems?

3. Evaluate the insertion site dressings. If there is a hemothorax, is the dressing dry and intact? Does it need to be reinforced or changed? Follow facility policy for changing the dressing to the chest tube insertion site.

Sample Documentation

10/12/12   1825   Dr. Chapman inserted one chest tube for hemothorax. Attached to Pleuravac drainage system with wet suction at −20 cm. Water seal established with 2 cm water. Chest tube draining mod amt of dark red fluid, less than 100 mL/hr. All connections double-taped. Drsg at insertion site clean, dry, and intact. Resting quietly in bed in semi-Fowler's position eating ice chips. States he "can breathe better" after chest tube insertion. Requests pain med for incisional pain. ————————
————————— *Nurse's signature and credentials*

🌐 Post Conference

You were really worried when you walked into your patient's room the first morning and saw him with his tracheostomy, sounding all bubbly and coughing frequently. He pointed to the tracheostomy and mouthed the word "suction." Without much time to think, you grabbed a suction catheter and glove kit and set up quickly but without contaminating your sterile field or sterile supplies. You remembered as you suctioned to hold your own breath and not suction for longer than 10 seconds. It was obvious to you that the suctioning procedure tired your patient and made him a little short of breath. However, once you had suctioned his tracheostomy several times, he could breath considerably better and mouthed "thank you." After that, you weren't afraid to suction him. His tracheostomy collar stayed in place pretty well, and you were able to clean his inner cannula the first day with your instructor's guidance. By the second day, you were feeling far more confident about all of his care. By the third day of clinicals, you were showing other students how to suction him.

KEY POINTS

- Muscles, nerves, and chemicals all play a role in causing and controlling respirations.

- Impaired oxygenation may be due to hypoxia or hypoxemia caused by airway obstruction, secretions in the alveoli, chronic lung disease, and trauma.

- Respiratory assessment of the patient with impaired oxygenation must be very thorough to avoid missing subtle signs of hypoxia or hypoxemia.

- Crepitus indicates air under the skin, or subcutaneous emphysema, and the source of leaking air must be found and treated.

- Diagnostic tests for which you will obtain specimens include sputum testing and throat cultures.

- Patients with impaired oxygen need to expand the lungs fully, which can be accomplished by turning, coughing, and deep breathing; use of an incentive spirometer; and nebulizer treatments with bronchodilators.

- Supplemental oxygen is available from different sources and with a variety of delivery devices. All require use of stringent safety precautions to prevent fire.

- The patient with chronic lung disease needs to conserve energy and preserve accessory muscles for breathing.

- Artificial airways vary from small plastic devices inserted in the mouth to tubes inserted through the nose, mouth, or an incision into the trachea.

- When caring for patients with artificial airways, you will suction to keep them patent. For tracheostomies, you will remove the inner cannula to clean or replace it.

- Chest tubes are inserted to re-establish intrathoracic pressure, remove air and drainage, and reinflate the lung.

- Chest tube drainage systems generally have three chambers: one for suction, one to create a water seal, and one to collect drainage.

- You are responsible for marking output for your shift, keeping the drainage unit upright and below the level of the chest, and keeping the tubing free from kinks and loops.

- You must know how to troubleshoot air leaks and what to do if the chest tube accidentally comes out or becomes disconnected from the closed drainage system.

REVIEW QUESTIONS

Select the answer that is most appropriate for each of the following questions. Some questions may have more than one correct answer. Check all that apply.

1. Which is (are) true of chemical regulation of respirations?

   a. Chemoreceptors are located in the carotid and aorta and the brain.

   b. The cerebellum is responsible for brain control of respirations.

   c. The chemoreceptors in the brain cause an increase in the rate and depth of respirations in response to changes in blood pH.

   d. If the carbon dioxide level is higher than normal in the blood, the blood becomes more acidic and the pH falls below 7.35.

   e. If the oxygen level in the blood falls, this provides the stimulus to breathe in people who do not have chronic lung disease.

   f. Chemoreceptors in the carotid and aorta respond to decreased oxygen in the blood and send the message to the medulla.

2. A patient who has chronic lung disease is stimulated to breathe because the chemoreceptors detect:

   a. low oxygen in the blood.

   b. high oxygen in the blood.

   c. low carbon dioxide in the blood.

   d. high carbon dioxide in the blood.

3. You are caring for a patient who has lung disease. Yesterday, the patient was pleasant and cooperative. Today, the patient is irritable, restless, and a little confused. She is also complaining of a headache. What concerns you the most about this situation?

   a. The patient's complaint of headache. Along with her other symptoms, it could indicate an impending stroke.

   b. All of the symptoms concern you because they could all be signs of early hypoxia.

   c. The confusion concerns you the most because it could indicate the beginning of Alzheimer's disease.

   d. None of these symptoms concerns you greatly because the patient is probably just having a bad day.

4. You listen to the patient's lungs and hear adventitious breath sounds bilaterally. You note a frequent productive cough of thick yellow sputum. Which other assessments will you quickly make?

a. Perform pulse oximetry to determine SaO_2.

b. Assess color of the lips, nailbeds, and mucous membranes.

c. Assess respiratory rate, character, and quality.

d. Palpate for crepitus.

e. Determine how much fluid intake the patient has had in the past 24 hours.

5. Incentive spirometry is used to:

a. deliver moisture and medication deep into the lungs.

b. help prevent pneumonia and atelectasis.

c. measure the rate and amount of air in a forceful exhalation.

d. help the patient conserve energy when performing ADLs.

6. Your patient has a blood pH of 7.48 and is on oxygen at 8 L/min. Which oxygen delivery device is best for this patient?

a. A simple face mask

b. A Venturi mask

c. A partial rebreathing mask

d. A face tent

SHORT ANSWER QUESTIONS

7. The physician asks for a stat pulse oximetry reading on a patient wearing dark nail polish. What will you do?

8. When you look at the arterial blood gas results on your patient, you see that his pH is 7.32. What condition does this patient have?

CRITICAL THINKING EXERCISES

9. Your patient had a chest tube inserted yesterday to drain a hemothorax and has been doing well. Suddenly the patient becomes restless and agitated, and respirations become more labored. When you take vital signs, you find the BP has dropped to 96/60, pulse is up to 110, and respirations are increased to 26 per minute. What will you do next?

10. Your patient with a tracheostomy is on a ventilator. His neck looks swollen this morning and it has not been that way previously. What are your concerns?

ADDITIONAL RESOURCES

For additional Resources, Questions, and Activities, please see:

 Student Resource Disk

DavisPlus **http://davisplus.fadavis.com**

 Student Study Guide

REFERENCES

Beattie S. Drawing blood for ABGs. *RN* [serial online]. 2006;April 1. Available at: http://www.modernmedicine.com/modernmedicine/Acute+Care+Focus/Drawing-blood-for-ABGs/ArticleStandard/Article/detail/315021.

Editors of *Nursing2008.* Photo Guide: Monitoring your adult patient with bedside pulse oximetry. *Nursing 2008.* 2008;38(9):42-44.

Halpin AP, Bunting JM, Selecky PA, Bosveld SG, Hong D. Nursing assessment for predicting obstructive sleep apnea: community hospital approach. *Topics Adv Pract Nurs eJournal* [serial online]. Feb 15, 2008;8(1). Available at: http://www.medscape.com/viewarticle/568404.

Hoch DB. Cerebral hypoxia. 2008. Available at: http://www.nlm.nih.gov/medlineplus/ency/article/001435.htm. Accessed October 16, 2009.

Lasater M. When a pulse ox reading doesn't tell the whole story. *RN* [serial online]. 2006;July 1. Available at: http://www.modernmedicine.com/modernmedicine/Consult+Stat/When-a-pulse-ox-reading-doesnt-tell-the-whole-story/ArticleStandard/Article/detail/339914.

Mancini MC. Hemothorax: follow-up. 2008. Available at: http://emedicine.medscape.com/article/425518-followup. Accessed October 16, 2009.

Regan EN, Dallachiesa L. How to care for a patient with a tracheostomy. *Nursing2009.* 2009;39(8):34-39.

Roman M, Mercado D. Review of chest tube use. *MedSurg Nurs.* 2006;15:41.

Rushing J. Clinical do's & don'ts: Managing a water-seal chest drainage unit. *Nursing2007.* 2007;37(12):37.

Scanlon V, Sanders T. *Essentials of Anatomy and Physiology.* Philadelphia: FA Davis; 2007.

Smyth M. Critical care extra: Acute respiratory failure: Part 1. Failure in oxygenation: when a patient loses the ability to oxygenate the blood. *Am J Nurs.* 2005;105(5):72GG-72OO.

University of Pittsburgh Medical Center. Chest tube insertion and care. October 2007. Available at: http://www.upmc.com/HealthAtoZ/patienteducation/Documents/Chesttubes.pdf.

Venes D, ed. *Taber's Cyclopedic Medical Dictionary.* 21st ed. Philadelphia: FA Davis; 2009.

Wilkinson JM, Van Leuven K. *Fundamentals of Nursing: Theory, Concepts, and Applications.* Philadelphia: FA Davis; 2007.

Williams L, Hopper P. *Understanding Medical Surgical Nursing.* 3rd ed. Philadelphia: FA Davis; 2007.

Fluids, Electrolytes, and Acid-Base Balance

Key Terms

Acidosis

Aldosterone

Alkalosis

Antidiuretic hormone (ADH)

Ascites

Bicarbonate

Buffer

Dehydration

Diffusion

Extracellular fluid (ECF)

Filtration

Fluid volume deficit

Interstitial space

Intracellular fluid (ICF)

Intravascular space

Osmosis

pH

Third-spacing

Objectives

1. Define key terms associated with fluids, electrolytes, and acid-base balance.
2. Describe the functions, distribution, and regulation of body fluids.
3. List normal ranges of electrolytes.
4. Identify important dietary sources of electrolytes.
5. Explain primary functions of key electrolytes.
6. Identify normal and imbalanced pH.
7. Describe the role of buffer systems in acid-base balance.
8. Identify primary causes of fluid, electrolyte, and acid-base imbalances.
9. Identify key assessment findings of fluid, electrolyte, and acid-base imbalances.
10. Explain nursing care for fluid, electrolyte, and acid-base imbalances.
11. Restate key areas of concern for fluid, electrolyte, and acid-base imbalances.

🌐 Clinical Connection

Your Assignment: You have been assigned the care of a patient admitted to the hospital with hyperkalemia. She has been in the intensive care unit and had repeated Kayexalate enemas. You will be caring for her on the first day on the nursing unit after being moved out of intensive care. This seems a bit frightening to you, because you are unsure what symptoms will indicate that she is having a problem with hyperkalemia again. In fact, you are not exactly sure what hyperkalemia is. You know that she has been seriously ill and is on telemetry, so you think it must have something to do with her heart.

Your Actions: Before you care for this patient, you decide to do some serious research. You determine that hyperkalemia is an electrolyte imbalance, and you remember that you never did understand electrolytes very well in your anatomy and physiology class. It all seems confusing to you. And you aren't sure if those Kayexalate enemas were to bring down a level that was too high or bring up a level that was too low. You decide to spend some time reading about electrolyte imbalances. You want to find out how to assess this patient for worsening symptoms, and what the blood levels should be now. You also want to know about foods she should or shouldn't eat to prevent further imbalances. You want to find out why she is on telemetry and what could happen with her heart rhythm.

Oxygen is your body's number one requirement to sustain life, with food, water, and physical safety following it in close order. In this chapter you will learn why water is the second most critical substance for sustaining life. You will learn that, wherever you find water within the body, you will also find substances called *electrolytes*. You will also learn about the forces and processes that regulate the movement of water and electrolytes, as well as the role they play in maintenance of the body's acid-base balance. Then you will learn how to apply this information to care for patients who have disturbances of acid-base or fluid and electrolyte balance.

Water

Water normally accounts for 50% to 70% of the body's total weight and serves as the liquid in which the body's solid components are dissolved. Age affects the percentage of water that comprises total body weight. For example:

- **Adult males:** 60% to 65%
- **Adult females:** 55% to 60%
- **Older adults:** 50% to 55%
- **Children:** 50% to 55%
- **Full-term infant:** 65% to 70%
- **Premature infant:** 65% to 80%

Within the body, the lungs are composed of approximately 90% water while the brain is 70% water. Each individual's blood is 80% to 83% water. The body has such a high requirement for water that fluid losses can interfere with homeostasis and impair certain bodily functions to such an extent that an individual can only survive a few days without water intake.

Knowledge Connection
What percentage of body weight is made by water in the following age groups: Newborns? Adult male? Older adult female? Teenager? Adult female? What is the most important to survival, water or food?

Distribution and Movement of Body Fluids

Body fluids reside in one of two water compartments: intracellular space and extracellular space. In healthy patients, approximately two-thirds of body fluids reside inside of the individual cells, which are individual living units that require their own water, nutrients, and oxygen. Cells comprise the water compartment that holds **intracellular fluid (ICF)**. The other one-third of the body's fluid is located in the compartments outside the cells; this fluid is known as **extracellular fluid (ECF)**.

The extracellular compartment is further divided into two main spaces: the interstitial space and the intravascular space. The **interstitial space** is that space surrounding and between cells, which holds fluid known as either tissue fluid or interstitial fluid. Lymph fluid is also considered to be part of the interstitial fluid. The **intravascular space** includes the blood vessels and the heart and holds the plasma. ECF also includes the cerebrospinal fluid surrounding and cushioning the brain and spinal cord, specialized fluids such as aqueous humor within the eye chambers, and synovial fluid that lubricates joints. However, because these fluids constitute such a small percentage of the ECF, we do not include them when we are discussing fluid and electrolyte balance.

Even though fluids are distributed within the interstitial space and the intravascular space, they are never static. Fluids are continually moving across membranes to other compartments in an effort to maintain equilibrium between the compartments. This movement of fluid is controlled by several processes, including osmosis, diffusion, and filtration, all of which are partially related to fluid volume. The volume of fluid is directly affected by the amount of water ingested and absorbed from the gastrointestinal (GI) tract.

Fluid volumes are very closely related to the concentration of the molecule sodium chloride, also know as *table salt*. If individuals take in or retain too much sodium chloride, they will also retain excess water. Water will travel back and forth between ICF spaces and ECF spaces dependent upon where there is more sodium chloride. One way to think of it is *where sodium goes, water follows*. That is why, after eating a large bag of buttered, salted popcorn, you find yourself thirsty and drinking lots of liquids.

The fluid inside cells is called the *cytoplasmic matrix* and contains about 70% water. The concentration of certain elements inside of cells is much higher than that outside of cells. The electrolyte potassium and protein molecules are found in much higher concentrations inside of cells than outside of cells, whereas sodium, chloride, and bicarbonate normally occur in higher concentrations outside.

Knowledge Connection
Which water compartment contains approximately two-thirds of the body's water content? What are the two subdivisions within extracellular compartment? How much of the fluid inside each cell is made up of water? What follows sodium?

Osmosis
The membranes that form the various fluid compartments include the vessel walls that hold the blood within the vasculature and the cellular membranes that contain the cell's contents. These membranes are described as *semipermeable*, which means that they allow passage of certain substances, but not all.

Body fluids consist of a water-based *solvent* and various particles of *solute*, substances that will dissolve in the solvent. The number of solutes present in the solvent determines the fluid's *osmolality* or concentration. When a difference in osmolality exists in the fluid on two sides of a semipermeable membrane, the body's homeostatic mechanisms kick into action in an attempt to balance those differences.

Osmosis is the process in which water moves through a semipermeable membrane from the side where the fluid is lowest in solute concentration to the side where the fluid is highest in solute concentration (Fig. 29-1). The goal of osmosis is to balance out the two fluid concentrations until they are equal on both sides of the membrane. This could be the difference between the concentration of the blood within a capillary and the concentration of the interstitial fluid outside of the capillary in the interstitial space, or it could be the difference between the concentration of the cellular fluid and the concentration of the interstitial fluid on the other side of the cell membrane.

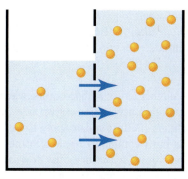

Figure 29-1   Osmosis is the movement of water across a semipermeable membrane from the less concentrated solution to the more concentrated solution. The purpose is to dilute the more concentrated solution to equal that of the lesser concentrated solution.

Knowledge Connection
Which does osmosis move: water or solute?

To envision this process, picture a clear container that is divided down the middle by a semipermeable membrane that will allow water to pass through but not solute. On each side of the membrane, there are 8 ounces of water. You pour 4 ounces of table salt into the water in the right side, but only add 1 ounce of salt to the water in the left side. Now the fluid on the right side has a great deal more solute, making it much more concentrated than the water on the left side. The difference in the solute content would cause the less dense water on the left side to permeate through the membrane into the right side until the two concentrations were equalized on both sides. *Osmotic pressure* is the amount of power that is exerted by the concentration of solutes, such as sodium chloride, which works to prevent water from moving out of the specific compartment. Because the osmotic pressure of the fluid on the right side is greater due to the higher concentration of solutes, it prevents the water from flowing out from the right to the left side. This same increased concentration of solutes draws or pulls the water through the semipermeable membrane (osmosis) in an attempt to effect dilution of the right side.

Blood plasma is the liquid portion of the blood that remains after removing the blood cells; it is approximately 90% water and normally contains plasma proteins that are too large to pass through the semipermeable capillary walls. An important function of the primary plasma protein albumin is to assist in the maintenance of fluid balance within the intravascular spaces. Albumin works similarly to solutes, such as electrolytes, in that the higher the concentration of albumin, the greater the osmotic pressure in that particular compartment. When we are referring to the osmotic pressure exerted by and related to the albumin level of the blood plasma, it is termed the *oncotic pressure*.

When there is an increased concentration of waste components excreted into a patient's urine, such as glucose or contrast dye, the increased osmotic pressure will draw an extra volume of water to go with it to be eliminated. This is known as *osmotic diuresis.* Box 29-1 presents an example of an osmotic diuretic.

Diffusion

Diffusion is another process that occurs when there is a difference in solute concentration on two sides of a semipermeable membrane. Diffusion can apply to either solute or solvent, but is most commonly applied to the solute particles; **diffusion** allows a substance to flow over naturally from an area of higher concentration into an area of lower concentration (Fig. 29-2).

To envision this process, think about what happens when you pour a colored powdered substance, such as a flavored drink mix colored red, into a clear pitcher of water. The colored particles initially group in a small, bright red, dense pile on top of the water before sinking into the water, making an area of intense bright red just below the water's surface. Then as the particles continue to seep toward the bottom of the pitcher, they begin to spread out to the areas where there are no red particles, coloring the water as they go. Eventually, as the drink mix particles spread evenly throughout the water, the water becomes a lighter, evenly colored red liquid.

An example of how diffusion is utilized in the body would be the exchange of oxygen and carbon dioxide. When you inhale room air into your lungs, it fills the alveoli with air concentrated with oxygen. The capillary that surrounds each alveolus carries venous blood, from which most of the oxygen has been depleted as it was used by the cells in the body, as well as a high concentration of carbon dioxide, the waste product that is left over after oxidation within the tissues. That makes a higher concentration of oxygen molecules on the alveolar side of the alveolar-capillary membrane than there is on the capillary side. Plus, it makes the concentration of carbon dioxide higher on the capillary side of the alveolar-capillary membrane than on the alveolar side. The more highly concentrated oxygen molecules within the alveoli diffuse across the alveolar-capillary membrane into the capillary blood, where they can bind with hemoglobin and be transported to the cells all over the body. The more highly concentrated carbon dioxide molecules within

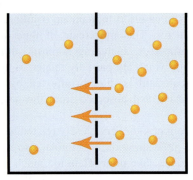

Figure 29-2 Diffusion is the movement of solute across a semipermeable membrane from an area of higher solute concentration to the area of lower solute concentration.

the capillaries diffuse across the alveolar-capillary membrane into the lungs, where they can be exhaled from the body.

Knowledge Connection

Which does diffusion most commonly move, water or solutes? Compare the differences in osmosis and diffusion.

Filtration

Filtration is the passage of fluid through a partial barrier separating the fluid from certain particles that are too large to pass through the semipermeable membrane. One place where filtration occurs is between the intravascular and interstitial spaces, where fluid movement is affected by *hydrostatic pressure,* the force the volume of fluid exerts against the capillary walls. When the fluid volume within the intravascular space increases, so does the hydrostatic pressure. Each time the heart beats, more blood is pumped out of the left ventricle into the systemic circulation, which increases the pressure the blood physically exerts against the walls of the vessels. This pumping action of the heart forces the increased hydrostatic pressure through the arteries, through the arterioles, and into the capillaries, forcing fluid and electrolytes through the capillary walls into the interstitial space, but not allowing larger molecules such as albumin to leave the intravascular space. The end result is the filtration of fluid from the intravascular space into the interstitial space, which if excessive results in edema.

Movement of Absorbed Water From the Gastrointestinal Tract

When you drink a glass of water, the water you swallow passes through the esophagus and into the stomach. The bloodstream absorbs some of the water from the stomach and small intestine, but most is not absorbed until it reaches the large intestine. Approximately 80% of the volume of water entering the first section of the large intestine, the *cecum,* is absorbed there. The water molecules must cross through the intestinal wall and capillary wall to enter the bloodstream.

Box 29-1

Mannitol: An Osmotic Diuretic

A highly concentrated sugar alcohol called *mannitol* is sometimes administered intravenously to patients suffering with increased intracranial pressure, which if poorly controlled can result in brain damage. The purpose of the mannitol is to cause *osmotic diuresis,* which means to increase the osmolality of the blood so that water will be pulled from the interstitial spaces into the intravascular space, where it can then be eliminated by the kidneys. This will lower the fluid content within the brain and thereby reduce the intracranial pressure.

Once the water has entered the bloodstream, it becomes part of the plasma and is circulated throughout the vasculature until reaching the capillary beds, where semipermeable capillary walls allow passage of necessary fluid, required nutrients, and oxygen from the intravascular to the interstitial spaces. This is the same place where carbon dioxide and other waste products are diffused from the interstitial fluid across the capillary wall into the bloodstream to be carried away and removed from the body. Hydrostatic pressure pushes plasma out of the vascular space and across the capillary wall, into the interstitial space where the fluid is now known as interstitial fluid or *tissue fluid,* which differs from plasma because it does not contain blood cells as does the plasma. This fluid normally moves in and out of the vascular space to maintain a balance. Waste products from the cells travel via the interstitial fluid into the bloodstream to the kidneys, where the waste products can be filtered out into the urine.

Dependent upon the concentration of solute and the degree of osmosis, the fluid in the interstitial space may or may not be moved across another membrane, the cell membrane, into the cell's intracellular space. If the concentration of solute is higher inside the cell than outside, osmosis will cause fluid to move from the interstitial spaces across cell membranes into the cells to dilute the higher concentration of solutes and maintain a balance of fluids and electrolytes. This can result in swelling of cells if too much water is moved inside the cells. If the concentration of solute is higher outside the cells in the interstitial spaces, osmosis will cause water to move from the intracellular space across the cell membrane into the interstitial spaces to attempt to dilute the solute concentration, resulting in edema.

The movement of fluid also occurs in the opposite direction as intracellular fluid is drawn from the cell through the cell membrane into the interstitial space, and then once again into the intravascular space inside the capillaries. These movements of fluid are effected by various pressure processes, including the hydrostatic pressure from blood pressure and osmotic pressures from solute dissolved in fluid. The goal of all the fluid movement back and forth between water compartments is to maintain constant *relative* proportions of fluid and solutes. This means that, if the water is balanced on both sides of a semipermeable membrane, then the electrolytes are also balanced, known as *fluid and electrolyte homeostasis.*

Abnormal Movement of Fluids

When, for some reason, the body is unable to maintain fluid and electrolyte balance, normal fluid-moving processes are impaired. One of the possible results of this imbalance is **third-spacing** of fluids, meaning the fluids are shifted to areas where they can no longer contribute to fluid and electrolyte balance between ICF and ECF. The fluids are still within the body but they are unavailable for normal use. For example, when excessive fluid has moved into the interstitial space, such as you might have with severe congestive heart failure, edema results. Another example includes liver diseases that result in increased blood pressure in the *portal circulation,* or the circulation that supplies the liver with blood. The fluid is forced out of the circulation and into the peritoneal cavity, where it is no longer available for use by the body. The diseased liver fails to produce adequate levels of protein to maintain oncotic pressure within the blood plasma, allowing excessive volumes of fluid to leave the intravascular space and move to the interstitial space. This third-spacing of fluid results in edema and **ascites,** a large collection of fluid within the peritoneal cavity. The effects of third-spacing include the following:

- Lowering the volume of the blood, thereby lowering the blood pressure
- Increasing the volume of fluid in the interstitial spaces, thereby possibly causing excessive edema, which can result in compression of nerve endings, capillaries, and cells
- Lowering the solute concentration of the interstitial fluid, thereby causing excessive amounts of water to move into the cells, resulting in overhydration and possible rupture of the cells, better known as *cellular death*

Knowledge Connection
What are three effects of third-spacing?

Functions of Water in the Body

Water is required by the body for various functions, including the following:

- **Maintaining temperature:** Water helps to maintain body temperature, whether warm or cold. Because it takes longer for the temperature of liquid to change than it does for solid matter, the body's water protects from extreme changes. For example, when you step out of a warm house into a blizzard, your body fluids help to preserve heat. When the body is overheating, evaporation of fluid from sweat and from breathing will keep the body cool. Of course, there are limitations to this ability. Water can only help the body to preserve heat for a certain length of time, depending upon factors such as the clothing a person is wearing. Also, water's ability to cool the body can deteriorate when the body becomes dehydrated after large amounts of sweat are lost and not replenished. When patients are dehydrated, they can lose the ability to regulate their own temperature.
- **Transporting electrolytes, minerals, vitamins, and waste products:** Water transports electrolytes such as sodium and potassium, minerals such as zinc and copper, and vitamins such as vitamin C and the B-complex vitamins to all the individual cells throughout the body. Water also serves to transport waste products from the cells to the blood so that they can be eliminated in the urine.
- **Protecting the brain and spinal cord:** Water, as a component of spinal fluid, acts as a cushion for organs such as the brain and spinal cord, protecting these organs from damage from outside forces.

• **Lubricating the joints and digestive tract:** As one component of synovial fluid, water helps to lubricate joints such as the knees and elbows, reducing friction and allowing for smoother movement. It also provides for the smooth passage of food through the digestive tract, from the mouth through the large intestine.

Knowledge Connection

Explain four functions of water in the body.

Regulation of Body Fluids

The most important factor determining water intake is thirst. The hypothalamus in the brain receives information from *osmoreceptors,* which are receptors that are able to detect when there is an elevated concentration of solutes in the blood, increasing the blood's *osmolality,* or plasma concentration. Increased osmolality results in low fluid levels. When the hypothalamus detects these conditions, it stimulates thirst. However, if there is too much fluid or if there is a problem with the osmoreceptors, the body will not stimulate thirst.

Water Intake

As you learned in Chapter 23, the average adult needs to consume somewhere between 1,440 and 1,920 mL of water per day. Depending upon lifestyle and activity, some individuals may need larger water intakes, such as pregnant or nursing women, those individuals who work or exert in extremely hot environments, and athletes. The body can also make 100 to 300 mL of water per day from hydrogen (H^+) and oxygen (O_2).

Body Composition

Fatty tissue contains less water than muscular tissue, allowing one's body composition and size to influence the volume of water carried by the body. Men, typically more muscular than women, tend to have a higher percentage of body weight due to water. Obese individuals and elders, who commonly have lost much of their muscle mass, have a lower percentage of body fluid than that of the younger and more lean individuals.

Hormonal Regulation

Several hormones work to keep fluid in the body and to produce an appropriate volume of urine output. Antidiuretic hormone (ADH) and aldosterone both work on the kidneys to decrease urine production and increase body fluid level. Atrial natriuretic factor (ANF) causes the kidneys to excrete more urine to decrease the body fluid level.

Antidiuretic Hormone

The hypothalamus produces antidiuretic hormone, also known as *vasopressin,* which is stored in the posterior pituitary gland to be released as needed. When the osmoreceptors that are located within the hypothalamus are able to detect increased osmolality of the blood, the hypothalamus stimulates the posterior pituitary to release more ADH.

Antidiuretic hormone directs the kidney tubules to increase water reabsorption independently of solids, which helps to dilute the concentration of the blood. This suppression of volume of urine production results in a more concentrated urine. Therefore, ADH probably plays the most significant role in determining whether the urine that is excreted is dilute or concentrated.

Aldosterone

When kidney *baroreceptors* (Box 29-2) sense a low blood volume flowing through the kidneys, the kidneys release an enzyme known as *renin.* Renin begins a cascade of enzyme-induced conversions, the end product of which stimulates the adrenal cortex to produce its primary mineralocorticoid called aldosterone. **Aldosterone** regulates fluid and electrolyte balance by stimulating the kidneys to retain more sodium and excrete potassium. By increasing the amount of sodium that is reabsorbed, the water reabsorption naturally increases. Remember *where sodium goes, water follows.* This retention of water increases the blood volume and raises blood pressure. Figure 29-3 presents a more detailed description of this cascade of conversions.

Atrial Natriuretic Factor

When baroreceptors in the vena cava and atrial chambers of the heart detect that there is too much pressure, meaning that there is excessive blood volume, the atrium produces atrial natriuretic factor (ANF). This hormone inhibits renal secretion of renin, interfering with the cascade of hormones that increases sodium and water retention by the kidneys. The kidneys proceed to excrete more sodium, and this increase in sodium causes more fluid to be lost. The end result is increased urinary production and a decrease in the level of body fluids, which also lowers the blood pressure.

Normal Fluid Losses

The most obvious ways in which the body loses fluid is through elimination of urine and feces. Fluid losses through excretion of urine are controlled by ADH, aldosterone, and the extent of insensible fluid loss. *Insensible fluid loss* is that which cannot be directly measured, such as fluid lost during respiration and perspiration. Normal fluid loss for healthy

---

BOX 29-2

Baroreceptors

A baroreceptor is a sensory nerve ending that detects, or is stimulated by, changes in pressure due to the blood volume. Another term for baroreceptor is *pressoreceptor.* These receptors are located in the atrial walls of the heart and in the inferior and superior venae cavae, as well as in the aorta and the carotid sinus located at the base of the internal carotid artery. When pressure changes are detected, the baroreceptors send a message to the central nervous system to either increase or decrease arterial diameter and increase or decrease heart rate.

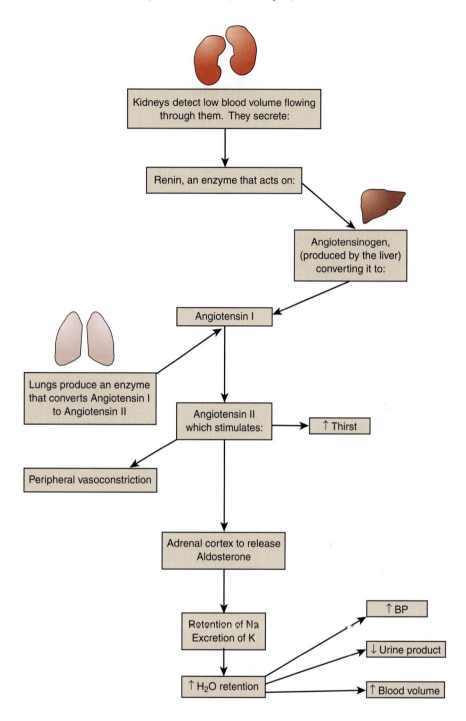

Figure 29-3 Renin-angiotensin-aldosterone system.

patients varies from about 1 to 3 L/day, depending on fluid intake (Table 29-1).

Fluid Volume Disturbances

Determining the type of fluid volume disturbance is not a simple measurement of just the fluid lost or gained. It must be determined if the patient has lost both water and electrolytes, or has lost more fluid than electrolytes, or has experienced an increase in both fluids and electrolytes or in body fluid only.

Fluid Volume Deficit

A true **fluid volume deficit**, also known as *hypovolemia*, only results when there is an equal loss of both fluid and

Table 29-1 Estimates of Adult Fluid Loss and Gain per 24 Hours

Loss or Gain	Fluid Source	Volume
Loss	Urine	1,200–2,100 mL
	Diuretics can cause loss up to:	*6,000 mL*
Loss	Insensible respirations	200–300 mL
Loss	Gastrointestinal tract	100–200 mL
	Vomiting can cause loss up to:	*6,000 mL*
Loss	Insensible perspiration	400–600 mL
	If environmental temperatures are high enough, can cause loss up to:	*1,000 mL/hr*
Gain	Water production through metabolism of ingested food	100–300 mL
Gain	Oral liquids	1,000–2,000 mL
Gain	Water in food	800–900 mL

the electrolytes contained in that fluid. The water-to-solute ratio in the body must remain balanced even though there is a loss, as would be the case when an individual hemorrhages. With blood loss, there is equal loss of water as well as solid components of the blood, such as electrolytes, protein, red blood cells, white blood cells, and thrombocytes. If there is loss of fluid only, resulting in the increase of electrolyte concentrations in the remaining body fluid, it is called **dehydration**. It is pertinent that you are able to detect the differences as they require different treatments. We will cover dehydration later with the electrolyte disturbances.

Causes of fluid volume deficit can be related to prolonged insufficient fluid intake or loss of fluid. There are some patients who experience a lack of thirst, called *adipsia*. This is a common problem for elderly individuals who lose their sense of thirst over time. This can also occur for patients with brain injuries. Young children, dependent upon others to provide them with fluids, can develop a fluid

volume deficit if they go without fluids for a prolonged time. Extreme nausea, even though there is no vomiting, may prevent someone from drinking fluids for several days.

Another source of fluid deficit might be abnormal fluid losses. Losses can be due to bleeding, prolonged tachypnea, excessive sweating, fever, diarrhea, vomiting, or excessive urination due to diuresis. Severe depletion of fluid volume can also occur in hot climates or with extreme amounts of exertion or exercise. It is important to understand that fluid volume deficit can occur in varying degrees of seriousness based on the degree of loss, ranging from mild to life threatening.

Knowledge Connection
What is the difference between fluid volume depletion and dehydration? What causes fluid volume depletion?

People and Places Connection
Fluid Intake in Elders
Seniors, whether living independently or with caregivers at home or living in a long-term care facility, are at high risk for dehydration. Many seniors experience a declining sense of thirst due to changes in the brain. When this occurs, either the senior or the caregiver will need to ensure that the senior is drinking water, even when not feeling thirsty. The recommended amount of fluid intake per day is about 1,800 mL, or 2 quarts. Alcohol and dietary supplements are less hydrating than water. Some liquids such as coffee and tea can also have a diuretic effect.

Elderly patients with cardiac or kidney disease, however, may be placed on a fluid restriction. These seniors will need to monitor how much fluid their physician or nurse practitioner has prescribed for them to take daily, monitor their daily weight, and watch for increased or decreased amount of urine production.

Assessment and Diagnostic Findings
It is important that you assess the patient who might be at risk for fluid volume deficit as well as the patient who has already been diagnosed with the problem. Box 29-3 provides a list of signs and symptoms that may be indicative of fluid volume deficit. Diagnostic test results supporting fluid volume deficit may include the following:

• Urine specific gravity is high or concentrated.
• Hemoglobin and hematocrit, due to the increased concentration, may appear to be elevated, or in the case of hemorrhage may actually be decreased. *Note: It may take a while for the test values to drop in response to hemorrhage.*
• Blood urea nitrogen (BUN) may appear to be elevated due to the increased concentration.
• Electrolytes may be within normal ranges if losses have been equal.

Box 29-3

Signs and Symptoms of Fluid Volume Deficit

Be alert for signs and symptoms that may indicate the presence of or risk for developing fluid volume deficit. Be especially vigilant when monitoring infants, children, and older adults, who are at increased risk of fluid imbalances.

- Patient reports of little or no fluid intake or urine output
- Patient reports of significant number of occurrences of vomiting or diarrhea
- Flushed, pale, hot, dry skin with nonelastic turgor (nonelastic turgor is a very late sign)
- Complaints of thirst or nausea
- Dry, cracked tongue and lips
- Elevated heart rate
- Weak pulse
- Fever
- Low blood pressure
- In young children, soft feel of eye globe when gently palpated through the eyelid or eye globe sunken into the face
- In newborns, sunken or depressed fontanels
- Decreased level of consciousness (severe fluid volume deficit)
- Confusion (severe fluid volume deficit)

Knowledge Connection

List at least six signs and symptoms of fluid volume depletion. Explain how volume depletion affects urine specific gravity and hemoglobin results.

Treatment and Nursing Care

Cautious fluid and electrolyte replacement is a priority. Infusion of IV fluids with appropriate electrolytes is the primary treatment. However, rapid infusion of IV fluids can result in electrolyte imbalance and place stress on the heart and kidneys. Oral fluids, including electrolyte fluids, may also be ordered if the patient is able to keep them down without vomiting or diarrhea. However, a patient may not be able to absorb fluid through the GI tract with extreme fluid volume deficit. In this case, only IV fluids will be administered.

If the source of loss is from the GI tract, antiemetic medications may be ordered for nausea or vomiting, or antidiarrheal medication for loose stools. Once the patient is able to tolerate oral fluids, a clear liquid diet advanced as tolerated is generally ordered.

Monitor vital signs for low blood pressure, elevated pulse rate, and elevated temperature. Measure and monitor intake and output for balance. Normally, the output total should be equal to or within 300 to 500 mL of the total intake. So in a patient with fluid volume deficit, the urinary output will *initially* be absent or less than the intake, but should gradually increase as the patient becomes more hydrated. Persistent urinary output below 30 mL/hr may be indicative of renal failure if the deficit was severe and prolonged.

Make certain each patient voids at least every 8 hours and notify the physician if a patient fails to void. Continue to assess for further losses by observing for profuse diaphoresis, measuring volume of emesis and liquid stools.

Even though a patient who has fluid volume deficit needs fluids, if the IV fluids are infused rapidly, it is possible to cause fluid volume excess, or overload. Monitor all patients who receive IV fluids for signs and symptoms of fluid volume excess, including auscultation of breath sounds, noting adventitious sounds, to ensure that the patient is not developing signs of fluid overload. Also monitor for rapid increase of blood pressure, increased pulse volume, and tachypnea. Observe for dyspnea and cough.

Assess the patient's oral mucous membranes for dryness and provide mouth care as needed. If oral fluids are not allowed, the physician may order ice chips as long as the patient is not vomiting.

Knowledge Connection

What assessments should be made for possible or actual fluid volume depletion? What diagnostic tests would be ordered? What is the primary treatment for this problem? What is the danger of infusing IV fluids too rapidly?

Fluid Volume Excess

Most fluid volume excess, also known as *hypervolemia,* is caused by retention of sodium and water in the ECF spaces. This may be due to intake of dietary sodium, administration of IV fluids containing sodium, or the retention of sodium or fluid as a result of medication or kidney, heart, or liver diseases. The result is the same for all these causes: decreased urinary output and expansion of fluid volume within the intravascular and interstitial spaces.

In rare cases a patient may develop excessive thirst, or *polydipsia,* related to various medical conditions such as diabetes mellitus, diabetes insipidus, or mental illness. This can result in ingestion of tremendous volumes of fluid, even several thousand milliliters. Retention of fluids may occur due to the poor pumping mechanism of congestive heart failure that reduces cardiac output and kidney perfusion. Renal failure with decreased glomerular filtration rate can result in inadequate excretion of urine.

Infants, small children, frail elders, and patients with congestive heart failure or renal failure are more susceptible to fluid overload than the average adult patient. Fluids administered orally or intravenously may place the patient in fluid overload and cause serious problems if the health care provider is not alert to the signs and symptoms of fluid overload.

What is generally the etiology of a fluid volume excess? What type of patients are considered more susceptible to fluid overload problems?

Assessment and Diagnostic Findings

For patients at risk for or with a known diagnosis of fluid volume excess, assess the renal and digestive systems as well as the respiratory and cardiovascular systems (Box 29-4). Diagnostic test results supporting fluid volume excess may include:

- Low hemoglobin or hematocrit due to hemodilution
- Low urine specific gravity due to dilution
- Fluid or pleural effusion noted on chest x-ray
- Low partial pressure of oxygen in arterial blood (PaO_2) in arterial blood gases (ABGs)
- Decreased BUN due to hemodilution
- Decreased sodium or other electrolytes due to hemodilution

Knowledge Connection
Name at least eight signs and symptoms of fluid volume excess. What diagnostic test results might support this diagnosis?

Box 29-4

Possible Assessment Findings Related to Fluid Volume Excess

Signs and symptoms of fluid volume excess may appear suddenly. Assess the potential of each patient receiving IV fluids for medical history or current conditions to identify if the patient might be at risk for fluid volume excess. Monitor intake and output, auscultate breath sounds, and evaluate vital signs of all patients receiving IV fluids.

- Increased respiratory rate, shortness of breath with exertion, or labored respirations
- Sudden onset of coughing
- Jugular vein distention
- Increased blood pressure, pulse pressure, or central venous pressure
- Full, bounding pulse
- Edema of extremities or dependent areas, such as sacrum
- Auscultation of rales or wheezes, and muffled or distant heart sounds
- Weight gain
- Increased urine production in an attempt to rid body of excess fluid
- Pink or frothy sputum
- Decreased oxygen saturation level
- Anxiety or fear that is unexplainable by the patient
- Ascites (distention of the abdomen due to fluid collection in the peritoneal cavity)

Treatment and Nursing Care

You should carefully monitor intake and output for both acutely and chronically ill patients who have been diagnosed with fluid volume excess or are at risk for the disorder, including those receiving tube feedings and those who have IV fluids infusing. Administer ordered diuretics and monitor for effectiveness. Assess daily weights at the same time of the day, preferably before breakfast, using the same scales and with the patient wearing the same type of garment.

A low-sodium diet may be ordered to restrict dietary intake of sodium, or the patient may be instructed to avoid adding salt to food. Monitor meal trays to ensure there are no extra salt packets or high-sodium foods. If the physician has ordered fluid restriction, determine the volume of fluid allowed on each shift and monitor it closely. Post the volume of fluids allowed for each shift above the patient's bed or on a marker board to serve as a reminder for patient, family, and staff. Collaborate with the dietary service to limit fluids sent on meal trays. Provide patient and family teaching to ensure understanding and cooperation with intake and output, documentation, and ingestion of sodium and fluids.

Assess vital signs, including the oxygen saturation by pulse oximetry (SpO_2), every 4 hours unless severity requires more frequent assessment. Monitor for elevated blood pressure, increased pulse rate and volume, and elevated temperature. Auscultate breath sounds and heart sounds at least every 4 hours, noting adventitious, decreased, or absent breath sounds and muffling of S_1 and S_2. Assess the extremities and dependent body sites for edema. Monitor urine output every 2 to 3 hours, or evenly hourly if inadequate urine excretion is suspected. A continuous indwelling Foley catheter must be in place if you need to monitor hourly output. Monitor laboratory and x-ray results as previously mentioned.

It is usually necessary for the physician to order one or more diuretics. Some diuretics such as furosemide, a loop diuretic, are known to deplete the serum level of potassium, making it necessary that you monitor the laboratory results for changes in potassium level. If the potassium level drops below normal, supplemental potassium will have to be administered. If the patient has respiratory difficulties, supplemental oxygen can be ordered. Severely impaired renal function that does not respond to diuretics and standard treatment may require dialysis to remove the waste products along with the excess sodium and fluid.

Knowledge Connection
Describe the basic assessments you should make when fluid volume excess is suspected or diagnosed. What nursing interventions would be appropriate for fluid volume excess?

Furosemide

Many patients are prescribed diuretics to assist with elimination of excess fluids. Patients often call these drugs their "water pills." Some types of diuretics, such as osmotic diuretics cause the patient to lose potassium and sodium. Furosemide (Lasix), a common osmotic diuretic, can also cause magnesium and calcium losses. Because hypokalemia is common when patients take daily furosemide, the physician may also prescribe extra dietary potassium or potassium supplements. According to the Institute of Medicine (IOM), adequate intake of potassium for adults is 4,700 mg/day. Most patients will take 20 milliequivalents (mEq), equal to about 1,500 mg/day (10 mEq is equal to 750 mg), and receive the rest of their potassium intake through their diet.

Teach your patients taking furosemide to follow up for their blood work as ordered. It is very important that electrolyte levels be checked regularly. Encourage them to eat foods high in potassium, such as bananas, which provide about 500 mg each. Other foods high in potassium include yellow and orange fruits such as oranges and apricots, avocados, baked potatoes, sweet potatoes, yogurt, white beans, and halibut.

Electrolytes

Electrolytes are chemical substances that, when dissolved in water, release either their positive or negative electrically charged particles, called *ions*, which are capable of conducting electrical current. An *anion* is a negatively charged ion such as chloride (Cl^-). A *cation* is a positively charged ion such as sodium (Na^+) or potassium (K^+).

Electrolytes play various roles, including helping to transmit electrical impulses through nerve and muscle fibers and assisting to maintain balance between the ICF and ECF compartments. Table 29-2 presents the normal ranges, functions, and sources of the various electrolytes.

Sodium

Sodium (Na^+) is the most abundant cation in the ECF compartments, including the blood, with the serum level ranging from 135 to 145 mEq/L. It is also the primary electrolyte involved in determining ECF volumes and controlling the osmolality of the fluids, which in turn controls fluid distribution throughout the body. Sodium also stimulates conduction of electrical impulses, thereby helping to maintain the neuromuscular irritability that is required for skeletal and heart muscles to function. Even certain medications work to increase either fluid excretion or fluid retention by causing sodium to move across cellular membranes and capillary walls (see Table 29-2).

In the blood, sodium in measured in milliequivalents (mEq); in food, it is measured in milligrams (mg). The American Heart Association recommends that healthy adults consume no more than 2,300 mg/day. This is about 1 teaspoon of table salt, or sodium chloride. *Safety: For those individuals falling within the following population groups,*

Table 29-2   Electrolyte Ranges, Functions, Regulation, and Nutritional Sources

Electrolyte, Cation or Anion	Location in Body	Normal Blood Range	Regulation of Blood Level	Functions	Sources for Intake
Sodium (Na^+) Cation	ECF*	135–145 mEq/L Changes in direct proportion to Cl^-	Regulated by ADH and aldosterone Reabsorbed and excreted by kidneys Requires active transport to cross cell membranes	Controls fluid osmolality and volume of blood Stimulates conduction of electrical impulses along nerves Works with calcium to regulate muscle contraction	Salt: most individuals obtain 90%–94% from packaged, processed foods, including bacon, ham, canned vegetables, soy sauce, steak sauces, other sauces, salad dressings, processed cheeses, sandwich meats, salty snacks such as chips, jerky, pretzels, canned soups, broths Adding table salt to prepared foods

(table continues on page 656)

Table 29-2 Electrolyte Ranges, Functions, Regulation, and Nutritional Sources (continued)

Electrolyte, Cation or Anion	Location in Body	Normal Blood Range	Regulation of Blood Level	Functions	Sources for Intake
Chloride (Cl⁻) Anion	ECF* (mostly interstitial compartment) Part of HCl in gastric juices	98–106 mEq/L Changes in direct proportion to sodium Has inverse relationship with bicarbonate	Reabsorbed and excreted by kidneys Regulated by ADH and aldosterone Low level of potassium will lower Cl⁻ level	Assists sodium in regulating fluid osmolality and volume Important for acid-base balance Production of gastric HCl	High-sodium-content foods listed above Lettuce, tomatoes, celery, olives, seaweed
Potassium (K⁺) Cation	98% ICF* 2% ECF	3.5–5.0 mEq/L	Diuretics cause loss GI disturbances cause loss Reabsorbed and excreted by kidneys Regulated by aldosterone	98% in ICF helps regulate fluid balance 2% in ECF is important for neuromuscular functions, *especially for the heart's contractility and rhythm*	Dried fruits, tomatoes, potatoes, spinach and other leafy greens, oranges, bananas, cantaloupe, red meat, chicken, fish, nuts, soy products
Magnesium (Mg²⁺) Cation	99% bones & ICF (2nd most abundant ICF cation) 1% ECF	1.5–2.5 mEq/L	Amount present in diet Malabsorptive conditions Small bowel resection Excreted by kidneys Low albumin level decreases Mg²⁺	Assists neuromuscular function; dilation of arteries and arterioles; enzyme function; carbohydrate and protein metabolism	Leafy green vegetables, whole grains, beans, fish (halibut), almonds, soybeans
Bicarbonate (HCO₃⁻) Anion	ICF and ECF Kidneys excrete and reabsorb it	22–26 mEq/L Has inverse relationship with Cl⁻	Reabsorbed and excreted by kidneys Diuretics cause loss Renal disease causes loss GI disturbances cause loss	Primary buffer for acid-base balance	Primary dietary source: baking soda Produced by body

Table 29-2   **Electrolyte Ranges, Functions, Regulation, and Nutritional Sources** (continued)

Electrolyte, Cation or Anion	Location in Body	Normal Blood Range	Regulation of Blood Level	Functions	Sources for Intake
Calcium (Ca^{2+}) Cation	99% bones and teeth (ICF) 1% ECF Half of this 1% being *ionized* Ca^{2+} and half being *protein-bound*	*Total Ca^{2+}*: 9.0–10.5 mg/dL *Ionized Ca^{2}*: 4.5–5.1 mg/dL	Combines with phosphorus in bones and teeth Inversely proportional with phosphorus Vitamin D Calcitonin lowers blood level Parathyroid hormone raises blood level	Strengthen skeletal bones and teeth *Ionized Ca*: stimulates conduction of electrical impulses via nerves, which controls muscle contraction and relaxation, includes heart muscle Initiates enzyme action Cellular membrane permeability	Dairy products, green vegetables, shellfish, salmon, dried beans
Phosphorus (PO_4^{3-}) Anion	Located in every cell of the body	2.5–4.5 mg/dL May be higher in children	Combines with phosphorus in bones and teeth Inversely proportional to calcium Parathyroid hormone	Vital for all tissues; muscle and red blood cell functions; metabolism of fat, protein, carbohydrates; manufacturing ATP energy source	Meats, fish, egg yolks, dairy products, nuts, beans, legumes, whole grains, soft drinks

Note: An asterisk (*) indicates the most abundant cation and anion found in the intracellular and extracellular compartments.

it is recommended they should consume no more than 1,500 mg/day:

- *Individuals with hypertension*
- *Individuals who are 40 years of age or older*
- *African Americans*

Sodium Imbalances: Deficiency and Excess

Hyponatremia occurs when the serum level of sodium falls below normal. This can be caused by decreased sodium intake, a loss of body fluids containing sodium, or an excessive intake of water that does not contain sodium, which is known to result in *dilutional hyponatremia*. As sodium levels in the extracellular compartments decrease to a lower level than that which is inside the cell, an imbalance develops. In an attempt to equalize the sodium concentration on both sides of the semipermeable membrane, water is pulled into the cells to dilute the sodium concentration to the same concentration as that on the outside of the cells. This results in swelling of the cells and causes potassium to be shifted out of the cells.

Safety: Dilutional hyponatremia can be inadvertently caused by medical health care providers by administration of multiple tap-water enemas, repeated irrigation of nasogastric tubes with tap or distilled water, and infusion of excessive sodium-free IV fluids. A patient can also develop dilutional hyponatremia due to compulsive drinking of abnormally high volumes of tap water, usually attributed to mental illness.

Hypernatremia is the condition of a higher-than-normal concentration of sodium in the blood, which can lead to death if not corrected. Most sodium excesses are caused by eating too much sodium chloride, or salt. Most individuals think of sodium intake as "only that salt they have sprinkled on their food." However, that is not the case, as there is significant sodium found in canned and processed foods. Even some prescription and over-the-counter medications contain sodium in the form of sodium bicarbonate.

Sometimes hypernatremia is caused by severe dehydration that decreases the solvent (water) level without decreasing the sodium level. Thus, the same number of sodium ions in a smaller volume of water simply increases the concentration of the sodium, disrupting the normal fluid and electrolyte balance. As discussed earlier in the chapter, the various imbalances impair the normal functions of the specific electrolyte that is out of balance. Hypernatremia causes fluid to shift from the cells to the interstitial spaces, which causes the cells to dehydrate. The dehydrated cells are then unable to function optimally, ultimately affecting the function of every body system. Signs and symptoms of sodium imbalances are listed in Table 29-3.

Treatment and Nursing Care

Correction of a patient's sodium imbalance must be done slowly and carefully to prevent further damage. Trying to correct sodium levels too rapidly can lead to further swelling or shrinking of cells, especially brain cells.

Table 29-3 Electrolyte Imbalances

Electrolyte Imbalance and Name	Signs and Symptoms	Causative Factors
Sodium		
Deficit: hyponatremia	Anorexia, nausea, vomiting, headache, lethargy, muscle weakness or twitching, nonelastic skin turgor, tremors, seizures, swelling of optic nerve	GI suctioning, vomiting, diarrhea, ↑ blood sugar, congestive heart failure, renal disease, adrenal insufficiency, oxytocin, excessive infusion of D5W IV fluid, disease known as SIADH, administration of more than one tap-water enema, excessive diaphoresis
Excess: hypernatremia	Thirst, ↑ T, sticky mucous membranes, dry mouth, flushed skin, lethargy, restlessness, oliguria, ↑ irritability, hallucinations, seizures; pulmonary edema	Diabetes insipidus; heat stroke; watery diarrhea; ingestion of excessive corticosteroids, sodium chloride, or bicarbonate
Chloride		
Deficit: hypochloremia	Signs of hypokalemia and metabolic alkalosis: ↑ muscle excitability, tetany, ↓ R, shallow R, agitation, irritability, seizures, coma	↓ intake of Cl⁻ or Na⁺ such as sodium-restricted diet; potassium deficiency, excessive diaphoresis, diarrhea, vomiting, diuretics, gastric suctioning, congestive heart failure, IV fluids without Cl⁻, Addison's disease, metabolic alkalosis
Excess: hyperchloremia	Signs of metabolic acidosis, hyperkalemia, and hypernatremia: ↑ R rate and depth, dyspnea, ↑ P, ↓ cardiac output, arrhythmias, weakness, severe edema, ↓ LOC and coma	↑ Na⁺ serum level, respiratory alkalosis, hyperparathyroidism, severe diarrhea, sodium retention caused by head trauma & ↑ intracranial pressure, renal failure, salicylate overdose, corticosteroid use, diuretic use, dehydration, metabolic acidosis, administration of Kayexalate
Potassium		
Deficit: hypokalemia	Weak, rapid, or irregular P, ↓ BP, anorexia, nausea, vomiting, ↓ deep tendon reflexes, fatigue, muscular weakness and cramps, numbness, abdominal distention, ↓ peristalsis, ileus	Diarrhea; gastric suctioning; vomiting; bulimia; starvation; diuresis due to osmotic diuretics; digoxin toxicity; administration of carbenicillin, corticosteroids, and amphotericin B

Table 29-3 **Electrolyte Imbalances** (continued)

Electrolyte Imbalance and Name	Signs and Symptoms	Causative Factors
Excess: hyperkalemia	Bradycardia and other arrhythmias, nausea, intestinal cramping, diarrhea, anxiety, muscle weakness, numbness or prickly sensations, flaccid paralysis	Renal failure, ketoacidosis, large burns, excessive use of K^+-sparing diuretics, too-rapid IV administration of K^+, severe dehydration _Safety: Both severe deficit or excess can result in life-threatening arrhythmias._
Magnesium		
Deficit: hypomagnesemia	Vomiting, anorexia, insomnia, arrhythmias, mood swings and hyperirritability, dizziness, ↑ neuromuscular irritability, muscle weakness and tremors, positive Chvostek's and Trousseau's signs	Starvation, malabsorption disorders, ketoacidosis, alcoholism and alcohol withdrawal, administration of gentamicin, hyperparathyroidism, vomiting
Excess: hypermagnesemia	↓ BP, ↑ P, ↓ R, hypoactive reflexes, muscle weakness and paralysis, drowsiness, lethargy, flushing, diaphoresis, cardiac arrest, death	Late renal failure, adrenal insufficiency, excessive administration of IV Mg^{2+} or oral antacids
Calcium		
Deficit: hypocalcemia	Muscle cramps and tremors; tetany; ↓ BP; tingling or numbness of fingers, toes, around the mouth; bronchospasm; carpopedal spasms; ↑ deep tendon reflexes; prolonged Q-T interval on EKG; positive Chvostek's and Trousseau's signs	Inadequate vitamin D consumption, malabsorption disorders, pancreatitis, peritonitis, alkalosis, hypothyroidism or hypoparathyroidism
Excess: hypercalcemia	Severe constipation, anorexia, nausea, vomiting, polydipsia, lethargy, fatigue, headache, polyuria, ↓ deep tendon reflexes, muscular weakness, bone fractures without trauma, confusion, slurred speech, psychosis, ileus development	Prolonged bedrest, excessive ingestion of calcium or vitamin D supplements, excessive serum level of digitalis, cancer, metabolic acidosis
Phosphorus		
Deficit: hypophosphatemia	Muscle weakness, bone pain, paresthesia of extremities and around the mouth, stuttering, chest pain, confusion, irregular P, ↑ susceptibility to infection, respiratory failure	↓ K^+ or ↓ Mg^{2+} serum level, vomiting, diarrhea, hyperventilation, burns, hyperparathyroidism, bone disease, diabetic ketoacidosis, alcoholism and alcohol withdrawal, bowel disorders, poor dietary intake
Excess: hyperphosphatemia	↑ P, tetany, anorexia, nausea, tingling of fingers and toes, irritability, carpopedal spasms, ↑ deep tendon reflexes, muscle twitching, tetany, seizures, ↓ cardiac output, coma	Renal failure, excessive intake of vitamin D or phosphorus, fluid volume depletion, conditions causing breakdown of large amounts of tissue

Treatment for hyponatremia involves the administration of additional sodium, either orally, via nasogastric tube, or intravenously. Mild hyponatremia is often remedied with consumption of foods with high sodium content. If the patient is unable to absorb fluids via the digestive tract, the physician will probably order an isotonic IV fluid such as 0.9% sodium chloride or lactated Ringer's solution. You will need to assess vital signs, noting hypotension and increased pulse rate or weakening pulse volume. Monitor intake and output, evaluating balance. If the patient has orthostatic hypotension, assist with ambulation to prevent injury or falls. Always use normal saline 0.9% for nasogastric tube irrigations. If a physician orders tap-water enemas, restrict the number of enemas to one. If more than one is required, such as bowel preparation for a procedure or surgery, consult with the physician regarding use of normal saline to prevent electrolyte problems.

If hyponatremia is severe, assess the patient for signs and symptoms of increased intracranial pressure (Box 29-5). An extreme case of hyponatremia may require infusion of a hypertonic IV solution, such as 3% or 5% sodium chloride, to pull the excess water from the brain. These hypertonic IV fluids are rarely used in general medical-surgical settings due to the fact that they require constant, stringent observation throughout infusion. *Safety: Infusion of hypertonic IV solutions requires extremely close monitoring and generally is carried out in an intensive care unit.* For information regarding tonicity of IV fluids, see Chapter 38. These patients may also require supplemental oxygen and antiseizure medications.

For the patient with hypernatremia, monitor intake and output to be certain the excess fluid begins to be eliminated.

Box 29-5
Signs and Symptoms of Increased Intracranial Pressure

The earlier the signs and symptoms are detected, the better the patient's chance of escaping brain damage and permanent neurological deficits. Observe for even subtle changes in level of consciousness.

Early Sign
• Changes in level of consciousness (LOC)*

Late Signs
• Rising systolic blood pressure to hypertensive levels**
• Widening pulse pressure**
• Decreasing pulse rate to bradycardia**
• Pupillary changes
• Impaired body temperature control by the hypothalamus

---

* Decreases in LOC may be very subtle, such as decreased attentiveness or mild drowsiness, or obvious, such as profound unresponsiveness. Changes in LOC are also exhibited as excitement, from subtle signs of increasing nervousness, anxiety, or agitation to strong unexplained anger or outbursts and erratic body movements.

** When seen together, these three signs are known as Cushing's triad.

Monitor vital signs for elevated blood pressure and bounding pulse. It is important to teach patients to monitor their dietary sodium intake in an effort to prevent future problems. They should be encouraged to read labels carefully, limit salty snacks, eat fresh foods that have not been cured by salts, and ask about low-salt alternatives when dining out.

Chloride

Chloride (Cl^-) accounts for approximately two-thirds of the body's anions and is commonly bound with sodium or potassium ions. It shares a direct relationship with sodium and an inverse relationship with bicarbonate. The majority of chloride is bound to sodium in dietary sources as well as in the body, and is usually consumed in the form of table salt. Much of the remaining chloride is bound to potassium in the form of potassium chloride.

Chloride is found in interstitial fluid, lymph fluid, sweat, and gastric and pancreatic digestive juices, with lesser amounts in the blood. Chloride combines with hydrogen to form hydrochloric acid in the gastric juices of the stomach, which is used to break down foods. Other functions of chloride include regulating the osmolality of the ECF and assisting in maintaining the body's acid-base balance. The daily dietary requirement of chloride for adults is 2,300 mg/day. The primary route of excretion is through the kidneys, while a small amount is lost in the feces (see Table 29-2).

Chloride Imbalance: Deficiency and Excess

Chloride is nearly always chemically bonded to another electrolyte in the body. As a result, chloride imbalances are most commonly seen in combination with other electrolyte imbalances, such as hyponatremia or hypernatremia, with similar signs and symptoms, and caused by the same factors. A below-normal serum level of chloride is known as *hypochloremia*. When the chloride level continues to drop, the kidneys attempt to balance the loss by conserving sodium and bicarbonate, which may result in an increased bicarbonate level in the ECF. This raises the pH and leads to metabolic alkalosis, which you will read more about later in this chapter.

Hyperchloremia describes a serum chloride level above normal and its occurrence is rare except when it accompanies metabolic acidosis. Because it is so directly related to the sodium level, it may be associated with hypernatremia, as well as bicarbonate loss due to the inverse relationship. Its association with metabolic acidosis that is usually due to renal or gastric loss of bicarbonate, which increases reabsorption of chloride that forms acidifying salts. As the level of acidified salts increases and bicarbonate continues to decrease, metabolic acidosis is the result (see Table 29-3).

Treatment and Nursing Care

Dependent upon the severity of hypochloremia, treatment to restore the chloride level to normal may range from an increase in dietary sodium chloride to infusion of IV fluids, such as 0.9% sodium chloride or 0.45% sodium chloride. (See Table 29-2 for a list of foods high in sodium chloride.) If the patient has been receiving a diuretic, the physician will determine whether to change it to a different diuretic or to discontinue it. It will be important that you monitor intake and output. If the patient routinely drinks water without electrolytes or bottled water, the physician may restrict the patient from drinking it.

Fluid loss through vomiting or diarrhea must also be measured to monitor appropriate replacement. High and low levels of chloride can change the acid-base balance of the body and cause serious neurological and respiratory changes, so these conditions must be managed carefully.

When hyperchloremia is associated with metabolic acidosis, the primary treatment is to correct the acidosis by administering diuretics to lower blood levels of chloride. It may be necessary to administer IV sodium bicarbonate to help raise the serum (blood) level of bicarbonate and decrease the acidity. For mild hyperchloremia, lactated Ringer's solution is administered because it converts to bicarbonate in the liver. This serves to increase the base bicarbonate level, which helps to correct acidosis. It is important to monitor the patient's intake and output and laboratory results.

Potassium

Potassium (K^+) is represented by the letter "K" because of its ancient name, Kalium. It is the most abundant cation in the ICF. Potassium functions in transmission of nerve impulses and muscle contraction. It assists in building proteins and muscles as well as in the breakdown of carbohydrates. It contributes to the osmolarity of body fluids, therefore playing a major role in keeping fluids inside of cells.

Although 3.5 to 5.0 mEq/L is considered to be the normal serum range for potassium, some physicians prefer to keep the serum potassium above 4.0 mEq/L in patients with heart problems to reduce risk of arrhythmias. The IOM reports that most people who follow a typical Western diet take in the minimum amount of potassium, but do not eat enough to stay in optimum health. The IOM is now supporting the idea that a dietary intake of 4.7 g/day may decrease long-term health problems (see Table 29-2).

Potassium Imbalances: Deficiency and Excess

Hypokalemia is defined as a potassium level that is below normal range, and *hyperkalemia* is an elevated level. Hypokalemia can cause muscle weakness and *tetany,* or severe muscle spasms. More importantly, because potassium is a key electrolyte in controlling nerve transmission of the electrical impulses that cause the heart to contract, both low and high levels of potassium can affect the heart rhythm and cause life-threatening arrhythmias.

In patients with renal failure, the kidney functions become impaired and the kidneys do a poor job of filtering out the excess potassium, which raises the serum potassium level. (See Table 29-3 for further information regarding potassium imbalances.)

Treatment and Nursing Care

In patients with hypokalemia, low levels of serum potassium can be increased with supplemental potassium chloride (KCl) as oral tablets, liquids, powders, or IV formulations. A patient who routinely takes medications such as furosemide, a diuretic that increases excretion of sodium, potassium, and water volume in the form of increased urination, is likely to take a daily oral dose of potassium in order to prevent hypokalemia from occurring. It is your responsibility to monitor the serum potassium levels of all your patients, but especially be mindful of the serum potassium levels in a patient who:

- Is vomiting or having diarrhea
- Has a nasogastric tube to suction
- Is suffering from malnutrition or dehydration
- Is taking osmotic diuretics
- Has renal disease

Hyperkalemia must be treated to prevent problems. In some cases a patient may require emergency treatment for a dangerously elevated level of potassium. This may include administration of medications such as sodium polystyrene sulfonate (Kayexalate), which binds with potassium and stimulates potassium elimination through stools. For treatment of hyperkalemia in patients with impaired renal function, it is common to restrict the dietary intake of potassium-rich foods such as potatoes.

In severe hyperkalemia, it may also be necessary to administer IV glucose and insulin, to help drive potassium back into the cells. *Safety: KCl is never administered by IV push or intramuscularly. Because of a high potential for death associated with IV potassium, most institutions require that it be mixed into a diluted IV solution by the pharmacy and then be double-checked by the nurse before it is administered to the patient.* It should be administered over several hours at the preferred rate of 10 to 20 mEq/hr. The infusion rate should never exceed 40 to 60 mEq/hr. *Safety: When KCl is added to a 1,000-mL bag of solution, the KCl will concentrate at the bottom of the bag of IV solution. Agitate the solution well before infusing.*

Real-World Connection

The Dangers of Potassium Chloride

Potassium chloride is a dangerous drug—so dangerous, in fact, that in some states it is used for death-by-injection death penalties—which is why it is so very important to be careful when administrating it to a patient. The following story illustrates just how careful you should be:

A student nurse on a medical-surgical clinical was administering medications. One of the patients was scheduled to receive a daily dose of potassium chloride (KCl) via the IV route. After the student read the order, she interpreted the order to mean IV push, which means to inject the drug directly into the IV line over a couple of minutes, rather than to dilute the KCl in a 1,000-mL bag of IV solution and infuse it over several hours. The student administered the KCl via direct IV push. The concentrated dose of KCl interrupted the electrical conduction in the patient's heart. The patient arrested and died.

This tragic but true event could have been prevented by using basic safety measures. Always make certain you are familiar with any medication you are going to administer, no matter what it is: over-the-counter or prescription, narcotic or vitamin supplement, or an electrolyte. If you are not familiar with the specific medication, look it up in your drug reference book, always. *Safety: When administering an electrolyte in less than 1,000 mL of fluid via the IV route, a second nurse should be asked to double-check and confirm the prepared medication, route, and rate of administration prior to administration.*

Calcium

Calcium (Ca^{2+}) is the most common mineral in our bodies; 99% of it is combined with phosphorus and located in the bones and teeth, with the remaining 1% located outside the skeletal system in the blood. This 1%, known as the *total serum calcium level,* easily and rapidly exchanges back and forth between the blood and bone. The serum calcium level is controlled by calcitonin, excreted by the thyroid gland, and parathyroid hormone (PTH), excreted by the parathyroid glands. When the serum calcium level becomes low, PTH is excreted, which causes release of calcium from the skeletal system into the blood to maintain adequate serum level. When the serum level of calcium elevates above normal, the thyroid excretes calcitonin, which acts to increase resorption of calcium from the blood into bone, lowering the serum level.

Approximately half of the total serum calcium is ionized, meaning that it is physiologically active for use in various body functions. Ionized calcium helps control the permeability of cellular membranes and assists with blood coagulation. Ionized calcium stimulates transmission of electrical impulses along nerve pathways, including the electrical conduction pathways of the heart that control contraction and relaxation of the heart. This control of electrical impulse conduction regulates contraction and relaxation of muscles throughout the body as well. Initiation of various essential chemical processes depends on ionized calcium to activate the appropriate enzymes. The remaining half of the serum ionized calcium is bound with protein, mostly with albumin. Use care to differentiate between the total serum calcium and the ionized calcium values when you review laboratory results in the medical record. Normal ranges for total serum calcium should be twice as high as those for ionized calcium (see Table 29-2).

It is estimated that we need 1,200 mg of calcium each day. Children require higher levels due to the rapid metabolism of calcium by their growing bones. Because vitamin D is required for the absorption of calcium from the GI tract, individuals who consume enough calcium but are not getting adequate vitamin D may not be absorbing their dietary calcium. Individuals who do not normally expose their skin to the sun are at high risk for vitamin D deficiency. Less calcium is absorbed from the GI tract and an increased level of calcium is excreted by the kidneys as we continue to age.

Calcium Imbalances: Deficiency and Excess

Hypocalcemia is defined as having lower-than-normal serum calcium. It is common with diseases that cause poor digestive absorption, such as anorexia or inflammatory bowel disease. Because calcium is necessary for adequate blood clotting and control of excitable tissues, hypocalcemia may increase bleeding and result in cardiac arrhythmias. Chronic low calcium levels can cause loss of bone and high blood pressure.

You may recall that weight-bearing exercise increases bone strength due to stimulating serum calcium to be deposited into the skeletal system. The opposite occurs when a patient remains on bedrest for extended periods of time. The lack of weight-bearing exercise increases the rate of resorption, removing more calcium from the bones and absorbing it back into the bloodstream. This can result in an excessive serum calcium level known as *hypercalcemia,* which can affect the electrical rhythm of the heart. Chronic high levels of calcium can contribute to kidney stones, which are often undetected until the patient complains of severe flank pain (see Table 29-3).

A disease known as *osteoporosis* causes a higher level of calcium resorption than the level being deposited in the bones. *Resorption* is the process of removing calcium from the bones and absorbing it back into the bloodstream. The higher level of resorption leaves the bone structure weakened, with tiny holes or gaps within the bone, giving it a honeycomb appearance. Because of their weakened structure, the affected bones are easily fractured, sometimes without a stimulus such as a fall.

For example, a patient may present for treatment reporting that he or she fell. Upon examination, a femur fracture is identified. Your first thought may be that the fall caused the fracture, which is normally the case. However, a patient with severe osteoporosis may experience a fracture without trauma, which then causes the individual to fall because the broken bone is no longer able to bear the person's weight. This is known as a *pathological fracture.* It is important to remember that, even though a patient has a healthy serum calcium level, he or she may have a severe deficit of total body calcium.

Treatment and Nursing Care

Hypocalemia is treated with oral tablets or IV calcium along with vitamin D to increase gastrointestinal absorption of calcium. Certain forms of IV calcium are extremely irritating to veins and can cause serious problems if allowed to extravasate into the subcutaneous tissues. *Safety: Intravenous infusion of calcium also can cause bradycardia and death if administered too rapidly, thus making it a necessity to use a volumetric infusion pump and assess the IV site and rate of infusion every 30 to 60 minutes.* You should keep the patient receiving IV calcium on bedrest during infusion and monitor the blood pressure for hypotension, a side effect of IV calcium.

You will need to monitor the patient with hypocalcemia for muscle twitching and tetany as well as for cardiac irregularity. You will need to assess for spasms of the facial muscles and the arms and legs, and tingling around the mouth or tips of the fingers. The patient may become disoriented and confused. Some have even been known to have hallucinations. It is common to find the patient with hypocalcemia experiencing depression. There may also be electrocardiogram changes: the lengthening of the interval between the onset of the QRS complex and the beginning of the T wave.

Patients suffering from hypocalcemia may also present with Trousseau's sign (Fig. 29-4) and Chvostek's sign (Fig. 29-5).

If hypocalcemia is due to a problem with the kidneys or the parathyroid gland, then the treatment is focused on those organs. Extreme hypocalcemia requires immediate treatment to stave off death, and may need IV administration of calcium to raise the serum level and of bisphosphonates to prevent further bone breakdown.

Treatment of severe hypercalcemia is focused on reducing the excessive calcium in the blood due to the 50% mortality rate if not resolved promptly. Encourage fluids and monitor IV infusions, if ordered, to help dilute the blood level of calcium. If IV normal saline solution is administered, it may be in conjunction with furosemide, a diuretic that increases urinary excretion of sodium and calcium. Calcitonin may also be ordered to increase calcium exchange from blood to bone, thus lowering the blood level. If the patient takes digitalis, a drug that increases the strength of cardiac contractions and slows the pulse, it will be important for you to assess for signs of digitalis toxicity as hypercalcemia *potentiates* (or magnifies) the digitalis effects. Monitor the patient for bradycardia, digestive complaints, and visual disturbances.

Figure 29-5 To check for Chvostek's sign, tap the face in front of the ear and below the zygomatic bone. Facial twitching constitutes a positive sign.

Magnesium

Like calcium, magnesium (Mg^{2+}) is also part of the bone structure. About 50% to 60% of the body's magnesium is located within bone cells, and the rest works to actively assist with the metabolic work of other cells and metabolizing ATP for energy. These include cells of the heart, vascular system, skeletal muscles, nerves, and immune system. Magnesium has a role in activating enzymes and metabolizing protein and carbohydrates. It also helps to lower blood pressure by dilating the peripheral blood vessels and reducing peripheral vascular resistance. New research shows that magnesium can help protect the heart and support the immune system. Magnesium is important for neuromuscular function and is sometimes used by patients who experience twitching and uncontrolled movements of their legs while trying to sleep. The magnesium works at the neuromuscular junctions, producing somewhat of a *sedative effect,* reducing the excitability and twitching of the muscles. It also serves to depress the central nervous system. To maintain an appropriate blood level and prevent deficiency, the Food and Drug Administration (FDA) recommends a daily intake of 400 mg magnesium (see Table 29-2).

Magnesium Imbalances: Deficiency and Excess

Hypomagnesemia refers to a blood level of magnesium that is below the normal range. It is believed that most Western diets do not contain enough magnesium. Although hypomagnesemia may not cause severe symptoms, over time it can have a negative affect on the individual's overall health. In general, low levels of magnesium will increase nervous system irritability and muscular contractility. Patients with alcoholism frequently develop hypomagnesemia along with other nutritional deficiencies. When an individual with alcoholism experiences alcohol withdrawal, treatment commonly requires IV infusion of glucose as well as other nutrients in which the patient is deficient. Administration of the glucose will cause magnesium to shift back into the cells, further

Figure 29-4   To check for Trousseau's sign, inflate a sphygmomanometer above systolic pressure. Flexion of the wrist and hand constitutes a positive sign.

worsening of the low magnesium blood level. This makes it necessary to provide either oral or IV magnesium supplementation along with the glucose and other nutrients.

A high level of magnesium, known as *hypermagnesemia,* will slow the nervous system responses, including the respiratory rate, and generally depress neuromuscular junctions. Hypermagnesemia may be caused by adrenal or thyroid gland disease, excessive magnesium-containing antacid or laxative use, and hypothermia. However, the two most common sources of excess magnesium are diabetic ketoacidosis and kidney failure. During ketoacidosis, when fat and protein are broken down for energy rather than glucose, intracellular magnesium is moved outside the cells into the intravascular spaces, raising the blood levels. When the kidneys functions are impaired, they do not remove adequate levels of magnesium from the blood, leaving a higher than normal blood level (see Table 29-3).

Treatment and Nursing Care

Both deficient and excessive levels of magnesium are closely linked to potassium and calcium imbalance. Therefore when one imbalance is present, you will want to assess for the same imbalance in the other two electrolytes, as returning magnesium levels to normal will require treatment of the imbalance of these other electrolytes. Hypomagnesemia can be treated with oral magnesium tablets if it is not too severe. With critically high levels of magnesium, IV calcium may be given and diuretic medications or dialysis may be ordered to promote excretion of magnesium. Patients with hypermagnesemia should be assessed for the use of over-the-counter antacids and laxatives containing magnesium, as well as their knowledge of other methods of maintaining bowel regularity.

Phosphorus

Phosphates are ions of the element *phosphorus,* but the two names are generally used interchangeably. Phosphate (PO_4^{3-}) is the primary intracellular anion and is essential to all body tissues, especially red blood cells and muscle cells. Phosphorus is used in the formation of adenosine triphosphate (ATP) and energy exchange by cells, and serves as part of the acid-base buffering system. Similar to magnesium, 70% to 80% of phosphorus is stored in the bones and teeth. Approximately 10% is located in nerve tissue and another 10% in muscle cells. The phosphorus level is inversely proportional to the level of calcium, which means that dropping phosphorus levels in the blood will cause calcium blood levels to rise proportionately and vice versa. A high phosphorus level causes calcium to leave the bloodstream and can cause calcium to be deposited in organs rather than the bones (see Table 29-2).

Phosphate Imbalances: Deficiency and Excess

When there is a low magnesium level or a high calcium level, you will want to assess for a low phosphorus level, known as *hypophosphatemia.* Dietary hypophosphatemia is rare, since phosphorus is abundant in the Western diet, though a diet that is deficient in vitamin D can decrease blood levels of phosphorus. A severely low level of phosphorus is dangerous for the patient and must be treated as soon as possible.

Hyperphosphatemia is the name for excessively high blood levels of phosphorus; few signs or symptoms accompany the elevation. Children generally have slightly higher levels of phosphorus than adults (see Table 29-3).

Treatment and Nursing Care

Nurses should assess for a history of malnutrition and laxative use, then educate the patient on phosphorus requirements. If phosphorus is chronically high, as with patients with chronic kidney disease, oral medications can be prescribed over a long period that will bind phosphorus. Patients may also be prescribed a low-phosphorus diet. If phosphorus is low, dietary changes or supplements may be ordered; for more severe cases, it is common to use the IV route for replacement. However, when administered via the IV route, phosphorus should not be infused any faster than 10 mEq/hr.

Bicarbonate

Bicarbonate (HCO_3^-) is a main anion of the ECF that is controlled by the kidneys. It is also present in lesser amounts in the ICF. Its normal range is 22 to 24 mEq/L. Its primary function is to serve as a buffer in regulating the acid-base balance of the blood. Because bicarbonate is an alkaline buffer, it helps to decrease acidity of the blood. Bicarbonate is not generally consumed in the diet except in minute amounts in the form of sodium bicarbonate, commonly known as baking soda. Therefore, it must be produced by the body.

Bicarbonate Imbalances: Deficiency and Excess

Because bicarbonate and chloride work together to keep an overall electrical equilibrium, a chloride imbalance can affect the bicarbonate level. Bicarbonate acts as an acid buffer, and therefore deficiencies or excesses can result in acid-base imbalance. Medical treatment and nursing care for bicarbonate imbalances are focused more on resolving the underlying problem that caused the imbalance, rather than just correcting the imbalance. Bicarbonate will be discussed more fully in the acid-base balance section of this chapter.

> *Knowledge Connection*
> Which electrolyte is the Western diet lacking? Which two electrolytes play a role in muscle contraction and relaxation? Which electrolyte can be depleted by furosemide? Which electrolyte is an acid buffer?

Acid-Base Balance

All components of the human body function together with the intent of maintaining *homeostasis,* a state of balance essential to maintain basic cellular functions and sustain life. One area of homeostasis that must be maintained is the acid-base balance of body fluids. An *acid* is a substance that can donate a hydrogen ion (H⁺), and by doing so helps to increase the hydrogen concentration of a solution, making it more acidic. A *base* or *alkaline* substance is one that can accept an H⁺ ion or donate a hydroxyl ion (OH⁻), both of which help to decrease the concentration of hydrogen ions and increase alkalinity. Acid-base balance refers to the balance of the acids and alkaline bases of body fluids. A prolonged or extreme imbalance between the two will lead to death.

pH Scale

The status of acid-base balance is determined by comparing the number of acidic free hydrogen ions (H⁺) to the number of alkaline hydroxyl ions (OH⁻) present in body fluids. The OH⁻ is simply one oxygen and one hydrogen that have bonded together. Because the H⁺ is no longer a *free* ion of hydrogen but is bonded with the oxygen ion, it is no longer an acid. A solution that is acidic contains a higher concentration of hydrogen ions than hydroxyl ions. If a solution has an equal concentration of the two ions, the solution is neutral. When the hydrogen ion concentration is less than that of the hydroxyl ions, the solution is alkaline.

The scale that is used to determine this acid-base balance is known as the *pH scale;* **pH** stands for *parts hydrogen.* The scale ranges from 0 to 14, with a pH between 0 and 6.9 being acidic, and 0 being the most acidic; 7 is neutral; and 7.1 to 14 is alkaline or base, with 14 being the most alkaline. If you look at Figure 29-6, it is easy to see that a pH below the neutral 7 has more hydrogen ions than hydroxyl ions, making it acidic. On the other end of the scale, you can discern that a pH above neutral 7 contains more hydroxyl ions than hydrogen ions, making the solution alkaline. *Safety: An individual's blood pH must stay within a very narrow range that is slightly alkaline to ensure survival: between 7.35 and 7.45.* Other body fluids each have a different pH (see Fig. 29-6).

Knowledge Connection

What do the "p" and the "H" in pH stand for? What is the normal range of pH of human blood? Explain how the pH scale works, including what happens to both components involved in pH measurement.

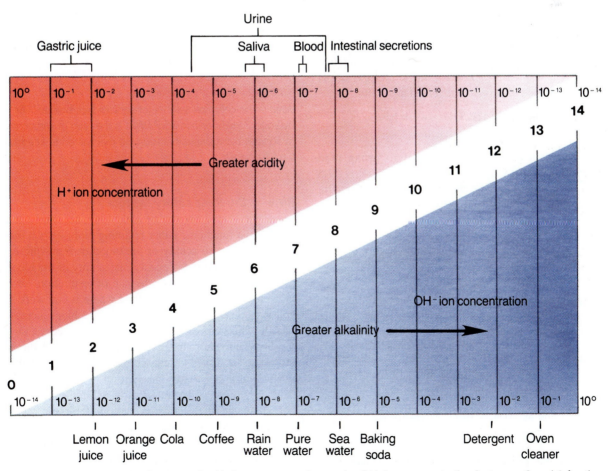

Figure 29-6 The pH scale. Compare the H⁺ ion concentration to the OH⁻ ion concentration between 0 and 1 for the most acidic pH. Then compare the H⁺ ion and OH⁻ ion concentrations between 13 and 14 for the most alkaline pH. The neutral pH of 7 shows an equal concentration of H⁺ ions and OH⁻ ions. Note the pH of various common household items indicated along the bottom edge. Then compare their pH to the pH of different body fluids indicated across the top edge.

Regulation of Acid-Base Balance

There are three basic systems that work together in the body to regulate and maintain acid-base balance. Each system does its part to compensate for alterations in pH caused when one of the three systems becomes impaired and is unable to perform its normal functions to maintain acid-base balance. The three systems include the:

- Bicarbonate buffer system
- Respiratory system—the lungs control retention and elimination of carbon dioxide (CO_2), an acid
- Renal system—the kidneys control retention and elimination of hydrogen (H), an acid, and sodium bicarbonate ($NaHCO_3$), a base

Note: *Sodium bicarbonate ($NaHCO_3$) is commonly used interchangeably with bicarbonate (HCO_3^-) when discussing blood gases, as you will notice in this chapter. It is also important to note that there are other metabolic processes and diseases, besides diseases of the kidneys, that can also impair acid-base balance.*

Bicarbonate Buffer System

A **buffer** is a substance that can bind, or form an ionic bond, with a strong acid or base to prevent large changes in the pH of body fluids. Another way to look at it is that a buffer binds with a strong acid to decrease acidity; or the buffer binds with a strong base to decrease alkalinity of the body. The bicarbonate buffer system consists of the following two chemicals that help to prevent the extreme changes in pH that cause increased acidity and increased alkalinity:

- **Sodium bicarbonate ($NaHCO_3$):** a weak base
- **Carbonic acid (H_2CO_3):** a weak acid

To maintain acid-base balance, the following ratio must be met: 1 part H_2CO_3 to 20 parts $NaHCO_3$. (Box 29-6 presents an explanation of the chemical symbols for sodium bicarbonate and carbonic acid.) Both sodium bicarbonate

---

Box 29-6

Symbol Similarity

As you may have already noticed, there is some similarity between the chemical symbol for the weak base sodium bicarbonate ($NaHCO_3$) and the symbol for the weak acid carbonic acid (H_2CO_3). Let's look at the sodium bicarbonate symbol and break it down: Na and HCO_3. You probably already know that the Na represents sodium. The remaining HCO_3 represents bicarbonate. Here is where you may have noticed the similarity. The symbol for carbonic acid, H_2CO_3, is the same as the symbol for bicarbonate, HCO_3, except that it has a "2" after the hydrogen symbol. This means that the carbonic acid has two hydrogen atoms, noted as H_2, while bicarbonate has only one hydrogen atom, noted as H. Otherwise, both symbols have the same one carbon atom, noted as C, and three oxygen atoms, noted as O_3.

---

and carbonic acid have the ability to react with another substance to create either a weaker acid or base.

Buffer and Strong Acid Produces Weaker Acid
When sodium bicarbonate, a weak base, combines with a strong acid (such as hydrochloric acid, HCl) in an attempt to reduce the acidity caused by the strong acid, it yields two chemicals that cannot maintain the previous higher level of acidity. These two chemicals are sodium chloride and a much weaker acid you are familiar with: carbonic acid. In other words, the weak base combines with a strong acid to make a weaker acid.

$$NaHCO_3 + HCl \rightarrow NaCl + H_2CO_3$$
(Sodium bicarbonate, a weak base + hydrochloric acid, a strong acid → harmless sodium chloride + carbonic acid, a weak acid)

Buffer and Strong Base Produces Weaker Base
When carbonic acid, a weak acid, combines with a strong base (such as sodium hydroxide, NaOH) in an attempt to reduce the alkalinity caused by the strong base, it yields two chemicals that cannot maintain the previous higher level of alkalinity. These two chemicals are water and a weaker base you are familiar with: sodium bicarbonate.

$$H_2CO_3 + NaOH \rightarrow H_2O + NaHCO_3$$
(carbonic acid, a weak acid + sodium hydroxide, a strong base → water + sodium bicarbonate, a weaker base)

Knowledge Connection
What is the chemical symbol for sodium bicarbonate? For hydrogen? Hydrochloric acid? What is the ratio of carbonic acid to sodium bicarbonate that must be maintained to keep acid-base balance?

Role of the Respiratory System

In relation to acid-base balance, the lungs are responsible for one of two functions: either retaining more carbon dioxide (CO_2) to increase acidity of the blood or removing excess CO_2 from the blood to decrease the acidity of the blood. To retain CO_2, the lungs slow the rate of respiration, allowing more CO_2 to remain in the blood where it can work to increase acidity. To remove excess CO_2, the lungs increase the rate of respiration so they can exhale the excess CO_2 from the body into the atmosphere. The decrease in the blood level of CO_2 serves to also decrease the acidity. This relatively simple respiratory mechanism helps to maintain the balance between acids and bases, keeping the pH within the normal range between 7.35 and 7.45. These chemical changes occur very quickly but can correct a limited variance in pH, plus the correction is somewhat short lived.

To further explain the relationship of CO_2 to the level of acidity of the blood, let's see how CO_2 becomes an acid. When the lungs are unable to exhale *all* of the CO_2 that body cells create during metabolism, excess CO_2 molecules remaining in the blood form ionic bonds with molecules of water (H_2O). Each ionic bond of CO_2 and H_2O results in formation of carbonic acid (H_2CO_3). Carbonic acid is a weak acid that can only increase acidity of the blood by releasing free hydrogen (H^+) ions. As you have already learned, excess H^+ ions increase the acidity of the blood and drop the pH so that the acids and bases are no longer balanced. The above chemical reaction is demonstrated here:

$$CO_2 + H_2O \rightarrow H_2CO_3 \rightarrow H^+ + HCO_3^-$$
(carbon dioxide + water $\rightarrow$ carbonic acid $\rightarrow$ hydrogen bicarbonate)

Knowledge Connection

What happens when carbon dioxide bonds with water? When does CO_2 become an acid? What does the chemical symbol H_2CO_3 represent?

Role of the Kidneys

In relation to acid-base balance, the kidneys have the ability to perform four basic functions as needed to assist in maintaining the proper blood pH:

1. Retain hydrogen (H^+)
2. Excrete H^+
3. Retain sodium bicarbonate ($NaHCO_3$)
4. Excrete $NaHCO_3$

When the body fluids become too acidic, the kidneys' job is to remove H^+ from the blood and excrete it into the urine to be carried out of the body, and to reabsorb more $NaHCO_3$ back into the blood. Each of these two actions will make the blood less acidic and increase its alkalinity, helping to return the pH back to normal. When the kidneys sense that the blood is too alkaline, they will retain more H^+ in the blood to increase the acidity and excrete more $NaHCO_3$ into the urine to further decrease alkalinity of the blood, once again helping to return the pH back to normal.

The kidneys work more slowly than the lungs, changing the pH balance over a period of days rather than hours. However, while taking longer to make pH adjustments, the kidneys are capable of making much more significant changes in the pH than are the lungs, making the kidneys the most effective of the three systems for balancing blood pH.

Knowledge Connection

Which two body organs are involved in managing acid-base balance? What are the specific functions of each system that affect acid-base balance? Which system works most effectively to make pH adjustments?

Acid-Base Imbalance

An uncorrected acid-base imbalance will lead to either acidosis or alkalosis. **Acidosis** means an increase of acids, while **alkalosis** means an increase in bases or alkaline substances.

Normally, there are subtle shifts back and forth in the blood pH between slightly acidotic and slightly alkalotic as situations and conditions change minute amounts; however, the buffer, respiratory, and renal systems are able to accommodate these shifts and, through compensation, bring the blood back to a normal pH. When patients are ill from chronic or acute diseases, their bodies are sometimes unable to respond quickly enough or strongly enough to prevent extreme changes in pH, resulting in additional and possibly more serious health problems. The illness may involve either the pulmonary or the renal system, and by impairing its normal functions, make the system the actual source of the acid-base imbalance. However, there are other metabolic problems that can cause the metabolic imbalances. Some of these problems will be discussed a little later in this chapter.

Anatomy and Physiology Connection

The Brain and Acid-Base Balance

There are chemoreceptors located in the aorta, carotid arteries, and medulla that have the capability to sense or detect changes in blood levels of O_2 and CO_2, as well as disturbances in the pH. Upon sensing a lowering pH, meaning increasing acidity, receptors send a message to the brain indicating that the blood's pH is too acidic. The medulla then signals the lungs to increase the rate of respiration, which will blow off more CO_2, helping to reduce acidity of the blood. Upon sensing a higher pH, meaning increasing alkalinity, receptors send a message to the brain indicating the blood's pH is too alkaline. The brain then signals the lungs to decrease the rate of respirations, which will allow retention of more CO_2 so that it can bond with H_2O and make more H_2CO_3, which can release more H^+ ions. This raises the acidity of the blood toward a more normal pH.

Respiratory Imbalances

Respiratory conditions and disease can create either alkalosis or acidosis. If an illness causes a patient to breath too rapidly or too deeply, the effect will be excessive loss of CO_2, thereby decreasing acidity of the blood. If the condition continues, it results in excessive alkalinity, which raises the blood pH above 7.45 and is known as *respiratory alkalosis*. If disease processes make a patient unable to take deep breaths, decrease the rate of respirations, or somehow interfere with the exchange of CO_2 and O_2 gases, excessive CO_2 will be retained, causing the blood's pH to become increasingly acidic. If allowed to continue until the blood pH is sufficiently acidic and the pH drops below 7.35, a condition known as *respiratory acidosis* results. When the lungs are the source of either acidosis or alkalosis, the kidneys do what they can to compensate for the impaired lungs (Box 29-7).

Metabolic Imbalances

Metabolic diseases that cause excessive loss of H^+ or excessive gain of bicarbonate can result in an elevated pH above 7.45, known as *metabolic alkalosis*. Severe vomiting and

Box 29-7

Compensation for Respiratory and Metabolic Acid-Base Imbalances

The renal system (kidneys) and the respiratory system (lungs) work together, along with the buffer system, to compensate for each other's impaired functioning during illness or injury. If one system's impairment causes acidosis, the other system will perform its part to "get rid" of components that it can control that would contribute to further acidosis. If one system is impaired in such a manner that it results in alkalosis, the other system will do whatever it can to get rid of the components that it controls that would further contribute to the alkalosis. These compensatory actions are listed below.

- **If the lungs cause respiratory alkalosis:** The kidneys retain H^+ and excrete $NaHCO_3$ into the urine to decrease alkalinity and increase acidity of the blood.
- **If the lungs cause respiratory acidosis:** The kidneys retain $NaHCO_3$ and excrete H into the urine to decrease acidity and increase alkalinity of the blood.
- **If any metabolic condition causes metabolic alkalosis:** The lungs retain CO_2 to decrease alkalinity and increase acidity of the blood. If the kidneys are NOT the source of the imbalance, they will conserve H and excrete $NaHCO_3$ into the urine to increase acidity of the blood.
- **If any metabolic condition causes metabolic acidosis:** The lungs increase respiratory rate/depth to blow off more CO_2 to decrease acidity and increase alkalinity of the blood. If the kidneys are NOT the source of the metabolic imbalance, they will conserve $NaHCO_3$ and retain H^+ to decrease acidity and increase alkalinity of the blood.

nasogastric suctioning are two of the most common causes of metabolic alkalosis, both due to loss of potassium (K^+) and hydrochloric acid (HCl) in the gastric juices. HCl contains hydrogen and chloride, so the loss of this acid contributes to development of alkalosis.

The loss of gastric K^+ contributes to alkalosis in two ways. Loss of gastric K^+ due to vomiting or suction causes decreased absorption of K^+ from diet, which results in hypokalemia. When the blood level gets low, it causes intracellular K^+ to move out of the cells and into the blood in an attempt to maintain adequate blood levels. When a cation leaves the cells, it must be replaced by another cation to maintain neutrality of electrical charges, so H^+ is moved into the cells. Hypokalemia also stimulates the kidneys to conserve K^+ and excrete H^+, causing further loss of acid.

Other situations that can give rise to metabolic alkalosis include long-term use of a diuretic such as furosemide that causes K^+ loss in the urine; a gastrostomy tube draining gastric contents; or administration of excessive amounts of sodium bicarbonate during resuscitative efforts. Diseases that can cause metabolic alkalosis include Cushing's syndrome and hyperaldosteronism because they cause abnormal electrolyte metabolism.

Metabolic acidosis is the condition of excessive H^+ concentration or an excessively low level of bicarbonate that is caused by a metabolic disease or condition that results in a pH below 7.35. Diseases and conditions that affect the lower intestinal tract and result in excessive losses of bicarbonate, such as diarrhea, ulcerative colitis, and surgical colectomy, all serve as common causes of metabolic acidosis. Renal failure reduces the kidney's ability to adequately filter wastes and excess electrolytes from the blood. This can cause hyperkalemia, elevated blood levels of creatinine, and excessive H^+ retention and can result in metabolic acidosis. Any cardiovascular diseases that impair blood flow to the kidneys can lead to varying degrees of renal failure and metabolic acidosis as a result. Critical levels of metabolic acidosis can occur rapidly due to changes in the cell's metabolism related to a diabetic crisis, alcohol or medicine poisoning, crushing bone injuries, or burns.

Compensation by the Lungs

The respiratory system responds quickly to minute changes in pH and works very rapidly, continuously adjusting as needed to help balance the pH, but is only capable of making small adjustments in the pH. When a larger pH adjustment is required, especially for a longer period of time, the lungs' ability to compensate will be limited and they will require the assistance of the kidneys to return the pH to normal ranges (see Box 29-7).

Treatment and Nursing Care for Acid-Base Imbalances

Because there are various respiratory illnesses that can cause pH imbalance, it is key that you understand the pathophysiology of the disease process causing the problem. If you do not understand how the disease changes either the structure of the respiratory system or the way that the system functions, you will not understand what you must do to intervene and correct the problem. Monitor vital signs for tachypnea and bradypnea, tachycardia, and fever. Assess characteristics of the patient's respirations, including depth and pattern, dyspnea, length of inspiration versus expiration, use of accessory respiratory muscles, and level of difficulty. Are there substernal or costal retractions? Assess skin, mucous membranes, and nailbeds for cyanosis. Assess O_2 saturation and need for supplemental O_2. Monitor laboratory results of arterial blood gases (ABGs). Seriously ill patients may require endotracheal intubation and mechanical ventilation.

In Chapter 28, you were introduced to the laboratory diagnostic test called arterial blood gases (ABGs). See Table 28-2 to review the normal ranges for ABGs and the significance of abnormal levels. Box 29-8 provides steps to follow while interpreting ABG results, with examples.

Knowledge Connection

Which two body systems are key in managing acid-base changes? What functions can each of these organs perform in efforts to maintain acid-base balance? Explain at least two causes of metabolic acidosis and two causes of metabolic alkalosis.

Box 29-8

Arterial Blood Gases Interpretation Steps

Arterial blood gas results are useless you understand what they mean. Interpretation of arterial blood gas results must be done systematically, following the steps below closely and in the order they are presented. It is important to understand each step and be able to apply the information, not just regurgitate the normal ranges of the various components. Begin by evaluating the pH, followed by the PCO_2 (referred to as CO_2 in the rest of this box), and then the HCO_3^-. After having evaluated all three components, you should be able to determine whether there is an imbalance and, if so, which system caused the problem and whether there is compensation or not.

Normal ranges:

> pH = 7.35–7.45
> CO_2 = 35–45 mm Hg
> HCO_3^- = 22–26 mEq/L

CO_2 is considered an acid. HCO_3^- is considered a base, or alkaline. If the pH is below 7.35, it is acidic. If the pH is above 7.45, it is alkaline. If the CO_2 is elevated, it will increase acidity, and if it is below normal, it will increase alkalinity. If the HCO_3^- is elevated, it will increase alkalinity, and if it is below normal, it will increase acidity. Both systems will attempt to compensate for any deviations from normal that the other system might have made.

1. View the pH result and determine whether it is within normal limits, acidotic, or alkalotic.
2. Analyze the CO_2: Is it within normal limits; elevated, meaning acidosis; or low, meaning alkalosis?
3. Analyze the HCO_3^-: Is it within normal limits; low, meaning acidosis; or elevated, meaning alkalosis?
4. If all three are within normal range, you have normal ABGs.
5. **If the pH shows acidosis:** Determining which of the CO_2 (lungs) or HCO_3^- (kidneys or other metabolic process) values also indicates acidosis should identify the source of the imbalance.
   Examples:
   a. pH=7.30, CO_2=48, HCO_3^-=26: The lungs have retained excessive CO_2 *(acid)*; now pH is acidic (= respiratory acidosis).

   b. pH=7.30, CO_2=44, HCO_3^-=20: The kidneys excreted extra HCO_3^- *(base)* and retained too much H^+ *(acid)*; now pH is acidic (= metabolic acidosis).

   c. pH=7.49, CO_2=31, HCO_3^-=23: The lungs have blown off excess CO_2 *(base)*; now pH is alkalotic (= respiratory alkalosis).

   d. pH=7.49, CO_2=41, HCO_3^-=30: The kidneys have retained extra HCO_3^- *(base)* and excreted extra H^+; now pH is alkalotic (= metabolic alkalosis).

6. **If both lungs and kidneys indicate they are the source of alkalosis (or acidosis):** Both respiratory and metabolic alkalosis (and acidosis) are present.
   Example: pH=7.30, CO_2=49, HCO_3^-=19
   The lungs retained too much CO_2 *(acid)*; the kidneys retained too much H^+ *(acid)* and excreted too much HCO_3^- *(base)*. Therefore, pH=acidic, CO_2=acidic, and HCO_3^-=acidic, giving you respiratory acidosis and metabolic acidosis.

7. **If one system is the cause of the imbalance:** If the lungs, for example, have caused acidosis by retaining too much CO_2 *(acid)*, but the kidneys have really worked at compensating by getting rid of as much H^+ *(acid)* and retaining as much HCO_3^- *(base)* as possible, the end result is that the kidneys may successfully bring the pH back to normal range, even if it is only barely within the range. This is known as *compensation*.
   Example: pH = 7.45 (close to alkaline end), CO_2 = 32 (alkaline), HCO_3^- = 20 (acidic)
   The pH is just barely within normal range (close to the alkalotic end). The lungs show evidence of causing the alkalosis by blowing off too much CO_2 *(acid)*. This produces CO_2 = 32 (decreasing acidity and increasing alkalinity). This indicates that there was respiratory alkalosis; but the kidneys excreted extra HCO_3^- *(base)* and retained extra H^+ *(acid)*, which increased acidity and decreased alkalinity, bringing the pH back into normal range (just barely). This is known as respiratory alkalosis with compensation.

Nursing Care Plan for a Patient With a Fluid Imbalance

When you plan care for a patient with a fluid volume deficit or fluid volume excess, it is important to assess for signs and symptoms of electrolyte imbalance as well. To develop a thorough care plan, you will be thinking about many potential problems as well as those that you identify.

You have arrived at the hospital to work the day shift from 0700 until 1530 and you are assigned to provide nursing care for a 26-year-old female with Crohn's disease. She was admitted to the hospital around 0400 with dehydration secondary to persistent diarrhea for 3 weeks. At home, she had gotten up to go to the bathroom and fainted, so her husband called an ambulance.

After receiving report, it is time to assess the new patient and begin developing her plan of care. You know that it will be important to be particularly alert to signs and symptoms of electrolyte imbalance as well as fluid imbalance.

Assessment

As you perform the head-to-toe assessment on this patient, you find that her skin and mucous membranes are very dry. Her lips are cracked and chapped, her tongue shows deep furrows, and her eyes appear to be sunken in the orbital frame. Her pulse is 102 and is weak but regular. Her supine blood pressure is 96/52. When you check her skin

(care plan continues on page 670)

Nursing Care Plan for a Patient With a Fluid Imbalance (continued)

turgor, it remains tented for longer than 3 seconds. She weighs 120 lbs. (54.5 kg) and is 5 feet 2 inches (157.5 cm) tall. She informs you that her normal weight is 131 lbs. (59.5 kg). Her husband tells you that she seemed confused earlier when the ambulance arrived, but she is now oriented to all four spheres and answering your questions appropriately. She tells you that she has not voided since before she went to bed at 2300. Her lab work shows elevated sodium and low chloride in the blood. She tells you that in the past she had had short episodes of diarrhea due to her Crohn's disease, but that she has never had it for this long and nothing she has taken stopped it for very long.

Nursing Diagnosis

As you analyze your assessment findings, you must determine which nursing diagnoses apply to this patient. It is obvious that she did not call the physician as she should have when the diarrhea continued for so long. You know that she is dehydrated, and that she has had diarrhea for too long and it must be stopped to improve her dehydration. You are concerned about the appearance of her dry, cracked mouth, but more so regarding the fact that she has not voided in 9 hours, because you know the minimum output indicating adequate kidney function is 30 mL/hr. You determine that the following nursing diagnoses are appropriate for her:

- Fluid volume deficit
- Diarrhea
- Risk for impaired oral mucous membranes
- Knowledge deficit regarding management of her chronic disease

The first two nursing diagnoses are addressed in this care plan, but the other diagnoses are appropriate to be added as well.

Planning

Planning interventions requires you to first determine what outcomes you want and what patient responses are desired. You determine that the desired outcomes include adequate fluid volume, as evidenced by adequate intake of between 1,800 and 2,500 mL/day, and output that is within 200 to 300 mL of the intake; moist oral mucus membranes; and elastic skin turgor by the time she is discharged from the hospital. The priority outcome is that she receives adequate fluids that will be evidenced by the kidneys producing urine within the next 8 hours. Another desired outcome is that she will have four or fewer formed bowel movements per day before she leaves the hospital. Now you are ready to plan the interventions you need to perform to help bring about the desired outcomes for this patient.

Interventions

Your nursing interventions are designed to help meet the needs identified in each nursing diagnosis. Table 29-4 presents the interventions to perform.

Evaluation

As you evaluate your patient's responses to your interventions, you can decide if the action is effective, if it needs to be continued, or if it needs to be changed. Table 29-4 includes evaluations of each intervention.

Table 29-4 Nursing Care Plan for a Patient With a Fluid Imbalance

Nursing Diagnosis: Deficient fluid volume related to prolonged diarrhea as evidenced by decreased BP, and decreased skin turgor and dry mucus membranes
Expected Outcomes: BP will stabilize with no signs of orthostatic hypotension, I/O balanced prior to discharge

Interventions	Evaluation
Monitor vital signs every 4 hours or more frequently, with blood pressure taken in lying, sitting, and standing positions, noting orthostatic hypotension; note elevated temperature, tachycardia, weak or thready pulse.	10/16/11: 0800 – Supine BP 98/62, sitting BP 90/58, standing BP 78/50. Requires assistance to sit on side of bed. Not able to ambulate due to dizziness accompanying BP drops. T – 100.4°F; P – 104 weak. 10/16/11: BP stability better by evening. 2015 – BP 108/78 supine, 104/66 sitting, 102/64 standing. T – 99.2°F; P – 82 reg & strong. No c/o dizziness. Able to be up to bathroom with assistance. 10/17/11: BP supine 128/76, sitting 126/78, standing 128/66; T – 98.8°F; P – 81 and regular. Alert and oriented. Able to be up unassisted. No dizziness.

Table 29-4 **Nursing Care Plan for a Patient With a Fluid Imbalance** (continued)

Nursing Diagnosis: Deficient fluid volume related to prolonged diarrhea as evidenced by decreased BP, and decreased skin turgor and dry mucus membranes
Expected Outcomes: BP will stabilize with no signs of orthostatic hypotension, I/O balanced prior to discharge

Interventions	Evaluation
Maintain careful intake and output record. Offer the patient 8 ounces of fluid every hour. She likes Sprite, hot tea, and water. Measure loose stools and include all IV fluids in intake.	10/15/11: 24-hr Intake – 3,350 mL. Output – 1,175 mL (700 mL was from 8 loose stools). IV @ 125 mL/hr. Drinking some fluid each hour when cued. Taking Sprite better than other fluids. 10/16/11: 24-hr Intake – 3,420 mL. Output – 1,400 mL (250 mL was 5 loose stools). IV rate ↓ 80 mL/hr. Drinking fluids well. 10/17/11: Intake – 2,555 mL. Output – 2,400 mL (3 loose stools – 160 mL). IV has been discontinued.
Weigh the patient every morning.	10/15/11 Weight 125 lbs. (56.8 kg) 10/16/11 Wt. down @ 124.5 lbs. (56.6 kg) 10/17/11 Wt. up @ 126 lbs. (57.2 kg)
Administer IV fluids and assess for signs and symptoms of fluid volume overload (shortness of breath, pedal or sacral edema, and increasing blood pressure or full bounding pulse).	10/15/11: Tolerated IV NS 1,000 mL w/ 20 mEq KCl at 125 mL/hr without s/sx of fluid volume excess. Site without erythema/edema. 10/16/11: IV ↓ 80 mL/hr; no signs of FVE. Site without erythema/edema. 10/17/11: IV discontinued.

Nursing Diagnosis: Diarrhea related to bowel inflammation as evidenced by many liquid stools per day
Expected Outcomes: Number of stools will decrease to less than 3/day by discharge.

Interventions	Evaluation
Administer antidiarrheal medications as ordered and evaluate their effectiveness.	10/16/11: Med helping; stools decreased to 8 in 24 hours; 5 loose BMs.
Auscultate bowel sounds every 4 hours and note any decrease in hyperactivity.	10/16/11: Bowel sounds remain hyperactive. 10/17/11: Bowel sounds active; stools slowed to 3 in 24 hours, semiformed.
Assure the patient that you will respond to her call light promptly or place a bedpan within her reach.	10/16/11 No anxiety noted. Uses call light. No accidents. 10/17/11 Up to BR unassisted. Denies weakness/dizziness. Up to bathroom prn.
Place an incontinence pad beneath the patient to keep the bed clean.	No incontinence. Linens clean.
Demonstrate compassion and understanding regarding the patient's diarrhea.	No anxiety exhibited.

🌐 Post Conference

You learned how serious hyperkalemia can be. Your patient did well the first day you cared for her, but on the second day you noticed during your assessment that her heart rate was irregular, with a pattern of two beats and a skipped beat. You also noted that her urine output over the last 12 hours was less than 30 mL/hr. The monitor tech called and said your patient was having premature ventricular contractions. The patient told you that she felt weak and like her heart was "flip-flopping." You notified your instructor and the supervising nurse, who called the physician. Stat orders for a potassium level and basic metabolic profile (BMP) were received. Her blood work showed that her potassium level had risen from 4.8 to 5.6 mEq/L in 36 hours. Her BMP showed high levels of creatinine. The physician was again notified and ordered the patient transferred back to the ICU with acute renal insufficiency and hyperkalemia. You understood the need to act quickly and helped with the transfer. The ICU nurse told you that he would be administering Kayexalate enemas to the patient and that, if they do not effectively bring the patient's potassium back into normal range, dialysis may be necessary. You felt really good, like a contributing part of the nursing team, because you had picked up on a key assessment indicating a potentially serious problem for this patient.

KEY POINTS

- Proper balance of body fluids and electrolytes is essential for functions of cells, organs, and each of the body systems.

- Changes in fluid level are dependent on intake, output, illness, environmental factors, energy expenditure, and internal regulation.

- Electrolytes are key to maintaining body fluid balance and correct functioning of body systems.

- Adequate electrolytes are typically taken in through a balanced diet.

- Poor diet, medications, and diseases can deplete electrolytes.

- Overingestion of electrolytes, certain medications, and diseases can create excess levels of electrolytes.

- Correcting electrolyte and fluid imbalances requires assessment and careful intervention.

- The lungs retain CO_2 (acid) to increase acidity of the blood and blow off more CO_2 (acid) to decrease acidity and increase alkalinity of the blood.

- The kidneys retain HCO_3^- (base) and excrete extra H^+ (acid) to increase alkalinity of the blood; they also excrete more HCO_3^- (base) and retain more H^+ (acid) to increase acidity of the blood.

REVIEW QUESTIONS

Select the answer that is most appropriate for each of the following questions. Some questions may have more than one correct answer. Check all that apply.

1. You will expect to find which of the following during the skin assessment of a patient with dehydration?

   a. Redness

   b. Dryness

   c. Dependent edema

   d. Blisters

   e. Prolonged skin tenting

2. The nurse is completing an intake and output sheet for the patient. Which will the nurse include in the output?

   a. Sweat

   b. Peritoneal fluid

   c. Liquid stool

   d. Emesis

   e. Interstitial fluid

   f. Urine

3. The patient complains of shortness of breath and is expectorating pink frothy sputum. The nurse would assess for further signs and symptoms of:

   a. hyperkalemia.

   b. hypomagnesemia.

   c. fluid overload.

   d. fluid deficit.

   e. dehydration.

4. When teaching a patient about ways to avoid fluid overload, the nurse explains it is best to eat a diet that is low in:

   a. potassium.

   b. calcium.

   c. magnesium.

   d. sodium.

   e. phosphorus.

5. You know that your patient with chronic kidney disease will need more teaching if she says:

   a. "I will eat more oranges to prevent potassium buildup."

   b. "I will increase my milk intake to keep my calcium levels in the normal range."

   c. "I will avoid bananas so my potassium level will not get too high."

   d. "I can have scrambled eggs for breakfast as long as my calcium is not too high."

6. Your patient has a low potassium level, uncorrected by oral medications. The physician orders 30 mEq of KCl added to the IV of 1,000 mL of normal saline to infuse at 80 mL/hr. Which nursing intervention is of the most importance to perform today?

   a. Serve a diet with potassium-rich foods.

   b. Restrict sodium in the diet.

   c. Monitor blood levels of all electrolytes.

   d. Make certain urine output is at least 30 mL/hr.

   e. Monitor for fever and tachypnea.

7. Your patient is admitted with alkalosis. Which laboratory finding would you expect?

   a. pH of 7.30

   b. pH of 7.48

   c. Decreased HCO_3^-

   d. Elevated PCO_2

8. A patient has severe first-, second-, and third-degree burns. Intravenous fluids were initiated upon admission 2 hours ago. You are preparing to review her electrolyte results. Which electrolyte do you anticipate will be elevated?

   a. Chloride

   b. Potassium

   c. Magnesium

   d. Calcium

9. The patient for whom you are providing care has been receiving furosemide, a diuretic, in an effort to remove the excess water that has been retained as a result of congestive heart failure. When you are preparing to assist the patient with a shower, she tells you that she is so tired today and that she just does not feel that her legs will hold her up long enough to take a shower. You know that she took a shower each of the past 3 days and wonder to what you might attribute this change. Which of the following laboratory results could explain her fatigue and muscle weakness?

   a. Hypokalemia

   b. Hyperchloremia

   c. Hypocalcemia

   d. Hypernatremia

10. If ABG results are pH = 7.32, CO_2 = 47, and HCO_3^- = 26, which of the following would be a correct analysis?

   a. Respiratory acidosis

   b. Respiratory alkalosis

   c. Metabolic acidosis

   d. Metabolic alkalosis

11. If ABG results are pH = 7.47, CO_2 = 43, and HCO_3^- = 29, which of the following would be a correct analysis?

   a. Respiratory acidosis

   b. Respiratory alkalosis

   c. Metabolic acidosis

   d. Metabolic alkalosis

12. If ABG results are pH = 7.33, CO_2 = 37, and HCO_3^- = 19, which of the following would be a correct analysis?

   a. Respiratory acidosis

   b. Respiratory alkalosis

   c. Metabolic acidosis

   d. Metabolic alkalosis

CRITICAL THINKING EXERCISE

13. The patient is a 79-year-old male with chronic heart disease. His wife calls his physician's office to report that he is short of breath and not feeling well. She reports that he doesn't have a fever and his heart rate and blood pressure readings on their home monitor were normal. You suspect congestive heart failure, which can cause fluid retention. What assessment question should you ask that could best confirm your suspicion?

ADDITIONAL RESOURCES

For additional Resources, Questions, and Activities, please see:

 Student Resource Disk

DavisPlus http://davisplus.fadavis.com

 Student Study Guide

REFERENCES

American Heart Association. Sodium. 2009. Available at: http://www.americanheart.org/presenter.jhtml?identifier=4708. Accessed November 27, 2009.

American Nurses Association and the National Council of State Boards of Nursing. Joint statement on delegation, American Nurses Association (ANA) and the National Council of State Boards of Nursing (NCSBN). 2006. Available at: http://www.ncsbn.org/Joint_statement.pdf. Accessed November 27, 2009.

Doenges ME, Moorhouse MF, Murr AC. *Nursing Diagnosis Manual: Planning, Individualizing, and Documenting Client Care.* 2nd ed. Philadelphia: FA Davis; 2008.

Mayo Clinic Staff. Caffeine: how much is too much? 2009. Available at: http://www.mayoclinic.com/health/caffeine/NU00600. Accessed November 27, 2009.

National Cancer Institute. Hypercalcemia PDQ®, Health Professional Version. 2008. Available at: http://www.cancer.gov/cancertopics/pdq/supportivecare/hypercalcemia/. Accessed November 27, 2009.

Nuget PM, Vitale BA. *Fundamentals Success.* 2nd ed. Philadelphia: FA Davis; 2008.

Scanlon VC, Sanders T. *Essentials of Anatomy and Physiology.* 3rd ed. Philadelphia: FA Davis; 2007.

Society of Neuroscience. The neural regulation of thirst. Brain Briefings. 2008. Available at: http://www.sfn.org/index.cfm?pagename=brainBriefings_thirst. Accessed November 27, 2009.

Van Leeuwen AM, Poelhuis-Leth DJ. *Davis's Comprehensive Handbook of Laboratory and Diagnostic Tests with Nursing Implications.* 3rd ed. Philadelphia: FA Davis; 2009.

Venes D, ed. *Taber's Cyclopedic Medical Dictionary.* 21st ed. Philadelphia: FA Davis; 2009.

Wilkinson JM, Van Leuven K. *Fundamentals of Nursing: Theory, Concepts, and Applications.* Philadelphia: FA Davis; 2007.

30

Bowel Elimination and Care

Key Terms

Colostomy

Constipation

Defecation

Diarrhea

Distention

Fecal incontinence

Flatus

Guaiac test

Ileostomy

Impaction

Kayexalate enema

Melena

Normal flora

Occult blood

Peristalsis

Siphon enema

Steatorrhea

Stoma

Tenesmus

Objectives

1. Define key terms related to bowel elimination and care.
2. Explain the digestion, absorption, and metabolism of nutrients.
3. Differentiate between normal and abnormal function in digestion and bowel elimination.
4. Differentiate between normal and abnormal characteristics of feces.
5. Explain how different factors affect bowel elimination.
6. Enumerate independent nursing interventions to promote bowel elimination.
7. Accurately assess bowel elimination problems.
8. Describe interventions that help to prevent and treat bowel elimination problems.
9. Contrast different types of enemas.
10. Describe the possible complications of bowel elimination and treatment of problems.
11. List signs and symptoms of vagal stimulation.
12. Prioritize nursing actions to perform when vagal stimulation is suspected.
13. Explain how to obtain stool specimens for culture and sensitivity and for ova and parasites, and how to test for occult blood.
14. Compare the different types of bowel diversions.
15. Discuss ostomy care and patient teaching regarding care.
16. Describe the steps necessary to develop a care plan for a patient with a bowel diversion.

Skills

30-1 Administering an Enema

30-2 Obtaining a Stool Specimen for Culture, and Ova and Parasites

30-3 Performing Guaiac Testing: Testing Stool Specimen for Occult Blood

30-4 Removing a Fecal Impaction

30-5 Applying/Changing an Ostomy Appliance

30-6 Irrigating a Colostomy

 ## Clinical Connection

Your Assignment: You are assigned to care for a 58-year-old male who had a total *colectomy* (removal of the colon) yesterday as a result of colon cancer. He has a permanent ileostomy as well as an abdominal incision with staples. You learn in report that his pain medication has been increased to better manage his discomfort.

Your Actions: As you prepare to care for this patient, you will need to know how to care for a new ileostomy. You will also need to know how to assess the stoma for evidence of adequate blood supply, as well as what type of output to expect from the ileostomy. You will need to assess his surgical wound for bleeding, approximation, and signs and symptoms of infection. In addition, you will need to manage his pain to keep him comfortable and perform routine postoperative care.

Some nurses may view assisting with bowel elimination as nurse's aide work and low on the list of nursing priorities. However, understanding the importance of proper bowel elimination and the extent to which it can affect how a patient feels cannot be overstated. Problematic bowel elimination can cause mild to extreme discomfort as well as major health problems. In this chapter, you will learn the importance of proper bowel elimination, physical assessments related to bowel elimination, alternative methods of bowel elimination, abnormal patterns of elimination, and the appropriate nursing skills to promote proper bowel elimination.

Bowel Elimination

Bowel elimination occurs after nutrients are moved through the gastrointestinal (GI) tract, also known as the alimentary canal; this process begins in the *os,* or mouth, and ends as the waste products are eliminated as *feces,* or stool, via the anus. The process of bowel elimination is known as **defecation**.

Anatomy and Physiology Connection

Gastrointestinal Tract

The propulsion of a bolus of food through the GI tract is due to the rhythmic wave-like movements that begin in the esophagus and continue to the rectum, termed **peristalsis**. The mechanism of peristalsis is contraction of the circular and longitudinal muscles in the walls of the GI tract. As the muscles contract, the food bolus is pushed forward through the GI tract. In the stomach, enzymes break down the bolus of food, converting it into a semiliquid mass of partly digested food and digestive secretions known as *chyme.* There is some absorption of water and alcohol that occurs while food is in the stomach, but the stomach serves mostly as a reservoir allowing chyme to slowly be emptied into the small intestine for further digestion and absorption. The chyme passes through the outlet of the stomach called the *pyloric sphincter* and into the small intestine, which is composed of the duodenum, jejunum, and ileum. It is here that most nutrients are absorbed into the blood via capillaries located in the villi and microvilli of the walls of the intestinal mucosa. The remaining chyme that is unable to be broken down for absorption passes through the ileocecal valve into the cecum portion of the colon, or large intestine. The ileocecal valve prevents backflow from the colon into the small intestine.

In the colon reside bacteria known as **normal flora**, whose purpose it is to prevent infection and maintain health. The bacteria interact with the chyme, which produces a gas called **flatus**. As peristalsis moves the GI contents and flatus through the colon, it results in gurgles, clicks, and tinkling sounds, known as *bowel sounds.*

Most water absorption occurs in the colon, beginning in the cecum, followed by the ascending colon, transverse colon, descending colon, and finally the sigmoid colon, leaving a soft, formed mass of fecal material. As fecal material moves through the sigmoid colon into the rectum, the intestinal walls distend to accommodate the fecal mass. This **distention**, or stretching out of the intestinal walls and making them appear inflated, stimulates the walls' stretch receptors and sends impulses to the central nervous system, which in turn signals the muscular walls of the sigmoid colon and rectum to contract. This is known as the *defecation reflex* and is under voluntary control of the individual. The mass of waste will then pass through the internal and external anal sphincters, where it is expelled as feces.

Frequency of Elimination

Frequency of bowel elimination changes throughout the life span. Infants will normally have between three and six bowel movements daily. Children accomplish voluntary control of elimination between the ages of 2 and 3 years after their neuromuscular structures are developed. The frequency of bowel movements usually decreases to one or two bowel movements per day. This pattern is usually maintained throughout adulthood. However, peristalsis decreases as the individual ages, making elderly individuals more prone to constipation, or hard stools that are difficult to pass.

Some patients will normally have one bowel movement daily, while others may go several days between movements, and yet others may have several bowel movements each day. The goal of your elimination care is to maintain the patient's normal frequency pattern of bowel elimination, or as close to it as possible. At the very least, you must make certain the patient has a bowel movement at least every 3 days to prevent constipation.

Knowledge Connection

Describe what happens during peristalsis. Explain the importance of normal flora in the GI tract. Explain the defecation reflex. What is the longest length of time a patient should be allowed to go without having a bowel movement?

Timing of Elimination

Because peristalsis begins with the introduction of food into the GI tract, the urge to defecate commonly occurs 30 minutes to 1 hour after eating. If the patient ignores the reflex and puts off going to the bathroom for a bowel movement until a later time, the stool remains in the intestines longer than necessary and can become dry and hard, contributing to the development of constipation. It is helpful to provide the patient free time after each meal for toileting, offering assistance as needed.

Characteristics of Feces

Characteristics of stool include color, shape, consistency, odor, and frequency. A normal stool will vary depending on diet, amount of fiber and fluids, exercise, medications, and other habits. When there is a disease process occurring in the GI tract, the changes in the characteristics of stool may provide clues as to the medical diagnosis, which is one of the reasons that assessment of bowel function is important. Table 30-1 presents a summary of normal and abnormal characteristics of stool.

Normal Characteristics

The typical stool is soft, formed, light yellowish-brown to dark brown, and slightly odiferous, and falls into a slightly curved shape. Sometimes a normal stool may be a different color, such as red or green, simply due to variations in dietary intake. For example, eating green foods such as spinach may result in greenish-black streaks in the feces, while eating beets may result in red-tinted stools. Ingestion of iron supplements normally causes stools to be very dark brown or black.

Like frequency, the expected color and consistency of stool is also different across the life span. Normally newborns have black, shiny, sticky stools called *meconium.* Infants who are breastfed will usually have a bright yellow, pasty, seedy-appearing stool, while babies who receive formula or cow's milk will have a darker yellowish-brown or tan-colored stool that is much more firm and formed.

Abnormal Characteristics

If the patient has inadequate fluid intake or transit time is prolonged, meaning stool is held in the body longer than usual, the stool may be a harder consistency and be passed in smaller balls or clumps, rather than a softer, longer, curved shape. If transit time is extremely short due to increased peristalsis, little or no water will be absorbed and the stool will be liquid or semiliquid. Several liquid or watery stools per day are classified as diarrhea.

The stool consistency or shape may change due to variation in amount of fiber intake, an increase in amount of ingested fat, or changes in the structure of the intestine. Fiber intake will affect the bulk of the stool. **Steatorrhea** refers to stool containing an abnormally high amount of undigested fat. This stool will appear fluffy, float on water, and have a foul odor. Steatorrhea may occur as a result of a malabsorption disorder, such as

Table 30-1 **Normal and Abnormal Characteristics of Stool**

	Normal Characteristics	Abnormal Characteristics
Consistency	Soft, formed consistency	Liquid or semiliquid, watery, unformed, very hard and dry
Shape	Longer curved shape, cylindrical	Balls, clumps, or broken-off chunks, flat or ribbon-like, pencil-like
Color	Yellow in infants Light brown to dark brown in others	Bright red blood, black, coffee-grounds appearance, pale, white, gray, or clay-color
Presence of infection	Absence of pus, mucous, fat	Presence of pus, excessive mucus, foamy, or floating on water
Presence of parasites	Absence of parasites	Presence of worms or eggs
Odor	Slight odor	Foul odor, strongly odiferous, bloody or old-blood smell, metallic smell

Crohn's disease. Compression of the colon by a tumor can result in ribbon-shaped stools, which are sometimes the first clue to the presence of a colon malignancy. Mucus, blood, and pus in the stool generally indicate inflammation or infection of the intestinal mucosa, such as ulcerative colitis. Stools may appear to be coated with mucus or look slimy and show traces of blood or pus. Parasites, or worms, and their eggs may be observed in the stools of an infected patient. Any of these abnormalities should be reported to the physician.

Clay-colored or pale white stools are indicative of an absence of bile in the intestines, usually due to a blockage in the bile ducts of the liver and gallbladder, and should be reported to the physician. Antacids and x-ray barium, which is used to help visualize organs for radiological tests, will both cause the stools to be white. Abnormal color may also include red or black from blood. *Frank blood* in the stool is bright red blood visible with the naked eye, while **occult blood** is hidden or not visible. To determine the presence of occult blood, a **guaiac test** must be performed on the stool sample. Specks or traces of bright red blood may be the result of a torn hemorrhoid. Larger amounts of frank blood indicate bleeding or hemorrhage from the colon. Smaller amounts of blood that come from higher in the digestive tract, such as the stomach, having been partially digested, will have a distinctive *old blood* odor and a black, tarry appearance known as **melena**. Bleeding from the small intestine will often result in a maroon-colored stool. A large hemorrhage from the stomach or intestines can cause a large volume of bright red, or frank, blood. All bleeding is considered serious until proven otherwise and should be reported to the physician.

Knowledge Connection
Compare normal and abnormal characteristics of feces. Name at least two reasons that a stool may be pale or white. What is the term denoting excessive fat in the stool? What is the difference between frank and occult blood in a stool?

Alterations in Bowel Elimination

The most commonly seen alterations in bowel elimination include constipation, diarrhea, impaction, and fecal incontinence.

Constipation

Constipation is the term used for less frequent, hard, formed stools that are difficult to expel. Constipation may include a bloated feeling, as it occurs in degrees of severity. A person may be mildly constipated or severely constipated, which can lead to **impaction**, the blockage of the movement of contents through the intestines by a bulk mass of very hard stool. A patient with an impaction may complain of loss of appetite, known as *anorexia;* bloating; cramping; malaise; or not feeling well. Other patients may voice no complaints at all, making it important to identify the length of time since the last bowel movement. It is also not uncommon to find that an elderly patient from a long-term care facility who is admitted to the hospital for other health issues is constipated or has a fecal impaction.

Diarrhea

Loose or watery stools occurring three or more times a day are classified as **diarrhea** and may or may not be accompanied by cramping or **tenesmus**, which is identified by increased rectal pressure and a feeling of the need to defecate. Loose stools can cause excoriation of perianal skin. Protracted diarrhea can result in dehydration and electrolyte imbalance. Elderly patients, infants, and small children dehydrate much quicker than young or middle-aged adults, making it pertinent to accurately assess the fluid volume loss that occurs with diarrhea.

Some patients have conditions that cause intermittent diarrhea and constipation. Once the diarrhea leads to an empty bowel, peristalsis decreases and transit time is slowed. This allows more time for absorption of water, leading to formed and dryer stools, which may then result in constipation.

Causes of Constipation and Diarrhea

Both constipation and diarrhea can be caused by many things. Possible causes include:

- Change in activity level
- Change in dietary and fluid intake
- Side effects of medication
- Side effects of surgery
- Pregnancy
- High stress levels and emotional problems
- Laxative abuse
- Aging process
- Structural changes
- Chemical changes
- Food allergies

Changes in Activity Level

One of the benefits of physical activity is that it stimulates peristalsis. Most hospitalized patients experience a change in their level of physical activity. Even if there are no activity restrictions and the patient is allowed to ambulate, he or she is certain to get less activity and exercise than at home. Many patients have physician's orders to limit activity to bathroom privileges only or even complete bedrest. The decrease in physical activity results in slower peristalsis and increased risk of constipation, making it very important that you carefully track and document patients' bowel movements.

Changes in Dietary and Fluid Intake

Certain foods slow peristalsis, including processed sugar products and other low-fiber foods. Inadequate fiber intake decreases stool mass as well as decreasing peristalsis, lending to development of constipation. Too much fiber can result in excessive flatus, and too much fiber without adequate fluids can contribute to constipation. Eating at irregular times tends to lead to irregularity of bowel movements and constipation, while individuals who eat three meals daily at regular intervals tend to have more regular patterns of bowel elimination. *Lactose intolerance,* the inability to digest dairy products, can cause diarrhea when dairy products are ingested.

The amount and type of fluid intake also impact bowel elimination. Too little fluid leads to harder stools as the body absorbs the majority of the fluid intake in an attempt to maintain fluid and electrolyte balance, leaving inadequate fluid in the colon to keep the stool soft. Some individuals find that hot or cold drinks help to stimulate peristalsis. A common example is the individual for whom a cup of coffee or tea early in the morning stimulates the daily bowel movement. This individual may have difficulty with constipation if he or she is forced to miss one or two mornings' hot coffee.

Side Effects of Medication

Antibiotics administered to treat infection can also kill some of the good bacteria that the body needs to stay healthy, specifically the normal flora found in the bowel. When the level of normal flora decreases, other microorganisms such as fungi are allowed to grow disproportionately, causing what is called an *opportunistic infection.* Opportunistic infections take control of the bowel, causing diarrhea.

One of the more severe opportunistic infections is *Clostridium difficile,* otherwise known as *C. diff.* If *C. difficile* starts in a long-term care facility, it is difficult to keep it from spreading among the residents, who often have compromised immune systems.

Some over-the-counter medications, such as Maalox, an antacid containing magnesium, can cause diarrhea, while the aluminum present in Amphogel or the calcium carbonate present in Tums may cause constipation. Iron supplements cause constipation in many people. Narcotic pain medications, especially opioid analgesics such as morphine, meperidine, and codeine, are among the worst offenders to slow intestinal peristalsis, which increases the risk of constipation. Certain classifications of medications, such as anticholinergics, calcium channel blockers, and nitrates, may contribute to gastroesophogeal reflux disease. Both steroids and nonsteroidal anti-inflammatory drugs (NSAIDs) may cause symptoms of gastritis, such as diarrhea.

The liver is one of the primary organs that breaks down, or metabolizes, medications and alcohol. Over a period of time certain drugs, as well as the use of multiple drugs at the same time, can damage the liver, contributing to development of liver disease, which in turn affects digestive processes. Some of the medications that fall into this category include certain antibiotics and antipsychotics, immunosuppressive agents, anti-tuberculosis drugs, and anticonvulsants. Even common over-the-counter medications such as acetaminophen and niacin, a B vitamin, can harm the liver when overused or taken in high dosages.

Side Effects of Surgery

Surgery, especially surgery on the GI tract, will decrease peristalsis and increase the risk for constipation. Anesthesia drugs can slow or completely halt peristalsis. Manipulation of the bowel changes the chemistry of the intestinal muscle cells, resulting in slowing of peristalsis. Postoperative pain can also suppress the urge to defecate. All postoperative patients should be assessed for adequate bowel elimination to prevent constipation. Surgery, anesthesia drugs, and pain medication can also cause nausea, vomiting, and problems with ingestion, digestion, and absorption. (See Chapter 33 for more information about postoperative patient care.)

Pregnancy

A decrease in the stimulation of muscles of the digestive tract and crowding of the sigmoid colon by the enlarging uterus both lend themselves to development of constipation.

High Stress Levels and Emotional Problems

High levels of stress or anxiety, as well as other emotional problems, can cause increased peristalsis and intestinal mucus production, which may result in diarrhea. Depression may inhibit peristalsis, contributing to constipation.

Laxative Abuse

Patients who use laxatives to ensure daily bowel movements can become physically, as well as psychologically, dependent upon the medications to have a bowel movement.

Aging Process

The natural aging process brings changes in bowel function that contribute to constipation, making it a greater risk for elders. Esophageal emptying and peristalsis slow as we age. The muscle tone of the smooth muscles of the GI tract and the control of the two rectal sphincters both decrease, contributing to constipation and **fecal incontinence,** or loss of voluntary control of rectal sphincters.

Structural Changes

One example of a structural change occurs with a disease process known as diverticulosis. This condition occurs when the muscular wall of the colon weakens and separates, allowing small pouches or pockets of the inner wall to protrude outward. These pouches easily trap fecal material and become inflamed. Such a pouch is called a *diverticulum.* When they become inflamed, the condition is referred to as *diverticulitis,* which can cause diarrhea and severe cramping sufficient to force a visit to a physician. Diverticuli have also been known to rupture, or *perforate,* allowing fecal material and bacteria to enter the sterile peritoneum and cause peritonitis, a life-threatening infection. Common signs and symptoms of peritonitis include malaise, anorexia, nausea, vomiting, abdominal distention, decreased or absent bowel sounds, and fever (or hypothermia if more advanced). Abdominal pain may be mild to severe; the classic sign of peritonitis being a *constant intense pain that worsens with movement.*

The nerves of the sigmoid colon, rectum, and both anal sphincters must be intact in order for the patient to sense the presence of the stool in the rectum and the need to defecate. If these nerves are damaged or there is an interruption in communication between these nerves and the brain, as with a severed spinal cord, the patient will be unable to identify when defecation is imminent, and will not possess control over the sphincters to voluntarily retain or expel stool. This can result in constipation, impaction, or fecal incontinence.

Other structural changes include surgical alterations such as colostomies and ileostomies, which will be discussed later in this chapter.

Chemical Changes

Inflammatory processes within the GI tract can be initiated by autoimmune diseases such as Crohn's disease or by infectious microorganisms such as bacteria or viruses. The common name for bacterial or viral infections of the GI tract is *gastroenteritis.* Inflammation causes the mucosal lining and musculature of the intestinal tract to become edematous and increase mucus production. The edema and excessive mucus inhibit absorption and increase peristalsis. The result can be nausea, vomiting, cramping, or diarrhea. The transit time can be shortened dramatically, meaning that nutrients and water do not remain in the intestinal tract long enough to allow for absorption, resulting in dehydration and malnutrition.

Food Allergies

Food allergies, and even some seasonal environmental allergies, can cause edema and inflammation of the intestinal walls with increased mucus production. The inflammation increases peristalsis, which decreases transit time, inhibits absorption, and results in diarrhea.

Knowledge Connection

Describe at least eight factors that influence bowel elimination. Explain specifically how opioid analgesics affect bowel elimination. What is meant by laxative abuse? What is meant by increasing transit time?

People and Places Connection

Bowel Elimination and Aging

As healthy people age, it is common to find that their level of exercise and physical activity naturally declines. Those with health problems and debility may find their level of physical activity further hindered—and when an individual is less active, the need for the body's fuel, which is food, also decreases. When an individual eats less, he or she sometimes becomes more selective in what is eaten, leaning more toward favorite foods rather than focusing on maintaining a balanced and more nutritious diet.

Even issues such as improperly fitting dentures or *edentia,* the lack of teeth, decrease the ability to consume adequate levels of fiber. Any of these factors alone can result in decreased peristalsis and constipation, but when combined with the previously noted natural changes of aging, the increased risk for constipation in elders becomes obvious.

Diarrhea can result in fluid volume depletion in all ages, but is more serious in infants and elders. A sudden water loss of as little as 5% of body weight requires treatment, while an 8% to 10% weight loss is considered to be a critical level of

(connection continues on page 681)

dehydration. If the water loss from diarrhea is not abated before the loss reaches 13% to 15% of the body weight, death is likely. Seventy-five percent to 80% of an infant's weight is due to body water content, whereas an adult's is 65% to 70%, and the older adult's decreases to 55% to 60%. Elders also suffer a reduced sense of thirst. The combination of these two factors places the older adult at a higher risk for dehydration as a result of diarrhea. Infants and small children will dehydrate from diarrhea the fastest of any age group, due to their small size. Even though their percentage of body-water weight is higher than adults, their small size and weight cause even small losses of fluid to have a greater impact.

Fecal Impaction

Fecal impaction may occur in the rectum, the sigmoid flexure, or any part of the large colon and is more common in elders, patients on bedrest, and severely dehydrated patients. Any cause of constipation may lead also to impaction. One common cause, especially in elders, is the abuse of laxatives. When laxatives are taken over a period of months and years, the bowel loses some of its natural contractibility, making bowel movements dependent upon taking laxatives.

Sometimes small amounts of diarrhea are an indication of an impaction. In some situations, liquid stool from higher in the rectum or colon may seep around the solid impaction. When this happens, the patient may think he or she has diarrhea, or may notice smears of liquid stool in the underwear or incontinence briefs. It is very important for the nurse to differentiate between diarrhea and the seepage of stool around an impaction. If stool seepage is reported and treated as diarrhea, it will make the impaction worse. If an impaction is not relieved, obstruction or perforation of the bowel wall can occur.

Fecal Incontinence

Continence, or rectal compliance, is the ability to voluntarily maintain the stool in the rectum until a convenient time for a bowel movement, as opposed to bowel or fecal incontinence where the voluntary control is lost. The degree or severity of incontinence may range from an occasional seepage of stool while passing flatus to continuous rectal seepage. If the nerves innervating the rectal sphincters have been damaged or severed, as in a spinal cord injury, the patient loses the ability to sense when the rectum is distended, necessitating expulsion of fecal material. Voluntary control of having a bowel movement is lost, resulting in fecal incontinence. Disoriented patients and those with arrested mental development may exhibit fecal incontinence.

Even though incontinence is beyond the patient's control, it can still be a source of guilt, serious embarrassment, and destruction of self-esteem. It can result in social isolation and loss of sexuality.

Promotion of Bowel Elimination

Promotion of bowel elimination begins with thorough assessment and data collection upon admission to the hospital. Then assessment of bowel movements should be performed and documented every shift thereafter. Documentation should always include:

- Color
- Amount
- Consistency
- Unusual shape
- Unusual odor

Other interventions you should perform to promote bowel functions include increasing activity, ensuring adequate fluid and fiber intake, providing privacy, and positioning for elimination. Box 30-1 lists independent nursing interventions to promote bowel elimination.

Subjective Assessment

Admission to the hospital should begin with collection of subjective information regarding the patient's normal bowel habits and any current problems the patient may be experiencing. Inquire of the patient regarding:

- Frequency of normal elimination pattern
- Whether there are current problems such as diarrhea or constipation, and their date of onset
- Frequency of stools
- Amount of stools
- Color of stools
- Consistency of stools

Box 30-1

Independent Nursing Interventions to Promote Bowel Elimination

There are various interventions that you may perform without a physician's order. The following are examples of independent nursing interventions that are useful in promoting bowel elimination:

- Determine the patient's normal bowel movement frequency pattern.
- Carefully track and document frequency, amount, color, and consistency of bowel movements.
- Assess bowel sounds at least once a shift, noting hypoactive, hyperactive, or absent sounds.
- If on bedrest: Reposition the patient at least every 2 hours and perform passive or active range-of-motion exercises at least twice a day (see Chapter 16).
- If ambulatory: Increase activity by ambulating three to four times daily, getting up in chair for meals.
- Encourage fluids, including water and fruit juices, as allowed by physician's orders.
- Encourage fiber intake as allowed by the patient's diet order, including whole grains, fruits, and vegetables.

- Shape of stools
- Abdominal cramping
- Anal burning or itching
- Pain with defecation
- Presence of tenesmus
- Allergies
- Routine medications and medications taken for the elimination problem, both prescription and over-the-counter
- Changes in appetite
- Dietary habits, including amount of fiber and regularity of mealtimes
- Amount and type of fluid intake
- Nausea or vomiting
- Food intolerances
- Presence of hemorrhoids

Objective Assessment

Perform a physical assessment to determine the objective signs. First, assess the shape of the abdomen. The shape should be rounded or flat, but not distended or inflated. Distention related to the GI tract may be a sign of excessive gas, fluid, or stool.

Next, auscultate the bowel sounds using the diaphragm surface rather than the bell of your stethoscope to better hear the sounds. Listen in all four quadrants. Bowel sounds should be assessed at least once per shift and more often as indicated. Normal bowel sounds are heard as soft gurgles and irregular clicks, between 5 and 30 per minute. If there are fewer than five per minute, they are described as hypoactive bowel sounds. If the patient has more than 30 per minute or if they are continuous, this is described as hyperactive bowel sounds, as with diarrhea. If sounds are excessively loud and gurgling, with a noise like splashing, they are termed *borborygmi*. Sometimes they are related to hunger and may be described as a *growling stomach*. When these increased sounds are not related to hunger, they may indicate possible bowel blockage, especially if they are high pitched and tinkling in one area and absent or decreased in the distal portion of the colon, which is heard in the left lower quadrant of the abdomen.

Bowel sounds may decrease when constipation is occurring. However, as constipation progresses to the point at which an impaction or intestinal blockage occurs, the peristalsis may increase or become hyperactive proximal to the blockage. The intestinal contents will churn and mix as the peristalsis pushes against the blockage. The intestine proximal to the blockage will distend while the intestine distal to the blockage may empty. The area distal to the blockage may have very distant or even absent bowel sounds. *Safety: An absence of bowel sounds indicates a problem and should always be reported to the physician.* It is important to be aware that some individuals have very quiet and difficult-to-hear bowel sounds, necessitating that you listen carefully and for an adequate period of time. If you think that bowel sounds are absent, be certain to listen for at least 3 to 5 minutes in each of the four quadrants before declaring this.

Avoid palpating the abdomen until after you have assessed the bowel sounds, as palpation may stimulate bowel sounds that were not there naturally. Normally, one's abdomen is soft when palpated, but it may become firm or hard with excessive gas, constipation, or obstruction of the bowel.

Knowledge Connection

Contrast subjective and objective assessment of bowel elimination patterns. What information should be documented after each bowel movement?

Increased Activity

Physical activity stimulates peristalsis. When a patient enters the hospital, it is probable that his or her activity level will be decreased from the normal activities of home life. If allowed, the patient should be ambulated in the hallways at least three to four times daily and sat up in a chair for meals. When patients are ordered to remain on bedrest or to have limited ambulation, it is important that you do what you can to increase their physical activities within the restrictions of the physician's orders. Make certain that the bedridden patient is turned, or repositioned, at least every 2 hours to help stimulate the normal peristalsis of the intestinal tract. Range-of-motion exercises should also be performed at least twice daily if the patient is not allowed to ambulate at all. Refer to Chapter 16 for further information regarding range-of-motion exercises.

Adequate Fluid and Fiber Intake

When there is inadequate fluid intake, the water that has been ingested is absorbed from the bowel into the bloodstream in an attempt to prevent dehydration. Without enough water to keep the stools soft, they become hard and difficult to expel. Unless contraindicated, fluid intake should be maintained between 1,500 and 2,500 mL/day in most adults. Teach your patient how much fluid intake he or she should have and why it is important.

If your patient is not drinking adequately, do not simply chart the lack of fluid intake; find out what the patient likes to drink and then provide an adequate supply of those fluids. Water intake should be encouraged, but other fluids such as coffee, tea, carbonated drinks, juice, sports drinks, flavored drink mixes, milk, flavored bottled water, and broth are acceptable replacements if the patient fails to drink adequate amounts of water. If the patient is debilitated, it will be your responsibility not only to encourage fluids, but to provide the patient with whatever assistance is required to drink the fluids. This may include use of a straw, assisting to a sitting position, or holding the cup for the patient. Debilitated, elderly, or confused patients may not be able to drink more than a few sips at a time, thus making it necessary to provide a drink every 15 to 20 minutes in an attempt to provide adequate intake. This task may be delegated to the CNA or UAP.

It is important that the patient also has adequate fiber intake, generally 25 to 35 g/day. Encourage fiber intake as allowed by the patient's diet order, including whole grains, fruits, and vegetables. Again, you must educate your patient as to why fiber is needed and how much is required for normal bowel elimination. A patient is generally more compliant when he or she understands the purpose of an intervention. Box 30-2 lists foods high in fiber.

Privacy

Be certain to provide patient privacy for elimination. As a nurse, you will become comfortable with and view elimination as a natural function and see no reason for embarrassment. However, that probably does not reflect how your patient will feel about it. It will be helpful for you to consider how you would feel if you had to expel a bowel movement in the presence of a stranger. Would you want to do this? Or would you prefer privacy? There are some individuals who believe they are unable to have a bowel movement in the presence of family, let alone a stranger. Some patients will do everything possible to prevent bowel elimination except when they are in the privacy of their own home.

If the patient requires use of a bedpan or bedside commode (BSC), shut the room door, pull the privacy curtain, place the bedpan or assist the patient to the BSC, provide toilet tissue, and wait outside the curtain if at all possible. If the patient can be left unattended, leave the room and tell the patient you will return in a few minutes. Make certain the patient can reach the call light before you leave. If you must stay in the room, try to be as unobtrusive as you can.

Box 30-2

Foods High in Fiber Content

Adequate fiber intake is important for healthy bowel elimination. Processed foods have little or no fiber. Some fruits and vegetables, especially raw, have high fiber content, as listed below:

- Apples, unpeeled
- Artichokes
- Beans
- Blueberries
- Broccoli
- Cabbage
- Carrots
- Cauliflower
- Cherries
- Corn
- Dried fruits
- Flaxseed
- Legumes
- Nuts
- Oatmeal
- Oranges
- Pears, unpeeled
- Plums
- Popcorn
- Prunes
- Raisins
- Raspberries
- Strawberries
- Sunflower seeds
- Whole-grain breads
- Whole-grain cereals
- Whole-grain flour

If the patient is allowed bathroom privileges (BRP) and it is safe for him or her to sit unassisted in the bathroom, make certain the call light is within reach and the patient knows how to use it, and close the bathroom door as well as the room door before leaving the patient's room. If you must remain present for standby assistance, make yourself busy straightening the room and making the bed. Provide whatever privacy can be safely afforded.

Privacy should also be provided when discussing elimination with the patient. Avoid asking a patient in the presence of visitors if he or she has had a bowel movement or to describe the characteristics of the stool.

Positioning

The most comfortable and natural position for bowel elimination is the upright sitting position. If the patient is allowed to ambulate or have BRP, assist the patient to the bathroom. If the patient is unable to walk that far, use a BSC. When the patient is restricted to the bed, use a bedpan and place the patient in high or semi-Fowler's position. For details regarding placement of a bedpan, refer to Chapter 31.

Management of Alterations in Elimination

It is important to remember to use universal precautions when contact with feces is possible. This means that you must wear gloves when changing the linens of an incontinent patient, emptying a bedpan or bedside commode, removing a fecal impaction, obtaining a stool specimen, administering an enema, providing colostomy care, or performing any other nursing care that may place you in direct contact with feces.

Management of constipation, diarrhea, and fecal incontinence may be as simple as educating the patient and convincing him or her to improve dietary and fluid intake habits. If this does not correct the problem or the patient is unwilling to make these changes, further intervention may be necessary.

Dietary Considerations

While constipation is the condition most commonly managed by altering dietary intake, sometimes diarrhea can also be treated with certain foods and fluids. Many physicians will order clear liquid diets during the first 24 hours of diarrhea caused by infection and inflammation. The clear liquids help to decrease the GI tract's digestive workload, allowing it time to rest and heal. Decaffeinated green or black teas, which contain tannin, and herbal teas such as chamomile may be used to soothe an inflamed colon and slow peristalsis. Sports drinks containing electrolytes, such as Gatorade, help to replace fluid and electrolytes lost with diarrhea. Pedialyte is an over-the-counter electrolyte replacement drink designed for infants and small children. (Refer to Chapter 29 for further details regarding fluid and electrolyte balance.) During the first 24 hours, avoid serving extremely hot or cold liquids, both of which can increase peristalsis. During this time, fluids are best tolerated if you serve them at room temperature or only slightly warmed or cooled.

If diarrhea lasts longer than 24 to 36 hours, full liquids along with any type of *cooked* fruits and vegetables, such as applesauce or carrots, may be given. Apple pectin is a common treatment for diarrhea. It is the primary ingredient found in over-the-counter antidiarrheal medications such as Kaopectate. *Safety: Avoid serving apple juice because it will increase diarrhea.* Aged cheeses and bananas are also considered therapeutic dietary additions for patients with diarrhea. Mashed bananas, applesauce, and cooked carrots are popular choices for infants with diarrhea. When diarrhea is due to loss of normal flora, yogurt containing active bacteria helps to replace normal flora and promote healing. It can also be used concurrently while taking prescribed antibiotics to prevent the loss of normal flora.

Medications

Various medications are available to treat diarrhea and constipation. Many are over the counter and others are only obtained by prescription. Medications to treat diarrhea may coat the mucous membranes of the bowel, inhibit peristalsis, or treat the disease or infectious process causing the diarrhea. Some medications stimulate absorption of intestinal fluids into the bloodstream and actually bind the toxins of the diarrhea-causing microorganisms so they are removed during defecation. This not only helps to slow the diarrhea but also helps in prevention of dehydration.

Lactobacillus acidophilus is a supplement that comes in several forms and can be used to replace normal flora or used concurrently with antibiotics to prevent loss of normal flora. It is also used as treatment for diarrhea caused by a virus known as *Rotavirus*.

Medications for constipation may work by directly stimulating peristalsis, softening the stool, or adding bulk to the stool. Stool softeners and those that add bulk are safer than the laxatives that stimulate peristalsis. Patients may have already attempted to treat themselves with medications at home, so it is important to collect information regarding medications used at home, from either the patient or family members.

Enemas

When medication does not relieve the problem of constipation, the physician may order an *enema,* the instillation of a solution into the colon via the rectum, to relieve the problem. There are several types of enemas, and each has a specific purpose. Water temperature of enemas should be between 105°F and 110°F to avoid burning the intestinal mucosa. Use a bath thermometer to check water temperature. If one is not available, pour a small amount of the solution on the inner side of your bare wrist. It should feel warm but never hot. Water that is too cold will cause abdominal cramping and may restrict the patient's ability to retain the water. Figure 30-1 shows examples of enema administration equipment and supplies.

Always preserve the patient's modesty and provide privacy for administration and elimination of an enema. Before beginning actual administration of the enema, position the patient in a Sims' or left lateral side-lying position (Fig. 30-2). Skill 30-1 (page 698) provides the steps for administering an enema.

Safety: Never attempt insertion of the tip of the tubing into the patient's rectum while the patient is in a sitting position, as on the toilet. The angle of the natural curve of the rectum and sigmoid colon changes when sitting. This can cause the tip of the tubing to scrape the intestinal wall, possibly damaging the mucosal lining, and increases risk of perforating the intestinal wall.

The normal length to insert the tip of the tubing is 3 to 4 inches for administration of a cleansing enema to an adult. This generally allows instillation of enema solution into the

Figure 30-2 Patient positioned on left side in left-lateral position for enema administration. Note the internal diagram of the colon.

rectum, sigmoid colon, and descending colon for lower bowel cleansing. However, in certain cases the physician may order what is termed a *high enema* as opposed to a normal *low enema.* When the physician feels that more of the colon beyond the sigmoid colon needs to be cleansed, he or she may order the higher instillation. The procedure is initiated the same way, with the patient lying on the left side. After instillation of about half of the enema solution, reposition the patient first to a supine position and then to the right lateral side-lying position to administer the remaining solution. The repositioning aids the flow of water backward through the intestinal tract. It flows from the rectum into the sigmoid colon, then into the descending colon, and finally into the transverse portion of the colon.

Cleansing Enemas

Cleansing enemas are most commonly administered to relieve constipation, but are also used to empty and cleanse the bowel prior to surgery or tests. Several solutions may be used for cleansing enemas. Large volumes of solution, 500 to 1,000 mL for an adult, are introduced into the rectum, distending the bowel, which stimulates peristalsis and rapid evacuation of the bowel. Small-volume enemas, less than 250 mL and usually only 90 to 120 mL, are easier and quicker to administer, as well as being less tiring for the patient.

For preparation for colon surgery, colon visualization, or radiological tests, the physician may order *enemas til clear.* This means that enemas are administered until the expelled solution no longer contains feces and is relatively clear, but within a limit of three 1,000-mL enemas. In other words, avoid giving more than three large-volume enemas consecutively. Administering more than three can result in excessive patient fatigue and excessive irritation of the mucosal lining of the intestine.

Types of Solution

Numerous types of solutions are used in administration of enemas. The most commonly used types include tap water, normal saline, soapsuds, and commercially prepackaged small-volume oil or sodium phosphate solutions. Table 30-2 presents types of solutions and volumes.

Figure 30-1 An enema bag, commercially prepared enemas, and an enema bucket with supplies for administration.

Table 30-2 Types and Volume of Solution Used in Enemas

Solution Type	Volume for Adults	Purpose	Restrictions for Use
Tap water	500–1,000 mL	Cleansing	Hypotonic. *Safety: Do NOT use for infants, children, or patients with congestive heart failure.* Could result in fluid volume overload.
Normal saline (NS) (0.9%)	500–1,000 mL	Cleansing	Isotonic. Safe for use in children and congestive heart failure patients. Infants: use 50–150 mL Toddlers: use 150–350 mL School-age children: use 350–500 mL
Soapsuds (use castile soap only)	Add to tap water or NS at a ratio of 5 mL soapsuds per 1,000 mL	Cleansing	*Safety: Mix castile soap in saline, not tap water, for infants, children, or patients with congestive heart failure.*
Hypertonic sodium phosphate	120 mL	Cleansing	Normally used only for adults.
Oil retention	120 mL	Softens stool	Normally used only for adults.

Soapsuds

Soapsuds (SS) enemas work not only through distention of the intestine, but also by irritating the walls of the intestine, providing further stimulus to increase peristalsis. Only pure castile soap or a soap designated by facility policy should be used. Other soaps are too harsh and can cause damage to the mucosal lining of the intestines. An SS enema should be mixed using a concentration of 5 mL of pure castile soap for each 1,000 mL of water or normal saline.

Tap Water

Tap water is hypotonic, which allows a portion of the instilled solution to diffuse from the intestinal lumen into the interstitial spaces and vascular system, putting infants, children, and patients with fluid balance issues, such as congestive heart failure, at risk for fluid volume overload. Therefore, tap water should only be used in adults without fluid volume problems.

Normal Saline (0.9% Sodium Chloride in Water)

Normal saline is isotonic and is the only solution considered safe to administer to infants, children, and patients with congestive heart failure or any other condition that places the patient at risk for fluid volume overload. (Refer to Chapter 29 for further details regarding tonicity of fluids.)

Hypertonic Solutions

Hypertonic solutions may be used in small volumes for adults. The most commonly used are commercially prepackaged and may be known as a sodium phosphate enema or Fleet enema. These commercially prepackaged enemas require no preparation, are easy and quick to administer, and are less uncomfortable and fatiguing for the patient

(Fig. 30-3). Hypertonic solutions are rarely used for large-volume enemas, because the high tonicity of the solution can pull water from the interstitial spaces and cells into the colon for expulsion. This increases the risk of fluid and electrolyte imbalances such as dehydration.

Some physicians may order a special type of enema, such as a *milk and molasses enema,* another type of hypertonic solution that is sometimes used for persistent constipation and impaction removal. It is an extremely effective, but quite messy enema to administer. Follow the facility policy for mixing and administering this type of enema.

Oil Retention Enemas

Oil retention enemas are administered to soften the hard stool of an impaction so that it can be removed more easily and with less discomfort for the patient. A smaller volume,

Figure 30-3 Administration of a commercially prepackaged enema.

usually 90 to 120 mL, should be instilled approximately an hour prior to removal of the impaction to allow sufficient time for the oil to be effective.

Medicating Enemas

Medication may be given by way of an enema as well. A steroid may be given to decrease the inflammation of the walls of the rectum and colon. A medicated enema may also be given for the purpose of exchanging substances. An example of this type is a **Kayexalate enema**, administered for the purpose of lowering a very high potassium level. The Kayexalate is instilled and retained for a time, allowing potassium to be pulled from the bloodstream and absorbed into the Kayexalate. Then, when the enema is expelled, excess potassium is removed. Refer to facility policy for administration instructions.

Return Flow Enemas

A *return flow enema,* also known as a *Harris flush,* is administered for the purpose of removing flatus, or gas, and not specifically for the removal of stool as with other types of enemas. When a Harris flush is ordered by the physician, you will prepare a tap-water or saline enema and instill a small amount of solution, usually 100 to 200 mL, into the patient's rectum. The enema container is then lowered below the level of the rectum, allowing flatus to siphon back through the same tube and be expelled into the enema container in the form of gas bubbles. This process is continued until there is no longer any gas returned. In a patient who is postsurgery, sterile water is used. You may also hear this type of enema referred to as a **siphon enema**.

Knowledge Connection
Which enema solution is safe for administration to infants and patients with congestive heart failure? What is the normal enema volume for a cleansing enema for an adult? A 3-year-old child?

Contraindications to Enemas

There are numerous conditions that may preclude you from administering an enema. It is your responsibility to assess for these conditions. Contraindications may include:

• Rectal surgery
• Severe bleeding hemorrhoids
• Ulcerative colitis or Crohn's disease
• Rectal fissure
• Rectal cancer
• Excessive bleeding potential due to disease or medication
• Certain heart conditions such as myocardial infarction or unstable angina

Complications of Enemas

Enemas are normally viewed as simple procedures not requiring much knowledge or experience, but this is a myth. Administration of an enema can have serious consequences

if the person administering it is not aware of the potential risks. Two serious complications include the vagal response and perforation of the intestinal wall, which can result in hemorrhage and infection.

Vagal Response

Anytime you insert an enema tube into a patient's rectum, there is the possibility of stimulating the vagus nerve, which innervates not only the GI tract, but also the heart and bronchioles. *Safety: When stimulated, it can drop the heart rate as low as 30 to 40 beats per minute (bpm) and cause constriction of the bronchioles of the lungs. As you know, a heart rate of 30 or 40 bpm is insufficient to support adequate blood pressure and circulation for longer than a few minutes, making it important to know the signs and symptoms to watch for (Box 30-3).*

If the patient complains of or exhibits any of these symptoms, you should immediately:

• Stop the enema.
• Remove the tube from the rectum.
• Place the patient in the supine position.
• Assess pulse rate, skin color, and whether or not the patient is diaphoretic.
• Call for immediate assistance, but do not leave the patient.
• If the pulse rate is below 60 bpm, place the patient in the shock position, with the head lower than the feet.
• Assess blood pressure as soon as a cuff is available.
• Supply oxygen if needed.

Box 30-3

Signs and Symptoms of Vagus Nerve Stimulation

During administration of enemas and impaction removal, you should constantly assess the patient for the following signs and symptoms of vagus nerve stimulation:

Symptoms
• Complaints of:
  • Chest pain
  • Chest heaviness or pressure
  • Shortness of breath or inability to breathe
  • Dizziness
  • Feeling like he or she is going to faint
  • Nausea

Signs
• Pallor
• Clammy skin
• Pulse rate under 60 bpm
  Please note that the patient does not have to exhibit all of the signs and symptoms; even one sign or symptom requires you to **stop administering the enema or removing the impaction** until it is established whether or not the patient can tolerate resumption of the enema.

The patient will usually recover quickly, increasing the heart rate back to the normal range and raising the blood pressure, but you must be prepared to react quickly and correctly if recovery is not immediate. When necessary, the drug of choice for raising the heart rate is *atropine.*

Perforation of the Colon

Always be gentle when inserting an enema tube; never force it or insert it further than 4 to 6 inches. You should direct the tip of the tubing toward the umbilicus to follow the natural direction of the sigmoid colon. If you are not careful, it is possible to *perforate,* or go through, the intestinal wall. This can result in introduction of bacteria into the sterile peritoneal cavity, bleeding, and even hemorrhage. Again, never force the enema tubing if you meet resistance.

Knowledge Connection

Explain what to do if signs or symptoms of a vagal response are noted during enema administration. What can you do to reduce risk of intestinal perforation?

Supervision/Delegation Connection

Delegating Administration of an Enema

There will be times when you will need to delegate administration of an enema to a UAP or a CNA. Because you are held responsible for safe and competent administration of the enema, it is very important that you can verify that the UAP or CNA has received specific training and is competent in performance of the skill. The training should be documented in writing for your best protection. It is your responsibility to assess the patient's condition and determine whether it is safe to have the UAP or CNA perform the skill. Make certain that the UAP or CNA clearly understands the vagal response, including the signs and symptoms and the actions to take if signs or symptoms are noted, and specifically to notify you immediately. It is also your responsibility to determine that the UAP or CNA understands appropriate steps to take to decrease the risk of perforating the intestinal wall.

Perineal Care

If the patient has diarrhea or is incontinent of stool, it is very important that you provide good perineal care to prevent the complications caused by feces on the skin. Feces are damaging to the skin and will result in irritation and excoriation if allowed to stay on the skin for extended periods of time. This destruction of skin results in loss of the body's first line of protection from infection.

Cleanse the skin around the perineum, rectum, and buttocks after each incontinent stool, with soap and warm water. Rinse the skin well and pat dry. If incontinence of stool is frequent, it may be necessary to add the protection of a topical barrier cream to help prevent skin breakdown.

Obtaining a Stool Specimen

It will be your responsibility to collect a stool specimen when one is needed for testing. Skill 30-2 (page 700) shows the steps for collecting a stool specimen. Stool samples may be tested for the presence of parasites, parasitic eggs called ova, blood, and microorganisms. As required by universal precautions, you will need to wear examination gloves while collecting the specimen. The stool specimen must be collected in a clean bedpan, a specimen pan that sits under the rim of the toilet, or a clean bedside commode. For an alert and oriented patient, you will need to explain the procedure in order to elicit his or her cooperation in the collection. It is important to use terminology that the patient understands when giving instructions about collecting the stool specimen. Include step-by-step instructions on how to collect the specimen, including washing of the hands. If the patient is an infant or is incontinent, collect the stool specimen directly from the diaper or incontinence brief.

If you are instructing a nonhospitalized patient in how to obtain a stool specimen for occult blood testing, it is important to educate the patient regarding not only how to collect the specimen, but dietary restrictions that should be followed for 1 to 2 days prior to specimen collection. Box 30-4 provides a list of specific food, medications, and supplements to avoid.

Depending on facility policy, you may be the one to perform the test for hidden, or occult, blood while other tests will be performed by laboratory personnel. The test for blood may be referred to as a hemacult test, a guaiac test, or simply as an occult blood test and can be performed in the patient's bathroom. For further details, refer to Skill 30-3 (page 701).

Digital Removal of Impaction

When your patient has a fecal impaction, it usually requires digital removal before administering a cleansing enema. This involves insertion of the gloved index finger into the

Box 30-4

Substances to Avoid Prior to Stool Occult Blood Testing

Certain foods and medications can cause *false-positive* results and should be avoided for 48 hours pretesting. Anything containing red dye or food coloring should also be avoided.

- Alcohol
- Antacids
- Antidiarrheals
- Gastric irritants such as NSAIDs or steroids
- Red jello
- Red meats
- Red popsicles
- Vegetables and fruits high in peroxidase, an enzyme found in apples, bananas, grapes, and broccoli
- Vitamin C and iron supplements

anus to manually break the fecal mass into small pieces and remove them from the rectum. This procedure may be embarrassing as well as painful for the patient. To make the procedure less uncomfortable, it is helpful to instill an oil retention enema about 1 hour prior to digital removal. Some patients may even require mild pain medication to better tolerate the procedure. Skill 30-4 (page 702) presents the steps required to remove a fecal impaction.

There are several things you must consider before actually removing the impaction. First, review the facility's policy and procedures to determine which personnel are permitted to perform the procedure and whether or not a physician's order is required. Most hospitals do not allow delegation of this procedure to a CNA or UAP. Next, review the patient's medical record for all of the patient's diagnoses. The same conditions that may contraindicate an enema may also contraindicate digital removal of impaction by the nurse. Once you have determined it is safe, you may proceed. Remember to monitor for signs of vagal nerve stimulation, just as you do with enema administration.

Treatment of Fecal Incontinence

If the incontinence is caused by diarrhea, antidiarrhea medications may be ordered. If it is caused by seepage of stool around an impaction, the physician may order removal of the impaction, enemas, and possibly stool softeners.

When incontinence is chronic, bowel training may be initiated. The goal of bowel training is to establish regular bowel elimination. The patient should be placed on the commode or bedpan upon arising daily, after each meal, and anytime the patient says that his or her bowels have to move. Maintain a record of the patient's bowel activity. Once the time of day for the patient's normal bowel movement has been established, attempts are made to trigger defecation at that time. When a pattern of bowel elimination cannot be established, it is recommended to attempt to train the bowels to move within 1 hour after breakfast. This is an ideal time because the first meal of the day stimulates the strong peristalsis of the defecation reflex. A bowel training program involves ensuring adequate dietary intake of fiber from whole wheat products, fruits, and vegetables; adequate intake of water and other fluids; and physical exercise. Because exercising and ingestion of food and fluids requires patient participation, it is important to have the patient's agreement and cooperation. Bowel training is a long and involved process, but the return of a patient's self-esteem makes it worth the effort.

Patients with fecal incontinence of uncontrolled diarrhea stools are at risk for skin breakdown. Topical barrier creams help to prevent excoriation, but if it is not possible to keep the patient clean and dry most of the time, a fecal incontinence pouch may be the best choice to protect skin integrity. Generally the plastic bag–like pouch has a peel-off backing around its opening. A moisture-proof barrier ring is generally used to attach the pouch to the patient's skin. The barrier ring also has a peel-off backing that must be removed before applying the ring to the skin around the anus. The peel-off backing on the pouch opening is then removed so that the pouch can be adhered to the barrier ring. Apply carefully, ensuring that there are no leaks. Once the pouch is secured, fecal material drains into the pouch, which should be emptied before it is half full to prevent spills. Most systems are designed to be changed every 2 to 3 days unless a leak requires the pouch to be changed earlier.

Whether or not the incontinence can be resolved, it is so important that you not only be professional and kind, but try to add an extra dose of compassion when you care for these patients. Teach nursing staff members and the patient's family members to avoid criticism or judgmental comments that may be hurtful. Teach them to be cautious in nonverbal communication as well, to avoid actions or body language that may imply that the patient is to blame or that cleaning the patient is offensive. That includes maintaining a neutral or even pleasant facial expression. Never refer to the pads used to protect the patient from fecal waste as *diapers,* as this can be traumatizing to the adult patient. It is best to call them incontinence pads or briefs, or by a brand name such as Depends. Help to preserve your patient's dignity. Remember to consider: How would you feel if you were in the patient's situation?

Knowledge Connection

Summarize perineal care and its importance. What risks exist when you digitally remove an impaction? Explain possible methods for managing fecal incontinence.

Alternative Bowel Elimination

Certain disease processes and injuries can necessitate that a patient be provided with an alternative form of bowel elimination by surgically creating a bowel diversion. A bowel diversion is the redirection of the contents of the small or large intestine through an alternate exit site made through the abdominal wall. The fecal material, known as effluent, empties into an ostomy appliance, otherwise known as a bag or pouch. A need for a bowel diversion may be due to:

- Cancerous tumor
- Infarcted area in which the bowel walls have become ischemic and died
- Disease process such as Crohn's disease
- Ruptured diverticulum
- Ulcerative colitis
- Traumatic abdominal injury

When the diversion is brought to the outside of the body through the abdominal wall, the new opening is called an *ostomy* and the mouth of the ostomy is called a **stoma**. The name of the ostomy is determined by the area of the bowel that is brought out through the abdominal wall. If a part of the small intestine, such as the ileum, is used, it is called an **ileostomy**. If a part of the large intestine, or colon, is used, it is called a **colostomy**. A colostomy is further identified based on the section of the large bowel utilized to form the stoma: ascending, transverse, descending, or sigmoid colon (Fig. 30-4).

Colostomy

A colostomy stoma will have a single opening, termed a *single-barreled* or *end stoma*, if the distal colon is permanently removed, as with cancer of the descending or sigmoid colon. When a colostomy is performed due to severe inflammatory disease, such as Crohn's disease, the distal portion of the colon may not need to be removed, only allowed time to rest and heal the diseased portion. In this situation, the colon may be completely incised, or cut into two pieces. Both ends of the dissected colon are brought to the surface and two stomas are formed, a proximal and a distal stoma. This is known as a *double-barreled* colostomy stoma (see Fig. 30-4c). The stool will empty from the proximal stoma, and the distal stoma leads to the portion of the colon that is rested and allowed to heal. The only drainage from the distal stoma will be mucus produced by the mucosal lining of the intestine. The rectum and anus remain intact. After the distal portion of the colon heals, the loop is *anastomosed,* or surgically reconnected, and placed back into the abdominal cavity, and the abdominal wall closed. Normal elimination is then restored.

Another type of stoma seen in treatment of inflammatory disease is the *loop stoma.* A loop of bowel, usually the transverse colon, is brought to the surface of the abdomen. A plastic rod known as a *bridge* or *stay* is positioned under the loop of colon to keep it outside the body, and it is stitched to the abdominal wall. A slit is made in the loop and the colon is cuffed back on itself and also stitched to the abdominal wall. Stool will be expelled from the proximal opening. Occasionally the stool will seep from the proximal stoma into the distal stoma, and the patient will still have small amounts of stool coming from the rectum.

Stool Consistency

The stool consistency will depend upon the section of the colon in which the stoma is located. If a colostomy is created in the ascending colon, effluent will be liquid to mushy with a foul odor. A right transverse stoma will expel mushy to semiformed effluent, while feces from a left transverse stoma will be semiformed to soft in consistency. A stoma created in the descending or sigmoid colon will produce soft to hard formed stools.

Ileostomy

A diversion created in the ileum portion of the small intestine is known as an ileostomy (see Fig. 30-4e). This type of stoma is created at the end of the ileum due to removal of the large colon. Effluent from an ileostomy is liquid, as the majority of the water is not absorbed until it reaches the large bowel. The expulsion of effluent is continual, requiring constant wearing of a pouch. The effluent contains enzymes, making it corrosive to the skin surrounding the stoma. A loss of a large amount of ileostomy drainage can lead to symptoms of malnutrition and electrolyte imbalance.

Kock Pouch

A *Kock pouch* is a diversion that uses the terminal portion of the ileum to form an internal pouch, or reservoir, to collect and store the effluent prior to evacuation from the body. A flap is formed that closes the reservoir, preventing leakage of the thin and watery effluent. Several times a day, the patient inserts a catheter to drain the reservoir. This type of stoma is also known as a *continent ostomy* because the patient has control over when the reservoir is drained. There are also several modified versions of the Kock pouch.

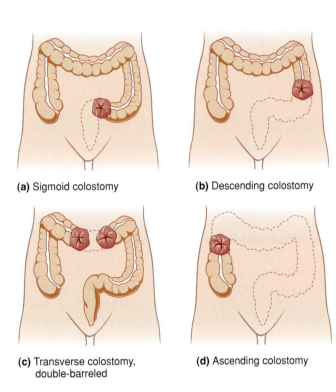

(a) Sigmoid colostomy

(b) Descending colostomy

(c) Transverse colostomy, double-barreled

(d) Ascending colostomy

(e) Ileostomy

Figure 30-4 Locations of bowel diversion ostomies: (a) Sigmoid colostomy. (b) Descending colostomy. (c) Transverse colostomy, double-barreled. (d) Ascending colostomy. (e) Ileostomy.

Contrast single-barrel, double-barrel, and loop stomas. Describe how an ileostomy is different from a colostomy located in the descending colon. Explain what a Kock pouch is.

Nursing Care of Ostomies

Many hospitals are now utilizing nurses who have been specially trained to provide ostomy care. These enterostomal therapy nurses not only provide direct patient care and teaching, but also offer encouragement and emotional support, introduce the patient to ostomy support groups, serve as a resource person regarding different types of ostomy supplies, and serve as patient advocates. Their goal is to assist the patient to return to a normal life. However, even if ostomy nurses are available in your facility, it is still necessary that you are able to assess and care for the patient with an ostomy. The ostomy nurse may not be available 24 hours a day, 7 days a week.

As with all nursing care, care of an ostomy begins with assessment or collection of data. Begin with the subjective data:

• What was the reason for the ostomy?
• When was the ostomy performed?
• What type of ostomy is it?
• What type of appliance, or ostomy bag, is in use?
• When was the appliance last emptied or changed?
• How much of the care is the patient able to perform, if any?

Once subjective data have been obtained, you will want to assess the patient and the stoma for objective data, noting:

• Contour and color of the abdomen, scars, and the surgical site; the presence of a dressing, sutures/clamps, and drains
• Appearance of the stoma, including size and edema, color, moisture level
• Appearance of *peristomal skin,* the skin surrounding the stoma
• Characteristics of the effluent/fecal drainage
• Intactness of the faceplate and fullness of the appliance bag

If the ostomy is new, assess the patient for postoperative pain as well as how the patient is dealing with the new stoma. Does the patient look at the new stoma or avert his or her eyes? Does the patient make eye contact with you? Ask questions regarding care of the stoma? Verbalize desire to learn about stoma care? This can be a blow to a patient's self-esteem, and the patient's attitude may depend largely upon your reactions during provision of nursing care. Be careful to exhibit acceptance.

A new stoma should be pink to red, shiny, and moist (Fig. 30-5). Pallor, cyanosis, or a dusky color indicates impaired blood supply, while black depicts necrosis. Any impairment of blood supply should be reported to the physician

and may require surgical intervention. Initially, there may be edema of the stoma, but the stoma should shrink to a small size over the first 2 to 3 weeks postsurgery. An established stoma will be smaller, pinkish-red, and drier in appearance. The peristomal skin should be free of irritation, excoriation, and erythema.

What assessments should be made for a new colostomy? What abnormal findings would require reporting to the physician?

Applying an Appliance

Ostomy appliances come in different sizes. To determine the correct size flange and opening on the ostomy bag to use, the stoma must be measured. The stoma size is determined using a stoma measuring device made of card stock. The card has different sizes of holes cut out, each labeled with its corresponding size. The measuring device is held to the stoma to determine the size that best fits the stoma. The correct size will fit around the stoma and allow only $\frac{1}{8}$ to $\frac{1}{4}$ inch of peristomal skin to show (Fig. 30-6). Once the correct size has been determined, it is used to select the correct size flange on the ostomy bag.

Ostomy appliances also come in different types (Fig. 30-7). Some appliances are designed as a one-piece

Figure 30-5   This healthy stoma is shiny, moist, and red.

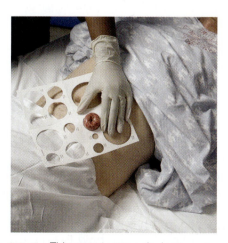

Figure 30-6   This nurse uses a device to measure the stoma size.

Figure 30-7 Ostomy supplies.

unit that has an attached adhesive disk that applies directly to the patient's abdomen after peeling the protective backing off the adhesive disk. Others are designed as two-piece units; the bag attaches to an adhesive disk called a *wafer faceplate* that adheres to the abdomen. The bag flange snaps onto the plastic flange on the wafer faceplate, somewhat like Tupperware lids attach. The faceplate is changed every 3 to 5 days or sooner if the adhesive backing begins to loosen from the skin. Once the adhesive on the faceplate begins to lose contact with the skin, it allows effluent to leak underneath the faceplate, which can cause severe excoriation of the skin. If leakage continues unheeded, infection and further ulceration of tissue can occur.

The ostomy appliance bag should be emptied when one-third to one-half full to prevent leakage and odor. Most bags have a drain located on the bottom edge of the bag that can be opened to empty the bag. Some patients prefer to remove the bag and apply a new one, while yet others prefer to empty the bag, rinse it in cool water, dry it, and reapply. Ostomy supplies are generally expensive, making it difficult for some patients to afford them. This may limit how often the patient is willing to apply new bags. For further details regarding changing an ostomy appliance, refer to Skill 30-5 (page 703).

Skin Care

When applying or changing an appliance, assess the stoma and the skin around it to make certain there is no irritation, excoriation, or ulceration. Then use a soft washcloth, warm water, and mild soap to wash the stoma and skin, rinse thoroughly, and pat dry. Numerous products are available for use to help protect the skin around the stoma. An example is a protective barrier cream that may be used around the stoma to protect the small area of skin that shows after the appliance is in place.

Irrigating a Colostomy

A colostomy irrigation is similar to an enema. Colostomies may be irrigated to evacuate stool due to constipation, or irrigation may be used postoperatively for stomas located in the descending or sigmoid colon. When irrigating a descending or sigmoid colostomy, the goal is to train the ostomy to evacuate at the same time each day. Because the stool is formed, it is possible to train the bowel to evacuate in the morning right after breakfast when peristalsis is naturally stimulated by eating breakfast. If the bowel is trained to move early in the day, some patients even find it unnecessary to wear an appliance for the remainder of the day, providing the patient with a great sense of control. Skill 30-6 (page 705) provides more information on colostomy irrigation.

> ### Knowledge Connection
> How do you determine which size of colostomy bag opening would best meet the patient's needs? How often should an appliance bag be emptied? How often should you change the faceplate and appliance bag? Explain two purposes for colostomy irrigation.

Nursing Care Plan for a Patient With a New Colostomy of the Descending Colon

Your patient is a 39-year-old male who had severe ulcerative colitis that necessitated removal of the distal portion of his colon 1 day ago. He now has a permanent colostomy in the descending colon. He has refused to look at the stoma or drainage bag, but has verbalized that he knows that he will have to learn how to take care of the colostomy. He has a very supportive wife and two teenage sons.

Assessment

Your first step in planning care for a patient with a colostomy is to gather all available data, including physical assessment of the colostomy stoma. Begin by seeking the answers to these questions:

- Is the colostomy located in the ascending, transverse, descending, or sigmoid colon?
- How is the patient coping with the new colostomy? Has the patient looked at the stoma yet? Verbalized

Nursing Care Plan for a Patient With a New Colostomy of the Descending Colon (continued)

feelings about the new colostomy? Demonstrated interest in learning how to care for a colostomy? Is there a strong support system?
• What type of appliance is being utilized?
• What patient teaching has already been done?
• Has referral to a support group been made?

Now it is time to physically assess the patient, colostomy stoma, peristomal skin, and effluent characteristics, noting the following information:

• Does the patient make eye contact when you converse about the colostomy?
• Does the patient look at the colostomy and drainage bag while you are assessing them?
• What are the characteristics of the effluent? Color? Consistency? Amount? Odor?
• What does the stoma look like? Location? Color? Moist? Edematous? Bleeding?
• What size is it? Measure it with the stoma sizing card to determine the exact size of hole to cut in a faceplate when a new one is needed.
• What is the condition of the skin around the stoma? Is it intact? Excoriated? Erythematous? Blistered? Bleeding?
• Is there any pain or discomfort?
• Does the patient have any questions or concerns?

The data you collect tell you that the patient's stoma is still edematous and a reddish color. It is moist and shiny with a heavy coating of clear mucus. It is located on the left side of the abdomen where the left upper quadrant and left lower quadrant meet. The abdomen is fairly flat without fat folds or scarring near the stoma site. As you assess the stoma and effluent, you notice that the patient glances down at the stoma briefly a couple of times and then looks away. The rest of the time, he looks directly at you. The effluent is brown and semiformed with lots of mucus. The bag is about one-quarter full. A 1½-inch flanged colostomy bag with a drain in the bottom is currently in use and still fits appropriately, exposing only ⅛ inch of peristomal skin. The peristomal skin is intact, but slightly erythematous. There are no blisters or signs of bleeding. The patient acknowledges current incisional pain at a level of 7 on a scale of 1 to 10. He states that he has been trying to avoid asking for pain medication, because he does not like to take it. No patient teaching or referral to an ostomy support group has been done. Toward the end of your physical assessment, he asks you if the "thing" will always look this gross, and how a person ever overcomes the feelings of disgust when caring for the colostomy.

Nursing Diagnoses

Now that you have collected the data, you will need to analyze this information and determine what type of problems this patient actually has and what problems he seems to be at risk for developing. The process for determining these actual problems and potential problems involves reviewing the data you have learned about this particular patient during your assessment. Then you can determine the appropriate nursing diagnoses.

You are encouraged because the patient at least glanced at his stoma while you were performing the assessment. Having noted that he was looking at you most of the time, you were careful to make frequent eye contact with him, so that he was able to observe your level of comfort and acceptance while looking at his stoma. You were careful to avoid making any type of facial expression that could be interpreted as unpleasant, unaccepting, or disgusted. He also asked you about overcoming feelings of disgust when caring for the colostomy, indicating that he is able to express at least some feelings about the stoma. This may indicate that he is ready to ask for help in adjusting to the change in body image.

Though the skin integrity is impaired due to the new stoma, physical assessment showed that the stoma is red and edematous, as you would expect in a fresh stoma. There are no signs of infection or bleeding. The peristomal skin is intact but slightly pink.

The effluent is brown and mushy without form, with a moderate amount of clear mucus. Because the colostomy is located in the descending colon, you know that the effluent will become at least semiformed once the colon heals enough to absorb the extra water from the stool. You also expect the amount of mucus to decrease over the next 1 to 2 weeks as the inflammatory process of healing gradually comes to an end. The flange on the bag is the correct size for the stoma at this stage of edema, but you know that the stoma will continue to shrink with time and healing.

After reviewing your NANDA-I list of nursing diagnoses, you are able to determine that he has at least six nursing diagnoses:

• Impaired skin integrity
• Knowledge deficit
• Readiness for enhanced knowledge
• Disturbed body image
• Impaired comfort
• Impaired walking due to his discomfort

(care plan continues on page 694)

Nursing Care Plan for a Patient With a New Colostomy of the Descending Colon (continued)

Now you can begin planning how to care for these problems.

Planning

When planning what nursing interventions should be provided, you remember that not only are patients' needs different, but the interventions that will work best for each individual patient are different as well. You know that you will want to provide interventions that will best apply to this specific man.

You begin with his discomfort. When one is in pain, it is difficult to deal with an altered body image and next to impossible to learn something new. What pain medications are ordered for him? Are the medications working effectively? Has he been requesting pain medication at all? Reviewing his physician's orders, you find that he does have pain medications ordered. You also review the medication administration record and find that he has not had anything for pain since late on the day of surgery. When you ask him about it, he tells you that he does not like to take pain medications, that "only wimps need drugs for pain." He also tells you that he has not been out of bed since surgery. You explain to him that pain impedes or slows the healing process, and that it is important to relieve his pain so he can better deal with other aspects of his care, as well as to speed the healing process so he can go home as soon as possible.

Because you know that ambulation will not only help to increase his strength, stimulate circulation, prevent pneumonia and blood clots, and stimulate peristalsis, it will also help to work out the soreness, you plan to teach him why ambulation is so important. You also plan to make certain he ambulates in the hallway at least four times a day, gradually increasing the distance, and gets up in a chair for all meals.

You plan to document the erythema in his care plan and assess the surgical site and peristomal skin at least once per shift for signs of infection. To prevent further erythema and skin breakdown in the peristomal skin, you plan to clean the area with warm soap and water at least once per shift and make certain the colostomy bag is emptied as soon as it is one-third to one-half full, and to teach him to do the same.

Because the colostomy is new to both the patient and his wife, you plan to introduce them to the different supplies that are available as well as how to apply and change the ostomy appliance. You also plan to teach them how to irrigate the colostomy in an attempt to give the patient more control over the evacuation time of his bowels. Your hope is that he will be able to train the bowel to empty only once a day after breakfast, enabling the patient to go without an appliance bag during the day. This plays a key part in maintaining good self-esteem.

You know that he will need emotional support even after he is discharged, so you ask him if you may refer him to the local ostomy support group and schedule the first visit for the next day. While discussing the advantages of a support group, he tells you that his wife has voiced interest in learning how to care for his colostomy, and you encourage her participation. You plan to begin teaching him colostomy care as soon as the wife arrives this morning. You know that his acceptance of the change in his body image is greatly dependent upon his wife's acceptance as well as your reactions while caring for the colostomy.

Implementation

You are now at the stage of the nursing process to implement, or actually perform, the interventions that you have planned, as described in Table 30-3.

Evaluation

Once the interventions, or nursing actions, have been performed, you will want to evaluate whether they were effective or not (see Table 30-3). Did they accomplish what you intended? Did they help the patient's problem?

It seems that the patient and his wife are learning quickly how to care for his colostomy. They have met with a male member of the ostomy support group each day and plan to be active participants. The patient is exhibiting more acceptance and says that it is not nearly as gross as he had feared it would be. He expresses gratitude to you for introducing him to the support group and for being patient while he learned how to care for his new ostomy. Even though he is to be discharged in a day or two, you understand the patient will still have to deal with self-image disturbance as he and his wife are able to resume sexual activity; however, you feel confident that he will continue to adapt with the support of his wife and the support group.

Table 30-3   Care Plan for a Patient With a New Colostomy of the Descending Colon

Nursing Diagnosis: Impaired comfort, related to surgical incision, as evidenced by c/o pain and reluctance to get out of bed.
Expected Outcomes: Analgesic will effectively reduce pain below 4 within 90 minutes of administration of injection. Patient will ambulate in hall a minimum of three times per day by tomorrow. Patient will demonstrate proper splinting of abdomen when coughing and ambulating by tomorrow

Interventions	Evaluations
Use a pain scale of 1–10 to assess for pain and discomfort several times per shift; describing characteristics of pain.	Day 2: Initial c/o pain @ 7. Day 3: C/o pain @ 5. Day 5: C/o pain @ 4.
Encourage the patient to ask for pain medication before pain becomes severe enough to limit movement.	Day 2: Waited until pain was 7 before asking for meds, reminded to call earlier to try to keep pain below 4. Day 3: Called for med at level 5 pain.
Ambulate the patient in the hall at least 3–4 times/day, splinting his abdomen as needed.	Day 2: With assistance, ambulated 30 ft. in hallway twice and 50 ft. twice, tolerated with minimal increase in pain, states splinting helped; passed some flatus. Day 3: With standby assistance, ambulated 50 ft. once and 100 ft. three times. States he now feels much better after each ambulation.
Get the patient up in a chair for all meals and prn.	Day 2: Assisted to chair for all meals, tolerated w/o complaints. Ambulated w/ assist in room. Day 3: To chair w/ standby assistance. Tolerated w/o complaint. Then amb in hall twice w/o assistance. Day 5: Gets up for meals and walks ad lib without assistance or prompting

Nursing Diagnosis: Impaired skin integrity, related to surgical procedure, as evidenced by abdominal incision.
Expected Outcomes: Stoma will remain pink and moist until discharge. Edema will begin to decrease within 2 days.

Interventions	Evaluations
Assess the stoma for color, moisture, edema, and size daily on the 7/3 shift.	Day 2: Red, moist, lots of mucus, moderate edema, measures 1¼ in. diameter. Day 3: Red, moist, lots mucus, decreasing edema, 1¼ in. diameter. Day 5: Healing, pinkish-red, moist, less mucus today, diameter is 1¹⁄₁₆ in. Day 6: Pinkish red, moist, less mucus, 1 in. diameter.
Assess peristomal skin for erythema, edema, and intactness of skin at least once per shift.	Day 2: Slight erythema, no edema, skin intact. Day 3: Slight erythema, no edema, skin intact. Day 5: No erythema or edema, skin intact.
Gently cleanse the stoma and peristomal skin each time the appliance bag is emptied and at least once per shift if the bag does not have to be emptied.	Day 2: Cleansed 3 times on 7/3. Day 3: Cleansed 4 times on 7/3. Day 5: Cleansed once on 7/3.
Empty the appliance bag when ⅓ to ½ full to prevent constant contact of stool on skin.	Day 2: Emptied 3 times on 7/3. Day 3: He emptied bag twice, emptied twice by nurse. Day 5: Emptied once on 7/3.

(table continues on page 696)

Table 30-3 **Care Plan for a Patient With a New Colostomy of the Descending Colon** (continued)

Nursing Diagnosis: Knowledge deficit, related to new colostomy and care, as evidenced by questions regarding how to care for colostomy

Expected Outcomes: Verbalizes understanding of basic ostomy care within 3 days; correctly demonstrates ostomy irrigation within 4 days; empties ostomy bag without assistance by 4th day.

Interventions	Evaluations
Determine the patient's baseline of knowledge regarding normal bowel anatomy and physiology (A&P) and his new colostomy's function.	Day 2: No knowledge of normal bowel A&P or colostomy function.
Determine the patient's baseline of knowledge regarding care of a colostomy.	Day 2: No knowledge.
Determine teaching methods the patient prefers: verbal, written, video, or hands-on. Prepare an appropriate plan.	States he likes to listen to verbal explanation while observing hands-on demonstration. Does not like learning from video or written material.

Nursing Diagnosis: Readiness for enhanced knowledge, related to self-care of colostomy, as evidenced by asking nurses questions regarding self-care

Expected Outcomes: Both patient and wife will attend teaching sessions as scheduled; will be able to verbally explain the purpose of and how to care for ostomy by day 3; will correctly demonstrate changing appliance by day 3 and irrigation by day 5.

Interventions	Evaluations
Arrange times when the patient and wife can both be present for teaching sessions, avoiding late evenings when the patient may be too fatigued to learn.	Wife plans to be here each morning @ 900 a.m. for teaching. Both prefer 2–3 short sessions/day rather than 1 longer session.
Present teaching in segments to avoid overwhelming the patient or wife. a. Colostomy structure and function b. Availability of different type supplies c. How to apply and change appliance d. Stoma/skin cleansing and care e. Purpose of and how to perform colostomy irrigation Demonstrate each aspect of the colostomy while verbally explaining what you are doing, allowing the patient and wife to simply observe one or two times before implementing the teaching plan you have designed for them. When ready, have the patient perform a return demonstration of colostomy care and irrigation. Allow the wife to perform the skills as well.	Day 2: Explained colostomy A&P. Demonstrated changing appliance and emptying bag, while explaining verbally. He asked a few questions; wife asked many questions. Both verbally expressed understanding of answers. Both able to explain colostomy function. Day 3: Both are still able to explain colostomy function & how to empty & change bag. Both deny readiness to attempt return demonstration, but observed while nurse performed colostomy care & irrigation. Asked lots of questions about irrigation. Variety of supplies discussed, including advantages/disadvantages. Day 4: Has selected Style #212 bag that attaches to faceplate on abdomen & has a drain and plug in the bottom of bag. Emptied bag correctly. Said he thought he was "actually going to be able to take care of it" and that he wants to "observe one more irrigation" before attempting to do it himself. Wife performed irrigation without difficulty. Day 5: With wife's help, he emptied & changed bag w/o difficulty. Also demonstrated proper irrigation procedure.

Table 30-3   Care Plan for a Patient With a New Colostomy of the Descending Colon (continued)

Nursing Diagnosis: Disturbed body image, related to new colostomy, as evidenced by avoidance of looking at stoma.
Expected Outcomes: Patient will agree to visit with support group by day 4. Patient will observe stoma care by day 2. Patient will be able to explain various steps to prevent flatus and accidental spillage of effluent by discharge.

Interventions	Evaluations
Obtain the patient's permission to refer him to the local ostomy support group and make arrangements for visits to begin ASAP.	Day 2: Permission granted. Support group notified, will be here this afternoon.
Provide the patient with ample time to verbalize his concerns. Make time to sit with the patient 5–10 minutes a couple of times a day to encourage him to talk.	Day 2: Sat with him twice before support group came, he asked few questions; sat with him once after group, he asked more questions. Day 3: Sat with him; he verbalizing concerns RE: odor control, other people "knowing" about ostomy. Discussion lasted 20–25 min. Day 5: Definitely more optimistic.
Make frequent eye contact during provision of colostomy care. Maintain a pleasant facial expression, smiling when appropriate.	Day 2: Makes eye contact only briefly. Day 3: Making much better eye contact. Smiled a couple of times during care & teaching.
Teach the patient that irrigating a colostomy located in the descending colon may allow him to regulate bowel movements and maybe even eliminate the need to wear an appliance during the day.	Day 3: Says this gives him "more hope." Day 5: As frequency of evacuation decreases, expresses more satisfaction.
Teach the patient to avoid foods that cause excess flatus.	Day 3: Verbally verifies understanding.
Teach the patient about products that he can use to reduce odors.	Day 3: Verbalizes understanding.
Encourage the patient and his wife to talk about their feelings regarding sexual activity.	Day 3: States they have already discussed with support group and understand, optimistic.

Skill 30-1 Administering an Enema*

Assessment Steps

1. Review the physician's order for type and volume to administer. *This identifies what supplies are needed.*

2. *Safety: Review the patient's medical record for conditions that might contraindicate administration of an enema, such as glaucoma or increased intracranial pressure. If such a condition is noted, notify the physician for further clarification of the enema order.*

3. Determine whether there are physician's orders restricting the patient's activity level.

4. Assess the patient's cognitive level and level of mobility. *This determines whether a bedpan or bedside commode will be needed.*

5. Assess the patient's rectal sphincter control. *This identifies the need to administer the enema solution while the patient is on the bedpan.*

6. Assess for last bowel movement, abdominal distention, and the presence of bowel sounds. *This provides a baseline for evaluation of effectiveness.*

Planning Steps

1. Gather needed equipment and supplies: several pairs of clean examination gloves, disposable protective gown, waterproof pad, water-soluble lubricant, "do not enter" sign to place on room door, toilet tissue, washcloths and towel, bath blanket, bedpan with cover or bedside commode if needed, enema administration set and solution for type enema ordered, IV pole.

Implementation Steps

1. Follow the Initial Implementation Steps located on the inside front cover.

2. Close the clamp on the administration set tubing *to prevent fluid from escaping before you begin the procedure.*

3. Prepare solution as needed and fill the container to the desired volume. *Safety: Water temperature should be between 105°F and 110°F (40.5°C to 43.3°C) to prevent burns and cold water cramping. Never heat water in a microwave oven.* If preparing an SS enema, add castile soap at a ratio of 5 mL per 1,000 mL normal saline (NS) or tap water. If the enema volume is 500 mL, then add only 2.5 mL of soap.

4. Prime the enema administration tubing: open the clamp and allow solution to dispel all the air in the tubing. Then close the clamp. *This prevents air from entering the colon, causing painful gas for your patient.*

5. Hang the administration set on an IV pole, adjusted to a height of 12 to 18 inches above the patient's hip level with the bed positioned at working height for you. *This level allows the solution to flow at the correct amount of pressure.*

6. Position yourself on the patient's right side *to easily visualize the anus before inserting the enema.*

7. Position the patient in the left lateral side-lying position or Sims' position. *This allows gravity to assist with the retention of the solution by pulling the solution directly into the sigmoid and descending colon.*

8. If a bedside commode is to be used, position it close to the bed where it is accessible. *Safety: Arrange furniture and equipment to provide a clear pathway to the commode; if the patient is able to ambulate to the bathroom, open the bathroom door and clear the pathway. Position nonskid slippers and toilet tissue close by.*

9. Cover the patient with a bath blanket, exposing only the buttocks and rectum, *to provide privacy and preserve modesty.*

10. If the patient does not have good sphincter control, position a bedpan close to the patient's buttocks, *ready to slide into position when needed.*

11. Lubricate 4 to 6 inches of the distal end of the tubing with a water-soluble lubricant such as K-Y jelly *to facilitate easy insertion into the rectum.*

12. Carefully and slowly insert the tip of the tubing 3 to 4 inches into the rectum, directing the tip toward the umbilicus *so that it enters the rectum without causing trauma.*

13. While holding the enema administration container at the patient's hip level, release the tubing clamp and begin instillation of the solution. Gradually raise the container to a height of 12 to 18 inches above the patient's hip level. Instill the solution

---

*For all enemas except commercially prepackaged small-volume enemas.

Skill 30-1 (continued)

slowly. *Raising the height of the enema container too fast or too high increases the rate at which solution is instilled. The faster solution is instilled, the less the patient is able to receive and retain the solution. It will also result in more cramping and discomfort for the patient.*

14. If the patient complains of cramping, clamp the tubing and instruct the patient to take slow deep breaths through pursed lips. Proceed only after the patient reports that cramping has stopped. *This will help the patient be more comfortable and be able to retain the solution longer.*

15. Continually monitor the patient for signs and symptoms of vagal stimulation. Do not administer more than 1,000 mL at a time *to prevent overdistention of the colon.*

16. Upon completion of instillation, clamp the tubing and carefully and slowly remove it from the patient's anus, covering the dirty tip with paper towels or a washcloth.

17. Place a disposable administration set in the trash according to facility policy. Reusable sets may be rinsed with tap water and hung in the bathroom to drain and dry until used again.

18. Remove contaminated gloves. Wash hands.

19. Instruct the patient to hold the solution for 15 to 20 minutes if possible. *This will improve the effectiveness of the enema.*

20. When the patient is ready, apply clean examination gloves and assist the patient to the bathroom or bedside commode if allowed. Otherwise, place the patient on the bedpan and raise the head of the bed to 80 to 90 degrees, making certain toilet tissue and the call light are within the patient's reach. *This puts the patient in a natural positon for defecation.*

21. Remove gloves and protective gown. Wash hands.

22. Provide as much privacy as possible for expulsion of the enema *so that the patient is not embarrassed by sounds or smells.*

23. If the patient was able to get up to the bathroom, instruct the patient not to flush until you or another nursing staff member has time to observe the results. *This allows you to observe the color, consistency, and amount of return and to document it.*

24. After expulsion of the enema, apply clean examination gloves and assist the patient as needed to cleanse the anus and buttocks. Be certain to rinse and dry skin thoroughly *to prevent chapping.*

25. Before flushing the toilet, or emptying the bedpan or bedside commode into the toilet, be certain to assess the results of the enema.

26. Follow the Ending Implementation Steps located on the inside back cover.

27. Document the administration procedure, including the type and volume instilled, the patient's tolerance, and the return results, including the characteristics of the stool.

Evaluation Steps

1. Assess returned enema results, including amount, color, and consistency.

2. Assess the patient's abdomen for distention and bowel sounds. Make certain the patient is comfortable and has no further needs before leaving the room.

Sample Documentation

12-29-10   9:30 a.m.   *Bowel sounds hypoactive in all 4 quadrants. Abdomen slightly distended, but soft. States last BM was 3 days ago and complains of a sense of "fullness and bloating" in abdomen. 1,000-mL NS enema administered rectally per physician's orders. Received and retained full volume without difficulty or complaints of cramping. Assisted to bathroom. Expelled large volume of brown, soft, formed stool without difficulty. Perineal care performed. Bowel sounds active in all 4 quadrants. Abdomen now flat and soft. Expresses feelings of relief and improved comfort.* ————————
————————— *Nurse's signature and credentials*

Skill 30-2 Obtaining a Stool Specimen for Culture, and Ova and Parasites

Assessment Steps

1. Review the physician's orders for type of test and stool specimen to obtain.

2. Review the patient's chart for activity restrictions, level of mobility, and cognition. *This helps to determine if the patient can get up to the bedside commode or bathroom or requires use of a bedpan for collection of the specimen.*

3. Review facility policy and procedure and printed instructions accompanying the specimen testing supplies to be used *to ensure that you are performing the procedure correctly.*

Planning Steps

1. Gather needed equipment and supplies: specimen container; tongue blade; bedpan if on bedrest, or specimen pan for toilet or bedside commode if patient is able to get up; examination gloves; plastic bag in which to place the specimen container after specimen collection; laboratory requisition.

2. Instruct the patient to notify you as soon as he or she has the urge to defecate *so that you can obtain a stool specimen.*

Implementation Steps

1. Follow the Initial Implementation Steps located on the inside front cover.

2. Provide privacy during elimination.

3. If the patient is able to get up, place the specimen pan under the rim of the toilet or bedside commode *to catch the feces.*

4. Place the patient on the clean and dry bedpan, or assist to the bedside commode or toilet.

5. Instruct the patient to empty the bladder if necessary before defecation *to avoid contamination of stool specimen with urine.* Tell the patient that toilet tissue should not be placed in the specimen pan or bedpan, whichever is used, *to prevent contamination of the specimen.*

6. After the bowels have moved, remove the bedpan if one is in use; wear gloves to assist the patient to clean the perineal area as needed.

7. If the patient got up for the bowel movement, assist the patient back to bed and make him or her comfortable.

8. Wear gloves for collection of the stool specimen *to prevent contact with blood or body fluids.*

9. Using a clean tongue blade, collect 1 to 2 inches of formed stool and place inside the appropriate specimen container for the ordered test. Take the stool specimen from at least two areas of the feces, collecting any abnormal specimen findings such as blood, mucus, or visible parasites or eggs. *This allows the laboratory to test any abnormalities in the stool.* If the stool is liquid, place 1 to 2 ounces of liquid stool in the specimen container. Close the container lid securely *to prevent leakage.*

10. Complete and apply a label to the specimen container, including the patient's name, ID number, and room number; the physician's name; the test to be run; and the date and time of specimen collection. Place the capped specimen container inside a plastic bag for delivery of the specimen to the laboratory. *This protects you and anyone else handling the specimen from contact with blood or body fluids.*

11. Empty the bedpan or bedside commode of any remaining stool. Flush the toilet and clean the bedpan or bedside commode.

12. Follow the Ending Implementation Steps located on the inside back cover.

13. Deliver the specimen to the laboratory within 15 minutes of collection *so that it can be tested while it is fresh, while any ova or parasites that may be present in the specimen are still alive.*

14. Document the type of stool specimen collected, including color and consistency of the fecal specimen, date and time of collection, and delivery time to the laboratory.

Evaluation Steps

1. Assess the patient for comfort and needs before leaving room.

Sample Documentation

11-10-11   9:15 a.m.   Assisted to bathroom for defecation. Stool specimen collected for culture and sensitivity. Feces yellowish-brown, liquid consistency. Delivery to lab at 9:25 a.m.
———————————————— Nurse's signature and credentials

Skill 30-3 Performing Guaiac Testing: Testing Stool Specimen for Occult Blood

Assessment Steps

1. Review the physician's order for type of test to be done.
2. Review the patient's chart to determine the patient's level of cognition and mobility. *This helps to determine if the patient can get up to the bedside commode or bathroom or requires use of a bedpan for collection of the specimen.*
3. Review facility policy for this procedure. Read guaiac test card instructions.

Planning Steps

1. Gather needed equipment and supplies: guaiac card with instructions for performing the test; tongue blade; bottle of developer; bedpan if on bedrest, or specimen pan for toilet or bedside commode if the patient is able to get up; examination gloves; plastic bag in which to place specimen test card after specimen collection; laboratory requisition.

Implementation Steps

1. Follow the Initial Implementation Steps located on the inside front cover.
2. Provide privacy during elimination.
3. Apply clean examination gloves.
4. If the patient is able to get up, place the specimen pan under the rim of the toilet or bedside commode *to catch the feces.*
5. Place the patient on the clean and dry bedpan, or assist to the bedside commode or toilet.
6. Instruct the patient to empty the bladder if necessary before defecation *to avoid contamination of stool specimen with urine.* Tell the patient that toilet tissue should not be placed in the specimen pan or bedpan, whichever is used, *to prevent contamination of the specimen.*
7. After the bowels have moved, remove the bedpan if one is in use; wear gloves to assist the patient to clean the perineal area as needed.
8. If the patient got up for the bowel movement, assist the patient back to bed and make him or her comfortable.
9. Use the wooden tongue blade for collection of the stool specimen. Select the specimen from two different areas of the stool, especially any part of stool that is red, maroon, black, or tarry in appearance. *This allows for testing of the areas most likely to contain blood.*
10. According to test card instructions, apply a thin smear of feces to the two sample areas on the back side of the test card and close the flaps. Wait the instructed length of time before applying drops of liquid developer *to ensure accurate results.*
11. Apply the designated number of drops of developer, usually 2, over each of the two feces smears and on the spot labeled "control." Apply the developer drops to the designated side of the card, usually the front side. *This allows the developer to penetrate the paper to the specimen.*

12. Wait for the designated length of time before reading the test results. The color on the control site will indicate a positive result by turning the paper a bluish color, *which is indicative of a positive result.* Compare the two feces sample sites to the control site. *The test results are positive for presence of blood if the feces smears turn a blue or bluish-purple color, similar to the control color. The test results are negative if the smears do not turn blue.*
13. Most facility policies require the guaiac test card to be placed in a plastic bag and delivered to the laboratory *for verification of the test results.*
14. Follow the Ending Implementation Steps located on the inside back cover.
15. Document the characteristics of the bowel movement, including color, amount, and consistency of the feces, and whether the results were negative or positive.

Evaluation Steps

1. Notify the physician according to facility policy regarding positive results for presence of blood.

Sample Documentation

11-23-11 8:35 a.m. Assisted to bedside commode for bowel movement. Specimen obtained and applied to guaiac test card. Feces were small amount of brown formed stool with small amount of bright red streaking throughout stool. Test results for presence of blood were positive. Specimen sent to lab for verification. Physician telephoned about positive results. ————————
———————————— Nurse's signature and credentials

Skill 30-4 Removing a Fecal Impaction

Assessment Steps

1. Review facility policy to determine who may perform this procedure and whether a physician's order is required. If required, review the physician's order.
2. Review the patient's medical record for conditions that might contraindicate digital removal of an impaction by a nurse.
3. Assess the patient's pulse rate and blood pressure to establish a baseline.

Planning Steps

1. Gather needed equipment and supplies: several pairs of clean examination gloves, disposable protective gown, water-soluble lubricant such as K-Y jelly, waterproof pad, cover for bedpan (a disposable pad similar to the waterproof pad to be placed under the patient works well), toilet tissue, washcloths and towels, wash basin, "do not enter" sign for room door.

Implementation Steps

1. Follow the Initial Implementation Steps located on the inside front cover.
2. Provide privacy and protect modesty as well as you can.
3. Position yourself on the right side of the bed. Position the patient in a left lateral side-lying or Sims' position *to facilitate access to the rectum and lower sigmoid colon.*
4. Cover the patient with a bath blanket, exposing only the rectum and buttocks, *to provide warmth and privacy.*
5. Place a waterproof pad underneath the patient's hips *to protect the linens.*
6. Position the bedpan on the bed close to the buttocks *to help prevent unnecessary soiling of linens.* Have toilet tissue within reach.
7. Generously lubricate your gloved index finger *to reduce the discomfort of the procedure.*
8. Gently insert the finger into the anus and past both the outer and inner rectal sphincters until the fecal mass is located.
9. Slide the index finger between the outside of the fecal mass and the intestinal wall. Flex the finger toward the center of the fecal mass. *This allows you to break up the mass so it can be removed. Safety: Never flex the finger toward the outside of the fecal mass, toward the intestinal wall. This increases risk of perforating the bowel wall.*
10. Using as little motion of the finger as possible, gently break up the fecal mass into small pieces and remove them from the rectum. *This relieves the blockage caused by the impaction and causes the least discomfort to the patient.* Place feces in the bedpan and repeat the process until the impaction is removed.
11. Continually monitor the patient for signs and symptoms of vagal stimulation. *Safety: If such symptoms are noted, stop the procedure immediately.*
12. After the impaction is removed, clean the anus area with toilet tissue and place used tissue in the bedpan.
13. Remove contaminated gloves and dispose of in trash according to facility policy.

14. Apply clean examination gloves.
15. Cover the bedpan and place it in the bathroom while washing the patient.
16. Use warm soap and water to wash the anus area and buttocks *to remove any fecal material and mucus.*
17. Remove the soiled pad from under the patient's hips and replace with a clean pad if needed.
18. Empty the contents of the bedpan into the toilet, noting characteristics of the feces before flushing.
19. Follow the Ending Implementation Steps located on the inside back cover.
20. Document the procedure; amount, color, and consistency of the feces; and the patient's tolerance of the procedure.

Evaluation Steps

1. Assess the patient's comfort level and any further needs.

Sample Documentation

12-31-10   8:30 a.m.   States last BM was tiny and hard, 3 days ago and has been constipated ever since. Complains of rectal and abdominal pressure. Fecal impaction digitally removed per physician's order without difficulty. Very large amount of brown, hard stool removed from impaction low in the rectal vault. Tolerated with only complaints of minor pressure in rectum. Perineal care performed. Bed returned to lowest position and call light within patient's reach. Instructed to notify nurse if further assistance or bowel elimination is required. ————————
——————————— *Nurse's signature and credentials*

Skill 30-5 Applying/Changing an Ostomy Appliance

Assessment Steps

1. Review the patient's medical record and care plan for type of ostomy care to provide, date of and reason for ostomy construction, type of supplies to use, current patient condition, degree of self-care for ostomy, identified patient problems (including psychosocial issues and response to ostomy), and last time the appliance bag and faceplate were changed.

2. Assess the patient's bowel sounds, appliance bag and faceplate, and characteristics and amount of effluent/fecal drainage *to verify type of supplies to use and determine whether the bag needs to be emptied before changing it.*

Planning Steps

1. Gather needed equipment and supplies: stoma size measuring device; type of faceplate, bag, and supplies being used; clean examination gloves; wash basin and soap, washcloths, and towels; toilet tissue; bath blanket; two moisture-proof pads; bedpan and cover or bedside commode as needed.

Implementation Steps

1. Follow the Initial Implementation Steps located on the inside front cover.

2. Provide privacy and protect modesty as well as you can.

3. If patient condition allows, assist the patient to the bedside commode. *Ostomy care is easier to provide on the commode. Plus, once at home, the patient will probably perform the procedure while sitting on the toilet.* If the patient is unable to get out of bed, position him or her in the low semi-Fowler's position.

4. Arrange supplies within easy reach.

5. Cover the patient with the bath blanket *to reduce soiling of linens.* If in bed, place a moisture-proof pad beside the patient and one across the patient's lap. In sitting on bedside commode, place one across the patient's lap. *This will help protect the patient from contact with feces during the appliance change.*

6. Apply clean examination gloves *to reduce contamination of hands.*

7. Unsnap the flange of the ostomy bag from the faceplate. Remove the bag and empty the contents into the bedpan if the bag is to be reused. If the bag is to be changed, place the entire bag in the bedpan and cover until through changing the appliance. *This allows you to remove the feces using a bedpan.*

8. If reusing the bag, rinse the bag out with tap water *to reduce residual fecal material within the bag.*

9. Gently clean drainage and feces from the stoma and peristomal skin. Gently wash with warm soap and water, using as many clean washcloths as needed. If the ostomy is oozing effluent, it is helpful to place a clean, dry washcloth or gauze 4×4s over the stoma *to prevent contamination of the cleansed area until a new faceplate or bag is reapplied.*

10. If the faceplate adhesive appears to be leaking or needs to be changed, gently remove it by pulling each edge toward the stoma, *to prevent tearing or stretching of the peristomal skin opening surrounding the stoma.*

11. Gently clean, rinse, and dry the surrounding skin well. *This helps to maintain the skin beneath the adhesive of the faceplate in good condition.*

12. Assess the stoma for color, moisture level, size, and edema. If the ostomy is new, use the card stock cut-out sizing device to measure the stoma. Select the correct size that will allow only ⅛ to ¼ inch of peristomal skin to show around the stoma. This helps to reduce the amount of skin exposed to feces and at risk for excoriation.

13. Assess the peristomal skin for breaks in integrity, erythema, drainage, and edema, *which would indicate potential infection.*

14. Verify the correct size of opening on the new appliance bag and faceplate with the new measurement obtained. *This helps ensure that the faceplate will fit correctly without leaking.*

15. Peel the backing off the adhesive disk of the wafer faceplate. Remove the dry washcloth covering the stoma and position the hole in the faceplate with the stoma centered in the middle of the opening. *This helps ensure that the faceplate is correctly positioned and will not cause pressure or allow leaking.*

16. Apply the adhesive side of the wafer faceplate by gently pressing it against the skin. Use care to make certain there are no wrinkles in the adhesive surface nor the skin under it. Gently rub the outer surface of the faceplate with your fingers *to smooth and warm the adhesive disk to body temperature for better adhesion to the skin.*

(skill continues on page 704)

Skill 30-5 (continued)

17. Reassess that there are no leaks before applying the bag to the faceplate. If not, gently press the

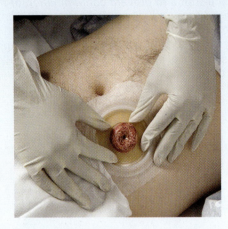

plastic flange onto the receiving flange on the faceplate. It works somewhat like a Tupperware lid seals. If the ostomy is new, avoid using excessive pressure on the newly traumatized area *to reduce discomfort for the patient.*

18. If the situation is right for teaching, explain the procedure to the patient as you go, maintaining good eye contact and a neutral facial expression. Avoid acting rushed. If the patient is sitting on a bedside commode, squat down while providing ostomy care. *It places you at eye level with the patient so that you can better observe the patient's responses. It also allows the patient to observe your accepting attitude and facial expression, and helps to build rapport while being on the same level physically as the patient rather than physically towering over the patient, looking down at and talking downward to the patient, which can be perceived as dominating and negative by some patients.*

19. Remove contaminated gloves and wash hands.

20. Apply clean gloves to clean up your work site, disposing of contaminated supplies according to facility policy.

21. Follow the Ending Implementation Steps located on the inside back cover.

22. Document the procedure, including assessment findings regarding the stoma and peristomal skin; amount, color, and consistency of effluent/fecal drainage; the patient's verbal and nonverbal responses; any abnormalities encountered or difficulties experienced; and patient teaching provided. Also document the effectiveness of teaching by noting the patient's response to the teaching. Make a note of the extent of patient participation in ostomy care.

Evaluation Steps

1. Assess the patient for comfort and needs before leaving the room.

Sample Documentation

12-27-10   10:00 a.m.   New colostomy of Left descending colon constructed 2 days ago. Stoma is red, edematous, moist and shiny. Peristomal skin is pink, intact, without edema or drainage. Bag ⅓ full of brown semiformed fecal drainage with clear mucus. Assisted patient to bedside commode for ostomy care. Stoma measured: 2-in. diameter. Bag emptied, rinsed with tap water, dried and reapplied. Patient observed procedure and asked questions regarding ostomy care, made good eye contact. Verbalized that she knew she could learn to take care of the new ostomy. Stated that she had originally thought the diagnosis of colon cancer meant an automatic death warrant and that she was glad to just be alive. Occasionally smiled during our interaction. Informed her that a representative from the local support group would be in to see her after lunch. Still up in chair with call light within reach. No complaints voiced. ————— —————————— Nurse's signature and credentials

Skill 30-6 Irrigating a Colostomy

Assessment Steps

1. Review the patient's medical record and care plan for type of ostomy care to provide, date of and reason for ostomy construction, type of supplies to use, current patient condition, degree of self-care for ostomy, identified patient problems (including psychosocial issues and response to ostomy), last time the appliance bag and faceplate were changed, and date of last irrigation.

2. Assess the patient's bowel sounds, appliance bag and faceplate, and characteristics and amount of effluent/fecal drainage *to verify type of supplies to use.*

Planning Steps

1. Gather needed equipment and supplies: new faceplate, bag, and supplies being used; clean examination gloves; ostomy irrigation sleeve; irrigation administration set with cone-tipped tubing; irrigation solution; wash basin and soap, washcloths, and towels; toilet tissue; bath blanket; moisture-proof pad; IV pole; bedpan and cover or bedside commode as needed.

Implementation Steps

1. Follow the Initial Implementation Steps located on the inside front cover.

2. Provide privacy and protect modesty as well as you can.

3. Prepare solution as needed and fill administration set container to the desired volume, usually between 500 and 1000 mL. *Safety: Water temperature should be between 105°F and 110°F (40.5°C to 43.3°C) to prevent burns and cold water cramping. Never heat water in a microwave oven.*

4. Hang the filled irrigation administration container on the IV pole to a height level with the patient's hips once he or she is in position *to provide for the least amount of pressure when beginning the irrigation.*

5. If patient condition allows, assist the patient to the bedside commode. Irrigation is easier to perform on the commode. If unable to get out of bed, position the patient in a left lateral side-lying position *to facilitate the best access to the colon.*

6. Cover the patient with the bath blanket *to reduce soiling of linens and maintain modesty.* Place moisture-proof pad across the patient's lap *to reduce soiling of gown.* If in bed, place a moisture-proof pad beside the patient underneath the stoma *to protect the patient's abdomen from irrigation fluid.*

7. Apply clean examination gloves *to reduce contamination of hands.*

8. Remove the appliance bag and clean feces from the stoma and peristomal skin with toilet tissue and warm wet washcloth as needed.

9. Place the elastic belt around the patient's waist and clip the irrigation sleeve to the belt *to more easily hold the sleeve in place.*

10. Place the open-ended tail of the bag in a bedpan if the patient is in bed, or between the patient's thighs into the bedside commode. *This will ensure that the irrigation solution and return go into the bedpan or bedside commode.*

11. Lubricate the tip of the insertion cone and your dominant gloved index finger *to reduce patient discomfort upon insertion.*

12. If the cone will not insert into the stoma, lift the top edge of the irrigation sleeve off the patient's abdomen and gently insert your lubricated index finger about 1 inch into the stoma opening. Give the stoma several seconds to relax and dilate. If the stoma opening is too tight for insertion of your index finger, use the smaller pinkie finger first. Then use the index finger to further dilate the opening. You will be able to feel the release of constriction around your finger. Once release is felt, remove the finger. *Stomas will sometimes contract and require gentle dilation before insertion of the administration cone.*

13. Insert the tip of the insertion cone into the stoma. The cone is graduated in size to be inserted until the cone fits snuggly inside the stoma opening. *This allows one cone size to fit any size of stoma and prevents leakage of solution while instilling irrigation solution.*

14. Release the tubing clamp, allowing solution to flow into the intestinal lumen. Gradually raise the height of the irrigation administration container to 12 inches above the patient's hip level *to slowly increase the rate of flow.*

(skill continues on page 706)

Skill 30-6 (continued)

15. Stop or slow solution flow as needed *to control retention and patient cramping.*

16. Once solution instillation is completed, remove the cone from the stoma and allow irrigation sleeve to set against the patient's skin *to receive returned contents.*

17. Return of solution may be immediate or may take up to 30 minutes. Wash, rinse, and hang the irrigation administration equipment to dry in the patient's bathroom. *The irrigation set can be reused by the same patient several times.*

18. Remove contaminated gloves, wash hands, and apply clean gloves.

19. After expulsion of irrigation, remove the irrigation sleeve and elastic belt. Wash, rinse, and pat dry the stoma and peristomal skin, reassessing its condition as you do this *to observe any changes that may have occurred during the irrigation.*

20. Apply a new faceplate and bag as needed.

21. Assess the characteristics of the returned contents before emptying into the toilet.

22. Assist the patient to return to bed or reposition as desired.

23. Follow the Ending Implementation Steps located on the inside back cover.

24. Document the procedure, including type and volume of solution, difficulties encountered, and characteristics of the returned contents, including color, amount, and consistency of effluent/fecal drainage. Also document assessment findings regarding the stoma and peristomal skin, including color, edema, skin integrity, and moisture level of the stoma.

25. Document any patient teaching performed and evaluate the effectiveness by noting the patient's verbal and nonverbal responses.

Evaluation Steps

1. Assess for patient comfort and needs before leaving the room.

Sample Documentation

> 11-10-11   8:00 a.m.   Assisted to bedside commode. Colostomy irrigated with 500 mL of 0.9% normal saline without difficulty. Stoma was pinkish red, moist and shiny, no edema. Peristomal skin was intact, and without erythema or edema. Large amount of soft formed brown stool returned within 2 to 3 minutes of instillation. Patient unable to assist with procedure due to severe contractures of both hands. Conversed with nurse and made good eye contact throughout procedure. Faceplate clean and intact. Clean bag applied. Assisted to return to bed. No complaints voiced. ———
> ——————— *Nurse's signature and credentials*

🌐 Post Conference

Your day turned out to be rather exciting in some ways. When you were assessing your patient, you noticed that his ileostomy was leaking under the faceplate, so you decided (with appropriate orders) to change the ostomy appliance. While you were doing so, you noticed that the stoma was a very pale pink. Remembering what you had learned, you pouched the ileostomy, then notified your instructor of your findings. He agreed with you that the stoma was too pale to be receiving good blood supply. The charge nurse was notified, who then called the physician. Because of your excellent assessment, the physician took the patient back to surgery to revise the stoma, ensuring that it would have good blood supply. The physician stated that, had the stoma gone for 24 more hours in this condition, even more intestine would have had to be removed. You also learned the difficulties of keeping an ileostomy pouch emptied in a timely manner, because it seemed to fill up quickly with liquid effluent.

KEY POINTS

- Patterns of bowel elimination frequency vary throughout the life span and from individual to individual.
- The most common types of abnormal bowel elimination are diarrhea, constipation, flatulence, and fecal incontinence.
- Diarrhea is defined as several loose, watery stools within 24 hours.
- Constipation is defined as difficulty having a bowel movement due to dry, hard stool.
- An impaction is the inability to evacuate a mass of dry, hard stool from the bowels.
- Diarrhea may indicate an impaction where the liquid stool above the impaction seeps around it.
- Hidden blood in the stool is known as occult blood.
- Visible blood in the stool may appear as black and tarry, maroon, or bright red frank blood.
- Alterations in bowel elimination may be caused by a change in activity level, diet and fluid intake, side effects of medication, side effects of surgery, pregnancy, psychological problems, the aging process, laxative abuse, inflammation or infection, structural changes in the bowel tissue, or food allergies.
- Signs and symptoms of vagal stimulation include chest pain, heaviness, or pressure, dyspnea, dizziness, fainting, nausea, pale or clammy skin, and bradycardia.
- Assessment of bowel movements includes color, amount, consistency, and odor.
- Types of bowel diversions include colostomies, ileostomies, and Kock pouches.
- It is important to provide privacy and preserve the patient's dignity and modesty during delivery of nursing care related to bowel elimination.

REVIEW QUESTIONS

Select the answer that is most appropriate for each of the following questions. Some questions may have more than one correct answer. Check all that apply.

1. Which of the following would be the most accurate statement about digestion and elimination?

   a. All individuals have at least one bowel movement daily.

   b. An infant may have up to six bowel movements daily.

   c. GI peristalsis increases with age, making incontinence a normal finding.

   d. A stool is only considered normal if the color is a shade of brown.

2. Several medications have GI side effects and may lead to diarrhea or constipation. Indicate which of the following medications would be most likely to cause constipation in the patient.

   a. Amphogel

   b. Maalox

   c. Magnesium citrate

   d. Meperidine

   e. Amoxicillin

   f. Ferrous sulfate (iron)

   g. Imodium AD

   h. Milk of magnesia

3. A female patient is recovering from abdominal surgery 2 days ago. Her abdomen is distended and firm and she complains of moderate to severe cramping and abdominal discomfort. As of yet, she has been unable to pass much flatus rectally. Which type of enema would be most helpful to this patient?

   a. Fleet Phospho-Soda enema

   b. Oil retention enema

   c. Harris flush enema

   d. Small-volume enema

4. Which of the following signs and symptoms may be an indication of vagal stimulation during the digital removal of an impaction?

   a. Complaint of rectal pressure

   b. Pulse rate of 42 beats per minute

   c. Complaint of difficulty breathing

   d. Moist skin

   e. Complaint of abdominal cramping

   f. Complaint of feeling faint

5. What of the following would be the best enema to administer to a patient before digital removal of an impaction?

   a. Siphon enema

   b. Oil retention enema

   c. Soapsuds enema

   d. Harris flush enema

6. Which of the following factors is most likely to result in diarrhea?

   a. Loss of intestinal normal flora.

   b. Drinking excessive fluids.

   c. Administration of opioid narcotics.

   d. Manipulation of intestines during colon surgery.

   e. Eating 10 to 15 grams of fiber per day.

7. The patient is to receive a cleansing enema for relief of constipation. Which of the following factors **must** be assessed prior to administration of the enema?

   a. Type of solution to administer

   b. Date of last bowel movement

   c. Type of diet the patient has been receiving

   d. Assessment of bowel sounds

   e. The patient's temperature

8. Which of the following assessment data might indicate the patient is having difficulty accepting his or her new colostomy?

   a. Asks questions about how to take care of the colostomy.

   b. Observes as you irrigate the colostomy.

   c. Looks at stoma and makes good eye contact with you during ostomy care.

   d. Refuses to attempt care, and tells you to "just do it."

CRITICAL THINKING EXERCISES

9. You are caring for a 62-year-old female admitted to a hospital 45 miles from her hometown with a right mid-femur fracture. Surgical repair was performed yesterday under general anesthetic. She has a history of arteriosclerosis and is very hard-of-hearing. Her dentures are at home and there is no one to retrieve them for her until her daughter arrives in 3 days. She is an avid gardener and usually works in her gardens about an hour each morning before the temperature gets too hot. Each evening, she spends 30 minutes to an hour walking through the park admiring the trees, shrubs, and flowers. Her physician's orders include the following:

   • Bedrest
   • Assess circulation to right lower leg every 2 hours
   • Edentulous diet
   • Morphine sulfate 6 mg intramuscularly every 3 to 4 hours prn severe pain
   • Acetaminophen 50 mg or 2 tabs orally every 4 to 6 hours prn lesser pain

   Which of the above factors puts this patient at risk for constipation?

10. Gerome Flygenhall has a new permanent colostomy located in the ascending colon. What teaching or services would be appropriate to provide for this patient? Be inclusive.

ADDITIONAL RESOURCES

For additional Resources, Questions, and Activities, please see:

 Student Resource Disk

 DavisPlus **http://davisplus.fadavis.com**

 Student Study Guide

REFERENCES

Arai R. What does shape of stool mean? Available at: http://www.yourtotalhealth.ivillage.com/what-does-shape-stool-mean.html. Accessed October 28, 2009.

Barr JE. Assessment and management of stomal complications: a framework for clinical decision making. *Ostomy Wound Manage.* 2004;50(9):50-52, 54, 56 passim.

Bloodindex. Normal laboratory values. 2008. Available at: http://www.bloodindex.org/normal_laboratory_values.php. Accessed October 28, 2009.

Coffin CM. Stool tests. 2006. Available at: http://kidshealth.org/parent/general/sick/labtest8.html. Accessed October 28, 2009.

Convatec. Postoperative stoma assessment and pouching. 2008. Available at: http://www.convatec.com/en/cvtus-postoprsus/cvt-portallev1/0/detail/0/1580/1913/postoperative-stoma-assessment-and-pouching.aspx. Accessed October 28, 2009.

Dillon PM. *Nursing Health Assessment: A Critical Thinking Case Studies Approach.* 2nd ed. Philadelphia: FA Davis; 2007.

GlobalRPh.com. Common lab values. 2008. Available at: http://www.globalrph.com/labs.htm. Accessed October 28, 2009.

Gould B. *Pathophysiology for the Health Professions.* 3rd ed. Philadelphia: Saunders; 2006.

Harvard Health Publications. What is a healthy bowel movement? Available at: http://health.msn.com/health-topics/digestive-health/ibd-and-crohns/articlepage.aspx?cp-documentid=100098792. Accessed October 30, 2008.

Herlihy B. *The Human Body in Health & Illness.* 3rd ed. St. Louis: Saunders Elsevier; 2007.

Mosby's Dictionary of Medicine, Nursing & Health Professions. 8th ed. Philadelphia: Mosby; 2009.

National Cancer Institute. Gastrointestinal complications. 2008. Available at: http://www.cancer.gov/cancertopics/pdq/supportivecare/gastrointestinalcomplications/healthprofessional/allpages. Accessed October 28, 2009.

National Cancer Institute. Normal blood values. 2008. Available at: http://training.seer.cancer.gov/start_here.html. Accessed October 28, 2009.

Scanlon VC, Sanders T. *Essentials of Anatomy and Physiology.* 3rd ed. Philadelphia: FA Davis; 2007.

Wilkinson JM, Van Leuven K. *Fundamentals of Nursing: Theory, Concepts, and Applications.* Philadelphia: FA Davis; 2007.

Williams LS, Hopper PD. *Understanding Medical-Surgical Nursing.* 3rd ed. Philadelphia: FA Davis; 2007.

Zychowicz M. Abdominal assessment. 2008. Available at: http://www.wiziq.com/educational-tutorials/presentation/3689-advancedabdominalexam. Accessed October 28, 2009.

Urinary Elimination and Care

Key Terms

Anuria

Blood urea nitrogen (BUN)

Dialysis

Dysuria

Hematuria

Incontinence

Indwelling catheter

Nocturia

Oliguria

Polyuria

Renal calculi

Residual urine

Specific gravity

Straight catheter

Stress incontinence

Urge incontinence

Urinary diversion

Urinary retention

Urinary tract infection (UTI)

Void

Objectives

1. Define key terms related to urinary elimination.
2. Describe normal and abnormal urine output.
3. Discuss characteristics of normal urine and the significance of abnormal characteristics.
4. Explain the causes and complications of urinary retention.
5. Describe the treatment for urinary retention and residual urine.
6. Enumerate types of urinary incontinence.
7. Describe nursing interventions to help manage incontinence.
8. Identify steps in bladder training.
9. Discuss methods of assessing urine.
10. List the steps for collecting a 24-hour urine sample.
11. Explain ways to assist patients with toileting.
12. Identify purposes, types, and sizes of urinary catheters.
13. Discuss the care of patients with an indwelling urinary catheter.
14. Identify types of urinary diversions.
15. Describe the occurrence, risk factors for, and prevention of UTIs.
16. Plan care for a patient with urinary incontinence.

Skills

31-1 Assisting the Male Patient With a Urinal

31-2 Assisting With a Bedpan

31-3 Obtaining a Clean-catch Midstream Urine Specimen

31-4 Inserting an Indwelling Urinary Catheter

31-5 Obtaining a Urine Specimen From an Indwelling Urinary Catheter

(skills continue on page 710)

Skills (continued)

31-6 Inserting a Straight Catheter
31-7 Performing Continuous Bladder Irrigation
31-8 Applying a Condom Catheter
31-9 Irrigating a Closed Urinary Drainage System
31-10 Discontinuing an Indwelling Urinary Catheter

Clinical Connection

Your Assignment: You are assigned to care for a 24-year-old male with a spinal cord injury due to a boating accident. He has an indwelling catheter. In report, you hear that there are physician's orders to irrigate the catheter every 8 hours prn for decreased output because he sometimes has mucus that blocks the catheter. The order is for a closed system irrigation. Also ordered is a 24-hour urine collection.

Your Actions: Your first thought is to wonder what a closed system irrigation means. Then you try to remember what you know about performing a 24-hour urine collection. You remember something about keeping the specimen container on ice, but then you realize that the patient has an indwelling catheter. You wonder how to keep that cold for 24 hours.

You may not have thought about the importance of normal urinary function until you entered nursing school. Now, however, you are learning how important it is for the body to rid itself of waste products. In this chapter, you will learn how to assist patients who are unable to urinate normally as well as those who need assistance with normal voiding. You will learn how to collect urine specimens in a variety of situations and how to insert and manage catheters.

Normal Urinary Elimination

You will hear various terms used in health care to refer to the elimination of urine. You may hear a nurse say that a patient has voided 300 mL of urine. **Void** is another word for urinate. An older term that you may also hear is *micturate,* which also means to void or to urinate.

Urinary elimination cleanses the blood of anything the body does not need. Urine is made up of approximately 95% water, with the remaining 5% being the solutes that are dissolved in the water, such as mineral salts and nitrogenous waste products. Nitrogenous waste products result from the body's cellular metabolism and tend to accumulate in the bloodstream. The kidneys eliminate these waste products before the blood levels rise high enough to be damaging,

or toxic, to the body. Three waste products that must be removed are:

1. *Urea,* which results from amino acid metabolism
2. *Uric acid,* which results from breakdown of ribonucleic acid (RNA) and deoxyribonucleic acid (DNA)
3. *Creatinine,* which is the waste product of muscle metabolism

The kidneys filter these waste products from the blood and eliminate them in the urine, along with the excess water that is excreted, the excess electrolytes, any hydrogen ions that need to be eliminated, toxins, and other substances that result from illnesses.

Characteristics of Urine

The characteristics of urine that can be determined with only the use of your senses include color, clarity, amount, and odor. With the use of supplies and equipment, pH and specific gravity of urine can also be determined.

Color and Clarity

Normal urine is straw-colored, and clear without sediment. The color of urine is a primary indicator of whether or not the patient has had adequate fluid intake: the more yellow the color, the lower the patient's hydration level. As dehydration worsens, the urine color may become darker yellow and then amber.

Urine can be cloudy, or have increased *turbidity,* due to the presence of fat globules, red or white blood cells, or bacteria. When blood is present in the urine—either visible or microscopic blood—it is referred to as **hematuria**. When the pH of urine is excessively alkaline, it can result in turbidity and the formation of certain types of crystals; however, an excessively acidic pH can also result in turbidity and formation of other types of crystals. *Sediment* is any substance that settles to the bottom of a liquid. Components that may produce urine sediment include uric acid, bacteria, mucus, and phosphates.

Urine can also increase in turbidity if it is left sitting after the specimen has been collected, because the components in the urine start to break down. If a specimen is not going to be analyzed within 1 hour, it should be refrigerated.

Odor

Urine does have a very mild odor described as *slightly aromatic*. Other odors, such as a sweet or fruity smell, a strong ammonia-like smell, or a foul odor, indicate possible problems.

Amount

The amount of urine an adult produces in a day is a result of many metabolic occurrences in the body. The normal range of urine production is 1,000 to 3,000 mL in a 24-hour period. The acceptable *minimal* amount of urinary output per hour is 30 mL. Partially dependent upon the amount of fluid taken in, the volume of urine excreted by a patient whose fluids and electrolytes are balanced should be within a difference of approximately 300 to 500 mL from the total intake. As a nurse, you can make the decision to monitor a patient's intake and output any time it is indicated. For example, if you are concerned that a patient is not making as much urine as you think he or she should, or you see beginning signs of fluid overload, you would want to begin strict monitoring of the intake and output.

Oliguria

Oliguria, defined as urinary output of less than 30 mL/hr, can be caused by decreased fluid intake, dehydration, illness, urinary obstruction, or renal failure. Oliguria may also be caused by hemorrhage or by the severe loss of body fluids, such as occurs when a patient has sustained burns through all skin layers, losing large amounts of intracellular and interstitial fluid.

Polyuria

Increased urinary output, or **polyuria**, defined as output greater than 3,000 mL/day, can be caused by excessive fluid intake or the consumption of alcohol, which affects the kidney's ability to reabsorb water. Certain medications also can affect the amount of urine output. Diuretics, or "water pills," increase urine production and should be given early in the day. If administered in the evening, the patient will most likely be up several times during the night to urinate. This not only disturbs the patient's sleep, but increases the risk of falls in elders. Two commonly prescribed diuretics are furosemide (Lasix) and hydrochlorothiazide, also known as HCTZ.

Because some diuretic medications also increase the amount of electrolytes that are filtered from the blood and excreted in the urine, you should always monitor the patient's laboratory results for abnormal electrolyte levels in the blood. For example, furosemide is known for depleting the potassium level and often requires that a potassium supplement be administered to prevent electrolyte imbalance. Chapter 29 further explains fluid and electrolyte levels.

Anuria

Anuria is the absence of urine or minimal urine production and can be the result of a temporary illness or urinary tract obstruction, or be a symptom of a serious underlying condition, such as kidney failure, that must be diagnosed and treated. If anuria is caused by a temporary illness such as vomiting and diarrhea due to a virus, the kidneys may start producing urine on their own when the illness is treated and hydration restored; however, when the kidneys fail, dialysis must be started. **Dialysis** is the process of using a machine to filter waste products and salts, and to remove excess fluid from the blood. This treatment may be temporary or long term depending on the cause of the anuria.

pH

The pH of urine is normally 4.6 to 8.0, depending largely on diet. A diet high in protein or cranberries will cause the pH to be lower, or more acidic; a diet high in citrus fruits, dairy products, or vegetables will cause the pH to be higher, or more alkaline. Determining the pH of the urine is helpful in the diagnosis and management of urinary tract infections (UTIs), which tend to make the urine more alkaline; and in diagnosing some types of renal calculi, also referred to as *kidney stones.*

Specific Gravity

Specific gravity is the result of comparing the weight of a substance with an equal amount of water. The normal specific gravity for urine is 1.010 to 1.025. When the specific gravity is high, it means that the urine is more concentrated. When the specific gravity is low, the urine is more dilute. A low specific gravity may be caused by excessive fluid intake or impaired kidney function. A high specific gravity can be the result of dehydration, hemorrhage, or diabetes mellitus.

Anatomy and Physiology Connection

Urinary System

The urinary system is a multiorgan system, consisting of the two kidneys containing millions of nephrons that filter the blood. The blood flows through the renal arteries into the kidney, into the nephron, and into the glomerulus, where filtration takes place. The blood pressure forces substances

(connection continues on page 712)

through the porous walls of the glomerulus to produce the filtrate. As the filtrate travels on through the proximal convoluted tubule, loop of Henle, distal tubule, and collecting tubule, most of the filtrate is reabsorbed, leaving only the waste products, toxins, excess electrolytes, and water to be excreted as urine.

Urine leaves the kidney by way of the ureter and travels by peristaltic action to the urinary bladder for storage. The ureters from both kidneys attach to the posterior base of the bladder, allowing urine to actually enter the bladder from the inferior or bottom side, not from the top or superior side of the bladder. Because of this, urine can *reflux,* or back up, into the kidneys if the valve at the cystoureteral junction does not close properly.

Urine is stored in the bladder, a sac made of smooth muscle, until the urge to void is felt when approximately 200 to 400 mL of urine has collected. The bladder can hold 1,000 mL or more of urine but is usually emptied long before it reaches that amount. The detrusor muscle in the walls of the bladder contracts, causing the bladder to empty. Urine leaves the bladder by way of the urethra and passes through two sphincters: the internal urinary sphincter at the neck of the bladder and the external urinary sphincter near the end of the urethra. In males, as the urethra leaves the bladder, it passes through the prostate, which surrounds the urethra and neck of the bladder, explaining how an enlarged prostate can inhibit or prevent urination. The urine then exits the body via the urinary meatus.

An important point to remember is that there is one continuous membrane that lines the urinary system; it extends from the external urinary meatus all the way to the kidneys. This membrane allows bacteria to spread from outside the urinary meatus through the urethra into the bladder, to ascend up the ureters and into the kidneys, where the individual's total volume of blood perfuses through the kidneys many times each day to be filtered. This direct pathway allows bacteria to spread to the blood, leading to a very serious systemic infection known as *urinary sepsis.* For this reason, proper perineal care and hygiene are very important to prevent UTIs.

Knowledge Connection

How much urine do the kidneys normally make in a 24-hour period? When reviewing laboratory results for a patient, what would a specific gravity of 1.005 tell you about the patient's hydration status? A specific gravity of 1.033? What is the difference between anuria and oliguria?

Normal Voiding Patterns

The average individual urinates four to six times per day and does not routinely get up during the sleeping hours to void. Urinary frequency and volume of output are directly related to fluid intake. Because some individuals drink a large amount of fluid in a 24-hour period, you would expect them to urinate more frequently and have a larger output than those who have minimal fluid intake.

Assisting With Toileting

When normally independent patients are in acute or long-term care settings, they often need assistance with personal hygiene and elimination. All members of the nursing team need to respond to patients' toileting needs in a timely manner to foster continued independence. When assisting patients with toileting, follow these guidelines:

- Offer the opportunity to use the bathroom or bedpan before and after meals, and at bedtime.
- Male patients may use a urinal for voiding (Fig. 31-1). Some men find it difficult to void while sitting or lying in bed. If allowed, the male patient may stand at the bedside to void into the urinal. Skill 31-1 (page 731) describes how to assist a male patient with a urinal.
- Use a fracture pan, which is smaller and flatter, for patients who have had hip or back surgeries. The pan slips more easily under the buttocks and does not require that the patient be rolled from side to side. A fracture pan may also be used for patients who are very thin or if a regular bedpan causes back discomfort. In that situation, the patient may be rolled from side to side to place the fracture pan (see Fig. 31-1).
- Provide patients with privacy and avoid rushing them.
- Offer patients the opportunity to perform hand hygiene after toileting.

Patients who are unable to ambulate to the bathroom will use a bedside commode. A bedside commode is a portable chair with a toilet seat and collection bucket beneath it, which is removed for cleaning. The commode is placed near the patient's bed for easy access.

Patients with orders for bedrest are not allowed to be out of the bed to go to the bathroom or to use a bedside commode. These patients will need to use a bedpan for elimination (see Fig. 31-1). It may be embarrassing to them to ask for assistance, and they may delay as long as possible before asking for help. Always respond quickly to every patient's request for the bedpan to prevent incontinence or accidents. Skill 31-2 (page 731) shows the steps for assisting a patient with a bedpan.

Figure 31-1 The urinal, bedpan, and fracture pan are all used to assist patients with urination.

Assessing Urine and Urinary Output

You will find that you are constantly assessing the function of the urinary tract, whether it is simply using your physical assessment skills, evaluating the results of diagnostic tests, or possibly even performing a test on the urine.

Physical Assessment

Nearly every day you will assess the urine's characteristics. What color is it, and what is the clarity, which simply means *is it clear or not?* You should always be alert to any odor that urine may emit, because normally the urine only presents a very mildly aromatic odor, so it is important to note if the urine smells sweet, foul, or like ammonia. The volume or amount of urine produced is always pertinent. A decrease in volume of urine voided may be a sign of dehydration, infection, or renal impairment.

It is necessary to monitor for *edema,* or swelling, due to water retention. Edema due to kidney problems may be found in the hands, legs and feet, sacrum, and face. The quickest way to assess whether or not a patient is retaining water is to perform daily weights, at the same time each day, with the same scales, and with the patient wearing approximately the same amount of clothing. Remember, a gallon of water weighs approximately 8 pounds (3.6 kg), making it easy to determine how much water is actually retained or excreted.

The frequency of urination is important also. The average individual urinates four to six times per day and does not routinely get up during the sleeping hours to void. So extra trips made to the bathroom during the night or more or less frequent episodes of urination may be cause for further assessment. Increased frequency of urination may be a sign of UTI, bladder inflammation, or diabetes mellitus.

If a patient complains of burning or of difficulty starting the stream of urine, you will want to take note of that. Painful or difficult urination is called **dysuria**. Urination should not burn, and the patient should have voluntary control over the starting and stopping of the stream of urine. Burning during urination may be indicative of UTI or bladder or urethral inflammation.

Collecting Specimens and Testing Urine

In a hospital setting, you may not perform urinalysis or urine cultures yourself, but you will be responsible for reviewing the laboratory reports for abnormalities and alerting the physician to them. Therefore, you will need to know the significance of the tests and the possible results.

Some nursing positions may require you to assess specific gravity rather than send a specimen to the laboratory. You will, however, collect urine specimens for laboratory testing as ordered by the health care provider. You may find it common practice to perform some urine testing if you work in community health or in a physician's office.

Urinalysis

One of the most common diagnostic tests ordered in the health care setting is a urinalysis (UA). Components of a urinalysis are found in Table 31-1. This test is done to determine the presence of renal calculi, UTI, malignancy, and diseases affecting the kidneys. You will be responsible for obtaining urine specimens for urinalysis. Skill 33-3 (page 732) lists the steps of obtaining a clean-catch midstream urine specimen. *Safety: When you obtain a specimen, transport it to the laboratory immediately or store it in a refrigerator. Urine that is left standing longer than 1 hour starts to break down, and the test becomes ineffective.*

Timed Urinary Collection

Another type of microscopic urine diagnostic test is a timed urinary collection; the most common timed urine specimen is a 24-hour urine collection. This type of specimen is helpful in evaluating kidney function by measuring the levels of various components in the urine, especially protein levels. The amount of protein the kidneys allow to pass into the urine can help diagnose kidney disease. It is very important that *all* the urine produced within the 24-hour collection time is added to the specimen jug. If urine from a single voiding is inadvertently flushed down the toilet, the 24-hour collection must be restarted. Follow these guidelines to correctly obtain the timed urine specimen:

- Ask the patient to void and discard the urine. This ensures that the 24-hour specimen begins with the patient having an empty bladder.
- Note the exact time that the urine is voided and discarded. This begins the 24-hour period.
- Post signs in the patient's room and on the door stating that the 24-hour urine collection is in progress. Include the date and time the collection started and the date and time it is to end.
- Collect every drop of urine that is voided during the next 24 hours and pour it into the specified large-volume container. This container is kept on ice or refrigerated to prevent the urine from decomposing.
- If the patient has an indwelling urinary catheter, place the collection bag in a basin with ice. Empty the collection bag into the 24-hour urine container.
- If any urine is discarded during the 24-hour period, the entire specimen must be restarted.
- Exactly 24 hours after the collection began, ask the patient to void one last time and add the urine to the collection container. Then take the 24-hour specimen to the laboratory for testing. Remove the signs and inform the patient that the collection is completed.

Reagent Testing

Sometimes urine is tested with reagent sticks, or dipsticks, to obtain immediate results (Fig. 31-2). When dipped into urine and the excess tapped off, each reagent pad changes color to indicate values of pH, specific gravity, protein,

Table 31-1 Urinalysis Results

Characteristic	Normal Findings	Abnormal Findings	Possible Cause
Color and appearance	Straw-colored to pale yellow	Lighter or totally clear	Increased fluid intake, diabetes insipidus
		Dark yellow	Concentrated from decreased fluid intake or dehydration Medications and diet can also affect the color of urine
	Clear	Cloudy or increased turbidity	Phosphate precipitation from setting, blood, epithelial cells, pus, fat droplets, bacteria, RBCs, WBCs
		Milky	Pus, fat globules
		Red or reddish-brown	Blood, sulfa drug
		Bright orangey-red	Pyridium (anesthetic drug for urinary burning)
		Yellowish- or greenish-brown	Bile in urine
		Green	*Pseudomonas* infection of urinary tract
pH	4.6–8.0	High pH (alkaline)	Vaginal discharge, diet high in citrate
		Low pH (acidotic)	Diet high in protein, cranberry juice
Specific gravity	1.010–1.025	Less than 1.010	Overhydration; dilute urine due to kidney impairment
		Greater than 1.025	Dehydration, hemorrhage, diabetes mellitus
Odor	Slightly aromatic	Strong fruity odor	Diabetes mellitus, starvation, and dehydration all cause formation of ketone bodies
		Fetid or foul odor	*Escherichia coli* infection
		Maple syrup odor	Maple syrup urine disease
		Fecal odor	Rectal fistula
Bacteria	Negative	+1 to +4 TNTC (too numerous to count)	Urinary tract infection

Table 31-1 **Urinalysis Results** (continued)

Characteristic	Normal Findings	Abnormal Findings	Possible Cause
Protein	Usually none	Increased	Decreased renal function, some drugs, contamination with vaginal secretions
	Transiently 2–8 mg/dL	Above 8 mg/dL	Transient elevation may be due to excess exercise, emotional stress, or cold bath
Leukocyte esterase	Negative	Present	Pyuria
Nitrites	Negative	Present	Infection
Glucose	Negative	Positive	Diabetes mellitus, Cushing's syndrome, liver and pancreatic disease
Ketones	Negative	Positive	Uncontrolled diabetes mellitus, pregnancy, carbohydrate-free diet, starvation
White blood cells (WBCs, leukocytes)	3–4	Increased number	Urinary tract or vaginal infection
White blood cell casts	Negative	Present	Upper urinary tract infection
Red blood cells (RBCs)	1–2	Increased number	Damage to renal tubules, tumors, renal calculi, or infection
Red blood cell casts	Negative	Positive	Upper urinary tract infections
Crystals	Few/negative	Positive	Renal stones

glucose, ketones, bilirubin, urobilinogen, blood leukocyte, and nitrite levels. This information can be used to screen for evidence of a UTI or the presence of abnormal substances in the urine. There are chemically impregnated pads on the stick that react to the urine. Each reagent pad must be read at specific times. The color changes on the pads are compared to a chart on the side of the dipstick bottle. If abnormal results are found, they should be confirmed by a urinalysis. These dipsticks are often used to test urine quickly in physicians' offices and clinics. Box 31-1 lists the steps used in performing a urine dipstick test.

Straining Urine

Renal calculi, commonly referred to as *kidney stones,* can occur anywhere in the renal system from the kidneys to the urethra. When a stone passes out of the body, it is important

to retain it and send it to the laboratory for analysis. The health care provider may write an order to strain all urine. You will use a special urine strainer, shaped like a cone with a fine wire mesh at the narrow end (Fig. 31-3). Once the patient voids into a specimen pan placed in the toilet, pour the urine through the strainer. If a stone is collected, send it to the laboratory for analysis if ordered.

Measuring Intake and Output

It is very important for you to know whether the amount of urine produced by a patient is adequate or not. Remember that minimum acceptable output is 30 mL/hr, or 240 mL in 8 hours. For knowledge of the urine output to be most useful, you will also want to measure the intake of fluid, otherwise known as measuring intake and output (I&O). Not only

Figure 31-2 Urine dipsticks are used for quick testing at the bedside.

Box 31-1

Performing a Urine Dipstick

You may do a quick test of urine for abnormal findings using reagent strips, commonly referred to as urine dipsticks. To use these dipsticks correctly, follow these guidelines:

• Read the manufacturer's instructions before performing the test.
• Check the expiration date on the bottle of test strips.
• Put on clean gloves for the test.
• Remove one strip from the bottle and recap the bottle immediately to prevent contamination of other strips.
• Dip the test strip into the urine and begin timing.
• Hold the strip next to the bottle label, lining up the strip's small colored square pads to the corresponding ones on the bottle label.
• At each specified time, read the appropriate colored pad and note the results.

Figure 31-3 The urine strainer is used to detect the presence of stones; the specimen pan allows you to collect urine for testing or measurement.

will you measure the amount of fluid going in and fluid coming out, but you will assess the balance between the intake and output; which means to compare fluid intake to urine output for each shift as well as the totals for each 24-hour period. When intake is greater than output, the patient is at risk for fluid overload. When output is greater than intake, the patient is at risk for fluid deficiency or dehydration. These fluid imbalances are discussed in Chapter 29.

To measure urine output of an ambulatory patient, place a specimen pan underneath the rim of the toilet or bedside commode to catch the urine. The inside of the specimen pan is marked in milliliter increments (see Fig. 31-3). Males generally use the urinal to void, and it too is marked in milliliter increments. If a bedridden patient voids in the bedpan, you will pour the urine into a graduated receptacle or a specimen pan to be measured before emptying it into the toilet.

Supervision/Delegation Connection

Monitoring Intake and Output

Monitoring intake and output is a task that can be delegated to unlicensed personnel. As a nurse, if you are depending on someone else from the health care team to aid you in assessing I&O, it is important to make sure he or she performs this assignment accurately and understands the importance of the task. Make sure you provide parameters to be reported to you during the shift if they occur. For example, you may need to know if the patient with a Foley catheter has less than 30 mL/hr of output for 2 consecutive hours; or if the patient without a catheter does not void at least every 4 hours. If oliguria is overlooked and goes unreported for several hours, the patient may experience complications. Although the task of monitoring output can be delegated, licensed personnel are ultimately responsible. When working with assistive personnel, provide clear instructions and expectations; never make the assumption that they know what needs to be reported to you. This is especially important when new members are added to your health care team. Monitor I&O when a patient has an indwelling urinary catheter even if the health care provider does not write an order for it.

Real-World Connection

Monitoring Urinary Output

Patients who have had abdominal surgery usually return to the medical-surgical floor with an indwelling urinary catheter in place. During morning report, the night shift nurse reported that Mrs. J, who had a cesarean section the night before, had only 240 mL of urinary output for the previous 8 hours. Standard orders are to discontinue the urinary catheter the following morning, usually done at 0600 by the night shift nurse. Because the night nurse was concerned that the amount of urine was barely adequate, he made a clinical decision after emptying the drainage bag to leave the catheter in place until the health care provider made rounds.

When the day shift nurse went into the room to assess the patient at 0800, there was 60 mL of clear, dark amber urine in the drainage bag. When the patient's physician made rounds at 0900 there was only 90 mL of urine in the bag. After reviewing the I&O record from the previous shift, the physician wrote the order to cancel the catheter removal that had been written the day before, as well as writing several new orders.

Nursing judgment constantly compels us to think critically about everything we encounter, especially before we take further action. Even though the patient had produced the minimum acceptable amount of urine, other factors were taken into consideration by the nurse before he made the correct decision regarding discontinuing the catheter. The physician appreciated and praised his clinical judgment. Eventually, the patient was taken back to the operating room and was found to have a large hematoma, or blood clot, in her abdomen that had to be removed.

Knowledge Connection

You have asked assistive personnel to collect a final specimen from a patient who is in the process of collecting a 24-hour urine specimen. What instructions will you provide? When might reagent strips be used to test urine? What is the purpose of an order to strain all urine?

Alterations in Urinary Function

Any single structure of the urinary system can malfunction, or a combination of structures can cause alterations in function of the system. The bladder may not empty completely or it may not empty at all. The patient may be unable to control the urine as it leaves the bladder for various reasons. In addition, there may be blockages that prevent the urine from traveling from the kidneys to the bladder to then be expelled, or the prostate gland in the male may be so enlarged that the patient is unable to empty his bladder.

Altered Bladder Function

When the bladder does not contract and empty, the patient may experience painful bladder spasms and distention. The nurse must take action to remove the urine from the bladder. When the patient cannot empty the bladder completely, the urine that remains in the bladder can become a good medium for bacteria growth leading to infection. When the patient cannot control his or her urine output, it can be upsetting and embarrassing.

Urinary Retention

Urinary retention is the inability to empty the bladder at all or the inability to completely empty the bladder. It can be acute or chronic. With urinary retention, the kidneys are functioning normally and producing urine and the ureters are transporting the urine to the bladder to be stored, but for some reason the bladder is not emptying. An obstruction such as a kidney stone, an enlarged prostate gland, a tumor, a pregnant uterus, an infection, or scar tissue may cause retention. Other causes of urinary retention include UTIs, disorders or diseases of the nerves that regulate the bladder and urinary sphincters, postoperative complications due to anesthesia, inflammation, edema from surgery, and medications. An enlarged prostate is a frequent cause of urinary retention in older men. The prostate gland surrounds the urethra and, when the gland enlarges, it constricts the urethra and can prevent the bladder from emptying. After a period of time, the urine in the bladder can reflux into the kidneys, causing *hydronephrosis*, which is the stretching of the renal pelvis due to the obstruction of the flow of urine from the bladder. If the obstruction is not relieved, hydronephrosis can lead to kidney atrophy and chronic renal failure.

Residual Urine

Residual urine is urine that remains in the bladder after the patient voids. It may be caused by bladder outlet obstruction or problems with the detrusor muscle's contractility. Normally, the maximum amount of urine left in the bladder after voiding is 100 mL. To determine if a patient has residual urine, begin by palpating the bladder just above the symphysis pubis to evaluate if there is any bladder distention, as there might be with a large volume of residual. Then you may perform a bladder scan for an accurate estimation of the volume of urine that is present. A bladder scan is a noninvasive procedure that uses ultrasound to measure the amount of residual urine (Fig. 31-4).

Nocturia

When a person wakes often during the night to urinate, it is known as **nocturia**. Occasional nocturia may be caused by ingesting large amounts of fluid in the evening. If a

Figure 31-4   The bladder scan is used to detect the presence of residual urine in the bladder.

patient has persistent nocturia, it may be due to an underlying disease process, such as congestive heart failure, uncontrolled diabetes mellitus, a UTI, an enlarged prostate, or kidney disease. Nocturia should not be dismissed as a normal part of aging and should be evaluated by a health care provider.

Urinary Incontinence

By 2 to 3 years of age, children have full control of their bladder; this control continues through adulthood for most people. However, there are situations in which this bladder control is lost during adulthood; this inability to control the passing of urine is urinary **incontinence**.

Incontinence is more common in women, though the incidence increases for both men and women as they age; however, this does not mean that it is a normal part of the aging process. When a patient experiences incontinence, he or she may be affected emotionally as well as physically. Patients may be forced to make lifestyle adjustments, giving up activities and social situations they once enjoyed due to loss of bladder control and the fear that people will be able detect the smell of urine. Incontinence can cause hardships in the workplace as well. To make matters worse, because people often perceive it as a normal part of the aging process, they may not seek treatment; patients may also be too embarrassed to seek treatment.

Types of Incontinence

Stress incontinence occurs with increased abdominal pressure, causing urine to leak out of the bladder. Stress incontinence is seen more in women than in men. Increased abdominal pressure can be caused by coughing, laughing, sneezing, vomiting, and heavy lifting or straining—anything that elicits a "bearing down" effect. Factors that may contribute to the development of stress incontinence include vaginal births, previous pelvic or vaginal surgery, genetics, hormone levels, and chronic medical conditions. When pelvic floor muscles become weak, they do not support the bladder and urethra, leading to urine leakage.

Urge incontinence, also known as *overactive bladder,* is the inability to keep urine in the bladder long enough to get to the restroom. Normally, most people void five to six times a day. When a patient experiences urge incontinence, he or she may urinate more frequently than normal in the daytime and experience nocturia two or three times per night. The patient may have urine leakage because of the inability to get to the bathroom quickly. This type of incontinence is caused by bladder spasms or contractions that lead to involuntary passing of urine. Triggers that may lead to urge incontinence include the sound of running water, drinking liquid, or placing your hands in warm water. Urge incontinence is often caused by a UTI, but many times the cause is not known. Muscle toning and strengthening exercises are sometimes successful treatments for urge incontinence. *Mixed incontinence* is diagnosed when a patient experiences both stress and urge incontinence.

Overflow incontinence occurs when the bladder is distended due to an obstruction, preventing it from emptying normally. Some urine may then leak past the blockage, causing overflow. The most common cause of this obstruction is an enlarged prostate gland in men.

Other types of incontinence are less common. These include functional, total, and neuropathic incontinence. *Functional incontinence* occurs when the person is unable to reach a bathroom to urinate. This may be due to the unavailability of bathroom facilities or the person's inability to get on the toilet before urination occurs. *Total incontinence* is the loss of urine with no warning. In this situation, the person is unaware of the need to void and makes no effort to get to a bathroom. *Neuropathic incontinence* occurs when the nerves that control the bladder and surrounding structures are not getting the message to the brain that the bladder is full.

Managing Incontinence

One treatment for stress incontinence involves teaching the patient to perform Kegel exercises, which will strengthen and tone the pelvic floor muscles. The exercises must be done regularly and indefinitely to be effective. Box 31-2 provides a description of how to teach a patient to perform Kegel exercises.

Encourage women to engage in a moderate exercise program on a regular basis to help decrease the incidence of incontinence. Studies have shown that women who engage in regular, moderately intensive physical activity have less urinary incontinence than women who lead sedentary lifestyles.

Bladder Training

Nurses can initiate a bladder training program without a physician's order to assist the patient in managing urinary incontinence. Bladder training involves assisting the patient to the bathroom at set times throughout the day, even if the urge to urinate is not recognized. For example, you would assist the patient to the bathroom after meals and every

Box 31-2

Kegel Exercise Instructions

You may need to explain how to perform pelvic floor exercises to help prevent or control certain types of urinary incontinence. Instruct the patient using these guidelines:
- Have the patient lie supine.
- Have the patient place the hands on the lower abdomen to ensure that the abdominal muscles stay relaxed.
- Tell the patient to tighten the pelvic floor muscles (the muscles that stop the flow of urine or prevent you from passing gas) without tightening the abdominal or thigh muscles.
- Encourage the patient to hold the contraction for 5 to 10 seconds, then relax for 5 to 10 seconds. The patient should perform 40 to 60 exercises spread throughout the day.
- Advise the patient to not perform the exercises while urinating because it can cause urinary retention.

2 hours during the day to increase awareness of the need to void. Follow these guidelines to increase the effectiveness of bladder training:

- Ensure that the patient is taking in adequate amounts of fluid, at least 64 ounces per day, to help maintain a healthy urinary tract and facilitate the elimination of waste.
- Teach patients to avoid caffeinated beverages and to drink more during the day and less in the evening to avoid nighttime incontinence.
- Offer fluids throughout the day, avoiding a large volume of fluid all at one time. Find out which fluids the patient prefers and offer an 8-ounce glass of fluid every 2 hours.
- If bladder training is being done in a health care facility, provide opportunities for toileting on a regular schedule.
- Assist the patient to the bathroom or offer a bedpan every 2 hours and assess the patient frequently for incontinence. If the patient has been incontinent between toileting, decrease the length of time between offering the bedpan or assistance to the bathroom.
- Most people void in the morning, after meals and before bed. Try to mimic the patient's normal voiding patterns.

In some circumstances, bladder training is not appropriate. If the patient is not able to understand the program or does not wish to participate, he or she is not a candidate for bladder training. In this situation, good skin care is very important to prevent skin breakdown. *Safety: Clean the skin as soon as urinary incontinence is detected. When urine is left on the skin, the liquid portion evaporates and the chemicals left behind can cause skin irritation and skin breakdown.* Change the patient's incontinence briefs and perform perineal care at least every 2 hours. In general, indwelling urinary catheters are not placed for long-term urinary incontinence because they can lead to UTIs, sepsis, urethral strictures, prostatitis, and the potential development of bladder cancer.

Knowledge Connection

During data collection, you ask a male patient about problems with urination. He replies, "It seems to take me longer to pee than it used to." What is the patient experiencing? What are the differences in managing stress versus urge urinary incontinence?

Laboratory and Diagnostic Connection

Assessing Kidney Function and Failure
Two blood tests, **blood urea nitrogen (BUN)** and serum creatinine, reflect kidney function. Urea nitrogen in the blood is a waste product normally eliminated from the body when the kidneys filter it out of the blood and excrete it into the urine. The normal levels of BUN are 10 to 20 mg/dL in adults. Abnormal elevations in BUN may reflect infection or some degree of renal impairment. Creatinine is another waste product produced by the body and excreted by the kidneys.

The normal level of creatinine in the blood is 0.6 to 1.2 mg/dL in an adult male and 0.5 to 1.1 mg/dL in an adult female. An increase in creatinine in the blood usually indicates decreased or impaired renal function. A health care provider can use the serum creatinine level to determine the glomerular filtration rate (GFR) to determine the stage of renal disease that a patient is in. A GFR less than 60 mL/min when tested over 3 months indicates chronic kidney disease. A GFR less than 15 mL/min indicates renal failure. Physicians monitor the BUN, serum creatinine, and GFR over several months to determine the extent of chronic kidney disease and treat the patient to prevent further progression of the disease.

Caring for Patients With Altered Urinary Function

Over your career, you will probably care for many patients with altered urinary function. The alteration may be related to the patient's original diagnosis and admission, or it may be due to an additional issue that developed after admission.

Urinary Catheters

One of the most common situations you will encounter is caring for patients with an indwelling catheter in place, or the need to insert a straight catheter to obtain residual urine or a sterile urine specimen. A *urinary catheter* is a tube usually made of rubber, plastic, latex, polyvinyl, or silicone that is inserted through the urethra into the bladder. It may be inserted and then quickly removed after the bladder is emptied, as in the case of a straight catheter, or it may remain in place when an attached balloon is inflated, anchoring it in the bladder.

Types of Catheters
There are many different types of catheters, including straight catheters, indwelling catheters, three-way catheters, and condom catheters. Box 31-3 describes different types of urinary catheters and their uses. Figure 31-5 shows cross sections of different types of catheters.

Indwelling Catheters
When you care for a patient with urinary retention, you will expect to receive orders to insert an **indwelling catheter**, also known as a *double-lumen catheter* or *Foley catheter*, to empty the bladder. The catheter will remain in the bladder, usually for a few days, and drain the urine on a continuous basis. Skill 31-4 (page 733) provides more information on inserting an indwelling urinary catheter. Skill 31-5 (page 736) provides information on obtaining a urine sample from an indwelling urinary catheter.

An indwelling catheter may be ordered when an accurate measurement of urine output is required, for a patient undergoing surgery to keep the bladder empty during

Box 31-3

Types of Catheters and Their Uses

Some catheters may be called by several different names. It is important to be familiar with the type of catheter, its function, and the names it may be called.

- **Straight Catheter:** Also known as a *single-lumen catheter.* Used only for insertion into the urinary bladder to obtain a sterile urine specimen or a one-time drainage of urine from the bladder. It is aseptically inserted into the bladder through the urinary meatus, where either all the urine is drained or just enough urine for a specimen is obtained. Then the straight catheter is removed.
- **Indwelling Catheter:** Also known as a *double-lumen catheter* and a *Foley catheter.* Remains in the urinary bladder for a designated period of time. After insertion, one lumen is used to inflate a balloon near the tip of the catheter with 5 to 30 mL of sterile water; the amount of water is dependent upon the size of the balloon. This inflated balloon sits at the junction of the bladder and the urethra, to hold the catheter in place and help seal the exit from the bladder so urine does not leak around the catheter (see Fig. 31-6). Urine continually drains out of the bladder through the lumen of the catheter into a drainage bag that hangs low on the side of the patient's bed. Indwelling catheters are inserted when the patient will need urine drainage for 1 or more days.
- **Three-way Catheter:** Also known as a *triple-lumen catheter* and an *Alcock catheter.* Used in only one specific situation: After a male patient has had a transurethral resection of the

prostate, the surgeon will insert a triple-lumen catheter with a 30- to 60-mL balloon to provide traction and help control bleeding. The third lumen in the catheter allows instillation of sterile fluid into the bladder during continuous bladder irrigation to help evacuate tissue and clots from the urinary bladder.
- **Coudé Catheter:** Used specifically to accommodate an enlarged prostate in male patients. It has a curved tip, allowing it to more easily pass through an enlarged prostate gland and enter the bladder.
- **Suprapubic Catheter:** Placed following trauma or surgery to the urethra or if an indwelling catheter cannot be inserted into the bladder. The physician makes a small incision above the pubic bone, passes an instrument through the abdominal wall and into the bladder, then places the catheter. This procedure requires that the patient be given mild sedation or a local anesthetic.
- **Condom Catheter:** Also known as a *Texas catheter.* Used for males who are incontinent of urine to avoid the risk of infection related to insertion of an indwelling catheter. It is similar to a regular condom and is applied by rolling it onto the penis. It is a condom-like sheath with a 2-inch drainage tube connector on the tip that connects to a urinary drainage bag. The sheath collects the urine and allows it to drain through the drainage tube into the drainage bag, either a regular urinary drainage bag or a smaller bag that can be strapped to the thigh.

Figure 31-5 Types of catheters: (a) Straight catheter, also called a single-lumen catheter. (b) Indwelling catheter, also known as a double-lumen or Foley catheter. (c) Three-way catheter, also known as a triple-lumen catheter, used for continuous bladder irrigations.

the surgery to prevent accidental damage, for patients who are unable to tolerate getting up to the bathroom, and for patients who are comatose to prevent incontinence and skin breakdown. It is not uncommon for patients to return from surgery with an indwelling catheter in place. It is

your nursing responsibility to assess urinary output, including color, clarity, and amount, during your shift. Figure 31-6 shows indwelling catheters in both male and female patients.

In some circumstances, special catheters must be used to achieve placement of an indwelling catheter. If an

(a)

(b)

Figure 31-6 Placement of indwelling catheters: (a) Location of an indwelling catheter with the balloon inflated in a male. (b) Location of an indwelling catheter with the balloon inflated in a female.

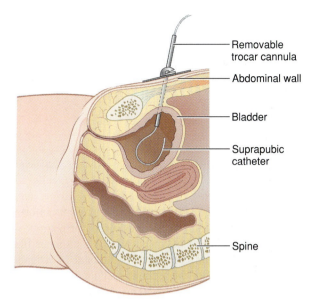

— Removable trocar cannula

— Abdominal wall

— Bladder

— Suprapubic catheter

— Spine

Figure 31-7 A suprapubic catheter is inserted through the abdominal wall directly into the bladder.

obstruction in the urethra or neck of the bladder is present, it may be difficult to pass the catheter into the bladder. If the obstruction is due to an enlarged prostate, a Coudé catheter may be the best choice (see Box 31-3).

If the catheter cannot be advanced into the bladder, a physician may have to insert a suprapubic catheter (see Box 31-3). Once the suprapubic catheter is inserted, the catheter is advanced about an inch into the bladder, and the balloon is filled with 5 mL of sterile water to hold it in place. Figure 31-7 shows insertion of a suprapubic catheter.

Straight Catheters

If you are caring for a patient who is unable to fully empty his or her bladder, and you have found residual urine in the bladder using a bladder scan, you could expect to receive orders to insert a **straight catheter**, also known as a *single-lumen catheter,* to empty the bladder. A straight catheter is a single tube with holes at the end. It is generally made of red rubber. The physician may or may not also order a sterile specimen from the bladder for a urinalysis or culture and sensitivity testing. Straight catheters are also used by patients who must catheterize themselves on a regular basis to empty the bladder. An example of this would be the patient with a condition called *neurogenic bladder,* where the nerves to the bladder have been permanently damaged. The patient cannot control the nerves that

cause the bladder to empty. The patient or a caregiver must insert a straight catheter to empty the patient's bladder several times per day, usually about every 4 hours.

In the hospital setting, you will use a sterile catheter insertion kit and a sterile straight catheter every time you insert a catheter. The hospital environment is full of pathogens and you must take every precaution to prevent contamination of your sterile field or the sterile catheter, which would then introduce harmful pathogens into the patient's bladder. See Chapter 22 for a review of sterile technique. Skill 31-6 (page 737) provides more information on inserting a straight catheter.

Three-Way Catheters

When the prostate gland enlarges in a male patient, it obstructs the urethra, causing the opening through which urine can pass to narrow significantly. In this situation, the enlargement of the prostate is not due to cancer, but is a benign condition called benign prostatic hypertrophy (BPH). A surgical procedure called transurethral resection of the prostate (TURP) is performed to remove the parts of the prostate that are blocking the urethra.

After this surgery, a *three-way catheter,* also known as a *triple-lumen catheter* or *Alcock catheter,* is inserted through the newly cleared urethra and into the bladder to allow for irrigation of the bladder. Because cutting has occurred, it is normal for blood and blood clots to pass through the three-way catheter and into the urinary drainage bag. The goal of nursing care after this procedure is to prevent any blood clots from obstructing the flow of the irrigation fluid into the bladder and back out again.

Continuous Bladder Irrigation

Irrigation fluid in large bags is hung from an IV pole and the tubing is aseptically attached to the third lumen of the three-way catheter. The irrigation fluid runs continuously at a slow rate to wash out blood and prevent clots from forming (Fig. 31-8). If the urine in the collection bag becomes red or clots are evident in the tubing, increase the rate to flush them out. *Safety: Assess for fluid return into the drainage bag frequently. It is possible for a blood clot to clog the urine drainage lumen, blocking urine and irrigation fluid from leaving the bladder. This is extremely important due to the fact that irrigation fluid continues to flow into the bladder via the irrigation lumen, filling the bladder fuller and fuller. This can result in overdistention of the bladder and could potentially rupture the bladder if the urine lumen remains clogged.* Skill 31-7 (page 739) presents information on how to perform a continuous bladder irrigation.

To correctly calculate output with a continuous bladder irrigation, you must subtract the amount of irrigation solution instilled from the amount of fluid in the urinary drainage bag. For example, if 750 mL of saline was instilled during irrigation and a total of 1,000 mL of fluid has collected in the drainage bag, the amount of urine output would be 250 mL, because you subtracted 750 from 1,000.

Figure 31-8 A continuous bladder irrigation consists of irrigation fluid from the large bag on the IV pole flowing through the triple-lumen catheter into the bladder, then out to the drainage bag on the side of the bed.

Labels on figure:
- Irrigation bag
- Drip chamber
- Clamp
- Tubing to irrigation port
- Bladder
- Inflation port
- Triple lumen catheter
- Drainage tubing
- Drainage bag

Condom Catheters

Condom catheters are not inserted into the bladder through the urethra, so they pose less of a risk for causing a UTI. Most condom catheters are held in place with a double-sided adhesive strip applied to the penis. It is important to apply the adhesive strip in a spiral. This prevents the strip from encircling the penis and potentially interfering with circulation. It is also important to keep the foreskin in place when applying a condom catheter to an uncircumsized male patient. Skill 31-8 (page 740) shows the steps for applying a condom catheter.

Catheter Size

Urinary catheters come in different sizes gauged by measuring the outer diameter of the catheter: the larger the number, the larger the catheter. The size is denoted with a number followed by *French (Fr),* which is the scale of measurement for urinary catheters. A child may need a size 8 French, an adult a size 14 or size 16 French. When a patient in long-term care or home care has had an indwelling catheter for several years, it may be necessary to use even larger sizes, such as 20 or 22 French because the urethra and cystourethral junction stretch over time. Catheters also come in different lengths according to their purpose. A 22-cm length would be appropriate for a female, a 40-cm for a male. However, in most health care settings, a standard length of 40 cm is used. Catheters also come with different sizes of inflatable balloons, from 5 to 30 mL.

Inserting Catheters

Insertion of any type of catheter requires a physician's order, which should be reviewed prior to the procedure. It is important to assess a patient for allergies to latex before inserting an indwelling urinary catheter. Always check for allergies to povidone-iodine (Betadine) as well, as it is provided in most catheter insertion kits for cleansing the meatus and surrounding area prior to insertion. If the patient is allergic to Betadine, you will need to obtain a different cleaning agent according to your facility policy. The type of catheter and the reason for catheterization will determine which supply kit you use. There are different kits for insertion of straight catheters and indwelling catheters. Figure 31-9 shows the contents of a straight catheter kit, and Figure 31-10 shows the contents of an indwelling catheter kit.

Insertion of a urinary catheter, in the hospital or another medical setting, requires stringent asepsis. Your sterile technique helps to prevent hospital-acquired UTIs; if you contaminate the catheter, your gloves, your sterile field, or sterile supplies, you must stop the procedure and start over with uncontaminated supplies. Failure to do so may cause your patient to experience infection, discomfort, added expense, and potentially death from sepsis. You may be the only person who knows if you have contaminated your sterile field or the sterile catheter during insertion. If that occurs, you must discard your supplies and begin again. *Safety: Contamination of the catheter or sterile field can lead to a*

Figure 31-9 A prepackaged straight catheter kit.

Figure 31-10 A prepackaged indwelling catheter kit.

hospital-acquired UTI. Refer back to Chapter 22 for review of sterile technique. Box 31-4 contains information regarding hospital costs associated with UTIs.

Before you begin the procedure of inserting a catheter, you will need to examine the patient's perineal anatomy. The female urinary meatus is normally located between the clitoris and the vagina; however, you may not see an obvious "opening," unless the patient has had many urinary catheters in the past. The female urinary meatus often resembles a small dimpling of the tissue, almost like a tiny slit or crease, rather than the easily detectable opening that you will see in the manikin in the skills laboratory. In an elderly female, you may even find the urethral meatus in a slightly different

location than indicated in textbook anatomy. The urinary meatus is generally located just below the clitoris, midway between the clitoris and the vaginal opening, or *introitus.* In some elderly females, you may find the urinary meatus at the edge of or slightly inside the vaginal opening. A lack of hormones causes the tissue of the vulva to *atrophy,* or shrink. This results in pulling the urinary meatus into the vaginal introitus, making it more difficult to access with a catheter. These two facts often surprise students during the first catheterization at clinicals.

In certain circumstances, you may find that you are unable to separate the female patient's legs due to severe contractures or other conditions. In these instances, a possible alternative may be to insert the catheter while the patient is lying on her side. Turn the patient to the lateral position and view the urinary meatus from that angle before you prepare to insert the catheter. Patients who have long-term indwelling catheters may be easier to catheterize from this position.

Male patients may exhibit anomalies as well. The urethra may open on the dorsum of the penis rather than at the tip of the penis, a condition known as *epispadias.* If the urethral meatus is located on the underside of the penis, the condition is termed *hypospadias.*

Some men have been circumcised, meaning that the foreskin that covers the glans penis has been surgically removed. This may be done due to cultural or religious preferences. For patients who have not been circumcised, you must retract the foreskin, or move it back from the glans, during catheterization. *Safety: It is extremely important that you replace the foreskin to its original position after you have inserted the indwelling catheter. Failure to do so can cause the glans penis to be deprived of adequate blood flow, leading to swelling and possible necrosis.*

When you try to insert a standard catheter in a male patient with an enlarged prostate, you may meet resistance. When this occurs, try twisting the catheter slightly as you attempt to advance it. It may be helpful to use your non-dominant hand, which is holding the penis, to shift the shaft of the penis in an attempt to better line up the distal portion of the urethra with the proximal portion that goes through the prostate. Avoid attempting to insert the catheter while holding the penis with only your index finger and thumb. Make certain you have a full-handed grasp of the shaft. Now shift the penis shaft just *slightly* to change the angle of the penis and urethra: *slightly* toward the patient's feet or toward his head, not big movements. This will sometimes be adequate to allow the catheter tip to enter the portion of the urethra that passes through the enlarged prostate. If that does not advance the tip beyond the prostate gland, the procedure may need to be attempted again using a Coudé catheter. Notify the physician and review your facility policy and procedure for use of a Coudé catheter, as some facilities require that a physician or even a urologist insert it.

Draining Urine From the Bladder

Once the catheter is inserted into the bladder, you will need to observe how much urine returns. When a full bladder is emptied too rapidly, the patient may experience bladder spasms. It is recommended that you always empty the bladder slowly, draining no more than 1,000 mL at one time; then clamp the catheter and waiting 30 minutes before allowing additional urine to drain.

Urine drains from the catheter through tubing attached to a drainage bag, where it is stored until emptied. When caring for the patient with an indwelling catheter, monitor the drainage bag that collects the urine as it drains from the bladder several times during your shift. Empty the bag at the end of the shift and more frequently if it becomes full. The numbers on the bag will provide you with only an approximate volume. Measure the exact volume of urine by emptying it into a graduated container. The task of emptying the catheter drainage bag can be assigned to assistive personnel, but monitoring urinary output during the shift is your responsibility. Unless otherwise ordered, output is normally recorded at the end of the shift. If the health care provider has ordered hourly output readings or you are concerned about the amount of urine, a catheter with a urometer can be inserted, which will give you an accurate reading. A *urometer* is a small plastic measuring device attached to the urine drainage bag that accurately measures very small amounts of urine.

Follow these guidelines for care of the urinary drainage bag:

- Empty the catheter bag every 8 hours or when it is full and document the amount in the medical record.
- When emptying the bag, do not touch the drainage spout to any surfaces, and wipe it with an alcohol swab before closing the spout.
- Always empty urine into a graduated container to obtain an accurate measurement. *Safety: Each patient must have his or her own graduated container for measurement. Sharing these containers among patients can lead to cross-contamination and increase the incidence of hospital-acquired UTIs.*

- Maintain the drainage bag below the level of the bladder at all times. If the bag is elevated, the tubing should be clamped first to prevent urine in the tubing from flowing back into the bladder, potentially causing a UTI.
- Keep the tubing free of kinks and coils.
- Hang the drainage bag on a moveable part of the bed; it should not lay on the floor. Avoid hanging it on the bed rails, however, as it could be raised above the level of the bladder when the rails are raised.

Troubleshooting Low Output

If there is no urine collecting in the drainage bag, palpate the urinary bladder above the pubic bone to assess for a full bladder. Check for kinks in the catheter tubing. Ensure that the patient is not lying on the catheter or drainage bag tubing. Manipulate the drainage bag tubing so that the urine flows in a downward manner by gravity. If the tubing is looped downward, urine will pool and back up because it cannot run uphill. Have the patient change positions and see if the bladder will empty.

If the bladder feels full, indicated during your assessment by palpating a firm area above the pubic bone, it is appropriate to perform a bladder scan. It is possible that the catheter is blocked by sediment or mucus. If none of the troubleshooting techniques improves output and the bladder definitely contains urine, notify the health care provider to obtain orders to irrigate the catheter.

Intermittent Catheter Irrigation

A catheter can be irrigated, or flushed, with sterile saline to rinse out sediment or mucus that may be blocking the openings on the tube in the bladder. It is important to use good aseptic technique to prevent introducing pathogens into the closed urinary drainage system. This is accomplished by using a sterile syringe and noncoring blunt needle or other needleless access device (Fig. 31-11). The sterile saline is drawn up as ordered from a sterile container into a 20-mL syringe. The tube on the drainage bag contains an access port for this purpose. Clamp the drainage bag tubing below the port. This causes the saline to go into the bladder and not simply drain into the bag. Skill 31-9 (page 741) lists the steps of irrigating a closed urinary drainage system.

Figure 31-11 This nurse is irrigating a catheter using a noncoring blunt needle, maintaining the closed system.

Catheter Care

Perform catheter care at least once a shift and anytime the catheter becomes contaminated by a bowel movement to prevent UTIs. Hold the catheter in your gloved hand to prevent traction on the tubing as you clean the catheter using a soapy washcloth, using downward strokes from the insertion site toward the catheter bag. Upward strokes encourage the movement of microorganisms into the bladder. Rinse the catheter and provide perineal care when you perform catheter care. See Chapter 15 for further information on perineal care.

Discontinuing Catheters

Indwelling catheters inserted for surgical patients may remain in place for several days. You must have a physician's order to discontinue an indwelling catheter. Skill 31-10 (page 742) shows the steps required to remove an indwelling urinary catheter. Upon removal of the catheter, it is important that you monitor for urinary retention, making certain that the patient urinates within a maximum of 8 hours after discontinuation of the catheter. Be certain to document when the patient voids and how much is voided. *Safety: If a patient has not voided in the 8 hours after removing an indwelling catheter, or has voided less than 240 mL, notify the health care provider.* The health care provider may then order a straight catheterization to empty the bladder or reinsertion of an indwelling catheter if the bladder scan reveals an excessive amount of residual urine.

Urinary Diversions

In some situations, it is not possible to empty the bladder by draining it with a catheter due to obstruction or interruption of the normal urine pathway. A **urinary diversion** means that the urine is eliminated by an alternative route rather than traveling through the bladder. These diversions may be established when there has been trauma to the bladder or the bladder has been removed as a result of bladder cancer. Occasionally, the ureters or bladder did not form correctly before birth, leading to a congenital condition requiring a urinary diversion.

One type of urinary diversion is the *ileal conduit,* wherein the ureters are attached to a section of the small intestine that has been used to create a pouch and stoma. The urine drains continuously from the stoma. The patient wears an appliance over the stoma to collect the urine. Application of appliances to a stoma is discussed in Chapter 30. One of the greatest challenges with an incontinent urinary diversion is skin care. If the patient has a problem with irritation or skin breakdown, an enterostomal therapist or nurse can recommend protective skin wipes or an ostomy powder to help protect the skin.

Additional types of urinary diversions include the *continent urostomy* and the newer *orthotopic bladder substitution.* For the continent urostomy, a pouch is created from the intestine, the ureters empty into the pouch, and a nipple

valve is constructed (Fig. 31-12). The patient performs self-catheterization intermittently during the day to empty the pouch (Fig. 31-13). For the orthotopic bladder substitution, a part of the intestines are used to make a new bladder. The ureters drain into it, and the urethra drains the substitute bladder. The patient is able to void through the urethra but may experience incontinence and may have to perform self-catheterization intermittently (see Fig. 31-13).

Urinary Tract Infections

A **urinary tract infection (UTI)** is caused by the presence of pathogens within the urinary tract. Any structure in the urinary tract may become infected, and the infection can

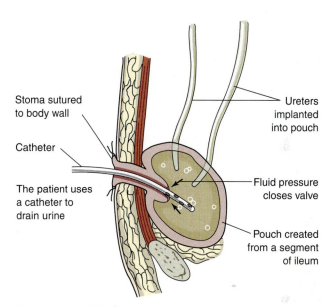

Figure 31-12 One type of urinary diversion, an ileal conduit: The ureters are implanted into a pouch made from a segment of the ileum that holds urine and opens to a stoma.

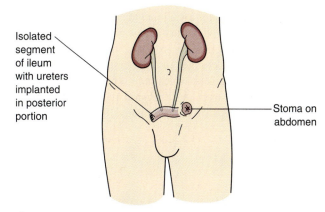

Figure 31-13 The continent urinary diversion: The pouch formed from intestine contains a valve that can be entered with a catheter to drain urine.

spread from one structure to another. An infection in the urinary bladder is called *cystitis*. If the infection is left untreated, it can travel from the bladder up the ureters and into the kidneys. An infection in the kidney is called *pyelonephritis*, which can cause renal scarring and eventually lead to loss of kidney function. Approximately 80% of UTIs are caused by bacteria from the bowel, or *enterobacteria*. UTIs are more commonly seen in women than men because of the close proximity of the urethral opening to the anus, allowing bacteria to travel from the perianal area into the urinary tract.

The body's defense mechanisms help prevent UTIs. The pH of urine is acidic to help kill bacteria. Vaginal secretions are also acidic, which inhibits microorganisms from the rectum from migrating into the bladder. When a person voids, it flushes bacteria from the urinary tract. As women age, the changes to the reproductive tract increase the risk of acquiring a UTI. The pH of the vagina becomes more alkaline, which is less hostile to invading pathogens. Sexual intercourse, the use of diaphragms, and the use of spermicidal gels can also increase the incidence of UTIs. Encourage female patients who have recurrent UTIs to empty the bladder after intercourse and use a method of birth control other than a diaphragm or spermicides.

In addition, if female patients have recurring UTIs, encourage them to avoid baths with the use of bath salts, perfumes, or bubble bath as these can irritate the urethra and cause infection that can migrate to the bladder. It is also important to empty the bladder frequently throughout the day to prevent pooling of urine in the bladder.

Symptoms of UTI include dysuria, urinary frequency, urgency, nocturia, low abdominal pain, and incontinence. If the patient has fever, chills, malaise, nausea, vomiting, and flank pain, the infection has most likely spread to the kidneys, causing pyelonephritis. In a physician's office, the diagnosis of UTI may be made using a urine dipstick test. The presence of nitrites and leukocyte esterase indicates a UTI. Nitrites can only be present if there are bacteria in the urine. A midstream clean-catch or straight catheter urine specimen may also be obtained for the purpose of performing a urinalysis to diagnose a UTI.

The treatment for a UTI includes rest, increased fluid intake, antibiotics, and urinary analgesics. The treatment for pyelonephritis may include hospitalization for IV antibiotics. Patients are encouraged to drink cranberry juice or take cranberry extract tablets, which inhibit bacteria from adhering to the urinary tract. As a general rule, patients should consume 64 ounces of noncaffeinated fluid a day unless contraindicated.

Knowledge Connection

What kind of bedpan would you obtain for a patient who has a fractured hip and is in traction prior to surgery? The UAP tells you that the output of a patient with a continuous bladder irrigation is 4,000 mL for an 8-hour shift. What additional information do you need to determine the amount of urine that was produced?

People and Places Connection

Home Health Care and Catheterizations

In the home health care setting, patients may need to perform self-catheterizations. Unlike in the acute care setting, self-catheterization at home is a clean rather than sterile procedure. Catheters are often washed and reused; patients wash their hands and put on nonsterile gloves when they perform the procedure. Those who may perform self-catheterization include patients with urinary retention, residual urine, or neurological conditions that prevent the bladder from emptying, or those who have a history of a spinal cord injury.

Long-term Care and Catheterizations

The Centers for Medicare and Medicaid Services of the U.S. Department of Health and Human Services states that only residents with appropriate justification should have indwelling urinary catheters. Appropriate use would include residents who have intractable urinary retention, stage III or stage IV pressure ulcers, terminal illness, or severe impairment such that positioning and clothing changes are uncomfortable or are associated with intractable pain.

Pediatric Considerations for Urinary Care

Urinary tract infection is second only to respiratory infections in children. The symptoms a child displays may be different then those seen in adults. Poor feeding, vomiting and diarrhea, and sleeplessness may occur. Children who were once toilet trained may have accidents. Children may also have personality changes. A child should be evaluated for a UTI if he or she presents with any of these symptoms. UTIs occur more often in girls than boys. Girls should be taught from a young age to wipe from front to back. If a young girl does have recurrent UTIs, instruct her parents to have her shower rather than bathe and avoid bubble baths, which can lead to UTIs. To obtain a urine specimen from a child who is not yet toilet trained, you may use a sterile plastic urine collector bag with an adhesive patch placed over the genitals. Another type of device for collecting a urine specimen from a child may have the catheter extending from a test tube–like collection device.

Nursing Care Plan for a Patient With a Urinary Tract Infection

Your patient assignment is a 22-year-old female college student who was admitted with a severe UTI and possible pyelonephritis. She tells you that she is very busy with school, work, and a new boyfriend, and that she does not have time to be sick. However, she states that she feels so awful with fever, chills, back pain, and painful urination that she knows she cannot keep up her schedule feeling this way. Figure 31-14 presents a concept map care plan for this patient.

Assessment

Your first step is to gather data regarding her symptoms and current complaints. Her vital signs are outside of normal limits, with a temperature of 101.4°F (38.6°C), pulse rate of 106, respirations of 24, and BP of 116/70. She is also complaining of pain in her back. As you question her more closely, you learn that the pain is just below her rib cage on both sides, which you know is also referred to as *flank pain.* When you ask about her voiding patterns, she tells you that she is urinating "constantly" but only in small amounts and that she feels pain and burning when she urinates. She tells you that she got little sleep the past 2 nights because she was "up and down" all night long and because of the pain in her back, which she rates at an 8 on a 0-to-10 scale. While you are talking with her, she experiences chilling and asks for another blanket. Upon palpation, you find mild tenderness over her bladder area. Her skin turgor is adequate and she has no signs of dehydration. She also tells you that she never wants to go through anything like this again, and asks what she can do to prevent it from happening in the future.

As you review her history, you assess risk factors that would contribute to developing a UTI. You learn that she normally drinks diet cola only, and rarely ever drinks water or juices. When she is well, she usually only voids two to three times per day and "holds it as long as she can" because she has little time between classes for bathroom breaks. She denies nocturia until the current symptoms began.

When you review her laboratory and diagnostic testing, you learn that her white blood cell (WBC) count is elevated to 16,000/mm³, indicating the presence of bacterial infection. Her urinalysis shows cloudy yellow urine with a strong ammonia smell, with abnormal contents of casts, few WBCs, few red blood cells (RBCs), and bacteria too numerous to count.

Nursing Diagnosis

After collecting your data, you have to analyze this information and determine what kind of problems this patient has or may be at risk for developing. In other words, what are her nursing diagnoses? If you are an LPN/LVN, you will assist the RN in this process of identifying the patient's problems, also known as her nursing diagnoses. In order to assign nursing diagnoses, you need to review what you have learned about this patient. She has several indications of UTI:

- She has frequency with pain and burning on urination.
- She has an elevated temperature, pulse, and respirations.
- She is experiencing nocturia, which is not normal for her.
- She is experiencing chilling.
- Her urinalysis shows the presence of WBCs, RBCs, and bacteria, as well as abnormal appearance and smell of urine.

In addition to these findings, you also have learned that she has additional complaints most likely related to a kidney infection, including the fact that her WBC is elevated to 16,000/mm³ and she is complaining of bilateral flank pain.

You also realize from her lifestyle that she does not know how to prevent further recurrence of UTIs because she drinks only caffeinated and carbonated beverages and she does not empty her bladder as frequently as needed.

After analyzing the data, you can identify several nursing diagnoses and prioritize them. The diagnosis with the highest priority is related to her discomfort and frequency of urination. The remaining nursing diagnoses focus on her pain, nausea, and lack of knowledge about UTIs. The nursing diagnoses you choose are:

- Impaired urinary elimination related to UTI as evidenced by dysuria and urinary frequency.
- Acute back pain related to probable kidney infection as evidenced by rating the pain at 8 and sleep disturbance
- Deficient knowledge of causes of UTI related to lack of exposure as evidenced by request for information

(care plan continues on page 728)

Nursing Care Plan for a Patient With a Urinary Tract Infection (continued)

Planning

Now it is time to plan the interventions you might want to implement to help her with her problems. As you look at your options, you determine that improving her urinary functioning so that she can urinate without discomfort and with decreased frequency is a priority. You know that you need to take steps to help relieve her back pain so she can rest, and that she must enhance her fluid intake to improve her urinary status. You also realize that you need to provide patient teaching about prevention and causes of UTI to help her from experiencing recurrent urinary problems.

Interventions

At this stage of the nursing process, you can now implement the interventions that you have planned. Table 31-2 provides nursing interventions for these nursing diagnoses.

Evaluation

The last step in the nursing process is to evaluate whether the interventions you have been implementing are helping the patient. Table 31-2 provides evaluations of those interventions. Continued follow-up should take place, but it looks like you are on the right track with your plan of care.

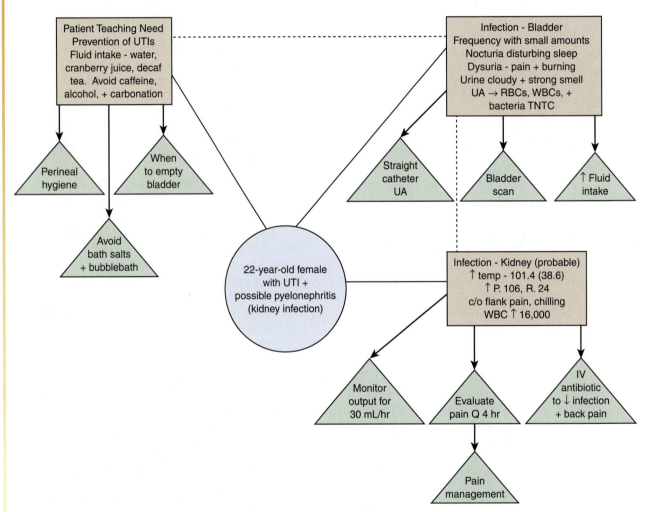

Figure 31-14 Concept map care plan for a patient with a UTI.

Table 31-2   **Nursing Care Plan for a Patient With a Urinary Tract Infection**

Nursing Diagnosis: Impaired urinary elimination related to UTI as evidenced by dysuria and urinary frequency.
Expected Outcomes: The patient will exhibit normal elimination patterns of voiding clear yellow urine in amounts of 200 mL or more before discharge.

Interventions	Evaluations
Encourage intake of fluids that do not irritate the bladder, such as those without alcohol, caffeine, and carbonation. Encourage cranberry juice because it inhibits bacteria from adhering to the urinary tract. Determine the patient's fluid preferences and offer those that she likes.	Day 1: Unable to take fluids at first due to nausea. Later in day was able to take 120 mL of apple juice and 100 mL of grape juice. Day 3: Taking fluids better, as nausea resolves. Verbalizes understanding of importance of fluids and took 200 mL of cranberry juice even though she does not like it much.
Keep the call light within reach and ask the patient to call for assistance to the bathroom. Observe urinary output with each void for color, consistency, and amount. Evaluate discomfort with each void.	Day 1: Up to bathroom approximately every hour. Urinated 50–80 mL each void of strong-smelling, dark yellow, cloudy urine. Day 3: Urinating approximately every 2–3 hr, 150–200 mL at each void of light yellow urine. Cloudiness and odor have improved.
Administer antibiotics as ordered to treat the UTI. Assess for effectiveness by testing the urine with reagent strips at bedside, according to facility policy.	Day 3: Antibiotics administered IV as ordered. Reagent strips show decrease in nitrates to normal levels.
Obtain straight catheterization urine specimen for culture and sensitivity (C&S) as ordered to determine infective organisms. Use meticulous sterile technique to prevent introduction of further infection.	Day 1: Straight cath performed using meticulous technique. Obtained 800 mL of cloudy, strong-smelling, dark yellow urine. Specimen for C&S sent to lab. Day 3: C&S shows presence of *E. coli* and *Staph. aureus* bacteria in urine; both are sensitive to prescribed antibiotic.
Perform a bladder scan to determine if the patient has residual urine in the bladder after emptying.	Day 2: Bladder scan done to check for residual urine. Less than 100 mL in bladder.

Nursing Diagnosis: Acute back pain related to probable kidney infection as evidenced by rating pain at 8 and sleep disturbance
Expected Outcomes: Patient will rate back pain at 0–4 within 24 hours. Patient will report improving back pain as pyelonephritis responds to antibiotic therapy.

Interventions	Evaluations
Evaluate pain levels every 4 hours using a rating scale of 0–10. Be prompt in administering pain medication.	Day 1: Consistently rates back pain at a 7–8. Meperidine (Demerol) and hydroxyzine HCl (Vistaril) administered as ordered at 4 p.m. and again at 8 p.m. Day 3: Rates pain at 3–5 and is taking hydrocodone/ acetaminophen (Lortab) every 6–8 hr.
Use distraction, gate theory techniques, or other methods to assist in pain relief.	Day 1: Watched TV for a brief period, but slept most of the time. Day 3: Distracted by friends visiting, then watching movie with boyfriend. Did not ask for pain medication for 8 hr.

(table continues on page 730)

Table 31-2 **Nursing Care Plan for a Patient With a Urinary Tract Infection** (continued)

Nursing Diagnosis: Acute back pain related to probable kidney infection as evidenced by rating pain at 8 and sleep disturbance
Expected Outcomes: Patient will rate back pain at 0–4 within 24 hours. Patient will report improving back pain as pyelonephritis responds to antibiotic therapy.

Interventions	Evaluations
Administer IV antibiotics as ordered to treat kidney infection, which is causing the back pain. Assess the patient's response to antibiotics, including temperature, pulse, and respiration changes as well as pain ratings.	Day 1: IV antibiotics administered as ordered through saline lock. Day 3: IV antibiotics discontinued and oral antibiotic started. Temp now 100.2°F (37.9°C), pulse 78, resp 18. Rates pain today at 3.
Monitor urinary output to ensure that the patient is producing amounts of at least 30 mL/hr to ensure adequate kidney functioning.	Day 1: Output total of 960 mL in 24 hr. Day 2: Output total of 1,600 in 24 hr. Day 3: Output total of 2,100 in 24 hr.

Nursing Diagnosis: Deficient knowledge of causes of UTI related to lack of exposure as evidenced by request for information
Expected Outcomes: Patient will verbalize understanding of causes of UTI and ways to prevent recurrence prior to discharge.

Interventions	Evaluations
Explain how a bladder infection can spread to the kidneys via the ureters. Emphasize the importance of early detection and treatment of a UTI to prevent spread to the upper urinary tract.	Day 3: Verbalized understanding when presented with visual aid drawing of the urinary system.
Review perineal hygiene: wipe front to back one time and dispose of toilet tissue. Wash front to back with a different area on the washcloth each time.	Day 3: Verbalized understanding of perineal hygiene and states that she always washes and wipes front to back.
Instruct the patient to avoid baths, especially with bath salts, perfumes, or bubble baths, which can irritate the urethra and lead to UTIs.	Day 3: Verbalized surprise that bath salts could irritate the urinary tract, stating she never thought about it before. States that she will stop use of them to help prevent recurrence of UTI.
Instruct the patient to avoid excessive intake of alcohol and caffeinated and carbonated beverages and to increase intake of water, fruit juices (especially cranberry juice), decaffeinated teas or coffee, and flavored waters.	Day 3: Verbalized understanding of the value of cranberry juice and has learned that mixing it with lemon-lime–flavored water makes it easier for her to drink. States she will continue to drink it daily to prevent recurrences. Also verbalized the need to change her habits from drinking diet cola all day. States that the hospital stay has helped her stop that habit and she will drink flavored waters or juices from now on.
Instruct the patient to empty the bladder every 3–4 hours throughout the day to prevent urine from pooling in the bladder.	Day 3: Verbalized surprise at this information and has decided when she can take bathroom breaks during her day to empty her bladder more frequently.
Instruct the patient to empty the bladder after intercourse and avoid the use of spermicides and diaphragm for birth control as these can lead to UTI in some people.	Day 3: Expressed gratitude for this information, stating she was completely unaware of the need to empty her bladder after intercourse to prevent recurrent UTIs.

Skill 31-1 Assisting the Male Patient With a Urinal

Assessment Steps

1. Check the physician's order for activity level *so you will know whether the patient can get out of bed or not.*
2. Determine if the patient prefers standing or sitting to urinate.
3. Determine if the patient is able to stand independently or with assistance at the side of the bed.

Planning Steps

1. Gather needed equipment and supplies: urinal, disposable wipes, clean gloves.

Implementation Steps

1. Follow the Initial Implementation Steps located on the inside front cover.
2. Apply clean examination gloves.
3. If the activity order allows, position the patient for comfort either standing beside the bed or sitting on the side of the bed. If the patient is on bedrest, elevate the head of bed as much as the patient desires.
4. Place the urinal between his legs and place the penis inside the opening to the urinal.
5. When the patient is finished, provide disposable antibacterial wipes *for patient hand hygiene.*

6. Measure the amount, color, clarity, and odor of the urine. In the older adult male patient, also note the size of the urine stream. Inquire if there was burning or difficulty starting the urine stream.
7. Empty the urinal, rinse it, and return it to the appropriate storage area.
8. Follow the Ending Implementation Steps located on the inside back cover.
9. If the patient is on I&O, record results on the I&O sheet at the beside.

Evaluation Steps

1. Note the patient's ability to perform the activity and how much assistance was required.
2. Note any abnormalities in color, amount, odor, or consistency of the urine.

Sample Documentation

12/9/11 1910 Assisted to stand at bedside to use urinal, voided 450 mL cloudy, blood-tinged urine. Denies burning or difficulty starting and stopping urine stream. Assisted back to bed. Complains of general soreness throughout entire body. States he feels it is due to laying in bed. Denies a need for pain med. ——————————————— Nurse's signature and credentials

Skill 31-2 Assisting With a Bedpan

Assessment Steps

1. Review the physician's order for elimination and activity level.
2. Determine what type of bedpan you will need. The patient's condition may determine whether or not a fracture pan is needed. *If the patient is unable to roll from side to side, is very thin, or if a regular bedpan causes pain, a fracture pan must be used.*

Planning Steps

1. Gather needed equipment and supplies: bedpan, clean gloves, toilet tissue, premoistened cleansing wipes or warm wet washcloth.

Implementation Steps

1. Follow the Initial Implementation Steps located on the inside front cover.
2. Apply clean examination gloves.

3. Position the patient on the bedpan or fracture pan.
   a. When using a regular bedpan, the patient should be assisted to roll to one side. Place the bedpan firmly against the buttocks and assist the patient to roll onto the back.
   b. A fracture pan can be placed under the hips when the patient raises the hips, without turning from side to side. If able, the patient can help by using a trapeze bar. The fracture pan can also be placed by turning the patient side to side, if the patient is able to do so.

(skill continues on page 732)

Skill 31-2 (continued)

4. Raise the head of the bed unless contraindicated.

5. Leave toilet paper or premoistened cleansing wipes and the call light within reach and pull the curtain *to allow for privacy.* If the patient is able to be left alone, step outside the room door *to provide additional privacy.* Inform the patient where you will be.

6. If you are monitoring intake and output, ask the patient to dispose of the paper in the trash *so you can accurately measure output.* Position the trash can close to the side of the bed.

7. Respond quickly when the patient signals that he or she is finished.

8. If the patient was unable to wipe and cleanse his or her perineal area, perform this task for the patient.

9. Carefully support the bedpan *to prevent spillage* while assisting the patient to either lift the hips off the bedpan or turn to the side *for removal of the pan.*

10. Offer hand sanitizer or a washcloth with soap *for the patient to wash his or her hands.*

11. Provide perineal care as required (see Chapter 15).

12. Clean the bedpan, dry, cover, and store in the bedside table or bathroom.

13. Follow the Ending Implementation Steps located on the inside back cover.

14. If the patient is on I&O, document appropriately on the I&O sheet at the bedside and on the flow sheet in the medical record.

Evaluation Steps

1. Note the amount, clarity, and color of the urine.

2. Evaluate the patient's response to being placed on the bedpan. Did he or she complain of pain or shortness of breath?

Sample Documentation

> 9/24/12 0725 Assisted onto fracture pan. Voided 325 mL clear yellow urine. Perineal care provided. No skin breakdown noted. Repositioned for comfort. ————————————
> ———————————————— *Nurse's signature and credentials*

Skill 31-3 Obtaining a Clean-catch Midstream Urine Specimen

Assessment Steps

1. Review the physician's order *to determine type of specimen needed.*

2. Review the patient's chart *to determine whether the patient can get out of bed for voiding.*

Planning Steps

1. Gather needed equipment and supplies: sterile urine cup, cleansing wipes.

Implementation Steps

1. Follow the Initial Implementation Steps located on the inside front cover.

2. Assist the patient with these steps, or if the patient is able to perform the procedure, instruct the patient regarding these steps:
   a. Take the cap off of the specimen container and place the cap on a flat surface, open side up.
   b. Avoid touching the inside of the specimen container or cap.
   For Female Patient
   c. Sit on the toilet. Spread the labia to expose the urinary meatus. Clean the meatus from front to back with a cleansing wipe without allowing the labia to close or contaminate the area being cleansed. Then dispose of the cleansing wipe. Repeat this process three times using the three

separate antiseptic wipes. *Using each wipe only once prevents cross-contamination.*
   d. Continue to hold the labia open and begin to urinate into the toilet. A couple of seconds after the urine stream has begun, place the specimen cup in the stream of urine, catching a sample of urine in the cup. It is not necessary to fill the cup more than one-quarter to one-third full.
   e. Remove the specimen cup and finish urinating into the toilet.
   f. Replace the lid on the cup without touching the inside of the lid.

Skill 31-3 (continued)

For Male Patient

c. Retract the foreskin if not circumcised. Clean the tip of the glans penis in a circular motion, moving from the meatus outward until the entire glans is cleansed. Dispose of the cleansing wipe. Use the second and third cleansing wipes and repeat the motion once with each wipe.

d. Begin to urinate in the toilet. A couple of seconds after the urine stream has begun, hold the specimen cup in the urine stream to collect the specimen.

e. Finish urinating into the toilet. *Safety: Replace the foreskin to its original position after you have completed the procedure.*

f. Replace the lid on the cup without touching the inside of the lid.

3. Apply a completed label to the specimen cup. It should include the patient's name, patient ID number, physician's name, patient's room number, date and time of specimen collection, and test to be performed.

4. Follow the Ending Implementation Steps located on the inside back cover.

5. *Safety: Place specimen cup in a biohazard specimen plastic bag and transport to the laboratory immediately. If the test is not performed immediately, the specimen should be stored in the laboratory refrigerator to prevent components from breaking down.*

Evaluation Steps

1. Note the amount, color, clarity, and odor of the urine.

2. Note any difficulties with urination or obtaining the clean-catch specimen.

3. Review test results when available and report abnormal findings to the physician.

Sample Documentation

10/23/13   0530   Midstream clean-catch urine specimen obtained for UA. 30 mL of dark amber, cloudy urine obtained. Labeled and sent to lab. ——————— Nurse's signature and credentials

Skill 31-4   Inserting an Indwelling Urinary Catheter

Assessment Steps

1. Assess the patient for allergies to latex, povidone-iodine (Betadine), or tape.

Planning Steps

1. Gather needed equipment and supplies: catheter tray, extra pair of sterile gloves, catheter leg strap, bath blanket for draping the patient.

Implementation Steps

1. Follow the Initial Implementation Steps located on the inside front cover.

2. Put on clean gloves and drape the patient for privacy. Provide perineal care and examine the urinary meatus. *This allows you to note any deviations from normal anatomy before you set up a sterile field.*

3. Position the patient before you set up the sterile field:
   • **For female patient:** Ask the patient to flex her knees and place her feet as far apart as possible.
   • **For male patient:** Position the male in the same manner or, if you prefer, have the patient lay flat with the legs close together. *These positions allow you to set up the sterile field either between the patient's legs or on top of the legs.*

4. Remove the catheter kit from the outside plastic packaging. Turn the edges of the plastic bag to the outside without contaminating the inside of the bag. Place toward the end of the bed *for use as a trash receptacle. The inside of the bag is still sterile, so if your gloves or forceps accidentally touch the inside as you discard items, they will not be contaminated.*

5. Position the catheterization tray:
   • **For female patient:** on the bed between the patient's legs.
   • **For male patient:** on the bed between the patient's legs or on the patient's lap, on top of the thighs.

6. Open the distal flap of the tray first, then both side flaps, and the flap closest to you last. *Safety: Touch only the 1-inch outer margin of the sterile wrapper with your bare hands to prevent contamination of your sterile field.*

7. Remove the sterile drape from the catheter kit without contaminating the contents of the tray.
   • **For female patient:** Place the sterile drape under the patient's buttocks, holding it by the 1-inch outer margin. *This extends the sterile field from the perineum to the catheter tray. Avoid touching any of the drape surface.* Remove the fenestrated drape (with a diamond-shaped opening in the middle) and lay it carefully over the perineum *to provide a sterile field around the urethra and labia.* **Note:** Some nurses do not use this drape. It is your preference.
   • **For male patient:** Place the sterile drape under the patient's buttocks or over the patient's lap, or thighs; holding it by the 1-inch outer margin. *This extends the sterile field from the perineum to the catheter tray.* Remove the fenestrated drape (with a diamond-shaped opening in the middle) and place it carefully around the penis *to provide a sterile field around the urethra and penis.*

(skill continues on page 734)

Skill 31-4 (continued)

8. Put on the sterile gloves provided in the catheter kit *to prevent introducing pathogens into the urinary tract during catheter insertion.*

9. Lift out the plastic tray, and place it on the sterile field, avoiding the 1-inch unsterile outer margin.

10. From the kit, pick up and open the lubricant and squeeze it onto a section of sterile plastic tray.

11. Open the package of Betadine and empty the contents over the cotton balls. **Note:** Some kits may be packaged with Betadine swabs instead of cotton balls and liquid Betadine. *Safety: Use another type of antiseptic cleanser if the patient is allergic to Betadine.*

12. Lift out the sterile catheter, which will be encased in a clear plastic bag or sheath to provide extra security for maintaining sterility of the catheter. Leave the plastic cover on the catheter while you test the catheter balloon. Hold most of the catheter in your nondominant hand, especially the tip and balloon that will be inserted into the sterile bladder. *This helps to control the sterility of the most important part of the catheter, because the rubber catheter will sometimes flex or move while instilling water to test the balloon.*

13. Using your dominant hand, pick up the syringe containing sterile water and screw the Luer-Lok tip to the colored port on the second lumen of the catheter. This second lumen is located at the Y-junction of the catheter.

14. While carefully holding the plastic-covered catheter in your nondominant hand, use your dominant hand to depress the plunger of the syringe *to instill the sterile water, inflating the balloon.* Observe the balloon for leaks. When balloon integrity is ensured, withdraw all the sterile water from the balloon back into the syringe, leaving the syringe attached to the catheter.

15. Carefully remove the plastic cover from the catheter, maintaining strict asepsis of the catheter. Drop the plastic off to the side of your sterile field. *Safety: Notice that this step says to "drop" it, rather than "lay it down," which would increase the risk of contaminating your sterile gloves.*

16. Now place the catheter with attached syringe into the sterile kit box within your sterile field. Use caution while you position the catheter. *After you let go of it, it tends to "flop" or "spring" from the inside of the box to the outside of the box, with the catheter tip sometimes landing outside your sterile field, contaminating the catheter.*

17. Cleanse the urinary meatus.
For Female Patient
a. Use your nondominant hand to spread the labia to expose the urinary meatus. *Safety: This hand is now unsterile because you have touched the patient's skin.*
b. While your nondominant hand continues to separate the labia, maintain exposure of the urinary meatus; with your dominant hand, pick up the Betadine swab or use the sterile forceps to pick up the Betadine-soaked cotton balls. Clean in the following order: Use one Betadine-soaked cotton ball or swab to clean the far labia minora from front to back. Drop the now-contaminated cotton ball or swab in the plastic bag you set up beyond your sterile field. *Safety: Do not remove your nondominant hand from the labia or let the labia close over the meatus. It will then be contaminated and must be cleansed again before proceeding with catheterization.*
c. Use forceps to pick up a second cotton ball or swab. Cleanse the near labia minora from front to back. Drop the now-contaminated cotton ball or swab into the plastic bag.
d. With the last cotton ball or swab, clean straight down from the clitoris over the urinary meatus and down past the vagina. Dispose of the cotton ball or swab as you have previously done.

Skill 31-4 (continued)

For Male Patient

a. Cleanse the urinary meatus and the entire glans penis, or head of the penis surrounding the meatus. Using your nondominant hand, grasp the penis shaft. Avoid using one or two fingers and the thumb; apply a full-handed grasp, retracting the foreskin if the man is uncircumcised. *Safety: This hand is now unsterile because you have touched the patient's skin.*

b. Hold the penis at a 90-degree angle to the body while applying gentle traction. With your dominant hand, pick up the Betadine swab or use the sterile forceps to pick up the Betadine-soaked cotton ball. Begin cleansing at the urinary meatus, moving in concentric circles until the entire glans penis is cleansed. Drop the now-contaminated cotton ball or swab in the plastic bag you set up beyond your sterile field. Use caution to avoid touching the sterile forceps or gloves to any potentially contaminated surface.

c. Repeat the same cleansing motion three times with three separate cotton balls or swabs. *Safety: Remember to use each antiseptic wipe only once, moving in a concentric circle over the meatus and entire glans. Do not remove your nondominant hand from the penis after cleaning it to prevent contamination.*

18. Pick up the sterile catheter with your dominant hand, dipping the tip in the lubricant you squirted on the plastic tray.

For Female Patient

a. Lubricate 1 to 2 inches of the catheter tip. Holding it about 1 inch from the tip of the catheter, insert it into the urinary meatus. Advance the catheter until you see urine flowing into the catheter tubing. At that time, advance the catheter another 1 to 2 inches to *ensure that the catheter is fully in the bladder. Safety: Do not let go of the catheter yet. Keep your dominant hand on the catheter to prevent it from sliding out of the bladder and urethra.*

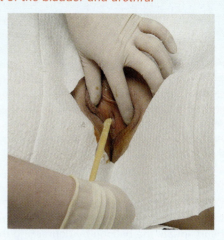

b. Release the labia and, with your nondominant hand, pick up the syringe and inflate the balloon by depressing the plunger on the syringe completely. Pull *gently* on the catheter *to seat the balloon at the cystourethral junction.*

c. Twist the syringe off of the connection port and dispose of it in the plastic bag.

For Male Patient

a. Lubricate approximately 5 to 7 inches of the catheter *to facilitate insertion and decrease discomfort to the patient.* **Note:** Some catheter kits include a sterile syringe containing lubricant rather than a package of lubricant. The tip of the syringe can be gently inserted into the urethra and the plunger depressed to fill the urethra with lubricant. Follow facility policy.

b. With your dominant hand, pick up the lubricated catheter and insert it into the urinary meatus. Advance the catheter 7 to 9 inches until you see urine flowing into the drainage tubing. Advance the catheter another 1 to 2 inches *to ensure that the catheter is fully in the bladder. Safety: If you inadvertently inflate the balloon while it is still in the urethra, you may damage the urethra.* Keep your dominant hand on the catheter *to prevent it from sliding out of the bladder and urethra.*

Note: If you meet resistance when inserting the catheter, the patient may have an enlarged prostate gland. Try gently twisting the catheter *to the right to facilitate the tip of the catheter passing the prostate. Safety: Do not force the catheter if you are unable to gently advance it.*

(skill continues on page 736)

Skill 31-4 (continued)

c. Release the penis and, with your nondominant hand, inflate the balloon by depressing the plunger on the syringe completely. Pull gently on the catheter *to seat the balloon at the cystouretheral junction.*

d. Twist the syringe off of the connection port and dispose of it in the plastic bag. Replace the foreskin if it was retracted. *Safety: If the foreskin is left in the retracted position, particularly with an indwelling catheter in place, it can cause a stricture-like effect, resulting in edema and possible necrosis of the head of the penis.*

19. Secure the indwelling catheter to the patient's thigh with a leg strap or tape. Some males may prefer to secure it to the lower abdomen. If you are not certain, simply ask the patient for his preference. To ensure adequate catheter length for patient movement, secure the catheter at the Y-junction. *Safety: This prevents tugging of the catheter, which in turn bangs the inflated balloon against the neck of the bladder where the urethra attaches. It also helps to prevent an ambulatory patient from stepping on the drainage tubing and accidentally pulling out the catheter.*

20. Cleanse all Betadine or other cleanser from the urinary meatus and surrounding area. *If left on the skin, it may cause irritation.*

21. Depending on the structure of the bed, hang the catheter drainage bag from a part of the bed that moves with the patient when raised or lowered, or hang on a stationary piece of the frame that remains static directly below the patient's hips. Avoiding using the bed rails. *Safety: If the drainage bag is hung on the bed rails, it can be elevated above the level of the bladder when the rails are raised.* Hanging the drainage bag on the side of the bed nearest the door allows you to do a quick visual assessment of the amount and color of urine in the bag. *Safety: The drainage bag should not be elevated above the level of the patient's bladder, unless it is first clamped close to the catheter connection to prevent urine from draining from the catheter tubing back into the bladder.*

22. Follow the Ending Implementation Steps located on the inside back cover.

Evaluation Steps

1. Evaluate how the patient tolerated the procedure. Did he or she complain of pain, burning, or other discomfort?

2. Evaluate the color, clarity, and amount of urine in the drainage bag after the procedure is completed. Avoid allowing more than 1,000 mL to drain at a time. Clamp the tubing in between drainings.

Sample Documentation

5/9/2011   0800   #16 fr foley catheter inserted with sterile technique without resistance or complaints. Patent and draining via gravity to drainage bag. Immediately returned approximately 400 mL clear, pale yellow urine. Secured to leg with leg strap. Denies discomfort. ——————————————
——————————— *Nurse's signature and credentials*

Skill 31-5   Obtaining a Urine Specimen From an Indwelling Urinary Catheter

Assessment Steps

1. Check the physician's order *to determine type of specimen to be obtained.*

Planning Steps

1. Gather needed equipment and supplies: sterile 10-mL syringe, sterile noncoring blunt needle or needleless access device (if unavailable, a sterile 22-gauge needle may be used) sterile specimen cup, alcohol wipes, clean gloves.

Implementation Steps

1. Follow the Initial Implementation Steps located on the inside front cover.

2. Clamp the tubing below the level of the port for 15 to 30 minutes and allow urine to collect in the tubing above the clamp.

3. Put on clean gloves; remove the cap from the specimen cup and place the lid on a flat surface with the open side up. Do not touch the inside of the sterile cup.

Skill 31-5 (continued)

4. Clean the port on the tubing with alcohol and allow it to dry. *This prevents the introduction of pathogens as the blunt needle penetrates the port.*

5. Using aseptic technique, insert the blunt needle or regular needle into the port at a 45- to 90-degree angle and pull the plunger back slowly and steadily. Withdraw between 5 and 8 mL of urine for an adequate amount of urine for testing. *Safety: The indwelling urinary catheter is a closed drainage system that should not be interrupted. Do not disconnect the catheter from the drainage bag tubing to obtain a specimen, as this will create a portal of entry for pathogens and increase the patient's risk of contracting an infection. Never obtain a urine specimen from the drainage bag.*

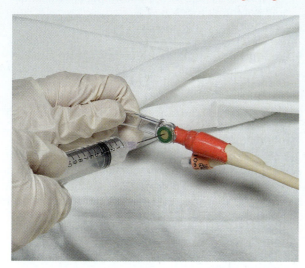

6. Hold the syringe over the specimen cup and carefully inject the urine into the cup using aseptic technique. Replace the lid on the specimen cup without touching the inside of the cup or lid.

7. Dispose of the needle and syringe in the sharps container immediately.

8. Unclamp the catheter tubing, *allowing free flow of urine.*

9. Apply a completed label to the specimen cup, with the patient's name and patient ID number, room number, physician's name, date and time of specimen collection, and name of test to be performed.

10. Follow the Ending Implementation Steps located on the inside back cover.

11. Place the specimen cup inside the plastic biohazard specimen bag and transport it to the laboratory. It must be taken to the laboratory promptly or refrigerated.

12. Document the procedure in the medical record, including the characteristics of the urine.

Evaluation Steps

1. Evaluate the color, clarity, odor, and amount of urine. Ensure that you have obtained an adequate amount for testing.

2. Evaluate whether aseptic technique was maintained correctly.

3. Review testing results as soon as available and report any abnormal findings to the physician.

Sample Documentation

6/20/11   1300   *Using aseptic technique, obtained 20 mL of clear yellow urine from port of indwelling catheter, placed in sterile specimen cup, labeled & hand-carried to lab for UA.* —————————
———————————— *Nurse's signature and credentials*

Skill 31-6   Inserting a Straight Catheter

Assessment Steps

1. Check the physician's order *to determine type of catheterization to be performed.*

2. Assess the patient for allergies to latex or povidone-iodine (Betadine).

Planning Steps

1. Gather needed equipment and supplies: washcloth, towel, straight catheter tray with specimen cup, extra pair of sterile gloves.

Implementation Steps

1. Follow the Initial Implementation Steps located on the inside front cover.

2. Put on clean gloves and drape the patient *for privacy.* Provide perineal care and examine the urinary meatus. *This allows you to note any*

deviations from normal anatomy before you set up a sterile field.

3. Position the patient as you did for an indwelling catheter (see Skill 31-4) before you set up the sterile field.

4. Position and open the sterile pack as you did for an indwelling catheter.

5. Set up your sterile field and place sterile drapes according to the way you did for the indwelling catheter.

6. Apply your sterile gloves.

7. Open the lid of the specimen cup that came in the catheter kit, and place the lid open side up on the sterile field. Leave the specimen container in the catheter kit basin *to prevent it from tipping easily on the bed.*

(skill continues on page 738)

Skill 31-6 (continued)

8. Open the package of lubricant and squeeze it onto the bottom of the catheter kit basin.

9. Lubricate approximately 2 to 3 inches of the catheter tip for a female and 5 to 7 inches for a male *to facilitate insertion and decrease discomfort to the patient.*

10. Open and prepare the package of Betadine cleanser as you did for the indwelling catheter. *Safety: Use another type of antiseptic cleanser if the patient is allergic to Betadine.*

11. Cleanse the urinary meatus (see Skill 31-4).
   For Female Patient
   a. Use your nondominant hand to spread the labia to expose the urinary meatus, just as you did for an indwelling catheter. *Safety: Remember this hand is now unsterile because you have touched the patient's skin.*
   b. Clean the far labia, near labia, and clitoris with antiseptic wipes as you did for an indwelling catheter. *Safety: Remember to use each antiseptic wipe only 1 time, cleansing from front to back. Do not remove your nondominant hand from the labia or let the labia close over the meatus because it will then be contaminated and must be cleansed again before proceeding with catheterization.*

   For Male Patient
   a. Hold the penis at a 90-degree angle to the body while applying gentle traction. *Safety: Once you grasp the penis with your nondominant hand and retract the foreskin if the man is uncircumcised, this hand is now unsterile because you have touched the patient's skin.*
   b. Clean the urinary meatus and the entire glans penis with antiseptic wipes as you did for an indwelling catheter. *Safety: Remember to use each antiseptic wipe only once, moving in a concentric circle over the meatus and entire glans. Do not remove your nondominant hand from the penis after cleaning it to prevent contamination.*

12. With your dominant hand, pick up the lubricated catheter and insert it into the urinary meatus. Advance the catheter until you see urine flowing from the end of the straight catheter into the catheter kit basin.

13. Once urine begins to flow, grasp the catheter close to the insertion site with your nondominant hand. Using same hand, pinch off the catheter to interrupt the urine flow while you use your dominant hand to place the end of the catheter into the specimen cup that is sitting inside the catheter kit basin. Allow urine to flow into the cup until it is one-half to three-quarters full.

14. Then pinch off the catheter again while you remove the end of the catheter from the specimen cup and lay it into the catheter kit basin. Still using your dominant hand, lightly screw the lid onto the specimen cup of urine. Then remove the cup from the catheter kit basin and set it nearby on the sterile field.

15. Now allow urine to flow into the basin until the bladder is emptied.

16. Remove the catheter from the urethra by gently pulling it straight out.

17. Tighten the lid on the specimen cup, wipe off any urine on the outside of the cup, and set it aside.

18. Cleanse antiseptic solution from patient's genitals and pat the skin dry. *Safety: Replace the foreskin to its original position after you completed the procedure.*

19. Pour the urine from the catheter kit basin into a graduated container to obtain an accurate measurement. Record the volume of urine and then pour the urine down the toilet.

20. Apply a completed label to the specimen cup, with the patient's name and patient ID number, room number, physician's name, date and time of specimen collection, and name of test to be performed.

21. Follow the Ending Implementation Steps located on the inside back cover.

22. Place the specimen cup inside the plastic biohazard specimen bag and transport it to the laboratory. It must be taken to the laboratory promptly or refrigerated.

Evaluation Steps

1. Evaluate how the patient tolerated the procedure. Did he or she complain of pain, burning, or other discomfort?

2. Evaluate the color, clarity, and amount of urine in the basin after the bladder has been completely drained.

Sample Documentation

5/9/2011   0800   #14 F straight catheter inserted using sterile technique. 400 mL clear yellow urine obtained. 40 mL of urine obtained for sterile specimen and sent to lab. Denies discomfort.
——————————————— *Nurse's signature and credentials*

Skill 31-7   Performing Continuous Bladder Irrigation

Assessment Steps

1. Check the physician's order for continuous bladder irrigation.

Planning Steps

1. Gather needed equipment and supplies: IV pole, sterile continuous urinary irrigation setup (includes a sterile spike on one end of the tubing and a length of connecting tubing that will connect with the third lumen of the triple-lumen catheter), a 3,000-mL bag of sterile normal saline (NS) irrigation solution, sterile drape.

   Note: Normally a triple-lumen catheter is inserted in surgery by the surgeon after a TURP. The patient would normally not have a triple-lumen catheter inserted, unless the irrigation setup was connected to the third lumen. Then you would only have to hang bags of solution and maintain the irrigation. However, it is possible to receive a patient from surgery with the third lumen plugged by a sterile catheter plug. Or you may receive an order to insert the catheter and connect it to an irrigation setup. If so, you would require the supplies for inserting the triple-lumen urinary catheter.

Implementation Steps

1. Follow the Initial Implementation Steps located on the inside front cover.

2. Close the roller clamp on the irrigation setup tubing.

3. Uncap the sterile spike on the end of the irrigation setup tubing. Aseptically insert the spike into the port on the bag of NS irrigation solution. Keep the cap on the other sterile end of the irrigation setup tubing.

4. Hang the bag on the IV pole and unclamp the roller clamp. Remove the cap on the end of the tube and allow NS to flow through the tube to displace all the air in the tube, otherwise known as *priming* the tube. Then replace the cap, still using aseptic technique, and close the roller clamp to stop the flow of NS.

   If Triple-Lumen Catheter Must Be Inserted
   - Insert the triple-lumen catheter using the same technique used for insertion of a double-lumen indwelling catheter (see Skill 31-4).
   - The urine drainage bag will be connected to the first lumen, which is the urine drainage lumen. The second lumen will be connected to the inflated balloon inside the bladder. The third lumen is the one that will connect to the irrigation setup tubing. It will allow sterile irrigant to flow into the bladder, where it will drain from the bladder along with the urine, via the urine-draining first lumen into the drainage bag.

5. Cleanse the outside of the third lumen and the plug with two alcohol sponges. Remove the plug from the third lumen of the catheter using aseptic technique and insert the other end of the irrigation tubing into the lumen. *Safety: Keep the roller clamp closed until the tubing is attached.*

6. Open the roller clamp on the tubing, allowing irrigation solution to flow into the bladder until urine returns clear to light pink, without blood clots. *Safety: Make certain that the solution is also returning through the catheter drainage tubing into the drainage bag.*

7. Once the returning urine and solution remain light pink to clear, without clots, the flow rate of the irrigation solution is set. Regulate the rate as necessary so that it keeps the returning urine and irrigant at this color. If the urine becomes dark pink or red, or contains clots, increase the flow rate until the light pink color is again achieved.

8. Monitor flow and bladder distention for several minutes before leaving the room. Return within 15 to 30 minutes to reassess the amount of return and its color. If the urine color remains good, then you may monitor the return about every hour to assess the color of the urine in the drainage tubing and drainage bag. Repeat Steps 7 and 8 as needed.

9. Follow the Ending Implementation Steps located on the inside back cover.

Evaluation Steps

1. Evaluate the effectiveness of the irrigation by noting the color of the urine/irrigant return.

2. Evaluate output for the presence of clots.

3. Evaluate the patient's response to the continuous bladder irrigation. Does he complain of pain, bladder fullness, or cramping? Immediately respond to patient complaints. Assess for a distended bladder regularly.

Sample Documentation

6/20/13   1530   20-Fr, triple-lumen catheter inserted without difficulty per physician's orders. Initiated continuous bladder irrigation with 3,000-mL bag of St. NS. Dark pink urine returned with dark red BB-size clots noted. Irrigant rate increased for 5 minutes until clots were no longer detected and urine was pale pink. Bladder palpated and nondistended. No complaints of cramping or discomfort. ——— Nurse's signature and credentials
6/20/13   1545   Urine remains light pink without clots. No complaints of cramping or bladder spasms voiced. ———
——————————— Nurse's signature and credentials

Skill 31-8 Applying a Condom Catheter

Assessment Steps

1. Assess the patient's genitals to determine size of catheter needed.
2. Assess for latex allergy.

Planning Steps

1. Gather needed equipment and supplies: correct-size condom catheter, clean gloves, cleansing wipes, urine collection bag, skin prep, washcloth, towel, bath basin, soap, scissors.

Implementation Steps

1. Follow the Initial Implementation Steps located on the inside front cover.
2. Place the patient in the supine position.
3. Position the sheet and towel so that there is no unnecessary exposure.
4. Provide perineal care *to ensure that the area is clean and reduce risk of introducing pathogens into the urethra.*
5. Apply skin prep around the shaft of the penis and allow drying according to package instructions *to increase adhesion of the adhesive strip.*
6. Apply the adhesive strip supplied by the manufacturer to the penis over the area of skin prep. Apply in a spiral pattern. Avoid wrapping a complete circle around the penis, *as it may have a tourniquet effect, cutting off circulation to the penis.*
7. Hold the penis in your nondominant hand; with your dominant hand, apply the catheter by slowly unrolling it over the glans penis and along the shaft of the penis. Leave 1 to 2 inches between the tip of the penis and the end of the condom catheter *to allow urine to drain without leaking from the condom and to prevent pressure on the head of the penis. Safety: Too much space left at the tip may allow the condom catheter to twist, causing urine to pool and loosen the adhesive. Constant urine contact with the skin can lead to maceration and skin breakdown.*

8. Attach the end of the condom catheter to the drainage bag and secure the tubing to the inside of the patient's thigh using a leg strap.
9. Follow the Ending Implementation Steps located on the inside back cover.

Evaluation Steps

1. Evaluate the catheter site within 30 to 60 minutes *to make sure urine is flowing freely and there is no leaking.* Also assess the penis for swelling and discoloration. Assess the urine for color, amount, clarity, and odor. Make these assessments every shift.

Sample Documentation

4/1/2011   1000   External condom catheter applied and attached to urine drainage bag. Skin intact. ——————————
————————————— Nurse's signature and credentials
4/1/2011   1045   Has drained 50 mL of clear dark yellow urine. No leakage. Penis without discoloration or edema. No C/O discomfort reported. ——————————— Nurse's signature and credentials

Skill 31-9 Irrigating a Closed Urinary Drainage System

Assessment Steps

1. Check the physician's order for amount and type of irrigant.
2. Assess the patient's need for catheter irrigation. Note color and clarity of urinary output. Assess for bladder distention by palpating the bladder above the symphysis pubis.
3. Assess the patient's pain level and the need for any pain medication before the procedure.

Planning Steps

1. Gather needed equipment and supplies: bottle of sterile normal saline (NS) irrigation solution or other ordered solution, irrigation tray, 60-mL syringe with a tip that will accommodate a blunt needle, noncoring blunt needle, alcohol wipes, clean gloves, waterproof drape.
2. Plan to keep the urinary drainage system closed during irrigation *to help prevent introduction of pathogens and prevent urinary tract infection.* Open irrigations are not recommended for this reason.

Implementation Steps

1. Follow the Initial Implementation Steps located on the inside front cover.
2. Apply clean gloves.
3. Empty the urine collection bag to allow for accurate output measurement.
4. Remove gloves, wash hands, and put on clean gloves.
5. Place the waterproof drape under the catheter port.
6. Open the sterile irrigation tray without contaminating the inside of it.
7. Pour approximately 100 mL of sterile NS irrigation solution into the sterile irrigation container.
8. Attach the blunt needle to the syringe using aseptic technique.
9. Clamp the urinary drainage tubing below the level of the irrigation port.
10. Aseptically draw up between 30 and 60 mL of sterile NS into the syringe.
11. Cleanse the irrigation port on the Foley drainage tubing with an alcohol swab.
12. Insert the blunt needle into the irrigation port and slowly inject approximately 30 to 60 mL of the solution, holding the port slightly higher than the level of the bladder so gravity will assist the solution to run into the catheter and bladder.
   Safety: If you meet resistance when irrigating the bladder, turn the patient slightly to the side and try

irrigating again. Do not force the solution. If you continue to be unable to irrigate due to resistance, stop the procedure and notify the physician.

13. After injecting the NS, remove the blunt needle from the port. If the physician has ordered more than 60 mL, unclamp the drainage tube and allow irrigation solution to drain into the drainage bag. Then refill the syringe with 60 mL of NS and continue irrigation until the ordered amount has been used. Be certain to wipe the port with another alcohol sponge before piercing the port each time.
   Note: If the physician has ordered a different solution and wants it to be left in the bladder as a bladder instillation, the solution will be instilled and then remain in the bladder for the length of time specified in the physician's order (for example, 30 minutes) with the tubing clamped. When the time has elapsed, return and unclamp the tubing.
14. After completion of the irrigation, wipe the port one last time with a new alcohol sponge.
15. Remove all contaminated supplies and dispose of them in appropriate biohazard container.
16. Empty the returned irrigant from the drainage bag, measure, dispose of it in the toilet, and record.
17. Follow the Ending Implementation Steps located on the inside back cover.

Evaluation Steps

1. Evaluate the ease of performing the irrigation or any resistance met during the irrigation/instillation.
2. Note color, amount, and characteristics of the irrigant return. Evaluate for the presence of clots or mucus.
3. Evaluate the patient's reaction to the procedure. Did he or she complain of pain, pressure, or cramping?

Sample Documentation

10/29/13   1300   C/O full bladder, bladder palpated above the symphysis pubis. No urine noted in Foley drainage tubing at this time. Physician notified. Order for catheter irrigation received. ———————— Nurse's signature and credentials
10/29/13   1325   Foley catheter irrigated with 60 mL of sterile NS per physician's order. No resistance noted. Returned 225 mL of blood-tinged yellow solution immediately upon unclamping drainage tubing, followed by darker yellow urine containing small strings of mucus and small flecks of clotted blood. No complaints of pain or cramping. States the bladder feels so much better now. ———————— Nurse's signature and credentials
10/29/13   1400   Urinary drainage bag now holds approximately 350 mL of blood-tinged urine. ————————
———————— Nurse's signature and credentials

Skill 31-10 Discontinuing an Indwelling Urinary Catheter

Assessment Steps

1. Check the physician's order to ensure catheter is to be discontinued.

Planning Steps

1. Gather needed equipment and supplies: clean examination gloves, 10-mL syringe with a Luer-Lok tip, towel or disposable drape.

Implementation Steps

1. Follow the Initial Implementation Steps located on the inside front cover.

2. Apply clean examination gloves and provide perineal care for the patient if needed.

3. Empty and measure the urine in the drainage bag.

4. Place the patient in the supine position and place a towel or disposable blue pad between the patient's legs underneath the perineum.

5. Attach the syringe to the colored port used for balloon inflation.

6. Pull back on the plunger to deflate the balloon. Withdraw until all fluid is removed and the catheter goes flat with further vacuum. Disconnect the syringe and empty it into a receptacle or trash can.

7. Reattach the syringe and pull back on the plunger again *to ensure that all the fluid has been emptied from the balloon.* Disconnect the syringe from the catheter.

8. Ask the patient to take a deep breath. As the patient exhales, gently give the catheter a slight twist *in case it is adhered to urethra,* and carefully but quickly withdraw the catheter and allow it to rest on the towel or blue pad.
   - **For male patient:** Use your nondominant hand to grasp the penis shaft using a full-handed grasp. Use your dominant hand to steadily withdraw the catheter straight out of the urethra.

9. Remove the disposable blue pad with the catheter wrapped inside and dispose of it along with the empty drainage bag directly into the biohazard bag in the trash.

10. Provide perineal care as needed.

11. Explain to the patient that the catheter is now discontinued and that he or she should call for assistance when the urge to void is felt. Instruct the patient to void into a specimen pan so that you can measure urinary output. *Safety: Monitor the patient closely to ensure that he or she is voiding in adequate amounts after the catheter has been removed. If the patient has not voided in the 8 hours following the catheter removal, notify the physician.*

12. Follow the Ending Implementation Steps located on the inside back cover.

13. Document the procedure appropriately, noting the time the catheter was removed.

Evaluation Steps

1. Evaluate urinary output and perform a bladder scan according to facility policy to ensure that the bladder is emptying adequately.

2. Evaluate the need for recatheterization due to inadequate output.

Sample Documentation

6/14/13   1215   #18 Fr indwelling catheter discontinued per order without difficulty. Instructed to urinate into specimen pan the first time so it can be measured. —————————————
—————————————— Nurse's signature and credentials
6/14/13   1500   Assisted to bathroom. Voided 350 mL of clear yellow urine. Bladder scan showed 25 mL of residual urine. —————————— Nurse's signature and credentials

 Post Conference

This has been one of your most interesting clinical experiences. Your patient was interesting and enjoyable. He seemed to enjoy having a student caring for him and said it gave him someone to talk with who was not so busy. The 24-hour urine specimen collection was a learning experience. You discovered that you had to keep the catheter drainage bag in a basin of ice during the collection period. You were rather relieved that he had a catheter, because then you did not accidentally flush any urine during the collection period. After the collection period was over, you took the large container to the lab. The catheter irrigation was a new experience as well, but you were able to insert the blunt needle without contamination and flush the saline through the catheter.

KEY POINTS

- Normal urinary output is 1,000 to 3,000 mL in 24 hours; the acceptable minimal output is 30 mL/hr. Anuria can be a symptom of kidney failure.

- Specific gravity can be used to evaluate hydration status.

- Because one continuous membrane lines the urinary system, infection can travel from the urinary meatus to the bladder, up the ureters and into the kidneys, where microorganisms are able to enter the bloodstream, causing sepsis.

- A variety of sizes and types of catheters exist. Catheters are sized by their diameter and measured in French units. Catheter types include straight, indwelling, and three-way catheters, each with a different purpose.

- After discontinuing an indwelling urinary catheter, it is important to monitor the patient for urinary retention. If the patient does not void within 8 hours after discontinuing the catheter, evaluate the need to recatheterize him or her. Call for physician's orders if no standing orders exist.

- Urinary incontinence is not normal after childbirth or with aging.

- Urinary incontinence may be due to increased abdominal pressure, such as with stress incontinence. It may also be due to urge incontinence, which occurs when the urge to urinate is very strong. Overflow incontinence is due to an obstruction that prevents the bladder from emptying normally.

- Nurses can help patients manage incontinence by initiating bladder training when appropriate, changing incontinence briefs every 2 hours, and providing excellent skin care whenever a patient has been incontinent.

- Urine is assessed in a variety of ways: urinalysis, timed urinary collections, straining for stones, and testing with reagent strips or dipsticks.

- Blood urea nitrogen and serum creatinine are blood tests used to diagnose renal insufficiency and renal failure.

- If a male patient is uncircumcised, you must retract the foreskin, or move it back from the glans, during catheterization. It is extremely important to replace the foreskin to its original position after you have inserted the indwelling catheter. Failure to do so can cause the glans penis to be deprived of adequate blood flow.

- After a male patient has had a transurethral resection of the prostate, he will have a triple-lumen catheter in place and a continuous bladder irrigation will be used to prevent blood clots from clogging the catheter.

- Monitoring intake and output can be done as a nursing decision.

- Urinary diversions are created when the bladder is damaged or removed.

REVIEW QUESTIONS

Select the answer that is most appropriate for each of the following questions. Some questions may have more than one correct answer. Check all that apply.

1. Which of the following may decrease the incidence of urinary tract infection?

  a. Using a diaphragm

  b. Increasing fluid intake

  c. Voiding after intercourse

  d. Frequent voiding

2. Indicate the path of the flow of urine through the following structures by numbering them in order.

  a. Ureter

  b. Urethra

  c. Bladder

  d. Kidney

  e. Meatus

3. Your patient has been diagnosed with an enlarged prostate. He is at risk for which of the following?

  a. Urinary suppression

  b. Urinary retention

  c. Urinary incontinence

  d. Urinary diversion

4. When reviewing the urinalysis results of a patient with the diagnosis of dehydration, which of the following would you expect to see?

  a. Specific gravity of 1.032

  b. pH of 7.0

  c. +Ketones

  d. +Nitrites

5. Which of the following statements made by a patient with incontinence would indicate a need for further teaching?

   a. "I can stop doing Kegel exercises when I no longer have a problem with leaking."

   b. "I can take medication that may help with my incontinence."

   c. "I may need surgery if other treatments don't work."

   d. "I should start a moderate exercise program."

6. You are initiating a 24-hour urine specimen collection for a patient as ordered by her health care provider. Which of the following will you do first?

   a. Post signs in the room and on the door stating that a 24-hour urine collection is in progress.

   b. Place ice inside a 24-hour urine container.

   c. Ask the patient to void, then discard the urine.

   d. Ask the patient to void, then pour the urine into the 24-hour urine container.

7. You have removed an indwelling catheter from a postsurgical patient. Which of the following would need to be reported to the health care provider?

   a. Eight hours after the catheter was removed, the patient has not voided.

   b. Bladder scan reveals 50 mL of residual urine.

   c. Voided urine is straw-colored without sediment.

   d. When assisted to the bedside commode, the patient complained of mild dizziness.

CRITICAL THINKING EXERCISES

8. You are caring for a patient who returned from the operating room several hours ago after having a transurethral resection of the prostate with continuous bladder irrigation. Thirty minutes ago you emptied the urine drainage bag, but now the amount of urine in the bag is decreased to 100 mL and it is dark red. What should you do?

9. A 67-year-old female patient is complaining of dysuria, frequency, and urgency when she urinates. She is diagnosed with a UTI. She asks you how this infection occurred. How will you respond?

10. You are working at a walk-in clinic. A patient is being seen with signs of dehydration and a UTI. She states, "I don't understand how I can be dehydrated, I drink all day long." What questions would you need to ask?

ADDITIONAL RESOURCES

For additional Resources, Questions, and Activities, please see:

 Student Resource Disk

 http://davisplus.fadavis.com

Student Study Guide

REFERENCES

Doenges ME, Moorehouse MF, Murr AC. *Nurse's Pocket Guide: Diagnoses, Prioritized Interventions, and Rationales.* 11th ed. Philadelphia: FA Davis; 2008.

Finnk HA, Taylor BC, Tackland JW, Rutks IR, Wilt TJ. Treatment interventions in nursing home residents with urinary incontinence: systemic review of randomized trials. *Mayo Clin Proc.* 2008;83: 1332-1343.

Fox S. Continence care for older adults in care homes. *Nurs Resident Care.* 2008;10(6):274-277.

Gray M. Assessment and management of urinary incontinence. *Nurse Pract.* 2005;30(7):33-43.

Hopkins TB. *Lab Notes.* 2nd ed. Philadelphia: FA Davis; 2009.

Kuklinski D, Koduri S. Predicting urinary tract infections in a urogynecology population. *Urol Nurs.* 2008;28:56-67.

Mangnall J. A guide to the management of incontinence in older people. *Gastrointest Nurs.* 2008;6(5):36-39.

Marchese K. Using Peplau's theory of interpersonal relations to guide the education of patient's undergoing urinary diversion. *Urol Nurs.* 2008;26:363-370.

Myers E, Hopkins T. *LPN Notes.* 2nd ed. Philadelphia: FA Davis; 2008.

Palmer MH. Urinary incontinence quality improvement in nursing homes: where have we been? where are we going? *Urol Nurs.* 2008;28:439-453.

Pellatt GC. Anatomy and physiology of urinary elimination. Part 1. *Br J Nurs.* 2007;16:406-410.

Pellatt GC. Anatomy and physiology of urinary elimination. Part 2—Retention, incontinence and catheterization. *Br J Nurs.* 2007; 16:480-485.

Peterson JA. Minmize urinary incontinence: maximize physical activity in women. *Urol Nurs.* 2008;28:351-356.

Pilcher KL. A multidisciplinary approach to improving urinary continence. *Nurs Standard.* 2008;23(8):42-46.

Rahn DD. Urinary tract infections: contemporary management. *Urol Nurs.* 2008;28:333-341.

Robinson J. Clinical skills: How to remove and change a suprapubic catheter. *Br J Nurs.* 2005;14:30-35.

Robinson J, Berry L. Insertion, care and management of suprapubic catheters. *Nurs Standard.* 2008;23(8):49-56.

Scanlon V, Sanders T. *Essentials of Anatomy and Physiology.* 3rd ed. Philadelphia: FA Davis; 2007.

Selby M. Dealing with incontinence. *Practice Nurse.* 2006;32(8):33-38.

Selius BA, Subedi R. Urinary retention in adults: diagnosis and initial management. *Am Fam Physician.* 2008;77:643-650.

Simerville JA, Maxted WC, Pahira JJ. Urinalysis: a comprehensive review. *Am Fam Physician.* 2005;71:1153-1162.

Venes D, ed. *Taber's Cyclopedic Medical Dictionary.* 21st ed. Philadelphia: FA Davis; 2009.

Ward SL, Hisley SM. *Maternal-Child Nursing Care.* Philadelphia: FA Davis; 2009.

Wilkinson JM, Van Leuven K. *Fundamentals of Nursing: Theory, Concepts, and Applications.* Philadelphia: FA Davis; 2007.

Williams L, Hopper P. *Understanding Medical-Surgical Nursing.* 3rd ed. Philadelphia: FA Davis; 2007.

Care of Elderly Patients

Key Terms

Ageism

Age-related macular degeneration

Alzheimer's disease

Aphasia

Cataract

Cerebrovascular accident (CVA)

Dementia

Dysphasia

Geri-chair

Glaucoma

Hallucination

Hemorrhagic stroke

Illusion

Ischemic stroke

Myocardial infarction

Resident

Transient ischemic attack

Objectives

1. Define key terms associated with care of elderly patients.
2. Discuss common myths and stereotypes about aging.
3. Differentiate between young-old, middle-old, old-old, and elite old adults.
4. Describe the physiological and psychosocial changes associated with aging.
5. Identify interventions to assist the older adult in adapting to age-related changes.
6. Discuss the significance of polypharmacy in the older adult.
7. Identify signs of elder abuse.
8. Discuss special considerations when assessing elderly patients.
9. Discuss nursing interventions and rationales to promote health and prevent illness and injury in the older adult.
10. Compare the differences between acute care nursing routines and those in long-term care.
11. Discuss long-term care safety issues that require intervention.

🌐 Clinical Connection

Your Assignment: You are preparing for your clinical experience in an acute care hospital. You have been assigned to care for an 86-year-old female patient with a diagnosis of urinary tract infection (UTI), confusion, congestive heart failure (CHF), and diabetes. She was found lying on the floor in her kitchen unable to clearly explain what happened. In addition, she is dehydrated. She lives alone. Her daughter lives out of town and tries to visit monthly. In report, the nurse says that there is some doubt that the patient has been purchasing and taking her medications for her CHF and diabetes. The daughter is coming today.

Your Actions: You feel somewhat overwhelmed by the number of problems this patient is facing. At first you think that, because she is so old, she should just go to a nursing home where they can give the medications to her or, if not that, move in with her daughter. You wish you had been assigned to a younger patient who was not confused. You need to review the effects of UTI and CHF on elderly patients. You realize that, without her medications, her chronic conditions could be out of control. You pretty much expect the worst when you walk into your patient's room.

This chapter contains information to help you relate to each of your older adult patients individually, not as simply "an old person." You will also learn about the physical and psychosocial changes of aging and how you can help prevent complications due to these changes.

A Description of Aging

Who are the elderly individuals in today's society? It is very easy for people to consider that anyone above a "certain age" is elderly. But how do we determine what that "certain age" is? Or is the term *elderly* to be associated with the ways in which one feels and behaves, as opposed to the actual chronological age that one is?

In the past, the age of 65 years has been associated with the time that a person becomes a senior citizen, or elderly. This is likely because 65 years was the magic age for retirement for many years. We now know that retirement can come at any age. Some people retire much earlier than 65, especially if they have the ability to support themselves. Others will work well past the age of 65, whether by necessity or by choice. Therefore, we no longer can identify an age as the marker for when someone becomes elderly. Many more criteria have to be assessed before that label can be assigned.

Classifications of Age Groups

For purposes of understanding how nurses care for the aging population, it is helpful to classify the different age groups of older adults. Each stage has its own nuances, in terms of physiological and psychosocial changes that take place. Individuals will also experience changes related to developmental, sociocultural, and spiritual issues that occur within these stages of older adulthood. These will be described in more detail later in this chapter.

It is important to realize that, in today's world, people live longer than ever before, particularly in Western society. This is due in part to changes in the health care system making it better equipped to manage chronic disease conditions. With that in mind, it is not unusual that people do not see themselves as old, as they continue to enjoy many of the same activities they enjoyed as a younger person, even though they are now older.

Young-old

The "young-old" are individuals ages 65 to 75 years. They may also be referred to as the young elderly. They have just started experiencing more of the physiological changes that are brought on by the aging process, although they may have experienced a somewhat gradual decline in physical health in the preceding decades. Common conditions seen in young-old individuals include elevations in blood pressure, higher cholesterol levels, and the onset of type 2 diabetes. Particularly in Western cultures, these conditions are prevalent due to sedentary lifestyles and the consumption of diets that are low in fiber, and high in fat and animal proteins. Although the young-old may experience some changes in health, it is not uncommon to find them still working in the public or private sector, or volunteering, while maintaining a social network of friends. It is within the next stage, middle-old, where physical and psychosocial changes begin to become more apparent.

Middle-old

The "middle-old" are individuals ages 75 to 85 years. These are people who have often retired from working and who are experiencing the losses of spouses, family members, and friends to death. Physical changes are more apparent, and often require that people refrain from doing things that formerly brought them pleasure, such as gardening, hobbies, and traveling. Although it is important to assess for depression in any patient, it is of particular importance to recognize that these individuals may be at higher risk for the development of a psychosocial disorder because of the implications of physical and social changes that affect their lives at this time.

Old-old

The "old-old" are those who are age 85 years and older. Often their health has significantly declined, leaving these people with the need for regular, and sometimes around-the-clock, assistance. The U.S. Census Bureau estimated in 2008 that 50% of elderly persons age 85 years and older require personal assistance with activities of daily living. The manner in which these needs are met is often determined by the person's culture. In Eastern cultures, elderly citizens are valued and most often the old-old will reside with family members. In Western cultures, many times younger family members are working as well as raising their own children, so it is more common for the old-old to live in long-term care or assisted living facilities. In Western civilization, when middle-aged individuals care for frail, elderly relatives, and are also raising their dependent children, it is commonly referred to as "sandwiching," meaning that the middle-aged generation is sandwiched between raising a family and caring for aging relatives. The U.S. Census Bureau projects that the old-old will be the fastest growing age group of the elderly populations into the next century.

Elite Old

The "elite old," also called centenarians, are 100 years of age or older. In 2004, 30 of the most developed countries were surveyed and found to have 130,000 centenarians living in them. This is more than twice the number reported only 14 years prior. Again, this is testimony to better medical management of chronic conditions.

The Aging Population and Nursing

By 2030, it is anticipated that 1 in every 5 U.S. citizens will be elderly, and that there will be 7 million citizens who are older than the age of 85 years, according to the National Institute on Aging. This means that there will be an increasing need for more nurses. Despite this, the Health Resources and Services Administration projects that the supply of nurses in the United States will fall by more than 1 million below the requirements needed to care for the population in the year 2020, unless extensive intervention is accomplished to recruit and retain more nurses.

Knowledge Connection

What are the differences between the young-old, the middle-old, and the old-old? Are there similarities you can identify?

Myths About Aging

It is not uncommon for others to categorize elderly people according to invalid assumptions. For example, some might stereotype elderly individuals as kind and nurturing, like doting grandparents. Other people, based on different experiences, might generalize that elderly people are confused, incompetent, or incapable of caring for themselves. Consider the many derogatory perceptions that people in today's society have of elders: old people are hard of hearing, senile, confused, unhappy, depressed, in poor health, forgetful, cranky, and boring. Elderly people are often seen as afterthoughts, incapable of having their own interests, desires, friendships, or activities. This practice of discrimination and prejudice against elders is referred to as **ageism**. The practice of ageism contributes to stereotyping, unequal treatment in the workforce, and denial of health care.

It is important to treat all patients as individuals, with unique characteristics and personalities, no matter the age of the patient. It is true that many of the patients you will care for will be elderly. Some may be confused and cranky, while others may be gentle and kind. In fact, your elderly patients will be quite similar to your younger patients, each one with different concerns and needs. It is never appropriate to practice ageism; rather, your purpose is to see your patients as individuals and provide whole-person care.

Some individuals may resort to ageism because of a lack of knowledge about elders. Many traditional myths about elders are easily proven to be incorrect. When you care for elderly individuals, first assess their state of health, their psychological well-being, and their own perceptions of their abilities. The old adage, "You are only as old as you feel" is true. Numerous people who fall into categorization of "young-old," "middle-old," or "old-old" are younger in health, mind, and spirit than people of a much younger chronological age. Your nursing care should always be personalized, based on the needs of the individual, not on your assumptions about a person based on his or her age.

Knowledge Connection

If you are working with another nurse who states, "All old people are the same—cranky and needy," what appropriate response could you make to educate the nurse and to help dispel the myths about older adults?

Physical Effects of Aging

Throughout a patient's life span, each day brings physical changes that contribute to the health of the individual. In the early, formative years, these changes are centered on development and growth of physical structures within the body. During middle age, the physical changes revolve around maintaining homeostasis for optimal functioning. As a patient ages beyond 65 years, the physical changes begin to shift toward a decline in performance. The specific types of changes, and the degree of change, are often related to genetics, lifestyle choices, and the effects of chronic illness. For those reasons, some individuals will experience more health problems with aging than others. In the following section, specific information about physiological changes and associated nursing considerations will be explored.

Changes in Neurological Functioning

As people age, they are less able to process information supplied by both the neurological system and the sensory system. Reflexes slow due to sluggish nerve transmission and synapses. These slower reflexes are often the cause of injuries in elders, because they may be unable to react quickly while walking, reaching, or driving. Falls are the most common form of injury related to diminished neurological function.

A **transient ischemic attack** is a temporary decrease in the blood supply to the brain, causing sudden symptoms of dizziness, visual changes, weakness, numbness in one or more limbs, and difficulty swallowing. These attacks are sometimes referred to as "ministrokes," although the patient regains full use and feeling after the attack has passed. They may last a few minutes or a few hours.

A **cerebrovascular accident (CVA)**, also known as *stroke* or *brain attack*, is also seen more often in the older adult. The cause of a CVA may be either a clot in a blood vessel or a bleeding blood vessel in the brain. When the cause of the CVA is a blood clot, it is referred to as an **ischemic stroke**; when the cause is a bleeding blood vessel, it is referred to as a **hemorrhagic stroke**. Either of these events interrupts normal blood flow to an area of the brain, resulting in death of brain tissue. Cerebrovascular accidents are often due to complications of conditions such as hypertension, atrial fibrillation, a diet high in saturated fats, elevated cholesterol levels, and diabetes. Depending on the portion of the brain affected by the stroke, the patient may be mildly to profoundly affected, based on the degree of blockage and the length of time the brain has gone without the necessary oxygen. A left-brain CVA affects motor functioning on the right side of the body, may impair speech, and may cause memory loss. A right-brain CVA affects motor functioning on the left side of the body, can cause visual disturbances, and also may cause memory loss. Cerebrovascular accidents can cause a variety of communication issues, including **aphasia**, or the inability to speak, and **dysphasia**, which is difficulty speaking or understanding the spoken word.

Behavioral patterns can be affected, without regard to the location of the CVA. Some behavioral changes exhibited after a CVA include depression, tearfulness, personality shifts, and apathy. Often these changes are permanent and can be quite distressing to the family. When you care for a patient who has had a CVA, focus on ways to promote and maintain safety, providing nonjudgmental, compassionate care, and support the family members as they adjust to changes in their loved one.

One of the most disturbing changes that may occur after a CVA or other neurological disorders is a decrease in alertness, awareness, and orientation. Confusion, delirium, dementia, and depression are often found in elderly patients, especially after a CVA or with other types of neurological illnesses. *Delirium* refers to a state of mental confusion that is usually accompanied by illusions and hallucinations. A **hallucination** is a false perception having no relation to reality; the person may believe that they see, hear, or smell something that is not really present. An **illusion** is a misinterpretation of sensory stimuli, such as seeing a coat rack but believing it is a human. The patient often is disoriented to time and place. **Dementia** is a decrease in intellectual functioning eventually resulting in the inability to care for oneself. It occurs gradually over months or years. Table 32-1 describes each of these conditions and the illnesses they often accompany.

Due to slowing of neurological processes, communication may be more difficult or take more time than with a younger adult. Speak slowly and be sure to face the patient when speaking to him or her. Allow plenty of time for the patient to respond. If you are in a hurry or feel busy, avoid seeming impatient as this may discourage the patient from attempting to communicate with you. Take the necessary time to engage in conversation with the patient; he or she just might have *something important to say*.

Table 32-2 provides information regarding the results of body system deficits, including neurological deficits, and the recommended nursing actions for these concerns.

Supervision/Delegation Connection

Caring for Confused Elderly Patients
In some states the RN or LPN/LVN can delegate certain tasks to UAPs when caring for confused elderly patients. These tasks may include performing hygiene routines, assisting with activities of daily living, transferring between bed and chair, answering call lights promptly, provision of adequate fluid intake and nutrition, and assisting the RN or LPN/LVN in maintaining environmental safety. If you chose to delegate when a patient is confused, be available to help the UAP since personal care may require two people under such circumstances.

Alzheimer's Disease

The most common type of dementia is seen in **Alzheimer's disease**, which is strongly associated with aging. The diagnosis of Alzheimer's disease is based on symptoms because the only way this disease can be confirmed is by finding the characteristic neurofibrillary tangles in the brain on autopsy. It is seen most commonly in middle-old and old-old adults, but has occurred in adults as young as 30 years.

Patients with Alzheimer's disease slowly withdraw from family and social interaction. They develop confusion that increases in severity until they reach a point where they

Table 32-1   **Changes in Orientation**

Disorder	Description	Reversible?	Associated Disorders and Conditions
Confusion	Cannot think clearly; considered a cognitive impairment	Sometimes	Drug side effect Cerebrovascular accident Trauma Metabolic disorders Alzheimer's disease and other dementias Excessive stimuli from around-the-clock nursing care in critical care unit and lights always on Hypoxia
Delirium	State of heightened awareness, hallucinations and vivid dreams present; often has emotional outbursts	Yes	Drug side effect Drug intoxication Drug or alcohol withdrawal Febrile state Hypoxia
Dementia	Deterioration of cognitive functioning without a disturbance in consciousness	No	Alzheimer's disease Cerebrovascular accident Head injury
Depression	Alteration in emotional state marked by intense sadness or despondency, hopelessness, powerlessness	Yes	After a loss of loved one, relationship, home, independence, or financial security Coupled with certain medications Lifestyle changes

Table 32-2   **Results of Body System Deficits and Recommended Nursing Actions**

Results of Body System Deficits	Recommended Nursing Actions
Neurological System Falls and broken bones	• Assess patient's safety in the environment. • Institute ways to improve safety.
Burns and other accidental injuries	• Assess risk for suicide or self-harm. • Refer to physician and appropriate mental health agencies.
Self-inflicted injuries	• Check on patient frequently. • Provide for sitters as needed and available. • Always explain what you are about to do before doing it. • Use calming tone of voice when interacting. • Leave light on at night if needed.
Confusion	• Recommend Alzheimer's disease support groups. • Refer to home health services and Alzheimer's disease residential facilities as appropriate. • Encourage respite services for family members taking care of confused patients.
Sensory System Decreased sensation	• Assess feet for injury, sores, or ingrown toenails, and encourage follow-up with physician. • Monitor temperature of bath water to prevent burns.

(table continues on page 750)

Table 32-2 **Results of Body System Deficits and Recommended Nursing Actions** (continued)

Results of Body System Deficits	Recommended Nursing Actions
Sensory System Poor vision	• Encourage to have regular eye examinations. • Provide adequate lighting for reading and moving about room. • Provide night-light as needed. • Keep pathways clear of objects. • Provide magnifiers for reading.
Impaired hearing	• Encourage regular hearing evaluations. • Teach patients about availability of systems that can activate flashing lights for smoke detectors, ringing telephones, and doorbells.
Cardiovascular System Elevated cholesterol and blood pressure	• Encourage a heart-healthy diet. • Assess blood pressure every 8 hours or more frequently.
Decreased peripheral circulation	• Assess peripheral pulses for weakness or absence; assess for slow capillary refill, decreased warmth of hands or feet, and pallor of extremities. • Assess for environmental temperature comfort: provide extra blankets as needed; raise room temperature prior to bathing to prevent chilling.
Decreased cardiac output	• Assess lungs for adventitious breath sounds, and heart sounds for irregular rhythm or indistinct heart sounds, every 8 hours. • Assess for shortness of breath with exertion, distended neck veins, pallor, bounding or thready radial pulse, tachypnea, pedal edema, weak or absent peripheral pulses; cold or pale extremities; confusion or restlessness; decreased level of consciousness; decreased urinary output. • Encourage regular, moderate exercise.
Respiratory System Chronic respiratory conditions	• Encourage patients to wash hands frequently and correctly, as well as use hand sanitizer if they are unable to wash with soap and water. • Instruct patients to stay 3 to 6 feet away from others who are ill with a respiratory illness. • Encourage compliance with respiratory medications and antibiotics. • Encourage patient to get flu and pneumonia vaccines. • Assure that bedridden patients are repositioned every 2 hours to prevent pneumonia. • Assess for fever, tachycardia, tachypnea; assess breath sounds, noting decreased, absent, or adventitious sounds.
Inadequate O_2 supply to meet body demands during activity	• Plan nursing care in manner to provide frequent rest periods. • Group nursing tasks together in short sessions to avoid constant interruption. • Observe for increases in respirations during activity. • Assess for pallor and cyanosis during activity. • Assess oxygen saturation level; apply and maintain supplemental oxygen as needed and ordered.
Gastrointestinal System Decreased peristalsis	• Encourage high-fiber foods, high fluid intake, activity, and appropriate use of laxatives and stool softeners.

Table 32-2 **Results of Body System Deficits and Recommended Nursing Actions** (continued)

Results of Body System Deficits	Recommended Nursing Actions
Gastrointestinal System Dryness of the mouth	• Perform mouth care every 8 hours or more often as needed.
Impaired sense of taste	• Encourage balanced, nutritional meals of foods the patient likes to eat.
Endocrine System Impaired blood sugar regulation	• Encourage balanced, nutritional meals and regular exercise. • Assess finger stick blood sugar as ordered and administer ordered antidiabetic medications.
Reproductive System Decreased estrogen production in females	• Educate about lubrication products and locally applied estrogen creams to decrease vaginal dryness.
Decreased circulation to genitalia in males	• Encourage discussion of erectile dysfunction if it is a problem. • Discuss blood sugar and blood pressure control, which can help decrease development of erectile dysfunction.
Genitourinary System Impaired emptying of bladder	• Scan bladder to detect urinary retention. • Assess for signs and symptoms of UTI: burning during urination, urgency, frequency, cloudy urine, foul odor to urine. • Encourage fluid intake of liquids patient likes to drink.
Decreased renal function	• Assess intake and output every 8 hours; observe for decreasing urine production, making certain that kidneys are producing the minimum of 30 mL/hr. Assess laboratory results for renal function: blood urea nitrogen (BUN), creatinine, glomerular filtration rate (GFR) • Assess intake and output every 8 hours; observe for decreasing urine production, making certain that kidneys are producing the minimum of 30 mL/hr.
Incontinence	• Implement bladder training when appropriate; assess for wet bed every hour; change wet linens as soon as detected; keep perineum and buttocks clean and dry. • If using adult waterproof underwear, avoid calling them diapers. • Treat incontinent patients with respect.
Musculoskeletal System Osteoporosis	• Encourage weight-bearing exercise. • Encourage increased calcium intake in foods and supplements. • Encourage compliance with other medications for bone strength. • Encourage installation and use of handrails in tubs and around toilets in patient's home. • Encourage use of commercial "emergency help signal devices" that can be worn around the neck and activated when patient falls or becomes seriously ill.
Contractures	• Perform range-of-motion exercises at least once or twice per day if a patient is unable to ambulate. • Encourage neck, arm, and leg exercises that can be performed while sitting in a chair. • Use hand rolls to prevent contractures of hands. • Maintain proper body alignment both in bed and when sitting in a chair. • Encourage patient to perform as much self-care as able.

(table continues on page 752)

Table 32-2 **Results of Body System Deficits and Recommended Nursing Actions** (continued)

Results of Body System Deficits	Recommended Nursing Actions
Integumentary System	
Skin easily damaged	• Encourage protection of skin, such as wearing only closed-toed shoes. • Assess and cover all skin tears or open areas. • Apply creams and lotions to prevent cracking of skin.
Increased capillary fragility	• Assess all injuries, even seemingly minor ones. • Ensure that bleeding is controlled and stopped. • Be careful to avoid bumping or scraping arms and legs on bed rails, bed frames, wheelchairs, or chair legs. • Be gentle when handling the patient; when applying tape to skin, use the least amount that will accomplish your goal. • Report bleeding gums.
Decreased circulation to skin and underlying tissue	• Turn immobile patients every 2 hours, and encourage frequent position changes in patients who can turn themselves. • Place pillows between knees and ankles when in side-lying positions. • Keep sheets as wrinkle-free as possible. • Avoid allowing patient to lay in a wet bed. • Change linens frequently. • Position heels so they do not constantly rest on the bed. • Use sheepskin elbow and heel protectors as needed. • Provide skin care several times per day if patient is bedridden. • Assess pressure points for erythema at least every 4 hours, sometimes as often as every 2 hours. • Encourage adequate fluids and nutrition; provide protein supplements if needed.

do not recognize their own family members. They often wander at night and sleep during the day. Eventually they are unable to walk and speak, making sounds rather than words. Patients with advanced Alzheimer's disease require complete care and are totally dependent on others. When family members are the primary caregivers, they may become overwhelmed; when this occurs, they, along with the patient, will need care and support.

It is difficult for family members to watch a loved one who has developed multiple medical problems "slip away" from them, particularly when one of the medical concerns is Alzheimer's disease or another form of dementia. Family members often describe this process as taking care of someone they feel like they do not know, because the cognitive changes seen in dementia seem to rob the patient of distinct personality features. While the nursing care for patients with dementia often focuses on maintenance of safety and assistance with activities of daily living, the care given to the caregiver is just as important, and focuses on preventing burnout.

Real-World Connection

Alzheimer's Disease

A 75-year-old woman was caring for her elderly husband who had multiple illnesses as well as Alzheimer's disease. She was devoted to him and was his sole caregiver. Eventually, hospice was called in to provide additional in-home care. His wife struggled with watching his decline and accepting help with his care. She felt as though she was losing her husband and best friend as he became more and more withdrawn. The hospice nurse answered her questions honestly and allowed her to verbalize her sadness regarding the fact that he would not get better.

As her husband's physical and neurological function continued to decline, it was suggested that he be moved to a skilled nursing facility. This was extremely difficult for his wife to allow, as she kept wondering if she could do more to be able to keep him home. Once again, the hospice nurse helped her see the reality of the situation. Using criteria recommended by the Alzheimer's Association (Box 32-1), the nurse assessed the wife's stress level and risk for burnout. The nurse also helped her understand that she was becoming overwhelmed, losing weight and sleep, and unable to keep her husband safe in the home setting. The nurse reassured the wife that he would be safe and attended to 24 hours a day, 7 days a week at the skilled nursing facility.

Three weeks after his admission to the facility, he passed away peacefully, and his wife was grateful for the care he was given prior to his death. Although her husband did not survive, she was at peace with her decision and valued those last days with him as she could completely focus on being with him, rather than trying to complete the innumerable tasks related to his care.

When you care for patients and family members in similar situations, it is important for you to help the family realize that it is not a sign of failure, but a sign of strength to tap into the help available for both them and their loved one.

Changes in Sensory Functioning

Encompassing vision, hearing, taste, smell, and touch, the senses are also affected by a slowing of the transmissions in the nervous system. Common visual disturbances in older adults include cataracts and glaucoma. **Cataracts** occur when the lens of the eye becomes cloudy, or opaque, causing visual blurring. **Glaucoma** is an eye disease characterized by increased intraocular pressure, which affects the optic nerve and can lead to blindness. **Age-related macular degeneration** is the destruction of the area in the retina where the optic nerve attaches, leading to the loss of central vision. In addition, many older adults complain of dry eyes due to less tearing, and changes in visual acuity related to complications of untreated hypertension and diabetes.

As with neurological changes, decreases in the sensory abilities predispose patients to injuries. *Presbycusis,* or the normal decrease in hearing that accompanies the aging process, can increase the risk for injury if people cannot hear alarms and sirens. They often are unable to hear even the telephone unless they are present in the same room as the

phone. When caring for a patient with decreased hearing, avoid shouting in an attempt to make them hear. It usually works best to lower the pitch of your voice, speak to the ear in which the patient hears the best, and slightly raise the volume of your voice. Another tactic that sometimes helps is to be on the same physical level as the patient and speak slowly, allowing him or her to read your lips. Inner ear disturbances can affect equilibrium, increasing the chance of falls. The number of olfactory nerves decreases, diminishing the sensation of smell, making it more difficult to detect such things as spoilage of food or gas leaks. Touch sensation can be decreased as peripheral blood flow decreases. The taste buds become less sensitive, requiring stronger flavors to stimulate the patient's sense of taste. This is why many older adults tend to eat more sweet desserts than when younger, because they can better taste sweets than other tastes.

When patients do not taste and enjoy foods, they are less likely to consume the needed amount of nutrients to maintain their appropriate body weight. So, if an older patient wants to eat his or her dessert first at mealtime, this should be allowed. Avoid treating them as children, telling them they cannot have their dessert until after they have eaten the other things on their plate. Table 32-2 provides information regarding sensory deficits and the recommended nursing actions for these concerns.

Changes in Cardiovascular Functioning

As patients age, the heart muscle loses elasticity, the blood vessels narrow as arteries collect fatty deposits, and peripheral pulses are less palpable. Circulation is decreased, resulting in complaints of feeling cold, especially at bath time. These patients require a warmer room and warmer clothes than younger people. These circulatory changes may all occur without the patient's awareness, which puts the person at a high risk for developing conditions such as coronary artery disease, hypertension, high cholesterol levels, **myocardial infarction** (also known as heart attack), or peripheral vascular disease. It is estimated that approximately two-thirds of individuals older than age 65 years have coronary artery disease. Table 32-2 provides information regarding the cardiovascular changes with aging and the recommended nursing actions for these concerns.

Changes in Respiratory Functioning

In an aging patient, you would expect that lung elasticity is decreased. As with many body systems, the flexibility of the normally elastic lung tissue is reduced over time. The alveoli do not expand fully, increasing the risk for pneumonia and bronchitis, and complications of underlying chronic pulmonary disease.

Older adults are also more vulnerable to infections, particularly respiratory infection due to decreased immune function. Therefore, be sure to educate patients about ways in which to protect themselves from easily-contracted

Box 32-1
Signs of Caregiver Burnout

When caring for a patient who has family members or friends involved in his or her care, it is important to pay attention for the signs of caregiver burnout. Even though caregivers are not necessarily sick, giving care to a loved one can be a very stressful experience. Ask these questions when assessing whether or not a caregiver is experiencing burnout:

- Does the caregiver feel that he or she must be the exclusive care provider?
- Does the caregiver feel that he or she is withdrawing from other friends, family, or activities because of the care he or she must provide for the loved one?
- Does the caregiver worry about the safety of the loved one?
- Is the caregiver anxious about finances and making health care decisions for his or her loved one?
- Is the caregiver denying the impact of the disease and its effects on the family?
- Is the caregiver experiencing grief or sadness that the relationship with the loved one is deteriorating?
- Does the caregiver get frustrated or angry when the loved one does not listen?
- Is the caregiver experiencing personal health problems in addition to caring for the loved one?

infections. Table 32-2 provides information about ways to help patients protect themselves from respiratory illnesses.

Changes in Gastrointestinal Functioning

As peristalsis slows in the older adult, the cycle of food digestion slows, which can lead to poor appetite and decreased food intake. This may then result in malnutrition, weight loss, and an overall decrease in immune function. It is very important that you investigate the cause of a loss of more than a few pounds or kilograms in patients who are not trying to lose weight.

Constipation may result from numerous factors. Many medications list constipation as a side effect. As patients grow older, their lack of activity may slow down the entire gastrointestinal functioning, including evacuation. Aging can affect peristalsis, increasing the amount of time that feces remains in the large intestine, causing more water to be absorbed, leaving the stool dry and hard. Some older adults become very focused on the frequency of their bowel movements and become distressed easily if constipation occurs. Administer ordered medications such as stool softeners and laxatives to help prevent this problem.

Xerostoma is the medical term for an excessively dry mouth. This is a common complaint of older adults, as many medications can dry normal secretions. The cells in the salivary glands, just as in the rest of the body, diminish in size and number, which compounds this problem. Table 32-2 provides information regarding deficits of gastrointestinal functioning and the recommended nursing actions for these concerns.

Changes in Endocrine and Genitourinary Functioning

As people age, the function of the pancreas decreases, which can lead to poorly controlled diabetes. Metabolism can slow, which means weight can increase. If patients are not able to exercise due to impaired mobility, the extra weight can affect their endurance.

As a complication of diabetes or other diseases, older adults may experience changes in renal function, leading to incomplete waste removal due to decreased efficiency of the filtering mechanism of the kidneys. This generally occurs gradually and may eventually lead to kidney failure. Figure 32-1 shows an elderly patient with renal changes.

With aging, the capacity of the bladder decreases due to loss of muscle tone. The bladder cannot hold as much urine as that of a younger adult, and older persons must go to the bathroom to empty the bladder more frequently. They often experience nocturia, which puts them at risk for falls and injuries when up at night. In addition, older adults are more at risk for developing UTIs due to more concentrated urine and decreased function of the immune response. Without proper attention, patients can develop urinary sepsis, a condition that warrants hospitalization and is often fatal. Table 32-2 provides information regarding endocrine and genitourinary system deficits and the recommended nursing actions for these concerns.

Figure 32-1 A patient with kidney failure does not necessarily look ill, but experiences lack of energy, anemia, and elevated BUN and creatinine levels.

Anatomy and Physiology Connection

Metabolization and Elimination of Medications

Most medications are metabolized and eliminated from the body via the hepatic and renal systems. After a medication is digested, it is absorbed into the bloodstream, where it can be transported through the portal vein to the liver, where most medications are metabolized, or broken down for use, leaving what is known as *by-products* or *end products*. The medication is then carried by the hepatic vein to the heart, where it is pumped out and circulated to the target organs. However, the drug is carried not only to the target organs, but through the entire body and eventually back to the liver, where any remaining drug can be processed further.

The end products of medications are filtered and removed from the blood as it flows through the kidneys and then excreted in the urine. If the liver or kidneys are not able to remove the toxins due to disease or impairment, they remain in the blood circulating through the body. Essentially, this can lead to cumulative effects similar to a drug overdose. The by-products of the metabolized medication are sometimes toxic to the liver. When the liver is exposed to excessively high levels or constant levels of a hepatotoxic drug, the liver can be seriously or even fatally damaged. An example of a drug that is toxic to the liver is acetaminophen, more commonly known as Tylenol. Many medications carry warnings that patients must have regular liver and kidney function testing while they are taking the drugs to detect damage to those organs that remove the medication from the body.

Changes in Reproductive Functioning

Older adults experience a normal decrease in hormone levels as they age. Men will experience a decline in testosterone, while women will experience a decline in estrogen. As this happens, men will still produce sperm, although they might not be as viable as sperm produced in younger years. Women will have gone through menopause during middle adulthood into early older age, which eliminates the possibility of childbearing.

This decrease in hormonal activity can change the older adult's sexual drive. Some older adults will gravitate toward less frequent sexual activity, while others will maintain an active sex life. Avoid stereotyping and assuming that seniors are uninterested in sexual relationships. Reassure patients about their own sexual needs and provide for privacy, caring for patients in a nonjudgmental fashion.

Erectile dysfunction (ED) is a condition in which men cannot achieve or maintain an erection. Medical disorders such as diabetes, kidney disease, chronic alcoholism, multiple sclerosis, atherosclerosis, vascular disease, and neurological disease can cause ED. Effective medications are available to treat ED.

It is most important for seniors to be educated about ways in which to protect themselves when they engage in sexual activity. The current generation of seniors did not grow up with the fear of sexually transmitted diseases, including HIV, AIDS, and hepatitis, so they may have questions about prevention. Table 32-2 provides information about reproductive system concerns and the recommended nursing actions for these concerns.

Changes in Musculoskeletal and Integumentary Functioning

As patients age, there is increased bone loss and muscle mass loss that increases the risk for injury. As calcium is lost from the bones due to decreased absorption (and estrogen loss that takes place in women), osteoporosis can develop. Figure 32-2 shows a resident with a musculoskeletal condition that requires the use of a wheelchair. A decrease in muscle fibers and motor neurons causes a decrease in muscle mass and strength. Skin becomes less elastic and more prone to drying, nails thicken, and the skin bruises easily. Because of these changes and changes related to diabetes, pay particular attention to the feet of patients with diabetes. They are less likely to be aware of dry, cracked skin on their heels, which can lead to an infection. They may also be unaware of a developing foot ulcer due to compromised blood flow that is often associated with diabetes.

The loss of subcutaneous fat and the decrease in sweat gland density over time change the older adult's ability to thermoregulate, meaning that they may chill more often than other individuals. Table 32-2 provides information regarding musculoskeletal and integumentary system deficits and the recommended nursing actions for these concerns.

Figure 32-2 A patient with musculoskeletal disorders uses a wheelchair for mobility.

Assessment Considerations for Older Adults

Although the physical assessment that you learned to do in Chapter 21 is identical to what you will perform for older adult patients, there are still elements that you need to focus on more intently to make this process as comfortable as possible. Box 32-2 provides tips for when you are performing a physical assessment on an older adult.

Knowledge Connection

In what ways is the assessment for the older adult the same as an assessment for anyone else? In what ways might the assessment differ? What might you teach an older adult about preventing UTIs?

Box 32-2

Tips for Performing Physical Assessment on Older Adults

When you obtain a health history, be certain to consider the patient holistically. Beyond the physical presentation of the patient, there are often emotional, psychological, spiritual, or sociocultural needs that are pressing to an older adult. Before you perform the physical examination, consider which accommodations might make this process easier for the patient. These may include:

- **Extra attention to safety:** Because elderly patients may not be as steady, consider how to make the physical assessment a safer experience. This may include assisting with transfers, helping the patient to move in the bed, and assisting the patient with disrobing and dressing as necessary.
- **Sessions:** Older adults may not be able to tolerate an entire physical assessment performed at once due to excessive fatigue. Plan your assessment to avoid tiring the patient. You may need to do part of the assessment, then allow the patient to rest a bit before you complete it.

Psychosocial Problems of Aging

When you perform an assessment on an older adult, keep in mind the numerous psychosocial concerns that he or she may have. Some of these were discussed earlier in this chapter, such as the loss of connection with loved ones that occurs in different types of dementia. Other concerns of older adults and their caregivers include:

• Fears about the dying process, as some people may struggle with spiritual beliefs
• Loss and grief as friends and family die or leave
• Safety concerns, including scams and crimes
• Elder abuse by caregivers
• Financial concerns regarding retirement and living arrangements

Loss, Grief, and Dying

It is a common misconception that, because a person is older, he or she is consumed with thoughts of death. Like most of us, thoughts of mortality do arise and are more prevalent if we receive a diagnosis of a terminal or untreatable disease. Figure 32-3 shows an elderly resident toward the end of her life. Older people may also feel their own mortality more strongly because of losing friends and family members to death with increasing frequency. One middle-old couple moved to a retirement center and made many new friends, but in the first year of residency, approximately half of them died. While other people moved in and took their places, this change was difficult for the couple. Chapter 10 discusses the stages of grieving and therapeutic approaches you can use with your patients who are dealing with grief. Chapter 8 provides information regarding the spiritual aspect of your nursing care.

When you care for older patients dealing with loss and grief, you can include the following when planning and delivering nursing care:

• **Refer to support groups:** Numerous support groups exist in most communities, focused on different types of losses. Some types of groups include those designed to support surviving spouses, those who have lost children, and those who have experienced any type of loss.
• **Educate about the importance of proper nutrition and exercise:** Older adults, especially those who live alone, may lose interest in food during an episode of loss and grief. Explain the importance of proper nutrition to keep the body strong and to help prevent new illnesses or worsening existing conditions. Exercise helps relieve stress and tension, and can provide a time for focusing on something other than grief.
• **Encourage rest:** Because the grieving process can be exhausting, it is important for older adults to have the opportunity to rest when needed.
• **Help find comfort and meaning:** Sometimes this is as simple as sitting with the patient and allowing him or her to express feelings about the loss just experienced. There is no magic formula for helping the patient find comfort, but the presence of another human being who allows him or her to express feelings can prove to be quite comforting, particularly if the older adult has lost a close friend or spouse. Chapter 10 provides additional information about ways to help grieving patients.
• **Encourage spirituality, if the patient desires:** Older adults may find comfort in their spiritual beliefs during times of loss. You may contact an appropriate person to assist the patient, such as a pastor, chaplain, priest, or shaman to assist them. Figure 32-4 shows an elderly person practicing his faith.

Figure 32-3 This patient is terminally ill and has been bathed, dressed, and made comfortable by the nursing staff.

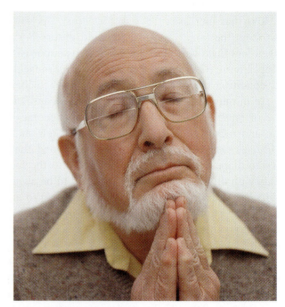

Figure 32-4 To meet the spiritual needs of elderly patients, provide opportunities for them to practice their faith.

• **Allow the patient to grieve:** Provide privacy or sit in silence with the patient, as indicated, to allow the patient time to grieve. Recognize that each person may grieve differently, so be supportive and nonjudgmental during this time.

Safety From Scams and Crime

Older adults are considered easy prey, as they are less skeptical about solicitations for money than younger individuals, making them frequent victims of those trying to defraud them of money.

It is not uncommon for such scams and crimes to take place over the telephone. The older adult does not know the caller, and sometimes it is easy for scammers to talk an elder into giving them credit card numbers or other identifying information, which they then use to defraud him or her. Because elderly people are often homebound and socially isolated, callers have an easy time gaining their trust, often because the caller is personable and sounds official. Older adults should be cautioned about giving personal information over the telephone, via the mail, or over the Internet, since so many of these schemes are indeed ways to pilfer money from unsuspecting people.

Other scams involve people who come to an older adult's home, representing themselves as repairmen or utility workers. These people are often dressed for the part and, when they gain entry into the home, they physically harm and rob the elderly person. Or they may give the false impression of having supplied the appropriate service, when in fact, only small portions of the work were actually completed or shoddy work was done. Then exorbitant amounts of money are paid to them and they disappear, leaving false contact information with the elderly individual. Caution older adults not to allow anyone in their home that they are not expecting, and to always ask for identification before allowing an expected worker in. It is sometimes helpful if the elderly individual will consult a trusted family member or friend who might assist in determining the legitimacy of the workers who are being considered for hire. However, many elderly individuals are struggling to maintain their sense of independence and are resistant to others helping them make their decisions.

Elder Abuse

It may come as a surprise to most to learn that it is estimated that between 1 and 2 million seniors have been injured, exploited, or otherwise mistreated by a caregiver, according to the National Center on Elder Abuse. This type of abuse can take place in many forms: *neglect,* which means that the caretaker has omitted providing basic, necessary care such as food or fluids, hygiene, or a safe environment; *psychological abuse,* which entails manipulation or mental cruelty; *physical abuse,* which involves any kind of physical harm done to the patient; and *exploitation,* which involves using the older adult for personal gain, such as gaining access to the older adult's bank account and using it without their knowledge.

Physical abuse is more recognized because of the outward signs that this type of abuse leaves behind. Be alert for these findings that could suggest abuse:

• **Excessive bruises in unexpected places:** This could be the caregiver's attempt to hide abuse by hurting the victim in places that would not normally be visible.
• **Bruises in multiple stages of healing:** This finding could potentially indicate that the older adult has been abused on an ongoing basis. When bruises are found in multiple stages of healing, it could be an indicator of infrequent abuse that occurs at different times or of frequent and varying kinds of abuse.
• **Bite marks:** Although less common than bruises and lacerations, bite marks may also be found and be indicative of abuse.
• **Burns:** Burns in varying locations over the body are often indicators of abuse. More frequent types of abusive burns are those from cigarettes, which produce small round burns. When found, they are commonly seen on the palms of the hands or the soles of the feet, or on the abdomen.
• **Lacerations:** Like burns, the finding of multiple lacerations, particularly in various stages of healing, may indicate that the older adult is living in an unsafe environment where he or she is repeatedly brushing against objects that cut, or that he or she is being purposely cut by a caregiver.
• **Fractures or dislocations:** Although there are no classic patterns of fractures that indicate elder abuse, keep in mind that repeated or multiple fractures or dislocations may be cause for concern.
• **Sedation:** Patients who are sedated may have been overdosed on medication. A caregiver may knowingly administer too much medication as a way to manage an elderly person, or a caregiver may accidentally be administering too much of a certain medication.
• **Dehydration or malnutrition:** These may be signs of poor dietary intake, and may not indicate abuse. However, continued or repeated admissions for dehydration or malnutrition may indicate that the patient is not being provided with proper nutritional intake.
• **Excessively poor hygiene or unsuitable clothing:** This finding may indicate that the patient is not being cared for appropriately. Some elderly people are unable to see that their clothing is not clean and may show a lack of interest in personal hygiene. Therefore, be sure to investigate the situation before assuming that abuse is taking place.

Financial Concerns

While many people are ready to retire at age 62 or 65, others prefer to remain in the workforce until age 70 or older. As they contemplate this change in work status, older people may express concerns about how they will provide for themselves, and if there will be enough money in the future when their income is fixed. Between the financial implications of older age and the physical changes that may take place, older adults may also have concerns about living arrangements. Many people wonder if they will have enough money to pay for a nursing home should they ever have to be admitted to one.

While you cannot solve these problems, you can provide empathetic, therapeutic listening, and refer the patient to appropriate resources for assistance. These resources may include social services, the local Area Agency on Aging, and other senior assistive facilities.

Positive Aspects of Aging

In this chapter, we have discussed all the changes that aging brings, both physical and psychosocial. However, with those changes, aging also brings wisdom and insight. It is often within this stage of life that people have so much knowledge to share with younger generations. Over the years, they have developed social skills, successfully raised families, excelled at a trade or business, learned from their own mistakes, experienced many things that others have yet to experience, and mastered concepts that younger adults have not yet grasped. They can utilize these rich pieces of knowledge as grandparents, civic leaders, volunteers, church workers, neighbors, and friends.

Be respectful of this special time in the life of an older adult, and work to promote self-esteem as physical, psychosocial, and spiritual changes take place. Avoid stereotypes and meet each patient where he or she is in the aging process, and you can effectively care for the patient's needs personally and professionally, while promoting dignity in the aging years. Figure 32-5 shows how allowing an elderly person to groom himself or herself can promote dignity.

Figure 32-5 When you care for elderly patients, help promote dignity by assisting them to look their best.

Long-term Care

While the aging process has the advantages of wisdom, more life experiences, and new and different opportunities, it also sometimes involves the loss of ability to live independently due to health problems, whether physical or mental. Many older adults may find it necessary to live in assisted living facilities or long-term care (LTC) facilities, more commonly known as nursing homes. You will probably have the opportunity to perform some of your clinical experiences in an LTC, and you will find that providing nursing care for these individuals is vastly different from the care you provide in an acute care setting. One difference is how you will refer to those for whom you provide care.

Patient or Resident?

You typically refer to the population within acute care facilities as patients or clients, and those individuals are in the facility temporarily because they require some type of diagnostics or treatment for health problems. Most individuals for whom you will provide care in LTC facilities are not there temporarily; they reside, or live, there. The facility is their actual home, their residence, and their place of refuge from society, although many of them would prefer to live somewhere else if they could. It is considered more appropriate to refer to these individuals as **residents** rather than patients.

Residents' Needs

Using the term *resident* may help you to maintain the focus of your role in providing nursing care. Even though an acute care patient and an LTC resident may have some of the same needs, you will have additional opportunities to meet more needs in the LTC setting. In acute care, you prioritize needs according to Maslow's hierarchy of needs, but it is performed within a much smaller time frame than in LTC, and may not require you to address needs from every level. When you care for patients in LTC, your primary focus will be to provide ongoing life services for the residents—those things we all need and desire, which address all levels of Maslow's hierarchy of needs:

- Oxygen and fresh air, water and nutrition, healthy elimination
- Rest and sleep, comfort and pain relief
- Optimal health
- Safety and security
- Spiritual edification
- Freedom from anxiety and fear
- Love and affection, acceptance by others
- Self-respect and being respected
- Self-esteem and self-confidence
- Productivity and self-worth
- Simple enjoyment and fulfillment in daily life

Helping to Meet These Needs

You will have ample chances to meet more of these needs than you will probably ever realize. When you enter an LTC facility, you have a unique opportunity to impact the lives of the residents and a chance to make their days brighter and more fulfilling. You have the opportunity to bring compassion, respect, comfort, and affection while you provide nursing care. One of the benefits for you is the opportunity to learn from a wealth of wisdom that the residents have to share. Many of them will have lived and experienced decades of life beyond that of the typical student. We can all learn from the older and wiser generations if we are willing. Encourage residents to reminisce and tell about events they have experienced. Listen attentively as you get to know the resident better, and you may gain knowledge or develop a better appreciation for the past. You might also enjoy it.

The LTC setting is different from acute care in a variety of ways: the contents of rooms, personal attire, personal care, nutrition and hydration, elimination and toileting, immobility and activity, medications, assessment, and documentation.

Resident Rooms

Because LTC residents live in a facility rather than spending a day or two there, it is important to remember that their rooms are their personal residences. It is even more important that you knock before entering their room, just like you do before entering someone's house. Residents may bring personal items, sometimes even pieces of furniture, to personalize their residence. Encourage residents to hang photographs and the artwork of grandchildren or other significant young ones. Use personal blankets, pillows, and afghans when available. Provide whatever assistance is required to keep the room, floor, and bathroom clean, but allow the resident to arrange his or her possessions as desired. It may look cluttered to you, but be just the way he or she wants it. Offer to help organize or straighten articles if the resident requires or desires assistance. If the resident is immobile or has severe dementia, it will be your responsibility to maintain the room's appearance and organization so that safety is not sacrificed.

Personal Attire

Residents wear their own clothing and shoes, unless the resident's condition is such that he or she requires continual medical and nursing intervention that is hindered by wearing personal clothing. Assist the resident as needed to get dressed each morning. If the resident is incontinent, change his or her clothing immediately. Families of residents may or may not prefer to do the resident's personal laundry. Some residents will require that the LTC facility employees launder their clothing. If this is the case, it is important for the resident's name to be written with a permanent marker on the label or inside the neck of the garment. Even socks and underwear must be marked to prevent misplacing articles of clothing in another resident's laundry. *Safety: Make certain that residents' shoes have nonskid soles to decrease risk of falls. If the soles are somewhat slick, it is helpful to apply several strips of adhesive tape across the soles of the shoes. The cloth side of the tape helps prevent slipping on a tile floor.*

Personal Care

Some residents may be able to perform their daily hygiene without assistance, but many will need assistance. For these residents, you will provide personal care, but on a slightly different schedule than in acute care. For example, most residents will not take a complete bath every day. Aging skin becomes drier and more fragile, so many residents will prefer to take a complete tub bath or shower only two to three times per week. On nonbath days you will wash the resident's face, hands, feet, and perineal area daily and as needed. Most facilities have shower rooms or tub rooms, with several tubs and shower stalls, which must be shared by all the residents. *Safety: You will need to disinfect shower chairs, tubs, and mechanical lifts after each use. This is paramount to prevent cross-contamination.* Without stringent disinfection between residents, it is possible to spread diseases caused by highly contagious organisms such as *Clostridium difficile* (*C. diff.*). This bacterium causes severe diarrhea that has the potential to be fatal in elderly and immune-suppressed individuals, and it can spread quickly throughout a facility.

Provide privacy for the residents by pulling the curtains between the bathing stations and ensure that the doors are kept closed while bathing facilities are in use. *Safety: Immediately mop up all water that is splashed or dripped onto the floor to prevent falls.* Whirlpool tubs are commonly used for bathing, providing the additional benefit of stimulating the circulation and débriding any wounds the resident may have. Safety is a real issue when bathing residents. It would be easy for residents with impaired mobility or dementia to drown in a whirlpool tub due to the depth of water. *Safety: Never leave a resident unattended while bathing! Environmental temperature must be kept warm enough that residents will not become chilled.*

Some residents are unable to stand or access the bathtub or whirlpool tub without the use of a mechanical lift. You learned about safe usage of this equipment in Chapter 16. *Safety: Remember to obtain an adequate number of coworkers to provide safe handling while transferring residents via a mechanical lift.*

Provide hair care for residents on a daily basis, and wash their hair at least once a week, or more often if needed. Many LTC facilities have beauty and barber shops, allowing residents to schedule appointments with professional stylists. If the facility does not have these types of services available, or if residents do not have someone who assists them in these matters, you will assist with styling their hair. It will help you to meet this need more easily if you think how you would feel if you were unable to perform these activities and no one else cared enough to assist you. Everyone wants to look their best to receive friends and loved ones when they come to visit; appearance is part of self-esteem.

Male residents may require assistance with shaving, some daily and others only two to three times per week. *Safety: If a resident has supplemental oxygen being delivered, turn it off for at least 10 minutes before shaving with an electric razor to allow the higher oxygen levels in the room air to dissipate.* If the resident cannot tolerate the removal of oxygen for that length of time, you will use a safety razor. *Safety: Before using a safety razor, assess whether the resident is taking anticoagulants such as warfarin (Coumadin), which would put the resident at risk for excessive bleeding in the event you should accidentally nick his skin.* Follow the facility policy regarding use of electric and safety razors.

You will perform nail care more frequently in LTC than in acute care. Follow facility policy carefully regarding who may cut or trim nails, especially those of a resident with diabetes or peripheral vascular disease (refer to Chapter 15).

Nutrition and Hydration

While you provide meals, snacks, and fluids to patients in acute care, the responsibility is more extensive in LTC. It is your responsibility to make certain that each resident maintains adequate dietary intake by:

- Ensuring that dentures are inserted for meals
- Assessing whether the food needs to be finely chopped or pureed

- Feeding or assisting the resident to eat, as needed
- Monitoring and recording the percentage eaten at each meal
- Ensuring that adequate fluids are ingested, usually a minimum of 1,500 mL/day
- Providing supplemental protein and carbohydrate drinks as needed
- Monitoring for weight loss on a weekly or monthly basis

Most LTC facilities have a policy addressing interventions to implement when a resident eats 50% or less of the food served for a meal. The most common intervention is to provide a supplemental nutrition drink, such as Ensure, between meals. Accrediting agencies look for documentation that this is done.

It is important that all residents who are able be taken to the dining room for each meal. Meals are a social event for most people, and this gathering allows residents to see, greet, and converse with their neighbors. Figure 32-6 shows residents socializing during a meal. For residents who are immobile, it is even more important to transfer them to the dining room for all three meals each day so they have more opportunity to interact with others. You may transfer residents via a wheelchair or a special chair called a geri-chair. A **geri-chair** is a recliner with side arms, a lap belt, and wheels so that it can be navigated through the hallways. It is used for residents who are unable to sit unassisted.

The dining room in most facilities contains multiple tables with assigned seats for each resident. This allows the staff to deliver special diets to the correct residents. *Safety: Always check the resident's meal card and diet before delivering the tray to the resident.*

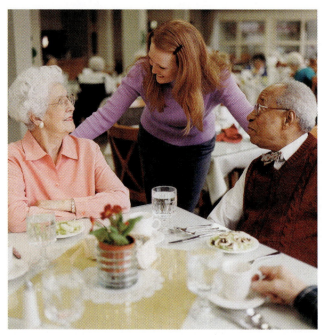

Figure 32-6 These residents are socializing during a meal.

When a resident is unable to feed himself or herself, you must assist him or her. It is important to sit in a chair next to the resident, rather than to stand. This puts you at eye level with the resident, improving communication and allowing the resident to see your face. Some residents are unable to look upward to see someone standing, towering above them. It is important to make mealtimes as pleasant as possible: Converse with the residents and include them in conversations whether or not they are able to verbalize. Try to make the mealtimes a happy and social time, as it can be in the home with one's family.

Elimination and Toileting

Not all residents in an LTC facility are incontinent of bowel and bladder, but many will be. Check incontinent residents every 1 to 2 hours for the need to be changed. Avoid allowing a resident to lie or sit in wet or dirty clothes or linens. Change them as needed and provide scrupulous perineal and skin care to prevent skin breakdown. Some residents may require barrier ointments to aid in protecting the skin from urine and feces. Avoid using the term *diaper* for incontinence briefs. Treat the resident with respect when you are changing the brief and washing the perineum after incontinence.

It is important to monitor and record whether or not each resident has a bowel movement on every shift. Residents with impaired mobility are particularly at risk for constipation. Most facilities have a policy requiring that each resident is provided with a stool softener or laxative if the resident does not have a bowel movement at least every 3 days. Careless tracking of daily bowel movements can result in fecal impaction, which is a very uncomfortable condition for the resident. (See Chapter 30 for more information about fecal impaction.)

Immobility

Residents can develop impaired mobility if you do not take action to prevent it. Encourage residents to get out of their rooms and to ambulate as much as possible. Encourage participation in exercise sessions and outdoor walks; encourage those with gardening interests to help tend to the flower gardens if they are physically able. Lead groups of residents in chair exercises, which can help prevent loss of strength and preserve joint mobility.

Frequently reposition bedfast residents and those who are restricted to sitting in a chair and unable to walk. The longest any resident should remain in any one position is 2 hours. Repositioning, assessing pressure points for erythema, and applying lotion as needed, are paramount to prevent pressure ulcers. Encourage residents, if they are able to do so, to sit in a chair for meals and to attend social events.

Provide passive and active range-of-motion exercises for bedfast residents to increase circulation and to prevent atrophy of muscles and contracture formation. Exercises should be performed at least once or twice per shift during daytime hours.

Also encourage the resident to do as much as he or she is able to do with regard to activities of daily living (ADLs). For example, if a resident is only able to wash his or her face and hands and brush his or her teeth and hair, encourage the resident to do so. Avoid doing it all yourself in an effort to "get done" because you are busy. Participation in self-care helps to increase activity but also fosters confidence, independence, and self-esteem.

Activity and Entertainment

Most LTC facilities schedule regular activities for the residents to participate in as they are able. Some examples may include:

- Craft-making sessions
- Manicure sessions
- Domino tournaments
- Group singing and karaoke
- Movie time
- Current event discussion groups
- Daily reading aloud of the newspaper or Bible
- Paint-by-number pictures, watercolors, and finger painting
- Bingo
- Ice cream socials
- Story time, where a novel is read aloud each session until completed

Some LTC facilities may even include music sessions in which residents are provided with instruments to play in accompaniment to someone playing the piano. Instruments may include triangles, cymbals, sticks, bells, tambourines, small hand drums, kazoos, or harmonicas. Encourage residents to participate in as many of these activities as possible. One of the best incentives is to include staff and family members who may be visiting at that time.

LTC facilities seek assistance from the local community to provide scheduled activities for residents, such as church services to be held in the facility chapel, vocal and instrumental talent sessions, monthly birthday celebrations, holiday parties, and visits by children's groups, such as school classes, Bible-school classes, and Girl Scout and Boy Scout troops. Visits by children seem to be especially enjoyed and appreciated by the residents. Another good activity that has proven to be very therapeutic is pet therapy. Kittens, puppies, baby lambs, rabbits, or other small animals are scheduled to be brought in for petting and cuddling once or twice a month. Aquariums set up in the lobby or television area are another treat for residents and sometimes have a calming effect on a resident experiencing an emotional event.

Medications

As with acute care, most LTC residents will have ordered medications that you will administer and document. Remember that elders will often have stronger reactions to medications and are more at risk for toxicity as the kidneys and liver are unable to rid the body of the drug as quickly as in younger adults. Be vigilant in assessing for oversedation and toxicity in these residents.

Assessment

When you care for acutely ill patients in the hospital setting, you perform a head-to-toe physical assessment at the beginning of each shift on each patient, and additionally as the patient's condition warrants further assessment. This is one of the biggest differences you will find in LTC. A complete head-to-toe assessment is generally performed once a month unless the resident exhibits signs or symptoms of illness or suffers an injury, in which case assessment is performed based upon the resident's condition and the frequency cited in facility policy. However, the assessments that are performed once a month include additional data beyond the traditional head-to-toe physical assessment. Some of the additional assessments that are made include:

- **General appearance:** characteristics such as emaciation, dry hair, or drooping on one side of the face
- **Adaptive equipment:** hearing aids, eyeglasses, dentures, and any prosthesis such as an eye or a limb
- **Ability to communicate:** includes verbal communication or nonverbal communication, with the method that is used if resident is unable to speak
- **Level of cognition:** including degree of dementia if present
- **General eating habits:** how well resident generally eats at mealtimes, dentition and ability to chew, type of diet, snacks, supplements, level of hydration, swallowing or aspiration problems, required use of thickening agent in liquids
- **Special nutritional assistance:** nasogastric or percutaneous endoscopic gastrostomy feeding tubes, type and amount of formula, frequency of instillation, tolerance of feedings, special body positioning required for feeding, frequency of assessment of tube placement
- **Bowel and bladder elimination status and habits:** continent or incontinent, presence of Foley catheter or ostomy, problems with diarrhea or constipation
- **Ambulatory status:** bedridden; whether one- or two-person assist or total assist is required for transfers; ambulates independently; able only to sit in a chair or lie in bed; requires use of cane walker, rolling walker, quad cane, single-prong cane, or gait belt to ambulate; or transferred with a wheelchair or geri-chair
- **Sleep habits:** how well the resident sleeps at night, whether or not the resident wanders, whether the resident is routinely awakened by pain
- **Medical equipment:** such as oxygen, suction machine, splint, cast, feeding pump
- **Activities:** include frequency of participation in activities, type of activities attended, as well as frequency of visitors

Vital Sign Assessment

Rather than assessing vital signs a minimum of three times per day as in acute care, vital signs are routinely assessed once a week or once a month, according to facility policy. If the resident exhibits signs or symptoms of illness or suffers an injury, vital signs are assessed more frequently for a period of time, as determined by the resident's condition and facility policy. When you administer medications to residents that require assessment of blood pressure or pulse, you will always check to be sure these vital signs fall within stated parameters before administering the medication.

Documentation

Documentation for residents in LTC facilities is less frequent and detailed than that done in acute care. Routinely, the nurse makes one entry in each resident's record once per week or according to facility policy. Additional entries must be made for any change in condition, signs or symptoms indicating possible problems, and when an accident occurs or injury is sustained. It will be your responsibility to know your employer's facility documentation policy. In addition, you will document medications according to facility policy.

Knowledge Connection
Discuss at least three safety issues about which you must be concerned when providing nursing care in a long-term facility. Explain why we refer to the long-term care population as "residents" rather than "patients."

The Problem of Polypharmacy in Elders

When a patient is taking multiple medications, a potential concern exists for polypharmacy complications. The term *polypharmacy* refers to the ingestion of many medications. It is common for the older adult to have more than one physician as he or she has developed various conditions over time. For example, the individual may have a primary family doctor, a cardiologist for heart problems, a pulmonary specialist for respiratory disease, and an internal medicine physician for diabetes. All of these physicians may prescribe medications to treat separate conditions; even though all of these medications are prescribed, their cumulative effects may cause adverse reactions or may result in drug-drug interactions because they are being taken together.

Ideally, each physician should inquire regarding other medications the patient is already taking, but this does not always happen. Even when a physican does ask a patient about medications he or she is currently taking, the physician may still order a same-type drug, but by a different name, thus putting the patient in jeopardy of overdose or drug toxicity.

Patients are often unaware of the reason for each of the different medications. They may also lack knowledge about the function of each medication and the possible interactions between drugs. Too often, health care workers hear patients say "I take a little white pill, and a blue pill, and a pink pill," but they cannot identify the names of the medications or the reasons for taking them. It is paramount that you teach patients and family members to maintain a complete list of all medications and the dosages being taken. This list should accompany the patient anytime he or she goes to the physician's office or to the hospital.

Patient Teaching Connection

Teaching Patients About Medications for Multiple Conditions

When working with a patient who takes multiple medications, teach the patient the details of the drug regimen, including:

- Reasons for taking each medication
- Dosage for each medication; for example, 1 pill or 2 pills, or the number of milligrams
- How often each medication is taken; for example, twice or three times a day
- Whether the medication should be taken on an empty stomach or with food

- Safety precautions associated with each medication
- How to tell if the medication is effective
- Potential side effects of each medication
- Interacting substances; for example, if the medication would interact with alcoholic beverages

Also teach the patient how to store medications for maximum safety and how to devise an administration system, as some patients do very well if they have a system for medication administration. Suggestions include a check-off calendar for each dose of each medication and a storage device that separates each dose for each day of the week.

Nursing Care Plan for an Elderly Patient

A 78-year-old female patient is admitted to the medical-surgical floor of an acute care hospital with the following medical diagnoses: bradycardia, nausea, congestive heart failure, mild dehydration, and hypokalemia. She lives alone but has family members who live in the same town. Figure 32-7 presents a concept map care plan for this patient.

Assessment

During your assessment, you discover that the patient has been taking the following medications at home: digoxin, Lasix, furosemide, Caduet, and Klor-Con. She has seen several different physicians, and one prescribed the Lasix while another prescribed the furosemide. You know that these are two different names for the same medication, so she is in effect taking double the needed dose. She tells you that she ran out of the Klor-Con and it has not arrived from her mail-order medication service yet. She estimates she has been without the medication for about a week. She also tells you that she has "no earthly idea" why she takes all these medicines, but assumes that they "will make me better someday."

When you assess her vital signs, her temperature is 98.8°F (37.11°C), pulse 52 and irregular, respirations 20, and blood pressure 106/64. She is alert and oriented to time, place, and person, and her pupils are equal and reactive to light and accommodation. She is weak and unsteady on her feet when you assist her to the bathroom. She states she has been weak and has not felt well for the past few days.

When you review her lab work, you find that her potassium is low at 3.1 mEq/L and her

digoxin level is elevated at 2.2. Her urine specific gravity is slightly elevated as well, indicating dehydration.

Nursing Diagnosis

After collecting all the data, you analyze this information and determine the primary nursing diagnoses for this patient. In order to determine this, you need to review what you have learned about this particular patient:

- She is taking two medications that are the same, prescribed by two different physicians, so she is probably getting too much diuretic.
- She has not taken her potassium supplement in a week, which is a further problem with the high dose of diuretic causing depletion of potassium.
- Her digoxin level is high and her heart rate is low, indicating digoxin toxicity.
- She is weak and unsteady on her feet, probably as a result of dehydration and hypokalemia.

You can identify that this patient has a significant risk associated with polypharmacy. After reviewing your NANDA-I list of nursing diagnoses, you are able to determine that she has the following nursing diagnoses:

- Risk for falls related to weakness as evidenced by unsteady ambulation, bradycardia, and hypokalemia
- Deficient knowledge related to medication purposes and schedules

Additional nursing diagnoses you might have identified also include deficient fluid volume and self-care deficit, toileting. For now, you will focus on the bulleted nursing diagnoses.

(care plan continues on page 764)

Nursing Care Plan for an Elderly Patient (continued)

Planning

You know that all patients are different, so you will only provide the interventions that will apply to this specific patient—and for this patient, you need to provide nursing care that will help her remain safe when ambulating and help her manage her medications appropriately to prevent further medication-related hospitalizations.

You need to consider that the patient is not aware that she is taking two medications that are the same, prescribed by two different physicians. It would be important to plan to teach about the medication regimen so that she would have a working knowledge of why she takes these medications, and what each should be doing for her. It would also be critical to consider teaching her how often each medication should be taken, and how much she should take at each dosing interval.

You must also consider that she is weak and unsteady on her feet due to her dehydration, digitoxin toxicity, bradycardia, and hypokalemia. All these together place her at high risk for falls. It is very important that you protect her from injury while she is in the hospital, and you must take immediate steps to prevent potential falls.

Possible short-term goals for this patient would include the following:

• Patient will be steady during ambulation and have increased muscle strength by discharge.
• Patient will verbalize purposes and schedules for medications by discharge.

Implementation

At this stage of the nursing process, you can now implement the interventions that you have planned. Table 32-3 provides nursing interventions for this nursing diagnosis.

Evaluation

The last step in the nursing process is to evaluate whether the interventions you have been implementing are helping the patient ambulate safely and master her medication regimen (see the evaluations in Table 32-3). Continued follow-up should take place, but it looks like you are on the right track with your plan of care.

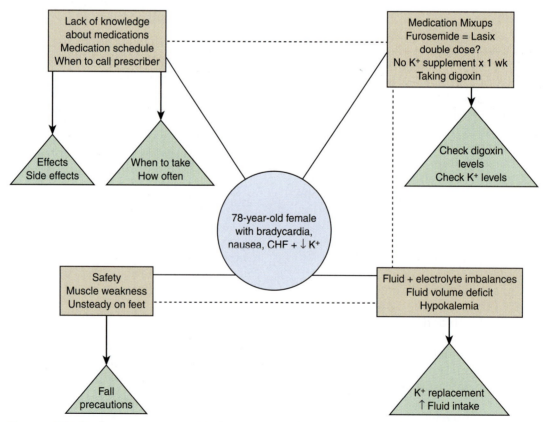

Figure 32-7 Concept map care plan for a 78-year-old female patient with bradycardia, nausea, congestive heart failure, and hypokalemia.

Table 32-3   Care Plan for an Elderly Patient

Nursing Diagnosis: Risk for falls related to weakness as evidenced by unsteady ambulation, bradycardia, and hypokalemia
Expected Outcomes: Patient will ambulate 20 feet with standby assistance by discharge. Patient will experience heart rate of 60 or above consistently before discharge. Patient will have confirmed potassium levels within normal range within 2 days.

Interventions	Evaluations
Evaluate the patient's fall risk using the Morse Fall Scale (see Chapter 13). Institute fall precautions. Post fall precautions on the door to the patient's room, in the Kardex, and in the patient's chart according to facility policy.	Day 1: Rated at a 35 on Morse Fall Scale and was identified as a medium fall risk. Placed on fall precautions immediately after admission and signs were posted on her door to indicate this. Day 3: She had experienced no falls or other injuries.
Instruct the patient not to get up alone. Check on the patient every 30 minutes to assist with any problems. Encourage the patient to use the call light—ensure that she knows where it is and how to use it. Keep needed items within her reach. Answer her call light promptly so the patient will not tire of waiting for help and attempt to get up alone. Respond to the bed/chair/leg monitor alarms immediately to prevent a fall. Assist the patient to ambulate to the chair or the bathroom when needed. Do not leave the patient alone while in the bathroom or on the bedside commode. Stay nearby to assist the patient back to bed.	Day 1: Was on bedrest and used the bedpan. Nursing staff checked on her every 30 min and she did not try to get up alone. Most of the time she would use the call light to ask for assistance, but occasionally she would call out to a staff member who walked by her room. Day 2: Able to get up to the bathroom with assistance. She was still weak but less unsteady on her feet and understood that she was not to get up alone. Day 3: She was able to go to the bathroom with standby assistance and was able to use her call light when she needed assistance.
Monitor vital signs every 4 hours. Assess heart rate and report pulse below 60. Monitor telemetry readings once per shift and anytime you are notified by the monitor technician. Assess blood pressure in three positions because heart rate is low and patient is at risk for falls.	Day 1: Heart rate remained below 60. The physician was aware and felt it was due to digitalis toxicity. Blood pressure showed a significant drop (> 30 mm Hg) when her position changed from sitting to standing. Day 3: Heart rate was 60. Telemetry readings remained in sinus rhythm throughout her hospital stay. Blood pressure was stable in all three positions.
Monitor potassium levels. Administer oral potassium as ordered. Administer IV potassium as ordered. Assess for signs and symptoms of hyper- or hypokalemia.	Day 1: Potassium was very low. The physician ordered potassium added to her IV drip and started her on oral potassium. Tolerated both without difficulty. Day 3: Potassium level was back up to 3.5.

Nursing Diagnosis: Deficient knowledge related to medication purposes and schedules
Expected Outcomes: Patient will verbalize medication purposes and administration within 3 days. Patient will verbalize criteria for notifying the prescriber regarding medication side effects prior to discharge.

Interventions	Evaluations
Teach the patient about her drug regimen, including brand names and generic names. Explain the importance of informing all physicians about all the medications she is taking. Review medications with the patient, explaining names, doses, and purposes of each.	Day 2: Able to verbalize the names of her medications when looking at a list. Able to identify the correct doses and times of day to take each medication. Verbalized understanding of the need to inform all physicians about each medication she is taking.

(table continues on page 766)

Table 32-3 **Care Plan for an Elderly Patient** (continued)

Nursing Diagnosis: Deficient knowledge related to medication purposes and schedules
Expected Outcomes: Patient will verbalize medication purposes and administration within 3 days. Patient will verbalize criteria for notifying the prescriber regarding medication side effects prior to discharge.

Interventions	Evaluations
Ask the physician for an order for home health care to follow the patient upon discharge to ensure that she has a system for setting up and taking her medications correctly.	Day 3: The physician ordered home health care follow-up for this patient. The home health nurse will visit after discharge from the hospital to ensure medication compliance.

Post Conference

During Post Conference, you shared about caring for your patient. The first day, you simply felt overwhelmed by all her medications: 13 pills for her 9 a.m. meds. She was less confused that day, as she had received IV fluids for dehydration and her UTI was responding well to antibiotics. She really looked happy when her daughter arrived. The second day was much better. While you understood more about her medications, it was clear that she did not and that she had not been taking them correctly. You were able to begin teaching her about her medicines and how to take them. Her confusion was better by her second day in the hospital, and her daughter was also learning about the medications so she could help her mother with them in the future. Your patient turned out to be an interesting and lively 86-year-old who offered to teach you how to knit. You confessed that your ideas about her at the beginning were quite wrong, and that you had unconsciously practiced ageism.

KEY POINTS

- Older adults are classified as "young-old," "middle-old," "old-old," and "elite old."

- The number of older adults in the United States will continue to increase substantially in the coming years.

- Older adults are all unique individuals with different states of health, different psychosocial dynamics, and different needs.

- Nurses should be active in dispelling the practice of ageism.

- Physical changes take place in all of the major organ systems as patients age. Most of these involve a slow decrease of the organ system functioning.

- Nursing care of the older adult should always include a component for patient safety.

- Patients should be monitored for risks associated with polypharmacy.

- Older adults are prone to experiencing fear or concern about the dying process. During this time of questioning, patients may struggle with their spirituality, and the meaning of their life in relation to what lies in the hereafter.

- Older adults may experience more loss and grief than younger adults, as friends and family of the same age category die.

- Older adults are at risk for elder abuse, scams, and crimes. The nurse should work with the patient and the caregivers to decrease the risks associated with these events.

- Questions about retirement, living arrangements, and fixed incomes may occupy the thoughts of older adults as they watch their lives changing.

REVIEW QUESTIONS

Select the answer that is most appropriate for each of the following questions. Some questions may have more than one correct answer. Check all that apply.

1. A nurse is caring for an elderly client. Which physiological change is of the highest concern?

   a. Urinary retention

   b. Slowing of metabolism

   c. Impaired visual acuity

   d. Development of age spots on the skin

2. An elderly client with dementia is brought to the primary health care provider's office. The client's daughter asks the nurse "What is dementia?" Which nursing response is appropriate?

   a. "The deterioration of all cognitive functions."

   b. "The inability to think with usual clarity, speed, and coherence."

   c. "A feeling of intense sadness, helplessness, and hopelessness."

   d. "A perceptual disorder characterized by dreams and hallucinations."

3. An elderly clients states "I can't afford to eat and buy all these medications." What nursing intervention would be most appropriate?

   a. Refer to chaplain's services.

   b. Refer to social services available.

   c. Help the client choose between food and medicine.

   d. Give the client $100 of your money to help buy medicine.

4. A nurse working in the hospital complains about his assignment, saying, "I don't have a single patient younger than 70 years old. I'll be babbling and confused by the end of my shift!" These comments reflect:

   a. humor in the workplace.

   b. the practice of ageism.

   c. an honest assessment of the assignment.

   d. caregiver burnout.

5. An elderly patient with diabetes is admitted with low blood sugar and a syncopal espisode. He is confused and unable to give clear answers to most questions. He is noted to have multiple decubiti, poor hygiene, and several old and new lacerations with varying areas of ecchymosis. Which is of most concern to you, the nurse?

   a. The possibility that elder abuse is occurring.

   b. Obtaining an accurate medical history.

   c. The need for diabetic teaching.

   d. The need for a tetanus shot because of his lacerations.

6. The nurse is assessing an "old-old" client. Which assessment finding should the nurse consider as highest priority?

   a. Slowing of peristalsis

   b. Decreased sense of smell

   c. Loss of skin elasticity

   d. Temperature of 94°F.

7. Which comment by the caregiver of an older adult patient with Alzheimer's disease would concern you the most?

   a. "I get tired, but my daughter comes to relieve me each day."

   b. "I can't sleep because I am afraid he will get out of the house."

   c. "This illness has affected the entire family, not just him."

   d. "The disease is progressing about the way we were told to expect that it would."

8. An 80-year-old patient is hospitalized with a urinary tract infection and peripheral vascular disease. In addition, he has glaucoma and diabetes. Which nursing actions would be appropriate for him?

a. Assess finger stick blood sugar as ordered.

b. Assess peripheral pulses, capillary refill, warmth, and color of extremities.

c. Assess risk for suicide or self-harm.

d. Perform mouth care every 8 hours or more often as needed.

e. Protect from injury due to impaired vision.

f. Encourage weight-bearing exercise and increased calcium intake.

g. Scan the bladder to detect urinary retention.

h. Encourage fluid intake of liquids the patient likes to drink.

i. Administer antidiabetic medications as ordered.

j. Assess for improvement of signs and symptoms of UTI.

CRITICAL THINKING EXERCISES

9. Describe how you might benefit from providing nursing care for residents in a long-term facility.

10. Describe how a young-old patient may differ from an old-old patient regarding physiological and psychosocial considerations. How would your approach in caring for both of these patients differ? How would your approach in caring for both of these patients be similar?

11. An elderly patient in an assisted living facility where you work tells you about a person he has recently met who is helping him invest his money. This person wants to be introduced to other residents for the same purpose. You have concerns that this could be a scam. What will you do?

ADDITIONAL RESOURCES

For additional Resources, Questions, and Activities, please see:

 Student Resource Disk

 http://davisplus.fadavis.com

 Student Study Guide

REFERENCES

American Stroke Association. Learn to recognize a stroke. 2009. Available at: http://www.strokeassociation.org/presenter.jhtml?identifier= 1020. Accessed November 11, 2009.

Anderson MA. *Caring for Older Adults Holistically.* 4th ed. Philadelphia: FA Davis; 2007.

Cuddy AJC, Norton MI, Fiske ST. This old stereotype: the pervasiveness and persistence of the elderly stereotype. *J Social Issues.* 2005;61:267-285. Retrieved March 13, 2009, from Research Library database (Document ID: 848146391).

DiFrancesco V, Zamboni M, Dioli A, Zoico E, Mazzali G, Omizzolo F, et al. Delayed postprandial gastric emptying and impaired gallbladder contraction together with elected cholecystokinin and peptide YY serum levels sustain satiety and inhibit hunger in healthy elderly persons. *J Gerontol A Biol Sci Med Sci.* 2005;60:1581-1585.

Grundy E, Henretta J. Between elderly parents and adult children: a new look at the intergenerational care provided by the "sandwich generation." *Ageing Society.* 2006;5:707-722. Retrieved March 13, 2009, from Research Library database (Document ID: 1223471711).

Hobbs FB. Population profile of the United States. 2008. Available at: http://www.census.gov/population/www/pop-profile/elderpop.html. Accessed November 11, 2009.

International Longevity Center. Ageism. 2007. Available at: http://www.ilcusa.org/pages/projects/ageism.php. Accessed November 11, 2009.

Kübler-Ross E. About grief and bereavement. 2008. Available at: http://www.ekrfoundation.org/about-grief.php. Accessed November 11, 2009.

Kübler-Ross E. *On Death and Dying.* New York: Scribner Classics; 1997.

National Center on Elder Abuse. Elder abuse prevalence and incidence. 2005. Available at: http://www.ncea.aoa.gov/ncearoot/Main_Site/pdf/publication/FinalStatistics050331.pdf. Accessed November 11, 2009.

National Institute on Aging. Aging in the United States: past, present and future. 2008. Available at: http://www.census.gov/ipc/prod/97agewc.pdf. Accessed November 11, 2009.

National Kidney and Urologic Diseases Information Clearinghouse. Erectile dysfunction. 2009. Available at: http://kidney.niddk.nih.gov/kudiseases/pubs/impotence. Accessed November 11, 2009.

Passel JS, Cohn D. Immigration to play lead role in future U.S. growth: U.S. population projections: 2005–2050. 2008. Available at: http://pewresearch.org/pubs/729/united-states-population-projections. Accessed November 11, 2009.

Rau R, Soroko E, Jasilionis D, Vaupel JW. Continued reductions in mortality at advanced ages. *Popul Dev Rev.* 2008;34:747-768. Retrieved March 13, 2009, from Research Library database (Document ID: 1608496431).

Sparks S, Taylor C. *Nursing Diagnosis Reference Manual.* 7th ed. Norristown, PA: Lippincott Williams & Wilkins; 2008.

Stowkowski L. Forensic issues for nurses—elder abuse. 2008. MedScape Nurses Web site. Available at: http://www.medscape.com/viewarticle/578859. Accessed November 11, 2009.

U.S. Department of Health and Human Services. What is behind HRSA's projected supply, demand, and shortage of registered nurses? Available at: ftp://ftp.hrsa.gov/bhpr/workforce/behindshortage.pdf. Accessed November 11, 2009.

Venes D, ed. *Taber's Cyclopedic Medical Dictionary.* 21st ed. Philadelphia: FA Davis; 2009.

CHAPTER

33

Care of the Surgical Patient

Key Terms

Anesthesia

Antiembolism hose

Approximation

Bier block

Conscious sedation

Corrective

Cosmetic

Dehiscence

Epidural anesthesia

Exploratory

Extubation

General anesthesia

Intubation

Laparoscopic

Local anesthesia

Malignant hyperthermia

Palliative

Postanesthesia care unit (PACU)

Regional anesthesia

Sequential compression devices (SCDs)

Objectives

1. Define key terms related to care of the surgical patient.
2. Differentiate between types of surgery by purpose, degree of urgency, and degree of risk.
3. Identify factors that increase the risks of surgery and anesthesia.
4. Describe the process of informed consent.
5. Explain the purpose of various preoperative laboratory tests.
6. Specify the important components of preoperative patient teaching.
7. Explain the various purposes of preoperative medications.
8. Explain the purpose for and the various data included on a preoperative checklist.
9. Compare the various roles and responsibilities of operative personnel.
10. Differentiate between the different types of anesthesia and rationales for selection.
11. Explain nursing procedures that may take place in the operating room and their rationales.
12. Prioritize nursing care during immediate postoperative and postanesthesia care.
13. Describe the admission process of a postsurgical patient to the hospital unit.
14. Accurately describe the assessment of the postsurgical patient on the hospital unit.
15. Identify potential postsurgical complications, with emphasis on prevention and intervention.
16. Develop a care plan for a patient who has had abdominal surgery.

Skills

33-1 Applying Antiembolism Hose

33-2 Applying Sequential Compression Devices

769

Clinical Connection

Your Assignment: You will be caring for a 58-year-old female patient who has recently been diagnosed with a cancerous tumor in her ascending colon. She will be going to surgery today at 0900 to have the tumor removed and the remaining intestines will be anastomosed, or reconnected surgically. Your instructor tells you that you will be responsible for completing most of the preoperative checklist and performing preop teaching. You will then care for this patient postoperatively after she returns to the nursing unit.

Your Actions: You are not sure what part of the intestines will be reconnected to what. You are also unsure of what you will need to do for the preoperative checklist because you have never seen one before. You are unsure what to include in your preop teaching. You also realize that you know nothing about colon cancer. Will the surgery be "curative?" Or will the patient also need chemotherapy or radiation therapy? Then you realize that you have never taken care of a patient immediately after return from surgery, but rather 1 to 2 days postoperative. You wonder what special care you may need to give her. You begin to research all of your questions, but you especially are concerned about your responsibilities for the preoperative checklist and what you need to do when your patient returns from surgery to the nursing unit.

This chapter will alleviate some of the mystery regarding what happens during surgery. You will learn how to provide nursing care in each phase of the surgical experience, including preoperative, intraoperative, and postoperative. You will learn how to assess and prepare your patients for surgery, the roles of the various operative personnel, and how to safely prioritize postoperative nursing care.

You have already learned that anxiety and fear are second priority *only* to basic physiological needs such as oxygen, food, and water. This chapter will supply you with the knowledge necessary to alleviate much of your surgical patient's anxiety and fear, one of the easier yet more helpful interventions that you can perform for a perioperative patient.

Purposes of Surgery

Surgery is performed for a number of reasons, including for treatment of a disease or injury, such as removing the gallbladder to treat inflammation and gallstones, termed a *cholecystectomy*. Surgical procedures that treat or cure disease are classified as *curative surgeries*. Other purposes for surgery include:

- **Correction:** Corrective surgery is done to repair an anatomic or congenital defect, such as repairing a cleft palate so a child can nurse or eat normally.
- **Cosmetic:** Cosmetic surgery may be performed to change or improve one's physical appearance. Examples of this type of procedure might include a face-lift or breast augmentation.
- **Exploration:** Exploratory surgery is done to provide further data and determine a diagnosis for a problem. For example, abdominal pain sometimes requires exploratory surgery to determine the cause.
- **Palliation:** Palliative surgery alleviates symptoms and provides comfort but does not necessarily cure the disease or heal the injury. An example of palliative surgery is removing as much of a tumor as possible, known as *debulking* a tumor, which can decrease pain and relieve pressure, though it will not cure the cancer.

Knowledge Connection

Compare curative surgery to palliative. Explain how cosmetic surgery is different from curative, corrective, and palliative. Which one do you think would be least likely to be covered by health insurance? What does exploratory surgery mean?

Degrees of Urgency

Correlating with the various reasons to perform surgery are degrees of urgency, meaning how quickly the surgery must be scheduled. The degrees of urgency include:

- **Elective surgery:** Any surgery that is voluntary and scheduled a week or more in advance. Elective surgery includes those surgeries intended to improve a patient's quality of life, either physically or psychologically. The surgery may be medically necessary, such as a cataract removal, or may be patient desired, such as breast augmentation.
- **Urgent surgery:** Surgery required within 24 hours of diagnosis to prevent complications that may occur with

waiting. An example of urgent surgery would be a hip pinning following fracture to prevent complications associated with immobility and emboli formation.

- **Emergency surgery:** Surgery that cannot be delayed, and is usually scheduled within 2 hours to prevent serious complication or death. Examples include a stable gastrointestinal bleed or subdural hematoma evacuation.
- **Salvage surgery:** Surgery required when cardiopulmonary resuscitation is in progress on the way to the operating room, or the patient's life or limb is threatened. Examples of this type of surgery include such things as a gunshot wound or a ruptured aneurysm.

Knowledge Connection

Classify the following surgeries for purpose and degree of urgency:

- Repair of hand after exploding fireworks almost blew the thumb off
- Liposuction of abdomen
- Appendectomy due to acute severe right-sided, lower abdominal pain
- Tonsillectomy for history of repeated strep infections of the throat and tonsils
- Open reduction of fractured femur with excessive bleeding into thigh
- Removal of cancerous tumor wrapped around the spinal cord in a patient with advanced metastatic cancer of the brain and bone, who suddenly lost all function and sensation below the waist.

Various Surgical Settings

In the past, surgery was only performed in hospitals, but improved technology has allowed health care professionals to safely perform certain surgeries in a number of different settings. This allows for reduced expenses and decreased time away from home for the patient. It also reduces hospitals' demands for nursing personnel to provide postoperative patient care, decreasing their costs.

Outpatient Surgery

Outpatient surgery is that which is performed on a patient who is not admitted to the hospital as an inpatient: the patient arrives at the site prior to surgery, has the procedure, spends certain hours in the recovery room, and returns home the same day. The perfect candidate for outpatient surgery is a patient with few to no pre-existing medical conditions. The surgeries that are performed on an outpatient basis include only minor surgical procedures with minimal postoperative risk of complications. They may be performed in a stand-alone surgery center, in a medical office, or in a hospital outpatient surgery department where the patient is

not admitted as an inpatient and generally does not stay overnight.

Stand-alone Surgery Center

A stand-alone surgery center is a facility designed to only provide perioperative care for minor surgical procedures during the day; it is generally open for a specified length of time each day, such as from 0700 to 1900. All types of anesthesia can be administered as needed and postoperatively, and recovery room services are provided until the patient is awake and stable enough to be discharged to home. An example of a surgery well suited for a surgery center would be a knee arthroscopy on a young adult. The patient is scheduled to arrive at the surgery center 1 to 2 hours prior to surgery, undergoes the procedure, and after several hours in recovery is released to go home. Procedures in this setting may be described as *day surgery*.

Medical Office

Certain procedures that are considered very minor and do not require anesthesia other than an injection of a *local anesthetic,* an agent that will numb the site, may be performed in the physician's medical office. An example of a surgery well suited for a medical office would be a *vasectomy.*

Hospital Outpatient Surgery Department

Many hospitals now offer surgery on an outpatient basis as well as on an inpatient basis. The patient comes to the facility for the surgical procedure, but is not admitted as an inpatient and generally does not spend the night there. When compared to the freestanding surgery center or medical office, a hospital-based outpatient surgery allows for more extensive surgery on higher risk patients who may have to be given general anesthesia that puts the patient to sleep. The difference is that the hospital has readily accessible personnel and laboratory facilities, as well as the ability for overnight stay should the patient develop complications. An example of surgery well suited for hospital-based outpatient surgery would be a tonsillectomy on an 8-year-old, where the risk of bleeding is highest between 6 and 8 hours after surgery.

Inpatient Surgery

Inpatient, hospital-based surgery is performed on patients who have been admitted to the hospital; the patient is sent to surgery from an inpatient bed, emergency room, or intensive care unit. These patients may require hospitalization before surgery to stabilize a pre-existing or acute condition, which requires surgical intervention. An example of this type of surgery would be a patient admitted for abdominal pain, who required insertion of a nasogastric tube and IV therapy. Once the nasogastric tube was inserted, the patient was diagnosed as having a gastrointestinal bleed, which will require surgical intervention to prevent hemorrhage.

Preoperative Care of the Surgical Patient

When most new nursing students think of caring for the surgical patient, they may think of just caring for the patient during surgery or postsurgery, but it is important to realize that there is a tremendous amount of care to be provided preoperatively as well. Patients presenting for surgery bring with them a personal history of medical problems and prior surgeries, family histories of disease or illness, and personal indications for surgery. Your job is to help optimally prepare the patient and, where appropriate, the patient's family, for the surgery and anesthesia.

Presurgical Assessment

Presurgical assessment includes a preliminary process of assessment and preoperative testing to ensure that the patient is healthy enough to undergo surgery and **anesthesia**, which is the loss of sensation, with or without loss of consciousness, accomplished by the administration of inhaled or injected medications. Presurgical assessment also helps the surgeon determine if the patient should or can be scheduled for surgery at a freestanding surgical center or medical office, or if the patient would be better cared for in a hospital setting.

After assessment and testing, a patient judged to be a safe candidate for surgery is said to have received *presurgical clearance*. Patients may have their presurgical clearance done in the surgeon's office, a freestanding laboratory facility, or the hospital's laboratory. This process helps to identify pre-existing medical conditions such as hypertension and diabetes that need to be optimized before adding the threat of surgery and anesthesia. A physician may also decide to delay portions of the presurgical assessment until the patient arrives at the surgical site.

Safety: The primary goal of the presurgical assessment is patient safety.

Patient History

You will want to begin your preoperative assessment with the goal of obtaining a detailed patient history. The history is one of the best measures of patient status, so it is important that your questioning be targeted, specific, and complete. Taking the patient's history has eight steps:

1. **Exploring the patient's understanding of the need for surgery to be performed:** This will help you to make sure the patient knows what procedure is being performed and why. Be certain the patient understands his or her options as well as the expected results of the surgery.

2. **Asking about any previous surgeries and anesthetics:** This will help you find out about any problems that may have occurred with previous surgeries, such as severe nausea or an allergic reaction.

3. **Asking about the patient's family health history:** This includes asking about any family history of anesthetic problems.

4. **Asking about current medication use, including prescription medications, over-the-counter medications, and herbal medications:** This may provide clues to pre-existing medical problems, as well as identifying potential drug interactions that may occur with anesthetic exposure.

5. **Asking about medication allergies and intolerances:** This is necessary to prevent exposures to known harmful medications and should remind you to see that the patient has an allergy band applied and the chart correctly labeled for allergies.

6. **Asking about alcohol and illegal drug use, abuse, and addiction:** This will help you anticipate potential drug interactions and problems with pain management after surgery. It can also alert you to observe for withdrawal signs and symptoms related to abuse of and addiction to illegal drugs.

7. **Asking about tobacco use:** Tobacco use can contribute to intraoperative and postoperative problems with oxygenation and ventilation. This information directs care toward prevention of postoperative hypoventilation and pneumonia.

8. **Asking females about the possibility of pregnancy, specifically to determine the date of the patient's last menstrual period:** Unless an emergency, surgery during pregnancy should be avoided.

Review of Systems

The review of systems is designed to identify the presence or absence of pre-existing diseases that may affect either the surgical procedure or the administration of anesthesia. Pre-existing disease may also be the cause for surgery, as in the case of severe arthritis and the need for a joint replacement, or it may be a factor that increases perioperative risks. It is especially important to assess organ systems that can be affected by the anesthetics, such as the central nervous and cardiovascular systems, as well as organ systems that affect the actions of anesthetics, such as the pulmonary and renal systems, and the accessory gastrointestinal organs such as the liver.

Cardiovascular System

Ask about pre-existing *arrhythmias,* which are heart rhythm irregularities, chest pain, and myocardial infarction, the medical name for a heart attack. This is important, because of the risk of reinfarction during surgery. Ask about hypertension, and if present ask about medications used and compliance; also assess the degree of control of the blood pressure. A patient with poorly controlled hypertension may have begun to develop end-stage renal damage, meaning the kidney function has deteriorated to minimal functioning. This would clue you to the need for preoperative testing of renal function. If the patient has a history of heart failure, you would be clued to assess for edema in the extremities; auscultation of heart sounds, noting muffled S_1 and S_2; and auscultation of breath sounds, noting crackles or rhonchi. If there are signs and symptoms of heart failure, surgery will probably be cancelled until the patient's symptoms abate.

Respiratory System

Ask the patient about dyspnea, both exertional and at rest. This can provide clues about pulmonary and cardiac disease. If the patient has a history of asthma or other chronic obstructive pulmonary disease (COPD), inquire about inhaler and oxygen use. These patients will be at a higher risk for airway irritation intraoperatively and postoperatively. It would also be pertinent to inquire if the patient takes corticosteroids because they tend to inhibit wound healing.

Central Nervous System

As you are asking questions of your patient, assess if your patient is able to follow commands and understand your teaching. If the patient does not follow simple requests or answer your questions, make certain that the lack of response is not due to a language barrier. Evaluate any neurological deficit so that you have a clear understanding of adjustments that need to be made in delivering care. For example, a patient with dementia might benefit from having a family member remain at the bedside in the preoperative holding area and immediately after surgery in the **postanesthesia care unit (PACU)**. Normally this might not be allowed, but for a patient with severe dementia it might make the difference in reducing stress, confusion, or lack of cooperation.

Renal System

As many anesthetic agents and medications are eliminated through the kidneys, it is important to assess for pre-existing renal disease, as failure to eliminate medications can result in toxicity. In addition, the patient with renal dysfunction is almost always anemic, which has the potential to compromise oxygenation. Coagulation deficits may also be present in patients who are on dialysis. Tests that will help determine the health status of the kidneys are the *creatinine* and

estimated glomerular filtration rate (eGFR). Creatinine, which is an end waste product of metabolism, is removed from the blood by the kidneys. Therefore, an elevated serum level of creatinine points toward kidney problems. The creatinine levels are also used to calculate an eGFR, which provides data about kidney function. However, the eGFR is only applicable to nonpregnant patients between 18 and 70 years of age, who are not obese and who do not have severe nutritional deficiencies.

Musculoskeletal System

Arthritis is the most common musculoskeletal disease found in the older surgical patient. Arthritis can compromise positioning, and medications taken for arthritis, such as aspirin and nonsteroidal anti-inflammatory drugs (NSAIDs), such as ibuprofen and naproxyn, affect platelet function, which increases the risk of bleeding.

Gastrointestinal System

Malnutrition and anemia can compromise wound healing, while obesity increases the risk of pulmonary and cardiac compromise. Malnutrition is characterized by several laboratory tests including low serum *prealbumin, albumin, transferrin, hematocrit* (Hct), and *hemoglobin* (Hgb) levels. Prealbumin, a protein produced primarily by the liver, is good evidence of the patient's protein status and serves as one of the best indicators of malnutrition. Albumin, a protein produced in the liver, is a good indicator not only of nutritional status, but also of liver function itself. Transferrin is a glucoprotein produced by the liver that carries over half of the body's iron. When the serum level of transferrin remains low, it can interfere with production of hemoglobin, which can lead to anemia. Together low Hgb and Hct results serve as the primary determinant of anemia. Obesity is a risk factor for hypertension, coronary artery disease, stroke, reflux and aspiration, and airway difficulties.

The liver is the primary organ for drug metabolism, so any pre-existing hepatic disease such as hepatitis, cirrhosis, or alcoholism has the potential to decrease the rate and efficacy of drug clearance. In addition, the liver is responsible for the production of clotting factors to assist with clotting of blood and bile for digestion. It regulates carbohydrate, amino acid, and lipid metabolism, and it stores the fat-soluble vitamins A, D, E, and K, the water-soluble vitamins A and D, and iron and copper, so liver disease increases the risk of bleeding and malnutrition as well as poor wound healing. The tests that provide clotting information are the *prothrombin time* (PT) and the *international normalized ratio* (INR), which are ordered together. When the clotting sequence is prolonged, it provides information regarding the status of the liver as well as an elevated risk for bleeding. Another test called the *activated partial thromboplastin time* (APTT) provides further data indicating whether or not the patient has an increased risk for bleeding.

Endocrine System

Although most patients with pre-existing endocrine disease will have the disease well controlled before surgery, the patient with diabetes is at the greatest risk for sudden increases and decreases in blood sugar levels due to NPO status, emotional stress preoperatively, and the physical stress of surgery itself.

Hematological System

The patient with a low *red blood cell* (RBC) count or Hgb level is at risk for problems with oxygenation, as the RBCs carry the hemoglobin that is responsible for carrying oxygen to cells throughout the body. Patients with low platelet counts are at risk for excessive bleeding and hemorrhage. Even when the platelet count is normal, if the PT, INR, and APTT are excessively long, the patient may still be at risk for bleeding during surgery. Patients with low *white blood cell* (WBC) counts have decreased immunity and are at more risk for infection than an individual with a normal WBC level.

Physical Examination

A complete physical examination may or may not have been done in advance of the day of surgery by the surgeon or medical provider. If it was not performed prior to admission, the admitting physician and/or surgeon should perform the examination to ascertain patient stability. The anesthesia provider may also perform an assessment to determine whether the patient is a good candidate for anesthesia.

Knowledge Connection
Which body systems are important with regard to the metabolism of anesthesia agents? Which laboratory test results provide you with data regarding the patient's nutritional status? Which tests are significant for a patient who has chronic respiratory problems and requires surgery? What significance would a low WBC count have for a patient about to have surgery? How might having severe arthritis affect a patient who undergoes surgery? Which laboratory tests provide you information regarding the patient is at risk for bleeding/hemorrhage problems?

Preoperative Diagnostic Testing

The ordering of preoperative laboratory tests should be based on the patient's individual history and physical examination, with consideration of the specific surgery to be performed. Also, most facilities have standing orders requiring that certain laboratory tests be performed on all surgical patients.

Laboratory and Diagnostic Connection

Standard Preoperative Laboratory Tests
Most facilities require the following basic tests as the minimum for all preoperative patients:

- **Complete blood cell count (CBC):** Done to detect low hemoglobin and hematocrit indicating anemia, which could place the patient at risk for hypoxia if there is heavy blood loss. It is also important to ensure that the WBC count does not indicate a current infection and that the platelet count is within normal range. A low platelet count would put the patient at risk for coagulation problems. *Safety: A patient with a normal platelet count is not ensured to be free of coagulation problems, as there are various other components that also affect the clotting process.*
- **Urinalysis (UA):** Done to rule out urinary tract infection and to look for protein, which could indicate impaired renal function. An elevated specific gravity could also indicate that the patient is dehydrated, which would require infusion of IV fluids prior to surgery.
- **Electrocardiogram (EKG): Done to detect cardiac arrhythmias or signs of ischemia,** which is lack of oxygen delivery to the heart muscle via coronary arteries.

Some facilities have a standing policy to perform a preoperative pregnancy test, known as the *human chorionic gonadotropin (hCG) test,* on all females of childbearing age. It is imperative to know whether or not a woman is pregnant prior to performing surgery on her, especially in the first trimester when anesthesia medications as well as postoperative medications may interfere with fetal development.

Laboratory tests should be ordered in correlation to the history and physical examination findings to evaluate the extent and control of disease progression; to detect imbalances that require preoperative correction, such as a low serum potassium (K^+) level; and as an assessment of perioperative risk. Box 33-1 provides an example of a checklist that can be used to help determine the need for specific preoperative laboratory testing.

Prior to going into surgery, the anesthesia provider and often the surgeon or internist will evaluate preoperative laboratory tests and the preoperative EKG for any abnormality that requires correction before surgery. Sometimes, scheduled surgery must be cancelled. For example, if the patient has been taking warfarin to prevent blood clots, clotting times will be assessed before surgery. Although the warfarin will have been stopped in advance to prevent surgical bleeding, the return to normal clotting values may not have yet occurred, which might require surgery to be postponed. If a new abnormal finding is seen on EKG, surgery may be postponed for a cardiologist evaluation.

Knowledge Connection
What three diagnostic tests are generally performed on every preoperative patient? How might routine medications that a patient has been taking be a problem for the surgical patient? Which test is sometimes performed preoperatively, but only on women?

Preoperative Patient Teaching

Research has shown that a patient who receives good preoperative teaching tends to do better postoperatively and have

Box 33-1

Checklist for Ordering Preoperative Laboratory Tests

Note: If one or more conditions are present, it is sufficient indication for the physician to order the associated laboratory test.

Hemoglobin (Hgb)/Hematocrit (Hct)/Red Blood Cell Count (RBC)

_____ Routinely performed prior to ALL SURGERIES
_____ Potential for heavy blood loss due to type of surgery
_____ Known anemia
_____ Bleeding disorder
_____ Receiving radiation or chemotherapy
_____ Severe, chronic disease
_____ Excessively heavy menstrual periods
_____ Chronic respiratory disease

White Blood Cell Count With Differential (WBC with Diff)

_____ Routinely performed prior to ALL SURGERIES
_____ Infection
_____ Known disease of bone marrow
_____ Radiation/chemotherapy
_____ Aplastic anemia
_____ Unexplained fever

Platelets (PLT)

_____ Known platelet abnormality
_____ Excessive bleeding identified
_____ Known blood disease: anemia, leukemia
_____ History of radiation or chemotherapy
_____ Use of nonsteroidal anti-inflammatory drugs, aspirin, clopidogrel (Plavix), warfarin (Coumadin)
_____ Unexplained bruising

Prothombin Time (PT)/Activated Partial Thromboplastin Time (APTT)/International Normalized Ratio (INR) (all are clotting function tests)

_____ Known or suspected clotting abnormality
_____ Anticoagulant therapy
_____ Hemorrhage
_____ Anemia
_____ Liver disease
_____ Thrombosis
_____ Malnutrition or poor nutrition
_____ Presence of excessive bruises

Electrolyte Panel/Blood Urea Nitrogen (BUN)/Creatinine

_____ Age older than 40 years
_____ Use of diuretics
_____ Renal disease
_____ History of fever, diarrhea, or vomiting
_____ Syndrome of inappropriate antidiuretic hormone secretion (SIADH)
_____ Liver disease
_____ Diseases resulting in malabsorption
_____ Diabetes mellitus

Blood Chemistry

(entire panels of tests or specific individual tests, such as glucose, uric acid, total bilirubin, total protein, prealbumin, albumin, cholesterol, serum glutamic-oxaloacetic transaminase [SGOT], lactate dehydrogenase, alkaline phosphatase, serum glutamic-pyruvic transaminase [SGPT])

_____ Age older than 40 years
_____ Diabetes mellitus
_____ Hypoglycemia
_____ Pancreatic disease
_____ Pituitary disease
_____ Adrenal disease/steroid therapy
_____ Liver disease
_____ Radiation/chemotherapy
_____ Malnutrition

Electrocardiography

_____ Age older than 40 years
_____ Known cardiac abnormality
_____ Family history of cardiac problems

Urinalysis

_____ Unexplained fever
_____ Hematuria
_____ Flank tenderness
_____ Complaints of frequency/urgency/dysuria
_____ Dehydration
_____ Fluid and electrolyte imbalance

Chest X-ray (CXR)

_____ Productive cough
_____ Decreased, adventitious, or absent breath sounds
_____ History of congestive heart failure (CHF)

a smoother, shorter recovery period. Preoperative teaching provides the patient and family with information, skills, and instructions that will support optimal healing, be conducive to the shortest recovery period, and serve to prevent or reduce postoperative complications.

It is common and expected that the patient and the patient's family will feel anxiety in relation to a scheduled surgery. Keep in mind that the average layperson does not have even the _basic_ knowledge related to nursing

and medical care that you now have and may take for granted. By assisting the patient and family to understand what will happen and what the patient will and may experience, you can relieve some of these "fears of the unknown." There may also be legitimate fear related to the results of the surgery, including possible disfigurement or death. This fear is a preoperative issue that can impair communication, alter one's cognitive ability to process information, and immobilize one's ability to function. In order to limit the patient's anxiety prior to surgery, provide the following:

- Information regarding preoperative preparations, including diagnostic tests, NPO status, skin shave or scrub, intestinal preparation, insertion of tubes or IVs, and administration of preoperative medications
- What the patient can expect in the operating room (OR), including equipment, bright lights, cold temperatures, and masked staff members wearing caps and gowns that make it difficult to identify each one
- A description of the general roles of the various OR team members who will be responsible for the patient's care
- What the patient will and may experience postoperatively once in the PACU, also known as the *recovery room*
- Actions the patient can take to help prevent complications, decrease discomfort, shorten recovery time, and optimize healing

Sometimes a little knowledge allows the patient or family to feel they have a little bit of control over the situation. Your skill in anticipating and assessing their knowledge needs and providing the appropriate teaching to meet those needs will help to allay their fears, reduce their anxiety, and increase active participation in and compliance with medical advice and recommendations. (Refer back to Chapter 12 for further details regarding patient teaching.)

Knowledge Connection
What are the benefits of performing preoperative teaching? List the types of things that should be taught preoperatively.

Patient Teaching Connection

Preoperative Teaching for Outpatient Laparoscopic Cholecystectomy
A patient is scheduled for an outpatient **laparoscopic** cholecystectomy, which is removal of the gallbladder using a specialized scope and instruments. Rather than opening the abdominal cavity with a standard 4- to 6-inch (10.16- to 15.24-cm) incision, the scope is inserted into the abdominal cavity via three or four tiny incisions between ½ and ¾ inch (1.27 to 1.85 cm) in length. This laparoscopic approach reduces risk of infection, decreases postoperative pain, and shortens recovery time. Initial teaching should be done in the physician's office during the same visit at which the decision was made to schedule the surgery. The following is the information that the patient needs to know prior to arrival at the outpatient surgery center on the day of surgery:

1. Do not eat or drink anything for a specified period of time (according to the physician's protocol, generally 6 to 12 hours) before surgery.
2. Avoid smoking 24 hours preoperatively. Advise to ask physician for nicotine patches if desired.
3. Arrange for a driver to take the patient home afterward.

4. Shower with antibacterial soap the night before surgery.
5. Bring the completed registration/admission packet supplied preoperatively as well as any advance directives the patient may have.
6. Confirm the date, time, and physical location and phone number of the surgery center.
7. Leave jewelry and valuables at home.
8. Discuss any medications or herbal supplements that must be held preoperatively.

Along with these instructions, an explanation of what will occur on the day of surgery should be included (Box 33-2). Additional specific preoperative teaching topics will be taught the morning of surgery before the patient goes to the OR. These topics would include:

- Turn, cough, and deep breathing exercises, which are addressed below
- The specific device the patient's surgeon uses to stimulate venous return from the lower extremities, such as antiembolism hose, ankle and leg exercises, or a sequential compression device, which are discussed in the following section of this chapter
- The approximate length of time the patient will be in the OR and recovery
- The importance of asking for pain medication before the pain becomes severe
- The importance of informing staff of nausea as soon as it is detected in an attempt to prevent vomiting
- Showing the family where they can wait for the physician's report

Turn, Cough, and Deep Breathing Exercises
One important risk reduction strategy is promotion of optimal ventilation to prevent pneumonia and atelectasis. The most common things you will teach to help prevent these respiratory complications is how to effectively cough and deep breathe and why it is important to turn from side to side every 1 to 2 hours. Turning from side to side prevents secretions from pooling in one area of the lungs, known as *stasis*. Pooled secretions provide the perfect medium for bacterial growth which leads to hypostatic pneumonia. Turning also stimulates deeper inhalation, which along with coughing and deep breathing helps with the elimination of anesthetic gases. Deep breathing helps to expand the lungs more fully and works to prevent *atelectasis*, or collapse of one or more lobes of the lung.

Explaining the rationale behind the repeated instruction to "take a deep breath" will help the patient understand that this intervention is designed to aid in the elimination of anesthetic gases and to promote gas exchange. The deep breathing and coughing should be initiated as soon as the surgical procedure is completed and anesthesia is discontinued. (See Chapter 28 for more information about respiratory care.)

Incentive Spirometry
Incentive spirometry may also be instituted to promote deep breathing, to increase lung volume, and to encourage coughing

Box 33-2

Example of Outpatient Surgery Teaching

The following dialogue is an example of preoperative teaching you might provide for a patient scheduled for an outpatient surgery:

"Feel free to stop me at any point during this teaching session and ask any questions that come to mind. Otherwise, you may forget them by the time I am through speaking. Okay? Your surgery is scheduled on Tuesday, March 9, 2011, at 7:30 a.m. Be certain you do not eat or drink any type of fluid, including water, after 10 p.m. on Monday night, the night before your surgery. Bring all your completed paperwork and preoperative lab results with you and arrive at the surgery center by 6 a.m. Give the paperwork to the receptionist. She will take you to the holding area, where we will prepare you for surgery.

You will change into a hospital gown, and be asked a lot of questions, and your IV will be started. Your chart will be reviewed and consent for surgery explained and signed. Bring a written list of any questions that you may have so that you do not forget any of them. We will do some preoperative teaching, show you how to deep breathe and cough to prevent pneumonia, discuss postoperative pain and nausea medications, and start your IV. You will meet the anesthesiologist, Dr. Nancy Blehm, and talk with her and your surgeon before being taken into surgery. You will be given medication in your IV to decrease the likelihood of nausea postoperatively as well as medication to relax you and probably make you drowsy. You may have up to two family members accompany you while in the holding area, where you typically will be for 30 to 60 minutes.

We will then take you from holding to the OR, where you will again be asked more questions; some will be the same ones you have already answered, such as 'Are you allergic to any medications?' This part of a protocol we do for your safety. The room will probably feel cold but we will provide you with as many blankets as you need. Everyone in the OR will be dressed in scrubs and will be wearing masks. The anesthesiologist will place electrodes on your chest so that she can monitor your heart and a blood pressure cuff on your arm to monitor your blood pressure. She will then administer sedative medication into your IV line to make you drowsy. Dr. Blehm will monitor your breathing, oxygen levels, heart rhythm, and all your vital statistics that are necessary to keep you safe and well. You will have your own personal circulating nurse whose primary responsibility will be to act as your advocate and see that everything runs smoothly for you. You will be asleep in no time, and when you begin to wake up you will probably be in the recovery room.

This type of surgery typically lasts between 30 and 60 minutes, and combined with the recovery time, you will probably be ready to go home within 3 to 4 hours. We will direct your family to the waiting room where the surgeon will come to find them after surgery. We will keep your family informed of your condition and notify them if there are delays. If you wish, you may have one family member at the bedside while in recovery. If you are not nauseated after waking up, you will be allowed ice chips first; if you tolerate them, you will be allowed to sip dark cola or lemon-lime sodas and munch on saltine crackers. Once you are fully awake, able to take fluids without nausea, and have urinated, you will be discharged to go home. A prescription for pain medication will be provided prior to discharge. Do you have any questions I might answer for you?"

---

to clear mucus from the airway. This skill should also be taught and practiced before surgery and reinforced after surgery. (See Chapter 28 for more on incentive spirometry.)

Stimulation of Lower Extremity Circulation

One of the most common and serious complications of surgery is formation of a *thrombus* or blood clot. Normally, the contractions of the leg muscles help to compress leg veins and stimulate venous return of blood to the heart. When a patient is less active or restricted to bedrest, the result is less contraction of the leg muscles. This allows venous blood flow to slow, and blood to pool in the veins and, eventually, coagulate and form clots.

The condition of forming these clots is commonly referred to as *deep venous thrombosis* (DVT). Research shows that even traveling on long air flights allows sufficient slowing of venous return to increase an individual's risk of blood clots in the legs.

The clots impair circulation in the legs, cause inflammation of the vein at the site of the attached clot, and can break loose from the vein wall to be carried into the circulation that is returning blood back to the heart and pulmonary circulation to be reoxygenated. Once the clot is carried to the lungs, it becomes known as a *pulmonary embolism* (PE). Pulmonary embolisms cause severe respiratory distress and have the potential to be fatal. Therefore, prevention of thrombus formation is key.

Prevention involves stimulation of the venous return of blood to the heart so that it does not begin to pool. The patient should be instructed regarding three ways to stimulate lower extremity circulation: leg exercises, antiembolism hose, and sequential compression devices (SCDs).

Leg Exercises

You will want to teach leg exercises to your patient as a method of preventing clot formation. The exercises are designed to flex and extend the leg muscles so that, as the muscles contract, they compress the leg veins, assisting them to return blood back to the heart. The exercises are the easiest and most natural way to stimulate peripheral circulation and prevent venous stasis and deep venous thrombosis or clots. Teach your patients to perform the following exercises:

- Ankle circles with the toes extended, 10 times in each direction, both clockwise and counterclockwise
- Ankle pumps, alternating ankle flexion and extension for a total of 10 times each
- Leg flexion and extension: Bend the knees, placing the feet flat on bed. Keeping the plantar surface of the foot on the bed, bring one foot at a time as close to the buttock as possible. Then slide the same foot toward the foot of the bed until the leg is fully extended. Repeat this using the other leg. This should be done 10 times for each leg.

Antiembolism Hose

Antiembolism hose or stockings are often called AE hose or TED hose. TED stands for *thromboembolic disorder*, the primary diagnosis for use of the hose. They are a pair of strong support hose that are applied to compress the leg veins, assisting them to return blood back to the right side of the heart where it can be sent through the pulmonary artery to the lungs to be reoxygenated. This helps to prevent blood from pooling in the leg veins from inactivity and bedrest. Instruct the patient preoperatively regarding the purpose and importance of the hose. The hose are sometimes applied preoperatively, dependent upon physician's orders and facility policy.

It is pertinent that the TED hose fit the patient's legs properly, so measure the appropriate leg dimensions before selecting the size to apply. For thigh-high hose, measure the length of the leg from the gluteal fold to the bottom of the heel. Then measure the circumference of the calf and the thigh at their largest diameters. Cross-reference these measurements on the TED chart to determine which size to select.

It is important to prevent the hose fabric from bunching together, especially at the ankle and knee joints (Fig. 33-1). The tops of thigh-high TEDs also tend to roll down. If the fabric is allowed to bunch together or the tops to roll down, those areas will work like a tourniquet and restrict venous blood return, exacerbating pooling of blood. Monitor the TEDs every couple of hours to ensure that they are kept smooth and are not restricting circulation. Assess pedal pulses each shift to ensure arterial blood flow to the feet.

Remove the hose at least twice per day to prevent excessive pressure or tension on any one spot. Good times to remove the TED hose are during the morning bath and during delivery of bedtime care. This allows you the opportunity to assess the skin of the legs and feet for areas of erythema, breaks in the skin, and edema. Wash and dry the legs and feet well before reapplying the hose. Performing this again before bedtime helps to make the patient comfortable for sleep. Skill 33-1 (page 799) provides more information on application of TED hose.

Sequential Compression Devices

Sequential compression devices (SCDs) may also be known by brand names, such as Pneumatic Air Stockings (PAS). They consist of compression sleeve pads capable of having air pumped into and out of them. They are designed to wrap around the legs and come in thigh-high or knee-high lengths. The sleeve pads connect via tubing to a compression pump, which intermittently pumps air into the sleeves until filled and then empties the air, deflating the sleeves around the legs (Fig. 33-2). This process results in intermittent compression of the legs, aiding venous return of blood to the heart. You will want to teach the patient the purpose and significance of their use in order to gain compliance and cooperation in reapplying them after ambulation or toileting. Skill 33-2 (page 801) provides more information on application of SCDs.

Knowledge Connection

What are the purposes for turning, coughing, deep breathing, and use of an incentive spirometer? Why do we use sequential compression devices? What must be done prior to applying a pair of TED hose? Which body system do TED hose help? Explain what a PE is and why it is dangerous. Which body system will leg exercises stimulate?

Postoperative Pain and Discomfort Control

Teach your patient that medication will be ordered for pain, nausea and vomiting, and various other discomforts that may be anticipated postoperatively. Explain to the patient that it is always best to keep pain under control by asking for medication before the pain gets too severe. Explain the pain scale that you will be using to assess the patient's level of discomfort. Look and listen for verification of understanding. Never assume that it is understood just because you said

Figure 33-1 Antiembolism hose should be worn pulled all the way up and kept smooth, without wrinkles, bunching, or the top edge rolling down.

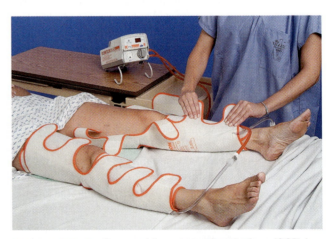

Figure 33-2 Sequential compression devices (SCDs) are applied by wrapping the compression sleeve pads around the legs, then connecting them to the pump unit via connecting tubes.

it. If the patient voices concerns regarding addiction to pain medications, carefully explain that addiction is rarely an issue when there is a medical need and the medication is taken according to physician's orders.

Knowledge Connection

Once you have *taught* something to a patient, what must you do to determine its effectiveness? What phase of the nursing process would this be? What phase of the nursing process would taking a medical history be? And patient teaching?

Preoperative Medications

The administration of preoperative medications is designed to address a specific patient need, based on the patient history, examination, laboratory tests, or surgery. The purpose and goal of premedication will dictate the specific medication choice. One purpose for administering preoperative medications is a safety issue: prevention of aspiration during anesthesia and recovery. Anticholinergics such as atropine, scopolamine, and glycopyrrolate may be given preoperatively to dry secretions, thereby decreasing the risk of aspiration and increased airway irritability. These drugs are indicated for patients who have:

- Pre-existing problems with secretions
- Previously had a stroke
- Parkinson's disease

as well as for:

- Toddlers
- Small children
- Patients whose surgery will result in stimulation of oral mucous membranes, because stimulation of the oral mucosa can increase salivation 10-fold, potentially placing the airway at risk

Other indications for premedication include the desire to decrease intraoperative anesthesia requirements and the need to induce analgesia, especially when preoperative patient preparation may prove uncomfortable, as may be the case with placement of IV lines or the injections associated with regional blockade.

Antibiotics may be given prior to surgery to decrease the risk of infection, particularly of the surgical incision. Antibiotics are also used to prevent bacterial endocarditis in patients with a history of congenital or rheumatic heart disease and valve disease with regurgitation. Many hospitals have developed written protocols regarding the use of antibiotic prophylaxis, both to ensure use in appropriate patients and to prevent inappropriate use when unnecessary.

Box 33-3 presents a comprehensive list of purposes for which preoperative medications may be administered. Most will be administered intravenously when the patient arrives in the holding area before surgery.

Box 33-3

Purposes and Goals of Premedication

There are various reasons for administration of preoperative medications. The most common ones include the following:

- Relieve apprehension and anxiety
- Provide sedation
- Provide analgesia
- Provide amnesia
- Decrease anesthetic requirements
- Decrease gastric volume and acidity
- Prevent nausea and vomiting
- Dry secretions and prevent aspiration
- Prevent bradycardia
- Facilitate induction
- Decrease allergic reaction
- Decrease stress of parental separation
- Prevent infection
- Prevent clot formation

Knowledge Connection

What determines which preoperative medication will be ordered?

Informed Consent

As you learned in Chapter 3, an informed consent must be completed and signed by the patient prior to performing surgery, which means that the patient must be informed and understand the procedure for which he or she is about to give consent. The consent form should list the correct surgical procedure that is to be done, and most will include a partial list of possible risks or complications, some of which are life threatening. The physician is responsible for providing explanation of the:

- Procedure to be performed
- The expected or desired outcome of the procedure
- Alternatives that are available in place of the procedure
- The expected outcomes of the alternatives or simply not having the procedure at all
- Risks of the procedure and anesthesia

Once the physician has explained all these things, the patient must be allowed to ask questions and register any concerns. Once all of the patient's questions and concerns have been addressed, it is required that the patient acknowledges verbally that he or she understands the procedure and risks. Some consent forms include an area in which the patient writes, using layperson's terminology, what he or she understands the surgery to be. For example, the patient who is having a cholecystectomy might write "take out my gallbladder." Figure 33-3 presents an example of a surgical consent form.

The patient or authorized person then signs the form granting permission for the surgery. The nurse generally

REQUEST AND CONSENT FOR SURGICAL, MEDICAL OR DIAGNOSTIC PROCEDURES
AND ACKNOWLEDGMENT OF RECEIPT OF INFORMATION

Patient: _____Emma May_____

Patient NO: _____#48476006110_____ DATE: ____2/12/13_____ TIME: _____1645_____

The hospital and your physician are required by law to obtain your consent to perform the surgical, medical or diagnostic procedure(s) listed below. Signing this form will acknowledge that you request and consent to your physician performing the recommended procedure(s). Your signature also confirms that your physician has explained to you the procedure(s), the risks of the procedure(s), the alternatives, if any, and risks of the alternatives and the risks or consequences of foregoing all treatment. **Please READ THIS ENTIRE FORM CAREFULLY** and then before signing it, ask your physician any additional questions you may have. Your request and consent is valid until you withdraw it.

1. I hereby request and authorize _____Dr. Brad Monett_____ with hospital personnel and/or other trained persons of his/her choice and/or Medical/Physician Assistant/Nursing Student _____ to perform upon (patient) _____me, Emma May_____ the following surgical, medical or diagnostic procedure(s) _____Left total knee replacement_____ _____ to include any necessary or advisable anesthesia and disposal of tissue removed during surgery. I further request and authorize my physician and his assistant(s) to perform any other procedure that in his or their judgment is advisable for my well-being. This additional request and authority is extended as I recognize that during the above listed procedure(s), unforeseen conditions may require different or additional procedures.

2. I hereby request and consent to the administration of such anesthetics as are necessary. I further request that the choice of anesthetic to be used shall be made by professional anesthesia personnel.

3. I acknowledge that some of the risks known to be associated with surgery and anesthesia and which may be applicable to the proposed procedure(s) are:

INFECTION	**LOSS OF AN ARM OR LEG**
SEVERE BLOOD LOSS	**LOSS OF BLADDER FUNCTION**
IMPOTENCE	**LOSS OF BOWEL FUNCTION**
DISFIGURING SCARS	**PARALYSIS BELOW THE WAIST**
LOSS OF FUNCTION OF AN ORGAN	**PARALYSIS BELOW THE NECK**
LOSS OF FUNCTION OF AN ARM OR LEG	**BRAIN DAMAGE**
LOSS OF AN ORGAN	**DEATH**

4. I am aware that the practice of medicine and surgery is not an exact science and acknowledge that no guarantees or warranties have been made to me concerning the results of the procedure(s). I acknowledge that even though my physician has advised me of all known risks, up to and including the rare but possible severe risks as revealed in item 3 of this form, that additional unforeseeable and unpreventable situations could arise in the course of my care which might result in injury.

5. I HEREBY STATE THAT I HAVE READ AND UNDERSTAND THIS REQUEST AND CONSENT AND THAT ALL MY QUESTIONS ABOUT THE PROCEDURE(S), ALTERNATIVE PROCEDURE(S), AND RISKS OF EACH HAVE BEEN ANSWERED IN LANGUAGE THAT I UNDERSTOOD AND THAT ALL BLANKS WERE FILLED IN PRIOR TO MY SIGNATURE.

Signed: ____Emma L. May_____
Patient or person authorized
to request procedures for patient:_____

Relationship or Capacity: _____

Witness to signature: ____K. Gann, LPN_____

I have explained the procedure(s), alternative(s) and risks to the person or persons whose signature or signatures are affixed above.

____Dr. Brad Monett_____
Signature of Physician

Figure 33-3 Surgical consent form.

signs it only as a witness to the fact that it was the patient or authorized person's signature (Fig. 33-4). The physician also must sign the consent form acknowledging that it was he or she who explained everything to the patient.

As part of this informed consent process, for procedures involving either a left or right designation for the surgery (such as left leg or right ear), you should mark the correct side and site of the planned surgical procedure with an indelible ink marker. Mark it right onto the patient's body to reduce the risk of error. For example, if the left breast is to be removed, a large "X" and something similar to "this side only" or "yes" is written on the left breast. Some physicians and nurses even write "Not this side!" or "no" on the nonoperative side in a further attempt to prevent removal of the wrong body part.

Knowledge Connection

What are your responsibilities as a nurse regarding obtaining consent for surgery? What should health care providers do to reduce risk of performing surgery on the wrong side of the patient's body when a left or right designation is required for the site procedure?

Preoperative Checklist

As a nurse, one of your final preoperative responsibilities to the patient is to confirm that all preoperative tasks have been completed and that the patient is ready to go into surgery. The use of a preoperative checklist can facilitate a last-minute confirmation as well as provide documentation. Placing the checklist on top of the chart makes it readily available for the anesthesia provider and the OR nurses. A quick look for a completed checklist will confirm that the patient is ready for surgery. An example of one facility's preoperative checklist may be seen in Figure 33-5.

Figure 33-4   This nurse is witnessing the patient sign a surgical consent form.

The Holding Area

The patient will be transported from his or her room via a gurney or a wheelchair to the holding area, where the patient will remain until taken into the surgery suite (Fig. 33-6). If the facility policy permits, allow the family to accompany the patient to the holding area and provide them a few minutes to hug or kiss each other good-bye. Depending upon facility policy, if the patient is a child, the parents may be allowed to accompany the child into the holding area. Direct the family to the appropriate waiting area where the physician will come to talk with them after surgery.

Once the patient is in the holding area, any remaining preoperative orders will be carried out. An IV may be initiated while in the holding area. The circulating nurse will confirm the identity of the patient, making sure that allergy and identification bands are in place. The nurse will confirm completion of preoperative orders and preparation, as well as checking for the presence of the signed consent form and ordered laboratory tests. Only when this has been completed will the patient be brought into the surgery suite.

Knowledge Connection

What types of things are on the surgery checklist? What are the circulating nurse's responsibilities in the holding area?

Intraoperative Care of the Surgical Patient

The OR is a specialized environment, created with one primary goal in mind: patient safety. To safely perform a surgical procedure requires numerous personnel and specialized equipment and instruments (Fig. 33-7). Each surgical team member has specific responsibilities that must revolve around that which is *in the patient's best interest*. The nurses working in the OR play a specialized role in patient care, advocating for the patient, who is unable to advocate for himself or herself due to the administration of anesthesia.

Surgical Team Members

Patient care is the responsibility of the entire surgical team, which at the minimum consists of the following:

• Anesthesia provider
• Surgeon
• First surgical assistant
• Circulating nurse
• Scrub nurse

Anesthesia Provider

The anesthesia provider has the responsibility for sustaining the patient's life and ensuring that the patient remains comfortable. The provider may be a physician or a registered nurse with specific anesthesia training. A *medical doctor*

SURGICAL CHECKLIST AND PREOPERATIVE NURSING RECORD

Date: _____

Patient Name: _____   Procedure: _____

Floor Check		Preoperative Checklist	OR Check		Preoperative Nursing Record
Chart			Chart		PRE-OP HOLDING AREA ADMIT TIME: _____ AM/PM
Yes	No		Yes	No	
		New Physician's Orders and Progress Sheets on Chart			PRE-OP HOLDING AREA VITAL SIGNS: T _____ BP _____ P _____ R _____ SaO$_2$ _____
		Surgical Consent: Correct, Signed and Witnessed			
		Sterilization Permit: on Chart: Correct, Signed, Witnessed			
		History and Physical on Chart			
		Skin Assessment Completed			
		Labs on Chart:			
		Blood Ordered T&C, WB, PC, FFP, PLT, No. Units:			
		Pregnancy Report on Chart Pos Neg			
		EKG on Chart			
		Chest Film Report on Chart			
		X-ray Report on Chart			
		Patient Stickers on Chart			
Patient			Patient		
Yes	No		Yes	No	
		ID Band on Patient and Correct			
		Prep: Shave and/or Skin Done Initial:			
		NPO Since: Time _____			
		Dentures: Plates Partials removed left in none			
		Glasses/Contact Lenses: removed left on/in none			
		Hearing aid: removed left on none			
		Patient voided or Catheterized Time: _____			
		Jewelry: Secured Removed None			
		Hairpins, makeup, nail polish Removed None			
		IV Site _____ Size _____ Solution _____			
		Patient verbalizes surgical procedure as_____			
		Patient verbalizes surgical site as _____			
		Surgical site marked			
		Will accept blood or derivatives (other than own or directed donor)			
		Has donated own blood or has a directed donor			

Allergies/sensitivities, reactions:

Pre-op Vital Signs: Time: _____ T _____ BP _____ P _____
R _____ SaO$_2$ _____

	Pre-op Medications			
Time	Medication	Dose	Route	Location

Nurses Notes:

Time	

Nurse Signature: _____

Figure 33-5 Sample Preoperative Checklist.

Figure 33-6   Surgical holding area.

Figure 33-7   An operating room in use. Anesthesia is on the right.

anesthesiologist (MDA) is a physician who has education, experience, licensing, and credentialing in administration of anesthesia. A c*ertified registered nurse anesthetist (CRNA)* is a registered nurse who has gone through extensive education and training to deliver anesthesia care, most commonly through completion of a master's degree in nursing. The CRNA administers anesthetics under the supervision of a physician, who may be an MDA or may be the surgeon performing the procedure. An *anesthesiologist assistant (AA)* is an allied health professional who works under the direction of a licensed anesthesiologist to develop and implement anesthesia care plans. All AAs possess a premedical background and a baccalaureate degree, and also complete a comprehensive didactic and clinical program at the graduate school level.

Surgeon

The surgeon is a physician who has been granted surgical privileges to perform a surgical procedure in a facility based on education, experience, licensing, and credentialing. The surgeon may perform the procedure independently or may have a first surgical assistant, which is common in more complex and lengthy surgeries.

First Surgical Assistant

The first surgical assistant may be another physician, a physician assistant, or a registered nurse. The *registered nurse first assistant (RNFA)* is a registered nurse who has received additional education and extensive training in the field of surgery. The RNFA directly assists the surgeon throughout the procedure, which may include controlling hemostasis, assisting with instrumentation, manipulating and incising tissue, and suturing or stapling and closing the incision. The RNFA may also be directly involved with patient care preoperatively and during recovery.

Circulating Nurse

The circulating nurse is a registered nurse; this role cannot be delegated to an LPN/LVN. The circulating nurse is responsible for management of the care of the patient throughout the surgical procedure. The circulator is the primary patient advocate and is responsible for ensuring that everything that is done in the OR is in the best interest of the patient, who can no longer speak for himself or herself once anesthesia has been administered. Besides ensuring that the correct procedure is performed, the circulating nurse also maintains the patient's rights, provides appropriate privacy and preservation of modesty, and preserves the patient's dignity. The circulating nurse, who is not scrubbed, can leave the room if needed or obtain supplies from cabinets within the room, opening them directly onto the sterile field.

The circulating nurse is responsible for coordination of the surgical team and any additional personnel who might be required for successful completion of the procedure. It is this nurse's job to maintain the safest environment possible for the patient while carefully observing the patient's condition from his or her arrival in the OR until the patient has been transferred to the PACU. This involves specifics such as calling a time-out before surgery (which will be addressed a little later) and taking sponge and needle counts to ensure that these items are not left inside the operative site.

Scrub Nurse

The scrub nurse can be an RN, an LPN/LVN, or a certified scrub technician. It is the scrub nurse's job to set up the sterile field with all the appropriate sterile instruments and supplies immediately prior to actually beginning the procedure. It is also the scrub nurse's responsibility to then ensure that sterility of the field is maintained while actively assisting the surgeons working within the sterile field during surgery. This includes passing sterile instruments, surgical sponges, suture and needles, staple guns, suction tips, or other equipment to the surgeons.

Knowledge Connection
Explain the various roles and responsibilities of the surgical staff.

Preparation of Surgical Suite

Before any surgical procedure begins, the OR nursing staff are responsible for preparing the surgical environment. This will first involve preparation of the room by making sure that the room has been disinfected and is ready to accept the patient. All equipment needed for the procedure will be brought into the room and set up as much as the room will allow prior to the introduction of both the patient and personnel. This is important, for once room setup begins it will be the responsibility of the OR nursing staff to make sure that the equipment remains sterile. Frequently, the OR nursing staff will work from both experience and prepared "cheat sheets" that contain information about equipment needed for a particular type of surgery, as well as individual surgeon preferences for equipment and glove sizes. To set the room up, the scrub nurse must first scrub, so that he or she is in a position to begin working with and setting up sterile supplies. The surgical scrub is designed with the primary goal of prevention of infection through the most cost-effective, simplest method known to reduce wound infection: handwashing.

As another step in patient protection, a *time-out* is called when a patient enters the OR. Initiated by the circulating nurse, a time-out is designed to prevent the risk of the wrong patient, wrong site, and wrong surgery. During the time-out, the RN will verify and document verification of the:

• Patient's identity and date of birth
• Presence of signed consent in the chart
• Correct site of surgery: if the surgery has a left or right distinction or involves multiple structures, such as fingers, or multiple levels, such as in spinal surgery, the surgical sites should be marked with a permanent marker
• Correct procedure
• Presence of correct x-ray or other films
• Presence of needed special equipment

Knowledge Connection
Who calls the time-out? What is its purpose?

Types of Anesthesia

Anesthetic agents are administered to decrease or completely block sensory perception; some agents either partially or completely decrease the level of consciousness. The different types of anesthesia include:

• **General anesthesia:** the patient is totally unconscious
• **Conscious sedation:** the patient is asleep but not totally unconscious
• **Regional anesthesia**: specific nerves and the region innervated by the nerves, such as a finger, an arm, or the lower half of the body, are blocked from sensory perception by injection of a local anesthetic numbing agent such as lidocaine

• **Local anesthesia**: a very small area of tissue is blocked from sensory perception by injection of a local anesthetic numbing agent such as lidocaine

The decision regarding type of anesthesia is based on the type of surgery to be performed, the patient's pre-existing medical conditions, and the preference of the surgeon and anesthesia provider. A patient having open heart surgery requires a general anesthetic. A patient having a knee arthroscopy may be a candidate for general or regional anesthesia. Depending upon the site, a biopsy can sometimes be done under local anesthesia. Conscious sedation is commonly used for diagnostic procedures such as a colonoscopy or an esophagogastroduodenoscopy (EGD), for closed reduction of fractures, and in medical and dental offices for certain anxiety-producing procedures.

General Anesthesia
General anesthesia has five objectives:

1. Loss of consciousness
2. Amnesia regarding the procedure
3. Pain relief
4. Skeletal muscle relaxation
5. Blocking reflexes such as coughing and gagging, as well as endocrine and autonomic responses

As no one medication is capable of meeting all of these objectives, general anesthesia requires the administration of multiple agents. Narcotics are used for pain relief. Benzodiazepines are used to reduce anxiety and to provide amnesia and sedation. Muscle relaxants are used for skeletal muscle relaxation and to facilitate placement of the endotracheal tube or laryngeal mask airway to control ventilation. Intravenous anesthetics are used for sedation and to induce and maintain anesthesia. Inhalation agents are used to induce and maintain loss of consciousness.

The advantages of general anesthesia are that it can be used for procedures that take longer to complete, reduces patient anxiety, reduces memory of the procedure, and provides complete comfort for the patient throughout the surgical procedure. Disadvantages include risk of aspiration due to vomiting, respiratory or cardiac arrest, brain damage, stroke, and death.

Conscious Sedation
Twilight sleep is a state of hypoconsciousness, or partial anesthesia, in which medications have reduced sensation so that less pain is experienced. **Conscious sedation** provides a controlled minimal level of sedation that allows the patient to be relaxed and in twilight asleep while still being able to maintain his or her own airway and yet respond purposefully. Various medications may be used to attain this state of decreased consciousness, such as opioids, hypnotics, and sedatives. Use of conscious sedation is dependent upon the procedure to be done, the patient's health, and both the patient and physician's preferences. The advantages include patient comfort, less risk, and that the

patient is easily wakened. The one disadvantage of conscious sedation is that it can only be used for certain short procedures.

Regional Anesthesia

Regional anesthetic techniques are used to isolate the administration of a local anesthetic, such as lidocaine, to a specific nerve or region to prevent transmission of sensory information to and from the section of the body. This results in numbness or loss of feeling as well as loss of ability to voluntarily move the area. Common types of regional anesthesia are spinal anesthesia, epidural anesthesia, peripheral nerve block, and local anesthesia.

Spinal Anesthesia

Spinal anesthesia, sometimes called a *spinal block,* involves injection of the anesthetic into the cerebrospinal fluid in the subarachnoid space (Fig. 33-8A). The nerves below the site of injection are blocked from central nervous system transmissions. It is commonly used for delivery of a baby, perirectal surgery, and abdominal or lower extremity surgery.

The advantages of spinal anesthesia include no loss of consciousness and more rapid recovery, reduction of aspiration due to vomiting, and potential for decreased need of pain medications in the immediate postoperative period. Disadvantages are that the type of surgical procedure may limit this as an option, and that the patient may require additional IV agents to be administered for anxiety, as the patient will potentially be awake with this type of anesthesia.

Side Effects

Possible side effects include urinary retention, hypotension, and headache. If the patient is unable to empty the bladder, it may be necessary to perform a catheterization to drain the bladder or place an indwelling catheter to be left until sensation returns to the lower half of the body.

The patient should be monitored for hypotension due to vasodilation of the peripheral blood vessels, which allows blood pressure to drop excessively. The vasodilation occurs due to the blocking of the sympathetic vasomotor nerves.

Some patients develop a post–spinal anesthesia headache due to leakage of spinal fluid during the spinal anesthetic. The anesthesia provider may participate in treatment of a spinal headache if necessary. These patients should be monitored closely.

Sometimes spinal anesthesia will affect a higher level of the spinal cord than intended due to the anesthetic seeping above the injection site rather than limiting sensation blockage to below the site. The danger with this side effect is that it may paralyze the respiratory muscles and decrease the heart rate. Monitor the vital signs closely and position the patient in a high Fowler's position if this becomes a problem. It is rare, but possible that the patient's ventilation may require ventilatory support until the anesthetic wears off.

Epidural Anesthesia

Epidural anesthesia differs from spinal anesthesia in that a small catheter is inserted into the epidural space of the spinal column to provide a continual administration of a stronger anesthetic agent. Some physicians utilize epidurals for postoperative pain control as well as during surgery. The second difference is the area of instillation of the anesthetic. Because the anesthetic agent is instilled into the epidural space, it does not come in contact with the spinal cord as it

(a)   (b)

Figure 33-8 A. Spinal anesthesia is the injection of a local anesthetic agent into the subarachnoid space. It blocks sensation and movement below the injection site. B. Continuous epidural anesthesia can be used to provide postoperative analgesia.

does with spinal anesthesia, thus making it safer for the patient (Fig. 33-8B). The advantages and disadvantages are similar to those of spinal anesthesia.

Side Effects

If the anesthesia provider inadvertently injects the anesthetic agent too deeply into the subarachnoid space, this too can result in respiratory depression and paralysis. This requires support of respirations until the respiratory nerves and muscles regain their ability to function.

Peripheral Nerve Block

If anesthesia is desired for an area such as an arm or leg, a peripheral nerve block may be the anesthesia of choice. The anesthetic is injected into a nerve or group of nerves to depress transmission of signals to and from the site. The advantages include no loss of consciousness and a lower risk of side effects. A common type of peripheral nerve block is the **Bier block**. A tourniquet is placed around an extremity to decrease venous return while continuing to allow full arterial delivery of oxygenated blood to the site. The anesthetic agent is injected intravenously in the extremity or portion of the extremity that is distal to the tourniquet. The anesthetic causes loss of sensation in the area as long as the tourniquet remains in place. The disadvantage of the Bier block is that the tourniquet cannot be left in place longer than 2 hours, thus limiting the length of time that anesthesia may be effective.

Local Anesthesia

Local anesthesia is supplied through the use of agents such as lidocaine, which may be administered by injection or applied topically to mucous membranes for loss of sensation of a very small area, such as the nose and throat or for a skin or soft tissue biopsy. The advantages are that the patient remains awake and alert, fewer risks are involved, and the anesthetic takes less time to wear off. The only disadvantage is that it can only be used for small areas.

Knowledge Connection

What type of surgery might be performed using a spinal block? Conscious sedation? Bier block?

Intraoperative Interventions

Numerous interventions must be performed in the OR besides the actual surgical procedure performed by the surgeon. Many of these interventions are related to safety of the patient.

Miscellaneous Interventions and Equipment

Sometimes the patient's IV is not started until the patient is in the OR. Many of the supplies and equipment that are used, as well as the interventions performed, are to provide safety for the patient. Cardiac monitor electrodes are applied to the patient's chest for monitoring cardiac rate and rhythm.

Grounding pads are applied to allow safe usage of electrical equipment. Safety straps are used to secure the patient to the operating table.

Automated vital sign machines and pulse oximeters are applied to monitor the patient's blood pressure, pulse, and oxygen saturation levels. The anesthesia provider also monitors the patient's temperature throughout the surgery to ensure that the patient does not become hypothermic or develop **malignant hyperthermia**, a rapid and severe rise in body temperature that occurs while under a general anesthesia due to an inherited genetic trait. The anesthesiologist or nurse anesthetist administers the appropriate anesthesia. For a general anesthesia, he or she will administer appropriate medications to sedate the patient, perform **intubation**, which is the insertion of an endotracheal tube into the patient's trachea to maintain an open airway and administer inhalant anesthesia and oxygen (Fig. 33-9), and attach the ventilator for use once the patient is sufficiently sedated to paralyze the respiratory muscles.

Specific interventions may be performed, such as insertion of a Foley catheter or a nasogastric tube. Suction is kept readily available for use by the anesthesia provider to maintain a clear airway and for use by the operating team to maintain visibility within the operative site. The suction is used to remove blood and other body fluids that pool within the operative site.

Placement of tube in airway

Figure 33-9   Endotracheal tube.

In an effort to protect the patient from microorganisms and infection, special ventilation systems have been installed to prevent air from the rest of the facility from entering the OR. Room temperature and humidity are controlled within tight ranges to decrease bacterial growth. Surgical hand scrubs are performed by the OR team members, who may not wear artificial nails or jewelry. Sterile instruments, equipment, overhead light handle covers, supplies, gowns, and gloves are also used to protect the patient, as are clean face masks and hair coverings. The gowns, gloves, masks, and hair coverings are accompanied by face shields or goggles as well as shoe covers to protect the OR team members from any blood-borne pathogens that may be carried in the patient's body fluids.

Positioning the Patient

Once the anesthesia has been initiated, an important task of the OR team is to provide appropriate and safe positioning of the patient. The team may use straps, wedges, pillows, and surgical table attachments to maintain positioning. Special surgical tables or extension pieces may be required for morbidly obese and extremely tall patients. Variables to be considered in positioning the patient include the need for:

• Access to the surgical site
• Access to the patient's airway
• Monitoring of vital signs
• Maintaining patient body alignment
• Patient safety
• Patient comfort

Surgical Shave

Shaving hair from the operative site is no longer routinely done. Research has shown that it increases the risk of infection by allowing microbes easier access through the patient's first line of defense, via microscopic nicks to the skin. Therefore, the hair on the operative site is generally just clipped very short unless it is necessary to remove all hair. If the hair is to be clipped, this may be done by the nurses caring for the patient preoperatively, while the scrub nurse is generally responsible for shaving the operative site if it is required.

Surgical Scrub

Once the patient has been positioned for the surgery, the operative site skin will be vigorously scrubbed with an antimicrobial wash and paint. The combination of an antiseptic agent and the friction of application helps to further reduce the microbial count. The antiseptic solution will be applied using a sponge or sterile instrument, working in concentric circles from the center of the surgical site to the periphery. A combination alcohol-iodine solution (DuraPrep) is the most commonly used agent. Alcohol is used for a rapid microbial kill with fast drying, while the iodine provides for a water-insoluble persistent film. Skin preparation should be documented by the circulating nurse on the intraoperative record.

Draping the Patient

After the skin is cleansed and dried with a sterile towel, surgical draping can begin. The drape allows for isolation of the surgical site and localizes the sterile field to the surgical site. Draping will also maintain patient privacy. Drapes should be applied in such a way as to allow for the full possibility of surgical incisions, for any potential additional incisions, and for the placement of surgical drains that might be placed at the end of surgery.

The Surgical Procedure

More and more surgeries are being performed using endoscopic techniques, which while more technically difficult, minimize surgical trauma, speed recovery and discharge, and reduce postoperative complications. However, there are many types of surgery that require an incision of several or more inches for introduction of instruments and performance of required maneuvers.

Although a detailed description of every surgical procedure is not possible in this text, it is possible to identify descriptors that help to explain the procedure. For example, some common descriptors are:

• **-ectomy:** To remove, as in tonsillectomy (removal of tonsils) or lobectomy (removal of lobe of the lung)
• **-otomy:** To cut or separate, as in craniotomy (cutting of bones of the cranium or skull)
• **-ostomy:** To create an opening, as in colostomy (opening into the colon for elimination of wastes)
• **Transplant:** To uproot and replant, as in kidney transplant (removal of kidney from donor to recipient)
• **Ablation:** To remove from, as in surgical ablation of heart tissue for atrial fibrillation

Tissue Specimens

If tissue samples are obtained for biopsy or other testing, or cultures are obtained for laboratory analysis, the scrub nurse will assist in placing the sampled tissue into collection medium and will make the transfer of collected specimens to the circulating nurse, who prepares patient labels for the containers and completes appropriate requisitions. The circulating nurse is responsible for the transfer of tissue specimens to the appropriate laboratory.

Needle, Sponge, and Instrument Counts

An additional intervention to promote patient safety is the counting and recording of numbers of sponges, needles and other sharps, and instruments used during a procedure to prevent the unintentional retention of foreign items in the surgical wound. The count is performed and documented between the scrub nurse and the circulating nurse:

• As the room is set up before the procedure is started
• When additional supplies are opened and added to the sterile field
• When the scrub nurse is replaced by a second scrub nurse at any point during the procedure

- Before closure of each surgical cavity
- At the end of the case prior to the closure of the surgical incision
- After skin closure

Final Intraoperative Interventions

At the end of the surgery, the anesthesia provider will lighten the anesthetic to the point that the endotracheal tube can be removed, called **extubation**, prior to transport, if possible. The circulating nurse completes documentation and then assists the anesthesia provider in the safe transfer of the patient to the PACU or to an intensive care specialty unit. Upon arrival to the PACU or intensive care specialty floor, the anesthesia provider or circulating nurse provides a verbal report, along with the written anesthesia record containing information about the patient's preoperative status, need for surgery, and intraoperative summary of the surgery and anesthetic course, to the nurse who will be providing postanesthesia nursing care. Any complications will be identified, as will any special needs. The report information will be documented in the PACU record.

While the circulating nurse transports the patient from the OR, the scrub nurse breaks down the room and takes instruments to central sterile (the area of the hospital the primary function of which is to sterilize supplies and equipment) for cleaning, disinfection, and resterilization. There instruments are cleaned and disinfected with an automatic instrument washer, similar to a dishwasher. Disinfection does not sterilize, it only reduces the microbial count, so once the clean instruments are sorted and grouped into specific surgery instrument packs, they are sterilized to render them free of all microorganisms in an *autoclave,* a machine that uses heat and steam pressure for a specified length of time to ensure that no microorganisms survive.

Postoperative Care of the Surgical Patient

Admission to the PACU begins the transition from the OR to postoperative care. In the PACU, the RN will maintain close observation and assessment of the patient, usually observing no more than two patients at a time, until the patient is ready to transfer back to his or her room, where other nurses provide further postoperative care.

Postanesthesia Assessment and Care

Patients are monitored continuously by the PACU nurse, with documentation of the assessments done on admission, every 15 minutes, and again upon discharge to the patient's room. Assessments and documentation may be more frequent, as often as every 5 minutes, if the patient is still intubated, deterioration occurs, or an intervention is initiated due to a change in condition.

In the PACU, the immediate priority is to maintain a patent airway and verify respiratory and cardiac function. This requires immediate application and observation of a pulse oximeter, EKG monitor, blood pressure monitor, and supplemental oxygen, as well as assessment of respiratory rate, depth, and characteristics. Anesthesia may compromise both cardiac and pulmonary function, and depending on type, the surgery itself may compromise both as well. Suction must be readily available for use in maintaining an open airway.

After the admission assessment is completed and the patient is deemed stable, the PACU nurse will develop a plan of care directed toward anesthetic and surgical recovery.

Potential Patient Problems and Complications

Postoperative problems and side effects are limitless as the patient is more vulnerable in the unconscious state. Respiratory problems, cardiovascular problems, gastrointestinal problems, hypothermia, and pain and discomfort are possible following general anesthesia.

Respiratory Problems

Potential respiratory problems common to the PACU after general anesthesia include obstruction of the airway, hypoxemia, and hypoventilation. Respiratory problems may be due to blockage of the airway by laryngeal edema, excessive secretions, or the tongue; anesthetic agents; narcotics given for pain; surgery; pre-existing medical conditions such as emphysema; or risk factors such as being a smoker.

Nursing Care

The best treatment for respiratory problems is to prevent them from occurring if at all possible. Most patients will have an oral or nasal airway placed once the endotracheal tube is removed to help maintain a patent airway until the patient is sufficiently awake to handle his or her own secretions. (See Chapter 28 for more information about artificial airways.)

To help prevent respiratory complications:

- Prepare suction equipment and suction the patient as needed.
- Monitor the respiratory rate, depth, and pattern at least every 15 minutes, or more often if necessary, until the patient is stable and more awake.
- Apply supplemental oxygen at the appropriate liter flow and with the appropriate delivery device.
- Monitor breath sounds and oxygen saturation level. Elevate the head of the gurney if necessary. Encourage the patient to take deep breaths as he or she becomes more awake.

By staying alert to patient condition and impending changes and being proactive with preventative nursing care, you can facilitate the elimination of inhalation agents and carbon dioxide, promote effective gas exchange, and reduce certain respiratory problems.

Cardiovascular Problems

Potential cardiac problems seen in the PACU include tachycardia and bradycardia and hypotension and hypertension. Both anesthetic agents and blood loss may compromise heart rhythm and function as well as affect the blood pressure. Respiratory problems can also affect cardiac status.

Nursing Care

As cardiac problems are common, an EKG monitor is applied for all patients during recovery, making it possible to monitor both the heart rate and rhythm for detection of bradycardia, tachycardia, and other arrhythmias. To help prevent cardiac complications:

- Auscultate heart sounds, noting muffled or distant S_1 or S_2.
- Monitor blood pressure closely, noting even small decreases.
- Administer IV fluids adjusted according to patient condition.
- Assess the patient's skin color and temperature, and whether moist or dry.
- Assess the strength of apical, radial, and pedal pulses; and capillary refill in all four extremities.
- Monitor for excessive bleeding from the surgical site and drains. Excessive blood loss may be visible or internal; because bleeding can be unseen, assess the size of the operative site and surrounding area for edema or, if the abdomen, distention.
- Always be alert to falling blood pressure and tachycardia that occurs suddenly, persists, or rapidly reoccurs even with fluid administration.

Real-World Connection

Postoperative Complications

The student nurse was caring for a postoperative patient who had just returned from having a laproscopic cholecystectomy (removal of the gallbladder). The student had performed an initial assessment and assessed vital signs upon the patient's return to the nursing unit; all findings were within normal limits except for incisional pain at a 7. The patient was drowsy but responded to voice and followed simple commands to take deep breaths and splint the incision while coughing. Pain control was provided by a patient-controlled analgesia pump with morphine. The pump was programmed for continual infusion of a low dose of the morphine as well as intermittent doses to be delivered according to the preset parameters and frequency of patient use.

The instructor entered the room about 90 minutes later to check the patient's status while the student was gone to lunch. Upon entering the room, the instructor observed the patient with circumoral cyanosis, cyanotic nailbeds, and erratic, shallow respirations at 5 per minute. The apical pulse was very irregular, beating at a rate in the 60s and 70s and then within seconds speeding up to rates over 130 per minute.

Supplemental O_2 was applied at 4 L/min via nasal cannula. Telemetry was applied for monitoring cardiac rate and rhythm. The physician was notified and the morphine discontinued. The patient required stimulation and was encouraged to turn, cough, and deep breathe every few minutes over the next hour to maintain the respiratory rate above 10.

Within 60 minutes the patient's vital signs had stabilized, again within normal limits except for a tachycardia of 110, and the patient had awakened enough to get up to the bathroom with assistance to void. The final outcome was positive, but these events serve to demonstrate how quickly a postoperative patient can deteriorate even after anesthesia has been discontinued, the patient has been extubated and has returned to the nursing unit from the PACU, and assessment findings and vital signs have indicated the patient was stable. A postoperative patient's condition can turn in the blink of an eye.

Gastrointestinal Problems

General anesthesia relaxes the smooth muscles as well as the skeletal muscles. This decreases and may completely inhibit peristalsis in the gastrointestinal tract, therefore slowing or stopping the passage of gastrointestinal contents through the alimentary canal intraoperatively and for a period of time postoperatively. Though much progress has been made to decrease postoperative nausea and vomiting by administration of medications, many patients still experience these complications. Some anesthetic agents are more prone to induce these symptoms than others.

Nursing Care

To help prevent gastrointestinal problems:

- Administer antiemetic medications ordered for prn use.
- Use suction as needed.
- Keep an emesis basin, washcloth, and towel within reach. A cool wet cloth on the forehead or neck may feel good to the patient experiencing nausea.

Hypothermia

Whether hypothermia occurs is dependent upon the length of time in surgery, the degree of exposure, and the age of the patient. Warming the patient is another priority of the PACU nurse.

Nursing Care

To prevent hypothermia, take the following steps:

- Monitor temperature and complaints of being cold, including teeth chattering, chilling tremors or shakes, and mottling of skin.
- Apply additional warmed blankets as needed. If cloth blankets are not adequate, use warm air flow blankets to raise the patient's body temperature.
- Assess patient temperature to differentiate between hypothermia and the tremors and shaking caused by general anesthesia as consciousness is regained, which the patient may interpret as being cold.

Pain and Discomfort

Probably the most common problems in the PACU are pain and discomfort. Discomfort may be due to incision or tissue manipulation during surgery, throat irritation due to use of an endotracheal tube for general anesthesia, the presence of drains or various tubes such as chest tubes, the presence of casts, or nausea and vomiting.

Nursing Care

Even if the patient received some pain medication in the OR, pain medications given there are usually short acting and may require additional doses in the PACU. Some tips to help relieve a patient's pain and discomfort include:

- Administering pain medication as ordered, generally via the IV route
- Treating pain according to the patient's evaluation of its severity

Other PACU Nursing Responsibilities

The PACU nurse must also note and carry out any postoperative physician's orders that are to be performed while in recovery, such as obtaining x-rays, administration of antibiotics, or applying ice packs.

Discharge From PACU

The patient can be discharged for transfer to his or her room or to go home *only* after meeting all the criteria for discharge, which include both recovery from anesthesia and the absence of any anesthetic or surgical complications. Prior to discharge, the nurse will make and document a final assessment and complete the PACU record documentation. The transfer report provides information about the patient's current status, pre-existing medical history, and a summary of the surgery, anesthetic, and PACU course. Complications will be identified, as will special needs. Then the PACU nurse will notify the receiving nurse on the floor of the impending transfer, reporting any special patient needs, which gives the receiving nurse time to gather and prepare any additional supplies or equipment so they are ready for use when the patient arrives.

Return to the Patient's Room

If the surgical patient is an inpatient before going to surgery and thought to be returning to the same room, it is best to prepare the room to receive the patient postoperatively as soon as the patient is transported to the OR. This prevents the patient being brought back to a room that is not ready to receive a postoperative patient. If the postoperative patient is to be transferred to a new floor and room, the recovery room nurse should notify the floor where the patient will be sent after surgery that a postoperative patient will be transferred to the floor. If this is done as soon as the patient is received in the PACU, this allows time for the receiving nurse to prepare the room and make it ready for the postoperative patient.

Room Preparation

Room preparation includes obtaining needed supplies and preparing a surgical bed with a lifting or draw sheet and disposable waterproof pads if needed. (Refer to Chapter 15, Skill 15-10, for steps of making a surgical bed.) In addition, the furniture should be arranged so the gurney can be positioned parallel to the bed so that the heads of the gurney and bed are aligned with each other. This better positions the patient so that, after transferring from the PACU gurney into his or her bed, the patient is properly positioned at the head of the bed (Fig. 33-10). It also prevents the staff having to lift the patient a second time to move him or her toward the head of the bed.

The room should be arranged to provide easy access with the gurney. Move chairs, the over-the-bed table, and the bedside table out of the way so that nothing impedes the direct path from the door to the side of the bed. Remove unnecessary clutter from both tables to accommodate the supplies you will be using immediately upon return of the patient. Store patient belongings in the closet and drawers until needed. Equipment and supplies that should be ready for use at the bedside may be found in Box 33-4. Postoperative patients may return with numerous pieces of equipment requiring space and reorganization of furniture to accommodate them. Failure to adequately prepare the room, supplies, and equipment can result not only in decreased efficiency of care but unsafe conditions should the patient suddenly develop problems.

Initial Postoperative Patient Assessment

Transfer the patient from the gurney to the bed using as much assistance as needed for safety. If the patient is able to help, allow him or her to do so. This is a good time to multitask. While transferring the patient to the bed, assess the patient's skin color and temperature and whether it is dry or moist, the color of urine in the Foley drainage bag, and whether the IV site is intact.

Figure 33-10 When transferring a postoperative patient from a gurney to a nursing unit bed, align the head of the gurney with the head of the bed before transferring the patient.

Box 33-4

Equipment and Supplies Needed for Postoperative Patient Care

There are many supplies and pieces of equipment that are required for proper postoperative care. Certain things will be needed as soon as the patient is transferred from the gurney to the bed, such as vital sign equipment. Some are safety related, allowing you to be prepared for an emergency situation that could develop, such as the suction equipment; others are needed simply to meet the patient's needs after surgery. Having all your supplies will also save you the footwork and time of making multiple trips to gather supplies, one or two at a time as you need each one. Additionally, the postoperative patient should not be left alone for at least the first 15 to 30 minutes after returning to the room. Equipment and supplies to gather include:

- Vital sign equipment, including pulse oximeter
- Penlight
- IV pole with infusion pump
- Suction equipment
- Oxygen setup with delivery device
- Emesis basin
- Washcloths and towels
- Clean patient gown
- Box of tissues
- Mouth care supplies with lip lubricant
- Several extra pillows for positioning
- Extra blankets
- Pen and paper to record vital signs
- TED hose and/or sequential compression device according to physician's orders
- Small pillow for splinting (for abdominal surgeries)
- Small cup of ice chips if physician's orders allow
- Specimen pan to measure urinary output
- Ice pack if ordered

First Priority

Once the patient is in the bed, your immediate priority is to complete an initial assessment with vital signs to determine the patient's condition and establish a baseline for subsequent comparisons. The assessment should begin with the number one priority: airway and gas exchange. Is the airway patent? Is there an oral or a nasal airway in place? Or is one needed? Assess respiration rate, depth, and pattern. Assess color of the skin, noting pallor or cyanosis. Assess oxygen saturation, noting if below 95%. Apply supplemental oxygen if ordered or if the patient's respiratory status indicates a need.

Second Priority

Determine the patient's level of responsiveness and ability to follow instructions by instructing the patient to take several deep breaths while you are applying the pulse oximeter, blood pressure cuff, and cardiac monitor if ordered or according to facility policy. Begin assessing for cardiac stability by obtaining a pulse rate and blood pressure; note a weak or thready pulse, tachycardia, bradycardia, or other arrhythmias as well as hypo- or hypertension. Auscultate heart sounds, breath sounds, and bowel sounds. Note muffled or distant S_1 or S_2; absent, decreased, or adventitious breath sounds; and hypoactive or absent bowel sounds (Fig. 33-11). Assess peripheral circulation by assessing peripheral pulses and temperature of all four extremities, noting weak or absent pulses and cool or cold hands or feet. Check pupils for equality of size and response to light stimulus.

Surgical Site

Assess the surgical site and dressing for bleeding and drainage. Using an ink pen, draw a circle around any area of drainage on the dressing, along with notation of the current date and time. This allows you to later gauge additional amounts of bleeding or drainage. Any drains should be assessed and attached, if ordered, to the appropriate suction. If Hemovac or Jackson-Pratt drainage devices are in use, ensure that they are activated. (Refer back to Chapter 26 to review care of drains.) Make sure you wear gloves when working with drains and dressings. If the dressing is saturated with blood, reinforce the dressing with sterile gauze 4×4s or larger abdominal combined dressings, also known as ABD pads, and notify the surgeon. You should not remove the initial surgical dressing without a direct physician's order. Assess for abdominal distention and rigidity, which may be indicative of internal hemorrhage.

Fluids and Related Equipment

Assess type of IV fluid hanging, IV patency, and rate of infusion, and assess the IV site for erythema, edema, and intactness of site dressing. If the patient has a Foley catheter connected to gravity drainage, assess its intactness, patency, color, clarity, and volume of urine output. Make certain the tubing is properly secured to the leg or, if a male prefers, the abdomen. This reduces trauma to the neck of the bladder and the internal sphincter, where the inflated balloon constantly tugs against them if allowed to dangle unsecured

Figure 33-11 Once a patient is returned to the nursing unit from the PACU, a complete assessment should be performed to determine the patient's condition.

from the urinary meatus. This can cause discomfort, such as a burning or pulling sensation, as well as increasing the feeling that the patient needs to void.

Pain and Discomfort

Thoroughly assess the patient's pain level using the facility's preferred pain scale. (See Chapter 19 for further information regarding use of pain scales.) Be certain not only to assess the site and the intensity of the pain, but also to include characteristics of the pain. For example, is the pain sharp or stabbing? Dull, aching, or cramping? Is it limited to the surgical incision site? Or is it, for example, in the shoulder from which the arm was extended during surgery? Determine what medications were administered during surgery and in the PACU to reduce risk of overmedicating the patient. Once you have completed the assessment, administer analgesics according to the physician's orders, evaluating the medication's effectiveness. Remember, the pain is as bad as the patient says it is, not as bad as you think it should be.

Safety Interventions

Make sure that the call bell is within reach of the patient, side rails raised for safety, and the bed is lowered to its lowest position. The head of the bed is generally raised for patient comfort, unless contraindicated by the type of surgery. The bedside table should also be brought within reach, with needed supplies, including water or ice chips if allowed.

Documentation

Document your assessment, including the six vital signs, as soon as possible. Begin an intake and output record.

Supervision/Delegation Connection

Postoperative Assessment

Delegation of postoperative assessment and vital signs to unlicensed personnel is not appropriate until the patient's condition is determined to be stable. You are responsible for observing the postoperative patient and assessing him or her according to the patient's individual responses to surgery and anesthesia. Even though vital sign assessment may be safely delegated to unlicensed personnel in certain other situations, this is not one of them.

Continued Assessments

You should remain at the bedside until you are certain that the patient is stable. After your initial assessment is complete, continue to monitor level of consciousness and respiratory and cardiac status—including vital signs—at 15-minute intervals for the first hour.

After the first hour of monitoring vital signs every 15 minutes, if they are stable, assessments can be lengthened to every 30 to 60 minutes according to facility policy. (See Box 33-5 for an example of a frequency schedule.) The assessments are performed at progressively lengthening intervals over the first 24 hours postoperatively. Most hospital

---

Box 33-5

Example of Postoperative Vital Sign Frequency

After a general anesthetic, it is necessary to monitor the patient's postoperative vital signs frequently to detect developing problems as early as possible. Each facility will have its own policy delineating vital sign frequency, but the following is a commonly used schedule:
- Every 15 minutes × 4
- Every 30 minutes × 4
- Every 1 hour × 4
- Every 2 hours × 4
- Every 4 hours × 4
- Then every 8 hours

---

units have a standardized postsurgical care plan in place that details postsurgical care routines, regardless of the type of surgery. If your patient shows any signs of instability, call for assistance without leaving the bedside.

Pain Control

Pain assessment remains a major priority throughout the entire postoperative period. The postsurgical orders will specify available interventions, which may include use of a patient-controlled analgesia (PCA) pump, IV administration, or administration of oral medications. Remember, you have a number of nonpharmacologic interventions available to assist with pain control as well, including repositioning, use of warm blankets, music, and touch. However, these alternatives do not replace pain medication when the patient needs medication, unless there are cultural or personal beliefs prohibiting use of analgesic pain medications.

Fluid and Electrolyte Balance

The patient's fluid and electrolyte balance should be monitored closely. If the patient does not have an indwelling Foley catheter, you should make certain the patient voids within 8 hours. If the patient cannot void within the specified length of time, it may be necessary to obtain a physician's order to either perform a straight catheterization or insert an indwelling urinary catheter. Be certain to measure all urine output as well as emesis and other drainage. The patient may still be NPO and dependent upon IV fluids for hydration. Keep the mouth and lips moist to reduce dryness, cracking, and discomfort due to dry mucous membranes. Monitor the IV fluid and rate of infusion and perform an IV site assessment at least every 2 hours. Make certain the intake and output are balanced to prevent fluid overload or dehydration.

Postoperative Orders

Postoperative orders may also include additional specific assessments to be made, such as hourly urine output or neurological examinations, and specific actions to be taken, including turning the patient every 2 hours, when to get the patient out of bed, and specific patterns that, if present, require notification of the surgeon, including parameters for blood pressure, pulse, temperature, and oxygen saturation. *Safety: All preoperative orders are discontinued when a patient goes to surgery. New ones must be written when the patient returns to the nursing unit.* Box 33-6 provides further discussion on preoperative versus postoperative orders.

Postsurgical Complications

While there are postsurgical complications that may occur that are specific to the type of surgery performed, there are also some complications that may occur independently of the type of procedure. It is your role to help prevent these complications with accurate and pertinent assessments and delivery of appropriate nursing actions or interventions, and to intervene promptly if signs of these complications are noted.

Fever

It is somewhat common for the postoperative patient to run a low-grade temperature, within the range of 99°F to 99.8°F (37.1°C to 37.6°C) after surgery. But more elevated temperatures of 101°F (38.3°C) or higher may be a sign of infection. The more commonly seen infections include pneumonia, wound infection, and urinary tract infection, particularly if an indwelling catheter is present.

Nursing Care

A fever of 101°F requires notification of the surgeon. The surgeon will frequently order blood, urine, sputum, and wound cultures to determine the source of infection before ordering antibiotics to treat the infection. The surgeon may also order acetaminophen, a medication that reduces fever

---

Box 33-6

Preoperative Orders Versus Postoperative Orders

The standard of care is that all preoperative physician's orders are automatically discontinued when a patient goes to surgery, requiring that new orders be written for any care that is to be delivered postoperatively. The following pointers will help to keep you a safe and accurate practitioner.

- All preoperative orders are canceled when the patient goes to surgery.
- The physician must write new postoperative orders, including orders for any medications taken preoperatively that are to be administered postoperatively.
- If the physician writes "resume preoperative meds," you must clarify with the physician which specific medications are to be resumed. Never assume that it really means all of the medications that were taken before surgery.
- After clarifying with the physician, list the specific medications individually on the physician's order sheet. Some facilities require that the order be written beginning with: "Clarification of previous order to resume preoperative medications...."

---

and is classified as an *antipyretic* medication. High fevers (greater than 102°F) may require application of cool wet cloths to the forehead, neck, axilla, and groin.

Atelectasis

Atelectasis can cause postoperative hypoxemia, due most commonly to excessive secretions or decreased lung volumes. Low blood pressure can also contribute to atelectasis. In addition to the nonspecific signs of hypoxemia, ranging from agitation to excessive sleepiness, tachycardia to bradycardia, and hypertension to hypotension, patients will present with diminished to absent lung sounds. Patients at risk for atelectasis include any patient who:

- Has received general anesthesia, particularly if a smoker
- Has abdominal surgery pain
- Is on bedrest or restricted activity
- Has chronic respiratory disease

Nursing Care

Once again, prevention is key. Implementation of treatment strategies early, before the patient becomes symptomatic, will help to prevent the development of atelectasis. Treatment includes humidified oxygen, coughing and deep breathing exercises, incentive spirometry, repositioning, and promotion of increased mobility with early ambulation.

Pulmonary Embolism

Pulmonary embolism (PE) occurs as the result of a venous clot that is released into the circulation, lodging in a vessel in the lungs and obstructing blood flow and gas exchange. It is a leading cause of perioperative morbidity, with deaths generally occurring within 30 minutes of an acute event (Fig. 33-12). The patient will complain of acute shortness of breath and will immediately develop tachycardia, increased respiratory rate, and hypoxemia, even if already on oxygen. If severe, the patient may go into cardiac arrest.

Patients at risk for PE include those who have venous stasis or blood pooling; *hypercoagulability,* which is increased risk of clotting; or abnormalities of the blood vessel walls. These risk factors are increased in elderly patients and obese patients, in those with varicose veins, immobility, malignancy, and congestive heart failure, and in patients who have had pelvic or long-bone surgery.

Nursing Care

As a PE can be life threatening, prevention is important. TED hose and sequential compression devices may have been applied before or after surgery. Maintain both until the patient is able to get out of bed and ambulate to promote blood flow. See that the patient performs postoperative leg exercises to stimulate venous circulation and prevent stasis. An anticoagulant may be ordered for subcutaneous administration for patients who must remain on bedrest or who had surgery on the skeletal system, such as repair of a hip fracture or knee replacement.

Pulmonary embolism

Figure 33-12 Pulmonary embolism.

Nausea and Vomiting

Nausea and vomiting, while not life threatening, is distressing for patients. It may be caused by the agents used in the OR, NPO status, pain medications used after surgery, or because of a nasogastric (NG) tube that is not functioning appropriately.

Nursing Care

Assess for nausea and treat as soon as possible to prevent vomiting. Surgeons commonly order an antiemetic to be available on an as-needed basis for patient comfort. For surgeries associated with nausea and vomiting, the anesthesia provider or PACU nurse may have given a dose of the antiemetic already, so check the OR and PACU records first, before administering the first dose.

Urinary Retention

Urinary retention following surgery may occur due to use of a regional anesthetic such as a spinal, or may be due to narcotics administered for pain after surgery.

Nursing Care

Monitor intake and output carefully and, if the patient is unable to void, assess the bladder for distention. If distention is present, try to assist the patient to void by helping him or her to the bathroom unless contraindicated; if the patient is male, you may help him stand to void. Running water may also be helpful. If the patient remains unable to void, the surgeon may order bladder catheterization. However, to decrease the risk of infection, the catheter is not usually left in place. For surgeries after which voiding is known to be difficult or output monitoring is critical, a catheter is placed in the OR.

Wound Infection

The edges of the surgical incision should meet and be aligned with one another, known as **approximation**. Wound **dehiscence** refers to a separation of the wound edges. Occurring most commonly 7 to 10 days postoperatively, it is seen in approximately 2% of all midline abdominal incisions. It is associated with 15% to 40% mortality, as the underlying cause is most commonly infection.

Patients at risk for alterations in wound healing include those with diabetes, malnutrition, suppressed immune function, advanced age, and infection. A patient taking corticosteroids for chronic conditions such as rheumatoid arthritis or obstructive pulmonary disease should be considered to be immunosuppressed, due to the medication's action to reduce the body's normal anti-inflammatory response.

Nursing Care

While dressing changes are routinely the responsibility of the nurse, sometimes a surgeon will prefer to remove the initial surgical dressing on the first postoperative day. Unless the physician orders otherwise, you should assess the wound daily, noting possible signs of infection such as poor approximation of incision edges, dehiscence, erythema, edema, and color, amount, and odor of drainage. *Safety: Perform proper handwashing prior to wound assessment or dressing change, and use clean or sterile gloves as appropriate.* If a surgical drain is present, look for erythema, edema, and drainage around the insertion site, as well as color, amount, and odor of the drainage from the drain itself. Accurate assessment allows for early detection of and intervention for infection. Document your assessment, noting changes from previous assessments. In addition to monitoring the wound, assess temperature for fever and monitor the WBC count for elevation related to infection. If dehiscence occurs, cover the wound with a large sterile dressing or sterile surgical towel moistened with sterile normal saline. Notify the surgeon immediately. (Chapter 26 details wound assessment and management.)

Nursing Care Plan for a Patient Who Is Postoperative Following Colectomy

You are assigned to care for Jeremy Lackey, a 67-year-old male admitted the previous evening with the diagnosis of inflammatory bowel disease. He has just returned from surgery where he underwent a segmental colectomy with anastomosis. This means the surgeon removed the diseased segment of his colon and rejoined the ends of the remaining portions. Now you need to get started developing Mr. Lackey's care plan. Figure 33-13 presents a concept map care plan for this patient.

Assessment

Development of a care plan begins by first gathering all the available data. You will need to determine postoperative problems you can anticipate for this patient. But you know that a physical assessment is your priority at this time.

- What is his LOC?
- Are his vital signs stable?
- What is the status of his respiratory system?
- What is the status of his cardiovascular system?

- What is the status of his neurological system?
- Is the patient comfortable or experiencing pain? Nauseated?
- What equipment is in use? IV pump? PCA? SCDs?
- What are the patient's postoperative needs?
- Have postoperative physician's orders been carried out yet?
- Did the patient receive preoperative teaching?

The physician's orders were being noted by the off-going nurse. You went directly to the patient's room and assessed him to determine his current status and establish a baseline. You have just documented the assessment. A synopsis of the assessment findings includes the following information:

Still groggy but responsive to voice and follows simple commands; oriented to 4 spheres. Pupils equal and responsive to light bilaterally. BP – 118/66, T – 98.2°F, AP – 96 regular and distinct, R – 19/minute shallow and even, SpO_2 – 95% with O_2 on @ 2 L/min per nasal

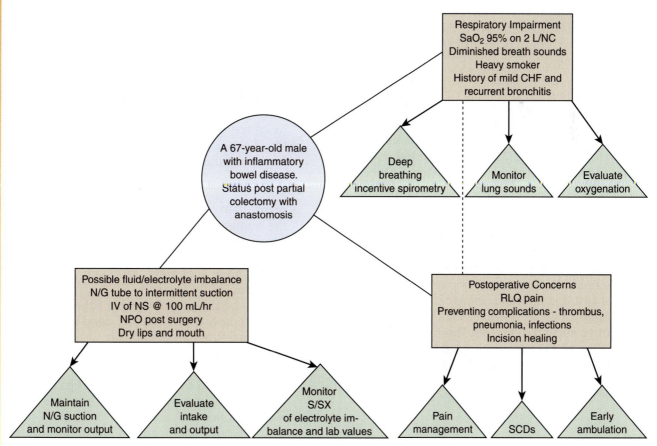

Figure 33-13 Concept map care plan for a patient having abdominal surgery.

(care plan continues on page 796)

Nursing Care Plan for a Patient Who Is Postoperative Following Colectomy (continued)

cannula. Breath sounds diminished in all 5 lobes, but improve when cued to take deep breath; no adventitious breath sounds. C/O dry lips and mouth. Requesting ice chips. Right lower quadrant abdominal pain @ 4, down from 9 before analgesic. NG tube to low suction patent, draining dark green contents. Denies nausea. Abdominal dressing dry and intact. Abdomen flat and soft. No bowel sounds auscultated. IV of 1,000 mL 0.45% NS infusing in left forearm @ 100 mL/hr via infusion pump. Site without erythema or edema. Has not voided since returning from OR. Bladder not palpable. SCDs on both legs with capillary refill time less than 3 seconds and strong pedal pulses bilaterally.

The chart reflects that preoperative teaching was done with the patient and family, and understanding of teaching was evidenced. You note that he is a heavy smoker and has had several bouts of bronchitis over the last 5 years. He has a history of mild congestive heart failure for which he takes a diuretic to prevent water retention. Postoperative physician's orders are now noted. There is no additional care to deliver at this time.

Nursing Diagnosis

Now that you have collected all the data, you need to analyze this information and determine what type of problems Mr. Lackey may have or may be at risk for developing. The first things that come to mind are his smoking, medical history of bronchitis, and diminished breath sounds—plus he had a general anesthetic and is currently experiencing decreased physical activity. He has supplemental O_2. The congestive heart failure could potentially cause some respiratory issues and will have to be watched. All this information leads to the presence of a breathing problem or *impaired gas exchange,* your first and priority nursing diagnosis.

Mr. Lackey has postoperative *pain,* another priority nursing diagnosis. The fact that he is NPO and has an NG tube connected to suction removing gastric juices and electrolytes tells you that he has a *risk for fluid and electrolyte imbalance,* your next nursing diagnosis.

Planning

Now you need to plan what nursing interventions should be performed to prevent the possible problems and actual problems that you know to expect. You want to individualize the plan of care, making certain the interventions meet Mr. Lackey's specific needs. Interventions that should help the patient's nursing diagnoses include:

- **Impaired gas exchange**
  - Assess respiratory rate, depth, and pattern and SpO_2 every 15 minutes $\times$ 4; every 30 minutes $\times$ 4; every 1 hour $\times$ 4; every 2 hours $\times$ 4; every 4 hours $\times$ 4; and then every 8 hours. If abnormal, modify to more frequent intervals.
  - Encourage the patient to turn, cough, and deep breathe 5 times every 2 hours, noting cough effort and whether or not there is sputum production. Auscultate breath sounds every 4 hours, noting any absent, decreased, or adventitious breath sounds. Assess for exertional dyspnea while repositioning.
  - Assist the patient to use an incentive spirometer every hour $\times$ 8, then every 2 hours; 5 inspirations with initial goal of 700-mL volume, increasing goal by 100 mL once able to meet each goal.
  - Maintain O_2 @ 2 L/min per NC.
  - Have suction equipment readily available at bedside.
  - Elevate the head of the bed 30 to 60 degrees as needed to assist breathing.
  - Assist the patient to dangle for 5 to 10 minutes twice tonight.
  - May have bedside commode.
  - Begin ambulation in room in a.m. Then in halls QID.
- **Pain**
  - Assess pain during each patient contact using the numerical pain scale of 0 to 10.
  - Assess site and characteristics of the pain.
  - Reposition the patient every 2 hours, ensuring proper body alignment, propping with pillows for support and comfort.
  - Encourage the patient to splint the incision with a pillow when moving, deep breathing, or coughing to lessen discomfort.
  - Provide back or foot massage one to two times per shift.
  - Provide mouth care and keep the lips moist with petroleum-free lip moisturizer at least every 4 hours.
  - Keep NG tube connected to low, intermittent suction, secured to nose so that it doesn't press

Nursing Care Plan for a Patient Who Is Postoperative Following Colectomy (continued)

against the naris. Pin tubing to gown to avoid hanging weight on nose.
- Give morphine 4 to 6 mg IV every 2 hours prn pain. Evaluate effectiveness within 20 to 30 minutes.
- Administer promethazine 50 mg IM every 4 to 6 hours prn N/V or to potentiate analgesic. Evaluate effectiveness of injection within 30 to 60 minutes.
- **Risk for Fluid and Electrolyte Imbalance**
  - Monitor I&O every shift, comparing total output to intake. Note if output is *less* than total intake by more than 300 mL.
  - Make certain the patient voids at least every 8 hours, noting cloudy, concentrated, or dark amber urine.
  - Continue IV infusion of 1,000 mL 0.45% NS with 30 mEq KCl @ 125 mL/hr per pump.
  - Assess NG tube connected to low, intermittent suction for patency and color, amount, and consistency of gastric contents every 2 hours. Measure and empty at end of shift.

- Assess for peripheral edema every 4 hours.
- Monitor laboratory results for elevated or decreased K^+, Na^+, and Cl^-.

Implementation

Now you can begin to carry out the interventions that you have planned. Table 33-1 lists nursing interventions for these nursing diagnoses.

Evaluation

The last phase of the nursing process is to evaluate whether the interventions you have been implementing are helping Mr. Lackey's respiratory efforts and preventing pneumonia. You will also want to evaluate whether or not the medications are keeping the patient comfortable and with a pain level less than 3 to 4 the majority of the time. What is the total I&O? Is he adequately hydrated? Are his electrolytes balanced? Table 33-1 provides evaluations of the nursing interventions.

Table 33-1 Nursing Care Plan for a Patient Who Is Postoperative Following Colectomy

Nursing Diagnosis: Impaired gas exchange, related to smoking, history of bronchitis, abdominal incision pain, and general anesthesia, as evidenced by diminished breath sounds and shallow respirations
Expected Outcomes: O_2 saturation will remain above 95%. Breath sounds will be clear to auscultation and will not be diminished by second postop day. Temperature will remain below 100.4°F. No evidence of pneumonia, supported by clear chest x-ray at discharge.

Interventions	Evaluation
Assess vital signs, noting increased respiratory rate, decreased depth, irregular pattern, decreased SpO_2, increased pulse rate, dropping blood pressure, and increased temperature. Use facility postoperative frequency schedule.	Day 1: Within normal limits all day. 10 p.m.: 122/74, 98.2°F orally, 88 reg & strong, 18 shallow & even. SpO_2 has remained above 95% since noon.
Encourage the patient to turn, cough, and deep breathe 5 times every 2 hours.	Day 1: Good resp effort, cough productive of small amount clear sputum.
Auscultate breath sounds every 4 hours, noting decreased, absent, or adventitious sounds.	Day 1: Diminished in 5 lobes; few fine crackles in RLL @ 10 p.m.
Assist the patient to use an incentive spirometer every 1 hour for 8 hours, then every 2 hours. Initial goal is volume of 700 mL; increase by 100 mL as patient meets each goal.	Day 1: Met 700-mL goal 2nd hr. Met 900-mL goal 5th hr. Met 1250-mL goal 12th hr. Still @ 1350 mL @ 10 p.m.

(table continues on page 798)

Table 33-1 **Nursing Care Plan for a Patient Who Is Postoperative Following Colectomy** (continued)

Nursing Diagnosis: Impaired gas exchange, related to smoking, history of bronchitis, abdominal incision pain, and general anesthesia, as evidenced by diminished breath sounds and shallow respirations

Expected Outcomes: O_2 saturation will remain above 95%. Breath sounds will be clear to auscultation and will not be diminished by second postop day. Temperature will remain below 100.4°F. No evidence of pneumonia, supported by clear chest x-ray at discharge.

Interventions	Evaluation
Maintain supplemental O_2 @ 2 L/min per nasal cannula.	Day 1: O_2 con't @ 2 L/min per nasal cannula. No dyspnea. Skin remains pink.
Elevate the head of the bed 30–60 degrees prn.	Day 1: Only needed head of bed up once for brushing teeth.
May use bedside commode.	Day 1: Only used urinal today.
Assist the patient to dangle for 5–10 minutes 2 times on day of surgery—ambulate in room tomorrow a.m.	Day 1: Dangled 5 min @ 3:00 p.m. & tolerated it without dyspnea, stated pain increased only while getting up to sitting position, felt good once upright.
Ambulate 4 times/day in halls—to begin 1 day postoperatively.	
Have suction setup ready in room.	Day 1: Handling own secretions.

Nursing Diagnosis: Pain, related to surgical manipulation of abdominal contents as evidenced by abdominal incision.

Expected Outcomes: Pain level below 5 within 60 minutes after analgesic administration; able to maintain below 3 with oral analgesic at discharge.

Interventions	Evaluation
Use 0–10 scale to assess pain at each contact with the patient.	Day 1: Highest pain rating was immediately after return from PACU @ 10. Maintained less than 5 remainder of day with analgesics.
Turn the patient every 2 hours, maintain proper body alignment, position & support with pillows for comfort.	Day 1: Erythema on sacrum resolves 5–10 min after repositioning. No other erythema noted. Skin remains intact over pressure points. Body alignment maintained with pillows. Does not like to lay on left side.
Encourage the patient to splint the incision when coughing or moving.	Day 1: Had to be reminded to splint while coughing, but said it does help a little.
Provide back or foot massage 1–2 times per shift.	Day 1: Reported that massages of back felt great and seemed to help him relax.
Provide mouth care and lip moisturizer every 4 hours.	Day 1: Applies lip moisturizer himself. Lips more moist than immediately postop.
Keep nasogastric tube connected to low, intermittent suction. Secure the tube to the patient's nose, avoiding pressure on naris. Pin the tube to the patient's gown.	Day 1: No erythema noted on naris.
Administer morphine 4–6 mg IV every 2 hours prn pain. Evaluate effectiveness within 20–30 minutes.	Day 1: 4 mg only controlled pain for 45–60 min. 6 mg kept pain less than 5 most of day.
Administer promethazine 50 mg IM every 4–6 hours prn nausea/vomiting or to potentiate morphine. Evaluate effectiveness within 30–60 min.	Day 1: Only required once for potentiation of first dose of morphine 4 mg. Decreased pain from 5 to 3.

Table 33-1   **Nursing Care Plan for a Patient Who Is Postoperative Following Colectomy** (continued)

Nursing Diagnosis: Risk for Fluid and Electrolyte Imbalance, related to NPO status and nasogastric suction.
Expected Outcomes: Electrolytes will remain within normal limits each day. Urine output will remain within 300 mL of IV intake.

Interventions	Evaluation
Monitor I&O every shift. Note if output is *less* than total intake by more than 300 mL.	Day 1: NPO. IV In – 3,000 mL; Out – 2,875 mL.
Make certain the patient voids at least every 8 hours. Assess characteristics.	Day 1: Voiding without difficulty; urine clear, yellow.
Continue IV infusion of 1,000 mL 0.45% NS with 30 mEq KCl @ 125 mL/hr.	Day 1: IV still @ 125 mL/hr. Site Rt. forearm, 18-gauge intracath, no edema/erythema, site dressing dry/intact.
Monitor laboratory results for elevated or decreased potassium, sodium, and chloride.	Day 1: Postop potassium 3.3 mEq; obtained order to increase IV potassium.
Assess nasogastric tube connected to low, intermittent suction for patency and drainage characteristics every 2 hours. Measure and empty at end of shift.	Day 1: Nasogastric tube patent, drainage thick, dark green. 24-hr Out – 525 mL.
Assess for peripheral edema every 4 hours.	Day 1: None.

Skill 33-1 Applying Antiembolism Hose

Assessment Steps

1. Review the physician's order to determine the type of hose ordered. *They come in knee-high and thigh-high lengths.*
2. Measure the patient's legs according to type ordered.
   • **For thigh-high:** Measure the length of the posterior aspect of the leg with the patient in the supine position, measuring from the gluteal fold to the plantar surface of the heel. Then measure the circumference of the largest part of the calf and the largest part of the thigh.
   • **For knee-high:** Measure the length from the posterior knee to the plantar surface of the heel.
   Cross-reference the measurements on the manufacturer's chart to determine the correct size. *This ensures proper fit.*
3. Assess skin integrity of both legs and feet. *This establishes a baseline against which you can measure future skin integrity and makes you aware of problems with the skin.*

Planning Steps

1. Gather needed supplies: antiembolism hose, powder. *Being prepared saves time and footwork.*
2. Plan to have your patient lie supine for a minimum of 15 minutes prior to application of hose. *This aids venous return of blood to the heart and reduces the risk of trapping pooled venous blood in the lower legs.*

Implementation Steps

1. Follow the Initial Implementation Steps located on the inside front cover.
2. Make certain that the patient's legs are clean and dry. *This reduces microorganisms and prevents maceration from applying the hose over moist skin.*
3. Grasp the top edge of the hose and slide your non-dominant hand into the hose and down to the heel of the hose, where you grasp the fabric of the heel with your hand.
4. Use your dominant hand to slowly pull the hose inside out, turning it down to the heel. *This enables you to slide the tight hose over the foot and calf more easily.*
5. With the patient's toes pointed down, grasp the turned foot of the hose and center it over the toes. Then ease the hose over the heel, making certain the heel is also centered in the hose before proceeding to slide it over the calf. *This helps to ensure more even compression over the foot and leg.*
6. Smooth all wrinkles from the hose and pull the hose up to its full length. Avoid allowing the hose to bunch, wrinkle, or fold over at its top. *This prevents constriction of venous circulation and pressure ulcers.*
7. If the hose style has closed toes rather than open toes, gently pull the hose at the end of the toes to provide more room for the toes and nails. *This helps to prevent capillary compression in the toes and sore toenails due to pressure at the corners of nail.*

(skill continues on page 800)

Skill 33-1 Applying Antiembolism Hose (continued)

8. Repeat the process for the other leg.

9. Follow the Ending Implementation Steps located on the inside back cover.

10. Remove hose at least twice per day: during bath and p.m. care. Wash and dry the legs; assess for pressure areas or impairment of skin integrity before reapplying hose. *This allows the skin to be exposed to air and stimulates circulation. It adds to the comfort of the patient and helps him or her to rest afterward.*

11. Assess pedal pulses each shift. *This ensures adequate arterial circulation to the feet.*
    Note: *Hose should be hand-washed daily and allowed to air dry to prevent soiled hose from smelling and irritating the skin. Therefore, the patient will require two pairs: one pair to wear while the other pair is drying.*

Evaluation Steps

1. Do the stockings fit smoothly without wrinkles? Do they come up to the correct height on the legs? *This ensures proper fit.*

2. Are you still able to palpate the pedal pulses? *This ensures that the stockings are not so tight that they block arterial blood flow to the feet.*

Sample Documentation

10-5-12 1930 Legs measured for thigh-high TED hose. Thigh = 29 in. Calf = 16 in. Length = 29 in. Skin of legs and feet intact and without erythema or edema. TED hose applied. Pedal pulses strong bilaterally. Purpose of TEDs explained. Verbalized understanding of purpose. States had worn them before. ———————————————— Nurse's signature and credentials

Skill 33-2 Applying Sequential Compression Devices

Assessment Steps

1. Verify the physician's order for length of device. *These devices come in different lengths.*
2. Measure circumference of the thigh if thigh-high length is ordered. *This ensures the proper amount of compression.*
3. Read the manufacturer's instructions for application and use of sequential compression devices. *Each trade-name SCD will work slightly differently.*

Planning Steps

1. Gather needed equipment and supplies: compression sleeves, compression pump or motor, connecting tubing. *Being prepared saves you time and footwork.*

Implementation Steps

1. Follow the Initial Implementation Steps located on the inside front cover.
2. Attach the pump unit to the foot of the bed according to the manufacturer's instructions. *Following the manufacturer's instructions ensures proper use and increases safety.*
3. Apply compression sleeves to the patient's legs according to the manufacturer's instructions. *Following the manufacturer's instructions ensures proper fit and use while increasing safety.*
4. Connect the tubings to the compression sleeves and the pump according to the manufacturer's instructions. *This allows air for compression to enter the compression sleeves from the pump.*

5. Assess to make certain there is room for you to insert two fingers between the compression sleeves and the patient's legs. *This prevents excessive compression.*
6. Turn on the pump.
7. Assess pedal pulses, skin color and temperature, sensation and movement of toes, presence of edema, and capillary refill of toes every 8 hours. *This ensures adequate circulation and nerve function.*
8. Instruct the patient to call for assistance to remove the SCDs if he or she is allowed to ambulate. *This helps to prevent falls.*
9. Follow the Ending Implementation Steps located on the inside back cover.

Evaluation Steps

1. Assess several cycles of inflation and deflation of the devices. Make certain the tubings are not kinked and preventing correct inflation. *This ensures proper function.*
2. Assess patient comfort *to validate correct placement and pressure of devices.*

Sample Documentation

9/7/12   1115   *Skin of legs and feet pink, warm, dry, intact. Pedal pulses strong and equal. Cap refill brisk bilaterally. Calf-high SCDs applied to legs. States they "feel good".*
———————————— *Nurse's signature and credentials*

🌐 Post Conference

You cared for the same patient, Ms. Baum, for all 3 days of your clinical experience. It was quite a time of learning for you. You listened as the staff nurse told the patient about the surgery. You taught her about turning, coughing, and deep breathing after surgery. You had to move very quickly to get everything done on the preoperative checklist before the OR transport came to take her to surgery. In fact, you had barely finished administering the ordered preoperative medications when the transport arrived. The nurse signed off with you on the checklist, though, and you felt good about getting it all done correctly.

You were not really prepared for how sick the patient was when she returned to the nursing unit after the surgery. She had a nasogastric tube, an IV, and a catheter in place, and she was moaning in pain. For just a moment or two, you nearly panicked. However, with your instructor's assistance, you calmed down quickly and went about caring for this lady. You focused on meeting her needs, assessing her status, monitoring her vital signs, and reassuring her family. Each postoperative day she was more improved, and you were able to remove the nasogastric tube and the catheter. By the third day, you learned, along with the patient, that no chemotherapy or radiation therapy would be necessary. You were relieved along with her, and you felt good about the care you had given her. She even told you that she wanted you to be her nurse if she was ever in the hospital again.

KEY POINTS

- Surgeries are classified by purpose, degree of urgency, and degree of risk.

- Surgery may be performed in freestanding surgery centers, medical clinics, or hospitals.

- Factors that increase risk of surgery and anesthesia include previous reaction to anesthesia, smoking, obesity, pre-existing medical conditions, malnutrition, immunosuppression, and impairment of the hepatic, renal, or pulmonary systems.

- Consent forms for surgical procedures must include the patient's or guardian's signature, but also imply informed consent, meaning the patient understood what was going to be done, what alternatives there were, risks and possible complications, and expected outcomes.

- Preoperative teaching should include steps of preparation for the surgery; what is going to be done; alternative choices; what will happen in the preoperative, intraoperative, and postoperative phases of surgery; availability of medications for pain and discomfort postoperatively; IVs; tubes and drains; dressings; fluid and food restrictions; activity restrictions; room temperature and equipment in the OR; and nursing routines such as frequent vital sign assessments.

- Preoperative checklist completion is the responsibility of the nursing unit nurse and the circulating nurse.

- The circulating nurse and the scrub nurse must perform several needle, sponge, and instrument counts.

- There are several types of anesthesia: general; conscious sedation; regional, which includes spinal and Bier block; and local.

- Patent airway and gas exchange are the top priority in the PACU and after return to the nursing unit.

- You should thoroughly assess each postoperative patient upon return from the PACU to the nursing unit.

REVIEW QUESTIONS

Select the answer that is most appropriate for each of the following questions. Some questions may have more than one correct answer. Check all that apply.

1. Which of the following patients is scheduled for palliative surgery?

   a. A patient scheduled for tonsillectomy due to repeated throat infections.

   b. A patient scheduled for repair of a gastric ulcer due to lack of healing with medication.

   c. A patient scheduled for removal of an untreatable cancerous brain tumor due to its impingement on the optic nerve.

   d. A patient scheduled for breast enlargement so her body shape will be better balanced.

   e. A patient scheduled for a hysterectomy (removal of female reproductive organs) due to severe endometriosis.

2. For which of the following patients would it be appropriate to schedule his or her surgery in a surgery center as opposed to a hospital setting?

   a. A patient with severe chronic respiratory disease who needs an appendectomy.

   b. A patient with an above-the-knee amputation who needs a breast biopsy.

   c. An elderly patient with hypertension and diabetes who needs a resection of the colon.

   d. A patient with hemophilia who needs a tonsillectomy.

3. Which of the following pieces of medical history would be pertinent regarding a patient being assessed to undergo a major abdominal surgery?

   a. Recent seizures

   b. History of rubella

   c. Has had multiple lacerations sutured

   d. Takes medication for cardiac problems

   e. Is allergic to milk

4. A male patient about to be scheduled for a major surgery tells the physician that he has been diagnosed with some kind of serious problem of his liver but can't remember the name of the disorder. About which of the following might the physician be concerned as a direct result of the patient's statement?

  a. The patient's ability to tolerate IV fluids.

  b. The patient's ability to urinate after surgery.

  c. The ability of the patient's blood to clot.

  d. The patient's ability to maintain adequate body temperature during anesthesia.

5. Which of the following tests are performed on most surgical patients preoperatively?

  a. Electrocardiogram (EKG), complete blood count (CBC), urinalysis (UA)

  b. Magnetic resonance imaging (MRI), serum sodium (Na^+) level, esophagogastroduodenoscopy (EGD)

  c. Lumbar puncture (LP), urine culture and sensitivity (Urine C&S), blood type

  d. Chest x-ray (CXR), finger stick blood sugar (FSBS), electrolytes (lytes)

SHORT ANSWER QUESTIONS

6. Discuss at least six categories or types of information you should teach preoperative patients.

7. What are three interventions you could perform to stimulate a postoperative patient's venous circulation?

8. Name at least three purposes for administering preoperative medication.

9. What are three of the primary responsibilities of the circulating nurse in surgery?

CRITICAL THINKING EXERCISE

10. Discuss five possible assessment findings you might detect in a new postoperative patient that would cause you concern, including what they might mean.

ADDITIONAL RESOURCES

For additional Resources, Questions, and Activities, please see:

 Student Resource Disk

 DavisPlus http://davisplus.fadavis.com

Student Study Guide

REFERENCES

Association of Operating Room Nurses. *Standards, Recommended Practices and Guidelines.* Denver: Association of Operating Room Nurses; 2007.

Drain C, Odom-Forren J. *PeriAnesthesia Nursing: A Critical Care Approach.* 5th ed. St. Louis: Mosby Elsevier; 2008.

Gundzid K. Nausea and vomiting in the ambulatory surgical setting. *Orthop Nurs.* 2008;27:182-188.

Hunter S, Thompson P, Langemo D, Hanson D, Anderson J. Wound and skin care: Understanding wound dehiscence. *Nursing2007.* 2007;37(9):28-29.

Litwack K. *Clinical Coach for Effective Perioperative Nursing Care.* Philadelphia: FA Davis; 2009.

McCarron K. Take a deep breath: Assessing atelectasis. *LPN2006.* 2006;2(3):20-25.

McGuire M, Gan TJ. Increasing patient safety while decreasing cost and aggravation: managing PONV (postoperative nausea and vomiting). January 31, 2007. Medscape CME Web site. Available at: http://cme.medscape.com/viewprogram/6226. Accessed November 20, 2009.

Rothrock J, ed. *Alexander's Care of the Patient in Surgery.* 13th ed. St. Louis: Mosby Elsevier; 2007.

Sharma S. Perioperative pulmonary management. June 30, 2006. Emedicine Web site. Available at: http://emedicine.medscape.com/article/284983-overview. Accessed November 20, 2009.

Spear M. Wound care management: Risk factors for surgical site infection. *Plastic Surg Nurs.* 2008;28:201-204.

Sussman C, Bates-Jensen B. *Wound Care: A Collaborative Practice Manual for Health Professionals.* 3rd ed. Philadelphia: Lippincott Williams & Wilkins, 2007.

Swaminathan A, Naderi S. Pneumonia, aspiration. March 26, 2008. Emedicine Web site. Available at: http://emedicine.medscape.com/article/807600-overview. Accessed November 20, 2009.

Wilkinson JM, Van Leuven K. *Fundamentals of Nursing: Theory, Concepts & Applications.* Philadelphia: FA Davis; 2007.

Williams LS, Hopper PD. *Understanding Medical-Surgical Nursing.* 3rd ed. Philadelphia: FA Davis; 2007.

Phlebotomy and Blood Specimens

Key Terms

Aerobic

Anaerobic

Anastomoses

Blood culture

Evacuated tube

Hematoma

Hemoconcentration

Hemolysis

Lymphostasis

Petechiae

Phlebotomy

Sclerosed

Septicemia

Syncope

Tortuous

Tourniquet

Objectives

1. Define key terms associated with phlebotomy and blood specimens.
2. Identify veins commonly used for venipuncture.
3. Describe situations in which certain veins may not be appropriate to perform venipuncture.
4. Explain how to find and access a vein.
5. Identify types of equipment used to perform venipuncture.
6. Compare the process of venipuncture using the evacuated tube method, syringe method, and butterfly infusion set.
7. Describe the types of blood collection tubes used in phlebotomy.
8. Designate the order of draw for collection tubes when performing venipuncture.
9. Describe how to properly label specimens.
10. Describe how to collect blood cultures.
11. Describe complications that can occur as a result of venipuncture.
12. Explain how to perform a skin puncture.

Skills

34-1 Applying a Tourniquet

34-2 Performing Venipuncture

34-3 Collecting a Blood Culture Specimen

34-4 Performing Skin Puncture for a Finger Stick Blood Sugar

Clinical Connection

Your Assignment: You have been assigned to clinical experience in a physician's office, where you will draw blood from several different patients throughout the day. The physician is a family practice physician, so the patients may be of different ages. You are concerned about being able to perform successful venipunctures on all of the patients, especially the elderly patients and the younger children. In addition, you have concerns about how to obtain specimens from patients whose veins tend to roll. One of your big concerns is the possibility of a patient fainting when you draw his or her blood.

Your Actions: You ask the clinical medical assistant in the office what types of experiences he has had performing phlebotomy. He assures you that you will do well, but you are not that sure. He offers to let you perform a venipuncture on him and draw a tube of blood using an evacuated tube system so you will feel more confident. As you perform this skill, you realize that a person's arm is very different from a phlebotomy practice arm, but you are able to draw his blood successfully. You still have concerns about elderly and young patients.

Phlebotomy is the practice of drawing blood samples. Though most hospitals and clinics hire specially trained individuals, known as *phlebotomists,* for this purpose, it is common for the nurse to draw blood samples as well. In this chapter, you will learn which veins are best to use and tips to make vein access easier. You will learn how to perform venipuncture, the correct labeling procedure for specimens, and how to perform skin punctures.

Phlebotomy

As you have already learned, protection from body fluids is always required when caring for patients. It is of particular importance when performing venipuncture, due to the potential for exposure to blood and blood-borne pathogens. Make certain that you wash your hands and wear gloves each time you perform venipuncture. You may occasionally see someone draw blood without gloves, but do not allow those bad habits to influence you negatively.

Why We Draw Blood

Blood contains white blood cells (WBCs), red blood cells (RBCs), platelets, oxygen, carbon dioxide, electrolytes, water, vitamins, minerals, proteins, hemoglobin, enzymes, hormones, antibodies, and waste products, which are the end products of cellular metabolism. The blood acts as the primary source of transportation for all of the substances required by body cells. After cells metabolize nutrients, the substances left are known as *end products of metabolism* or *waste products.* The blood transports these end products and the products of enzymatic reactions to the lungs and kidneys, where they can be eliminated from the body. Hemoglobin is carried by the RBCs, which bind with molecules of oxygen for transportation of the oxygen to cells throughout the body. Because blood has so many functions vital to life, blood samples provide a wealth of information regarding the condition of the body, help to identify problems with organ functions, and enable us to diagnose disease and measure its progression.

Preparation of the Patient

As with all interventions, identify your patient using two different methods, which is mandated by The Joint Commission. Usually this is done by asking the patient to tell you his or her name or the last four digits of his or her social security number, and by checking the patient's identification band against the laboratory requisition.

Explain the procedure to the patient in terms that the patient will understand. This helps to reduce anxiety and fear and allows the patient to cooperate with you as you draw the blood sample. Inform the patient that you will be as careful and gentle as possible, but never give false assurance that the venipuncture will *not* hurt.

The patient should be positioned in the supine or semi- or high Fowler's position for this procedure. If the patient has problems with hypotension or **syncope** (fainting), or if the patient voices or exhibits signs of anxiety regarding needles, place the patient in the supine position before attempting to draw blood. Never attempt phlebotomy while a patient is standing.

Knowledge Connection

Why is it important to explain what you are about to do before every procedure? What is the first step you must take to protect yourself from contact with body fluids during phlebotomy?

Selecting an Appropriate Vein for Venipuncture

The most commonly used site for venipuncture is the antecubital fossa, which is the shallow depressed area laying anterior to the elbow. However, other sites may also be used. Your selection will vary with each patient. Figure 34-1 shows the superficial veins of the inner aspects of the arm.

The median cubital is generally the vein of choice, followed by the cephalic vein and the basilic vein.

Anatomy and Physiology Connection

Veins and Arteries
There are some differences in veins and arteries. Veins carry deoxygenated blood and waste products from the capillaries back toward the heart, while arteries carry oxygenated blood and nutrients from the heart to the capillaries to be delivered to the body's tissues. The blood pressure is higher in arteries than in veins, thus necessitating that the artery walls be thicker than those of veins. Both arteries and veins have many **anastomoses**, or junctions where veins join other veins and arteries join other arteries, providing alternate routes for blood flow if one pathway should become obstructed.

Another difference is that veins have valves and arteries do not. The blood in veins must fight against gravity to return to the heart. These valves help to prevent backflow of blood, making it important to avoid damaging the valves when you access the vein for phlebotomy.

Veins on the dorsal side of the hand can also be used to draw blood if the antecubital areas are unavailable, but because they are not secured by as much tissue as the antecubital veins, they tend to roll more than arm veins. They also produce more discomfort with venipuncture than do veins in the antecubital area (Fig. 34-2). If the hand veins do not produce an appropriate site, the wrist veins may be used. As a last resort, veins in the feet are a possibility, but most facilities have strict policies regarding if and when they may be used. Some physicians believe puncture of the feet veins increases the risk of blood clots in the legs.

When a blood sample is required in newborns and infants younger than 2 years of age, skin puncture is used if at all possible. If a venipuncture is necessary, one of the veins on the dorsal side of the hand is preferred. When newborns do not have adequate hand veins, the scalp veins may be accessed by using a rubber band around the forehead in place of a tourniquet, but you must be specially trained to perform venipuncture of a scalp vein.

Sites to Avoid
Some veins should not be used for venipuncture due to certain conditions that can alter the quality of the blood specimen. For example, venipuncture should not be performed in an arm with IV access devices, because the fluids and medications may dilute or alter the specimen. Use the other arm.

If a patient has had a mastectomy on one side, avoid drawing blood from that arm. Once lymph tissue has been surgically removed, the lymph fluid does not move and remains static, a condition known as **lymphostasis**. To decrease risk of infection, use the opposite arm for venipuncture.

An arm with edema due to other causes should also be avoided because the fluid causing the edema may alter test results.

Sites with altered skin integrity should be avoided. This would include:

• Rashes
• Incisions or sutures
• Lesions
• Burns

Figure 34-1 Superficial veins of the forearm.

- Cephalic vein
- Basilic vein
- Median cubital vein
- Accessory cephalic vein
- Medial antebrachial vein

Figure 34-2 Superficial veins of the hand.

- Cephalic vein
- Basilic vein
- Dorsal venous arch
- Metacarpal veins
- Digital veins

- Severely macerated or softened, weeping skin
- New tattoos
- Abrasions
- Edema
- Contusions

To insert a needle in these areas might increase the risk of infection. To draw from an edematous area can result in dilution of the blood sample with serous tissue fluid. Do not perform venipuncture on scarred tissue, even though it is technically "intact." This includes scars from burns, trauma, surgery, and drug abuse.

Veins that are **tortuous**, or have many twists and turns, and veins that are **sclerosed**, which means that they feel hard and ropey, should not be used for venipuncture. These conditions can result in decreased blood flow through the area, which could alter the test results. Also avoid sections of veins where valves can be palpated to prevent damaging the valves.

Knowledge Connection

What is the first vein of choice to use for phlebotomy? The second choice? What veins or sites should be avoided?

Finding a Vein

When inspecting an arm or hand for detection of a vein to use for venipuncture, what you can *see* is not as pertinent as what you can *feel*. Selection of a vein should be based upon how the vein feels, not how it looks. Before palpating for a vein, apply a tourniquet around the upper arm several inches proximal to the antecubital area. A **tourniquet** is a rubber strap that can be snugly wrapped around the arm to occlude the venous return of blood toward the heart. This causes the vein to distend so that it may be better visualized and palpated. More description of tourniquets will be found later in this chapter under Equipment and Supplies.

Use your index or middle finger to palpate the skin over the areas of the arms or hands where you know the veins are located. Avoid using your thumb to palpate because it is less sensitive. A good vein will be elastic and feel bouncy when palpated. The vein should feel soft, not sclerosed. Feel for the shape and direction of the vein. The size of the vein, of course, is important—the larger the better. Box 34-1 provides a description of how you can learn to locate veins with your eyes closed.

Locating and Accessing Difficult Veins

Sometimes it is difficult to locate a suitable vein for phlebotomy or to access it once a vein is selected. Some of the situations in which this may occur include:

- Obesity
- Dehydration
- Tiny, fragile veins
- Rolling or collapsing veins

Box 34-1

Finding a Vein With Your Eyes Closed

While learning what a vein "feels like," a good exercise to improve your sensitivity to the feel is to practice with your eyes closed.

- Hold the hand and forearm of a classmate and close your eyes. The classmate will serve as your eyes while you get used to the feel of a vein versus the feel of an area without a palpable vein.
- Lightly bounce your index or middle finger up and down repeatedly on the skin surface, moving across the dorsal side of the hand, where the veins are usually the most easily detected. As you detect the difference in the elasticity and bounce indicating a vein, your partner can verify whether you are over a vein or not.
- After feeling the veins of the hand, move up the arm toward the wrist, then the forearm, and finally to the antecubital areas where the veins are usually not as prominent as they are on the hands.
- Then trade positions with the classmate and allow the classmate to feel while you serve as the eyes.

This exercise will also be useful when you learn to initiate IV access for infusion of fluids and PRN locks in Chapter 38.

Here are a few tips to try in these situations:

- Let gravity assist in filling the veins. Position the patient in such a way that the proposed arm is able to hang dependent, below the level of the heart, for several minutes.
- Apply warm packs. As you learned in Chapter 18, heat dilates veins, allowing more blood to fill them. A warm, wet towel can be applied to the arm and covered with plastic wrap to help hold the heat. Leave in place for 5 to 10 minutes.
- Use a blood pressure (BP) cuff to distend the veins. Asking the patient to clench and unclench his or her fist once or twice may also help, but avoid continuous opening and closing of the hand because it can alter the results of certain tests.
- Use an alcohol swab and apply rubbing friction to the area in an attempt to stimulate the vein to distend.
- Gently tap the site with your fingertips, but avoid slapping the skin because it stings and is very uncomfortable for the patient.

If the patient is obese, it may be very difficult to palpate a suitable vein through all the tissue. To exert adequate pressure to occlude the veins deep in the tissue will require the rather tight application of a tourniquet. If the tourniquet must be applied tighter than usual or the patient's skin is fragile, apply the tourniquet over the gown sleeve to reduce skin tears and discomfort.

If the vein rolls, use the index finger and thumb of your nondominant hand to anchor the vein both above and below the intended insertion site while making the puncture. If the veins are tiny, fragile, or collapsing, use a winged infusion set with a syringe, rather than an evacuated tube system in which the vacuum may be too strong for a fragile vein. Once access has been gained, pull back on the syringe plunger very gently and slowly to decrease the risk of rupturing or collapsing the vein. These different types of equipment are discussed later in this chapter.

The best antecubital vein to feel for is the median cubital vein, which is normally the most prominent, followed by the basilic and the cephalic veins. If you are unable to locate a vein in the antecubital area, try the hands and wrists. Most of all, be patient. Allow time for the heat, gravity, tapping, and friction to do their work. Be certain to remove the tourniquet frequently to avoid damage to tissue and veins.

Knowledge Connection
Which sense is most important in locating a suitable vein for phlebotomy, sight or sensation? List several tips that you can use when having trouble locating or accessing a vein.

Cleansing the Site

You have learned sterile technique in previous chapters and will be required to put it to use again when performing phlebotomy. You will cleanse the selected site with 70% isopropyl alcohol or chlorhexidine, or another bacteriostatic solution according to facility policy. Remember that, when drawing a specimen for blood alcohol level, alcohol should not be used to cleanse the site. Use povidone-iodine (Betadine) for cleansing the site prior to drawing blood for cultures and arterial blood gas analysis. Clean the site starting at the point where you intend to pierce the skin with the sterile needle, and moving outward in concentric circles until an area of 2 to 3 inches has been cleansed. Once you wipe the skin of the next larger concentric circle, do not go back over the previously cleansed center with the same antiseptic wipe, as this will bring contamination from the outer edges back to the center of the "cleansed" area. Make concentric circles small and tight so that you do not leave dry, contaminated areas between the circles where you cleansed. Allow the site to dry before making the initial puncture. When drawing blood for blood cultures and arterial blood gases, if you have excess povidone-iodine on the site, you may wipe if off using *only* a *sterile* gauze pad, such as a 2×2-inch gauze pad. The sterility of the needle must be preserved throughout the phlebotomy process.

Equipment and Supplies

A variety of access devices can be used for phlebotomy, each having its own advantages. The three types we will discuss include the evacuated tube system, syringe and needle, and butterfly or winged infusion set. There are also different types of tubes that you must use. Box 34-2 presents a list of equipment used in venipuncture.

Box 34-2
Venipuncture Equipment

It saves an extraordinary amount of time and energy to gather all needed supplies and equipment prior to initiating work at the patient's bedside. Make it a habit to be prepared before beginning venipuncture. The common items you will need to perform venipuncture include the following:
- Requisition for specific laboratory tests
- Labels for collection tubes
- Examination gloves
- Alcohol or povidone-iodine wipes
- Tourniquet or BP cuff
- Either:
  - A double-pointed needle and a plastic tube holder
    OR
  - A 1-inch, 21- or 23-gauge needle or a butterfly infusion set and a syringe
- Specific collection tubes for ordered tests
- 2×2-inch gauze pad
- 1-inch tape or bandage
- Plastic zippered or sealable bags for transportation of blood samples to laboratory

Requisition
A physician's order is required for each laboratory test to be done. When the order is noted, a laboratory requisition is completed that contains the patient's name and identifiers, the test to be performed, the ordering physician's name, and other data required by facility policy. Be certain to review the order and requisition prior to performing a blood draw.

Evacuated Tube System
To use the evacuated tube system, you will need a double-pointed needle, an evacuated tube, and a plastic barrel-shaped holder, which are diagrammed in Figure 34-3. The **evacuated tube** is a plastic or glass tube closed with a colored rubber stopper or a rubber stopper surrounded by a colored plastic top, from which a certain amount of air has been evacuated. Evacuation of the air leaves a vacuum inside the tube that will cause blood to flow into the tube once the tube is activated; the volume of blood that enters the tube equals the specific volume of air that was evacuated. The tube is activated by pushing the rubber stopper onto the sheathed pointed end of the needle that has been screwed into the plastic holder.

The rubber stoppers are color coded according to the type of additive the tube contains. Each laboratory test has a designated tube-top color and additive that must be used when drawing the blood sample (Fig. 34-4).

Needles
Needles come in different lengths from ½ to 2 inches. The common lengths used for phlebotomy vary from ½ inch for a newborn to 1½ inches for an obese adult. The diameter of the needle is known as the *gauge* of the needle. They range from 16 gauge to 30 gauge; remember that the larger the

Double-pointed Needle

Rubber-sheathed pointed end that pierces rubber stopper of evacuated tube

Safety device: covers needle after use

Needle bevel: pierces vein

Screws into plastic tube holder

Shaft of needle

A

Plastic Tube Holder

Luer-lock: needle screws in here

Tube goes in here

Phlange

Barrel

B

Evacuated Tube

Tube with vacuum pulls blood from vein into tube

Rubber stopper: Rubber-sheathed needle end inserts here

C

Assembled Evacuated Tube System

D

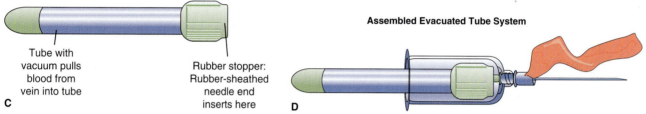

Figure 34-3 A. Double-pointed needle that screws into plastic tube holder; one end pierces the evacuated sample tube and the other end pierces the vein. B. Plastic tube holder into which the double-pointed needle will screw and that holds the evacuated tube. C. Evacuated sample tube that sits within the plastic tube holder; the rubber stopper top is pierced by the double-pointed needle, and the blood sample is pulled into the tube. D. Three pieces assembled and ready for use.

number, the smaller the size. Most phlebotomy is performed using between 20-gauge and 23-gauge needles. Preserve the sterility of the needle throughout the phlebotomy process. *Safety: Needles are used only once! Never restick a patient using the same needle.*

To use the evacuated tubes, you will need a special double-pointed needle designed solely for the evacuated tube system. One end of the needle is covered with a rubber sheath that screws into the needle end of the plastic tube holder. The other end of the needle is the portion that will be inserted into the patient's vein. Figure 34-5 shows the parts of a double-pointed needle compared to those of a regular hypodermic needle.

Plastic Tube Holder

You will also need a plastic tube holder, a round barrel that has a small opening on one end into which the needle is screwed, and that is open on the other end, allowing insertion of the evacuated tube (refer to Fig. 34-3). The tube is loosely inserted into the holder while the actual venipuncture is made. Then, once the needle tip is inside the patient's vein, the evacuated tube is activated by carefully pushing the rubber stopper of the tube onto the sheathed end of the needle. This movement forces the rubber sheath to scrunch up against the hub of the needle. Pushing the tube onto the needle activates the vacuum in the tube so that it will pull blood from the vein into the tube. Most plastic tube holders are designed to be disposed of after a single use to reduce risk of cross-contamination.

The advantage of this system is its ease of use and reduced risk of needle-stick injuries, especially when drawing blood for multiple tests. The contaminated needle is left uncapped, with the safety device engaged, and disposed of in a sharps container, which is made of hard plastic that is impervious to puncture by needles (Fig. 34-6). *Safety: Always use safety needles. Never recap a contaminated needle. Activate the safety device as soon as you withdraw the needle from the patient's arm (Fig. 34-7).*

Needle-and-Syringe Method

The vacuum in the evacuated tube system may be too strong and cause vein collapse of the smaller and more fragile veins in the elderly and children. For these veins, it may work better to use a needle and a syringe for venipuncture (Fig. 34-8). The syringe will allow you to control the rate at which the blood is pulled from the vein. The slower the extraction of the blood, the less chance there is of vein collapse. A small needle, such as a 1-inch length, 22- or 23-gauge needle, can be used for this method. Anything smaller can destroy the RBCs, releasing the hemoglobin and cellular contents into the plasma. This destruction of RBCs is known as **hemolysis**. A larger needle gauge, such as an 18- or 20-gauge needle, is then used to transfer the blood sample from the syringe into the evacuated tube so that it can be sent to the laboratory. The needle is inserted into the evacuated tube at an angle, and positioned so that the blood will run gently down one side of the tube in an effort to prevent hemolysis. Because of the extra handling of the blood specimen by having to

BD Vacutainer® Venous Blood Collection Tube Guide

Tubes with BD Hemogard™ Closure	Tubes with Conventional Stopper	Additive	Inversions at Blood Collection*	Laboratory Use
Gold	Red/Black	• Clot activator and gel for serum separation	5	For serum determinations in chemistry. May be used for routine blood donor screening and diagnostic testing of serum for infectious disease.** Tube inversions ensure mixing of clot activator with blood. Blood clotting time: 30 minutes.
Light Green	Green/Gray	• Lithium heparin and gel for plasma separation	8	BD Vacutainer® PST™ Tube for plasma determinations in chemistry. Tube inversions prevent clotting.
Red	Red	• None (glass) • Clot activator (plastic)	0 5	For serum determinations in chemistry. May be used for routine blood donor screening and diagnostic testing of serum for infectious disease.** Tube inversions ensure mixing of clot activator with blood. Blood clotting time: 60 minutes.
Orange	Gray/Yellow	• Thrombin	8	For stat serum determinations in chemistry. Tube inversions ensure complete clotting, which usually occurs in less than 5 minutes.
Royal Blue		• Clot activator (plastic serum) • K$_2$EDTA (plastic)	8 8 0 5 8	For trace-element, toxicology, and nutritional chemistry determinations. Special stopper formulation provides low levels of trace elements (see package insert).
Green		• Sodium heparin • Lithium heparin	8 8	For plasma determinations in chemistry. Tube inversions prevent clotting.
Gray		• Potassium oxalate/sodium fluoride • Sodium fluoride/Na$_2$ EDTA • Sodium fluoride (serum tube)	8 8 8	For glucose determinations. Oxalate and EDTA anticoagulants will give plasma samples. Sodium fluoride is the antiglycolytic agent. Tube inversions ensure proper mixing of additive and blood.
Tan		• K$_2$EDTA (plastic)	8 8	For lead determinations. This tube is certified to contain less than .01 µg/mL (ppm) lead. Tube inversions prevent clotting.
	Yellow	• Sodium polyanethol sulfonate (SPS) • Acid citrate dextrose additives (ACD): Solution A - 22.0 g/L trisodium citrate, 8.0 g/L citric acid, 24.5 g/L dextrose Solution B - 13.2 g/L trisodium citrate, 4.8 g/L citric acid, 14.7 g/L dextrose	8 8 8	SPS for blood culture specimen collections in microbiology. Tube inversions prevent clotting. ACD for use in blood bank studies, HLA phenotyping, and DNA and paternity testing.
Lavender		• Liquid K$_3$EDTA (glass) • Spray-coated K$_2$EDTA (plastic)	8 8	K$_2$EDTA and K$_3$EDTA for whole blood hematology determinations. K$_2$EDTA may be used for routine immunohematology testing and blood donor screening.*** Tube inversions prevent clotting.
White		• K$_2$EDTA with gel	8	For use in molecular diagnostic test methods (such as but not limited to polymerase chain reaction [PCR] and/or branched DNA [bDNA] amplification techniques).
Pink		• Spray-coated K$_2$EDTA	8	For whole blood hematology determinations. May be used for routine immunohematology testing and blood donor screening.*** Designed with special cross-match label for patient information required by the AABB. Tube inversions prevent clotting.
Light Blue	Clear	• Buffered sodium citrate 0.105 M (3.2%) glass 0.109 M (3.2%) plastic • Citrate, theophylline, adenosine, dipyridamole (CTAD)	3-4 3-4	For coagulation determinations. CTAD for platelet function assays and routine coagulation determination. Tube inversions prevent clotting.
Clear	Red/Gray	• None (plastic)	0	For use as a discard tube or secondary specimen collection tube.

Partial-draw Tubes (2 ml and 3 mL: 13 x 75 mm)	Additive	Inversions at Blood Collection*	Laboratory Use
Red	• None	0	For serum determinations in chemistry. May be used for routine blood donor screening, immunohematology testing,*** and diagnostic testing of serum for infectious disease.** Tube inversions ensure mixing of clot activator with blood. Blood clotting time: 60 minutes.
Green	• Sodium heparin • Lithium heparin	8 8	For plasma determinations in chemistry. Tube inversions prevent clotting.
Lavender	• Spray-coated K$_2$EDTA (plastic)	8 8	For whole blood hematology determinations. May be used for routine immunohematology testing and blood donor screening.*** Tube inversions prevent clotting.

Small-volume Pediatric Tubes (2 mL: 10.25 x 47 mm, 3 mL: 10.25 x 64 mm)	Additive	Inversions at Blood Collection*	Laboratory Use
Light Blue	• 0.105 M sodium citrate (3.2%)	3-4	For coagulation determinations. Tube inversions prevent clotting.

* Invert gently, do not shake

** The performance characteristics of these tubes have not been established for infectious disease testing in general; therefore, users must validate the use of these tubes for their specific assay-instrument/reagent system combinations and specimen storage conditions.

*** The performance characteristics of these tubes have not been established for immunohematology testing in general; therefore, users must validate the use of these tubes for their specific assay-instrument/reagent system combinations and specimen storage conditions.

BD Tube Guide. Courtesy and © 2008 Becton, Dickinson and Company.

Figure 34-4 BD Vacutainer Tube Guide.

Hypodermic Needle for Injections

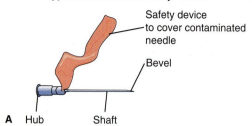

Double-pointed Needle for use with the Evacuated Tube System for Phlebotomy

Figure 34-5   A. Hypodermic needle for injections. B. Double-pointed needle for use with evacuated tube system for phlebotomy.

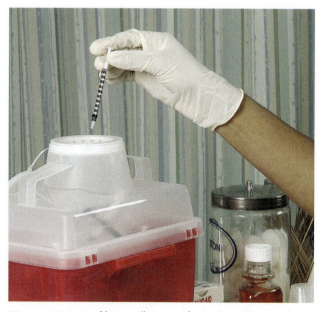

Figure 34-6   Always dispose of needles, glass, and other "sharps" in clearly labeled sharps containers; these must be puncture proof and clearly marked, and typically are red so they are easily identified.

transfer it from the syringe to an evacuated tube, there is an increased risk for needle sticks. *Safety: Always use safety needles. Activate the safety device immediately after withdrawing the needle from the tube into which you transferred the blood sample.*

Butterfly or Winged Infusion Sets

The butterfly or winged infusion set is especially useful for small or fragile veins (Fig. 34-9). The needle size may vary from 21 to 23 gauge and from ½ to ⅝ inch in length. The

Figure 34-7   Activate the safety device immediately to reduce risk of contaminated needle-stick injuries.

needle has two rubber wings at the base that fold upward to allow for easy holding. Tiny tubing extends from the needle for 6 to 8 inches and attaches to either a plastic holder or a Luer-Lok syringe. The advantage is that having the syringe farther from the needle allows for easier maneuvering. The winged needle also allows for stabilization of the needle with a piece of tape, making it ideal for use with children or elderly adults. The winged infusion sets also come with safety devices attached to the needle, which should be activated immediately after withdrawing the needle from the patient's skin.

Knowledge Connection

Beside wearing gloves, what steps should you take to protect yourself from possible contact with blood during phlebotomy? How do you activate an evacuated tube? What is hemolysis? What can cause hemolysis?

Tubes with Color-coded Tops

As mentioned previously, the tops of phlebotomy tubes are color-coded to designate the combination of additives that are within the tube. These additives are specific to certain laboratory tests, so that the different colored tops indicate different laboratory tests. Each manufacturer uses slightly different colors and additives. At the facility where you work, you will need to memorize the colors and the tests for which they are used. Table 34-1 lists tube-top colors and some of their designated tests.

Besides using aseptic technique, the order of draw is the most important aspect of phlebotomy. Additives from tubes that are drawn first can contaminate the subsequently drawn blood samples, requiring that certain tubes be drawn in a designated sequence. The color of tubes most commonly used should be drawn in the following order, unless the facility has a different policy that would override this sequence:

• **Yellow tubes or blood culture bottles:** used for blood specimens that must remain sterile during performance of test
• **Red:** no additives

Figure 34-8   Parts of a syringe and needle.

Figure 34-9   A butterfly infusion set.

- **Light blue:** contains sodium citrate
- **Red tiger-striped:** contains clot activators
- **Green:** contains heparin
- **Lavender:** contains EDTA, an anticoagulant
- **Gray:** contains sodium fluoride, an antiglycolytic agent
- **Orange or yellow/gray:** contains thrombin clot activator

Labels

All specimens must be labeled before sending them to the laboratory. Some facilities use computer-generated labels, while others use handwritten labels. If the label is to be written, use black ink or permanent marker. The labels should never be completed or applied before the specimen is drawn, nor should the label be attached after leaving the room. *Safety: The label should be completely filled out and attached to the collection tube in the patient's room after drawing the blood specimen.* Completion of the label and attachment to the collection tubes *before* actually obtaining the specimen allows for two errors to occur:

1. The labeled collection tube may be used for drawing blood from the wrong patient.
2. Completing the label ahead of time may lead to inaccuracy regarding time of draw.

Box 34-3 presents the required data for labeling specimens.

Tourniquet

There are several types of tourniquets made of rubber about 1 inch wide and 16 to 18 inches long. Some are designed to tie around the limb using a quick-release tie method, while

Table 34-1   Evacuated Tube-top Colors, Draw Sequence, and Designated Tests

Draw Sequence	Tube-top Color	Tests
1st	Yellow or blood culture bottles	Blood culture
2nd	Red	Chemistry tests, serology, blood bank
3rd	Light blue	Coagulation tests such as partial thromboplastin time (PTT), prothrombin time (PT)
4th	Red tiger-striped	Digoxin and other medication levels, vitamin B_{12}, folate, alcohol
5th	Green	Ammonia, stat electrolytes, arterial blood gases
6th	Lavender	Complete blood count (CBC), crossmatch, sedimentation rate
7th	Gray	Glucose, lactic acid, blood alcohol level
8th	Orange or yellow/gray	Stat serum chemistry

Box 34-3
Required Data for Labeling Specimens

Avoid labeling blood specimen tubes prior to the blood draw to reduce inaccuracy of time the blood specimen was drawn and inadvertently mismatching the labels to another patient's blood specimen tubes. There may be more than one patient with the same name, so be careful to include all needed identifying data. The label should include the following information:

- Patient's first and last name
- Hospital identification number
- Room number
- Physician's name
- Type of test ordered
- Date specimen was collected
- Time specimen was collected
- Your initials

others use Velcro to hold the ends. The rubber strap is placed around the limb 3 to 4 inches above the site you intend to stick. The loose ends of the tourniquet should dangle proximal to the tied portion of the tourniquet to avoid contaminating the needle insertion site. The tourniquet is applied tight enough to occlude the superficial veins that you will be using, but should allow blood to flow in the deeper arteries. This is assessed by ensuring that there is a palpable pulse distal to the tourniquet. For example, if using the antecubital site for drawing blood, the tourniquet should be placed about 3 to 4 inches above the antecubital area and there should be a palpable radial pulse. *Safety: The tourniquet should never be left in place for longer than 1 minute.* Leaving it on longer can cause hemolysis or **hemoconcentration**, a concentration of RBCs in the blood sample due to a decrease in the volume of plasma allowed to flow. If the tourniquet is applied too tightly, it can result in pinpoint areas of hemorrhage, known as **petechiae**, or cause bruises, called **hematomas**.

In patients whose veins are difficult to locate or are fragile, as is common in elderly patients, a sphygmomanometer or BP cuff can be used in place of a tourniquet. It allows for a more even distribution of the pressure applied to the arm to occlude the venous return. This prevents *rupture* or *"blowing"* of tiny and fragile veins. It also allows for better distention of the distal veins. The cuff is pumped above the diastolic pressure but below the systolic pressure. This is accomplished by palpating the radial pulse while inflating the cuff. Continue to inflate the cuff until the pulse is no longer felt, then deflate the cuff to the point where you can again feel the pulse. Tighten the screw valve at this point and proceed with the venipuncture.

Gloves

Nonsterile examination gloves are always worn when performing phlebotomy due to the risk of contact with blood, and are mandated by the Occupational Safety and Health Administration (OSHA). The gloves should fit tightly enough to aid with vein detection using your fingertips. *Safety: Always wash your hands before application and after removal of gloves. Change gloves between patients to avoid cross-contamination.*

Knowledge Connection

When should tubes of blood be labeled? What data should be on the label? How long can you safely leave a tourniquet on a patient's arm?

Performing Venipuncture

Once you have located a vein using the tourniquet, remove the tourniquet while you cleanse the site and make certain all supplies are positioned within easy reach. Some individuals prefer to apply clean examination gloves prior to cleansing the intended puncture site, while others prefer to apply the gloves after cleansing the site, giving the site time to dry. Using either alcohol or an antiseptic designated by facility policy, cleanse the site starting in the center and making concentric circles outward, until a 2-inch area has been prepared. Allow the site to dry. Make certain the site is not touched while it is drying and during reapplication of the tourniquet. If the site is accidentally contaminated before the skin puncture is made, the site must be cleansed again.

Reapply the tourniquet 3 to 4 inches above or proximal to the proposed site, tucking the tourniquet from the top so that the ends will not flop onto the cleansed area. (See Skill 34-1, page 818, for more on applying a tourniquet.) Aseptically uncap the needle. Hold the plastic tube holder or syringe in your dominant hand, with the needle bevel facing upward, your thumb on top, and your fingers underneath the holder to allow you to press fingers against the patient's arm for stabilization while changing tubes.

Use the thumb of your nondominant hand to hold tension, or traction, on the selected vein from a distal position, leaving adequate room to position the needle at an angle of 15 to 30 degrees without contaminating the needle. If the vein is shallow, use 15 degrees, and if the vein is deeper, increase the angle as needed up to 30 degrees. Make the skin puncture in a swift, smooth motion to decrease discomfort. As the needle enters the vein, you may feel a small *popping* or *giving* sensation or simply a lessening of resistance against the needle. If the vein is not successfully accessed with the initial puncture, *do not probe blindly.* Use the index finger of your nondominant hand to carefully palpate the vein proximal to the tip of the inserted needle to determine where the needle tip is in relationship to the vein. If the needle is not in the vein, it must be in one of four positions: either it is above the vein, to the right of the vein, below the vein, or to the left of the vein. You need to assess the position of both vein and needle tip to determine in which direction you need to move the needle. Blind probing with the needle in an attempt to find the vein is painful and can cause tissue damage or hematoma formation. While palpating, take care not to contaminate the needle or the needle insertion site. Once you have determined the relative position of the vein and needle, redirect the needle to enter the vein.

Once the needle enters the vein, press your fingers that are holding the plastic tube holder or syringe firmly against the patient's arm. Then use your nondominant hand to gently push the evacuated tube onto the needle. Use the index and middle fingers to grasp the barrel phlange and push the end of the tube onto the needle with your thumb, taking care not to push the needle through the other side of the vein. The evacuated tube will stop filling at a predesignated volume. If using a syringe, use your nondominant hand to slowly pull back on the plunger, allowing the syringe to fill to the required amount. Pulling the plunger back too quickly may result in collapsing the vein or hemolysis of RBCs.

When more than one tube is required, keep in mind the correct order of draw. As each tube is filled, continue to keep your dominant hand braced against the patient's arm while using your nondominant hand to gently remove the tube from the holder, place the next tube into the holder, and carefully push it onto the needle. Avoid moving the needle while removing or advancing the tube onto the needle. While the last tube is filling, remove the tourniquet. If tied correctly, this is accomplished by a gentle tug on the tucked end of the tourniquet. Remember that the tourniquet should stay on the arm no longer than 1 minute.

Once the last tube has filled completely, remove it from the holder, and withdraw the needle from the patient's arm. Immediately apply a 2×2-inch gauze pad to hold pressure on the puncture site. Activate the needle safety device promptly. Gently invert the tubes of blood two to three times. Avoid shaking the tubes.

Hold pressure on the site for a full 1 to 2 minutes until the bleeding stops, or longer if needed. It is best to refrain from *peeking* or lifting the gauze to see if the bleeding has stopped until at least 1 minute has passed. If you withdrew multiple tubes of blood or the patient is known to have a tendency to bleed longer, it may be helpful to have the patient elevate the arm above the heart level while holding direct pressure on the puncture site. Do not allow the patient to flex the elbow to hold the pressure on the site, as it tends to increase hematoma formation. The bleeding should always stop within a maximum of 3 to 5 minutes unless the patient is on anticoagulants, which may require you to hold pressure on the site for 10 minutes or longer. Do not be impatient, even though you may be very busy. After the bleeding has stopped, secure the gauze pad to the site with a piece of tape or a small bandage. Some facility policies dictate that a self-adhering wrap is to be wrapped around to the site to maintain pressure on the site for a longer period of time. Instruct the patient that the tape, bandage, or wrap should be removed after 1 to 2 hours.

Complete and inspect the labels for accuracy of information. Then attach the labels to each tube before leaving the patient's side to avoid accidental mismatching of specimens and patient labels. Place the specimens inside a designated container such as a plastic bag, along with the laboratory requisition, for transport to the laboratory. Dispose of contaminated items in the appropriate sharps container. Remove gloves and wash your hands. The specimens should be immediately transported to the laboratory. Document the procedure.

Skill 34-2 (page 819) details the steps in performing venipuncture.

Knowledge Connection

Describe the process of drawing a blood specimen. Where are contaminated items disposed of?

Laboratory and Diagnostic Connection

Drawing Blood Culture Specimens

Normally the blood is sterile within the vascular system. But when it is suspected that the patient has an infection in his or her blood, otherwise known as **septicemia**, blood specimens may be drawn to determine if organisms are present in the blood, and if so, which specific organism is the culprit. This test is known as a **blood culture**. Blood culture specimens are normally drawn during temperature spikes to better detect if organisms are present in the blood. When blood cultures are ordered, special care must be taken when drawing the blood specimen to ensure that no contamination of the specimen occurs.

Blood culture specimens are usually drawn in two separate long-necked bottles that fit into the plastic tube holder and advance onto the sheathed end of the needle. The first one that is drawn is used to determine if **anaerobic** organisms are present. Anaerobes are organisms that can live and replicate without oxygen. The second specimen drawn is for **aerobic** organisms, or those that grow and replicate in the presence of oxygen. When drawing blood culture specimens, it is critical to maintain asepsis and to also draw the correct volume of blood. Always check the facility policy for volume of blood to be drawn for the specific type of specimen bottles used. Skill 34-3 (page 821) details the steps in collecting a blood culture specimen.

Complications of Phlebotomy

Several complications may occur during phlebotomy. Leakage of blood out of the vein into the tissue around the needle insertion site will result in a hematoma. Care must be taken to remove the tourniquet prior to removing the needle from the vein, and pressure must be held over the puncture site for at least 1 to 2 minutes. Pressure should be routinely held

3 to 5 minutes on patients who are on anticoagulants, and up to 10 minutes if necessary. If a hematoma does form, it may ease the discomfort to apply a cold cloth or small ice pack. *Safety: Do not have the patient "bend the elbow" in an effort to keep pressure on the site.* Research shows that this increases the bleeding and bruising at the site. Ask the patient to raise the arm above the heart in an outstretched position, holding pressure on the gauze pad with the non-dominant hand, to decrease bleeding into the tissues after a blood draw.

When performing phlebotomy, the patient should be lying supine or sitting in the high Fowler's position. *Safety: Never draw blood from a standing patient.* If the patient complains of feeling faint, light-headed, or nauseated, the patient becomes pale, or the skin becomes cold and clammy, offer a cold cloth or compress to apply to the forehead and neck. Lower the head of the bed or, if the patient is sitting, have the patient lie down or put his or her head between the knees. If the patient experiences syncope during the blood draw, immediately remove the tourniquet and needle, holding pressure on the site.

Failure to obtain blood can be the result of several problems, which can be fixed as follows:

• **The needle is not in the vein:** Palpate the vein proximal to the needle and redirect the needle.
• **The needle is against a valve or wall of the vein:** Pull back on or rotate the needle slightly.
• **The evacuated tube has lost its vacuum:** Insert another tube.
• **The vein has collapsed because of use of an evacuated tube that was too large or pulling the plunger of the syringe back too quickly:** Remove the evacuated tube or cease pulling back on the syringe plunger. Remove the tourniquet to allow additional blood flow to the arm. Reapply the tourniquet and use a smaller tube or draw back on the syringe plunger more slowly.

If these attempts to fix the problem fail, remove the needle and perform venipuncture in the other arm using a fresh sterile needle. *Safety: Never use the same needle to make a second needle stick.*

Knowledge Connection
What are possible complications of phlebotomy? What nursing actions should you take to reduce risk of these complications? If they do occur, what should you do?

Skin Punctures

Skin or dermal punctures are a simpler way to obtain blood specimens for some tests, are used when veins are inaccessible, and are the preferred method of obtaining blood specimens from children younger than age 2 years. The site for

puncture in children older than age 2 years and adults is the fleshy portion just to the side of the center of the fingertip. Avoid the tip end of the finger as well as the sides, where there is less flesh between the skin and the bone. Do not puncture the index finger due to its high number of nerve endings, which makes puncturing it more painful. The pinkie finger has less flesh and is rarely used except on severely calloused hands, such as a farmer or oil field worker might have. Sometimes badly calloused hands will not bleed easily with a skin puncture. In this situation, the pinkie finger may be pierced because it is less calloused and will generally bleed better.

In children younger than 2 years, the heel is used rather than a fingertip. The puncture should be made on the medial and lateral aspects of the fleshy portion of the plantar surface of the heel. Avoid piercing the posterior edge or sides of the heel where the skin is closer to the calcaneus bone.

The skin is punctured using a spring-loaded lancet that is self-limiting regarding the depth and width of the puncture. The blood is dripped into a micro-collection tube or a capillary tube, or applied directly to a testing strip for a test such as a finger stick blood sugar (FSBS). Figure 34-10 shows one type of FSBS testing monitor, and Figure 34-11

Figure 34-10 Finger stick blood sugar monitor and lancet holder.

Figure 34-11 From left to right: Two styles of lancets to make skin puncture; two types of finger stick blood sugar strips upon which the drop of blood is placed; micro-collection tubes and capillary tubes in which the blood sample is placed.

shows lancets, a micro-collection tube, a capillary tube, and one type of FSBS strip.

Performing Skin Puncture

When a skin or dermal puncture is necessary, the hand to be pierced should be warmed if it is cold. This may be accomplished by washing the hands with soap and warm water or by applying a warm compress for several minutes. The heat will dilate the vessels, providing better blood flow when the skin is pierced.

Begin by cleansing the site with alcohol and allowing it to dry. Wearing gloves, hold the hand lower than the heart to allow for better capillary filling. Keep the fingertip lower than the palm of the patient's hand, holding it between your thumb and index finger. If using a spring-loaded lancet, place the device firmly against the sides of the fleshy aspect of the fingertip without pressing the device hard enough to indent the skin. Do not stick the sides or the tips of the fingers where the tissue is thin. Then press the lancet release button to activate the lancet. Wipe away the first drop of blood with sterile gauze to avoid alteration of the specimen by the dried alcohol on the skin or tissue fluid from the puncture site.

Now firmly squeeze the fingertip, alternately squeezing and releasing the pressure to express the blood sample. Avoid strenuously massaging or milking the puncture site to produce blood flow, as this can cause hemolysis and dilution of the sample with tissue fluids. If a capillary tube is being used to collect the specimen, hold the tube horizontally and touch the tip of the tube *lightly* to the drop of blood, but do not allow the tube to touch the puncture site itself. If the tube is not held horizontally, it will introduce air bubbles into the sample. When done correctly, capillary action will draw the blood into the tube. Avoid scraping the capillary tube against the skin in an attempt to collect the blood, as this can cause hemolysis. Once the tube is filled, tap the end of the capillary tube into the sealant clay to seal it.

If a micro-collection tube is used, hold the open end of the tube just beneath the dripping blood until the device is full. Then replace the cap to seal the tube.

If an FSBS is to be performed, use the designated strip for the specific monitor that will read the blood sample. Lightly touch the strip to the drop of blood, allowing capillary action to pull the blood onto the strip so that the monitor can read the glucose level. Skill 34-4 (page 822) provides more information on performing a skin puncture for an FSBS.

After collection of the blood sample, hold a 2×2-inch gauze pad over the puncture site with gentle but firm pressure to stop the bleeding. Dispose of contaminated items in the sharps container. Remove gloves and wash your hands. Document the procedure.

Figure 34-12 For infants, perform skin puncture on the lateral aspects of the plantar surface of the heel.

Figure 34-13 For older children and adults, perform skin puncture on the lateral aspects of the palmar side of the distal phalanx (fingertip).

Skill 34-1 Applying a Tourniquet

Assessment Steps

1. Assess the fragility of the patient's skin *to determine if the tourniquet should be placed over the sleeve of the patient's gown.*
2. Assess the antecubital areas of both arms *to evaluate the quality of the veins.*

Planning Steps

1. Select the vein that feels most suitable.

Implementation Steps

1. Follow the Initial Implementation Steps located on the inside front cover.
2. Place the rubber tourniquet under the upper arm, midway between the shoulder and the antecubital areas.
3. Bring the two ends around the arm and cross them over the upper arm, with the left end crossing below the right end.

4. With your left hand, grasp the tourniquet where it crosses over itself and grasp the lower tubing end with your right hand.

5. Pull the end in your right hand until it is taut and use your left hand to maintain the tension where the two ends cross.
6. Using your right hand, tuck the end of the tourniquet into the top side of the band that is now wrapped around the arm and held in place by your left hand.

7. Gently release your left hand's grasp and allow the tourniquet to tighten against the patient's arm. Both tails of the tourniquet should arise from the top of the band now surrounding the arm to prevent contamination of the site after cleansing.

Evaluation Steps

1. Evaluate if there is adequate distention of the intended vein. If so, proceed with venipuncture.

Skill 34-2 Performing Venipuncture

Assessment Steps

1. Review the physician's order *to determine the type of test for which blood is to be drawn.*
2. Obtain the requisition and compare it to the physician's order.
3. Determine whether special conditions such as fasting or specific times are required.
4. Assess the patient's veins *to determine which type of phlebotomy equipment will be best to use.*

Planning Steps

1. Gather needed equipment and supplies: tourniquet; clean gloves; alcohol sponges, chlorhexidine, or facility-specified antiseptic; laboratory requisition; correct colored-top tubes for ordered tests; labels; sterile 2×2-inch gauze pad; tape. *Gathering all needed supplies saves you time and effort.*
   - **Evacuated Tube System:** plastic tube holder, double-pointed needle or winged infusion set.
   - **Syringe and Needle System:** 5- or 10-mL syringe depending upon the amount of blood needed for the test(s), needle or winged infusion set.
2. Screw the needle or winged infusion set onto the plastic tube holder or syringe *so that it is ready to use.*

3. If more than one test is ordered, determine the order in which the tubes should be drawn.

Implementation Steps

1. Follow the Initial Implementation Steps located on the inside front cover.
2. *Safety: Wash your hands to prevent cross-contamination. This is particularly important due to the invasive nature of this skill.*
3. *Safety: Verify patient identity by checking the ID band and use a second method of identifying that this is the correct patient.*
4. Arrange supplies within arm's reach, positioned so that you do not have to turn around or lean to pick up the tubes once the needle is positioned in the vein.
5. Apply gloves.
6. Apply the tourniquet 3 to 4 inches above the intended puncture site, with the tails of the tourniquet extending from the top side *so they will not contaminate the site after cleansing it.*

7. Palpate the intended vein *to ensure that you have selected a good vein and that it is adequately distended.*
8. Cleanse the site with 70% alcohol, chlorhexidine, or as designated by facility policy. *Safety: If povidone-iodine is to be used, make certain the patient is not allergic to iodine or shellfish.*
9. Allow the site to dry for 30 seconds while you:
   - **Evacuated tube system:** Place the first tube loosely into the plastic tube holder. *Safety: Do not advance the rubber stopper onto the sheathed needle. This will result in loss of vacuum from the tube.*
   - **Needle and Syringe System:** Pull back and forth on the syringe plunger two or three times *to make certain it is not stuck.*
10. Uncap the needle. Position the needle so that the bevel is up.
11. *If you are using a winged infusion set known as a butterfly on either the plastic tube holder or syringe:* Fold the two wings just proximal to the needle upward. Hold the two wings together between your index finger and thumb.

If Using an Evacuated Tube System

12. Hold the plastic tube holder so that it rests on your fingertips and your thumb is on top of the holder, letting the tube lay loosely in the holder. If this does not feel comfortable, you may delay the insertion of the tube into the holder until you have gained access to the vein.

13. Using an angle between 15 and 30 degrees, pierce the skin in a swift, continuous motion.
14. Monitor for a slight "popping" sensation or release of resistance against the needle point, which you will feel when you enter the vein.

(skill continues on page 820)

Skill 34-2 (continued)

15. Once in the vein, brace your hand that is holding the phlebotomy device firmly against the patient's arm.

16. Using your nondominant hand, gently push the rubber stopper of the tube onto the sheathed end of the needle, using a slight pushing and twisting motion, making certain to maintain the stability of the needle *so that it will not be pushed through the vein.* Blood should begin to enter the tube.

17. When the tube stops filling, gently remove the tube from the holder with your nondominant hand, using a twisting motion as you pull the tube off the needle. Again, make certain to brace your dominant hand that is holding the plastic tube holder against the patient's arm *to stabilize the needle and prevent pulling it out of the vein.*

18. Gently invert the tube of blood two to three times and lay it aside. Pick up the next tube to be filled. Carefully repeat the process. Once the last tube is advanced onto the needle, using your nondominant hand, release the tourniquet while the tube fills.

19. When tube stops filling, remove it from holder as described above. Using your nondominant hand, place a 2 × 2-inch gauze pad over the needle insertion site while removing the needle from the patient's arm, applying firm pressure to the site immediately after the needle is withdrawn. *Safety: Immediately activate the needle safety device to prevent risk of needle stick.*

20. Place a piece of tape over the gauze pad to maintain pressure on the puncture site. You may want the patient to elevate the arm above the heart in an outstreched position, without bending the elbow, *to decrease bleeding.*

If Using a Needle and Syringe System

12. Hold the syringe so that it rests on your fingertips and your thumb is on top of the syringe.

13. Using an angle between 15 and 30 degrees, pierce the skin in a swift, continuous motion.

14. Monitor for a slight "popping" sensation or release of resistance against the needle point, which you will feel when you enter the vein.

15. Once in the vein, brace your hand that is holding the syringe firmly against the patient's arm.

16. Pull the plunger back slowly and gently begin drawing blood into the syringe. Avoid pulling the plunger back too quickly, *as this can collapse fragile veins.* Fill the syringe to the required volume.

17. Release the tourniquet using your nondominant hand.

18. Place the 2×2-inch gauze pad over the needle insertion site while quickly removing the needle from the patient's arm, applying firm pressure immediately after the needle is withdrawn. *Safety: Immediately activate the needle safety device to prevent risk of needle stick.*

19. Once bleeding has stopped, place a piece of tape over the gauze pad *to hold pressure on the site.* You may want the patient to elevate the arm above the heart in an outstreched position, without bending the elbow, *to decrease bleeding.*

20. Apply a clean 18- to 20-gauge needle to the syringe. Puncture the rubber stopper of the first tube to be filled. Enter the stopper at an angle, placing the tip of the needle against the inside of the tube to allow the blood to trickle down the side of the tube. *This helps prevent hemolysis.* The vacuum in the tube will pull the blood from the syringe, so you should not have to depress the plunger. Continue to fill the tubes in the correct order of draw.

For Either System

21. Dispose of the contaminated needle, syringe, and disposable plastic tube holder in the sharps container.

22. Label each tube of blood according to facility policy before leaving the patient's bedside. *This helps to ensure that the correct tests will be performed on the correct patient.*

23. Place specimens in a plastic bag or specified container, along with the requisition.

24. Follow the Ending Implementation Steps located on the inside back cover.

25. Deliver the specimens to the laboratory per facility policy.

Evaluation Steps

1. Reassess the puncture site to ensure that bleeding has stopped before leaving the room.

2. Remind the patient to remove the gauze pad and bandage in 1 to 2 hours.

Sample Documentation

9/19/10   1530   *Blood drawn for CBC from right antecubital and sent to the lab. Pressure dressing applied. No bleeding from site.*
——————————————— *Nurse's signature and credentials*

Skill 34-3 Collecting a Blood Culture Specimen

Assessment Steps

1. Review the physician's order *to verify the test to be performed and to determine whether the culture specimen can be drawn anytime or only during a temperature spike.*

2. Determine if blood for other laboratory tests is to be drawn at the same time as the blood culture specimen. *This may save the patient from an additional needle stick.*

3. Review facility policy regarding the correct volume of blood that is to be drawn for the blood specimens.

4. Obtain the requisition and compare it to the physician's order *to ensure correctness of order.*

5. Assess the patient's veins *to determine which type of phlebotomy equipment will be best to use.*

6. Assess whether or not the patient is allergic to povidone-iodine or shellfish. *This prevents unwarranted allergic reactions.*

Planning Steps

1. If multiple tests are ordered, plan to draw the blood culture specimen first.

2. Gather needed equipment and supplies: gloves, alcohol wipes, povidone-iodine swabs, tourniquet, double-pointed needle or winged infusion set, two evacuated tube system culture bottles, plastic holder, one clean 2×2-inch gauze pad, two sterile 2×2-inch gauze pads, labels, requisition, other tubes if further tests are to be performed. *Gathering all needed supplies saves you time and effort.*

3. Plan the sequence in which blood will be drawn. An anaerobic culture specimen is always drawn first, then an aerobic culture specimen, and then blood is drawn in the correct sequence for additional laboratory tests.

4. Screw the needle or winged infusion set onto the plastic holder *so that it is ready to use.*

5. Prepare two culture bottles. Remove the caps from each bottle. Cleanse each bottle top with at least two povidone-iodine swabs and allow to dry. Lay a sterile 2×2-inch gauze pad over each of the bottle tops.

Implementation Steps

1. Follow the Initial Implementation Steps located on the inside front cover.

2. Apply gloves *to protect yourself from blood-borne pathogens.*

3. *Safety: Verify patient identity by checking the ID band and use a second method of identifying that this is the correct patient.*

4. Apply the tourniquet and select the vein to be used.

5. Remove the tourniquet. *Safety: Avoid leaving tourniquet in place longer than 1 minute.*

6. Cleanse the site vigorously with alcohol wipes, using at least two separate wipes and cleansing at least a 2-inch circle. *This helps remove body oils from the skin's surface.*

7. Cleanse the site again using two povidone-iodine swabs if the patient is not allergic to iodine. (If allergic, cleanse the site again with a fresh alcohol wipe.)

Begin at the center and move outward in concentric circles. Allow the site to dry for 1 minute, allowing the iodine to dry. *This is necessary for the iodine to have adequate time to kill any bacteria on the skin's surface.*

8. Reapply the tourniquet, avoiding contamination of the site.

9. Wipe the tops of the bottles with the sterile 2×2-inch gauze pads *to wipe away any iodine residue.*

10. Uncap the needle. Holding the needle with bevel up and using a 15- to 30-degree angle, swiftly and smoothly insert the needle into the vein. Remember to inform the patient just prior to piercing the skin.

11. Once the needle is in the vein, use your nondominant hand to place the *anaerobic* culture bottle into the holder and push it onto the sheathed needle. Be certain to brace your dominant hand, which is holding the needle, against the patient's arm *to provide stability and prevent the needle from going through the vein.*

12. After the first bottle is filled, remove the bottle from the plastic holder and set aside.

13. Insert the *aerobic* culture bottle into the holder and gently push it onto the sheathed needle.

14. Remove the tourniquet while the second bottle is filling.

15. When the second bottle is filled, remove it from the holder.

16. Cover the puncture site with the clean 2×2-inch gauze pad and remove the needle from the patient's arm, applying firm pressure to the site as soon as the needle is withdrawn. *This prevents hematoma formation.*

17. Immediately activate the needle safety device and place the contaminated needle in the sharps container. *This helps to reduce risk of contaminated needle-stick injuries.*

18. When bleeding is stopped, apply a piece of tape over the gauze pad *to hold pressure on the puncture site.* Have the patient elevate the arm above the level of the heart *to reduce risk of hematoma formation,* but do not allow the patient to bend the arm at the elbow. *This is known to increase bleeding into the subcutaneous tissues.*

19. Complete and apply labels to both the anaerobic and aerobic specimen bottles before leaving the patient's bedside.

20. Follow the Ending Implementation Steps located on the inside back cover.

21. Transport specimens to laboratory per facility policy.

Evaluation Steps

1. Assess the site to make certain bleeding has stopped.

2. Remind the patient to remove the gauze pad and bandage in 1 to 2 hours.

Sample Documentation

3/5/11   2100   *Blood cultures drawn from left antecubital without difficulty. Specimens taken to lab. —————————————————— Nurse's signature and credentials*

Skill 34-4 Performing Skin Puncture for a Finger Stick Blood Sugar

Assessment Steps

1. Review the physician's order *to determine the type of test that is to be performed.*
2. Review the instructions for the correct use of the finger stick blood sugar monitor.

Planning Steps

1. Gather needed equipment and supplies: gloves, alcohol wipes, dry cotton balls, lancet, finger stick blood sugar monitor with correct strips, bandage, pen and paper.

Implementation Steps

1. Follow the Initial Implementation Steps located on the inside front cover.
2. Apply gloves *to protect you from blood-borne pathogens.*
3. Inquire if the patient has a preference as to which finger is pricked. *This is a simple choice that will allow the patient to feel that he or she has some control over the care received.*
4. Have the patient dangle the hand off the side of the bed or chair *to allow gravity to help fill the capillaries.* If the hand is cold, have the patient wash hands with warm water and soap *to increase blood flow to the hand.*
5. Cleanse the fingertip site with alcohol and let dry.
6. Hold the spring-loaded lancet against the fleshy fingertip pad, just slightly off-center, avoiding the very tip or the sides of the fingertip. Press the release button, causing the lancet to pierce the skin.

7. Apply gentle pressure to elicit a drop of blood, wiping away the first drop with a dry cotton ball. *This prevents the alcohol residue and tissue fluids from diluting the blood sample.*
8. Squeeze the next drop and touch the end of the monitor strip to the edge of the drop, allowing the strip to draw the blood into itself. Avoid scraping or touching the strip against the skin.

9. Use a cotton ball to hold firm pressure on the puncture site while waiting for the monitor to process the blood glucose level. Apply a bandage if the patient desires.
10. Dispose of the lancet in the sharps container.
11. Follow the Ending Implementation Steps located on the inside back cover.

Evaluation Steps

1. When the monitor produces the glucose level, write it down on paper. Do not rely on your memory.
2. Evaluate if the glucose level requires further action, such as notification of the physician or administration of insulin.

Sample Documentation

7/18/12   1630   FSBS – 213 mg/dL. Regular insulin 3 units given subcutaneously in left abdomen. —————————
————————————— Nurse's signature and credentials

🌐 Post Conference

When you met back with your instructor and fellow students, you were pleased to report that you were able to obtain all the blood specimens ordered in the physician's office. For one elderly patient, you had to try every tip you learned in this chapter, but you were finally able to get the specimen. No one fainted or even yelled, and you left feeling confident that you would be able to perform venipunctures in the future. The clinical medical assistant was very helpful and reminded you of tips to make the venipunctures and blood specimen collections easier to accomplish.

KEY POINTS

- The Joint Commission requires use of two methods to identify patients prior to procedures.
- The most common vein choice for phlebotomy is the median cubital.
- Sites where phlebotomy should be avoided include an arm with an IV, an arm on the side of a mastectomy, skin with altered integrity, scarred or edematous tissue, and tortuous or sclerosed veins.
- It is more important to be able to feel a vein than to see it.
- Use your index or middle finger to palpate for a vein.
- Tips to aid in accessing veins include application of warm moist compresses, hanging the arm dependently, applying friction using an alcohol wipe, using your finger for gentle tapping over the vein site, using a BP cuff instead of a tourniquet, and anchoring of the vein above and below the intended puncture site.
- The order of draw is yellow or culture bottles, red, light blue, red tiger-top, green, lavender, gray, and orange or yellow/gray.
- Always use safety needles. Never recap contaminated needles. Dispose of contaminated needles in the sharps container.
- Use between a 20-gauge and 23-gauge needle for phlebotomy.
- Wear gloves and maintain asepsis during phlebotomy.
- Label specimens after they are drawn, while still in the patient's room.
- Never leave a tourniquet on for longer than 1 minute.

REVIEW QUESTIONS

Select the answer that is most appropriate for each of the following questions. Some questions may have more than one correct answer. Check all that apply.

1. When selecting a vein for phlebotomy, which of the following are true?

   a. Use the vein that looks the largest, no matter what its condition.

   b. Avoid areas where the vein is crooked or feels hard and rope-like.

   c. The site of choice is the dorsal side of the hand.

   d. Use the right arm of a patient who has had a left mastectomy.

   e. Use the right arm of a patient who has an IV in the right arm.

2. Which of the following needle sizes would be an appropriate choice to use for phlebotomy in a 45-year-old patient?

   a. 16 gauge

   b. 19 gauge

   c. 21 gauge

   d. 23 gauge

   e. 30 gauge

3. The tourniquet should be applied where in relation to the intended puncture site?

   a. 6 inches distal to the site

   b. 3 inches distal to the site

   c. 6 inches proximal to the site

   d. 3 inches proximal to the site

4. A "good" vein for phlebotomy should meet which of the following criteria?

   a. It should feel bouncy.

   b. It should feel rigid.

   c. It should feel knobby.

   d. It should feel elastic.

5. When performing phlebotomy using a needle and syringe, drawing back on the plunger can result in which of the following complications?

   a. Collapse of vein

   b. Hematoma

   c. Infection of site

   d. Rolling the vein

   e. Blowing the vein

6. Activation of the needle safety device should occur when?

   a. Before the initial stick.

   b. During the draw of blood.

   c. Immediately after the tourniquet is released.

   d. As soon as the needle is withdrawn.

   e. After placing tape over the puncture site.

TRUE OR FALSE

7. Phlebotomy may be performed distal to an IV infusion.

8. Hemolysis results from drawing too large a volume of blood for a blood culture.

9. Electrolytes should be drawn before a CBC.

10. Light blue–topped tubes are used to draw blood for coagulation tests.

11. Each tube should be labeled with the patient's name, room number, date, and test to be done prior to drawing the blood to help prevent errors.

SHORT ANSWER QUESTIONS

12. Which test, when ordered, must always be drawn first when multiple tests are to be drawn?

13. When performing a finger stick blood sugar test, what do you do with the first drop of blood?

CRITICAL THINKING EXERCISE

14. Explain steps you should take to avoid hemolysis.

ADDITIONAL RESOURCES

For additional Resources, Questions, and Activities, please see:

Student Resource Disk

DavisPlus **http://davisplus.fadavis.com**

Student Study Guide

REFERENCES

Di Lorenzo MS, Strasinger SK. *Blood Collection: A Short Course*. 2nd ed. Philadelphia: FA Davis; 2010.

Garza D, Becan-McBride K. *Phlebotomy Simplified*. Upper Saddle River, NJ: Prentice Hall Professional Technical Reference; 2007.

Hoeltke LB. *The Complete Textbook of Phlebotomy*. 3rd ed. Clifton Park, NY: Cengage Learning; 2005.

Jewell S, Medves J, Duhn L, Boomhower K, Barrett JA, Rivoire E. Implementation and evaluation of a best practice initiative: venipuncture in the well baby. *Adv Neonatal Care*. 2007;7:222-229.

Leitch A, McCormick I, Gunn I, Gillespie T. Reducing the potential for phlebotomy tourniquets to act as a reservoir for methycillin-resistant staphylococcus aureus. *J Hosp Infect*. 2006;63:428-431.

Levine E, Budzikowski AS. Catheterization, axillary vein. Updated February 27, 2009. Available at: http://emedicine.medscape.com/article/1348912-print. Accessed November 13, 2009.

Rhoades J, Meeker J. *Davis's Guide to Clinical Nursing Skills*. Philadelphia: FA Davis; 2007.

U.S. Department of Labor, Occupational Safety and Health Administration. Enforcement procedures for the occupational exposure to blood-born pathogens. Directive CPL 2-2.69, November 2001. Available at: http://www.osha.gov/OshDoc/Directive_pdf/CPL_2-2_69.pdf. Accessed November 13, 2009.

Warekois RS, Robinson R. *Phlebotomy Worktext and Procedures Manual*. 2nd ed. Philadelphia: Elsevier Health Sciences; 2007.

Wener K. Venipuncture test. June 9, 2005. Available at: http://healthguide.howstuffworks.com/venipuncture-dictionary.htm. Accessed November 13, 2009.

UNIT
5

Medication Administration

Researching and Preparing Medications

Key Terms

Adverse effect

Allergic reaction

Brand name

Chemical name

Desired effect

Generic name

Medication administration record (MAR)

Mucosal route

Nursing drug guide

Oral route

Over-the-counter (OTC) medication

Parenteral route

Physician's Desk Reference (PDR)

Prescription medication

Side effect

Therapeutic level

Topical route

Toxicity

Objectives

1. Define key terms associated with researching and preparing medications.
2. Differentiate between the chemical, generic, and brand name of medications.
3. Explain when generic prescriptions might be used.
4. Discuss two general categories of medications.
5. Summarize the routes of medication administration.
6. Describe the schedule for controlled drugs, with an example of a drug in each schedule.
7. Contrast desired effects, side effects, and adverse effects of medications.
8. Describe allergic reactions, including anaphylaxis.
9. Identify resources to use when researching medications.
10. Discuss types of medication interactions that may occur.
11. Identify common classifications of medications and safety assessments to make prior to administering them.
12. Explain information and abbreviations found in prescriber's orders.
13. Calculate drug dosages using a formula.
14. Explain how to obtain medications for administration.
15. Determine the six rights, patient rights, and safety checks to perform to prevent medication errors.
16. Describe guidelines to use when preparing medications.
17. Discuss how to handle medication errors.

Clinical Connection

Your Assignment: You will be caring for a patient taking many medications, and you will administer medications for the first time in clinical tomorrow morning. You will need to administer eight oral medications, a nitroglycerin patch, and an insulin injection. You have no idea what most of the oral medications are for and cannot imagine how to say their names. You are a bit familiar with the nitroglycerin patch because your grandfather wears one. You are extremely nervous about administering the insulin injection because you can only think about all the things that can go wrong. You are fearful that you might make an error and harm your patient.

Your Actions: You must research each medication prior to administering it. You know that your instructor will expect you to know the classification, effect, and major side effects of each medication. In addition, you need to know if there are any lab values or vital signs you should assess prior to administering the medications. You are not sure where or how to find this information, and when you try to look it up in some reference books, you cannot find what you are looking for.

In this chapter, you will learn how to look up information about medications before you administer them. You will also learn general information about the classifications and effects of medications, as well as important assessment keys prior to administration of certain groups of drugs. In addition, you will learn the steps for preparing medications safely and in a way that helps prevent medication errors.

Fundamentals of Medications

A great deal of information about medications is available to you. There are thousands of medications that you could be administering, and new ones are continuously being developed. All that information is overwhelming to the average person. Even television commercials to promote a medication extol its virtues, then quickly follow with a list of side effects and cautions against its use. It is important to know about every medication before you take it or administer it to a patient. You will need to know about the names, categories, effects, and interactions of medications as well as the legal regulation of drugs and how to research a medication before you administer it.

Names, Categories, and Routes of Medications

A single medication actually may be called by three different names: its chemical name, generic name, and brand name. It is important to be aware of the overlap in the types of names of medications, as well as the differences in those names.

Names of Medications

The **chemical name** is the name of the exact ingredients of the medication. It reads like a chemical formula. For example, the chemical name for a common anti-inflammatory is (±)-2-(p-isobutylphenyl) proprionic acid. The chemical name is not used in prescribing or administering medications. Instead, the remaining two names are used.

The **generic name** is assigned by the U.S. Adopted Name Council (USANC). It is usually based, at least partially, on the chemical name, but is more of a shorthand version. In our example in the previous paragraph, the generic name of the common anti-inflammatory is *ibuprofen*. Generic names are not capitalized and are not owned by the pharmaceutical company that developed the drug, so they are also sometimes referred to as the *nonproprietary name*. All medications have a generic name, even if they are not available for purchase in generic form.

The **brand name**, also called the *trade name*, of a drug is usually shorter and easier to remember. This name is owned by the pharmaceutical company, so it is sometimes referred to as the *proprietary name*. One drug might have many brand names because it is made and sold by a variety of companies. In our example, the anti-inflammatory ibuprofen is sold under a variety of brand names such as *Motrin, Advil, Medipren, Pediaprofen,* and, in Canada, *Amersol*. Brand names are capitalized and often are registered, requiring the ® symbol to be used in print.

Generic Prescriptions

When a drug is first developed in the United States, it is patented by the pharmaceutical company that does the research and development. That company then sells the drug for a period of time with no competition from other manufacturers because it owns the patent; the price is designed to help offset the costs of the research and development. Approximately 10 years after the company begins selling the drug, the patent expires, which allows the drug to be sold as a generic medication and manufactured by other pharmaceutical companies under a different brand name. At this point, the generic medication will be less expensive than brand-name medication because it is no longer the exclusive property of the pharmaceutical company that developed it; therefore, the generic medication can be manufactured and offered at less expense, even though it is exactly the same medication as the brand-name medication.

Categories of Medications

Two general categories of medications exist: prescription and over the counter. **Prescription medications** are available with a written direction from a health care provider with prescriptive authority. This includes physicians, nurse practitioners, and in some situations physician assistants, depending on state laws. The prescription includes the patient's and physician's identifying information, the medication name and dose, instructions to the pharmacist, any special instructions, and directions to the patient.

Over-the-counter (OTC) medications are available without a prescription, and are also referred to as *nonprescription medications*. They may be purchased by the consumer for use at recommended dosages. Before a medication is offered as over the counter, it must be determined safe at the dose available. It may also be available in a stronger dose that requires a prescription. Our earlier example of ibuprofen is available over the counter in 200-mg tablets, but is available by prescription in a stronger dose of 800-mg tablets.

Routes of Medication Administration

Medications can be delivered by several routes. It is always important to know which route is ordered, as some medications can be given by more than one route. These routes will be discussed in more detail in the remaining chapters of this book.

- **Oral route**: Taken through the mouth, either by swallowing or by *sublingual* (under the tongue) or buccal (between cheek and gums) placement
- **Mucosal route**: Absorbed through the mucosa, such as medications applied through the rectum, vagina, eye, or ear, and inhaled into the lungs and bronchi
- **Topical route**: Applied to the skin; includes creams, ointments, lotions, and transdermal patches
- **Parenteral route**: Given beneath the skin; includes all injections, such as *intradermal* (between the layers of the skin), *subcutaneous* (beneath the skin), *intramuscular* (within muscle layers), and *intravenous* (into the vein)

Knowledge Connection
What is the difference between the generic name of a drug and a generic prescription? How might a drug be available both by prescription and over the counter? By which route would the pneumonia vaccine be delivered?

Legal Regulation of Medications

Over time, many laws have been enacted regarding the regulation of drugs. Several are designed to control the sales and use of narcotics, which are highly addictive. Some laws have been enacted to protect the public by regulating the manufacture and sale of all medications by the Food and Drug Administration (FDA). Box 35-1 gives a brief synopsis of the impact of several of these laws.

The Comprehensive Drug Abuse and Control Act categorized drugs according to their abuse potential using a schedule from I to V. All drugs in these schedules are considered controlled drugs and must be handled using specific guidelines. Box 35-2 provides a definition of each level and examples of the drugs in each. Schedule II drugs are kept under double lock and must be counted at the end of every shift. When medications are kept in a computerized cabinet, access is already limited and the count is automatically done by the computer. Other drugs may be included in the count as well, depending on facility policy. All of these medications given during the shift must be accounted for and signed out for administration to a patient.

Real-World Connection

Drug Abuse in Nursing
While no research shows that nurses abuse drugs at a higher rate than the general population, nurses certainly deal with high work-related stress and easy access to drugs.

One nurse began taking medications that were prescribed for her patients, known as *diverting drugs*, as a way to deal with the emotional pain of watching her sister die of cancer. The nurse could not relieve her sister's pain, but she could relieve her own. Over time, she diverted more and stronger medications until she was taking a tourniquet and a syringe filled with meperidine (Demerol) to the bathroom in the pocket of her scrubs. She would apply the tourniquet and inject the meperidine directly into her vein, then return to work in an impaired state.

One night, she apparently overdosed and was found unconscious in the bathroom, snoring loudly. Once she came to, the police escorted her off of the nursing unit in handcuffs. She faced a variety of criminal charges, including falsifying records, forging prescriptions, and possession of a controlled substance without a prescription.

This nurse's story ends well, though. She entered a drug treatment program and then continued in the Peer Assistance Program available through her state's board of nursing. As part of her recovery, she bravely told her story to nursing students to help them understand how easy it can be to abuse drugs. She also told the students about how difficult recovery can be, but that it is worth all the effort it takes. By complying with all the requirements of the Peer Assistance Program, she was able to get her nursing license back again and work in a setting without dispensing medications.

Effects and Interactions of Medications

Medications are prescribed to achieve a specific effect, such as pain relief. At the same time, other effects may occur that are not intended. Medications can interact with one another and cause a more intense effect or a decrease

B o x 3 5 - 1

Laws Regulating Medications

Many laws have been passed regarding medication quality and safety. These four laws impact the way drugs are developed, marketed, stored, and named today.

- **Food, Drug, and Cosmetic Act of 1938:** Established a government agency to approve all new drugs and determine that the drug was safe for humans. This agency became the U.S. Food and Drug Administration (FDA).
- **Durham-Humphrey Amendment of 1952:** Specified the criteria for prescription medications and over-the-counter medications.
- **Kefauver-Harris Amendment of 1962:** Established the FDA as responsible for giving drugs official (generic) names and specified criteria for deeming a drug safe and effective before it is offered for sale.
- **Comprehensive Drug Abuse and Control Act of 1970:** Established Schedules I through V, categorizing drugs according to their potential for abuse; set guidelines for manufacture, distribution, and sale of controlled substances; addressed the need for treatment for drug abuse and dependence; and made it illegal to possess a controlled substance without a legal prescription for it.

B o x 3 5 - 2

Scheduled (Controlled) Drugs With Examples

The Comprehensive Drug Abuse and Control Act of 1970 set up a classification of drugs by their abuse potential and medical usefulness and set guidelines for manufacture, distribution, and sale of controlled substances. Often referred to as the "drug schedule," this law sets the requirements for storing and handling controlled drugs.

- **Schedule I:** These drugs are highly addictive and have no medical purpose, therefore they are sometimes referred to as "street drugs." Examples: heroin, LSD, peyote, and mescaline.
- **Schedule II:** These drugs have high potential for abuse and do have accepted medical use. Examples: morphine, codeine, fentanyl, oxycodone, methadone, meperidine, amphetamines, and short-acting barbiturates.
- **Schedule III:** These drugs, while having potential for abuse, are at less risk to be abused than those in Schedules I and II. Examples: Lower doses of barbiturates, acetaminophen with codeine, paregoric, and anabolic steroids.
- **Schedule IV:** These drugs have a lower potential for abuse than Schedule I, II, and III medications. Examples: central nervous system depressants such as chloral hydrate, diazepam, lorazepam, meprobamate, and phenobarbital.
- **Schedule V:** These drugs have the lowest potential for abuse. Examples: medications with very small amounts of codeine and atropine, such as cough medications with codeine, and antidiarrheals such as diphenoxylate with atropine (Lomotil). A prescription may not be required, but the consumer will sign for the medication and provide identification when purchasing it.

in effectiveness. Medications can also interact with food and supplements such as vitamins and herbs, causing a response that is either greater or less than desired.

Medication Effects

The **desired effect** is the reason a medication is prescribed, or the purpose for which it is given. For example, if the patient has high blood pressure, the health care professional prescribes a medication to lower the blood pressure, which is the desired effect.

A **side effect** occurs when an unintended outcome also takes place. This outcome may not necessarily be unexpected, however. For example, a patient taking a high blood pressure medication may feel dizzy upon standing for a few seconds. When the patient stands, the effect of the blood pressure medication prevents the body from adjusting as quickly to a change in position, resulting in a momentary decrease in blood to the brain, causing dizziness. This type of side effect is minor and the patient may adjust to it. However, if the medication lowers the blood pressure too much, the patient may feel dizzy most of the time or even faint. The prescriber may need to adjust the dose or change the medication due to more severe side effects.

Adverse effects are also unintended, but are more severe or harmful than a side effect. Often these effects are unexpected at the normal medication dose. They may be due to the patient's inability to tolerate the normal dose or to his or her specific reaction to the drug. Some reasons that adverse reactions might occur include:

- Chronic illness that affects the body's ability to metabolize and excrete the drug
- Drug allergies
- Liver or renal impairment or failure
- History of previous drug reactions

Severe adverse effects are those that are life threatening, require medical intervention to prevent permanent damage or death, and could lead to hospitalization, disability, or congenital damage to an infant.

Allergic reactions occur when the patient's body reacts to the medication as a foreign invader to be destroyed. Generally, the first time the patient takes the offending medication, no reaction occurs. At this point, the body recognizes it as a foreign substance and forms antibodies against it. Then the next time the patient takes the medication, the body reacts with an allergic response. Sometimes the allergic response occurs much later, after the patient has taken the drug several times.

A typical mild allergic reaction causes a rash, hives, and itching. It usually resolves when the medication is discontinued. Sometimes the prescriber may have the patient take diphenhydramine (Benadryl) or another antihistamine concurrently with the drug and continue to take the drug as prescribed. The antihistamine helps prevent the mild allergic response.

Anaphylaxis

A more severe reaction, referred to as an *anaphylactic reaction,* is life threatening. It causes swelling of the airways, shortness of breath, respiratory arrest, decreased blood pressure, and eventually circulatory collapse. This type of reaction occurs as soon as the medication reaches the bloodstream, so if you are administering the medication through an IV line, the reaction will occur immediately. *Safety: If you suspect an anaphylactic reaction, stop the medication at once and follow facility procedure for responding to anaphylaxis.* The patient may have to be intubated and given ventilator support. Expect to administer IV fluids to increase blood volume and bring up the blood pressure. You may also be ordered to give additional IV medications such as epinephrine to stimulate the heart. *Safety: Always check the chart for allergies before administering any medication.*

Sometimes patients describe themselves as allergic to a medication, but when asked about the reaction, it is more typical of unpleasant side effects. For example, a patient may say, "Demerol makes me really sick. I vomit if I take it." This is most likely a description of the side effects of nausea and vomiting, common with meperidine (Demerol). Make sure the prescriber is aware, but he or she may still prescribe the medication along with another medication to relieve the side effects. *Safety: If the patient says he or she is allergic to a medication, you must record it as an allergy, along with documenting the patient's description of the reaction when the medication is taken.*

Classifications of medications that often cause allergic reactions include:

- Antibiotics, especially penicillin and sulfa drugs
- Iodine and dyes injected for certain procedures
- Vaccines
- Anticonvulsants, also known as seizure medications

Toxicity

When medications are administered as ordered, the goal is that the patient will have therapeutic levels of the drug in the bloodstream. A **therapeutic level** is the amount of medication in the blood that it takes to reach the desired effects on the target organ or organs. In many cases, the amount of medication required for the desired effect is far below the amount of medication that could cause harmful toxic effects. Most medications are not likely to cause a toxic effect unless they are taken in amounts greater than prescribed.

However, it is possible for patients to experience toxic effects of a medication. Certain medications can accumulate in the body rather than being completely excreted. As this happens, the patient will exhibit symptoms of **toxicity**, or too much of the medication in the body. If the patient continues to take the medication, severe toxic effects such as multiple organ failure and even death can occur.

Laboratory and Diagnostic Connection

Determining Digoxin Toxicity

One medication that can cause toxicity is digoxin, a cardiac glycoside that can accumulate in the body. Blood levels are drawn periodically to determine the amount of drug in the blood and whether the levels are elevated above therapeutic ranges. If the levels are elevated, the patient may develop symptoms of digoxin toxicity, which include nausea, vomiting, halos of light around objects, blurred vision, objects appearing to have a yellow cast, irregular heartbeat, and bradycardia. Blood levels greater than 2.0 nanograms per milliliter (ng/mL) of blood indicate toxic levels of digoxin. While the laboratory may notify the physician of toxic levels, nurses should be certain that the physician is aware of the laboratory results.

If the blood levels are elevated, the prescriber usually discontinues the medication for a few days to allow the medication to be removed from the bloodstream, then restarts it at a lower dose. *Safety: It is your responsibility to check the most recent blood levels of medications in the patient's chart and to hold any questionable dose until you speak with the prescriber.* For example, the patient is taking digoxin and you check the chart for the level drawn yesterday morning, and find that it is 2.1 ng/mL. You will not give another dose of digoxin until you notify the physician of the 2.1-ng/mL level and receive new orders. If you do not take the time to check this and just give the medication as ordered, you will make the patient even more toxic by administering another dose. Some common medications that may cause toxicity include:

- Digoxin
- Aminophylline
- Gentamicin
- Imipramine
- Phenobarbital
- Procainamide
- Valproic acid

Drug Interactions

Medications can interact with one another, causing increases or decreases in the desired effects. For example, the patient may be taking warfarin (Coumadin), an anticoagulant that prevents blood clotting. If the patient also takes a medication containing aspirin or ibuprofen, which also has anticoagulant properties, it will delay the ability of the blood to clot for longer than desired by the prescriber. This can lead to excessive bruising and spontaneous bleeding from the nose, gums, eyes, vagina, kidneys, and intestines. It can also lead to life-threatening hemorrhage if it is not reversed. Pharmacists keep close watch on prescribed medications to detect dangers of drug interactions, but patients must be educated to prevent interactions between prescription drugs and over-the-counter preparations.

Medications can also interact with certain foods. Patients are advised to avoid such foods while taking the particular drug, or advised to avoid taking the drug with specific foods or beverages. For example, the antibiotic tetracycline should not be taken with dairy products because proteins in these foods cause decreased absorption of the drug. Grapefruit juice should not be consumed with medications taken to lower cholesterol, because the juice interferes with the enzymes that break down the drugs, causing the blood levels of the medication to become too high.

Vitamins and herbal supplements can also interact with medications and interfere with their effectiveness. St. John's wort, a popular herbal supplement taken to relieve mild to moderate depression, can interact with many medications. It can interact with birth control pills by increasing the breakdown of estrogen, which will decrease the effectiveness of the medication. St. John's wort can also interact with narcotics, because it decreases the rate of excretion of these drugs from the body, leading to increased effects and side effects of some narcotics. *Safety: You are responsible to look up medications before you give them and be aware of any potential drug-drug, drug-food, or drug-supplement interactions.*

Knowledge Connection

Why might nurses be at risk for drug abuse? What would happen if you gave a patient a medication when his or her blood levels were already above therapeutic levels? List three types of drug interactions.

Researching Medications

No one can know or remember everything about all medications. A wealth of information is available about each individual medication, plus an overwhelming number of medications exist, with new ones being developed frequently. You must always look up medications to determine facts about them that you do not know or about which you are unsure. It is important to know how to obtain information about a medication when you need it. A variety of books are available, as well as downloads for smart phones, and websites that can be accessed with handheld computers. Pharmacists are also an excellent resource when you have a question about a medication or potential drug interaction.

Some of the more common books that you may use for medication research include the *Physician's Desk Reference* (PDR), nursing drug handbooks, and pharmacology textbooks.

Physician's Desk Reference

The *Physician's Desk Reference* (**PDR**) is a comprehensive book containing detailed information about a large number of medications. It contains the same information as that in

drug package inserts, which is provided by pharmaceutical companies. It also contains photographs of many oral medications if you need to identify a tablet or capsule. This book is found at the nurses' station in hospitals and is used by health care providers to prescribe medications, as well as by nurses to research medications.

The PDR can be confusing if you do not know how to use it. The information is very technical and detailed, making it more difficult to understand than some other references. It is divided into the following sections:

- **Manufacturer's Index:** This is the small section of white pages at the front of the book that lists in alphabetical order the major pharmaceutical manufacturers in the United States. It includes their addresses and contact people.
- **Brand and Generic Name Index:** These are the pink pages. The drugs are listed in alphabetical order by both brand and generic names, with the manufacturer in parentheses. Page numbers listed in bold locate prescribing information for that medication.
- **Product Category Index:** These are the blue pages. They provide a quick reference to drugs used to treat specific conditions. This is an index of prescribing categories; beneath each category is a list of all the medications with that particular therapeutic use.
- **Product Identification Section:** These are the glossy pages with colored pictures of selected medications. The drugs appear as their actual size with identifying marks on front and back.
- **Product Information Section:** This is the very large section of white pages, the main portion of the book. It lists the medications with the details of their chemical composition, indications for use, contraindications, warnings, routes, and administration guidelines.

Nursing Drug Guides

While the PDR is designed to be a comprehensive guide for physicians and prescribers, other references are more specific for nurses. **Nursing drug guides** include generic drugs listed in alphabetical order with information about the classification, brand names, absorption, indications for use, dosages, contraindications, cautions, interactions, nursing interventions, and patient teaching. Drugs that are a combination of two different medications must be looked up separately. For example, Zestoretic is a combination of lisinopril and hydrochlorothiazide. To obtain information about this drug, you would need to look up each component separately.

Nursing drug guides are smaller books than the PDR and can easily be kept on the medication cart or in the medication room for quick reference. The information is less detailed than that in the PDR and is more geared for nurse's needs. Figure 35-1 shows a nurse looking up a medication in a nursing drug guide.

Figure 35-1 This nurse is looking up a medication in a nursing drug guide prior to preparing the medication for administration.

Pharmacology Textbooks

You will probably use some type of pharmacology textbook in your nursing course. Most of these include classifications of drugs with explanations of the effects and uses for each class. As a nurse, you will often perform the same type of nursing interventions for all of the drugs in a particular classification. For example, all antihypertensive medications lower blood pressure. Therefore, you will always want to check the blood pressure before administering an antihypertensive to ensure that the blood pressure is not already so low that the medication will drop it too low.

Internet Resources

Many sites provide drug information. Be sure to use a reliable site, such as *www.pdrhealth.com.* Often, the drug information online is written for the patient, not for the nurse or other health care provider. These sites may be easier to read, but may omit important assessment and evaluation data.

Classifications and Effects of Medications

Because it is impossible to learn about every medication, you will find it helpful to learn information about groups of drugs that work in a similar manner and have similar effects and side effects. Table 35-1 includes some of the major classifications and their purposes.

(text continues on page 840)

Table 35-1   Classifications and Purposes of Medications

Classification	Purpose	Examples	Nursing Concerns
Cardiovascular Medications			
Antianginals	Increase blood flow and oxygen supplied to the heart muscle by causing the coronary arteries to dilate.	Beta blockers, calcium channel blockers, and vasodilators.	Because they dilate arteries, they also lower blood pressure. *Safety: Check blood pressure before administering them.*
Antiarrhythmics	Regulate an irregular heartbeat; act on the nerve impulses in the heart; often slow the heartbeat and decrease blood pressure.	Procanbid (procainamide), Cordarone (amiodarone), Betapace (sotalol), Calan (verapamil)	*Safety: Check vital signs before giving these medications. Hold if blood pressure or pulse is low and check with prescriber before administering.*
Anticoagulants	Delay blood clotting; sometimes called *blood thinners.* Prescribed to treat or prevent heart attack, stroke, and blood clot formation.	Heparin, given by injection or through an IV, and warfarin (Coumadin), given orally.	Because they delay blood clotting, side effects include internal or external bleeding. *Safety: Assess for tarry stools, bleeding gums, bleeding from the rectum or vagina, and nosebleeds.* Blood tests such as prothrombin time, partial thromboplastin time, and international normalized ratio are ordered to monitor anticoagulation.

(table continues on page 834)

Table 35-1 **Classifications and Purposes of Medications** (continued)

Classification	Purpose	Examples	Nursing Concerns
Cardiovascular Medications			
Antihyperlipidemics	Prescribed to treat high cholesterol and triglycerides in the blood, which contribute to plaque formation inside the arteries, causing narrowing and restriction of blood flow. This can contribute to heart attack, stroke, high blood pressure, and other conditions.	Reductase inhibitors such as atorvastatin (Lipitor), bile acid binding agents such as cholestyramine (Questran), fibric acid agents such as gemfibrozil (Lopid) and ezetimibe (Zetia).	Check liver function tests; assess for muscle pain and weakness, which could indicate myopathy.
Antihypertensives	Prescribed to lower blood pressure; often more than one drug is prescribed because they work in different ways.	Beta blockers slow the heartbeat and lower the blood pressure by blocking nerve messages from the brain. Calcium channel blockers act on the calcium in muscle cells to keep arteries dilated, which lowers blood pressure. Vasodilators cause the walls of arteries to open wider. Diuretics decrease the amount of excess fluid in the blood, which decreases blood pressure.	*Safety: Check blood pressure before administering to prevent hypotension.*
Cardiac glycosides	Prescribed to slow and strengthen the heartbeat; include all drugs that contain or are derived from digitalis. Used to treat congestive heart failure (CHF) and atrial arrhythmias, such as atrial fibrillation.	Most common is digoxin (Lanoxin).	Check digoxin blood levels before administering to prevent toxicity. *Safety: Because these medications cause the heart to slow, assess the apical pulse before administering them. If the rate is below 60, do not administer and notify prescriber.*

Table 35-1 **Classifications and Purposes of Medications** (continued)

Classification	Purpose	Examples	Nursing Concerns
Cardiovascular Medications			
Diuretics	Prescribed to decrease edema and fluid retention; rid the body of excess fluid through the urine. Are sometimes called *water pills*. Cause kidneys to increase salt and water output, which decreases excess fluid in the blood and lowers blood pressure.	*Thiazide diuretics*, commonly prescribed diuretics that have the side effect of depleting potassium. Furosemide (Lasix) is a commonly ordered *loop diuretic*. It is a stronger diuretic than thiazide diuretics and also causes potassium depletion. Patients on thiazide or loop diuretics may have a potassium supplement ordered as well. Other types of diuretics are potassium-sparing because they do not deplete potassium.	*Safety: Check potassium levels before administering thiazide or loop diuretics.* Patients taking potassium-sparing diuretics should not eat foods high in potassium or take potassium supplements.
Vasodilators	Prescribed to widen blood vessels, lower blood pressure, and increase circulation.	Diazoxide (Hyperstat) and nitroprusside (Nitropress) given IV. Hydralazine (Apresoline) and minoxidil (Loniten) given orally.	Side effects include headache, nausea, and hypotension. *Safety: Assess blood pressure before giving vasodilators to avoid causing hypotension.*
Gastrointestinal Medications			
Antacids	Used to neutralize stomach acid. Products contain aluminum, magnesium, calcium, or a combination of them.	Amphogel, Digel, Mylanta, and Maalox.	*Safety: Antacids interact with some medications. Ensure that you do not give them at the same time.* Most common side effects are either constipation or diarrhea.
Anticholinergics	Ordered to block the action of the parasympathetic nervous system; slow peristalsis and reduce stomach acid production. Sometimes called *antispasmodics,* prescribed for irritable bowel syndrome, ulcers, Parkinson's disease, and asthma.	Atropine, benztropine (Cogentin), dicyclomine (Bentyl), ipratropium (Atrovent).	Can reduce gastric motility, causing constipation, and can cause urinary retention. Assess frequently for distended bladder and abdomen.

(table continues on page 836)

Table 35-1   Classifications and Purposes of Medications (continued)

Classification	Purpose	Examples	Nursing Concerns
Gastrointestinal Medications			
Antiemetics	Ordered to relieve nausea and vomiting.	Ondansetron hydrochloride (Zofran), promethiazine (Phenergan), and prochlorperazine (Compazine).	May be given via injection or suppository, if patient is vomiting and unable to keep an oral medication down.
Gastroesophageal reflux disease medications	Given to reduce or block amount of acid produced by the stomach.	Esomeprazole (Nexium), omeprazole (Prilosec), and ranitidine (Zantac).	Check liver and kidney function tests for abnormal results.
Laxatives and stool softeners	Given to relieve constipation; stool softeners keep water in the feces of the large intestine. Some laxatives increase peristalsis to move the feces through the bowel quickly. Other laxatives, such as milk of magnesia, pull water into the intestine to prevent dry, hard feces.	Stool Softener: docusate calcium (Surfak). Laxatives: bulk forming such as Metamucil; mineral oil; herbal such as senna; stimulant such as bisacodyl (Dulcolax); osmotic such as polyethylene glycol (MiraLax)	*Safety: Assess the need before giving stool softeners or laxatives.* Do not continue to give regularly ordered stool softeners if the patient is having liquid stools. If the patient has not had a bowel movement for 2 days, it is appropriate to give an ordered prn laxative on the third day. This will prevent prolonged constipation or fecal impaction.
Endocrine Medications			
Antidiabetics	Oral hypoglycemics stimulate the pancreas to produce more insulin when it is not making enough to meet the body's needs. Insulin itself can only be given by injection because it would be destroyed by gastric acid. Insulin injections are prescribed when the pancreas no longer makes enough insulin, even in response to oral hypoglycemics. In some cases, both oral hypoglycemics and insulin injections are ordered.	Oral antidiabetics: Arcabose (Precose), Metformin (Glucophage), Glipizide (Glucotrol), Rosiglitazone (Avandia) Insulins: regular, NPH, insulin glargine (Lantus), insulin lispro (Humalog), insulin detemir (Levemir)	*Safety: Always check the patient's finger stick blood sugar prior to administering an antidiabetic medication.*

Table 35-1 **Classifications and Purposes of Medications** (continued)

Classification	Purpose	Examples	Nursing Concerns
Endocrine Medications			
Steroids	Ordered to relieve inflammation and to treat diseases such as asthma and bronchitis; may be ordered as skin cream, such as hydrocortisone, to treat local inflammations, and as injections directly into inflamed joints or into muscle to decrease systemic inflammation.	Prednisolone (Delta-cortef, Prelone, Inflamase), prednisone (Deltasone, Meticorten)	*Safety: Assess blood pressure before administering oral or injectable steroids as they cause hypertension.* Watch for signs of infection because steroids mask infections. Check fasting blood sugar levels because steroids increase blood sugar. Do not stop drug abruptly. Patient must be tapered off of steroids.
Thyroid replacement hormone	Ordered to replace thyroid hormone that is not being produced in sufficient amounts by the body.	Levothyroxine (Synthroid)	*Safety: Assess patient for excitability, tachycardia, irritability, and anxiety, which can indicate an excessive dose.*
Immune System Medications			
Antibiotics	Used to treat infections caused by bacteria by interfering with the way bacteria live and reproduce, allowing the immune system to more easily eliminate the infection. To be effective, antibiotics must be taken regularly for the prescribed amount of time. Bacteria must be completely killed or the infection can recur.	Aminoglycosides, cephalosporins, erythromycins, penicillins, quinolones, and tetracyclines.	*Safety: Check the patient's allergies before administering antibiotics. Assess for rash, itching, or hives.* Administer with food when appropriate to prevent stomach irritation, nausea, and vomiting. Tetracycline antibiotics should be given on an empty stomach and never administered with milk or dairy products.
Antifungals	Used to treat fungal infections such as athlete's foot and yeast infections.	Miconazole (Monistat).	Often in the form of topical creams or ointments, but some are given IV for severe systemic infections.
Anti-inflammatories	Prescribed to decrease the symptoms of inflammation, relieve pain from muscle strain/sprain and arthritis. Two types: steroids (see Endocrine Medications) and NSAIDs.	NSAID examples are aspirin-containing drugs (salicylates), ibuprofen (Motrin, Advil), indomethacin (Indocin), naproxen (Aleve), and nabumetone (Relafen).	Often cause gastrointestinal side effects such as heartburn, nausea, vomiting, and ulcers. *Safety: Assess for signs of bleeding ulcers such as tarry stools, especially in the elderly.*

(table continues on page 838)

Table 35-1 **Classifications and Purposes of Medications** (continued)

Classification	Purpose	Examples	Nursing Concerns
Immune System Medications			
Antivirals	Prescribed to treat viral infections.	Acyclovir (Zovirax), used to decrease the severity and number of outbreaks of genital herpes and shingles (herpes zoster). Zidovudine (AZT, Retrovir), used to treat HIV and AIDS.	These medications do not cure the diseases, but help minimize some symptoms.
Nervous System Medications			
Analgesics	Prescribed to relieve pain, often called *pain medicines;* include narcotics and non-narcotics. Narcotic analgesics act on the brain to relieve pain and are addictive; non-narcotic analgesics include NSAIDs and acetaminophen.	Example of acetaminophen is Tylenol. Examples of narcotic analgesics include oxycodone (OxyContin) and meperidine (Demerol). Sometimes narcotic and non-narcotic analgesics are combined in one medication; example is Percocet, combination of oxycodone (narcotic) and acetaminophen (non-narcotic).	Side effects of narcotics include nausea, vomiting, and slowing of respirations. *Safety: Assess patient for effectiveness of medication in relieving pain.*
Antianxiety medications	Antianxiety medications are prescribed to relieve anxiety, promote calm, rest, and sleep.	Barbiturates, benzodiazepine, and buspirone.	
Anticonvulsants	Ordered to decrease seizure activity due to epilepsy or other causes.	Phenytoin (Dilantin), valproic acid (Depakene), divalproex sodium (Depakote), and carbamazepine (Tegretol).	*Safety: Check blood levels of seizure medications before administering them to prevent toxicity.*
Antidepressants	Prescribed to relieve depression, and to treat certain types of pain, such as migraine headaches. Selective serotonin reuptake inhibitors (SSRIs) increase the function of neurotransmitters in the brain. Older drugs, particularly monoamine oxidase inhibitors (MAOIs), are prescribed for depression and to treat Parkinson's disease. These can interact with certain foods to cause severe hypertension.	Example of SSRI is fluoxetine (Prozac). Examples of MAOIs include phenelzine (Nardil) and selegiline (Eldepryl).	*Safety: Teach patients taking MAOIs to avoid foods high in tyramine, including smoked, aged, or pickled meat or fish, aged cheeses, aged sausages, and red wines, as ingesting these foods can lead to hypertensive crisis.*

Table 35-1   **Classifications and Purposes of Medications** (continued)

Classification	Purpose	Examples	Nursing Concerns
Nervous System Medications			
Sedative and hypnotic medications	Sedatives act on the brain to promote calm and sleep; hypnotics induce sleep and fall into two classes: benzodiazepines and nonbenzodiazepines. Benzodiazepines carry a higher risk for dependency, toxicity, and abuse.	Examples of sedatives include diphenhydramine (Benadryl), doxepin (Sinequan), and hydroxyzine (Atarax, Vistaril). Example of benzodiazepines is triazolam (Halcion). Examples of some nonbenzodiazepine hypnotics include zolpidem (Ambien) and eszopiclone (Lunesta).	*Safety: Caution patients not to get up alone after taking sedative or hypnotic medications.*
Respiratory Medications			
Antihistamines	Prescribed to block the action of histamine, which decreases allergy symptoms, including mild respiratory allergies such as hay fever and sinus conditions. Also used to prevent or treat motion sickness symptoms.	Examples include diphenhydramine (Benadryl) and loratadine (Claritin). Example of medication given to treat or prevent motion sickness is meclizine (Antivert).	These medications may cause drowsiness; patient should not drive or engage in potentially hazardous activities until the response to the drug is known.
Antitussives	Used to control coughing; nonprescription cough medicines usually contain dextromethorphan to suppress coughs or guiafenesin as an expectorant. Prescription-strength cough medicine may contain codeine, a narcotic, which also suppresses coughing.	Examples of nonprescription cough medicine containing dextromethorphan are Robitussin and Triaminic. Examples of prescription-strength antitussives are benzonatate (Tessalon) and hydrocodone (Hycotuss).	*Safety: If the cough is productive, an expectorant should be used rather than a cough suppressant.*
Bronchodilators	Prescribed to open airways to ease shortness of breath associated with asthma and emphysema. May be administered IV, orally, and as an inhalant.	Examples are aminophylline (Corophylline) and theophylline (Theo-24). Inhaler examples include albuterol (Proventil, Ventolin) and metaproterenol (Alupent).	Bronchodilators have side effects of nervousness, insomnia, tremors, anxiety, nausea, and vomiting. *Safety: Monitor theophylline and aminophylline blood levels because these drugs may cause toxicity.*
Expectorants	Used to thin mucus so it can be coughed out, to help prevent lung congestion leading to pneumonia.	Guaifenesin (Mucinex, Nortussin, Anti-Tuss)	Instruct patient to increase fluid intake to help loosen and thin mucus; drink at least 8 glasses of fluid daily.

Knowledge Connection
List four resources you can use to look up information about
medications you will administer. Why is it important to check
the patient's vital signs before administering an antiarrhythmic
medication? What laboratory value will you check before
administering a thiazide or a loop diuretic?

Preparing to Administer Medications

Anyone can remove a medication from the packaging and
hand it to a patient to swallow. This is not medication administration. Preparing medications is not a task you can
perform mindlessly. You must stay focused and think critically throughout the entire process.

Reading Medication Orders

Medication orders are written by health care providers with
prescriptive authority, such as physicians, nurse practitioners, and physician assistants. All medication orders must
include the:

- Date and time of the order
- Name of the medication, either generic or brand
- Dosage of medication
- Frequency for taking the medication (for example, twice
  per day)
- Route of administration, such as oral, intramuscular, or
  intravenous
- Patient's name (in the hospital setting, the order will be
  written on a physician order page, which is stamped with
  the patient's name)
- Signature of the prescriber

Figure 35-2 shows an example of a prescription written on a prescription pad.

Because medication names can be similar and hastily
written numbers may be unclear, it is very important to
verify any order that seems unclear. *Safety: If the dose,
route, or frequency is not appropriate for the medication,
notify the prescriber and verify the order.*

The frequency ordered for a medication may vary
greatly. It may be ordered several times per day, may be
ordered only as needed (prn), or may be ordered to be given
one time only. Read orders carefully to ensure that the frequency is appropriate, then follow the order. Box 35-3 provides details regarding specific ordered frequencies.

The medication order is transcribed from the physician's order sheet in the chart to the **medication administration record (MAR)**, which is usually kept in a notebook
on the medicine cart or computerized cabinet. The MAR
lists the medications and the times they are to be given. The
nurse initials in the correct box under the date and across
from the time to indicate that a medication has been administered. The MAR may be designed in such a way that the
nurse writes the time the medication is to be administered
beneath the date, then writes his or her initials next to the

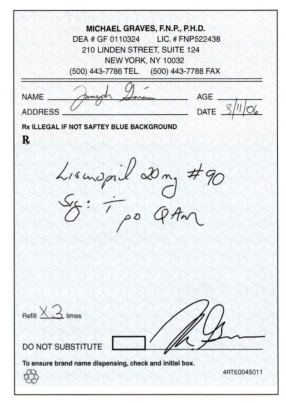

Figure 35-2 An example of a medication order written
on a prescription blank.

time as the medication is given (Fig. 35-3). Medications
given on a prn basis are documented in the nurses' notes, as
are medications that are withheld for some reason. An explanation is provided in the documentation. In long-term care
facilities, the back side of the MAR contains an area for

Box 35-3

Specific Ordered Frequencies

Medications are ordered at specific frequencies that are scheduled at routine times in the health care facility. Below are the
usually ordered frequencies for most medications. Pay close
attention to the frequencies written in medication orders and
do not confuse them.

- **Daily:** One time per day, may be morning or evening
- **Twice per day (bid):** Every 12 hours, or morning and evening
- **Three times per day (tid):** Every 8 hours or with meals
- **Four times per day (qid):** Every 4 hours; usually at 9 a.m.,
  1 p.m., 5 p.m., and 9 p.m.; for antibiotics, may be every
  6 hours, usually 12 a.m., 6 a.m., 12 p.m., and 6 p.m.
- **prn:** As needed within specified time limits. Example:
  Tylenol with codeine, 1 tab every 4 hours prn pain. Patient
  can take no closer together than every 4 hours.
- **Stat:** Immediately. Example: Nitroglycerin 0.4 mg sublingual
  stat.
- **One-time:** Give medication one time only and do not
  continue to administer it. Example: Mebendazole 100 mg
  1 tab to be given one time only.

HOSPITAL MEDICATION ADMINISTRATION RECORD

Codes For Injection Sites

A - Left Anterior Thigh
B - Left Deltoid
C - Left Gluteus Medius
D - Left Lateral Thigh
E - Left Ventral Gluteus
F - Left Lower Quadrant
G - Left Upper Quadrant

H - Right Anterior Thigh
I - Right Deltoid
J - Right Gluteus Medius
K - Right Lateral Thigh
L - Right Ventral Gluteus
M - Right Lower Quadrant
N - Right Upper Quadrant

Mary Smith 086432
age 46   John Miller, M.D.

ALLERGIES: PCN, Sulfa					DATE	DATE	DATE
DATE ORDERED	DATE REORD.	DRUG - DOSE - ROUTE - FREQUENCY		ADMIN. TIME	4.16.06	4.17.06	4.18.06
4.16.06		Lanoxin 0.25mg po Q D		0900	09 JW		
4.16.06		Rocephin 1 gm IV Q D		1200	1200 JW		
4.16.06		Zinacef 1 gm IV Q 8 hr		0800	08 JW		
				1600			
				2400			
SIGNATURE / SHIFT INDICATES				7-3	JW		
NURSE ADMINISTERING MEDICATIONS				3-11			
J Wilson, RN				11-7			

Figure 35-3 An example of a medication administration record (MAR).

documenting prn medications and medications that were not given. It is possible for errors to be made when orders are transcribed. When computerized ordering systems are used, there is less risk of human error, but mistakes can still occur. *Safety: Always compare the order on the MAR with the prescriber's original order to detect any possible errors before you prepare and administer medications.*

Abbreviations Used in Medication Orders

Standard abbreviations are often used to save time when prescribers write medication orders. Over the years, however, errors were made due to misinterpretations of some abbreviations. Therefore, The Joint Commission (formerly JCAHO) has determined that some medication abbreviations can no longer be used to prevent confusion and errors. In addition to that list, the Institute for Safe Medication Practices has compiled a list of Error-prone Abbreviations, Symbols, and Dose Designations. Box 35-4 includes acceptable abbreviations commonly used in medication orders along with their meanings.

Calculating Drug Dosages

Ideally, the dose of medication available to you will be the exact dose that the prescriber orders, but that does not always occur. If the available medication is in a different dose than what is ordered, you must calculate how much of the available medication to administer to your patient. For example, the prescriber may order 1,000 milligrams (mg) of an

antibiotic. However, the pharmacy may stock the medication only in 500-mg capsules. It will be your job to determine how many capsules to give the patient.

The same is true of liquid medications. When at home, you might take a teaspoon of a liquid, but in the hospital it may be ordered by milligrams, or the amount of the drug dissolved in liquid, expressed as milligrams per millili-

Box 35-4

Medical Abbreviations Commonly Used in Medication Orders

As you interpret medication orders, you will find medical abbreviations that are commonly used. Some abbreviations are officially not to be used and appear in a list in Chapter 5. Others are not encouraged by the Institute for Safe Medication Practices because they can be confused with other abbreviations and contribute to medication errors.

g	grams
gr	grains
h	hour
IM	intramuscularly
IV	intravenously
kg	kilograms
mg	milligrams
mL	milliliters
PO	*per os* in Latin, which means by mouth
q	every

ter (mg/mL). You will then be required to calculate how many milliliters of liquid to administer to give the desired milligrams of medication. For example, the physician may order amoxicillin liquid 250 mg per feeding tube every 6 hours. The bottle of amoxicillin might be labeled 250 mg/5 mL. That means that every 5 mL of liquid you pour out contains 250 mg of dissolved antibiotic.

If that is confusing, think of it this way: You add 4 teaspoons of sugar to 4 ounces of water and mix it well. When you measure out 1 ounce of water, it will contain 1 teaspoon of dissolved sugar, or 1 teaspoon/ounce. The same is true of medications dissolved in liquid, but the measurements are in the metric system rather than the household system, so the measurement is in milligrams/milliliter.

Systems of Measurement

Medication measurements are mostly made using the metric system. For example, most medications are ordered in milliliters, milligrams, or micrograms. Occasionally an older system of measurement called the *apothecary system* is used when medications are ordered that have existed for a very long time. For example, aspirin was originally measured in grains (gr), as was morphine. Grains are a measurement in the apothecary system (Table 35-2). The Joint Commission does not recommend use of the apothecary system due to the confusion it may cause.

The metric system is more accurate and standardized, so it has gradually replaced the apothecary system. The household system is the measurement system used with cooking: teaspoons, ounces, and pints. When a patient is discharged with medication orders, they are written in household measurements (for liquids) so the patient will be able to measure the medication at home.

Sometimes it may be necessary to convert between systems. This is not common, but in case you would need to do so, Table 35-2 provides equivalents between systems that

Table 35-3 **Converting Between Units of Measurement in the Metric System**

Micrograms	Milligrams	Grams
1,000,000	1,000	1
100,000	100	0.1
1,000	1	0.001

To change between units of measurement in the metric system, move the decimal three places to the **right** to convert to a smaller unit. Move the decimal three places to the **left** to convert to a larger unit.

will help you if you need to make such a conversion. Sometimes it is necessary to convert between different units of the metric system. Table 35-3 provides conversions between micrograms, milligrams, and grams.

Calculations

Calculations are not required often, but when they are, you need to have confidence that you can correctly perform them. It is recommended that you have your calculations checked by your instructor while you are a student and have a more experienced nurse check them when you first enter practice.

Many ways exist to arrive at the correct dose. There are several different formulas that you can use to calculate the correct amount of medication to administer. However, if you have math anxiety or get confused when using formulas, it may be easiest to learn one formula that can be used in the most common situations. This book utilizes one formula with several applications.

To correctly use a formula, you must know where to insert each number, then carry out the mathematical

Table 35-2 **Measurement Systems Equivalents**

Apothecary	Metric	Household
Weight Measures		
1 grain (gr)	60 or 65 milligrams (mg)	
½ gr	30 mg	
¼ gr	15 mg	
	1 kilogram (kg)	2.2 pounds (lbs.)
Volume Measures		
1 fluid dram	5 milliliters (mL)	1 teaspoon
3–4 fluid drams	15 mL	1 tablespoon
1 fluid ounce	30 mL	2 tablespoons

operations correctly. In this formula, the problem is set up as a fractional equation, and then cross multiplication must be performed to solve for the correct amount to administer, or *x*. The H stands for the dose you have on hand, or the dose available. The D stands for the dose that is ordered by the prescriber. The V stands for the vehicle, which is either a tablet or liquid. To set up the problem, arrange the information in this manner:

$$\frac{H}{V} = \frac{D}{x}$$

The next step is to cross multiply:

$$Hx = VD$$

Now you will solve for *x:*

$$x = \frac{VD}{H}$$

This is more easily understood when we use numbers in place of the letters. If the order is for amoxicillin liquid 500 mg per feeding tube every 6 hours, and we have on hand amoxicillin 250 mg/5 mL, we have to determine how many milliliters of liquid medication to administer (*x*). In this problem, H = 250, D = 500, and V = 5. When we plug those numbers into our formula, it looks like this:

$$\frac{250}{5} = \frac{500}{x}$$

When we cross multiply, it will look like this:

$$250x = 2,500$$

To get rid of the *x,* you must divide what is in front of it into both sides of the equation. In this case, we must divide 250 into 2500 to give us 1*x*.

$$1x = \frac{2,500}{250}$$

When you do the math, the answer becomes:

$$1x = 10 \text{ mL}$$

You will administer 10 mL of amoxicillin to the patient, to equal 500 mg of dissolved drug.

Converting Between Systems Using the Formula

You can also use this formula to convert between systems of measurement. For example, if your order is for 5 grains of aspirin, and the aspirin label on hand in the patient's medication drawer indicates that it contains 300 mg in 1 tablet, you can determine how much aspirin to administer. Because the aspirin that you have for use is labeled in milligrams, you need to know how many milligrams is equal to the ordered dose: 5 grains. In this situation, H = 300 mg, D = 5 gr, and V = 1 tablet. By looking at Table 35-2, you can see that 60 mg is equivalent to 1 gr. Set up the formula with numbers in place:

$$\frac{60 \text{ mg}}{1 \text{ gr}} = \frac{300 \text{ mg}}{x \text{ gr}}$$

When you cross multiply, you get $60x = 300$. When you divide both sides of the equation by 60 to solve for *x,* you get $x = 5$ gr. This tells you that the physician's order for 5 gr is equal to 300 mg, meaning that what you have available is equivalent to the amount the physician ordered. So you will give 1 tablet of aspirin to your patient.

To practice this skill, refer to the student workbook and CD for more problems.

Calculating Milligrams per Kilogram of Body Weight

Medications may be ordered in a different way to be more exact in the amount needed for the patient's body weight. You may see this ordered in pediatrics to prevent overdose of medications in different-sized patients, especially newborns. For example, the prescriber might order 50 mg/kg of ampicillin daily for a child who weighs 22 pounds. If the patient's weight is in pounds, you will need to convert it to kilograms using the formula above and the equivalent of 2.2 pounds equals 1 kilogram from Table 35-2:

$$\frac{2.2 \text{ lbs}}{1 \text{ kg}} = \frac{22 \text{ lbs}}{x \text{ kg}}$$

Now cross multiply: $2.2x = 22$
Divide each side by 2.2: $x = 10$

You are solving for the number of kilograms the 22-pound child weighs, so you know that the child weighs 10 kg.

Once you have the patient's weight in kilograms, you can determine how much medication to give. It is the physician's intent that the patient will receive 50 mg of medication for every kilogram of body weight. The patient weights 10 kg, so you must multiply that by 50 mg to determine the dose the patient will receive:

$$10 \text{ kg} \times 50 \text{ mg} = 500 \text{ mg total daily dose}$$

You will learn another formula for calculating IV flow rates in Chapter 38.

Knowledge Connection
List three systems of measurement used in preparing medications. Why were some abbreviations put on a "Do Not Use" list? If the physician orders digoxin 0.25 mg to be given PO and the Lanoxin tablets in the drawer are labeled 0.125 mg, how many tablets will you administer to your patient?

Obtaining Medications

In hospital settings, medications may be found in a variety of storage systems. These include computerized cabinets, carts, and locked bins in the patient rooms.

Computerized Cabinets
To provide inventory control as well as safe medication storage, many acute care facilities use a computerized cabinet. One type is called PYXIS®. You must have a password to enter the system, which records your identity as the person

who removed the medication. You then type in the patient's name and a list of ordered medications for that patient appears on the screen. When you choose a medication, the drawer containing it opens, allowing you to remove the medication. When you close the drawer, the medication is automatically charged to the patient. Narcotics are kept in this system as well. When the drawer opens, the count is automatically changed to reflect the removal of one dose. Figure 35-4 shows this type of computerized cabinet.

Medication Cart

A medication cart may be used in some acute and long-term care facilities. It is restocked by pharmacy staff every 24 hours in the hospital setting. In long-term care, the medications are packaged in 30-day punch cards and kept in the resident's section of the drawer. There is a separate locking drawer for narcotics storage, and the entire cart locks as well. *Safety: Always lock the medication cart when you are not obtaining medications from it.*

Locked Bins in Patient Rooms

In some settings, the patient's medications are kept in a locked bin built into the closet in the patient rooms. The bin can be unlocked and stocked from the hallway, and can be unlocked and accessed in the patient's room. This prevents nurses from having to run back and forth to medicine rooms or carts to obtain medications. Narcotics are kept in the medication room under two locks, however.

Figure 35-4 This is a type of computerized medication cabinet.

Rights Involving Medications

Prior to administering any medication, you must ensure that everything is correct, and that the patient is willing and able to take the medication. Six rights of administration help prevent you from making any errors. Patients' rights are established to protect them from being forced to take medications that they do not wish to take.

Rights of Medication Administration

To prevent medication errors, you need to check the six rights of administration prior to giving any medication to a patient. Ensure that you have the:

- **Right medication:** Remember that orders may have changed since the last time you administered medications to this patient. Check for new medication orders and orders to discontinue previous medications. *Safety: Always verify that you have the correct medication by reading the label and comparing it with the MAR. Do not identify medications by their size, shape, or color as many drugs have very similar appearances.*
- **Right dose:** You must carefully read the ordered dose and ensure that it is within appropriate range for the patient. Check the original prescriber's order to be certain about a dose. *Safety: Pay close attention to the placement of decimals, as this can cause over- or underdosing if you misread it.*
- **Right Route:** Ensure that you know the route by which you are to administer the medication. Some medications, such as hydrocortisone, may be given orally, topically, and as an injection. *Safety: Pay close attention to the ordered route. If you administer a medication by the wrong route, it is considered a medication error.*
- **Right Patient:** *Safety: Use two methods of identifying your patient.* Ask the patient to confirm his or her name, and check the patient's armband or other identifying information. If a patient is confused or hard of hearing, you may say, "Mr. Smith?" and he will answer with "Yes," even though he is not Mr. Smith. When two patients share a room, it is very important to identify each patient for each medication and procedure. Do not rely on "Bed A" and "Bed B" distinctions.
- **Right Date and Time:** Some instructors break this apart and have seven rights of medication administration. Orders may be written for a medication to be given every other day, so it is important to note the date and to administer the medication as ordered. Some drugs are given for a period of time, such as 10 days, then automatically discontinued unless reordered. If you give a medication on a day it is not ordered to be given, it is considered a medication error. To give a medication at the right time, it must be administered within ½ hour before or ½ hour after the scheduled time. For example, if a medication is ordered at 0900, you can give it between 0830 and 0930. *Safety: Be aware of when medications are due and administer them within the 1-hour window of time.*

- **Right Documentation:** You must document correctly and completely to meet this right. You will document on the MAR with your initials under the correct date and time. If the medication is a narcotic, you must also document the medication, amount, route, and patient's name in the narcotic record. If the medication is to be administered prn, you will write the date, time, medication, and reason for administering it on the back of the MAR or in the nurses' notes, depending on facility policy. You must also document the patient's response to it after a period of time has elapsed, usually an hour for oral medications. If you do not give a medication for some reason, such as a patient refusing a medication or feeling nauseated, you must circle your initials under the date and time on the MAR and explain why the medication was not given on the back. *Safety: Document all medications, given or not given, following facility policy.*

When you check these rights and confirm that they are correct, you decrease the chances of making a medication error.

Patient Rights

Patients also have rights regarding medication administration. They have the right to know what the medication is for and how it will affect them. They have the right to refuse a medication. The patient can choose not to take a medication and should not be judged negatively for his or her choice. For example, a patient on chemotherapy for cancer may choose to stop taking the medication due to the side effects. While you might not make that same choice, you need to respect the patient's choice.

Patients also have the right to question their medications. They are now encouraged to question a medicine if it does not look like what they take at home, or is not being administered at the frequency they normally take. Some patients know their own medications and routine far better than the nurse in the hospital does. *Safety: If the patient questions a medication, research it thoroughly before administering it. This is an important safety check regarding the correct administration of medications.*

Safety Checks

When you prepare medications for administration, it is very important for you to stay focused on the task at hand. Ensure that you have no distractions, such as idle conversations or interruptions. When you prepare medications, you will obtain all the medications ordered for a patient at the time they are to be given. It is best not to prepare medications for two patients at one time because it is too easy to get confused. To prevent errors as you prepare medications, perform these three safety checks:

1. Verify the medication, dose, route, patient, date, and time as you remove the medication from the cart, bin, or PYXIS® machine.
2. Verify the medication, dose, and route against the MAR prior to placing it in the medication cup and returning the container to the drawer, if applicable.

3. Verify the patient, medication, dose, and route at the bedside prior to opening it and administering it to the patient.

If you are administering a number of medications to a patient at one time, it is a good idea to count the number of ordered medicines on the MAR and count the number of medicines in the cup to ensure that you are giving the correct amount. For example, if a patient has eight oral medications ordered at 0900, you would count the number of medicines in the cup to be sure you have eight ready to administer.

Supervision/Delegation Connection

Medication Administration

You must always administer the medications that you prepare. Do not delegate that task to anyone. For example, you cannot prepare medications and then leave them at the bedside for the CNA or UAP to administer later, after the patient's bath. In hospitals, preparation and administration of medications is strictly a function of a licensed nurse and cannot be delegated to a CNA or UAP. In some states, specially trained medication aides are allowed to administer medications to the residents in a long-term facility. In that situation, it is your responsibility to oversee the medication administration if it is performed by a medication aide.

Guidelines for Preparing Medications

Before you administer any medication, whether oral, topical, inhaled, injectable, or intravenous, follow these guidelines:

- Check the orders on the MAR and compare them with the original prescriber's order. Check for any discrepancies and validate that the order is correct.
- Look up any medication with which you are unfamiliar. If you are unsure about the purpose or effect of a medication, look it up. As you review the orders, determine if you need to check the patient's chart for any laboratory values prior to administering the medications, then obtain the information required.
- Wash or sanitize your hands according to facility policy.
- Obtain the ordered medications from the computerized cabinet, medicine cart, or patient bin. As you do so:
  - Verify the six rights of medication administration.
  - Check medication allergies and compare with the ordered medication.
  - Perform the first two safety checks.
- Determine if all medications are provided in the same dose and unit of measurement as ordered. If not, perform drug calculations to ensure that you have the correct number of tablets or capsules, and that you have the correct amount of liquid medication.
- Place the unopened medications in a medicine cup.
- Close and lock the medication cart or patient medication bin. If you are using a computerized cabinet, clear your password.

- Immediately take the medication to the patient's bedside. If the patient is unavailable, store prepared medications according to facility policy. Label the medicine cup(s) with the patient's name and room number prior to storing them.
- Perform the third safety check at the bedside, prior to opening the individually packaged medications.
- Assess any required vital signs before administering the medications, such as blood pressure or pulse if the medication will decrease or increase those readings. Ascertain that it is safe to give the medication to the patient.
- Administer the medications to the patient. Stay with the patient to ensure that all medications are swallowed and no problems occur (see Chapter 36).
- *Safety: Do not leave medications at the patient's bedside or ask another person to administer them for you. Administer only what you prepare.*

Knowledge Connection

List the six rights of medication administration. What are the three safety checks to make when preparing a medication, and when do you perform them? How can you be sure that you have the correct number of medications for patients who take large amounts at one time?

Medication Errors

The best way to prevent medication errors is to be extremely careful during preparation, question anything that does not seem correct about the order, and know what you are giving, the expected effects, and the potential side effects. Check vital signs or blood levels of medications prior to administering them to prevent toxicity or adverse effects. Calculate drug dosages carefully and have them checked by another nurse before preparing the medication. Box 35-5 gives tips for preventing medication errors.

Handling a Medication Error

Although all staff make every effort to avoid a medication error, sometimes an error does occur. It may be that you discover the error or that you make an error. *Safety: The most important thing is that you are honest about the mistake so the patient can be protected from harm.*

If you find an error made by another nurse, follow the facility policy for reporting it. In most situations, you will report it to the unit nurse manager or his or her assistant. Because you found the error, you will fill out the incident report (see Chapter 3). Avoid making judgmental statements about anyone who makes a medication error, as it can happen to very good nurses at times. All it takes is distraction from the task at hand, lack of focus, or not being thorough in knowledge about the medication.

Box 35-5

Tips for Preventing Medication Errors

It is easy to confuse some medication names and doses. You must be very careful to read names and doses exactly to prevent errors. You must also focus completely on the task at hand when preparing medications for administration.

- **Read drug names carefully.** Many drug names are similar and can be confusing. Examples include Zantac and Xanax, baclofen and Bactroban, Phenergan and Phenapen, Zostrix and Zestril.
- **Read doses carefully, especially those with decimals.** Look for a 0 in front of the decimal to call attention to its presence so it will not be overlooked. Example: 0.125 mg and 0.25 mg are both doses of digoxin. Also, doses in different units of the metric system can be the cause of an error. Examples: thyroid hormone is provided in micrograms (mcg) but may be ordered in milligrams (mg); 0.1 milligram is equal to 100 micrograms.
- **Never administer a medication you are unknowledgeable about.** If you do not know what the medication is for or what the expected effects are, you must look it up. Even if it is inconvenient and time consuming, you must know what you are administering, and if the dose is within appropriate range.
- **Focus on medication preparation without distractions.** Prepare medications for one patient at a time.
- **Ask for clarification.** If an order is unclear, outside of usual dosage parameters, or seems inappropriate for the patient, clarify the order with the prescriber.

If you make an error, be honest and report it yourself following facility policy. Complete the incident report and notify the physician. This is a humbling experience, but you must put the patient's well-being above your own pride. Most hospitals have a nonpunitive approach to error reporting to prevent staff from failing to report incidents that could bring harm to a patient.

An example to illustrate this occurred to a nursing student on a leadership rotation toward the end of her practical nursing program. The student was administering medications to all the residents on one hall in a long-term care facility. She checked the MAR and prepared the medications for a male resident and administered them. She then prepared the medications for the roommate and administered them. When she returned to the MAR, she realized that she had made two errors: She had given each resident his roommate's medications. The student was extremely distressed and went to her instructor with the error. They notified the physicians for each resident and completed incident reports. The student monitored vital signs every hour and finger stick blood sugars every hour as ordered for 4 hours. Neither resident suffered any ill effects, but the situation could have been life threatening.

People and Places Connection

Age-Related Concerns of Medication Administration

When you prepare medications for children, you must be constantly focused on the correct dose for the weight of the child. You will give only a portion of an adult dose, and it is critical that your dosage calculations be correct. Have them checked by another health care professional to verify that you are administering the correct dosage. In addition, always be certain that you have the correct strength of the medication. An example of a potentially fatal error occurred when a nurse drew up heparin 10,000 units/mL instead of heparin 1,000 units/ml to flush an infant's IV line.

When you prepare medications for elderly patients, keep in mind that they are more at risk for toxicity due to impairment of liver and kidney function, causing the medication to build up in the blood. It is very important to check blood levels of medications and signs and symptoms of toxicity prior to administering medications to the elderly.

 ## Post Conference

Although you were nervous, you managed to prepare all of your patient's medications after looking them up in your nursing drug guide. When your instructor asked about each medication, you were ready with the answers. You even calculated a dose correctly. You check the patient's fasting blood sugar and finger stick blood sugar levels before administering the insulin. The patient's potassium level was 3.3, so you and your instructor talked with the PA prior to administering the ordered furosemide (Lasix). The PA told you to give the Lasix and wrote an order to increase the potassium supplement to 20 mEq bid. Your instructor had to remind you, once you got to the bedside, to assess the blood pressure before administering Lasix and another antihypertensive. You learned a great deal about your patient's medications and will know them well next time.

KEY POINTS

- Medications have three names based on chemical ingredients, generic assigned names, and brand names.
- Medications fall into two categories: prescription and over the counter. Sometimes a medication can be in both categories due to different strengths.
- Controlled drugs fall into one of five schedules based on their potential for abuse. Schedule II drugs must be kept under double lock and counted at the end of each shift.
- Medications are prescribed for desired effects, but may also cause side effects, which are usually mild and expected, as well as adverse effects, which are more severe and harmful.
- Allergic reactions to drugs may range from mild, causing itching, rash, and hives, to anaphylaxis, which causes swelling of the airways and shortness of breath, and can possibly lead to shock and death.
- Some medications can accumulate in the bloodstream and cause toxicity. Nurses are responsible for checking the most recent medication blood levels prior to administering medications known to cause toxicity. Hold any ordered dose if blood levels are elevated, and notify the prescriber.
- Drugs can interact with other drugs, with foods, and with supplements. Nurses are responsible for researching medications prior to administration to be aware of any potential interactions.
- Read prescriber orders closely and carefully, paying close attention to decimals and abbreviations. If the dose, route, or frequency is not appropriate for the medication or the patient, notify the prescriber and verify the order.
- The six rights of medication administration help prevent you from making medication errors while preparing medications.
- The three safety checks occur when you remove the medication from the storage area, before returning the container or remaining medication to the storage area, and at the bedside prior to opening and administering the medication.
- You must admit to any medication error you make for the sake of the patient's well-being.

R E V I E W   Q U E S T I O N S

Select the answer that is most appropriate for each of the following questions. Some questions may have more than one correct answer. Check all that apply.

1. The drug name that is assigned and is not owned by the pharmaceutical company that develops the drug is the:

   a. chemical name.

   b. proprietary name.

   c. brand name.

   d. generic name.

2. You are preparing to administer a Schedule II drug. What special considerations are necessary?

   a. It is kept under double lock or with limited access in a computerized medication cabinet.

   b. It has a lower potential for abuse than Schedule III drugs.

   c. The remaining medications must be counted.

   d. The count must match the total in the record book.

   e. If kept in a computerized medication cabinet, the count is automatically totaled by the computer.

3. When you administer an antihypertensive medication at a dose within normal ranges, the patient's blood pressure drops to 84/60. This is a/an:

   a. side effect.

   b. adverse effect.

   c. allergic reaction.

   d. anaphylactic reaction.

4. A patient tells you that he is allergic to a muscle relaxer because it makes him sleep all day. You know that this is a common side effect of this medication. What action will you take?

   a. Record it as an allergy in the chart only.

   b. Explain to the patient that he is not really allergic to the medication.

   c. Record it as an allergy in the chart with an explanation of the reaction.

   d. Notify the physician immediately of the allergy and check for blood levels of the drug in the chart.

5. A patient is taking a medication to lower cholesterol. You know that the patient needs more teaching about the medication when he says:

   a. "I will take my medicine each morning with grapefruit juice."

   b. "This medicine is to help lower the cholesterol level in my blood."

   c. "If I experience any adverse effects or problems, I will contact my doctor."

   d. "I need to eat a low-fat diet and exercise as well as take this medication."

6. A patient on birth control pills tells you that she is also taking St. John's wort as an herbal supplement for mild depression. Which response will you make?

   a. "You need to be on a prescription drug for depression, not treat yourself."

   b. "St. John's wort increases estrogen breakdown, so it can decrease the effectiveness of your birth control pills."

   c. "St. John's wort decreases the rate of excretion of estrogen, so it can increase the side effects of birth control pills."

   d. "Have you looked up the medications you are taking to see if it interacts with any of them?"

7. You are using the PDR to look up a medication to determine its effects and side effects. The best way to obtain information is to first look up the medication in the:

   a. Brand and Generic Name Index, then read about it in the Product Information Section.

   b. Product Identification Section, then read about it in the Product Information Section.

   c. Manufacturer's Index, then locate it in the Product Identification Section.

   d. Product Category Index, then the Manufacturer's Index.

SHORT ANSWER QUESTIONS

8. You read this medication order on the physician's order page stamped with the patient's name:

6-10-12   *Lopressor 50 mg bid.* —————— *J. Johnson, MD*

What, if anything, is missing from this order?

9. Calculate the dose to give the patient for this order. "Give ampicillin 1 g per PEG tube q 6 h." On hand you have ampicillin 500 mg/6 mL.

CRITICAL THINKING EXERCISE

10. You have prepared oral medications for your patient and taken them into his room. The patient is in the bathroom taking a shower. His wife says, "Just leave the medicine on the bedside table. I will see that he takes it." What will you do and why?

ADDITIONAL RESOURCES

For additional Resources, Questions, and Activities, please see:

   Student Resource Disk

   http://davisplus.fadavis.com

Student Study Guide

REFERENCES

Abood R. *Pharmacy Practice and the Law.* Sudbury, MA: Jones and Bartlett; 2008.

Broselow J, Luten R, Schuman J. Preventing medications errors in children: safeguarding children from medication errors in hospitals, office practices, and the home. Modern Medicine, June 1, 2008. Available at: http://www.modernmedicine.com/modernmedicine/Pediatrics/Preventing-medication-errors-in-children/ArticleStandard/Article/detail/522755.

Copp MA. Drug addiction among nurses: confronting a quiet epidemic. *RN.* 2009;72(4):40-44.

DaCosta P. Medication errors: what to do about look-alike/sound-alike drug names. Modern Medicine, July 1, 2009. Available at: http://www.modernmedicine.com/modernmedicine/Medication+Errors/Medication-errors-What-to-do-about-look-alikesound/ArticleStandard/Article/detail/608081.

Diehl-Oplinger L. Brush up on your drug calculation skills. Available at: http://nursesaregreat.com/articles/drugcal.htm. Accessed November 28, 2009.

Dugdale DC, Henochowitz SI, Zieve D. Drug allergies. MedlinePlus Web site. August 6, 2008. Available at: http://www.nlm.nih.gov/medlineplus/ency/article/000819.htm. Accessed November 28, 2009.

Greco FA, Zieve D. Therapeutic drug levels. Drugs.com Web site. August 24, 2009. Available at: http://www.drugs.com/enc/therapeutic-drug-levels.html. Accessed November 28, 2009.

Institute for Safe Medication Practices. Misidentification of alphanumeric symbols in both handwritten and computer-generated information. ISMP Medication Safety Alert! Nurse Advise-ERR [Newsletter]. July 2, 2009. Horsham, PA: Institute for Safe Medication Practices.

Maher-Brisen P. Addiction: an occupational hazard in nursing. *Am J Nurs.* 2007;107(8):78-79.

McCann J. *Best Practices: Evidence-Based Nursing Procedures.* 2nd ed. Philadelphia: Lippincott, Williams & Wilkins; 2007.

Silverman H. Trade name and generic drugs. Merck Manual Home Edition. April 2007. Available at: http://www.merck.com/mmhe/sec02/ch017/ch017a.html. Accessed November 28, 2009.

Venes D, ed. *Taber's Cyclopedic Medical Dictionary.* 21st ed. Philadelphia: FA Davis; 2009.

Wilkinson J, Van Leuven K. *Fundamentals of Nursing: Theory, Concepts & Applications.* Philadelphia: FA Davis; 2007.

Administering Oral, Topical, and Mucosal Medications

Key Terms

Buccal route

Capsule

Dry-powder inhaler (DPI)

Elixir

Enteric-coated

Metered-dose inhaler (MDI)

Narcotic

Oral route

Rectal route

Respiratory route

Solution

Sublingual route

Suspension

Sustained-release

Syrup

Tablet

Topical route

Transdermal route

Vaginal route

Objectives

1. Define key terms associated with oral, topical, and mucosal medications.
2. Differentiate between the use of oral, sublingual, and buccal routes of administration.
3. Describe the variety of oral forms of drugs.
4. Explain how to prepare liquid medications.
5. Describe special considerations for administration of narcotic medications.
6. Describe special precautions needed when administering medications to patients on tube feedings.
7. Discuss principles to use when administering medicines through an enteral tube.
8. Explain the differences in administering medications to children, adults, and older adults.
9. Discuss guidelines for administering medications via the topical and transdermal routes.
10. Describe guidelines to follow when administering eye, ear, and nasal medications.
11. Discuss vaginal medications and how they are administered.
12. Identify purposes of rectal medications and contraindications for this route.
13. Differentiate between the use of a metered-dose inhaler and a dry-powder inhaler.
14. Identify nursing responsibilities when administering oral, topical, and mucosal medications.
15. Explain how to document medication administration on paper and in electronic MARs.
16. Discuss ways to prevent errors in medication administration and documentation.
17. Explain what to do if a medication error occurs.

Skills

36-1 Administering Oral Medications

36-2 Administering Medications Through an Enteral Tube

36-3 Administering Topical and Transdermal Medications

36-4 Administering Eye and Ear Medications

36-5 Irrigating the Eye and Ear

36-6 Administering Vaginal Medications

36-7 Administering Rectal Suppositories

36-8 Administering Inhaled Medications

🌐 Clinical Connection

Your Assignment: You are assigned to care for a 22-year-old female with developmental disabilities and a seizure disorder. She suffered brain damage at birth and is unable to chew and swallow. She lives in a long-term care facility and was transferred from that facility to the hospital for management of her seizure disorder, as well as treatment of eczema, constipation, and a vaginal yeast infection. She has a PEG tube, and you will be administering her feedings and medications through it. You have never administered a tube feeding before, much less medications through a PEG.

Your Actions: You begin to review how to administer a tube feeding and realize that some medications are not compatible with tube feeding formulas. When you research the antiseizure medication ordered for your patient, you learn that its effectiveness is decreased by interaction with many tube feeding formulas. You are unsure how to administer the medication, but you know that your patient definitely needs it. Your instructor also mentioned something about one medication that must be mixed with apple juice, but you do not remember which one.

Administration of medications following the six rights is a huge responsibility. You must know not only the medication, dose, and route ordered, but how to correctly administer medications via every route. In this chapter, we will focus on administration of drugs via the oral, topical, mucosal, and inhaled routes. Injected and intravenous routes are discussed in Chapters 37 and 38, respectively.

Routes of Administration

Many drugs are available in multiple forms that can be administered by several routes. It is important to know the purposes, uses, and variations of each route. For example, variations of the oral route include the **sublingual route** (under the tongue) and the **buccal route** (between the cheek and gum). In addition to understanding how to administer the medications via all the routes, you will also need to learn which types of preparations are suitable for each route.

Oral Route

The **oral route** of administration is the method by which medications are taken through the mouth or oral mucous membrane. When you think of administering medications by the oral route, you most often think of medications that are swallowed. This route is commonly referred to as "by mouth" or PO (*per os* in Latin) and also includes drugs that directly enter the bloodstream through the oral mucosa. Medications enter the bloodstream through the oral mucosa when the sublingual and buccal routes are employed. Sublingual medications are placed beneath the tongue to be absorbed, and buccal medications are placed between the check and gum to be absorbed. Oral medications are available in various forms, including tablets, capsules, and liquid medications.

Tablets and Caplets

A **tablet** is made of powdered ingredients compressed into various sizes and shapes. Tablets are the most common form of oral medication, and the majority are designed to be swallowed. They are broken down by the digestive system and absorbed into the bloodstream. Caplets are similar to tablets but are oblong in shape, making them easier for some people to swallow. Tablets that are not swallowed whole may be in forms that can be chewed, or they may melt on contact with saliva. An example of the latter form is hyoscyamine sulfate (Levsin).

Chewable tablets, such as chewable low-dose aspirin, are an alternative for patients who have difficulty swallowing large capsules or tablets. Chewing also breaks down the medication for increased activity in the stomach, such as in chewable antacids.

Enteric-coated tablets contain an outer coating that does not dissolve until the medication reaches the intestines. This coating protects the stomach from ingredients in the medication that may be irritating, preventing nausea, vomiting, and ulcer formation. Some medications are destroyed by stomach acids, and the enteric coating prevents the acids from inactivating the drug before it reaches the intestines.

Another type of coated tablet is a film-coated tablet. This coating prevents contact with the active ingredient during normal handling, which could cause damage to the medication.

Sustained-release tablets, also called *controlled-release, delayed-release, extended-release,* or *modified-release tablets,* are designed to slow the absorption of the drug. These medications are absorbed slowly over time for a continuous effect. *Safety: Do not crush or break sustained-release or enteric-coated tablets.* Crushing a sustained-release tablet will cause the patient to receive all of the drug at one time, leading to severe adverse effects and possible overdose. Crushing an enteric-coated medication will cause the medication to be absorbed in the stomach rather than the intestine, leading to gastric irritation or possible destruction of the medication.

Buccal tablets are designed to dissolve between the cheek and gum. As it dissolves, the tablet is absorbed through the walls of the numerous blood vessels in the inner cheek. Similarly, sublingual tablets dissolve under the tongue and are absorbed by the blood vessels there. These medications do not have to be digested to enter the bloodstream.

Capsules

A **capsule** is a gelatin shell containing a powder or pellets of medication. It may be preferred over tablets because it is swallowed more easily. Capsules may contain sustained-release pellets that dissolve over time for lasting medication effect.

If the patient is unable to swallow the capsule, it may be opened and the contents mixed with 1 to 2 teaspoons of soft food, such as applesauce or ice cream. *Safety: Never put crushed tables or opened capsules in a full serving of ice cream or applesauce. The patient may refuse to eat the entire serving and you will not know how much medication has been ingested.* Not all capsules can be opened and safely administered in this way. Check your nursing drug guide or discuss with a pharmacist before opening capsules. Medications that should not be crushed are listed in Box 36-1. Skill 36-1 (page 863) provides more information regarding administration of oral medications.

Liquid Medications

Liquid oral dosage forms include syrups, elixirs, solutions, and suspensions. Health care providers often prescribe liquid medications to patients who cannot swallow solid dosage forms and for those with nasogastric or percutaneous endoscopic gastrostomy (PEG) tubes. Definitions for each type of liquid oral form are found in Box 36-2. *Safety: Always shake a suspension prior to administering it to mix the drug with the liquid. Failure to do so could cause*

Box 36-1

Medications That Should Not Be Crushed

Some medications should not be crushed because crushing can cause them to be absorbed too quickly or because they are designed to dissolve in the intestines rather than the stomach. In addition, some medications can irritate mucous membranes in the esophagus and stomach if they are crushed. Medications that should not be crushed include:

- Buccal or sublingual tablets
- Effervescent tablets
- Enteric-coated tablets
- Liquid-filled gelcaps
- Medications that may taste too bitter to swallow
- Mucous membrane irritants
- Neoplastic agents (chemotherapy for cancer treatment)
- Orally disintegrating medications
- Sustained-release tablets

For a complete list of each medication that should not be crushed, go to the Institute for Safe Medication Practices website at *www.ismp.org.*

Box 36-2

Forms of Liquid Medication

Liquid medications come in a variety of forms to make them easier to swallow. Some should be used with caution in certain circumstances.

- An **elixir** may contain sweeteners or flavorings. It may also contain water and alcohol and is generally clear in appearance, though some may contain colorings. Patients with a history of alcohol abuse or receiving disulfiram (Antabuse) should avoid elixirs due to the alcohol content.
- A **solution** is a liquid containing a dissolved substance.
- A **suspension** contains fine particles of medication mixed with, but not dissolved in, a liquid. When the mixture sits, the particles will drift to the bottom of the liquid.
- A **syrup** is a concentrated aqueous preparation of sugars, with or without flavoring agents, and medicinal substances.

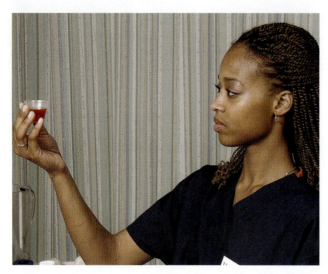

Figure 36-1   This nurse is measuring liquid medication at eye level.

ineffective medication action when doses are poured from the top of the bottle, and an overdose of medication when doses are poured from the bottom of the bottle.

When administering a liquid medication, shake the preparation if it is a suspension or if settling may have occurred. When you are pouring a dose from a bottle, you will usually use a plastic medicine cup. For infants and young children, you may use calibrated droppers or syringes. While pouring the liquid medication, hold the measuring device at eye level (Fig. 36-1). You will notice that the top of the liquid is not level, but instead it curves up on the sides and is slightly lower in the middle. This is called the *meniscus. Safety: When reading the amount of liquid in a medicine cup, read it at the lowest level of the meniscus.*

If you are pouring a liquid medication from a multiple-dose bottle, hold the label in the palm of your hand as you pour. In this way, no medication can accidentally be poured over the label and obscure the information on it.

In clinical settings, most liquid medications are packaged in single doses, also referred to as the *unit dose system.* It may not be necessary to pour out and measure liquid medications.

Some liquid medications, such as oral iron preparations, can stain the teeth. *Safety: Administer liquid medications that can stain teeth by having the patient drink it out of the medicine cup using a straw.* Have the patient drink a full glass of water afterward to prevent any of the medication from staying in contact with tooth enamel.

Holding Oral Medications

It is important to know when to withhold medications as well as when to administer them. *Safety: If the patient is NPO, do not administer routine medications unless ordered to do so.* For example, in some situations the

prescriber may write an order to give the medicines with a sip of water. If the patient is complaining of nausea or is vomiting, withhold the medication and notify the prescriber. If you give the medication, the patient may vomit all or part of it.

Administration of Oral Narcotic Medications

Narcotic medications are medications made with opium and opium derivatives that control and relieve pain. Narcotics are controlled substances, and may be formulated for oral, topical, injectable, and intravenous administration.

In the hospital setting, you may frequently administer oral narcotics to your patients. As you learned in Chapter 35, narcotics have a high potential for abuse and are regulated by law according to schedules. However, when narcotics are ordered by the prescriber for pain, it is appropriate to administer them. Often, the prescriber will order a strong narcotic for moderate to severe pain, and a less potent drug for mild to moderate pain. In those situations, you will use your nursing judgment as you assess the patient's pain level and how he or she rates the pain. Refer to Chapter 19 for information on assessing and managing pain.

Historically, nurses have undermedicated patients for pain rather than overmedicating them. It is important to assess the vital signs, especially respiratory status, prior to administering narcotics because they depress respirations and lower blood pressure. In addition to specific pain and vital sign assessments, obtaining narcotics for administration requires more steps than preparing other medications. See Chapter 35 for information on obtaining and preparing narcotics. *Safety: Remain with the patient until narcotic medications are swallowed to ensure that he or she does not "cheek" the medication. In rare situations, a patient might save up a number of narcotic medications to attempt suicide by taking them all at once.*

Counting Narcotic Medications

Nurses must count narcotics and other controlled substances at specific times, most commonly at shift changes. The on-coming nurse counts the narcotics with the off-going nurse. Any discrepancies must be accounted for and the narcotics record amended. If the count on the narcotics record does not match the number of narcotics in the drawer, report it immediately following facility policy, as federal law requires strict inventory and records with controlled substances compared to other prescription drugs. In some facilities, it is a policy that the off-going nurses cannot leave until the discrepancy is resolved. If it cannot be resolved, it may be policy for the nurses to participate in a urine drug screen to determine if diversion is occurring.

If you do not use a full dose of a narcotic, discard the unused narcotics and record the waste according to facility policies. For example, if you have an order for 50 mg of meperidine (Demerol) to be administered PO, and the meperidine in the drawer is in 100-mg tablets, you would administer only half of a tablet. The remaining half must be discarded according to facility policy. In most cases, you will dispose of it in a chemical waste container with another licensed nurse as a witness. Then you will record the narcotic drug wastage on the narcotic record and have the witness cosign with you. *Safety: In most situations, you will not dispose of wasted narcotic medications by flushing them down the toilet as this contributes to drugs in the environment.*

Knowledge Connection
What are narcotic drugs? How should you handle and administer narcotics? Describe the procedures for properly disposing of unused narcotics.

Enteral Tube Route

Patients who are unable to swallow food and medications may have a nasogastric or gastrostomy (PEG) tube placed. When that is the case, you will prepare oral medications and administer them through the enteral tube. For a review of feeding tubes and formulas, see Chapter 24.

Medication Considerations

Medications in tablet form will need to be crushed to a fine powder and mixed with 5 to 15 mL of water to be administered through the feeding tube. A mortal and pestle or a pill crusher may be used. When possible, the prescriber will order liquid medications, but if that is not possible, tablets will be crushed. Some medications, however, cannot be crushed because it will affect their absorption or desired effects (refer to Box 36-1).

Most capsules can be opened and mixed with water to be administered through the feeding tube. However, the contents of certain capsules must be mixed with juice rather than water and administered through a large-bore tube. *Safety: Always mix omeprazole (Prilosec) and lansoprazole (Prevacid) with apple or orange juice rather than water and flush the tube with juice.* This helps preserve the enteric coating on the granules and helps prevent clumping of the granules, which can then clog the tube. It is important to consult with the pharmacist before opening capsules and administering the contents through a feeding tube, especially with antireflux medications. Some timed-release capsules may be opened and mixed with 5 to 15 mL of water and then instilled via the tube. However, there are some timed-release medication capsules that cannot be opened for tube instillation. Timed-release medications that are crushed or capsules opened against recommendations by the manufacturer may result in not only a quicker onset of action, but a more intense or stronger effect, as well as severe adverse reactions.

Some medications should be taken on an empty stomach. Other medications can interact with the ingredients in tube feeding formulas and cause decreased effectiveness. Box 36-3 gives details about certain medications and their interactions with tube feeding formulas. Because such interactions are known to occur, it may be necessary to turn off a continuous tube feeding for a period of time before and after administering the medications. *Safety: Consult drug book references and the facility pharmacist to determine which medications may or may not be opened, crushed, mixed with formula, or administered via an enteral tube.*

Certain medications are known to cause clumping with tube feeding formula when given through an enteral tube. Small-bore feeding tubes can easily become obstructed if such clumping occurs. Although some of the medications that cause clumping are liquids, they should not be administered

Box 36-3

Common Medication and Enteral Formula Interactions

Always check for incompatibilities prior to administering medications through an enteral tube. The following medications are known to interact with tube feeding formulas. Recommendations of how to overcome those interactions are discussed.

Phenytoin (Dilantin) Suspension

If this antiseizure medication is given through an enteral tube and mixes with the formula in the patient's stomach, its absorption may be decreased by nearly 70%. When administering phenytoin, follow facility policy regarding stopping the continuous tube feeding. It is recommended that you stop the feeding for 1 to 2 hours prior to administering the phenytoin, then flush the tube with 60 mL of water after administering it to prevent the medication from adhering to the tube. Dilute phenytoin with 20 to 60 mL of water to improve its absorption before administering it through an enteral tube.

Carbamazepine (Tegretol) Suspension

This is another antiseizure medication that is not well absorbed when administered via enteral tube. This drug may adhere to the feeding tube itself. It is recommended that you dilute this medication with an equal volume of water or normal saline before administering it through an enteral tube to help prevent adherence to the tube. In addition, always flush the tube with at least 30 mL of water before and after administering any medication.

Warfarin (Coumadin)

This is an anticoagulant medication that is crushed and administered through an enteral tube. It can bind to the proteins in the tube feeding formula, decreasing its absorption and effectiveness. It is recommended that a continuous tube feeding be stopped for at least 1 hour before and 1 hour after warfarin administration to help prevent this interaction. If the medication is still less

(box continues on page 856)

Box 36-3 (continued)

Warfarin (Coumadin)

effective than required, it may be necessary for the physician to change the order to low-molecular-weight heparin (Lovenox), which is injectable only.

Fluoroquinolones

This is a class of antibiotics whose absorption is decreased by interactions with minerals in the feeding formula, such as calcium, magnesium, aluminum, and iron. It is recommended that you stop the tube feeding for at least 1 hour before and 2 hours after administering these types of antibiotics. It is also important to thoroughly crush the tablets and dilute them in 20 to 60 mL of water. *Safety: Do not administer ciprofloxacin (Cipro) suspension through a feeding tube because it may adhere to the tube and cause occlusion.*

Proton Pump Inhibitors

These medications help prevent symptoms of gastroesophageal reflux disease (GERD) by decreasing the amount of acid produced by the stomach. Because of their action, these medications are inactivated by gastric acid and are designed to dissolve in the duodenum. As discussed in the chapter text, omeprazole (Prilosec) and lansoprazole (Prevacid) may be opened and the granules mixed with apple or orange juice for administration down a large-bore enteral tube, then the tube should be flushed with more juice rather than with water.

If these medications must be administered through a small-bore enteral tube, you must dissolve the intact enteric-coated granules in a sodium bicarbonate 8.4% solution to prevent the drug from being destroyed by the stomach acid. Consult the pharmacist for assistance in this situation.

Another proton pump inhibitor, pantoprazole (Protonix), is available in a delayed-release suspension that contains enteric-coated granules. It is recommended that the suspension be drawn up in an oral syringe and mixed with apple juice for administration through an enteral tube.

However, another type of proton pump inhibitor, esomeprazole (Nexium), which is available in delayed-release capsules and a delayed-release oral suspension, should be mixed with water before administering through an enteral tube.

---

through an enteral feeding tube. Box 36-4 lists the medications that are known to cause clumping when administered with tube feeding formula.

Administration of Medication Through the Feeding Tube

When you administer medication through a feeding tube, it is important to keep several principles in mind. *Safety: Always flush the feeding tube with 30 to 60 mL of water before and after administration of medications to prevent interactions with formula in the tube, adherence of the drug to the tube, and clogging of the tube.*

It is ultimately your responsibility to know and follow the correct method of administration for each medication you give. Most medications will dissolve best in room-temperature or slightly warm water as opposed to cold water. There are conflicting theories regarding whether or not mixing medications together prior to administration will result in physical reactions that can alter or destroy their desired effects, so it is recommended that you administer each medication separately, never mixing the crushed pills or liquids together. This also makes it possible for you to identify each drug during administration; this is pertinent in case an interruption occurs during the administration process. For example, if you were administering medications through an enteral tube and accidentally spilled one medication, you could identify which medication the patient did not receive. Another situation might be that, while you are at the bedside preparing to administer the medications, the physician walks in and discontinues one of the medications that you have already crushed. In this example, you would be able to identify which medication to stop. If the medications were all mixed together in one cup, you would be unable to remove the discontinued medication.

When administering multiple medications, you must also flush the tube between medications with 5 to 15 mL of water to clear the medicine out of the tube before instilling the next medicine. This further reduces the risk of an adverse reaction occurring due to mixing two or more drugs together in a small amount of water. *Safety: Avoid mixing crushed pills or liquids together in the same cup to be as accurate as possible while administering medications.* Skill 36-2 (page 864) provides more information on administering medications through an enteral tube.

Box 36-4

Medications That Cause Clumping When Administered With Enteral Feeding Formulas

The following medications should not be administered with tube feeding formulas:

- Brompheniramine (Dimetapp)
- Ferrous sulfate (Feosol elixir)
- Guaifenesin (Robitussin)
- Lithium citrate (Cibalith-S)
- Monobasic sodium phosphate (Fleet Phospho-Soda)
- Potassium chloride liquid
- Pseudoephedrine hydrochloride (Sudafed syrup)

Supervision/Delegation Connection

Unlicensed Personnel and Medication Administration

If you are working in a setting where you supervise unlicensed personnel who administer medications, be very sure that they are knowledgeable about all aspects of medication administration in their scope of practice. Take time to observe each staff member when they prepare and administer medications. Ensure that the medicines are being administered correctly. Since you are the licensed person, you are responsible for the medications administered by those you supervise. Avoid assuming that your unlicensed staff members always know what to do.

Knowledge Connection

How much water should be used to flush an enteric tube before and after administration of medications? In how much water should a crushed medication be dissolved? How will you know if it is safe to crush a medication or open a capsule or administer a medication with a particular formula?

Administering Medications to Special Populations

Administration of medications to elders and to children can pose certain challenges. The elderly patient is more at risk for side effects and medication interactions, while children may be more resistant to swallowing medications. See Boxes 36-5 and 36-6 for tips on administering medications to these special populations.

People and Places Connection

Medication Organizers

Many elderly patients in home health care use medication organizers, which contain separate storage compartments for the medications to be taken at breakfast, lunch, dinner, and bedtime. These containers can be prepared for an entire week at a time. They offer the added benefit of allowing the client and the nurse to see if the medications have been taken.

Punch Card Systems

Most long-term care facilities use a punch card system for administering medications. Each card contains a 30-day supply of medication, which is numbered in descending order. Punch out the medication in order and you will be able to tell exactly how many tablets or capsules remain. Reorder resident's medications when a 7-day supply remains to avoid interruption in medication availability.

Topical Route

The **topical route** of administration involves applying a drug to the skin or mucous membranes. Topical drugs are typically used for their action at one specific site. In addition to the skin, other topical routes may include the vagina, anus, eyes, and ears; however, these are sometimes distinguished from topical drugs applied to the skin.

Topical drugs usually act locally, but may also have systemic effects. There are several different classes of

Box 36-5
Administering Medicines to Older Adults

Older adults may have problems taking medications due to difficulty swallowing. In addition, their reactions to and metabolism of medications may be different than those of a younger adult due to the effects of aging on different body systems.

It is important to keep the following considerations in mind when you are administering medications to the elderly:
- **Difficulty swallowing:** You may need to crush medications and mix them in 1 to 2 teaspoons of applesauce or ice cream for the older person to swallow. If medications cannot be crushed, you may need to obtain an order for a liquid medication.
- **Metabolism of medications:** Because aging causes patients to be more sensitive to medication effects and side effects, it is important to assess for toxicity and undesired effects frequently. Aging also affects the ability of the body to prevent medications from affecting the central nervous system, so assess for increased side effects of confusion or disorientation.
- **Multiple medications:** Many elderly people are taking a large number of medications for a variety of chronic conditions. Be alert to possible interactions of these medications with each other and with OTC medications, including supplements and herbal remedies.
- **Adverse drug reactions:** It is important to monitor laboratory results to know if medications should be held and the prescriber consulted. Monitor liver and kidney function tests for toxic effects of certain medications. When elderly patients are on multiple medicines, consider any new sign or symptom to be drug related until determined differently.

Box 36-6
Administering Medicines to Infants and Children

One major focus of administering medications to infants and children is getting them to take the medicine. Some devices and ideas to improve this include:
- **Administration devices:** Infants may spit out liquid medications. Use of an oral syringe is recommended because it offers more accurate dosing and is easy to use. Teach parents to remove the cap from the end of the syringe and to keep it out of the infant or child's reach to prevent choking. Place the syringe toward the back of the mouth in the cheek pouch and depress the plunger to administer the medication.
- **Small doses:** The amount of medication ordered for children is generally a fraction of an adult dose. Double-check the appropriate pediatric dosage for the patient's weight, usually ordered in milligrams per kilogram of body weight. Overdoses can easily occur. Some facilities require two nurses to check a pediatric medication dose before it is administered.
- **Objectionable taste:** If a child refuses a medication due to taste, speak with the pharmacist about adding a flavoring syrup to it. If the taste cannot be masked, you can offer a frozen juice bar to the child first, as it will help numb the taste buds. Praise the child when he or she takes the medication.

topical preparations, each with unique characteristics (Box 36-7).

When you administer topical medications such as creams and ointments, you will generally apply a thin coat of the medication to the affected area. Certain topical medications are ordered to be applied "liberally," or with a thick coat of medication. It is important that you know the appropriate application amount by researching the medication in a nursing drug guide. Use a cotton-tipped swab or a tongue depressor to apply the medicine. Avoid touching the opening of the tube or dispenser to the patient's skin to prevent contamination. Wear gloves when you administer topical medications to decrease the chance of contact with blood, body fluids, and medication.

Some topical medications should not be covered with an occlusive dressing because it can alter the absorption of the drug. If you are uncertain about covering a topical medication, check with the pharmacist before applying an occlusive dressing. Skill 36-3 (page 866) provides more information about administering topical medications.

Transdermal Route

The **transdermal route** is a method of applying a drug to the skin using a patch. The drug is absorbed through the skin into the bloodstream for a systemic effect (Fig. 36-2). The transdermal route delivers a slow, constant dose of medication. Transdermal patches are drugs bonded to an adhesive bandage and applied to the skin. Several drugs are now prepared in patch form, including nitroglycerin, nicotine, and oral contraceptives.

Safety: Before applying the patch, write the date, time of application, and your initials on the patch. When applying transdermal patches, avoid touching the medicated portion with your fingers. Wear gloves during the application, and apply each patch to a different place than the previous patch. Be sure to remove the previous patch first, to avoid giving the patient an overdose of medication. Try to

Figure 36-2 A transdermal patch is used for delivery of systemic medications.

choose a site that has the least amount of hair, for example, the upper arm or lower abdomen. It may be necessary to shave an area on the upper chest or arm so the patch will adhere. Do not cut patches to fit smaller areas. Skill 36-3 provides more information on applying a transdermal patch.

Knowledge Connection
Describe the different types of topical preparations. Why are certain drugs administered topically or transdermally?

Mucosal Route

Drugs may be absorbed through the mucous membranes in the eyes, nose, rectum, and vagina. This route is sometimes preferred because the drugs enter directly into the bloodstream, resulting in faster onset of action. For example, if a patient has nausea and vomiting, you may administer medication via a rectal suppository to relieve it. The drug is absorbed into the bloodstream for a rapid effect that could not be obtained by administering it orally. Some mucosal medications are administered for local effects, for example, a vaginal medication to treat a yeast infection or an eye medication to treat glaucoma.

Eye Medications
Drugs administered to the eye take the form of drops or ointments, and are usually applied in the lower conjuctival sac. Eye medications may be ordered to lubricate the eye, to prevent or treat conditions such as glaucoma or infection, or for diagnostic purposes. Examples of eye medications include timolol (Timoptic) for glaucoma, gentamicin (Garamycin) for bacterial infection such as conjunctivitis or "pink eye," and prednisolone (Inflamase) for inflammation.

When you administer eyedrops, you will place them into the middle part of the lower conjunctival sac. Have the patient tilt his or her head back and look upward. Gently pull the lower lid down to expose the sac. Gently brace your hand against the patient's forehead or cheek to prevent injury to the eye if the patient moves his or her

Box 36-7

Types of Topical Medication Preparations

The following is a list of the most common types of topical medications:
- **Creams** are typically *viscous* (thick) emulsions, with some *emollient* (moisturizing) ability. Creams are commonly used for topical steroids and in medications to relieve itching.
- **Gels** are not as thick as creams, and are usually clear, but may contain coloring. Phenergan gel is applied to the inner wrists to help relieve nausea.
- **Lotions**, like creams, are emulsions, but are less viscous and moisturizing. Some may be drying, such as calamine lotion for poison ivy.
- **Ointments**, like creams, are highly viscous and have an emollient base. They are often dispensed in tubes. Ointments are used for antibiotic and steroid topical medications.

head. Administer the drop of eye medication into the conjuctival sac.

To apply eye ointment, gently squeeze a line of ointment into the conjuctival sac. Instruct the patient to close his or her eyelids and move the eyes around while keeping the eyelids closed. Avoid applying pressure to the eyeball at all times. Also, avoid touching the tip of the tube or dropper to the patient's eye or skin to prevent contamination by pathogens. A tissue may be used to wipe from the inner to outer part of the eye along the eyelash. Advise patients not to rub their eyes after applying eyedrops or ointments.

In some situations, the drug that is administered for a local effect may be absorbed into the bloodstream and cause unwanted systemic effects. To prevent this, after you administer the eyedrops, press your gloved fingertip gently against the lacrimal ducts on either side of the nose for a few seconds. Skill 36-4 (page 867) provides further information about administering eye medications.

Ear Medications

Drugs administered in the ear are in the form of drops. These drugs may be used to soften cerumen, relieve pain, treat infection or inflammation, or facilitate removal of a foreign body, such as an insect or a small object. Examples of eardrops include ciprofloxin/hydrocortisone (Cipro HC) for infection and carbamide peroxide (Debrox) to soften earwax for removal.

To instill eardrops, position the patient lying on his or her side with the affected ear up. For adults and children older than 3 years of age, gently pull the pinna up and back. For children younger than 3 years of age, pull the pinna down and back. This helps straighten the ear canal, allowing drops to penetrate to the middle ear. Aim the dropper so that the medication drop rolls down the wall of the canal and does not drop directly onto the tympanic membrane, which would cause pain. *Safety: Avoid touching the dropper to the surface of the ear to prevent the introduction of pathogens into the bottle of ear medication.* Ask the patient to remain with his or her head positioned with the affected ear up for at least 2 minutes. A cotton ball may be placed loosely in the ear to absorb excess medication. *Safety: Do not administer eardrops to patients with damage to the tympanic membrane.* If in doubt, ensure that the tympanic membrane has been examined with an otoscope by a health care professional prior to administering the medication. Skill 36-4 provides more information about administering eardrops.

Eye and Ear Irrigations

You may have orders to irrigate a patient's eyes or ears with saline to flush away debris and contaminants. Sometimes you may be irrigating to remove a foreign body from the eye or ear, such as an insect in the ear or piece of sawdust in the eye. Occasionally, a small child will place a foreign body in a body orifice, including the ear. It is important to know that irrigation is contraindicated for the removal of a foreign body that could absorb fluid and enlarge. For example, a dry bean will absorb irrigation fluid and become even more securely wedged in the ear. Skill 36-5 (page 868) provides more information on eye and ear irrigation.

Nasal Medications

Nasal medications are administered to reduce inflammation, facilitate drainage, or treat infections in the nasal cavity. Drugs administered via the nasal mucosa are rapidly absorbed into the bloodstream. Some medications are administered for local effects on the nasal mucosa. Mucinex nasal spray (guaifenesin), for example, is used to promote sinus and nasal drainage by reducing swollen nasal membranes. Other drugs administered via the nasal route are given for systemic effects and are simply absorbed through the nasal mucosa. These medications include nicotine (Nicotrol Inhaler), calcitonin (Miacalcin), and sumatriptan (Imitrex).

Nasal decongestant sprays can be counterproductive if used for long periods of time. While they relieve congestion with administration, they can also cause a rebound effect with long-term use. This causes swelling of the nasal mucosa, leading to congestion, causing the need for more nasal spray. If long-term use continues, the arteries in the nasal passage will shrink and scar, causing lesions and nosebleeds. Generally, it is not recommended to use nasal decongestant sprays for more than 3 days. Steroid nasal sprays, such as budesonide (Rhinocort), generally do not cause these rebound effects.

To administer nasal sprays, it is very important to position the patient with the head flexed forward so that the spray enters the sinuses and does not go down the throat.

Vaginal Medications

Medications administered via the **vaginal route** come in the form of suppositories, creams, aerosol foams, or tablets that are inserted into the vagina and dissolve there. Some preparations come with a disposable tubular applicator with a plunger to insert the medication. Other medications come with a prefilled applicator that can simply be inserted and the plunger depressed. This route is typically used to treat local infections such as yeast infections, but may also be used for vaginitis, for endometrial atrophy, and for contraception with spermicidal agents.

When you administer creams using an applicator, you will attach the applicator to the end of the tube containing the cream. As you squeeze the tube, the cream will fill the applicator, pushing the plunger backward. When the applicator is filled with cream, you will detach it from the tube of medication, and insert it into the patient's vagina. Gently insert the applicator into the vagina along the posterior vaginal wall for approximately 3 inches (8 cm) and depress the plunger to disperse the cream. Always wear gloves when administering vaginal medications to prevent contact with blood and body fluids. Gently depress the plunger until all of the cream is inserted. Instruct the patient to remain lying down for between 5 and 15 minutes so the medication can be absorbed. Some medications are ordered to be given at bedtime to prevent loss of the cream when the patient stands upright.

When you administer a vaginal suppository, you will first lubricate the tip of the suppository with a water-soluble lubricant. Insert the suppository with the index finger. Vaginal tablets are diamond-shaped and fit into the end of an applicator with a plunger. After placing the tablet in the applicator, you may apply water-soluble lubricant to it. Gently insert the applicator into the vagina along the posterior vaginal wall for approximately 3 inches (8 cm) and depress the plunger. This will push the tablet deep into the vagina, where it will dissolve and the medication will be absorbed. The patient may wish to wear a perineal pad to protect clothes from drainage due to the cream, foam, or suppository. Skill 36-6 (page 869) provides more information about administering vaginal medications.

Rectal Medications

Rectal medications are typically available in suppository or enema form, but ointments and creams may also be administered. Medications given via the **rectal route** are inserted directly into the rectum and may be ordered when nausea or vomiting is present or when the patient cannot take anything by mouth. While it is a safe and convenient route, many people object to its use. Small children can be especially distressed by rectal administration of medications.

Rectal administration of medications may be used to directly treat local pain and inflammation. Hydrocortisone (Anucort-HC), for example, is a rectal suppository used for swelling and inflammation due to hemorrhoids. Sometimes seizure medications may be administered via the rectal route. Diazepam rectal gel (Diastat) is a medication approved for epilepsy. The rectal route may also be used for laxative purposes. Rectal suppositories are often administered to stimulate a bowel movement. One example is bisacodyl (Dulcolax) suppositories.

Medications may also be administered by enema. An example of this is a sodium polystyrene sulfonate (Kayexalate) enema, which is given to help decrease dangerously high potassium levels in the blood. See Chapter 30 for a more thorough discussion on enemas.

If a patient has cardiac dysrhythmia or had a recent myocardial infarction, avoid using the rectal route for medication administration, as insertion may stimulate the vagus nerve and trigger a dysrhythmia. Evaluate the appropriateness of administering medications via the rectal route to patients with undiagnosed abdominal pain or who have recently undergone surgery of the bowel, rectum, or prostate as the insertion of the medication could cause trauma or injury.

Rectal suppositories are bullet-shaped, with a rounded tip and a blunt end. When you administer a rectal suppository, you will first lubricate the tip with a water-soluble lubricant. Wear gloves to avoid possible contact with blood or body fluids. Insert the suppository rounded tip first and, with your index finger on the blunt end, push it past the internal anal sphincter so it will be retained in the rectum. Because rectal suppositories are made using a wax base, they are generally kept in the refrigerator to prevent melting. Skill 36-7 (page 870) provides more information about administering rectal suppositories.

Respiratory Medications

Medications administered by the **respiratory route** are dispersed in fine droplets and inhaled into the lungs and bronchial airways, usually through the use of inhalers or nebulizers (Fig. 36-3). The respiratory route of medication administration is often used to treat pulmonary conditions such as asthma and chronic obstructive pulmonary disease (COPD).

The onset of action following pulmonary administration is rapid. Nebulizers use compressed air forced through liquid medication, resulting in a fine mist inhaled into the bronchi and bronchioles to dilate them. Bronchodilators are given to open constricted airways and include albuterol (Ventolin, Proventil) and ipratropium bromide (Atrovent). Certain mucolytic drugs such as acetylcysteine (Mucomyst) may also be administered using a nebulizer. For more information on administering a nebulizer treatment, please refer to Chapter 28. Other methods of administering respiratory medications are metered-dose inhalers (MDIs) and dry-powder inhalers (DPIs).

Metered-Dose Inhalers

Metered-dose inhalers (MDIs) are pressurized medication dispensers that spray a premeasured amount of drug into the lungs. They are the most efficient way to get medications into the airways. Medications such as short-acting bronchodilators are delivered quickly to treat an acute asthma attack. MDIs are also used to deliver anti-inflammatory agents and bronchodilators for long-term management of asthma. *Safety: Instruct patients to avoid leaving MDIs in the car as heat may cause them to explode or rupture.*

Figure 36-3 Different types of inhalers: A. An ultrasonic nebulizer delivers medication and humidity as a fine mist. B. A metered-dose inhaler delivers measured doses. This one has a spacer. C. A dry-powder inhaler (Turbuhaler). D. A Diskhaler.

Some patients have difficulty using a MDI correctly, so it is important to teach the proper technique for administration. Skill 36-8 (page 871) provides more information on administering medication via an MDI.

Figure 36-4 How to tell if an inhaler is full, partially full, or empty.

Patient Teaching Connection

Using a Metered-Dose Inhaler

Instruct the patient to first shake the inhaler to mix the contents before delivery. Have the patient remove the mouthpiece cover and hold the inhaler 1½ to 2 inches away from the mouth. This prevents large droplets of medication from landing on the tongue and being rapidly absorbed, leading to increased severity of side effects such as nervousness, tremors, and tachycardia. Patients may be accustomed to placing the mouthpiece directly into the mouth, but newer research indicates that the 1½- to 2-inch distance is preferred.

Instruct the patient to inhale deeply as he or she depresses the canister, then hold the breath for 10 seconds. Teach the patient to then breathe out slowly through pursed lips. Frequently the order for MDI administration is to take 2 puffs. If that is the case, the patient should wait 1 full minute before taking the second puff to allow the medication to be completely absorbed.

In some situations, especially when the patients are elders or children, it may be difficult for them to coordinate depressing the canister with deep inhalation. In that case, a spacer may be used. This is a chamber that attaches to the inhaler mouthpiece and holds the medication after the canister is depressed. The patient can then inhale the medicine in several more shallow breaths.

Instruct patients to rinse their mouths with water and spit it out after using steroid inhalers. Steroids in the oral cavity can lead to a yeast infection called *thrush*. Rinsing out the mouth after use prevents the steroid from remaining in the oral cavity. If patients are using two types of inhalers, such as a bronchodilator and a steroid, instruct them to wait 5 minutes between the use of each inhaler. Instruct the patient to use the steroid inhaler last, then to rinse the mouth immediately after use.

MDI Maintenance
Wipe the mouthpiece of the MDI after use to remove excess medication. If a spacer is being used, rinse it daily in warm water, then allow to air dry. It can be difficult for patients to tell how much medication is left in an MDI. To help determine whether the canister is becoming close to empty, place it in a sink full of water (Fig. 36-4). As with other medications, discard expired inhalers and replace with new ones.

Dry-Powder Inhalers
Unlike MDIs, **dry-powder inhalers (DPIs)** do not contain a pressurized canister and do not spray medication out; rather, they rely on the force of the patient's own inhalation to dispense a dose of dry-powder medication. Common DPIs include the Rotahaler, Spinhaler, Diskus, and Handihaler.

Diskus inhalers are a frequently prescribed type of DPI. These are flat disks containing a number of small chambers, each loaded with an individual dose of dry medication. When you slide the thumb grip away from you, it reveals the mouthpiece and a lever. When the lever is pushed, it opens the door to the chamber. The patient must place the mouthpiece of the diskus directly into his or her mouth and close the lips around it. When the patient inhales deeply, the dry powder is breathed into the lungs. *Safety: Ensure that patient does not exhale directly into the DPI because the exhalation will disperse the powder.* Patients with severe asthma may not be able to produce enough air flow to successfully use these inhalers. Skill 36-8 gives more information on how to administer medication via a DPI.

Knowledge Connection
List four types of topical preparations. Under what circumstances might you question administering a medication rectally? Explain the differences between an MDI and a DPI.

Nursing Responsibilities for Administering Oral, Topical, and Mucosal Medications

As discussed in Chapter 35, you are responsible for assessing the patient, monitoring laboratory results, and evaluating the information before you administer any medications.

- Assess the patient for appropriateness of medication administration. For example, you have an order from a prescriber for a daily stool softener for a patient. When you question the patient about his or her bowel movements, you learn that the patient is having three or four soft stools each day, described as "almost diarrhea." In that case, it would not be appropriate to administer the stool softener without discussing it with the prescriber first.
- Check all laboratory results to determine if it is safe and appropriate to administer an ordered medication, as some medications can reach toxic levels or exceed the therapeutic effect. For example, if the patient is taking warfarin (Coumadin), it is important to check the prothrombin levels (pro time) or INR in the laboratory results first. This medication is an anticoagulant, and it is possible that the blood will not clot adequately if too much of the drug is in

the bloodstream. The patient may bleed from the vagina, rectum, nose, or gums. If the pro time or INR is above therapeutic range, you will hold the medication and notify the prescriber.

- Always check drug allergies prior to administering any medication. It is also important to check ingredients of combination medications in patients who are allergic to determine if a sensitivity exists. An example might be if you had an order to apply triple antibiotic ointment to an open area on a patient's arm. You will need to determine the names of the three antibiotics in the ointment and compare them to any allergies the patient might have. If the patient is allergic to neomycin, for example, he or she could react to the ointment as well as the systemic medication.
- Check the timing prior to administering medications and ensure that you are dispensing them appropriately. *Safety: For prn medications, you must check to see the last time the medication was given to ensure that the timing is within the ordered parameters.* If a medication is ordered every 4 hours prn, check the documentation to determine the last time it was given. Be sure that you administer the drug at least 4 hours from the last dose.

Laboratory and Diagnostic Connection

Coordinating Medication Administration With Blood Specimens

It is very important that you administer medications on time, especially when laboratory values are to be drawn. The laboratory staff plans to obtain blood specimens based on the expected time that medications are to be given. For example, a digoxin level is ordered to be drawn 8 hours after the medication is administered. If the patient is taken to another department for a diagnostic procedure and the medication is not given on time, alert the laboratory staff right away. Otherwise, the digoxin level may be drawn only 4 hours after administration, leading to an artificially elevated blood level and possible inappropriate changes in the medication dose.

Documentation of Medication Administration

Medication administration may be documented in one of two ways: on paper or electronically. More acute care hospitals are moving to the electronic version of medication administration records (MARs) because these systems help prevent medication errors due to built-in safeguards. The electronic system is expensive, however, and may be cost prohibitive for smaller facilities and long-term care facilities.

Documentation on a Paper MAR

Medication administration records provide documentation of the date and time a medication is administered, as well as the person who dispensed it. As discussed in Chapter 35, the record contains a grid with the date and time marked.

After you administer a medication in a hospital setting, you will immediately document it on the MAR. On most paper MARs, the ordered medications are listed on the left side with the times of administration. Across the top of the page, the dates are listed. You will initial in the appropriate section, across from the medication and time, and beneath the correct date, or write in the time followed by your initials. Some facilities have a policy that you write in the time you administered the medication followed by your initials. Then you draw a single line through the time to indicate the medication has been administered.

If a medication is not given for some reason, follow facility policy for documenting the omission. Often, the procedure is to initial in the section or box across from the medication, then circle your initials. This signals that an explanation will be found in the nurses' notes or on the reverse side of the MAR documenting why the medication was not given.

Paper MARs contain an area to correlate the nurse's initials with his or her full name and credentials. Figure 36-5 shows the area at the bottom of the MAR where the nurse writes his or her name to identify his or her initials.

Medications are transcribed from the prescriber's order sheet to the MAR. *Safety: There is potential for errors to occur during transcription of medication orders.* This is why it is always necessary for you to check the original prescriber's order to be certain that you are administering the medications as intended in that order.

Paper MARs also contain identifying information, including the patient's name and room number, patient identification number, physician's name, and the patient's allergies, which are listed in red ink. The medication listing includes the name of the medication (generic is preferred), and the dose, route, and frequency of administration.

When a medication is discontinued on a paper MAR, the entire section is highlighted in yellow all the way across the MAR and the word "discontinued" is written next to the medication on the list. Sometimes the abbreviation "disc" is used. The older abbreviation "d/c" is no longer acceptable because it could be mistaken for other words. *Safety: Always read the MAR carefully before administering medications.* Occasionally a medication may be marked as discontinued, but the section has not been highlighted in yellow, causing the potential for error.

Documentation of Special Situations

When a medication is ordered to be administered prn, or "as necessary," you will document it on the MAR in the section for prn medications. On some MARs, the prn medications are listed at the bottom of the MAR as they are given. Because these medications are not given at scheduled times, you must write in the time you have administered the medication. In addition, you must document the reason you gave the medication in the nurses' notes or other appropriate location, following facility policy.

HOSPITAL MEDICATION ADMINISTRATION RECORD

Codes For Injection Sites

A - Left Anterior Thigh	H - Right Anterior Thigh
B - Left Deltoid	I - Right Deltoid
C - Left Gluteus Medius	J - Right Gluteus Medius
D - Left Lateral Thigh	K - Right Lateral Thigh
E - Left Ventral Gluteus	L - Right Ventral Gluteus
F - Left Lower Quadrant	M - Right Lower Quadrant
G - Left Upper Quadrant	N - Right Upper Quadrant

Mary Smith 086432

age 46   John Miller, M.D.

ALLERGIES: *PCN, Sulfa*

DATE ORDERED	DATE REORD.	DRUG - DOSE - ROUTE - FREQUENCY	ADMIN. TIME	DATE 4.16.06	DATE 4.17.06	DATE 4.18.06
4.16.06		Lanoxin 0.25mg po Q D	0900	09 JW		
4.16.06		Rocephin 1 gm IV Q D	1200	1200 JW		
4.16.06		Zinacef 1 gm IV Q 8 hr	0800	08 JW		
			1600			
			2400			
SIGNATURE / SHIFT INDICATES			7-3	JW		
NURSE ADMINISTERING MEDICATIONS			3-11			
J Wilson, RN			11-7			

Figure 36-5   Documentation on a MAR.

It is very important to check back with the patient in 45 minutes to 1 hour to see if the medication relieved the problem. This is the evaluation phase of the nursing process. Document the patient's response to the medication. If the medication does not relieve the problem, you will then contact the prescriber and document that you have done so. Document any new orders received.

Narcotic medications are often given on a prn basis. In addition to the special documentation needed for prn medications, you must also sign out narcotic drugs in the narcotic record or narcotic book. As discussed in Chapter 35, it is extremely important to sign out these types of medications and ensure that the count is correct. In facilities that use electronic MARs, it is not necessary to sign out the narcotic medication separately, as the computerized system counts the drug for you. Skill 36-1 provides an example of documenting a prn narcotic medication.

Documentation on an Electronic MAR

Electronic medication administration records, or eMARs, are part of an electronic system designed to reduce administration errors. This system uses bar code reading technology to monitor the administration of medications. eMARs record patient health information into a computer database, including medication, allergies, past or present illnesses/injuries and hospital visits, and family history.

The principles of electronic documentation are the same as paper records. The physician orders the medication and the pharmacist dispenses it with a bar code attached, then delivers the medication to the computerized medication cabinet or medication cart. This offers a method of inventory control as well. The patient's identification band contains a special medication bar code. You can access your patient's ordered medications via a computer or handheld device. The screen will show the medications due at a particular time for a particular patient. When you scan the bar code of each medication with the scanner, similar to checking out at a grocery store, the computer screen shows any warning messages, interactions, or considerations before administering the medication. You will then determine if further action is needed before administering the medication.

When you go to the patient's room, you will still use two methods of identification for the patient, then scan the medication bar code on the patient's identification band. The administration of the medication is automatically recorded in the eMAR, and the medication is automatically charged to the patient. If you are using a handheld device, it may be necessary to download your administration of medications into a main computer. Follow facility policy as different software programs may require different pathways for documentation.

Documentation on MARs in Long-term Care

In many long-term care facilities, documentation of medications is done prior to taking the medication to the resident. This is known as the "PIG" method of administration, which stands for "Punch, Initial, Give." If for some reason the medication is not administered to the resident, you will circle your initials and document the reasons and results in the nurses' notes or on the MAR. Accurate and thorough documentation is vital for regulations, reimbursement, and quality of care.

Documenting Withheld or Refused Medications

Under certain circumstances, a drug may be withheld or refused. If a patient refuses a medication, take the time to ask the reason behind the action. If it is due to unpleasant side effects, you may be able to take some actions to minimize those side effects. If the patient believes the medication is not effective, document this and discuss it with the prescriber. Encourage patients and residents to take prescribed medications by explaining the desired effect of the drug. If the patient or resident continues to refuse, do not force the issue. Notify the prescriber and document in the nurses' notes the date, time and reason for withholding a drug. Then document the name of the prescriber notified and the prescriber's response. All actions must be documented to safeguard the patient.

Knowledge Connection
How do a paper MAR and an eMAR differ? What must be included in the documentation of a prn medication? How will others know which nurse is represented by the initials on the MAR? How will you document a medication that was not given?

Preventing Administration and Documentation Errors

It is your responsibility to do everything possible to prevent an error in administering and documenting the medications that you give to patients. It is extremely important to check and double-check each step of the medication administration process. To help you prevent administration and documentation errors, follow these guidelines:

- Always check the original prescriber's order against the order on the MAR. Investigate any discrepancies before administering any medications.
- Check for new or changed medication orders frequently. Avoid working solely off of a computer printout pulled at the beginning of the shift as medication orders often change throughout the shift.
- Read medication orders very carefully, being aware of drugs with similar names, and distinguishing between abbreviations.
- Look up any unfamiliar medication to ensure that you are administering the appropriate dose, and that you can assess for the intended effects and any side effects.
- Be certain that it is appropriate to administer the medication: check laboratory results, vital signs, or other parameters prior to administration.

- Always perform the three safety checks before administering a medication.
- Ensure that you follow the six rights of medication administration every time you prepare and give a medicine.
- Question any orders that require more than 1 to 2 tablets or capsules, or that exceed the recommended dose.
- Document medications as soon as you have administered them to prevent another nurse from coming behind you and administering them again.
- Check carefully for discontinued orders to avoid administering an incorrect medication.
- Ensure that you carefully supervise any unlicensed person whose job description includes administration of oral, topical, or mucosal medications.

Real-World Connection

Consequences of Medications Not Administered
The unlicensed staff members working in a group home for adults with developmental disabilities were responsible for administering oral, topical, and mucosal medications. A few residents had PEG tubes in place with medications ordered to be crushed and administered through the tube. One resident, a 19-year-old female, had a severe seizure disorder. She went into a seizure that could not be stopped, and eventually died.

When a family member was packing up her belongings, he noticed some of her medications had been dropped into the grill that covered the top of the heating and cooling unit next to her bed. When the grill was removed, many of the resident's pills were found there, including her antiseizure medications. Apparently one unlicensed staff member lacked the knowledge or the desire to crush the medicines and administer them through the PEG tube. All the medications were signed out as administered on the MAR for the past several months. While the family never knew who was responsible, they were still left to wonder if their loved one would not have died if she had received all of her medications correctly.

Remember that you are responsible for supervising unlicensed staff and ensuring that they are correctly performing medication administration.

If a Medication Error Occurs

Even when you are very careful, sometimes you make a medication error because you are human. The important thing is that you admit the error and take steps to protect your patient from injury or harm. Sometimes you may find an error made by another nurse. It is equally important to report that as well to protect the patient. Avoid being punitive or hypercritical of others if they make an error. Be supportive of other staff as it could be you making an error the next time. One very seasoned nurse explains that she worries more about new nurses who never make mistakes because they probably do, but are not admitting to them.

If you make a medication error, follow these steps:

- Put the patient first. Check for adverse effects from the medication. Take a set of vital signs and determine any abnormalities.
- Notify the prescriber and explain what happened.
- Carry out additional orders for assessing and monitoring the patient's response to the incorrect medication administration.
- Complete an incident report, following facility policy regarding further documentation or notification.
- Avoid being too hard on yourself or other nurses if an error occurs. It is very upsetting to make an error and

cause possible harm to a patient. It is so important for nurses to be supportive of one another and help solve the problems that might lead to future errors.

Knowledge Connection

List three ways to prevent making an error related to the order on the MAR. Give an example of a medication order that you would question. Explain what documentation is required if a medication error occurs.

Skill 36-1 Administering Oral Medications

Assessment Steps

1. Check the original prescriber's order, ensuring that it matches the order in the MAR, *to prevent oversight of a transcription error.*
2. Assess the need for measuring blood pressure, pulse, or finger stick blood sugar before administering the medication. *This prevents administering medications that are outside the parameters ordered.*
3. Assess laboratory results to determine appropriateness of medication administration *to determine if the patient has toxic levels of any medication or laboratory contraindications to administering the medication.*
4. For oral medications, assess whether the patient is able to swallow whole tablets or capsules *to determine whether to crush the medications or open the capsules prior to administration, if appropriate.*
5. For sublingual and buccal medications, assess the mouth for lesions, gum disease, and color of mucous membranes *to prevent administering medications that will not be well absorbed.*

Planning Steps

1. Plan to crush medications if patient is unable to swallow them whole. *Safety: Do not crush enteric-coated tablets as these drugs are irritating to the esophagus and stomach lining, and breaking their enteric coatings may lead to gastric irritation. Do not crush or break sustained-release drugs; doing so may lead to rapid absorption of large amounts of drug.*

Implementation Steps

Prepare the Medication

1. Wash hands and follow standard precautions.
2. Obtain the medication from the patient's drawer or from the computerized cabinet.
3. Follow the steps for preparing medications for administration, found in Chapter 35.
4. Verify the six rights of medication administration *to ensure that you have the right patient, right medication, right dose, right route, right date, and right time.*
5. Perform two safety checks *to ensure that you are obtaining the right medication for the correct patient.*

6. For liquid medications:
   a. Shake suspensions *to evenly distribute the medication in the liquid base.*
   b. Hold the bottle so the label is in the palm of your hand *to prevent drips from obscuring the label.*
   c. Hold the medicine cup at eye level and pour the liquid to the desired amount *to ensure accurate measurement.* Read the level at the center, or lowest point, of the meniscus.

Administer the Medication

7. Follow the Initial Implementation Steps located on the inside front cover.
8. Perform a third safety check *to ensure that you are administering the right medication to the correct patient.*
9. Tell the patient the name of the medication and explain its action, and explain how to take the medication, *to ensure the patient's cooperation.*
10. Pour water into a cup for the patient, if needed.
11. Assist the patient to a sitting position *to prevent choking or aspiration while taking medications.*
12. Open the unit dose packaging and drop the medication into the medicine cup without touching it with your fingers. *This prevents opening medications that will not be used and helps you identify each medication as you are about to administer it.*
13. Hand the medication to the patient. Hand water to the patient and offer more if needed, unless the patient is on a fluid restriction.
14. Remain with the patient until the medication is swallowed *to ensure that the patient does not choke or "cheek" the medication.*

(skill continues on page 866)

Skill 36-1 (continued)

For Sublingual and Buccal Drugs

• *For buccal administration,* instruct the patient to place the medication in the mouth against the cheek until it dissolves completely.

• For sublingual administration, tell the patient to open the mouth and lift the tongue. Place the medication under the tongue and instruct the patient to keep the medication there until it dissolves completely.
• Administer buccal or sublingual tablets whole; instruct the patient not to chew, swallow, or spit out these tablets before they dissolve completely.

15. Follow the Ending Implementation Steps located on the inside back cover.
16. Document the medication administration on the MAR and in the nurses' notes for prn medications. Document any medication that is withheld or refused in the nurses' notes.

Evaluation Steps

1. Assess the patient receiving medications via the buccal or sublingual route within 5 to 10 minutes *as the medication is rapidly absorbed via these routes.* Determine if the medication has been effective and follow orders for repeating.
2. Assess patients taking oral medications in 30 minutes after the medication is given. Assess for desired effects and adverse effects of the medications.
3. If the patient is experiencing adverse effects such as nausea or vomiting, notify the prescriber if no orders for an antiemetic are available.

Sample Documentation

7/09/13　1400　C/o rt shoulder pain. States the pain is at a 7 on a 0–10 scale and is sharp at times, throbbing at other times. Lortab 5 mg given PO for c/o rt shoulder pain. ————— ——————————— Nurse's signature and credentials
7/09/13　1440　States pain is better after medication. Rates it at a 3 now. ——————— Nurse's signature and credentials

---

Skill 36-2　Administering Medications Through an Enteral Tube

Assessment Steps

1. Check the original prescriber's order, ensuring that it matches the order in the MAR, *to prevent oversight of a transcription error.*
2. Assess for any contraindications to medication administration. Check laboratory results, check vital signs for results outside parameters, and check bowel sounds *to ensure that the medication will be digested and absorbed.*
3. Assess for the need for any prn medications *so you can prepare all medications at the same time.*
4. Assess the PEG tube insertion site for redness, edema, or purulent drainage, *which could indicate infection.*
5. Check placement of the nasogastric or PEG tube by aspirating stomach contents, checking the pH of stomach contents, and measuring the length of the tube as described in Chapter 24.
6. Check the amount of residual tube feeding in the patient's stomach. If you obtain 100 mL or more, delay administering the medication according to facility policy.

Planning Steps

1. Determine whether all nonliquid medications may be crushed or opened for administration through the tube. Consult with the pharmacist if you are unsure. *Safety: Do not crush enteric-coated tablets as these drugs are irritating to the esophagus and stomach lining, and breaking their enteric coatings may lead to gastric irritation. Do not crush or break sustained-release drugs; doing so may lead to rapid absorption of large amounts of drug.*
2. Determine the need to turn off the feeding pump before or after medication administration. (Refer to Box 36-3.)

Implementation Steps

Prepare the Medication

1. Wash hands and follow standard precautions.
2. Obtain the medication from the patient's drawer or from the computerized cabinet.
3. Follow the steps for preparing medications for administration, found in Chapter 35.

Skill 36-2 (continued)

4. Verify the six rights of medication administration *to ensure that you have the right patient, right medication, right dose, right route, right date, and right time.*

5. Perform two safety checks *to ensure that you are obtaining the right medication for the correct patient.*

6. Crush tablets that are safe to be crushed by placing in a mortar and crushing with a pestle or by using a pill-crushing device. Ensure that you get all the powder out of the mortar or out of the pill crusher.

7. For liquid medications:
   a. Shake suspensions *to evenly distribute the medication in the liquid base.*
   b. Hold the bottle so the label is in the palm of your hand *to prevent drips that could obscure the label.*
   c. Hold the medicine cup at eye level and pour the liquid to the desired amount *to ensure accurate measurement.* Read the level at the center, or lowest point, of the meniscus.

8. Place liquid medicines and crushed or opened medicines mixed with a small amount of water in separate medication cups. Do not mix the medications. *Safety: Mixing can cause medication interactions.*

Administer the Medication

9. Follow the Initial Implementation Steps located on the inside front cover.

10. Perform a third safety check *to ensure that you are administering the right medication to the correct patient.*

11. Tell the patient the name of the medication and explain the procedure, *to ensure the patient's cooperation.*

12. Ensure that tube placement and residual feeding have been checked (see Assessment Steps).

13. Clear the tube with 30 mL of water first. Follow the procedure in Chapter 24 for administering fluid through a nasogastric or PEG tube. *Clearing the tube removes formula that might adhere to the tube walls and interact with medications, as well as ensuring that the tube is patent before medications are administered through it.*

14. Administer the first medication through the tube and follow it with 5 to 15 mL of water. This may be done using a syringe with gentle pressure or by allowing it to flow in via gravity.

15. Administer the second medication through the tube and follow it with 5 to 15 mL of water.

16. Repeat Step 15 until all the medications have been given.

17. Clear the tube with 30 mL of water to ensure that all the medication is out of the tube and not adhering to the sides.

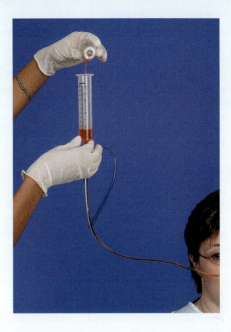

18. Restart the continuous tube feeding or hold the tube feeding for 1 to 2 hours, depending on the medications you have administered.

19. Follow the Ending Implementation Steps located on the inside back cover.

20. Document the medication administration on the MAR.

21. Document fluid given via tube on the intake portion of the I&O record. Include liquid medications and all water.

Evaluation Steps

1. Assess the patient 30 to 45 minutes after the medications are given. Assess for desired effects and adverse effects of the medications.

Sample Documentation

7/10/13 0900 Lansoprazole (Prevacid) 15 mg administered via PEG tube. Medication capsule opened and mixed with 15 mL of apple juice per pharmacist's instructions. Tube cleared with 30 mL of water before and after med admin. ————————
——————————— Nurse's signature and credentials

Skill 36-3 Administering Topical and Transdermal Medications

Assessment Steps

1. Check the original prescriber's order, ensuring that it matches the order in the MAR, *to prevent oversight of a transcription error.*

2. Assess the need for measuring blood pressure, pulse, or finger stick blood sugar before administering the medication. *This prevents administering medications that are outside the parameters ordered.*

3. Assess laboratory results to determine appropriateness of medication administration *to determine if the patient has toxic levels of any medication or laboratory contraindications to administering the medication.*

Planning Steps

1. For topical medications, determine if the area should be covered after application.

2. Gather needed supplies: gauze and tape or adhesive bandage *if topical medication is to be covered;* tongue blade or cotton-tipped swab *for application of a topical cream or ointment.*

Implementation Steps

Prepare the Medication

1. Wash hands and follow standard precautions.

2. Obtain the medication from the patient's drawer or from the computerized cabinet.

3. Follow the steps for preparing medications for administration, found in Chapter 35.

4. Verify the six rights of medication administration *to ensure that you have the right patient, right medication, right dose, right route, right date, and right time.*

5. Perform two safety checks *to ensure that you are obtaining the right medication for the correct patient.*

Administering the Medication

6. Follow the Initial Implementation Steps located on the inside front cover.

7. Perform a third safety check *to ensure that you are administering the right medication to the correct patient.*

8. Tell the patient the name of the medication and explain the procedure, *to ensure the patient's cooperation.*

For Topical Medications

9. Remove the existing dressing if one is in place.

10. Cleanse the area with sterile gauze and normal saline, or follow orders for cleansing with another solution. Pat dry. *Cleansing removes the previous layer of ointment or cream, and patting dry prevents irritation or abrasion to the injured area.*

11. Assess the appearance of the wound or lesion. Note redness, swelling, size, and drainage *to assess for infection and healing.*

12. Apply a small amount of topical ointment or cream to a cotton-tipped applicator or tongue blade *to prevent touching the tube of cream or ointment to the wound.* In some facilities, it may be required that you put a small amount of ointment or cream in a medicine cup, then take it to bedside.

13. Spread a thin coat of medication onto the affected area. *This allows the medication to penetrate the area and does not waste medicine.*

14. If the lesion is to be covered, apply sterile gauze without touching the area that will cover the wound *to prevent contamination.*

15. Write the date, time, and your initials on one piece of tape and apply it to the dressing as you tape it in place. *This identifies the last time the dressing was changed and by whom.*

16. Follow the Ending Implementation Steps located on the inside back cover.

17. Document the appearance of the wound or lesion and the type of dressing applied if one was used.

For Transdermal Medications

9. Locate and remove the existing patch.

10. Cleanse the area with an alcohol swab *to remove any remaining medication so it will no longer be absorbed.*

11. Select a new location for the patch you will apply. Choose an area with minimal body hair on the trunk or upper arms. Clip hair if necessary for the patch to stick.

12. If the area is oily or sweaty, cleanse it with an alcohol pad or soap and water.

13. Write the date, time, and your initials on the patch.

14. Remove the adhesive backing and apply the patch in the selected location.

15. Follow the Ending Implementation Steps located on the inside back cover.

16. Document the time, date, and site of application of the patch on the MAR according to facility policy.

Evaluation Steps

1. Assess the patient for any complaints of increasing discomfort 30 minutes after application of topical medication, *which could indicate a reaction to the medication.*

2. Notify the prescriber if there is no improvement visible over several days. *The medication may need to be changed.*

3. Assess the patient for adverse effects of transdermal medications *as they have systemic effects.*

Sample Documentation

7/12/13	1600	*Neosporin ointment applied to skin tear on L forearm. 2-cm × 3-cm open area; oozing serous fluid. Covered with sterile gauze and two strips of tape.* ——————— Nurse's signature and credentials
7/12/13	1645	*No complaints of pain or burning at wound site.* ——————— Nurse's signature and credentials

Skill 36-4 Administering Eye and Ear Medications

Assessment Steps

1. Check the original prescriber's order, ensuring that it matches the order in the MAR, *to prevent oversight of a transcription error.*

2. Assess the eye or ear. If discharge or crusting is present around the eye, clean with warm water and a washcloth before administering the medication. If wax or discharge is noted from the ear, gently wipe using a cotton ball.

3. Ensure that the tympanic membrane is intact prior to administration of ear medications. Check the health care provider's notes, or check the patient's ear with an otoscope if documentation is not available. *Medications should not be put into the ear of a patient with a nonintact eardrum as this causes them to enter the middle ear.*

4. Determine the patient's age *for correct administration of eardrops.*

Planning Steps

1. Gather needed supplies: tissues, cotton balls.

Implementation Steps

Prepare the Medication

1. Wash hands and follow standard precautions.

2. Obtain the medication from the patient's drawer or from the computerized cabinet.

3. Follow the steps for preparing medications for administration, found in Chapter 35.

4. Verify the six rights of medication administration *to ensure that you have the right patient, right medication, right dose, right route, right date, and right time.*

5. Perform two safety checks *to ensure that you are obtaining the right medication for the correct patient. Safety: Ensure that you are applying the medication to the correct eye or ear. Abbreviations for right, left, or both eyes and ears are no longer recommended for use due to medication errors related to them.*

6. Warm eardrops to room temperature by holding the bottle between the palms of your hands. *Administering cold eardrops can cause nausea.*

Administer the Medication

7. Follow the Initial Implementation Steps located on the inside front cover.

8. Perform a third safety check *to ensure that you are administering the right medication to the correct eye or ear of the correct patient.*

9. Tell the patient the name of the medication and explain the procedure, *to ensure the patient's cooperation.*

Administering Eyedrops

10. Assist the patient to a sitting position and ask him or her to tilt the head back slightly.

11. Gently pull the lower lid down to form a pouch, exposing the conjunctival sac.

12. Instill the prescribed number of drops and have the patient close his or her eyes for 30 seconds. Wipe off any excess medication with a tissue.

13. Follow the Ending Implementation Steps located on the inside back cover.

14. Document administration of eyedrops on the MAR.

Administering Eye Ointments

10. For eye ointments, assist the patient to a sitting position and ask him or her to tilt the head back slightly.

11. Gently pull the lower lid down to form a pouch, exposing the conjunctival sac.

12. Squeeze a ribbon of ointment into the pouch from the inner canthus to the outer canthus.

13. Instruct the patient to close the eyelids and gently move the eyes around under the lids to distribute the ointment. Wipe away any excess medication with a tissue. *Safety: Avoid touching the tip of the bottle or tube to the eye as this can cause pathogens to enter the medication.*

14. Follow the Ending Implementation Steps located on the inside back cover.

15. Document administration of eye ointment on the MAR.

Administering Ear Medications

10. Assist the patient to a lateral position with the affected ear up.

(skill continues on page 870)

Skill 36-4 (continued)

11. For adults and children over 3 years of age, gently pull the outer part of the ear (pinna) up and back. *This straightens the ear canal, allowing the medication to penetrate further into the ear.*

12. For children less than 3 years of age, pull the pinna down and back. *This straightens the ear canal, allowing the medication to penetrate further into the ear.*

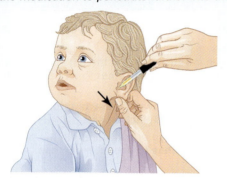

13. Instill the prescribed number of drops, making sure the drops fall against the side of the ear canal, not on the tympanic membrane, *to prevent pain.*

14. Place a cotton ball loosely in the ear for 20 to 30 minutes, if desired, then remove. *Safety: Do not leave the cotton ball in the ear as it provides a warm, dark, moist environment for pathogen growth.*

15. Follow the Ending Implementation Steps located on the inside back cover.

16. Document administration of eardrops on the MAR.

Evaluation Steps

1. Assess the patient for effects of the medication in 30 to 45 minutes.

2. Evaluate improvement in eye or ear discomfort. If the medication is not effective over a few days, notify the prescriber *as a different medication may be needed.*

Sample Documentation

7/14/12   1105   Timoptic 0.5% one drop administered to both eyes per order after return from surgery. No c/o pain or discomfort. Resting quietly, respirations even and unlabored at 18 per minute. ———————— Nurse's signature and credentials

Skill 36-5 Irrigating the Eye and Ear

Assessment Steps

1. Check the original prescriber's order, ensuring that it matches the order in the MAR, *to prevent oversight of a transcription error.*

2. Assess the purpose of the irrigation: removal of a foreign body, washing out excessive cerumen from the ears, removal of chemicals in the eyes.

3. Ensure that the tympanic membrane is intact prior to ear irrigation *to prevent damage to the middle ear.*

4. Assess the need for cleansing of the eye or ear prior to irrigation. If exudate is present, plan to cleanse the area with moistened cotton swabs.

Planning Steps

1. Gather needed supplies: irrigation solution (generally normal saline or tap water), basin for pouring irrigant, 35- to 60-mL syringe, basin for catching irrigant, clean gloves, waterproof pad.

Implementation Steps

1. Follow the Initial Implementation Steps located on the inside front cover.

2. Explain the procedure to the patient *to ensure the patient's cooperation.*

For Eye Irrigation

3. Assist the patient to lie on the side of the affected eye or to lie on the back with his or her head turned to the side of the affected eye, *allowing best access from the inner to the outer canthus.*

4. Place a basin along the side of the patient's head *to catch irrigant as flows from the eye.*

5. Draw up 30 mL of solution into the syringe, keeping the tip of the syringe sterile at all times *to prevent introduction of pathogens into the eye.*

6. Use your nondominant hand to hold the patient's eye open and ask the patient to look up.

7. Gently depress the plunger of the syringe, aiming a stream of irrigant toward the conjuctival sac flowing from the inner canthus to the outer canthus. *This prevents damage to the cornea.*

8. Repeat the irrigation process until the irrigation solution returns clear or the ordered amount of solution has been used.

Skill 36-5 (continued)

9. Dry the outside of the eyelids with swabs or tissue.

10. Follow the Ending Implementation Steps located on the inside back cover.

For Ear Irrigation

3. Warm the solution to body temperature by holding the bottle of irrigant under warm running water. *Safety: Instilling cold solution into the ear can cause nausea and dizziness.*

4. Assist the patient to sit up and tilt his or her head toward the unaffected ear. Ask the patient to hold the basin under the affected ear.

5. Draw up 30 mL of solution into the syringe.

6. Straighten the ear canal by pulling the pinna up and back, or if the patient is under the age of 3, pulling the pinna down and back.

7. Aim at the top wall of the ear canal and gently depress the plunger of the syringe. *Safety: Aiming the irrigation syringe directly into the canal can cause damage to the tympanic membrane.*

8. Repeat the irrigation process until no more debris returns in the irrigation fluid or until the ordered amount of fluid has been used.

9. Dry the outside of the ear with cotton swabs or tissue.

10. Follow the Ending Implementation Steps located on the inside back cover.

11. Document the type and amount of fluid used, the type and amount of debris obtained, and how the patient tolerated the procedure.

Evaluation Steps

1. Evaluate the patient's tolerance of the procedure. Determine if the procedure caused pain, discomfort, or nausea.

2. Evaluate the effectiveness of the irrigation; determine if the eye or ear is clear of debris or foreign body.

Sample Documentation

7/23/13   1325   L ear irrigated with 60 mL warmed normal saline to remove cerumen buildup. Mod amt of dark brown wax removed, then irrigation return clear. C/o mild pain during procedure, relieved after procedure completed. ——————
————————————— Nurse's signature and credentials

Skill 36-6 Administering Vaginal Medications

Assessment Steps

1. Check the original prescriber's order, ensuring that it matches the order in the MAR, *to prevent oversight of a transcription error.*

2. Assess the patient for complaints of itching, burning, or pain in the vaginal area.

3. Inspect the vaginal area for discharge and inflammation.

Planning Steps

1. Gather needed supplies: applicator for cream or tablet, washcloth and towel to cleanse the area if discharge is present. Obtain water-based lubricant if inserting a tablet.

Implementation Steps

Prepare the Medication

1. Wash hands and follow standard precautions.

2. Obtain the medication from the patient's drawer or from the computerized cabinet.

3. Follow the steps for preparing medications for administration, found in Chapter 35.

4. Verify the six rights of medication administration *to ensure that you have the right patient, right medication, right dose, right route, right date, and right time.*

5. Perform two safety checks *to ensure that you are obtaining the right medication for the correct patient.*

6. Attach the applicator to the tube of vaginal cream and squeeze until the applicator is filled and the plunger is pushed out, or insert the diamond-shaped tablet into the end of the appropriate applicator. Apply water-based lubricant to the tablet.

Administering the Medication

7. Follow the Initial Implementation Steps located on the inside front cover.

8. Perform a third safety check *to ensure that you are administering the right medication to the correct patient.*

9. Tell the patient the name of the medication and explain the procedure, *to ensure the patient's cooperation.*

10. Assist patient into the dorsal recumbent position, with the knees bent and feet apart.

11. Gently retract the folds of the labia *to expose the vaginal orifice.*

12. Cleanse the area with a washcloth and warm water if discharge is present.

13. Insert the applicator gently into the vagina. Depress the plunger completely *to distribute the medication.*

14. Withdraw applicator and wipe residual medication from the vaginal area.

(skill continues on page 872)

Skill 36-6 (continued)

Invert cap and pierce end of medication tube

Attach applicator

Squeeze medication into applicator

15. Encourage the patient to remain in the recumbent position for 20 to 30 minutes after administration *to allow for absorption of the medication.*

16. Apply a perineal pad *to prevent discharge of medication onto undergarments when the patient is upright.*

17. Wash applicator with soap and water, rinse, and dry. Store for future use.

18. Follow the Ending Implementation Steps located on the inside back cover.

19. Document the drug administered on the MAR.

Evaluation Steps

1. Evaluate the patient's response to the medication. Ask about relief of itching, burning, pain, and discomfort.

Sample Documentation

> 7/12/13 2010 Nystatin 100,000 units vaginal tablet inserted with applicator. Instructed to remain in dorsal recumbent position for 20 minutes. Peri pad given to protect underwear. ————
> ———————————— Nurse's signature and credentials

Skill 36-7 Administering Rectal Suppositories

Assessment Steps

1. Check the original prescriber's order, ensuring that it matches the order in the MAR, *to prevent oversight of a transcription error.*

2. Assess the need for the medication as this route can be used for a laxative, hemorrhoid treatment, or delivery of a systemic medication. If it is a systemic medication, assess the need for continued rectal administration, such as vomiting.

3. Assess bowel status. Do not administer if the patient has diarrhea without consulting the prescriber *as the medication will likely not be absorbed.*

Planning Steps

1. Obtain the suppository from the refrigerator. It will usually be stored there *to prevent melting of the wax base.* Obtain water-soluble lubricant.

Implementation Steps

Prepare the Medication

1. Wash hands and follow standard precautions.

2. Obtain the medication from the patient's drawer or from the computerized cabinet.

3. Follow the steps for preparing medications for administration, found in Chapter 35.

4. Verify the six rights of medication administration *to ensure that you have the right patient, right medication, right dose, right route, right date, and right time.*

5. Perform two safety checks *to ensure that you are obtaining the right medication for the correct patient.*

Administer the Medication

6. Follow the Initial Implementation Steps located on the inside front cover.

7. Perform a third safety check *to ensure that you are administering the right medication to the correct patient.*

8. Tell the patient the name of the medication and explain the procedure, *to ensure the patient's cooperation.*

9. Assist the patient to the left Sims' position. *This position allows best access to the rectum and sigmoid colon.*

10. Lubricate the tip of the suppository with a water-soluble lubricant *to make insertion more comfortable for the patient.*

11. Instruct the patient to take a deep breath to help relax the anal sphincters.

12. As the patient exhales, insert the suppository with the index finger, ensuring that it is past the internal anal sphincter *to facilitate retention.*

Skill 36-7 (continued)

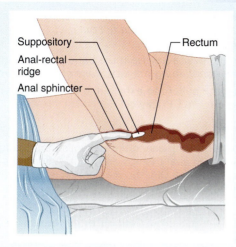

Suppository — Rectum
Anal-rectal ridge
Anal sphincter

13. Remove gloves and wash hands.

14. Instruct the patient to hold the suppository in the rectum as long as possible *to allow it to melt and the medication to be absorbed.*

15. Ask the patient to remain in the left Sims' or left lateral position for 10 to 15 minutes *to help him or her retain the suppository.*

16. Assist the patient to the bathroom, if needed, when the urge to expel the suppository is strong.

17. Follow the Ending Implementation Steps located on the inside back cover.

18. Document medication administration on the MAR. If it is a prn medication, document in nurses' notes the reason for the medication and the response.

Evaluation Steps

1. Evaluate the patient's response to the medication. If it is given as a laxative, note the color, amount, and consistency of the bowel movement and document it.

2. If the suppository is given for other purposes, evaluate the systemic response in 30 to 45 minutes and report any adverse effects.

Sample Documentation

07/13/13 2115 Dulcolax suppository administered via rectum for c/o constipation. States no B.M. in 2 days "but it feels like it is right there." Remains in L Sims' position to retain med. ———————————————— Nurse's signature and credentials
07/13/13 2200 Up to BR with assist. Expelled mod amt dark brown stool. States feels "much better now." ———————————————— Nurse's signature and credentials

Skill 36-8 Administering Inhaled Medications

Assessment Steps

1. Check the original prescriber's order, ensuring that it matches the order in the MAR, *to prevent oversight of a transcription error.*

2. Assess lung sounds *to determine respiratory status.*

3. Assess the need for measuring blood pressure or pulse prior to administering inhaled medications.

Planning Steps

1. Obtain a glass of water and emesis basin for the patient to use when rinsing his or her mouth after administration of inhaled medications.

Implementation Steps

Prepare the Medication

1. Wash hands and follow standard precautions.

2. Obtain the medication from the patient's drawer or from the computerized cabinet.

3. Follow the steps for preparing medications for administration, found in Chapter 35.

4. Verify the six rights of medication administration *to ensure that you have the right patient, right medication, right dose, right route, right date, and right time.*

5. Perform two safety checks *to ensure that you are obtaining the correct medication for the patient.*

Administering the Medication

6. Follow the Initial Implementation Steps located on the inside front cover.

7. Perform a third safety check *to ensure that you are administering the right medication to the correct patient.*

8. Tell the patient the name of the medication and explain the procedure, *to ensure the patient's cooperation.*

For MDI

9. Assist the patient into the upright position *to help expand the lungs fully when taking a deep breath.*

10. Remove the mouthpiece cap.

11. Shake the inhaler *to mix the medication and prepare it to spray.* If a spacer is to be used, attach it to the mouthpiece of the MDI.

12. Instruct the patient to tilt the head back slightly and breathe out completely.

13. Have the patient open his or her mouth while you hold the inhaler 1½ to 2 inches away. *This allows the spray that enters the mouth to be a fine mist rather than large droplets that may be absorbed by the oral mucosa and cause excessive side effects.* If a spacer is used, have patient close the lips around the mouthpiece of the spacer.

(skill continues on page 874)

Skill 36-8 (continued)

14. Press down on the inhaler to release 1 puff of medication as he or she takes a deep, slow breath in.

15. Once the medication is inhaled, instruct the patient to hold his or her breath for 10 seconds *to allow the medication to go into the lungs.*

16. If 2 puffs of medication are ordered, have the patient wait 1 minute before taking the second puff. *This allows the first puff to be absorbed before the second puff is taken.*

17. Have the patient rinse out the mouth after the last puff of medicine. Make sure the patient spits out the water and does not swallow. *This is especially important if the medication is a steroid as leaving it in the mouth can lead to thrush.*

18. Encourage the patient not to drink, eat, or brush the teeth immediately after using the MDI *as this can affect absorption of the medication.*

19. Follow the Ending Implementation Steps located on the inside back cover.

20. Document the administration of the MDI on the MAR and any other form according to facility policy.

For DPI

9. Assist the patient into the upright position *to help expand the lungs fully when taking a deep breath.*

10. For diskus-style DPIs, move the thumb grip away from you, *which will open the diskus and reveal the mouthpiece.*

11. Instruct the patient to hold the DPI upright *so that the powder drug does not fall out. Safety: Do not shake DPIs as they are in powder form.*

12. Move the lever away from the patient *to open the chamber containing the next dose of medication.*

13. Instruct the patient to exhale in a direction that is away from the DPI device. *Safety: If patient exhales into the DPI, it will cause the dose of powder to be dispersed so it is not available to be inhaled.*

14. Place the mouthpiece in the patient's mouth and tell him or her to seal the lips around it. A spacer is not necessary with a DPI; the medication is automatically inhaled when a breath is taken.

15. Have the patient inhale deeply and forcefully.

16. Instruct the patient to hold his or her breath for the count of 10.

17. Have the patient rinse out the mouth after the last puff of medicine. Make sure the patient spits the water out and does not swallow.

18. Follow the Ending Implementation Steps located on the inside back cover.

19. Document the administration of the DPI on the MAR and any other form according to facility policy.

Evaluation Steps

1. Assess lung sounds 30 to 45 minutes after the inhaler is administered to determine improvement.

2. Evaluate the patient for side effects of inhaled medications, especially nervousness, insomnia, restlessness, and nausea.

Sample Documentation

07-15-13   0915   Assisted with MDI. Required reminders not to put MDI mouthpiece in the mouth, but to hold it 1½ to 2 inches away. Also had difficulty coordinating spraying the MDI and inhaling at the same time. Able to perform correctly on the second inhalation with fewer cues. ————————————— ————————————— Nurse's signature and credentials

Post Conference

You learned a great deal about administration of medications in this clinical experience. You applied topical medication to the patient's eczema on her arms and legs. After contacting the pharmacist, you learned that you were not supposed to cover this type of medication. You gave a rectal suppository for constipation and a vaginal cream to treat her yeast infection. The patient was taking Tegretol suspension for her seizures. You knew that you had to dilute it with an equal volume of water and flush the tube carefully afterward to prevent it from adhering to the tube. The patient also had Prilosec ordered for acid reflux. You learned to open the capsule, then you mixed it with apple juice rather than water, and flushed the tube afterward with the apple juice. In your research, you learned that the potassium chloride liquid she was taking could cause clumping of the tube feeding formula. In the facility, the patient had had problems with her tube becoming obstructed easily. You informed the nurse, who talked with the doctor. The patient was discharged to the facility with new orders to discontinue the potassium chloride and to give the Prilosec with 8 ounces of orange juice daily to supply potassium.

KEY POINTS

- Drugs are available in a variety of forms, including tablets, capsules, liquids, eye and eardrops, nasal drops, rectal and vaginal suppositories, and inhalers.

- When you administer oral narcotic medications, you must be sure that the patient's vital signs are stable; you are also responsible for keeping an accurate count of narcotics and for disposing of any unused medications correctly with a witness and signatures.

- Several classifications of medications require special administration techniques when given via an enteral tube due to interactions with the tube feeding formula. You are responsible for knowing how to correctly administer these medications via the enteral tube.

- When preparing medications to administer through an enteral tube, prepare each separately in individual medication cups. When administering them, separate each medicine with 5 to 15 mL of water to prevent interactions between the medications or interactions with the formula, and to prevent drugs from adhering to the tube.

- Topical medications are often administered for local effects, while transdermal medications are given for systemic effects. You must evaluate the desired effects and side effects of both routes of medications.

- Eye medications are placed in the lower conjunctival sac to prevent damage to the cornea during administration.

- Ear medications should only be given to patients whose tympanic membrane is intact. Administer eardrops carefully, aiming the dropper so that the medication rolls down the wall of the ear canal and does not drop directly onto the tympanic membrane, which causes pain.

- Nasal medications are often given to reduce congestion, but some nasal sprays can cause a rebound effect with long-term use. This causes swelling of the nasal mucosa, leading to more congestion and the need for more nasal spray.

- Rectal medications are administered for local or systemic effects. This route is contraindicated in patients with certain cardiac conditions or those with bowel or rectal disorders.

- Metered-dose inhalers contain liquid medication delivered as a mist and inhaled into the airways. To avoid intense side effects, it is recommended that patients hold the mouthpiece 1½ to 2 inches away from the mouth during administration, which will prevent large drops of the drug from landing on the tongue and being rapidly absorbed.

- Dry-powder inhalers provide longer acting effects. These inhalers contain a dry powder that the patient inhales deep into the airways. Avoid allowing the patient to breathe into the DPI as it will disperse the powder and waste the dose.

- Document medications on the paper MAR according to facility policy. Include the medication, dose, route, frequency, date, time, and your initials. When an eMAR is used, the bar code technology documents and charges the medications as they are prepared and administered.

- Always check the six rights of medication administration and perform the three safety checks when preparing medications to help prevent making a medication error.

- If a medication error is discovered, you must document it on an incident report or according to facility policy, whether or not you made the error. Put the patient first and always admit to any medication error that occurs.

REVIEW QUESTIONS

Select the answer that is most appropriate for each of the following questions. Some questions may have more than one correct answer. Check all that apply.

1. The patient must receive timolol maleate (Timoptic) eyedrops. Where should you instill the eyedrops?

    a. The cornea

    b. The pupil

    c. The eyelid

    d. The lower conjunctival sac

2. Which of the following techniques is correct for the nurse when inserting a rectal suppository?

    a. Position the patient on his or her right side with the left leg flexed.

    b. During insertion, tell the patient to hold his or her breath.

    c. Lubricate the tip of the suppository.

    d. Gently insert the suppository, directing it with the index finger.

3. A patient has been prescribed a metered-dose inhaler (MDI) for the management of her asthma. Which of the following instructions should be given to the patient?

    a. Shake the inhaler before use.

    b. Breathe slowly and fully before administration.

    c. Administer by pressing the canister downward.

    d. Hold your breath as long as possible.

4. Buccal tablets are administered:

    a. under the tongue.

    b. between the upper lip and gum.

    c. by injection.

    d. through inhalation.

5. What steps will the nurse follow when administering a liquid cough syrup to the patient?

    a. Hold the medicine glass at eye level and pour the prescribed dose.

    b. The measurement line should be even with the fluid level at the base of the meniscus.

    c. Discard any excess.

    d. Dilute all liquids with water.

6. Which of the following drug administration routes is the safest and most convenient?

    a. Oral

    b. Topical

    c. Vaginal

    d. Nasal

7. Which of the following drug administration routes is through the epidermal layer of skin into the dermis?

    a. Oral

    b. Topical

    c. Inhalation

    d. Intravenous

8. Which of the following drug administration routes is rapid and across a large surface area?

    a. Oral

    b. Topical

    c. Inhalation

    d. Rectal

CRITICAL THINKING EXERCISES

9. A 54-year-old male patient with hypertension refuses to take the ordered beta blocker to lower his blood pressure. He states, "It does not work anyway, and I hate the way it makes me feel." How would you handle this situation?

10. A patient with a bleeding ulcer has a nasogastric tube in place that is connected to low intermittent suction. There is an order for Carafate suspension (to coat the ulcer) per tube. What concerns do you have and what will you do?

ADDITIONAL RESOURCES

For additional Resources, Questions, and Activities, please see:

 Student Resource Disk

 http://davisplus.fadavis.com

 Student Study Guide

REFERENCES

Beaman N. *Pharmacology Clear and Simple: A Drug Classifications and Dose Calculation Approach.* Philadelphia: FA Davis; 2008.

Broselow J, Luten R, Schuman J. Preventing medications errors in children: safeguarding children from medication errors in hospitals, office practices, and the home. Modern Medicine, June 1, 2008. Available at: http://www.modernmedicine.com/modernmedicine/Pediatrics/Preventing-medication-errors-in-children/ArticleStandard/Article/detail/522755.

Cohen H, Shastay AD. Getting to the root of medication errors. *Nursing2008.* 2008;38(12):39-47.

Deglin JH, Vallerand AH. *Davis's Drug Guide for Nurses.* 11th ed. Philadelphia: FA Davis; 2009.

Helmons PJ, Wargel LN, Daniels CE. Effect of bar-code-assisted medication administration on medication administration errors and accuracy in multiple patient care areas. *Am J Health Syst Pharm.* 2009;66:1202-1210.

Mitchell JF. Oral dosage forms that should not be crushed. Institute for Safe Medical Practices Web site. Available at: http://www.ismp.org/tools/donotcrush.pdf. Accessed December 1, 2009.

Wilkinson J, Van Leuven K. *Fundamentals of Nursing: Theory, Concepts & Applications.* Philadelphia: FA Davis; 2007.

Williams NT. Medication administration through enteral feeding tubes. *Am J Health Syst Pharm.* 2008;65:2347-2356.

Administering Intradermal, Subcutaneous, and Intramuscular Injections

Key Terms

Air-lock

Ampule

First-pass metabolism

Gauge

Insulin syringe

Intradermal (ID)

Intramuscular (IM)

Prefilled syringe

Subcutaneous (subcut)

Tuberculin (TB) syringe

Vial

Z-track

Objectives

1. Define key terms associated with intradermal, subcutaneous, and intramuscular injections.
2. Explain the significance of first-pass metabolism.
3. Describe the different types of syringes, including volume capacity and the units of measurement marked on each type.
4. Identify the different parts of a syringe and needle.
5. Describe the appropriate sites used for intradermal and subcutaneous injections.
6. Identify the anatomical landmarks and muscles used for intramuscular injections in adults and children.
7. Describe the volumes of medication that may be administered via the intradermal, subcutaneous, and intramuscular routes of injection.
8. Select appropriate needle gauge and length for the different routes of administration in the various injection sites.
9. Describe proper injection technique for intradermal, subcutaneous, and intramuscular injections, including Z-track.
10. Specify parts of the syringe and needle that must be kept sterile during preparation and administration of an injection.
11. Identify appropriate safety measures related to administration of injections.
12. Relate possible complications associated with different types of injections.
13. Explain the importance of compatibility of medications.
14. Identify appropriate steps to employ as you draw up and combine two types of insulin in a syringe, and administer via the subcutaneous route.
15. Correctly draw up medications from a vial and from an ampule.
16. Discuss diluents and any restrictions for use related to various age groups.
17. Identify medication classifications that require verification by more than one nurse prior to administration.
18. Discuss how the administration of insulin and heparin varies from other subcutaneous injection techniques.

Skills

37-1 Reconstituting and Withdrawing Medication From a Vial

37-2 Withdrawing Medication From an Ampule

37-3 Administering an Intradermal Injection

37-4 Combining and Administering Insulin Subcutaneously

37-5 Administering an Intramuscular Injection

37-6 Administering a Z-track Injection

Clinical Connection

Your Assignment: You will be caring for a 42-year-old male patient with poorly controlled diabetes and who has had a below-the-knee amputation 2 days previously. His medication orders include an injection of two types of insulin, NPH and regular insulin, every morning. In addition, he has meperidine ordered intramuscularly every 4 to 6 hours prn for incisional pain or phantom pain.

Your Actions: You are unsure about administering these injections, because you have only performed that skill in the lab. You prepare to research exactly how to administer insulin injections, and you are unsure about mixing two types of insulin in one syringe, so you will research that as well. As you think about administering insulin, you remember something about rotating sites, but you cannot remember for sure which sites are used for insulin, providing you with yet another topic for your research. You are excited about the opportunity to administer an intramuscular injection as well, but you are even less sure about finding those sites and wonder which would be most appropriate for this patient because he has an amputation. Then you start to wonder about what size of needle to use for the intramuscular injection. You begin researching the insulin and meperidine, their effects and side effects, and how to administer each type of injection.

This is the chapter that most student nurses have been waiting for: how to administer an injection, as injections are one of the skills that people most commonly relate to nurses. In this chapter, you will learn how to be a safe practitioner while administering medications via the intradermal, subcutaneous, and intramuscular routes. This includes more than just the technique of the injection itself. A safe practitioner must know how to select the proper syringe and correct gauge and length of needle, and know the sites where different medications may be administered, the potential complications, which medications are compatible, and much more that you may not have thought about until now.

Injections

Injections are considered to be administered via the parenteral route, which means not through the gastrointestinal tract. The parenteral routes of medication administration include intradermal (ID), subcutaneous (subcut), intramuscular

(IM), and intravenous (IV); all of these will be covered in this chapter except the IV route. You will learn about the IV route in the next chapter of this text.

The advantages of administration of medications by injection include:

- Bypassing the gastrointestinal tract, thereby preventing gastrointestinal irritation
- Rapid onset time compared to the oral route
- Ease of administration to uncooperative or unconscious patients
- Better absorption of drugs that are poorly absorbed via the oral route

However, parenteral administration also has it disadvantages, including that it:

- Is invasive and uncomfortable for the patient
- Is expensive
- Requires additional supplies and equipment
- Requires qualified personnel to administer
- Carries a risk of infection and nerve injury

Supplies and Equipment

Administration of medication per an injectable route requires various supplies and equipment, including a syringe, needle, alcohol prep pads, dry cotton ball or 2×2-inch (5×5-cm) gauze pad, needle disposal container, examination gloves, and bandage.

Syringes

A syringe is used to hold and introduce the medication into the needle, which will direct the medication into the body tissue. Medical syringes are typically disposable and made of plastic, while glass syringes are more prevalent in research settings. Syringes are available in numerous sizes, ranging from 0.3 to 60 mL, with the most common sizes being 1 mL and 3 mL. Each syringe has calibrations marked on the barrel in milliliters or units indicating the volume of medication to administer, depending upon the type of syringe and the type of medication to be injected with the syringe (Fig. 37-1).

Parts of a Syringe

A syringe has three main parts: a barrel, a plunger with a flange on the end, and a tip that connects to the needle (Fig. 37-2).

Barrel

The barrel is the hollow cylindrical chamber that holds the medication, and has graduated unit-of-measurement marks that indicate the various volumes of medication the syringe can hold. One end of the barrel has a tip that connects to the needle, and the other end of the barrel is open with a plunger inserted into it.

Tips

A syringe may have one of two types of tips (Fig. 37-3):

- **Luer-Lok tip:** has threaded grooves that screw onto the needle hub and lock it in place

(a)

(b)

(c)

(d)

(e)

Figure 37-1 Syringes: A. A U-100 syringe marked in units, of which there are 100/mL. B. A 1-mL tuberculin syringe marked in 0.01 mL (1/100th of a milliliter) and minims (16 minims equals 1 mL). C. A 3-mL standard syringe marked in whole milliliters and 0.1 mL (1/10th of a milliliter). D. A 5-mL standard syringe marked in whole milliliters and 0.2 mL (2/10ths of a milliliter). E. A 10-mL standard syringe marked in whole milliliters and 0.2 mL (2/10ths of a milliliter).

- **Slip-tip:** has a smooth, slightly tapered tip that inserts into the needle hub, requiring a slight twist of the syringe or needle to securely snug the needle and syringe together

Plunger

The plunger is a piston-like rod that fits inside the barrel and slides up and down the barrel to either draw up medication or push it out of the barrel. The end of the plunger that is inserted into the barrel is rubber tipped to provide traction against the barrel. On the other end of the plunger is a flange that allows you to grip the plunger to pull it back when drawing up medication (refer to Fig. 37-2).

Syringe Types

There are four major types of syringes, two of which are designed for administration of specific medications.

Regular Syringe

A *standard syringe* is most frequently used for intramuscular or subcutaneous injections. It is calibrated in milliliters (mL), and some also have minims (m) marked on them as well. Standard syringes are available in 1-, 3-, 5-, 10-, 20-,

Figure 37-2 Parts of a syringe and safety needle.

Figure 37-3 Syringe tips: A. Luer-Lok tip that screws on. B. Slip-tip that applies with a gentle push-and-twist motion.

and 60-mL sizes. You will use the 1-, 3-, and 5-mL syringes for most injections.

Tuberculin Syringe

The **tuberculin (TB) syringe** is a smaller diameter syringe that holds a total volume of 1 mL and is calibrated in tenths and hundredths of a milliliter as well as sixteenths of a minim, making it an excellent choice for administration of the small and precise volumes of medication required by newborns and infants as well as for the TB skin test for which it was designed (Fig. 37-4).

Insulin Syringe

The **insulin syringe** is similar in size and shape to a TB syringe, but it is calibrated in units of insulin and used only for injecting insulin. *Safety: It is no longer considered safe to abbreviate the word unit with "U". The Joint Commission has included it on the list of Do Not Use abbreviations. The word "units" must always be spelled out.* There are several sizes of insulin syringes that hold different total volumes of 0.3, 0.5, or 1 mL. A standard insulin syringe is 1 mL and holds up to 100 units of insulin. The smaller size

that holds only 0.3 mL is best for children who need very small doses of insulin and for people with poor eyesight. The calibrations are printed in a larger font, making it easier for patients with impaired vision to see the numbers more accurately.

An insulin syringe usually has a tiny-gauge, short, and permanently attached needle. The most common syringe size is marked for use with U-100 insulin, meaning the strength of the insulin is 100 units of insulin per 1-mL volume (see Fig. 37-4).

Prefilled Syringes

Prefilled syringes are single-dose, ready-to-use, disposable syringe cartridges, some with an attached needle and some to which you must attach a needle, that contain specific dosages of specific medications. The cartridge is loaded into a reusable plastic holder for administration. This drug-delivery device offers various advantages, including ease of use, convenience, and safety. Prefilled injection systems such as Carpuject® (Abbott) and Tubex® (Wyeth-Ayerst) are designed for safe and quick loading and unloading (Fig. 37-5).

Figure 37-4   Top: Insulin syringe. Bottom: Tuberculin syringe.

After using the cartridge, unscrew it from its holder and drop it vertically into a disposal container. *Safety: Do not recap the needle.*

Needles

The needle is a small, hollow, cylindrical tube with a sharp, beveled cutting-edge tip used to pierce the skin. It is usually made of steel or other metal. For administering injections, the needle must be attached to a syringe, which contains the medication.

Parts of a Needle

A hypodermic needle consists of a plastic *hub* used to attach the needle to the syringe, the *bevel,* the *cannula* or *shaft,* and a *safety guard* to cover the used needle as soon as it is withdrawn from the patient's body (see the orange safety needle guard in Fig. 37-6). All facilities should have both needle and syringe safety devices or use one of the needleless systems developed to reduce contaminated needle sticks.

The bevel is the slanted tip of the needle, designed to facilitate needle insertion and prevent *coring* (punching out a circular piece of skin) when inserting the needle. The bevel should *always* face upward when piercing the skin. The pointed tip entering the skin in front of the bevel limits the degree of tissue injury as the bevel allows for gradual increase in the size of the opening made in the skin. The shaft

denotes needle length. Maintain the sterility of the entire needle. Do not touch any part of it.

The needle has a plastic cap or cover that must be removed before use. *Safety: To prevent accidental needle sticks with contaminated needles, never recap a used needle.* Blood-borne pathogens can be transmitted from the patient to anyone stuck with the contaminated needle.

Gauge

The **gauge (G)** of a needle refers to the diameter of the needle and is indicated by numbers, typically between 14 G (2.1 mm) and 27 G (0.4 mm). The *higher* the gauge number,

Figure 37-5   Prefilled syringe cartridge with needle and three types of holders.

Figure 37-6   Standard syringe attached to a safety needle with orange guard, containing 1.7 mL of air.

the *smaller* the diameter of the needle. A 14-G (2.1-mm) needle is a very large-diameter needle while a 27-G (0.40 mm) is very tiny. The choice of needle gauge depends on several factors:

• Viscosity of the medication
• Route of administration
• Size of patient and muscle mass

A smaller gauge, from 14 G (2.1 mm) to 20 G (0.9 mm), has a larger diameter and because of this is required for *viscous,* or thick, medications; larger gauges, from 21 G (0.8 mm) to 30 G (0.3 mm) have smaller diameters and are used for thin medications. Smaller gauge needles generally cause less pain; however, the larger gauge needles such as 29 G (0.33 mm) and 30 G (0.3 mm) are so tiny that they are easily bent. The size of the muscle targeted for an intramuscular injection also affects the gauge somewhat. For example a thin, water-consistency medication might flow easily through a larger gauge (but smaller diameter) needle such as a 27 or 29 G. However, if the medication is to be injected intramuscularly into a 225-pound muscular male, a smaller gauge (but larger diameter) needle would be required in order to be strong enough to pierce a large muscle, whereas a 27-G needle would be appropriate to administer the same medication to a newborn with tiny muscles. Needle manufacturers may color-code needles according to gauge, though color coding is not universal and may vary between different manufacturers.

Length

Needles come in different lengths, ranging typically from $\frac{3}{8}$ to 2 inches (0.9 to 5 cm). The length is measured from the tip of the bevel to the junction of the hub and shaft. The choice of length depends on the weight, amount of fat, and muscle development of the patient; the site of injection; and the route of administration. A subcutaneous injection, injected into the layers of subcutaneous fat, is administered with a shorter needle, between $\frac{3}{8}$ and $\frac{7}{8}$ inch (0.9 to 2.2 cm) depending on the patient's size. An intramuscular injection, injected into the muscular layer below the subcutaneous layer, is administered in the body or largest portion of a muscle and requires a longer needle length, from 1 to 2 inches (2.5 to 5 cm).

Handling Syringes and Needles

Asepsis is a primary concern when handling syringes and needles. Always wash your hands before handling sterile injection supplies, and clean the work surface where you will be preparing the injection. Keep a facility-approved cleaning agent near the medication cart or counter where you routinely prepare medications, so that it will be handy to use.

Get Ready

Begin by reviewing the physician's order so you will know the type and volume of medication that you are to draw up and the route of administration. Assess your patient's age and size, the site you will use, and the amount of muscle mass or subcutaneous tissue at the site. Now you are prepared to select the appropriate syringe and the correct gauge and length of needle.

Gather all the supplies you will need prior to beginning the preparation of the injection. It will save you time and energy, make you more efficient and enable you to be more productive, make you appear more competent, and make it easier to maintain sterile technique required for proper preparation. If you have to stop what you are doing, lay down supplies and equipment, and possibly leave the patient room or medication cart in order to get something you forgot, this has the potential to require extra handwashing as well as repeated entering and exiting of the work site or patient room, and may force you to redirect your thoughts and focus, all of which reduce your organization and ability to be efficient and complete nursing care in a timely manner. It forces the patient to wait, and it may even require you to use additional sterile supplies, increasing costs. Taking the few extra minutes to assess which supplies you will need to administer an injection will save you time over the whole shift.

Maintain Asepsis

It is important to maintain sterility of the appropriate parts of the syringes and needles you work with. As you prepare the syringe, peel the sterile package open and lay the package down with the syringe still resting in one side of the package until you are ready to attach the needle. *Safety: Avoid taking the syringe out of the package and laying it on the bare countertop, where you risk contaminating the tip of the syringe.*

When handling a syringe, keep all parts that contact the medication or the patient sterile. This includes the syringe tip, the inside of the barrel, and the length of the plunger from the rubber tip inside the barrel to approximately 1 inch from the flange end. That keeps the portion of the plunger that comes in contact with the medication and goes in and out of the syringe barrel sterile. The outside of the barrel and the flange are the only parts that may be touched. It is not necessary to wear gloves for preparation of an injection, but always wear clean examination gloves for the actual administration of every injection to protect you from possible contact with body fluids and blood-borne pathogens.

The only part of a needle that may be touched is the plastic needle cap. The hub of the needle that attaches to the syringe must be kept sterile while preparing to attach it. Without touching the needle, peel the package open just far enough to expose the hub, fold the two package flaps down to the sides of the needle package, and hold them down with your nondominant fingers and thumb. With your dominant hand, pick up the sterile syringe from its wrapper, and if it has a cap on the syringe tip, aseptically remove it using both hands, one holding the syringe and one holding the cap, then attach the needle hub to the syringe. *Safety: Do not attempt to remove needle covers or syringe tip caps using a one-handed method. It is virtually impossible to push or flip the cover or cap off of the needle or syringe without contaminating it with the thumb that is pushing it off. Never use your teeth to pull off a needle cover.*

To attach the needle to a Luer-Lok syringe, place the hub of the needle against the threaded connector of the syringe and gently twist clockwise. The same type of needle will attach to a slip-tip syringe with a gentle push and twist. The needle and syringe are then ready for use.

Preventing Needlestick Injuries

Percutaneous injuries, commonly referred to as *needle-stick injuries,* are a significant occupational hazard for nurses and other health care workers. These injuries provide the perfect mode of transmission for blood-borne infectious diseases, including HIV, hepatitis B, and hepatitis C. Needle-stick injuries commonly occur when recapping contaminated needles, and may also result from improper needle disposal. *Safety: To prevent needle-stick injuries, never recap used needles. Do not bend, break, or cut needles before disposal.* Be vigilant to activate the needle safety guard immediately after use, as soon as the needle tip leaves the patient's body as you withdraw the needle after administering an injection. (See Fig. 37-7 for an example of two additional types of needle safety devices.) Drop the syringe and needle as one unit into the sharps container, which is made of a hard plastic that is nonpervious, or puncture proof (Fig. 37-8). Sharps containers come in various sizes from a small, approximately 8-ounce size all the way up to a 1.5-gallon size, and they are usually red. Some are designed to set on a countertop or medication cart, while others are designed to mount on the room wall.

Occupational safety guidelines published by the U.S. Centers for Disease Control and Prevention (CDC) and the Occupational Safety and Health Administration (OSHA) recommend against recapping any needles, both new and used, even when disposing of them. To maintain sterility of the needle, and because it is unsafe to carry an uncovered

Figure 37-8 Always dispose of needles and glass vials/ampules in a sharps container made of puncture-proof plastic, usually red.

needle while walking down the hallway, it is sometimes necessary to recap a clean needle after drawing up a medication so that you may carry it to the patient's room. When recapping a clean needle, use the *one-handed scoop technique.* Lay the cap on a flat surface with the open end extending a short distance beyond the edge of the flat surface. Maintaining sterility, scoop the cap onto the tip of the syringe needle held in your dominant hand (Fig. 37-9A). The free hand should be kept away from the exposed needle. Once the cap has been scooped up onto the needle, you may use your nondominant hand to pull the cap further onto the needle until it secures. An alternative method that works well for individuals whose hand might be shaking: First open a sterile package containing an alcohol pad, using care to touch only one corner of the alcohol pad to pull it out of the package. Lay the pad on the countertop and place the open end of the cap in the middle of the alcohol pad. Now scoop the cap onto the needle. The sterile alcohol pad provides an extra degree of sterility should you touch it on the way to the open end of the cap. *Safety: Never push on the end of the cap, as it is possible for a large needle to go through the end of the cap and into your finger. You should not use the two-handed method to recap even the sterile needle, as this develops a habit that can be performed with contaminated needles without even thinking about it.* There are also various recapping devices that can be purchased for one-handed recapping of sterile needles (see Fig. 37-9).

Ensure that proper needle disposal containers are conveniently located; this helps ensure proper needle disposal, and may reduce the inclination to recap used needles before disposal. There should be one in each patient room and on each medication cart or work counter where medications are prepared. *Safety: Never place needles in the garbage or in a recycling bin to prevent accidental needle sticks of*

Figure 37-7 Top Photo: A. Before injection. Safety device has not been activated. B. After injection and activation of safety device. Bottom Drawing: A. Needle before activation of retracting device. B. After needle retraction.

housekeeping employees and other department employees. It also decreases public access to disposed needles.

If a needle-stick injury occurs, immediately wash the punctured area with soap and water, encouraging bleeding from the site. Follow facility protocol and seek medical attention. Most facilities require testing for blood-borne pathogens—from both the individual on whom the needle was used and the recipient of the contaminated needle stick. The testing is normally done the same day of reporting and

Figure 37-9 The one-handed "scoop" method of recapping sterile needles. A. Without touching the sterile needle to the outside of the needle cap, scoop the cap onto the needle. B. Use the other hand to "pull" the cap down over the needle until secure. Do not place your finger on the end of the cap and "push" it on. C. Alternative: Needle recapping device.

two to three more times at specified intervals. Documentation, usually an incident or variance occurrence form, is completed according to facility policy and protocol.

Knowledge Connection
What are the parts of a syringe? What are the parts of a needle? How should you dispose of needles? How are needle-stick injuries prevented?

Medications

You must be knowledgeable about all medications that you are preparing to administer, but administration by the various injectable routes seems to increase the pertinence of knowing about the medication due to the simple fact that the effect will be quicker than with many other delivery methods. The injectable routes can result in an increased intensity, as well as an accelerated onset, of the drug's effect. It is helpful to note that the injected drug is not the least bit retrievable even immediately after administration, whereas an orally administered drug at least has a limited potential for retrieval of part or all of the dose by using gastric lavage or emetic medications to induce vomiting. Some topical medications can be at least partially removed with soap and water if caught quickly.

It will serve you well and make you a safer nurse to be vigilant in your research efforts regarding drugs to be administered per injection. The absolute minimum knowledge that you should acquire about each drug includes the following:

- Is the patient allergic to it?
- What is its classification?
- What does it do? How does it work?
- Why does this patient need this medication?
- Is the ordered dose within the safe dose parameters for this patient's age, size, and condition?
- Is the route appropriate for this particular drug? This patient?
- What assessments should you make prior to administering the medication? Afterward?
- How quick is the onset of drug action?
- For which side effects must you watch?
- Is there an antidote if one is needed?
- Is it compatible with other medications the patient is receiving?

Reconstitution and Drawing up Medications

Injectable medications may come in the form of a liquid or a powder that needs to be dissolved in a liquid. The powder form is used for medications that are not stable for very long once in solution. The process of dissolving powdered drugs with the use of a liquid or diluent such as sterile normal saline or sterile water is known as *reconstitution*. Some medication labels or inserts will provide more than one volume of diluent to use for the purpose of mixing different concentrations of the medication. It is always your responsibility to read the label and accompanying insert to determine the type and volume of diluent to use for reconstitution and the strength of the medication once it has been reconstituted.

Vials

A **vial** is a glass or plastic container of medication with a rubber stopper that must be punctured with a needle for medication removal (Fig. 37-10). If the label or insert indicates that the rubber stopper is designed for use with needleless systems, a needleless piercing device may be used in place of a needle (Fig. 37-11). However, do not use blunt needles or needleless piercing devices on any vial stopper or IV tubing injection port unless it specifies that it is designed for use with needleless systems. *Safety: Using non-sharps to pierce rubber stoppers that are not designed for such use allows the device to core the rubber. This means a round piece of the stopper is punched out and is now either in the medication or aspirated into the needle or syringe.*

Multiple- Versus Single-Dose Vials

Vials of parenteral solutions may be labeled as *single-dose* or *single-use* as well as *multiple-dose* or *multiple-use* vials. All multiple-dose vials contain bacteriostatic preservatives that reduce risk of microorganism growth, while the single-dose vials do not. *Safety: Avoid using single-dose vials more than once.* Upon opening a multiple-dose vial, write the date, time, and your initials on the label. Some medications are good for only 24 hours; others vary in the length of time for which the drug may safely be used after opening.

It is important to know that benzyl alcohol 0.9%, the bacteriostatic preservative used in multiple-dose vials of sterile water for injection and sodium chloride 0.9% for injection, is contraindicated for use in newborns. The warning is generally printed in red letters right on the label. Benzyl alcohol has been found to be toxic to neonates. Remember this when using multiple-dose vials.

Withdrawing Medication From a Vial

Wash your hands before handling medication and supplies. Remove the plastic cap from the top of the vial and then wipe the rubber stopper of the vial with an alcohol wipe. Using two hands, remove the needle cover from the needle attached to your syringe and lay the cover down or stand it

Figure 37-11   A syringe with a needleless piercing device.

in a needle-recapping device (refer to Fig. 37-9). Hold the syringe in your nondominant hand, and use your dominant hand to grasp the plunger, holding it only by the flange. Pull the plunger back, filling the syringe reservoir with air equal to the amount of solution to be drawn up. For example, if you are to draw up 1.7 mL of medication, pull back on the plunger to fill the syringe reservoir with 1.7 mL of air.

With the needle, pierce the rubber stopper of the medication vial at a 90-degree angle, allowing the pointed tip (the long side of the bevel) to enter the stopper first. Keep the needle tip above the fluid level and slowly inject the air from the syringe into the air space above the medication in the vial (Fig. 37-12). This slightly pressurizes the vial so the medication can be drawn out easily. *Safety: Do not inject air directly into the medication; doing so may introduce bubbles that will take up some of the space in the syringe and prevent you from drawing an exact dose of medication.*

Figure 37-10   Medication vials.

Figure 37-12   When instilling air into a vial, keep the needle tip above the fluid level.

After instilling the air into the vial, leave the needle inserted into the vial; invert both the vial and the syringe and carefully draw up the appropriate volume of medication by slowly pulling the plunger back (Fig. 37-13). Be certain to maintain sterility of the entire needle and the plunger that enters into the syringe barrel. Draw up the exact amount and inspect the syringe carefully for bubbles. If bubbles are present, pull back on the plunger and fill the syringe with approximately 1 mL of extra medication; most bubbles will then go to the top of the syringe, where they can be expelled from the syringe. If not, gently tap the side of the syringe to release the bubbles so they rise toward the needle (Fig. 37-14). Be certain to use care when tapping on the syringe; if you tap it too hard and do not have a secure hold on both the vial and the syringe, it is easy to bend the shaft of the needle. Slowly reinstill the air and any overfill of medication back into the vial. Withdraw the needle from vial. Skill 37-1 (page 900) provides more information on reconstituting and withdrawing medications from a vial.

Ampules

An **ampule** is a small, sealed glass drug container that must be broken to withdraw the medication. To prepare the ampule for withdrawal of medication, tap the top of the ampule to distribute the medication to the lower portion of the ampule. Wipe the neck of the ampule with an alcohol wipe to reduce bacterial contamination on the outside of the ampule. Use either a plastic device designed specifically for breaking an ampule, or an alcohol wipe or gauze pad held between your fingers and the neck of the ampule that you intend to break off. Snap the neck of the ampule, breaking it away from your body to avoid injury (Fig. 37-15).

Figure 37-14 If unable to get air out of a syringe, gently tap on the side of the syringe to free the air bubble so that it will rise to the top of the syringe, where it can be expelled.

Attach a *filter needle,* which has a device for filtering debris such as glass shards from ampules or rubber cores from vials, to the syringe you will use to draw up medication. Invert or tilt the ampule to facilitate withdrawal of the medication. Maintaining sterility of the filter needle and the medication in the ampule, insert the filter needle you attached to the syringe into the ampule without touching the needle to the outside of the ampule (Figs. 37-16 and 37-17). Unless you accidently instill air into the inverted ampule, medication will not leak out of the ampule even though it is upside down, due to surface tension of the fluid. Keeping the needle tip below the fluid level in the ampule, pull back on the syringe plunger until the appropriate volume of medication has been withdrawn, then remove the filter needle from the ampule. *Safety: You must change the filter needle after drawing up the medication and attach a new regular needle before administering the injection.*

If air is present in the syringe, tap the barrel of the syringe near the hub to move air toward the needle. Push carefully on the plunger to expel air or excess medication. Empty the unused portion of medication from the ampule. *Safety: Remove the filter needle from the syringe prior to administration of medication. Injecting the medication back through the same filter needle and into the patient will also instill any glass shards that the filter might have caught.* You must change the needle after withdrawing the medication from the ampule, then discard the ampule glass and filter needle in a puncture-resistant container to prevent accidental injury. Skill 37-2 (page 901) provides more information on withdrawing medication from an ampule.

Mixing Medications

Sometimes it may be appropriate to combine more than one drug in a syringe to avoid the discomfort of multiple

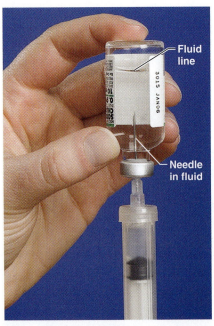

Figure 37-13 Invert the vial with the needle still inside the vial. Begin to pull back on the plunger to withdraw the desired volume of medication.

Fluid line

Needle in fluid

B

Figure 37-15 A. Use gauze or an alcohol wipe to protect your fingers when breaking an ampule. B. If available, break ampule necks with a special device designed for this purpose.

Figure 37-16 Invert the ampule and insert a sterile needle into the ampule, keeping the needle tip below the fluid level.

Figure 37-17 Tilting the ampule for medication removal.

injections. *Safety: It is crucial to check compatibility of medications before mixing and injecting them.*

Compatibility/Incompatibility of Medications

You must assess whether drugs are compatible with each other before you administer them together, and especially before you mix them together in the same syringe. *Incompatibility* is an unwanted reaction that occurs between the drug and the solution, container, or another drug. There are physical, chemical, and therapeutic type incompatibilities that can occur. Physical incompatibilities produce visible reactions such as color changes, precipitate formation, cloudiness, gas formation, or haze. A chemical incompatibility involves the degradation of the drug resulting from a chemical reaction. Therapeutic incompatibility occurs within

the patient, as the result of two concurrently administered drugs that interact. If there is a question about compatibility, review drug inserts and drug information texts, and consult with a pharmacist.

Ready to Mix

Once compatibility is established, cleanse both tops of the two vials with separate alcohol pads. Attach a filter needle to the syringe to draw up medications. If one or both of the vials are multiple-dose vials, fill the syringe with the amount of air equal to the medication dose needed from the first medication (for textbook purposes, we will call the first vial, *vial A,* and the second vial, *vial B*). Maintain the vial in an upright position and inject the air into vial A, but be careful not to touch the needle to the solution. This prevents medication from vial A from being transported on the needle and contaminating the medication in vial B when the needle is inserted. Remove the needle from vial A.

Then fill the syringe with the appropriate volume of air and inject the air into vial B. Without removing the needle from vial B, invert the vial and syringe and withdraw the required volume of medication into the syringe. Withdraw the needle from vial B and then reinsert it into vial A. Invert vial A carefully, and withdraw the required volume of medication, using caution to avoid drawing more than you need because you will be unable to inject any of it back into the vial now that the two medications are mixed. Replace the filter needle with an appropriate needle to be used for injection. The syringe then contains a mixture of medications from vials A and B.

The process is much easier when both vials are single-dose vials: Instill air in each vial, then withdraw medication from one vial and then the second vial. There is no need to protect the needle from contact with the first medication.

Mixing Medications From Prefilled Syringes

Medications from prefilled syringes may also be mixed. There are two ways to perform the task: both medications can be drawn into a separate syringe, or the second medication can be drawn into the prefilled cartridge if there is adequate room.

The first method is to draw the medication from the prefilled cartridge into a separate syringe. The end of the prefilled cartridge has a plastic adapter that may have its own attached needle or be designed so that a needle can be attached to it (refer to Fig. 37-5). For this method, apply gentle pressure to the entire plastic adaptor, bending it sideways, and it will slide easily off the end of the prefilled cartridge, exposing a rubber stopper at the end of the cartridge.

Cleanse the stopper with an alcohol wipe and then pierce the stopper with a hypodermic needle attached to a syringe, withdrawing the medication from the cartridge into the syringe. If the second medication is in a single-dose vial, first clean the vial stopper with alcohol. Pull into the same syringe a volume of air equal to the volume of medication to be withdrawn from the second medication vial. Insert the syringe needle into the vial and instill the air. Now withdraw the correct volume of medication into the syringe with the first medication, where they mix.

To mix both medications in the cartridge, place the cartridge in the plastic holder, retain the amount of air in the cartridge that will need to be instilled into the second medicine vial, and expel any excess air over that amount from the cartridge. Wipe the vial stopper with an alcohol wipe, then invert the vial prior to piercing the vial stopper with the needle on the prefilled cartridge. Hold the syringe with the first medication in a vertical position, with the needle tip pointing up. This allows air in the syringe to rise toward the needle and settle on top of the medication so that it can be injected rather than the medication in the syringe. Instill the

air from the cartridge and withdraw the appropriate volume of medication into the cartridge, where the two medications mix (Fig. 37-18).

Anatomy and Physiology Connection

Anatomy of the Tissues You Inject

The skin is the largest organ of the body. The skin regulates body temperature, provides a physical barrier for protection, prevents excess water loss or absorption, and contains nerve endings for sensory perception. The skin is divided into two main layers: the epidermis, which is the outermost layer of skin, and the dermis, which is the connective tissue layer of the skin located below the epidermis. The dermis, which is composed of collagen, elastic tissue, and reticular fibers, is attached to an underlying hypodermis, commonly known as the *subcutaneous connective tissue*. The subcutaneous connective tissue stores adipose tissue and contains larger blood vessels and nerves. The muscular tissue layer is deeper yet, beneath the subcutaneous layer. The dermal layer, the subcutaneous layer, and the muscle layer are each composed of different types of cells and tissue. The drug manufacturers design medications to work best in specific tissues; rarely is a drug compatible with all three layers of tissue. There are numerous drugs that are caustic and damaging when injected into the improper tissue layers.

Because the skin that covers all the layers underneath is the primary or first line of defense against microorganism invasion, any break in the skin's integrity places the patient at risk for infection, which is why it is imperative than you use stringent sterile technique when withdrawing medications from containers and during administration of injections. If you consistently use good technique, you will not find yourself responsible for an abscess or other infection due to an improperly administered injection.

Comparison of Routes of Administration

Generally oral administration is the safest and most convenient route; however, it has the slowest onset of action of all the routes. Before an oral medication can begin to work, it must first be absorbed from the gastrointestinal tract into the portal circulation that transports the medication to the liver. One of the liver's most important functions, protective in nature, is to metabolize potentially harmful agents in the blood, a process known as *detoxification*. The downside is that the process of metabolizing the drug decreases the amount of drug remaining in the blood after it leaves the liver to enter the systemic circulation, where it can perform its intended function. This process is known as **first-pass metabolism**. The routes of administration that escape first-pass metabolism include sublingual, buccal, and parenteral routes, because they all provide absorption directly into the systemic circulation rather than into the

Figure 37-18   Hold the syringe vertical, needle tip upward. This allows the air inside the syringe to rise above the medication so air can be instilled into the vial to maintain air pressure. Invert the vial before piercing the rubber stopper with the needle.

portal circulation of the digestive tract, where drugs are metabolized by the liver before entering the systemic circulation. Parenteral drugs elicit rapid responses because they circumvent first-pass metabolism, but because they cannot be retrieved, parenterally administered drugs may present more risks.

The most common parenteral routes are classified as **intradermal (ID), subcutaneous (Subcut),** and **intramuscular (IM)**. An ID injection deposits the medication into the *epidermis,* or the outer layers of the skin, while a subcutaneous injection is injected under the layers of the skin into the subcutaneous tissue layer. An IM injection is administered into the deep muscle tissue below the subcutaneous layer of tissue.

Intradermal Injections

An ID injection is the injection of a small amount of fluid into the dermis, or true skin layer immediately below the epidermis (Fig. 37-19). It is commonly used as a diagnostic tool, such as testing for allergies or tuberculosis. (Box 37-1 provides a description of administering an ID tuberculin skin test.) The left ventral forearm is the site most frequently used for tuberculin testing, using a substance called tuberculin purified protein derivative (P.P.D.). The right ventral forearm, upper chest, and upper back over the scapulae are the sites used for allergy testing.

The length of the needle for an ID injection should be ¼ to ½ inch, with a very small-diameter needle, between 25 and 30 G, and a length between ½ and ⅝ inch (1.27 to 1.58 cm). Position the needle bevel up and use a 15-degree angle for insertion of the needle. Instill the medication between the layers of the dermis to create a *bleb,* which looks somewhat like a small, raised, fluid-filled blister (Fig. 37-20). Avoid applying pressure or massaging the injection site. If a drop of blood or fluid leaks from the puncture site after withdrawing the needle, gently touch the corner of the drop with a dry cotton ball or alcohol wipe to remove it, but do not apply pressure to the site.

Safety: Activate the needle guard immediately after removal of the needle from the skin. You must be vigilant about this safety mechanism while you are still learning and perfecting your technique for this to become an automatic habit. Skill 37-3 (page 901) provides more information on administering an intradermal injection.

Figure 37-19   Intradermal injection delivers a small volume of medication into the dermal layer.

Box 37-1

Tuberculin Skin Testing

A substance known as tuberculin purified protein derivative, commonly called P.P.D., is used to test an individual for the presence of tuberculosis (TB). Inject a small volume (0.1 mL) intradermally on the ventral side of the left forearm. If correct intradermal injection technique is used, a pale elevation of the skin, called a wheal, that is approximately 6 to 10 mm in diameter will result, looking somewhat like a tiny blister that absorbs within a few minutes. Use an ink pen to circle the wheal and write the date and time next to the circle. Advise the patient to have the site read between 48 and 72 hours later for interpretation.

The interpretation involves determining if the site is indurated or not, and if so, the size of the induration. Induration is a palpable raised and hardened area where the P.P.D. was injected. If blisters are present, they also indicate a positive result. Any redness that may occur does not indicate a positive result. If induration or blistering is present, measure the size. Induration 2 mm or less diameter is considered negative. In a healthy individual, 15 mm is considered a positive reading. In a health care worker who has been exposed to TB, 10 mm is considered a positive reading. In some types of immunocompromised patients, even 5 mm may be considered a positive reading.

Figure 37-20 A small, discreet, pale, raised *bleb* should arise if you have the needle positioned correctly

Knowledge Connection

What is a P.P.D. skin test for? What volume of drug is administered for a P.P.D. test? Describe the range of needle gauges and lengths that are used for intradermal injections. What is meant by first-pass metabolism? Why is it important? What is a bleb?

Subcutaneous Injections

A subcutaneous (Subcut) injection deposits the medication into the subcutaneous layer below the skin and above the muscle layer (refer to Fig. 37-19). It contains fewer blood vessels than muscle, producing a slower absorption time compared to intramuscular injections. (*Note: The Joint Commission has mandated that previously used abbreviations for subcutaneous, including SC, SQ, and sub-q, increase the risk of medication errors and should no longer be used. The only abbreviation that may be used is Subcut.*) Sites for subcutaneous injection include the back of the upper arms, the abdomen (but stay a minimum of 2 inches away from the umbilicus), the anterior thighs, the area of the back just below the scapulae, and the upper buttocks (Fig. 37-21).

The subcutaneous route is useful when slow and continuous absorption is required. The abdomen provides more rapid absorption than the other subcutaneous sites and is the preferred sites for insulin and heparin, an anticoagulant. To prevent irritation and tissue damage, the medication must be isotonic and the same pH as that of the tissue.

To administer a subcutaneous injection, you will need a needle between ⅜ and ⅞ inch (0.95 to 2.22 cm) in length with a diameter between 24 and 29 G. You will administer the injection at a 45-degree angle. However, the angle of needle insertion and the length of needle may vary somewhat based upon the amount of fat and size of the patient. For example, if you are administering a subcutaneous injection into the abdomen of an extremely obese adult male, you could use any needle length between ⅜ and ⅞ inch (0.95 and 2.22 cm) and could use a 45-degree angle or even a 90-degree angle, because the layer of subcutaneous tissue would be thick enough that any of these would deposit medication within the subcutaneous tissue layer. This would not be the case if you were administering a subcutaneous injection in the abdomen of a petite, 101-pound, 22-year-old female. For this patient, you would need the shorter or ⅜- or ⅝-inch (0.95- to 1.58-cm) length of needle, and would use a 45-degree angle. Anything longer would deposit medication into the muscular tissue.

The maximum volume for subcutaneous injection according to most facility policies is 1 to 2 mL. It is your responsibility to know your facility's policy. You will pinch or bunch up the skin and underlying fat layer into a fold between your finger and thumb, which helps to lift the subcutaneous layer off the muscle, helping to ensure that you inject only subcutaneous tissue rather than muscle (Fig. 37-22).

Figure 37-21 Subcutaneous injection sites.

Figure 37-22 For subcutaneous injection, pull the skin taut as you pinch a large skinfold between your thumb and fingers, lifting the subcutaneous layer off the muscle.

As with all injection techniques, the insertion of the needle should be swift, piercing the skin and subcutaneous layer in one smooth motion. *Note: Avoid inserting the needle only a short distance and then having to push the needle further in to reach the proper depth, which results in additional discomfort for the patient.*

Do not aspirate before injecting medication, as there are few large blood vessels in the subcutaneous tissues, making it rare to hit a vessel. You will apply gentle pressure to the site after removing the needle and gently massage to distribute the medication into the tissue for better absorption, unless you are administering insulin or heparin. *Safety: Activate the needle safety device immediately after removal of the needle from the skin.* You must be vigilant about this safety mechanism while you are still learning and perfecting

your technique for this to become an automatic habit. *Safety: Do not massage the site after injection of insulin or heparin.*

Insulin and Heparin

Insulin and heparin are two commonly used drugs that are administered subcutaneously as well as intravenously. Both drugs, if administered incorrectly, can be life threatening; therefore, you must follow specific safety steps that are not necessary for other medications (Table 37-1).

Insulin

Insulin is a hormone that is necessary for transporting glucose from the blood into each individual cell of all the tissues in the human body. If insulin is not present to transport the glucose from the blood, the blood level of glucose elevates. Without glucose to utilize for energy production within the cells, all body processes and functions are impaired, which is what happens when an individual has diabetes mellitus: The pancreas does not produce adequate insulin to meet the body's needs.

Insulin types are designated according to their speed of action, including how long the interval is from administration of the insulin to the onset of its action, the timing of the insulin's strongest or peak action, and the duration of effect. Classifications generally are categorized as very rapid-acting, rapid-acting, intermediate-acting, long-acting, and very long-acting. *Safety: You will need to learn the onset, peak, and duration of the various insulins so that you can adequately assess patients for effectiveness of their insulin.* It is particularly important when a patient receives several doses or two or more types of insulin each day. The peak and duration times of multiple insulins will

Table 37-1   Tips for Safe Insulin and Heparin Administration

Medication	Tips for Safe Administration
Insulin	• Monitor finger stick blood glucose or serum glucose levels. • Use a syringe matching the strength of the insulin. • Have a second and third nurse verify that you have the correct type of insulin and the correct dosage drawn into the syringe. • Do not aspirate before injecting insulin. • Do not massage the site after removing the needle. • Monitor the patient for signs and symptoms of hypoglycemia and hyperglycemia.
Heparin	• Assess laboratory results—PT, INR, and APTT—before administering. • After checking the heparin label against the medication administration record three times, check it again. • Have a second and third nurse verify that you have the correct strength of heparin and the correct dosage drawn into the syringe. • Do not aspirate before instilling heparin. • Do not massage the site after withdrawing the needle. • Monitor the patient for bleeding gums, red blood cells in the urine, blood in the stools, and excessive bruising.

overlap with onset and peak times of previously administered insulins, compounding the effects on the patient's blood glucose level, which places the patient at increased risk for dangerously low glucose levels, known as *hypoglycemia* or *insulin shock*.

A patient whose blood glucose is elevated and unstable may require finger stick blood sugar (FSBS) measurements several times per day to monitor glucose levels, followed by administration of insulin, the dosage of which is determined according to a *sliding scale* that is dependent upon the FSBS results obtained at specified intervals (Table 37-2).

You will also need to know the signs and symptoms of both hypoglycemia and hyperglycemia so you can identify the problems quickly and prevent delay in treatment (Table 37-3). *Safety: It is important that you teach the patient with diabetes to wear a bracelet or necklace that states the patient has diabetes and uses insulin.* The bracelet or necklace should be easily seen so that the patient having a hypoglycemic reaction can be immediately identified as having diabetes, helping to ensure appropriate care for the patient.

Insulin preparations are measured in units and require use of specific insulin syringes for administration. Now most insulin is concentrated at 100 units per milliliter (U-100). Always confirm that you have the corresponding U-100 syringe to use with U-100 insulin. Rapid-acting insulin and short-acting insulin are often combined with intermediate-acting insulins. Not all types of insulins may be mixed. *Safety: Long-acting insulins, such as insulin glargine (Lantus), are never mixed with other insulins.* Some combination products come premixed in a single vial, such as Novolin 70/30, which is 70% intermediate-acting insulin and 30% short-acting insulin.

Knowledge Connection

What primary function of insulin makes it so important? What test result should you view prior to insulin administration?

Table 37-2 Example of an Insulin Sliding Scale

FSBS Results	Regular Insulin per Subcutaneous Route *Number of units to administer*
150–200 mg/dL	Give 2 units
201–250 mg/dL	Give 4 units
251–300 mg/dL	Give 6 units
301–350 mg/dL	Give 8 units
Greater than 350 mg/dL	Call physician

Insulin should be kept refrigerated. However, before withdrawing it, gently roll the vial between both hands for approximately 1 minute to resuspend and warm the medication. Avoid shaking or vigorously agitating the insulin. When mixing insulins in the same syringe, the *clear* rapid-acting insulin must be withdrawn into the syringe first, followed by the *cloudy* intermediate-acting insulin. Just remember "clear before cloudy." Skill 37-4 (page 902) provides more information on combining and administering insulin subcutaneously.

The preferred injection site for insulin is the abdomen because it provides faster and more consistent absorption, but the back of the upper arms, the thighs, and the buttocks may also be used. *Safety: Injection sites should be rotated to establish consistent blood insulin levels and reduce the risk of tissue damage, which will affect absorption.* If a patient is able to self-administer insulin, teach the patient to use a clock method on the abdomen; giving the insulin at the position of 12 o'clock, then 1 o'clock, then 2 o'clock, and so forth.

Patient Teaching Connection

Insulin Self-administration

It is important to help patients to be as independent as possible, including being adequately skilled to administer their own insulin. Part of your responsibility as a nurse will be to provide appropriate levels of patient education regarding this task. It helps to keep patient teaching as simple and straightforward as possible. The following steps provide simple but thorough instruction regarding self-administration of insulin.

- Wash your hands. (There is no need for the patient to wear gloves to self-administer.)
- Rotate injection sites with each dose to prevent tissue damage and increase absorption.
- Before drawing up the insulin suspension, gently roll and invert the bottle. Do not shake, as this can cause bubbles or foam to develop.
- Clean the rubber stopper of the vial with alcohol.
- Pinch the skin by squeezing a couple of inches of skin between your thumb and two fingers, pulling the skin and fat away from the underlying muscle.
- Cleanse the site with alcohol and allow to dry.
- Hold the syringe like a pencil in a vertical position, with the "eraser" end pointing toward the ceiling.
- Use a dart-like wrist action to make a swift puncture.
- Insert the needle at a 45-degree to 90-degree angle to the skinfold, depending upon the length of the needle and the thickness of the subcutaneous tissue layer.
- Push the plunger to inject the insulin.
- Release your grip on the skinfold.
- Remove the needle from the skin and activate the safety mechanism immediately. Do not recap used needles.
- Do not massage the site or cover the skin with a gauze pad.
- Dispose of the needle and syringe in a puncture-proof container.

Table 37-3   **Signs and Symptoms of Hypoglycemia and Hyperglycemia**

Condition	Signs and Symptoms	Immediate Actions to Take
Hypoglycemia	Pale, cool, clammy skin Tremors or palpitations Hunger or nausea Increased irritability Fatigue Difficulty concentrating Headache Dizziness or restlessness Drowsiness or lethargy	Assess finger stick blood sugar. If below 90 mg/dL and the patient is able to swallow, give a small glass of orange juice or other simple carbohydrates, followed by a protein source and complex carbohydrates such as peanut butter on wheat bread, cheese and crackers, or a glass of milk and a sandwich, to maintain glucose level.
Critically low hypoglycemia	Delirium Violent behavior Seizures Obtunded (diminished arousal/awareness) Coma Death	Assess finger stick blood sugar. Patients may vary dramatically in how low the glucose must go before exhibiting these serious CNS signs and symptoms: Some will exhibit them at 40 mg/dL while others may not until the blood glucose is down to 20 mg/dL. Treat these patients symptomatically. Notify the laboratory to draw a serum glucose level stat and then reassess the finger stick blood sugar within 30 minutes and prn. Assess vital signs and apply oxygen. Initiate an IV line if not already infusing. Notify the physician. Initiate standing orders until contact is established with the physician; this generally includes IV administration of dextrose 50%. If the patient is having a seizure, ensure a patent airway, protect from injury, and administer antiepileptic medication according to physician's orders.
Hyperglycemia	Hot, dry, flushed skin Thirst Fatigue or weakness Sleepiness Sweet or acetone odor to breath	Assess finger stick blood sugar. If glucose is above 200 mg/dL and there are no physician's orders specifying whether or not to administer insulin at this level of elevation, notify the physician. Administer rapid-acting insulin according to physician's orders. Reassess finger stick blood sugar in 1 hour and prn.
Critically high hyperglycemia	Vagueness Mental confusion Hypotension Coma Death	Assess finger stick blood sugar. As with extreme hypoglycemia, blood glucose may vary greatly from patient to patient: One may not exhibit these signs and symptoms even when glucose is 700 mg/dL or higher, while another may be already hypotensive or comatose at 500 mg/dL. Treat symptomatically as well as administering insulin to lower glucose. Notify the laboratory to draw a stat serum glucose. Reassess finger stick blood sugar in 1 hour and prn. Assess vital signs and apply oxygen. Notify the physician stat. Initiate an IV line if not already infusing. Administer rapid-acting insulin according to physician's orders.

Patients who require repeated insulin injections may develop *lipoatrophy*, the breakdown of subcutaneous fat at the site of repeated insulin injections, or *lipohypertrophy*, the buildup of subcutaneous fat at the site of repeated insulin injections. To avoid these complications, rotate injection sites around the abdomen, keeping them typically a fingerbreadth, or 1 inch, apart. *Safety: Do not massage after injecting insulin as this may cause erratic absorption of the drug.*

Heparin

Heparin is an anticoagulant drug that is administered to reduce and prevent formation of blood clots, which can cause cerebrovascular accidents (CVAs) and heart attacks, or myocardial infarctions (MIs). *Safety: Heparin comes in various strengths such as 1,000 units/mL, 5,000 units/mL, 10,000 units/mL, and 20,000 units/mL.* Heparin can be life threatening if an incorrect dosage is administered. *Safety: It is paramount that you always have a second nurse verify the strength of heparin and the dosage you have drawn into the syringe.* You should always monitor the laboratory results of the partial thromboplastin time (PTT), activated partial thromboplastin time (APTT), prothrombin time (PT), and international normalized ratio (INR) prior to administration. Heparin can be administered subcutaneously or intravenously, delivered by direct intravenous injection or a continuous intravenous drip. *Safety: Heparin should never be given IM. A continuous intravenous drip will require constant monitoring of the infusion rate.*

The abdomen is the preferred site for subcutaneous injection. Administer heparin slowly into the subcutaneous tissue and leave the needle in place for about 10 seconds before withdrawing it. Do not administer anywhere that has a scar or bruise. Do not rub or ice the site after injection as this can cause hemorrhage or bruising.

Laboratory and Diagnostic Connection

Prothrombin Time and Activated Partial Thromboplastin Time
The prothrombin time (PT) and the activated partial thromboplastin time (APTT) both assess the patient's own system of blood clot formation, evaluating the clotting factors I, II, V, VIII, IX, X, XI, and XII. Recall that factor I is fibrinogen and factor II is prothrombin. The only difference between these two tests is the activators that have been added to the reagent used to determine the PT. This results in a shorter clotting time using a more narrow normal range.

These tests are a measurement of the length of time that the body takes to complete the clotting process. Thus, a longer time result would indicate a slower clotting process while a shorter time result would mean the blood is completing its intrinsic clotting process faster than it should, contributing to the formation of clots, which are a source of problems for the patient. Heparin interferes with the intrinsic clotting process by inactivating prothrombin for several hours after administration of drug. This prolongs the clotting process.

The goal of heparin therapy is to lengthen both the PT and APTT to 1.5 to 2.5 times the normal range. The normal ranges and the therapeutic ranges desired for patients on anticoagulant therapy with heparin are as follows:

- **PT**
  - **Normal range:** 60 to 70 seconds
  - **Therapeutic range:** 90 to 175 seconds
- **APTT**
  - **Normal range:** 30 to 40 seconds
  - **Therapeutic range:** 45 to 100 seconds

Intramuscular Injections

Intramuscular injection is an injection directly into the largest portion of a muscle, called the *body* of the muscle. It is used for certain types of medications, particularly ones that are rapid and long lasting, such as vaccines, and those medication solutions that are irritating to the subcutaneous tissue.

Depending on the chemical properties of the drug, the medication may be absorbed either somewhat quickly or more gradually. Drugs in aqueous solution are rapidly absorbed. Drugs in oil or in other repository vehicles deliver a slow, constant absorption.

Intramuscular injections are administered in the larger muscles of the leg and hip, and smaller volume injections are administered in the deltoid of the upper arm. The maximum volume to inject intramuscularly is based on the site and the patient's muscle development:

- 2 to 3 mL for injecting a *large* ventrogluteal site (gluteus medius and gluteus minimus muscles) or a very large vastus lateralis muscle of the leg, in an adult
- 1 to 2 mL for a ventrogluteal (gluteus minimus and medius muscles), vastus lateralis, or rectus femoris site in a trim, average-size adult, older children with adequate muscle development, older adults, and thin patients
- 0.5 to 1 mL for small muscles in infants and small children
- 0.5 to 1 mL for the deltoid muscle in small children and up, through older adults

For average adults, the needle should be 1 to 1.5 inches (2.5 to 3 cm) in length, with a gauge size between 20 and

22 G (1.1 to 0.7 mm). If a medication is thin, use the smallest size needle that can be used for the injection, but if the medication is thick and viscous, you may have to use a larger 20-G (1.1-mm) needle. On occasion a medication is so thick and viscous that even an 18-G (1.2-mm) may be required, such as with gamma globulin.

Administer intramuscular injections at a 90-degree angle into the body of the target muscle. As with all injection techniques, the insertion of the needle should be swift, quickly piercing the skin and muscle in one smooth motion. *Note: Avoid inserting the needle only a short distance and then having to push the needle further in to reach the proper depth, which results in additional discomfort for the patient.*

Aspirate to ensure that the needle is not in a vessel. If blood returns into the syringe with aspiration, withdraw the needle, dispose of the medication-filled syringe in a sharps container, and draw up another dose of medication using a new syringe and needle. The IM route is generally used for irritating or caustic drugs and allows for administration of larger volumes of medication. Skill 37-5 (page 904) provides more information on administering an IM injection.

Some nurses prefer to use an **air-lock** for the purpose of reducing irritation of the tissue along the path the needle made through the skin, subcutaneous layer, and muscle. The air-lock technique is quite simple. After drawing up the exact volume of medication, continue to aspirate 0.1 to 0.2 mL of air into the syringe. When inverting the syringe to make the skin puncture and instill the medication, be certain to position the syringe so that it is vertical, allowing the air to rise above the medication in the syringe. This is necessary so that the air is not injected until after the medication, when it can help to lock the medication in the muscle (Fig. 37-23). The air clears any medication that remains in the needle, making it is less irritating to subcutaneous tissues during needle withdrawal. Medications such as interferon, iron dextran, or hydroxyzine hydrochloride (Vistaril), and vaccines such as diphtheria, tetanus toxoid, and pertussis, may be administered using the air-lock technique.

After withdrawing the needle from the tissue after an IM injection, hold pressure on the site with a 2×2-inch gauze pad or cotton ball, and massage the site to increase absorption. The exception is any intramuscular injection administered using the Z-track method; do not massage a Z-track. *Safety: Activate the needle safety device immediately after removal of the needle from the skin.*

Preventing Complications of IM Injections

Complications from intramuscular injection can arise from the needle puncture solution, incorrect technique, or the drug solution itself. To prevent infection of the injection site:

• Wash hands before you begin to prepare injections.
• Wash hands again after you enter the patient's room.
• Clean the injection site with alcohol or a facility-approved antiseptic; use adequate friction and clean the

Figure 37-23 A. Hold the syringe vertical so air is not trapped on the side of the syringe. Air should rise to the top of the medication solution. B. Once you invert the syringe to administer the injection, the air rises to the top, once more enabling it to enter the needle and patient after the medication has gone in.

site beginning in the center and wiping concentric circles outward until a 2-inch area is clean.
• Cover the puncture wound with a new bandage to allow the skin time to seal over.

Repetitive injections can cause bleeding, bruising, soreness, and muscle spasm. To prevent these complications:

• Make certain you review the patient's medical record and know whether the patient has any medical problems that might increase the risk of bleeding, such as hemophilia, anticoagulant therapy, or disease of the blood cell–producing tissue, or if the patient takes supplements or herbs that increase bleeding. Box 37-2 provides a list of common vitamins and herbs that increase bleeding.
• Rotate sites faithfully and document them to provide the next nurse with accurate data.

- Use the smallest gauge needle appropriate for the medication, site, and patient size.
- Make the needle puncture swiftly and at the correct angle.
- Apply a cotton ball, gauze pad, or alcohol wipe to the site immediately upon removal of the needle unless contraindicated, as for insulin and heparin.
- Apply a cool pack if bruising appears.

Z-Track

The **Z-track** method of intramuscular injection prevents irritating and dark-colored medications, such as iron dextran, from leaking out of the injection site into sensitive tissues or subcutaneous tissues that may stain. It also helps to reduce the inflammation and discomfort that can be caused by the medication irritating the subcutaneous tissue. The technique achieves this by closing the needle track in the tissue, preventing seepage of medication. Medications such as haloperidol (Haldol) and hydroxyzine (Vistaril) are typically administered by this method.

Place the lateral aspect of your nondominant hand against the patient's skin next to the intended insertion site, and pull or displace the skin and subcutaneous layer between 1 and 2 inches (2.5 and 5 cm) to one side, holding the tissue back while you use your dominant hand to swiftly pierce the skin and tissue with the needle to enter the muscle (Fig. 37-24). Without moving your nondominant hand from its tissue-securing position, close the index finger and thumb of that hand against the syringe to stabilize the needle; using your dominant hand, aspirate to ensure that

medication will not be injected into a vessel. If you obtain blood upon aspiration, recall that you discard the injection and prepare another dose using a new needle and syringe. Inject the medication over 10 to 15 seconds per milliliter of solution to reduce discomfort. Then wait 5 to 10 seconds to allow some of the medication to disperse away from the needle tip and track; swiftly withdraw the needle as you immediately release the skin and tissue being held back by your nondominant hand. This effectively closes off the needle track pathway and seals the medication within the body of the muscle. You may place an alcohol pad or cotton ball on the injection site and cover it with a bandage, but do not massage it, which can force medication into the subcutaneous tissue. *Safety: Activate the needle safety device immediately after removal of the needle from the skin.* You must be vigilant regarding performance of this safety mechanism while you are learning and perfecting your technique, so that it eventually becomes an automatic action that you do without having to consciously think about it. Skill 37-6 (page 905) provides more information on administering a Z-track injection.

Injection Site Identification

Correctly selecting the sites for IM injections requires you to know specific anatomical landmarks. Without this knowledge, you are at risk for causing discomfort, injury, and possibly permanent damage to the patient. Make it a priority to learn the correct anatomical landmarks and how to locate them for each IM injection site.

Ventrogluteal

The safest and most comfortable IM injection site for all patients older than 7 months is the ventrogluteal site. In the past, this was not the site of choice. In fact, nurses who trained prior to the 1990s were not taught about this site. Most were taught to use the dorsogluteal site, which is no longer recommended due to the risk of damaging

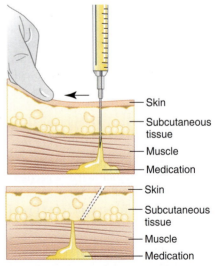

Figure 37-24 Z-track injection provides for closure of the needle track when you release the skin and tissue.

Box 37-2

Common Supplements That May Increase Bleeding

Even though supplements are easily obtained because they are considered "over-the-counter" drugs and do not require a prescription, this does not mean that they cannot cause dangerous problems. It is important to make the physician aware of all herbs, supplements, and even nonprescription drugs such as antacids, aspirin, or acetaminophen products that a patient takes.* Most surgeons will stop the following herbal supplements prior to a scheduled surgery due to their effect to increase bleeding:

- Cayenne
- Feverfew
- Ginkgo biloba
- Ginseng
- Omega-3 fatty acids
- St. John's wort
- Vitamins A and C
- Antiplatelet drugs

*Even though aspirin and acetaminophen are not herbal supplements, they are over-the-counter medications that most individuals feel free to take frequently, even on a daily basis. Both are known to have antiplatelet properties that increase bleeding and should be included on the patient's list of medications, herbs, and supplements if taken regularly.

the extremely large sciatic nerve that extends across the buttock and travels down the posterior aspect of the leg (Fig. 37-25).

This is your chance to help make a positive change in nursing by learning to use the ventrogluteal site as the site of choice. The dorsogluteal site should *only* be used if all other sites are not accessible.

The ventrogluteal site is the safest for IM injections because it is not close to any major blood vessels or nerves and there is little subcutaneous tissue overlying the gluteus medius and gluteus minimus muscles. To locate this site, have the patient assume a side-lying position with the foot on the top leg inverted to relax the hip muscles. Use your right hand for an injection on the patient's left hip and your left hand for an injection on the patient's right hip. Place the palm of your hand on the patient's greater trochanter with the index finger on the anterior superior iliac spine and your middle finger pointing toward the iliac crest. The "V" formed by your index and middle fingers marks your injection site. You should insert the needle in the center of the "V," slightly closer to the base of your two fingers (Fig. 37-26).

A

B

Figure 37-26 A. Diagram marking the number one choice for IM injections: the ventrogluteal injection site. B. Position the patient in a lateral side-lying position and place the palm of your hand over the greater trochanter. Point the index finger at the anterior superior iliac spine and the middle finger toward the iliac crest. The injection site is in the middle of the "V" form made by your fingers. If you are using the patient's left hip, you will use your right hand to make the "V"; if you are using the patient's right hip, you will use your left hand to make the "V."

Figure 37-25 The injection site must be accurately determined to avoid injury to the sciatic nerve.

Real-World Connection

Ventrogluteal Injection Site

The nursing instructor was taking weekly injections of vitamin B_{12} prescribed by her physician. Rather than give them herself, she thought it would provide the practical nursing students opportunity to get some injection practice. So she announced to the clinical students in Preconference that, for the next few months, a different student each week would get the opportunity to administer an IM injection to the instructor. Although somewhat good-naturedly reluctant to inject their instructor, yet wanting to take advantage of the opportunity, each week students would draw straws to determine which student received the honor of "sticking" the instructor. The students were allowed to select the injection site, and the second week, the student selected the ventrogluteal site, a site in which the instructor had never received an injection. The instructor was slightly apprehensive regarding use of the site, but agreed to allow the student to follow through with her selection. The student was nervous and shaking, but administered the IM injection

(connection continues on page 900)

into the ventrogluteal site using perfect technique. Not only was the instructor impressed with the total lack of discomfort, but she had not been able to identify when she was actually stuck due to the swiftness and perfect angle of insertion applied by the student. Through the following weeks, some students selected the vastus lateralis muscle and one other selected the dorsogluteal site, but the majority of the students followed suit and selected the ventrogluteal site for their turn at sticking the instructor.

Not only did the students receive the opportunity to administer an injection, but the instructor, who had never wanted to receive a ventrogluteal injection, was so impressed with the fact that she did not experience even minor discomfort from any of the injections at the site that she determined to use the ventrogluteal site as her primary injection site from that day forward, as did some of the students. This goes to show that using good technique when administering ventrogluteal injections will lead to minimal or no discomfort to the patient.

Deltoid

The most common site for injection of small volumes such as 0.5 or 1 mL is the deltoid muscle on the superior aspect of the upper arm. It is a smaller muscle than those of the other sites and is in close proximity to the brachial artery and radial nerve. Use the deltoid only for children with adequate muscle mass and adults. It is not suitable for newborns and small infants due to the lack of muscle development.

To select your site, locate the acromion process, place your little finger on the process and measure 3 fingerbreadths down. Inject into the fullest part of the deltoid (Fig. 37-27). Avoid going too low and posterior, where the radial nerve and artery are located. This site is appropriate for children ages 1 year to older adults. It is the most convenient to

access of all the IM injection sites, and the patient may be sitting up or lying in bed for the injection.

Vastus Lateralis

The vastus lateralis on the lateral aspect of the thigh is the second-choice site for injections larger than 1 mL if the ventrogluteal site cannot be accessed. It is the number one choice for newborns and infants who have not developed any of the gluteal muscles or the deltoid muscle. Absorption from this site is better than from other intramuscular sites.

To locate this site, have the patient assume either a supine position or a sitting position on the side of a bed or in a chair. Divide the thigh into thirds: Place one of your hands across the thigh next to the femoral crease (or next to the head of the trochanter) and your other hand across the distal aspect of the upper leg, just above the patella. The midpoint between your hands is the middle third of the thigh. Inject into the fullest portion of the muscle, just a little lateral to the longitudinal midline of the upper leg (Fig. 37-28).

Rectus Femoris

The rectus femoris is located in the longitudinal midline of the anterior thigh, but it is the last choice of sites to use and is for use in adults only, whenever rapid absorption is desired and other sites are inaccessible. *Safety: The rectus femoris site is not used in infants and children.* Many patients who self-administer injections at home use this site for its convenience. The disadvantage is that it is sometimes painful. It is near the vastus lateralis site, but lies more to the midline of the thigh. If you use this site, position the patient in the supine position and have the patient relax the thigh muscle as much as possible.

Dorsogluteal

The dorsogluteal site, as was mentioned earlier, is no longer the site of choice for IM injections—and it is never used in infants and small children. In adults, it should be used only as a last resort because of its proximity to the sciatic nerve, which can suffer injury and sometimes permanent damage when stuck by an errant needle. To identify the landmarks for this site, have the patient assume a prone position with the toes turned inward to relax the hip muscles. Palpate the posterior superior iliac spine and the greater trochanter.

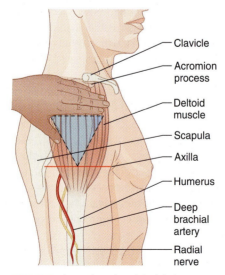

Figure 37-27 Locating the deltoid site.

- Clavicle
- Acromion process
- Deltoid muscle
- Scapula
- Axilla
- Humerus
- Deep brachial artery
- Radial nerve

Figure 37-28 Administering an IM injection in the vastus lateralis muscle.

Draw an imaginary line between the two landmarks. From the midpoint of this line, move approximately 1 inch above the line (toward the patient's head). This should place your finger in the upper, outer aspect of the buttock, where you are an adequate distance from the sciatic nerve (Fig. 37-29). This site is the last choice in adults when better sites are inaccessible, and is never a choice in infants and small children. For tips to decrease discomfort of injections, see Box 37-3.

People and Places Connection

Injection Variations for Infants, Toddlers, Children, and the Older Adult

- **Sites:** In newborns, infants, and toddlers, the vastus lateralis muscle on the anterolateral aspect of the upper leg is the muscle of choice for intramuscular injections. The gluteus muscles of the hip do not develop until a child begins to walk, and even then should not be used due to the proximity of the sciatic nerve in the tiny buttock. For school-age children through the older adult, the thicker gluteal muscle at the ventrogluteal site, where there are fewer nerves and blood vessels, is rapidly becoming the number one choice of sites, and the vastus lateralis or the deltoid muscle of the arm also may be used. The rectus femoris on the anterior thigh is no longer recommended in children of any age due to the increased discomfort of the site. However, the site is safe for IM injection in teenagers and adults if for some reason all other sites are deemed unsatisfactory.
- **Needle size:** For infants, use a ⅝-inch needle length in a 23- to 27-G needle. For children, older adults, or thin patients, use a ⅝- to 1-inch needle length in a 22- to 25-G needle. Always select length of needle based on the size of the muscle to be injected as well as the size of the patient.

Knowledge Connection

Describe the technique for intramuscular injection. Identify various needle lengths and gauge to use for IM injection. What is the maximum volume you may inject in the various muscles of each age group? How should a patient be positioned when administering an intramuscular injection? Describe the Z-track method for injection.

Box 37-3

Tips to Decrease Injection Discomfort

Sometimes needles and the medications themselves can be the cause of discomfort during an injection. Your knowledge and injection technique will also impact the level of discomfort accompanying your injections. But there are innumerable things you can do to improve your injection technique and make injections nearly "undetectable." There is nothing quite as rewarding after administering an injection as hearing the patient say, "You're already done? I didn't even feel the stick." This is the challenge that the authors pose to you. Try all of these tips, and you and your patients will be rewarded.

- Always use the smallest needle appropriate for the medication, site, and patient size.
- Be accurate in identifying landmarks for all injection sites: Just 1 inch off the correct site can cause unnecessary discomfort and injury to tissues and nerves.
- Know your medications: Identify those that are caustic and irritating to tissues. Make certain the correct route is ordered for the specific medication.
- Avoid administering a greater volume of medication than should be given at the site or that is too great for the size of the muscle.
- Avoid preparing the injection within the patient's view; this increases anxiety and discomfort.
- After inserting the needle through a vial stopper to draw up medication, change the needle for a new one that has not been dulled by the stopper and will not have medication on it.
- Explain what you are about to do to the patient to gain his or her compliance in holding still and relaxing the muscle.
- If the patient is a child, explain according to child's level of growth and development. Do not lie and say it will not hurt. Be truthful, but offer hope by including such things as "Try to hold real still and I'll try to be as easy as I can. It will sting for a minute and then it will be all over." Or "Hold on to your dolly real tight. I'll count to three and then you and I will both say OUCH together and then it will be over quickly."
- Distract the patient by engaging him or her in conversation.
- Assist the patient to assume the best position to relax the muscles of the site you select.
- Pull the skin over the site taut.
- Use the Z-track technique for all IM injections.
- Puncture the skin swiftly and to the proper depth to lessen the discomfort. Avoid shallow sticks where you then have to "push" the needle the rest of the way in.
- Stabilize the syringe and needle while injecting medication, not allowing any movement of the needle while it is within the tissues.
- Inject the medication slowly, no faster than 10 to 15 seconds per milliliter of medication.

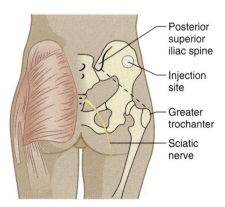

Figure 37-29 Locating the landmarks for the dorsogluteal site.

Posterior superior iliac spine

Injection site

Greater trochanter

Sciatic nerve

Skill 37-1 Reconstituting and Withdrawing Medication From a Vial

Assessment Steps

1. Review the physician's orders and the medication administration record (MAR) for the correct patient, medication, dose, route, and time. *This will ensure accuracy and currency of orders and prevent medication errors.*

2. Review a drug book for actions, required assessments, correct dosage, route, side effects, and expected results; review the drug insert for proper diluent, volume, and instructions for reconstitution. *This will ensure proper reconstitution steps are followed and will maintain stability of the drug.*

3. Assess the patient's allergies *to reduce risk of an allergic reaction.*

4. Select the correct medication vial, including medication name, dosage strength, dosage volume, dosage route and its appropriateness, and expiration, *to reduce the risk of medication error.*

5. Assess the vial contents for cloudiness, color changes, or particulate matter *to ensure quality of the medication.*

Planning Steps

1. Clean the workstation *to reduce microorganisms* before preparation of medication.

2. Gather needed supplies: appropriate syringes, needles, diluent, alcohol pads. *Being prepared saves time and energy. It also works to increase the patient's perception of your competence.*

Implementation Steps

1. Perform the Initial Implementation Steps located on the inside front cover.

2. Wash hands *to prevent cross-contamination.*

3. *Safety: Perform at least three medication label comparisons to the MAR to reduce the risk of medication error.*

4. Remove the cap from the medication vial and the diluent vial for access to the contents. Clean the rubber stoppers of both vials with separate alcohol swabs, rubbing in a circular motion, *to reduce microorganisms. Discard the swabs.*

5. Attach the needle to the syringe using aseptic technique *to reduce the risk of contamination of the medication.*

6. Draw up the specified volume of the specified diluent to ensure proper dissolving and concentration. *Safety: Note whether the diluent contains a bacteriostatic preservative or not, and correlate this with appropriateness of the patient's age.*

7. If using a multiple-dose vial, write the date, time, and your initials on the label *so staff will know when the vial was first opened.* If using a single-dose vial, dispose of it once you are through with it.

8. Wipe the stopper of the medication vial again with an alcohol wipe *to remove any contamination before puncturing the stopper again.*

9. Inject the diluent into the medication vial and mix until dissolved *to prevent particulate matter.*

10. Calculate the volume to withdraw from the vial to equal the physician's medication order, *to reduce the risk of medication error.*

11. Pull back on the syringe plunger to draw up an amount of air equal to the amount of medication you plan to withdraw from the vial. *This helps to maintain equal pressure inside the vial to ease removal of the medication.* Handle only the flange and the most distal 1 inch of the plunger *to avoid contaminating the portion of the plunger that will be reinserted into the sterile barrel with the medication.*

12. On a flat surface, hold the vial in one hand. Inject air through the rubber stopper into the vial, keeping the tip of needle above the fluid line *to prevent injecting air into the solution. Safety: Avoid using needleless piercing devices to access regular rubber stoppers, because they core the stopper. Obtain and attach a needleless vial adapter so that you can use a needleless piercing device, or use a safety needle to withdraw the medication from the vial.*

13. Invert the vial and move the needle tip below the fluid level *to avoid drawing up air.* Withdraw the ordered amount of medication. Keep the syringe at eye level *to ensure accuracy.*

14. Check the syringe for air bubbles. If bubbles are present, tap the syringe to remove them.

15. Remove the needle from the vial, holding the barrel of the syringe securely and maintaining sterility of the needle. *Activate the safety device to prevent needle stick.*

16. Change the needle *to prevent injecting the patient with a dull needle.* Before removing the needle from the tip of the syringe, pull back slightly on the plunger *to move the medication away from the tip of the syringe and reduce the risk of contamination or loss of medication.* Remove the needle and aseptically apply the new needle. Push the plunger gently *to dispel air from the syringe.*

17. Drop the contaminated needle into the sharps container *to reduce risk of needle sticks.*

18. Dispose of the vial or return it to the storage area if medication remains in a multiple-dose vial.

Evaluation Steps

1. Recheck your calculations and *evaluate if what you have drawn up is correct.*

Skill 37-2   Withdrawing Medication From an Ampule

Assessment Steps

1. Review the physician's orders and the medication administration record (MAR) for the correct patient, medication, dose, route, and time. *This will ensure accuracy and currency of orders and reduce the risk of medication error.*

2. Review a drug book and the drug insert for drug information *for accuracy.*

3. Assess the patient's allergies *to reduce the risk of an allergic reaction.*

4. Select the correct ampule, including medication name, dosage strength, dosage volume, dosage route and its appropriateness, and expiration, *to reduce the risk of medication error.*

5. Assess the ampule contents for cloudiness, color changes, or particulate matter *to ensure quality of the medication.*

Planning Steps

1. Clean the workstation *to reduce microorganisms* before preparation of medication.

2. Gather needed supplies: appropriate syringes, needles, alcohol pads, either a gauze pad or a commercial ampule-breaking device. *Being prepared saves time and energy.*

Implementation Steps

1. Perform the Initial Implementation Steps located on the inside front cover.

2. Wash hands *to prevent cross-contamination.*

3. *Safety: Perform at least three medication label comparisons to the MAR to reduce the risk of medication error.*

4. Attach the filter needle to the syringe. *This filters out shards of glass that may have fallen into the medication when breaking the ampule.*

5. If the medication is stuck at the top of the ampule, use your fingertip to gently flick the neck of the ampule. *This helps to ensure that an adequate volume of medication is available for withdrawal from the ampule.*

6. Clean the ampule neck with an alcohol wipe, using friction *to remove microorganisms.*

7. Holding the ampule below and away from your face, wrap a sterile gauze pad around the ampule neck *to protect your fingers* and snap the top off toward you *so that the ampule breaks away from you, helping any shards of glass to fly away from you.*

8. Holding the ampule with your nondominant hand, invert it or tilt it slightly. Insert the filter needle below the level of the liquid without contaminating the needle by touching it to the outside of the ampule; draw up the medication into the syringe. *This reduces contamination of the medication with glass shards.*

9. Pull back on the plunger, moving medication away from the end of the syringe *to reduce the risk of contamination or loss of medication.* Remove the filter needle and replace it aseptically with the injection needle, *so filtered glass within the needle will not be injected into the patient.*

10. Dispose of the ampule and filter needle in an appropriate container *to prevent needle sticks.*

11. Label the syringe with the drug name, dose, date, patient name, and time *to reduce chance of error.*

Evaluation Steps

1. Evaluate that the drug, dosage, route, and appropriate needle have been prepared.

Skill 37-3   Administering an Intradermal Injection

Assessment Steps

1. Review the physician's orders and the medication administration record (MAR) for the correct patient, medication, dose, route, and time. *This will ensure accuracy and currency of orders and help to prevent medication errors.*

2. Review a drug book and the drug insert for drug information *to ensure accuracy.*

3. Assess the patient's allergies *to reduce the risk of an allergic reaction.*

4. Assess the site to be used for injection, noting cuts, bruises, or other wounds that might contraindicate site usage. *Avoid injecting sites previously injected on the same day.*

Planning Steps

1. Gather needed supplies: 1-mL syringe, 24- to 28-G needles for drawing up an ID administration, alcohol wipes, dry cotton ball, black ink pen, examination gloves. *Being prepared saves time and footwork.*

Implementation Steps

Before Going to the Patient's Room

1. Wash hands *to prevent cross-contamination.*

2. *Safety: Perform two medication label comparisons to the MAR for right patient, right drug, right dose, right route, and right time to reduce risk of medication error.* Also check the expiration date of the medication.

3. Withdraw the medication from the ampule or vial, *maintaining sterility of appropriate pieces of equipment and medication.* Dispel any air from the syringe.

4. Recap the needle before walking to the patient's room *to maintain sterility of the needle.* Use the one-handed method of recapping or use a commercial recapping device *to prevent needle stick.*

(skill continues on page 904)

Skill 37-3 (continued)

After Entering the Patient's Room

5. Perform the Initial Implementation Steps located on the inside front cover.

6. *Safety: Perform a third medication label comparison to the MAR for right patient, right drug, right dose, right route, and right time to reduce risk of medication error.*

7. Explain the procedure to the patient *to reduce anxiety and increase cooperation.*

8. Wash hands again *to prevent cross-contamination* and apply clean examination gloves *to reduce risk of contact with body fluids.*

9. Select a site on the left inner forearm, if injecting P.P.D., for the intradermal injection. **Note:** *The left arm is used for P.P.D. testing.* Otherwise, you can use the right inner forearm, upper chest, or upper back for other intradermal injections.

10. Cleanse the area with an alcohol swab by wiping with a circular motion and moving outward from the injection site *to reduce microorganisms.* Allow the skin to dry.

11. Remove the needle cap with your nondominant hand by pulling it straight off to prevent contamination of the needle.

12. Spread the skin taut over the injection site *to ease piercing of the skin with the needle.*

13. Hold the syringe with the needle at a 15-degree angle to the patient's skin on the left inner forearm, bevel side up. Insert the needle into the skin to a maximum depth of $\frac{1}{8}$ inch (3 mm). Apply very GENTLE lift at the needle tip to ensure that you can see the bevel through the dermis, *which indicates you are not too deep.*

14. Slowly inject the medication while holding the GENTLE lift on the bevel, so that a $\frac{1}{4}$- to $\frac{1}{5}$-inch (6- to 10-mm) *wheal,* or discreet pale raised area of skin, forms at the tip of the needle. If a wheal does not begin to appear, withdraw the needle *very*

slightly and continue to inject until a wheal forms. *This ensures deposition of medication where it belongs, in the dermal layer.*

15. Remove the needle quickly at the same angle it was inserted, and release the skin. *This prevents the medication from leaking out.* Activate the safety device *to reduce the risk of needle stick.*

16. Do not massage the area after removing the needle. *Doing so may cause the medication to spread and alter its absorption.*

17. Discard the needle and syringe in the sharps container *to prevent needle stick.*

18. If injecting P.P.D., circle the site and write the date, time, and your initials by the circle.

19. Instruct the patient that the P.P.D. results must be read for interpretation at 48 and 72 hours. *This helps to gain patient compliance.*

20. Follow the Ending Implementation Steps located on the inside back cover.

21. Document the injection and site in the MAR and nurse's notes *for continuity of care.*

Evaluation Steps

1. Immediately following the injection, observe the injection site *for bleeding, swelling, or any signs of adverse reactions to the medication.*

2. Monitor the patient for at least 15 minutes after the injection *for signs of adverse reactions.*

Sample Documentation

11/1/12   0840   Administered 0.1 mL P.P.D. ID in lt. inner forearm, 8-mm bleb obtained. No reaction noted. Instructed that test must be read for interpretation at 48 and again at 72 hrs. for valid results. Verbally acknowledged understanding. ———————
——————————— Nurse's signature and credentials

Skill 37-4 Combining and Administering Insulin Subcutaneously

Assessment Steps

1. Assess an FSBS or check the last blood sugar reading for the patient *to ensure that the glucose level is not too low to safely administer insulin.*

2. Assess the patient for signs and symptoms of hypoglycemia and hyperglycemia.

3. Review the physician's order and compare with the medication administration record (MAR) *for accuracy and currency and to reduce the risk of medication error.*

4. Review the type of insulin to be injected in a drug text or resource to verify onset time, peak action time, and duration of insulin effect, *to reduce risk of failure to identify critical overlap times of multiple doses.*

5. Assess time and site of the last insulin dose *so you will know when to anticipate overlapping of multiple doses of insulin, which can cause sudden drops in blood glucose.*

Planning Steps

1. Determine the injection site. Rotate sites. Plan to use the abdomen for better absorption. Use the "clock" method of rotation of sites on the abdomen. Avoid using the same injection site as a previous injection on the same day *to reduce discomfort and excessive trauma to tissues.*

2. Clean the work area *to reduce microorganisms.*

3. Gather needed supplies: correct two types of insulin (check expiration dates), insulin syringe to match insulin strength (such as U-100 regular), alcohol wipes, gloves. *This saves time and footwork.*

Skill 37-4 (continued)

Implementation Steps

Before Going to the Patient's Room

1. Wash hands *to prevent cross-contamination.*

2. *Safety: Perform two label comparisons of each type of insulin to the MAR for right patient, right drug, right dose, right route, and right time to reduce risk of medication error.* Also check the expiration date of the insulin.

3. For NPH insulin, gently roll the vial between the palms of your hands *to warm and mix the insulin.* Do not shake.

4. Remove the needle cap and draw up air into the syringe equal to the total units of insulin to be drawn up from both vials *to maintain equal pressure.*

5. Clean the vial stoppers with a separate alcohol swab for each one *to reduce microorganisms.*

6. If regular insulin and NPH insulin are to be mixed, the *CLEAR* regular insulin should be drawn up first, after injecting air into both vials. *This sequence of drawing prevents regular (fast-acting) from being contaminated with NPH (intermediate-acting) insulin.*

7. Insert the needle into the stopper of the NPH vial and instill the number of units of air equal to the units of insulin to be removed. Then aseptically remove the needle from the stopper *to prevent contamination of the needle.*

8. Insert the needle into the stopper of the regular insulin vial and instill the remaining units of air to equal the units of insulin you plan to withdraw *to maintain equal pressure.* Do not remove the needle from the insulin vial.

9. Invert the vial with the needle still in the stopper. Carefully draw up the exact number of units of regular insulin ordered. Do not remove the needle from the insulin vial. *Safety: Take the MAR and written FSBS results along with the insulin to another staff nurse. Ask the nurse to tell you what you have.* The nurse should check the name on the MAR, name and type of insulin, and number of units drawn into the syringe; compare and verify that it is the amount indicated on the MAR for the patient's current blood sugar; and check the expiration date on the vial. The nurse should then initial the MAR *as the second witness of the insulin dose.* Dependent upon facility policy, you may be required to obtain a third nurse to witness the dose.

10. Withdraw the needle from the vial, taking care *to maintain sterility and to not bend the needle.*

11. Wipe the NPH insulin vial stopper again with an alcohol pad *to remove microorganisms.*

12. Insert the needle into the NPH insulin vial and invert the vial carefully *to avoid bending the needle.*

13. Withdraw slowly the *exact* number of units of NPH insulin. It must be exact, *because you are unable to reinstill any of it back into the vial as it is now mixed with regular insulin.* Do not remove the needle from the vial *so you can obtain verification of the correct dosage.*

14. Again, take it to the second nurse to compare and verify that you have what the MAR and blood sugar indicates you should administer. Have the nurse initial the MAR as the second witness. *This reduces chances of error.*

15. Remove the needle from the vial aseptically.

16. Recap the needle using the one-handed scoop method or a commercial recapping device *to prevent needle stick.*

17. Take the insulin to the patient's room.

After Entering the Patient's Room

18. Perform the Initial Implementation Steps located on the inside front cover.

19. *Safety: Perform a third medication label comparison to the MAR for right patient, right drug, right dose, right route, and right time to reduce risk of medication error.*

20. Explain the procedure to the patient *to reduce anxiety and increase cooperation.*

21. Wash hands again and apply clean gloves *to protect the patient from cross-contamination and you from blood-borne pathogens.*

22. Check the patient's identity using two methods according to facility policy *to reduce errors.*

23. Cleanse the skin site on the abdomen and allow to dry.

24. Pinch up a fold of skin and subcutaneous tissue, lifting it off the muscle layer *to prevent accidental injection into the muscle.*

25. Using a dart action, insert the needle at the appropriate 45- or 90-degree angle, as determined by the size of the patient and the length of the needle, *to ensure deposition of insulin into the subcutaneous layer.*

26. Do not aspirate. Inject the insulin and withdraw the needle using the same angle at which it was inserted.

27. Immediately activate the safety device *to prevent needle stick.*

28. Do not wipe the site.

29. Drop the syringe with the needle into the sharps container *to prevent needle sticks.*

30. Follow the Ending Implementation Steps located on the inside back cover.

31. Document insulin administration and site on the MAR *for continuity of care.*

Evaluation Steps

1. Immediately following the injection, observe the injection site *for bleeding, swelling, or any signs of adverse reactions to the medication.*

2. Monitor for signs and symptoms of hypoglycemia.

Sample Documentation

11/1/12   0750   FSBS 245 mg/dL. Reg insulin 4 units with NPH 10 units administered subcutaneously directly lt of umbilicus @ 3:00 position. Skin wd, alert, oriented ×4 spheres. ———

——————————————— *Nurse's signature and credentials*

Skill 37-5 Administering an Intramuscular Injection

Assessment Steps

1. Review the physician's orders and the medication administration record (MAR) for the correct patient, medication, dose, route, and time. *This will ensure accuracy and currency of orders.*

2. Review the drug book and drug insert for drug information *to increase safety of administration.*

3. Determine what assessments, if any, must be made prior to administration of the injection. If administering a prn medication, assess the length of the time interval since the last dose *to ensure an adequate time between doses.*

4. Assess the patient's allergies *to reduce chances of an allergic reaction.*

5. Determine the site of the last injection and where to inject this time, evaluating the patient's size and the length of needle to obtain *to ensure medication is deposited in correct muscle layer.* Avoid using the same injection site as used for a previous injection.

6. Ensure that the injection site area is not tender and is free of lumps.

Planning Steps

1. Clean your work surface *to prevent contamination of sterile injection supplies.*

2. Select a needle of the smallest suitable gauge and length based on the patient's size and muscle mass *to ensure the best IM deposition of the medication.* Gather needed supplies: correct size syringe, two needles, alcohol wipes, gauze pad, and gloves. *Being prepared saves time and effort.*

Implementation Steps

Before Going to the Patient's Room

1. Wash hands *to prevent cross-contamination.*

2. *Safety: Perform two label comparisons to the MAR for right patient, right drug, right dose, right route, and right time to reduce risk of medication error.*

3. Use aseptic technique to aspirate an amount of air into the syringe equal to the volume of medication you plan to withdraw from the vial *to maintain equal pressure in the vial.*

4. Wipe the vial stopper with an alcohol wipe *to reduce microorganisms.*

5. Use aseptic technique to inject the air into the vial, keeping the needle tip above the medication level *to prevent instilling air into the medication.*

6. With the needle still in the vial stopper, invert the vial and move the needle tip underneath the medication level *to avoid withdrawing air* while withdrawing medication from the vial.

7. Withdraw the appropriate dose, using care to remove any air from the syringe. Remove the needle from the medication vial.

8. Use the one-handed scoop method or a commercial cap holder to recap the needle. *This reduces risk of needle sticks.*

9. Pull back on the plunger to move medication away from the tip of the syringe *to avoid losing or contaminating medication.* Then remove the needle and drop the needle in the sharps container.

10. Open a new needle of appropriate gauge and length and apply it to the syringe without contaminating it. *This reduces the risk of contamination and provides the patient with a sharp needle that has not been dulled by going through stoppers.*

11. Take the medication to the patient's room.

After Entering the Patient's Room

12. Perform the Initial Implementation Steps located on the inside front cover.

13. *Safety: Perform a third medication label comparison to the MAR for right patient, right drug, right dose, right route, and right time to reduce risk of medication error.*

14. Explain the procedure to the patient *to reduce anxiety and increase cooperation.*

15. Wash hands again and apply clean examination gloves *to reduce cross-contamination and protect you from body fluids.*

16. Check the patient's identity using two methods as dictated by facility policy *to reduce medication errors.*

17. Position the patient comfortably *to allow access to the target site.* Use the ventrogluteal site as first choice in patients older than 7 months. Avoid using the dorsogluteal site unless it is the only choice *to reduce the risk of damaging the sciatic nerve.*

18. Wipe the site with alcohol and allow to air dry *to prevent burning.*

19. Pull the skin taut with your nondominant hand *to ease piercing the skin with the needle.*
    Note: It is considered by some nurses to be best practice to administer all intramuscular injections in sites other than the deltoid, using the Z-track method as an additional step to reduce discomfort of injections. *It helps to prevent medication from ascending back up the needle track after removal of the needle.* This is your choice. If you desire to use the Z-track method, see Skill 37-6.

20. Using your dominant hand, holding the needle so that the bevel is up, and using a 90-degree angle, swiftly pierce the skin and into the muscle with one smooth dart-like motion. *This reduces the discomfort of needle insertion.*

21. Secure the syringe with your nondominant hand *to prevent movement of the needle.*

22. Aspirate on the syringe before injecting the medication *to be sure you are not in a blood vessel.* (If there is blood in the syringe, withdraw the needle, activate the safety device, and discard the syringe and needle in the sharps container. Prepare a new injection.)

23. Hold the syringe steady while injecting the medication slowly, no faster than 10 to 15 seconds per milliliter of medication, *to prevent unnecessary discomfort by allowing the tissue to expand and the medication to disperse as the medication is injected.*

24. Swiftly withdraw the needle at the same angle you used to insert it, applying a gauze pad to the site with your nondominant hand as soon as the needle leaves the skin. Immediately activate the safety device *to prevent needle stick. Safety: If a sharps container is available at the bedside, drop the syringe and needle into it.*

Skill 37-5 (continued)

25. Massage the area gently *for better distribution and absorption.*
26. Follow the Ending Implementation Steps located on the inside back cover.
27. Document in the MAR and in nurses' notes if this is a new order, a one-time injection, or a prn injection.

Evaluation Steps

1. Immediately following the injection, observe the injection site *for bleeding, swelling, or any signs of adverse reactions to the medication.*

2. If this is first dose of a new medication, monitor the patient for at least 15 minutes after the injection *for signs of adverse reactions.*
3. Evaluate the effectiveness of the medication and document results.

Sample Documentation

11/1/12   1845   Third dose of Kefzol 500 mg IM given in Rt. ventrogluteal site without C/O of discomfort. ———————
——————————— Nurse's signature and credentials

Skill 37-6 Administering a Z-track Injection

Assessment Steps

1. Review the physician's orders and the medication administration record (MAR) for the correct patient, medication, dose, route, and time. *This will ensure accuracy and currency of orders.*
2. Review the drug book and drug insert for drug information *to increase safety of administration.*
3. Determine what assessments, if any, must be made prior to administration of the injection. If administering a prn medication, assess the length of the time interval since the last dose *to ensure an adequate time between doses.*
4. Assess the patient's allergies *to reduce chances of an allergic reaction.*
5. Determine the site of the last injection and where to inject this time, evaluating the patient's size and the length of needle to obtain, *to ensure the medication is deposited in the correct muscle layer.* Avoid using the same injection site as used for a previous injection.
6. Ensure that the injection site area is not tender and is free of lumps.

Planning Steps

1. Clean your work surface *to prevent contamination of sterile injection supplies.*
2. Wash hands *to prevent cross-contamination.*
3. Select a needle of the smallest suitable gauge and length based on the patient's size and muscle mass *to ensure the best IM deposition of the medication.* Gather needed supplies: correct size syringe, two needles, alcohol wipes, gloves. *Being prepared saves time and effort.*

Implementation Steps

Before Going to the Patient's Room

1. Wash hands *to prevent cross-contamination.*
2. *Safety: Perform two label comparisons to the MAR for right patient, right drug, right dose, right route, and right time to reduce risk of medication error.*

3. Use aseptic technique to aspirate an amount of air into the syringe equal to the volume of medication you plan to withdraw from the vial *to maintain equal pressure in the vial.*
4. Wipe the vial stopper with an alcohol wipe *to reduce microorganisms.*
5. Use aseptic technique to inject air into the vial, keeping the needle tip above the medication level *to prevent instilling air into the medication.*
6. With the needle still in the vial stopper, invert the vial and move the needle tip underneath the medication level *to avoid withdrawing air* while withdrawing medication from the vial.
7. After withdrawing the correct volume of medication, draw up 0.2 to 0.5 mL of air into the syringe to use for an air-lock. *This air-lock helps to prevent medication from reascending back up the needle track into the subcutaneous tissues, where it may be caustic.*
8. Remove the first needle and attach a second needle *to prevent tracking the medication through the subcutaneous tissue.*
9. Recap the new needle using the one-handed method *to reduce risk of needle sticks.*

After Entering the Patient's Room

10. Perform the Initial Implementation Steps located on the inside front cover.
11. *Safety: Perform a third medication label comparison to the MAR for right patient, right drug, right dose, right route, and right time to reduce risk of medication error.*
12. Explain the procedure to the patient *to reduce anxiety and increase cooperation.*
13. Wash hands again and apply clean examination gloves *to prevent cross-contamination and protect you from body fluids.*
14. Place the patient in the appropriate position *to expose the targeted muscle.*
15. Use appropriate landmarks to select the injection site and *reduce the risk of nerve injury.*

(skill continues on page 908)

Skill 37-6 (continued)

16. Cleanse the site with alcohol using concentric circles *to remove microorganisms.*

17. Just prior to injection, use the lateral aspect of your nondominant hand to pull the skin and underlying subcutaneous tissue to the side, displacing it laterally by 1 to 2 inches.

18. Using your dominant hand, hold the syringe with the needle bevel upward and swiftly pierce the skin, entering at a 90-degree angle, inserting the needle almost to the hub *to ensure deposition of medication in the muscle layer.*

19. Aspirate on the syringe before injecting the medication *to be sure you are not in a blood vessel.* (If there is blood in the syringe, remove the needle and discard the entire syringe. Draw up a new injection with a fresh syringe, needle, and medication.)

20. Without moving the needle, slowly inject the medication into the muscle, including instillation of the air-lock.

21. Wait for 5 to 10 seconds before withdrawing the needle. Release the tissue being held by your nondominant hand as the needle is withdrawn from the skin. *This allows the tissue to close the needle track at the muscle layer, preventing medication from entering the subcutaneous layer.* Activate the needle guard as soon as the needle leaves the skin *to reduce needle sticks.*

22. Do not massage the site. *Massaging the site after a Z-track injection may allow medication to be dispersed above the muscle as the needle track is manipulated.*

23. Discard the needle and syringe in the sharps container *to reduce needle sticks.*

24. Follow the Ending Implementation Steps located on the inside back cover.

25. Document the injection, technique used, and site in the MAR. Include any reactions to the injection.

Evaluation Steps

1. Immediately following the injection, observe the injection site *for bleeding, swelling, discoloration, or any signs of adverse reactions to the medication.*

2. If this is the patient's first exposure to the medication, monitor the patients for at least 15 minutes after the injection *for signs of adverse reactions.*

Sample Documentation

7/19/12 2115 *Cyanocobalamin 100 mcg administered IM using Z-track technique in Rt vastus lateralis without reports of discomfort.* ──────── *Nurse's signature and credentials*

 Post Conference

You shared with your classmates in Post Conference, allowing them to learn from your insights. Most of the injection procedure went well, especially when you were preparing the insulin. You were nervous, but you did remember to draw clear first and then cloudy insulin after you had injected the exact amount of air into each vial. You had difficulty recapping the needle to take it to the patient's room. You felt like you chased it all over the countertop. Your instructor helped you find a way to place it so that you did not do that the next time. Your intramuscular injection was rather nerve wracking for you, because the patient was in a great deal of pain after therapy when he asked for the meperidine. You were nervous and trying to hurry to get the pain relief to him. As a result, you accidentally touched the needle to your bare hand and had to change needles before you could give the medication. You identified the ventrogluteal site on his unaffected leg. You were so worried about hurting him with the injection, but he was just relieved to have the medication to relieve his pain. He assured you that any injection pain was quite minor to the pain he was experiencing in his amputated leg.

KEY POINTS

- Parenteral routes include intradermal, between the layers of the skin; subcutaneous, beneath the skin but above the muscle; and intramuscular, in muscle tissue.

- A syringe has three main parts: a barrel, a plunger on one end, and a tip on the other.

- The syringe tip will have either a slip-tip or a Luer-Lok connection, which attaches to a hypodermic needle.

- Syringes are available in numerous sizes, typically ranging from 0.5 to 60 mL.

- There are standard syringes, TB syringes, and insulin syringes.

- There are three parts of a needle: the bevel, or slant at the tip of the needle; the hub, or attachment point of the needle to the syringe; and the shaft or barrel, the main body of the needle.

- Needle sizes are designated by length and gauge. Gauges range from 14 to 30. The smaller the diameter of the needle, the higher the gauge number.

- The viscosity of the medication, the route of injection, and the size of the patient help to determine choice of needle gauge and length.

- Ampules contain single doses of medication in liquid form and require use of a filter needle to withdraw medication.

- Filter needles must ALWAYS be changed after drawing up medication from a glass ampule, before administering the injection.

- A vial is a container for parenteral medication that has a metal-enclosed rubber stopper on top. It can be a single-dose or multiple-dose vial.

- The site of choice for administering an IM injection for all patients older than 7 months is the ventrogluteal site.

- The site of choice for newborns and infants under 7 months of age is the vastus lateralis. The rectus femoris is not used on infants or small children.

- The maximum volume that can be injected in the deltoid muscle is 1 to 2 mL in older children and adults and 0.5 to 1 mL in infants.

- The maximum volume that can be injected in the ventrogluteal site is 1 to 2 mL in infants and children, the elderly, and the average-size adult.

- The maximum volume that can be injected into a very large individual's ventrogluteal site is 3 mL.

- Activate the safety device immediately after withdrawing the needle from the patient's skin.

- Dispose of needles in sharps containers immediately after use.

- Sterile needles should only be recapped using the one-handed method or a commercial recapping device.

- Never recap used needles.

REVIEW QUESTIONS

Select the answer that is most appropriate for each of the following questions. Some questions may have more than one correct answer. Check all that apply.

1. A parenteral route of medication administration is one that bypasses which of the following?

   a. Stomach

   b. Kidneys

   c. Skin

   d. Heart

   e. Liver

2. Injection of a drug into the upper layers of the skin is known as the _____ route of medication administration.

   a. intra-articular

   b. intradermal

   c. subcutaneous

   d. intramuscular

3. Which site of subcutaneous administration has the most rapid absorption of insulin?

   a. Vastus lateralis

   b. Dorsogluteal site

   c. Back of upper arm

   d. Abdomen

   e. Deltoid

4. Which of the following steps should the nurse perform when combining two types of insulin and administering them?

    a. Always withdraw intermediate-acting insulin first.

    b. When mixing insulins, remember "clear before cloudy."

    c. Inject with 20-G, 1-inch needle.

    d. Insert needle at a 45- or 90-degree angle.

    e. Mix Lantus with regular insulin.

5. A nurse needs to administer medication from an ampule. What of the following steps should the nurse take when drawing up this medication?

    a. Snap off the ampule neck using a sterile gauze pad.

    b. Hold the ampule away from the body when breaking.

    c. Tilt the ampule and place the injection needle into the liquid.

    d. Avoid tapping the top of the bottle.

    e. Use a filter needle to draw up medication.

6. What gauge and length of needle would you select to administer an IM injection of a nonviscous medication in the ventrogluteal site of a 40-year-old-male construction worker who is in good health and weighs 185 lbs?

    a. 25-G, 1-inch

    b. 18-G, 1.5-inch

    c. 22-G, 1.5-inch

    d. 24-G, 2-inch

    e. 20-G, ⅝-inch

7. You are about to administer a standard P.P.D. to a 31-year-old-male. Which of the following needles and syringes would be appropriate to use?

    a. Tuberculin syringe with 27-G, ⅝-inch needle

    b. 1-mL syringe with 20-G, 1.5-inch needle

    c. Insulin syringe with 25-G, ⅝-inch needle

    d. 3-mL syringe with 25-G, ½-inch needle

    e. 1-mL syringe with 18-G, 1-inch needle

8. In which of the following injections should you avoid aspirating before injecting the medication?

    a. Intramuscular injection of antibiotics

    b. Intradermal tuberculosis test

    c. Subcutaneous insulin

    d. Intramuscular pain medication

    e. Subcutaneous anticoagulant

9. Select the correct anatomical landmarks for the ventrogluteal site.

    a. Iliac crest

    b. Greater trochanter

    c. Acromion process

    d. Coccyx

    e. Anterior superior iliac spine

SHORT ANSWER QUESTION

10. A nurse is caring for an older adult female patient. What factors should the nurse consider when administering an intramuscular injection to the patient?

CRITICAL THINKING EXERCISES

11. Describe the differences between the intradermal, intramuscular, and subcutaneous injection routes, including any choice/most advantageous muscles or sites or restricted sites. Be thorough.

12. You are preparing to administer an antibiotic injection to a newborn that must be reconstituted before use. The medication label states that either Sterile NS for Injection, Sterile Water for Injection, or Sterile Bacteriostatic Water for Injection are appropriate diluents that may be used for reconstituting the antibiotic. When you go to the medication cart to obtain the diluent, you see three unopened vials to choose from: Sterile Normal Saline 0.9% (Multiple-Dose Vial), Sterile Water for Injection (Multiple-Dose Vial), and Sterile Water (single-dose vial). Which of the three diluents cannot be used in this particular situation? Why not, if the label says both NS for Injection and Water for Injection are both acceptable diluents?

ADDITIONAL RESOURCES

For additional Resources, Questions, and Activities, please see:

 Student Resource Disk

 http://davisplus.fadavis.com

 Student Study Guide

REFERENCES

American Association of Nurse Anesthetists. Enough is enough: health care leaders unite to launch injection safety campaign. February 11, 2009. Available at: http://www.aana.com/News.aspx?ucNavMenu_TS MenuTargetID62=&ucNavMenu_TSMenuTargetType4=&ucNavMenu_ TSMenuID=6&id1=9348. Accessed November 30, 2009.

Aziz AM, Ashton H, Pagett A, Mathieson K, Jones S, Mullin B. Sharps management in hospital: an audit of equipment, practice and awareness. *Br J Nurs.* 2009;18(2):92-98.

Buchholz S, Henke G. *Henke's Med-Math: Dosage Calculation, Preparation and Administration.* Philadelphia: Lippincott Williams & Wilkins; 2008.

Institute for Safe Medication Practices. Fatal outcome after inadvertent injection of topical epinephrine. March 26, 2009. Available at: http://www.ismp.org/Newsletters/acutecare/articles/20090326.asp. Accessed November 30, 2009.

Rhoads J, Meeker BJ. *Davis's Guide to Clinical Nursing Skills.* Philadelphia: FA Davis; 2007.

Scanlon V, Sanders T. *Essentials of Anatomy and Physiology.* 5th ed. Philadelphia: FA Davis; 2007.

Smeltzer S, Bare R, Cheever K, Hinkle J. *Brunner & Suddarth's Textbook of Medical-Surgical Nursing.* 11th ed. Philadelphia: Lippincott Williams & Wilkins; 2006.

The Joint Commission. 2000 National Patient Safety Goals. Available at: http://www.jointcommission.org/PatientSafety/ NationalPatientSafetyGoals/. Accessed November 30, 2009.

Wheeler AH. Therapeutics injection for pain management. Emedicine-Web MD Web site. July 29, 2009. Available at: http://emedicine. medscape.com/article/1143675-print. Accessed November 30, 2009.

Wilkinson JM, Van Leuven K. *Fundamentals of Nursing: Theory, Concepts & Applications.* Philadelphia: FA Davis; 2007.

Williams LS, Hopper PD. *Understanding Medical-Surgical Nursing.* 3rd ed. Philadelphia: FA Davis; 2007.

World Health Organization. Fact sheet No. 231: injection safety. Revised October 2006. Available at: http://www.who.int/mediacentre/ factsheets/fs231/en/.

Key Terms

Cannulation

Drug-drug interaction

Extravasation

Flange

Hemolysis

Hypertonic

Hypotonic

Hypovolemia

Infiltration

Isotonic

Nonvesicant

Packed red blood cells (PRBCs)

Parenteral

Patent

Plasma

Precipitate

Sclerosed

Thrombus

Vesicant

Objectives

1. Define key terms associated with preparing, initiating, and maintaining peripheral IV therapy.
2. Identify the purposes and benefits of peripheral IV therapy.
3. List the common components of IV fluids and their uses.
4. Compare the effects of infusing hypotonic, isotonic, and hypertonic IV fluids.
5. Describe equipment used for peripheral IV therapy.
6. Discuss the importance of asepsis during IV therapy.
7. Relate possible complications of IV therapy and their causes.
8. Contrast IV therapy in children, adults, and older adults.
9. Explain how to prepare, initiate, and maintain a peripheral IV infusion.
10. Calculate an infusion rate for a gravity infusion and a pump infusion.
11. Discuss peripheral IV therapy nursing care.
12. Summarize how to prepare, initiate, and monitor infusion of blood and blood products.
13. Apply knowledge of IV therapy in specific scenarios.

Skills

38-1 Administering IV Push Medication via PRN Lock or IV Line

38-2 Administering IV Piggyback Medication

38-3 Converting an IV Infusion to a PRN Lock

38-4 Calculating IV Infusion Rate

38-5 Adding Medications to Primary IV Solution

38-6 Initiating Peripheral Venipuncture

38-7 Adding a New Bag of IV Solution to Existing IV Line

38-8 Discontinuing an IV Infusion or PRN Lock

38-9 Preparing, Initiating, and Monitoring Infusion of Blood and Blood Products

Clinical Connection

Your Assignment: You will be caring for a 77-year-old male who was admitted with nausea, vomiting, and dehydration. The cause of his symptoms is not yet determined. He is NPO and has an IV infusion of D5 ½NS infusing at 60 mL/hr in his left forearm. According to his chart, it was difficult for the nurse to get the IV infusion started. When you go in to introduce yourself, he tells you that his arm is hurting and points to the IV site.

Your Actions: While there are many things you will need to do for this patient, your most immediate focus at this moment will be his IV infusion. You must decide if there is a problem with the infusion, and if so, what problem is occurring. Then you must decide what to do about the problem. And finally, if you need to restart his IV infusion, you need to know what size and type of device to use, how to insert it, what fluids to infuse and at what rate, and what additional complications to watch for.

As you learned in Chapter 29, fluid is one of the body's most essential substances, second only to oxygen. During illness or recovery from injury, the body is often unable to tolerate fluids and nutrition by mouth, thus necessitating infusion of fluids, electrolytes, and nutritional components by a route other than the usual route of the alimentary canal. Any other route, including the intravenous, subcutaneous, or intramuscular routes, is known as the **parenteral** route. This chapter is devoted to the *peripheral intravenous route,* which means to infuse directly into the vascular system by the way of a peripheral vein, as opposed to a larger central vein such as the subclavian or jugular. This chapter will introduce you to the entry-level knowledge and skills of peripheral IV therapy. Much skill and knowledge are required to prepare an infusion, initiate IV access, and maintain the infusion in a safe manner. Practice, and practice alone, will help you to develop stellar IV therapy skills and techniques.

Purposes of IV Therapy

Infusion of fluids intravenously may serve multiple purposes, including:

- Maintaining or providing daily body fluid and electrolytes due to inability to ingest fluids and nutrients by mouth
- Replacing abnormal or excessive loss of fluids and electrolytes
- Providing an avenue for IV administration of medications

Maintaining Fluids and Electrolytes

Whenever an individual refuses to drink adequate fluids or is unable to ingest fluids orally, whether it is due to nausea, inability to swallow, disease of the digestive tract, decreased level of consciousness, or NPO status for surgery, the body requires the necessary fluids be administered via a different route. Without maintenance of adequate fluid supply, the body can:

- Become dehydrated
- Develop imbalances between levels of fluid and electrolytes
- Develop impairment of cellular function, which impacts the functions of each body system
- In severe cases cease to function, resulting in death

Provision of maintenance fluids generally will include not only water, the primary need, but also electrolytes, glucose, and sometimes vitamins. The electrolytes are necessary to maintain homeostasis of fluids and electrolytes, which contribute to correct function of all body systems. Glucose is required for production of energy. It provides the calories, or fuel, that will be burned during all cellular functions. Glucose is also stored in the form of glycogen in the liver, to be converted back to glucose at a later time when energy needs require more fuel. Vitamins are required for various cellular functions such as growth of new tissue.

Replacing Fluid and Electrolyte Losses

There are numerous ways an individual can lose excessive amounts of fluids. Recall from Chapter 29 that fluids are normally lost on a daily basis through the kidneys, intestinal tract, skin, and lungs. Excessive losses in any of these areas, such as from high fever or working outside in extreme heat, require that the fluids be replaced to prevent dehydration. Diseases that cause excessive vomiting or diarrhea, require gastrointestinal suctioning, or simply prevent oral intake of fluids increase the fluid replacement needs. When the loss of water is accompanied by the loss of specific electrolytes, they must also be replaced. For example, gastric suctioning or vomiting can deplete sodium, chloride, potassium, and hydrochloric acid, resulting in hyponatremia, hypochloremia, hypokalemia, and metabolic alkalosis. Loss occurring with diarrhea includes loss of potassium, sodium, and bicarbonate. You may find it helpful to refer back to Chapter 29 regarding these imbalances.

Recall that, when fluids and electrolytes are lost in balanced proportions from extracellular spaces, the decrease in blood volume is called **hypovolemia**. The direct loss of blood from the cardiovascular system, in the form of hemorrhage, is another avenue of fluid and electrolyte loss along with the other components of blood. *It is important to remember that inadequate fluid within the cardiovascular system makes it impossible to provide adequate circulation to the cells, tissues, and organs, all of which are required to sustain life.* Replacement of lost fluids and electrolytes should be based upon actual fluid losses, increased metabolic needs, and laboratory results of serum electrolyte levels.

Infusion of Intravenous Medications

The administration of IV fluids provides an avenue through which we can assure the rapid and direct delivery of medications to the blood in the intravascular space when they are needed. Administering medications via the IV route delivers an increased potency of medication compared to the intramuscular or subcutaneous injection routes. Because of the increased drug potency and the immediacy of the drug's effects, the IV route of drug administration can be very dangerous if the person giving the drug does not have adequate knowledge of the drug's therapeutic effects, side effects, adverse reactions, and antidote, when appropriate.

Medications can be added to larger volumes of IV fluids, such as 500 or 1,000 mL, and infused continuously, or can be added to smaller volume of fluids, ranging from 50 to 250 mL, for delivery at specified intervals. Figure 38-1 shows the different IV container volume sizes.

Continuous IV Infusion

When continuous IV infusion of a drug is desired, the physician orders the dosage of medication to be administered. The pharmacist or nurse performs the calculations to determine the amount of drug to add to a specific volume of IV solution in order to achieve the desired concentration. The volume of solution may vary from 250 to 1,000 mL. Now the infusion rate that will deliver the prescribed dosage

must be calculated. All infusions of IV solution must be monitored closely to maintain the ordered rate of infusion, but it is doubly important if there is medication added to the solution.

IV Push

Some medications can be administered directly by a method known as *IV push,* which means the medication is injected directly into the vein using a needle and syringe. The IV push route of administration has two advantages: it produces an immediate therapeutic blood level and instantaneous effects of the drug. However, these same advantages serve as disadvantages as well. If the incorrect drug or dosage is administered, the unintentional blood level and effects of the wrong drug are immediate, sometimes harming the patient. It is also possible that the patient may suffer adverse reactions or be allergic to the drug. The immediacy of effects requires your vigilance in verifying that you are administering the right drug and dosage to the right patient at the right time, by the right route, and slowly according to the manufacturer's recommendations.

This route is commonly used in emergencies, surgery, and other situations in which immediate results are desired. If the patient has an intermittent infusion device, also known as a *PRN lock,* the medication can be administered IV push via the injection port without having the discomfort of another needle stick. Another way to administer IV push drugs is through the Y-injection port nearest the insertion site of a primary IV line with continuous infusion of IV fluids (Fig. 38-2).

Administration of IV push medication requires that the medication be compatible with the IV solution as well as any medications that have been added to the solution. Many facilities have policies in place requiring that all venous access devices (VADs) be flushed with 3 to 10 mL of

Figure 38-1 Intravenous solutions come in a variety of bag sizes/volumes: 50 mL, 250 mL, 500 mL, and 1,000 mL.

Figure 38-2 Administering IV push medication into the injection port closest to the insertion site of a continuously infusing IV. The nondominant hand pinches off the primary line between the Y-injection port and the IV bag to ensure that the medication infuses down-line toward the patient rather than up-line toward the IV solution bag.

sodium chloride, or normal saline (NS), prior to administration of IV push medications, and again after the IV push medication, regardless of compatibility or incompatibility. Other facilities may only require NS flushes if there is an incompatibility issue.

If the medication is not compatible, the flow must be stopped by pinching off the tubing just proximal to the injection port to be used. Three to 10 mL of NS are injected through the injection port, followed by the medication. Then the medication is flushed out of the line with another 3 to 10 mL of NS before resuming infusion of the incompatible IV solution. Most facilities stock prefilled syringes of NS flush, which save you the time of gathering supplies and drawing NS up each time you need a flush (Fig. 38-3). However, because some facilities charge what seem like exorbitant prices for the prefilled syringe of NS, it does significantly raise the cost to the patient.

Many medications must be diluted in 1 to 10 mL of NS prior to IV push administration. By diluting the medication, the level of vein irritation and patient discomfort are reduced. All IV push drugs must be administered over the manufacturer's recommended length of time. Some medications require an administration time of only 2 to 5 minutes; others require 7 to 10 minutes or more. *Safety: It is your responsibility to research the length of time over which you should give a medication.* This information can be found in the drug insert that comes with the drug or in a drug book, or can be obtained from the pharmacist. Skill 38-1 (page 944) provides more information on administering IV push medications.

Some state boards of nursing, some Nurse Practice Acts, and certain facilities place restrictions on who may administer IV push medications. Some designate that it is strictly the responsibility of the RN, while others allow both LPN/LVNs and RNs to perform this skill. Some facilities allow LPN/LVNs to administer IV push medications, but restrict administration of certain categories such as cardiac emergency drugs to the RN. It is your responsibility to know your own state board of nursing's philosophy and Nurse Practice Act scope of practice, as well as your facility's policy regarding this issue.

IV Piggyback

A third method of administering medications intravenously is called intravenous piggyback (IVPB). The medication is added to a smaller volume of IV solution, usually a volume between 50 and 250 mL of either 0.9% sodium chloride (NS) or dextrose 5% in water (D5W). The medication is then infused over a specified period of time between 15 and 90 minutes, depending upon the medication. A specially designed, shorter tubing connects the IVPB solution container to the most proximal Y-injection port located on the primary IV line, similar to *riding piggyback* on the primary line, thus the name. You will also hear it called *secondary tubing* as well as simply *piggyback tubing*. The terms are synonymous. The IVPB route is commonly used for administering medications that require intermittent infusion, such as every 4 hours or every 8 hours. Figure 38-4 identifies the parts of the primary and secondary IV tubings and shows how they work together. Skill 38-2 (page 946) provides more information on administering IVPB medications.

Some patients will no longer have a need for a continuously infusing IV solution but will still need the IV access for administration of intermittent IVPB or IV push medications. In such an instance, the physician may order to discontinue the IV fluids and convert to an intermittent infusion lock, termed a *PRN lock* or *saline lock*. The IV tubing is disconnected from the cannula in the vein and a PRN lock device is attached to the cannula. The PRN device is kept

Figure 38-4 IVPB medication infusing into the most proximal (closest to bag) Y-injection port on the primary administration set.

Figure 38-3 Prefilled syringes of normal saline with Luer-Lok tips and sterile caps; used to flush IV lines.

open, or **patent**, with IV flushes of NS administered at least every 8 hours. Skill 38-3 (page 949) provides more information on converting an IV infusion to a PRN lock.

If a patient has a PRN lock rather than a continuous primary IV solution, the shorter secondary tubing would not be long enough to administer an IVPB because it would not reach from the IVPB solution bag on the IV pole to the PRN lock injection port secured to the patient's arm or hand. Therefore, instead of using a secondary piggyback tubing, it would be necessary to use a basic primary IV tubing so that it would be of adequate length.

Knowledge Connection
What are three reasons for administration of IV fluids? Explain the difference in IV push and IVPB routes of administration. List four ways in which body fluids may be lost. What is the minimum time frame in which an IV push drug may be administered?

Compatibility Versus Incompatibility
Medications must be compatible with other drugs, additives, and IV solutions that are mixed or administered at the same time or immediately following each other. There are so many medications available today that numerous medications are incompatible and can result in **drug-drug interactions**. This means the interaction between the two drugs causes a change in the activity or components of one or more of the drugs. Some drug reactions may even produce a product that is totally unsafe to administer. Certain incompatible drugs, when mixed, cause a precipitate to form. A **precipitate** forms when one of the agents in a solution separates from the solvent and becomes a solid, insoluble product. It may or may not be visible to the naked eye, but when you can see it, it may look cloudy, hazy, or like fine floating crystals. Never allow an infusion to continue if you see precipitates forming in the fluid.

Some incompatible drugs require use of separate tubing sets to administer each medication, while others only require a specified interval of time to elapse between administrations of the two incompatible medications. When incompatible drugs require separate tubing sets for each medication, you must label the tubing with the date and time hung, name of the drug, and your initials. Other medications might only require that you flush the intermittent infusion lock or the primary IV line with NS both before and after giving each medication. This prevents the two medications from ever coming in contact with each other.

Safe Administration of IV Drugs

Knowledge required to safely administer IV medications includes:

- Patient's medication allergies
- Patient's disease or condition

- Sterile technique
- Integrity of the IV access
- Effects of the drug
- Correct form of medication for IV use
- Correct dosage for specific patient's age or weight
- Type of diluent to use if needed
- Volume of dilution required
- Rate of safe administration
- Expected effects of the medication
- Possible drug-drug interactions
- Possible adverse reactions, including the most common and those that are life threatening
- Appropriate nursing interventions to employ if an adverse reaction occurs

Knowledge Connection
Explain what drug incompatibility means. What does the term *precipitate* mean with regard to incompatibility? Identify at least 10 things you must know to safely administer IV medications.

IV Solutions

Intravenous fluids are made of water to which various percentages of components have been added. Common components found in different IV fluids include glucose, electrolytes, vitamins, and amino acids. The amounts of these solutes that are dissolved in the water determine the fluid's *tonicity* (the solute concentration of IV fluids) and the effect that it will have on the blood volume, cell size, and energy production.

Tonicity serves to meet the individual needs of patients as they are treated at different stages of diseases and conditions, each one of which may require differing volumes of water and solutes to provide or maintain homeostasis throughout the body. Intravenous fluids are responsible for saving lives every day. The danger that you need to understand is that the administration of improper amounts of water and solutes or the wrong concentration of the two components can cause complications and possibly patient death. It is important that you learn the differences between isotonic, hypotonic, and hypertonic fluids and what occurs physiologically after infusion of these solutions into the patient.

Isotonic Solution

As you learned in Chapter 29, an **isotonic** solution is fluid that contains an amount of solute that produces a concentration of dissolved particles equal to that of the intracellular and extracellular fluids of the human body. Because the concentration is equal, administration of the isotonic solution will not cause movement of water between the intravascular space, the interstitial space, and the intracellular space. In other words, there will be no movement of fluids across the semipermeable membranes of the blood vessels or cellular membranes as long as this ratio remains balanced (Fig. 38-5). Table 38-1 lists common isotonic fluids and their uses.

Hypotonic Solution

A **hypotonic** solution has a lower osmolarity than body fluids, which simply means there is less solute dissolved in the water, making the concentration of the dissolved particles less than that of the body fluids. Hypotonic solution infused into the intravascular space, or blood vessels, will cause shifting of body fluids out of the intravascular space and into the interstitial spaces, and then eventually into the intracellular spaces, rehydrating the cells (Fig. 38-6). (For further detail of this process, refer to the Anatomy and Physiology Connection below.)

This process makes a hypotonic solution good for use in patients who need simple water replacement due to lack of fluid intake or loss of body water without loss of electrolytes, known as *hypertonic dehydration*. For a list of common hypotonic fluids and their uses, refer to Table 38-1.

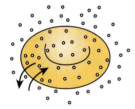

End result of infusing isotonic IV solution:

Figure 38-5 Fluid movement during infusion of isotonic IV solution. During infusion of isotonic IV solution, the body maintains balance as equal volumes of water cross back and forth continuously between the two extracellular spaces (blood inside the intravascular space and fluid in the interstitial spaces) and the intracellular spaces inside the cells. The end result is the balance shown inside and outside of a cell.

Maintaining Compartmental Fluid Balance

The body strives to maintain a homeostatic balance of fluids and electrolytes at all times. One of the mechanisms by which this is accomplished is the movement of the solvent, or liquid, component of body fluid. The fluid shifts described above result due to changes in *solute*, or particle, concentration dissolved in the solvent. By administering a hypotonic solution (one with a lower solute concentration than that in the body fluids) into the blood vessels, the solute concentration of the blood is lowered and the concentration in the interstitial space outside the blood vessels is now higher than that in the blood. Because of this imbalance, water then moves from inside the blood vessels, across the semipermeable membrane of the vessel walls, into the interstitial space in an attempt to balance the two levels of solute concentration. As this water moves into the interstitial space, the solute concentration in the fluid there is being diluted in an effort to equalize it to that of the fluid inside the blood vessels. As this process continues, the solute concentration of the fluid in the interstitial space now becomes less than that of the fluid within the cells. This imbalance causes water to move across the semipermeable cellular membrane from the interstitial space to the inside of the cells in an effort to maintain balance of the solute concentration of the interstitial and intracellular fluids. As water is moved from the interstitial spaces into the cells, the cells are rehydrated.

Recall from Chapter 29 that the movement of an excessive volume fluid from the vascular spaces into the interstitial spaces is known as third-spacing, which lowers both blood volume and blood pressure and causes edema. The increased volume of interstitial fluid dilutes the solute concentration, making the interstitial fluid hypotonic; excessive water then moves into the cells, causing them to swell and possibly rupture. *Safety: Infusion of an excessive volume of hypotonic IV fluids can result in cerebral edema, increased intracranial pressure, overhydration and rupture of brain cells, and death of the patient.* Box 38-1 lists early signs and symptoms of increased intracranial pressure.

Hypertonic Solution

If a fluid has a higher concentration of particles dissolved in it than the concentration in fluids of the body, it is known as **hypertonic** solution. Intravenous infusion of excessive hypertonic fluids causes water to be pulled from the interstitial space into the intravascular space in an attempt to balance the solute concentration on both sides of the semipermeable membrane, the vessel wall. This overloads the fluid volume within the vascular spaces, resulting in elevated blood pressure. The fluid movement does not stop here, however. The solute concentration of the interstitial fluid will increase as the water is pulled out of it to move into the blood vessels. Now the solute concentration of the interstitial fluid becomes greater than that found within the cells. The water will then be pulled out of the cells and into the

Table 38-1   **Common IV Solutions and Their Uses**

Solution	Uses	Special Considerations
Hypotonic		
Half-strength saline: may be written as ½ NS or 0.45% NaCl	Water replacement. Fluid and electrolyte replacement during gastric suction. Hypertonic dehydration. Depletion of Na^+ and Cl^-.	Avoid use in patients with liver disease, head trauma, burns. Can cause cerebral edema. *Safety: Should not be used in patients with hypotension, will further drop blood pressure.*
One-third strength saline: may be written as ⅓ NS or 0.33% NaCl	Free water replacement to aid kidneys in elimination of wastes.	*Safety: Should not be used in patients with hypotension, will further drop blood pressure.*
Isotonic		
5% Dextrose in water: may be written as D5W	Provide some calories for energy. Provide free water. Reduce protein breakdown for energy. Short-term treatment of dehydration, at controlled infusion rate. To administer medications by intravenous piggyback (IVPB) route.	*Safety: Do not use in patients who are allergic to corn.* Irritates veins, causing phlebitis. Use cautiously in patients with renal and cardiac disease; can result in fluid overload. *Safety: Observe for early signs and symptoms of fluid overload.* Continual infusion can result in electrolyte deficits. *After dextrose is metabolized, it becomes hypotonic.* Has been known to cause cerebral edema with continuous infusion. *Safety: Observe for early signs and symptoms of cerebral edema (increased intracranial pressure).* Avoid using for resuscitation; can cause hyperglycemia. Cannot be mixed with blood components; causes hemolysis.
Normal saline or sodium chloride: may be written as NS or 0.9% NaCl	Replacement of nutrients and electrolytes when no fluid shift is desired. *Only* fluid used to initiate and discontinue blood transfusion. Irrigant for IV access devices to prevent clotting. Vascular expander.	Can result in fluid volume excess. Use cautiously in patients with congestive heart failure. *Safety: Observe for early signs and symptoms of fluid overload.* Dilutes concentration of hemoglobin in the blood. May lower potassium levels.
Lactated Ringer's solution: may be written as LR	*Because it is most similar to electrolyte content of the blood,* it is used for fluid replacement in all types of dehydration and fluid volume deficits. Electrolyte replacement in intravascular fluid.	*Safety: Has some incompatibilities with medications. Check for compatibility before administering medication.* Can result in fluid volume excess.
Normosol-R: may be written as Normosol	Similar to LR.	Can result in circulatory overload.
5% Dextrose in 0.22% sodium chloride: may be written as D5 ¼NS	Supplies some calories. Treat dehydration. As a "fluid challenge" to assess kidney function.	*Safety: Do not use in patients who are allergic to corn.* Can result in circulatory overload. Fluid challenge: give 8 mL/m² of body surface area for 45 minutes to determine if kidneys begin to function by making urine.

(table continues on page 920)

Table 38-1 **Common IV Solutions and Their Uses** (continued)

Solution	Uses	Special Considerations
Hypertonic 5% Dextrose in 0.45% sodium chloride: may be written as D5 ½NS	Replace nutrients. Treat dehydration.	*Safety: Do not use in patients who are allergic to corn.* Can result in circulatory overload.
5% Dextrose with 0.9% normal saline: may be written as D5NS	Supplies calories. Used to expand blood volume.	*Safety: Do not use in patients who are allergic to corn.* Can result in circulatory overload.
10% to 50% Dextrose: may be written as D10W, D20W, D50W	Prefilled syringes of dextrose 50% in water are used to treat severe hypoglycemia, but dextrose 50% IV fluids are not used for continuous IV infusion.	*Safety: Any IV fluid with dextrose concentration greater than 10% cannot be given through peripheral veins. It must be administered via central veins.* *Safety: Do not use in patients who are allergic to corn.*
3% to 5% Sodium chloride: may be written as 3% NaCl and 5% NaCl	To treat severe sodium depletion and water overload. (Not commonly used.)	*Safety: Dangerous. Only small volumes are infused.* Irritates veins. Administer slowly. May cause circulatory overload.

extracellular spaces in an attempt to balance the solute concentration on both sides of the semipermeable cell membrane (Fig. 38-7). This reduction in cellular fluid can result in shrinking the cells. Cells in this condition will not function appropriately and can even die as a result. Table 38-1 lists common hypertonic solutions and their uses.

Knowledge Connection
Compare isotonic, hypotonic, and hypertonic fluids. Explain which direction fluid movement occurs when hypertonic fluid is administered intravenously. Explain the same for hypotonic fluid.

IV Equipment

A wide variety of IV equipment is available for use, and advancing technology provides new and improved choices of equipment at an amazingly rapid rate. The equipment that you learn to use in development of your IV skills probably will not be in use 10 years from now. The equipment of basic IV therapy includes numerous varieties of the following components:

- **IV needle cannula or catheter:** a needle covered with a flexible plastic cannula that is used to access a peripheral vein and through which IV fluid can enter the vein; once the plastic sheath has been advanced off the needle into the vein, the needle is removed (Fig. 38-8).

- **Winged butterfly:** a steel needle with plastic wings at the base of the needle, also known as a *scalp-vein needle* (Fig. 38-9). Used for shorter infusion times, usually less than 24 hours; phlebotomy; and when the longer, larger IV cannulas cannot be successfully inserted into a vein.
- **IV tubing:** tubing through which IV fluids may infuse from the IV bag to the patient.
- **IV infusion pump or controller:** an electronic or computerized pump/controller that is manually set to control the volume of solution to be infused and the rate of infusion.
- **Intermittent infusion IV access tubing or PRN locks:** devices that are designed to connect directly to the cannula and have an injection port on the opposite end through which medications can be intermittently infused without requiring a continuously infusing IV line (Fig. 38-10). The purpose of both PRN lock designs is to maintain venous access without continuously infusing fluids.
- **IV start kit:** a small kit containing generic supplies required to initiate an IV access device.

IV Needle Cannula

The IV needle cannula comes in many different designs, lengths, and *gauges* (G), which means the diameter size of the inner bore of the hollow needle. The needle is covered by a plastic sheath called an *IV cannula* or *catheter.* The cannula is slightly shorter than the needle, allowing the bevel at the tip of the needle to extend just beyond the end of the cannula (refer to Fig. 38-8). Once the bevel of

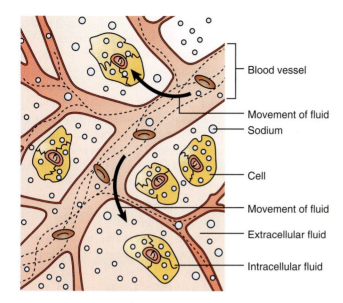

- Blood vessel
- Movement of fluid
- Sodium
- Cell
- Movement of fluid
- Extracellular fluid
- Intracellular fluid

End result of excessive hypotonic IV solution:

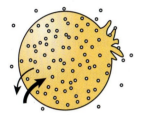

Figure 38-6 Fluid movement during infusion of hypotonic IV solution. The body tries to maintain balance when infusion of hypotonic IV solution dilutes the blood, making it less concentrated than the interstitial fluid. Osmosis pulls water from the blood to the interstitial spaces to dilute the more concentrated interstitial fluid. Once the interstitial fluid becomes less concentrated than the fluid inside the cells, osmosis will pull water from the interstitial spaces into the intracellular space inside the cells. If this is allowed to continue beyond the patient's specific needs, the cells will continue to fill with extra water, swelling until they eventually rupture and die, as seen in the diagram of a cell.

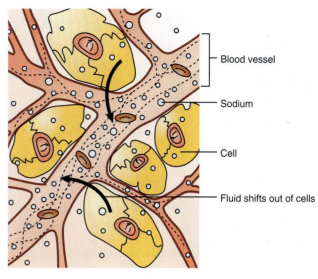

- Blood vessel
- Sodium
- Cell
- Fluid shifts out of cells

End result of excessive hypertonic fluid:

Figure 38-7 Fluid movement during infusion of hypertonic IV solution. The body tries to maintain balance when infusion of hypertonic IV solution raises the concentration of the blood. Then osmosis pulls the less concentrated interstitial fluid into the blood vessel to dilute the now more concentrated blood. This shifting causes the interstitial space to begin to dehydrate, increasing its concentration. This causes osmosis to pull the less concentrated intracellular fluid from inside the cells to the outside of the cells, where it can dilute the concentration of the interstitial fluid. The effect is cell shrinkage. If allowed to continue beyond the patient's level of need, the cells will eventually dehydrate, collapse, and lyse, ultimately destroying the cells, as seen in the diagram of a cell.

Box 38-1

Early Signs of Increased Intracranial Pressure

It is best to detect increasing intracranial pressure before it has progressed to the point that the vital signs deteriorate. Be alert to the following earlier signs:

- Change in level of consciousness
- Confusion
- Disorientation
- Headache increasing in severity
- Pupillary changes
- Purposeless movements
- Restlessness

- Over-the-needle plastic cannula
- Safety button: retracts needle when pushed
- Bevel of needle
- Hub of cannula
- Flash chamber: receives blood return
- Safety guard chamber: to receive retracted needle

Figure 38-8 The parts of a safety IV needle with over-the-needle cannula: needle, bevel of needle, over-the-needle cannula, flashback chamber, hub, needle retraction button, safety guard to receive retracted needle

Figure 38-9 Winged butterfly device, also known as a scalp-vein needle.

Figure 38-10 Various PRN lock injection port devices. At the top, one style of PRN lock device, commonly known as a "pigtail," has an injection port on one end of the PRN lock and on the other end a 4-inch extension tubing that ends in a Luer-Lok connection that screws directly onto the IV cannula hub. In the middle are three short PRN locks without attached extensions. They are about 1 inch (2.5 cm) in length and attach directly to the IV cannula hub. The PRN device on the bottom has an approximately 3-inch length extension tubing that is shaped like the letter "J." It is hard and does not flex like the "pigtail."

the needle, followed by the end of the cannula, has entered the vein, the cannula is carefully advanced off the end of the needle into the vein. Then the needle itself is removed. The process of advancing the IV cannula into the vein is known as **cannulation**.

Intravenous cannulas were found to be a better way to maintain IV access for a longer period of time than a regular steel needle. The plastic IV cannula does not irritate the vein as much as a steel needle. Neither does it become displaced by piercing through the other side of the vein as easily as a sharp steel needle.

The larger the gauge number, the smaller the diameter of the needle bore, and the smaller the gauge number, the larger the diameter. The cannula sizes include even numbers from the tiniest 24 G (0.6 mm) to very large 12 G (2.8 mm). They also come in different lengths from ½ to 2 inches (1.2 to 5 cm). The gauge and length to be used depend upon the size of the vein to be accessed, the viscosity or thickness of the solution to be infused through the cannula, and the rate at which it is to be infused (Table 38-2). Larger bore needles, such as 18 G (1.2 mm) to 20 G (0.9 mm), are used in the following situations:

- Administration of blood or blood product transfusions, so the viscous fluid can be rapidly infused
- When the risk of hemorrhage, fluctuation of vital signs, or shock exists, such as when a patient is scheduled for surgery
- When the patient has experienced some type of major trauma or disease and may need rapid infusion of fluids

Smaller bore needles, such as 22 or 24 G, are indicated in the following situations:

- When the patient has small veins, such as a young child or older adult
- When the patient has fragile veins, such as older adults or those who have had repeated IV medications
- When IV access is needed only intermittently, such as to administer IV antibiotics every 6 hours
- When the purpose is simply to maintain patency of the access device in case IV administration of medications or fluids should be necessary. The rate of infusion in this situation is known as TKO (to keep [the vein] open), which is 20 to 30 mL/hr, according to facility policy.

The most commonly selected gauges and lengths for use in adult patients are 20 to 22 G (0.9 to 0.7 mm), and 1 to 1.5 inches (25 to 40 mm) length. Figure 38-11 presents a variety of IV cannula sizes.

Winged Butterfly

The winged butterfly is also known as a *scalp-vein needle*. It has two small plastic wings, one extending from each side at the base of a steel needle. Both wings fold upward to provide a place for you to grasp the device while initiating IV

Table 38-2 **IV Cannula Gauge Infusion Capability**

IV Cannula Gauge	Fluid Volume Capability
20 G	Can infuse up to 3,900 mL/hr
22 G	Can infuse up to 2,200 mL/hr
24 G	Can infuse up to 1,400 mL/hr

Figure 38-11 Various sizes of IV needles with over-the-needle cannulas: 14 G, 16 G, 18 G, 20 G, 22 G, and 24 G.

access. The two wings are designed to lie flush to the skin surface. Tiny, flexible tubing extending from behind the wings attaches directly to the IV tubing. The winged butterfly sizes include the odd numbers from 19 to 29 G (1 to 0.3 mm) in diameter and from ⅜ to 1 inch (9.5 to 25 mm) in length (refer to Fig. 38-9).

Butterfly needles, though easy to insert and secure, infiltrate easier than a plastic over-the-needle cannula. The steel tip of the needle will more easily pierce the vein wall and allow seepage of solution into the interstitial tissues. Butterflies are mostly for short-term use such as administration of single doses of IV push medication and *phlebotomy*, which is drawing of blood samples. (Refer to Chapter 34 for further information related to phlebotomy.) Butterflies may be used to access scalp veins in newborns and infants up to 18 months of age, for infusion of IV fluids. The scalp veins are often selected in these infants due to the ease of securing the site on the head. Butterflies may also be used for patients in whom insertion of a typical IV cannula has been unsuccessful and IV therapy is required.

Knowledge Connection

Describe what a cannula is. What sizes and lengths do they come in? Which is smaller, an 18-G (1.2-mm) or a 24-G (0.6-mm) cannula? Which VAD is commonly used to access a newborn's scalp veins?

IV Tubing

Intravenous tubing is flexible, small-diameter tubing that either delivers IV solutions and medication from the solution bag to the cannula in the patient's vein or provides an avenue to deliver solution from a second bag to the primary IV line of a different solution. Intravenous tubing must have a sterile spike or piercing pin on one end to insert into the solution bag port. Just below the piercing pin is a **flange** that provides a place for your fingers to push the piercing pin into the solution bag port without contaminating the sterile piercing pin. Immediately below the flange is a drip chamber that holds a small volume of the IV solution before it enters the IV tubing. The drip chamber is filled one-third to one-half full and is the site you will observe to determine that solution is flowing. If the IV fluid is being infused by gravity, you will observe the drip chamber to count the number of drops per minute. Some IV tubing has an in-line filter to remove any foreign particles that might be found in the IV solution. There will be clamps on the tubing to shut off solution flow and control the rate of flow. Different types of clamps you may see include a *slide clamp*, which simply allows solution to flow or stops the flow, and a *roller clamp*, which allows you to not only start or stop the solution flow, but to regulate the rate of infusion by rolling the clamp either tighter or looser. Some IV pump tubing will have a cassette chamber that inserts into the pump mechanism. The opposite end of the tubing is the sterile end that inserts into the cannula hub. Both this end and the piercing pin are covered with caps when you take the tubing out of the package to help you in maintaining their sterility.

Intravenous tubing comes in many different styles, and it would be impossible to discuss them all here. We will discuss the basic types that are commonly used:

- **Primary IV tubing administration set:** The long, main tubing that allows continuous flow of IV fluids. It may be designed to flow by gravity or to be used with a pump or controller.
  - **Primary IV administration set for infusion by gravity:** The primary tubing for gravity flow has one or more Y-injection ports and a roller clamp to control the infusion rate (refer to Fig. 38-4).
  - **Primary IV administration set for infusion by pump:** Each primary pump tubing is designed and dedicated solely for use with the specific pump indicated by the manufacturer. These sets are not interchangeable with different brands of IV pumps. Some will have a small cassette chamber on them that inserts into the pump mechanism, and others will not.
- **Secondary medication (or IVPB) tubing administration set:** A shorter IV tubing, often termed *piggyback tubing*, that is used to administer medications at intervals; the tubing connects (piggybacks) to the most proximal Y-injection port of the primary IV tubing administration set (refer to Fig. 38-4).
- **Blood administration Y-set:** Tubing shaped like the letter "Y" (Fig. 38-12); two piercing pins on two upper ends insert into the bag of blood product and the bag of normal saline used to accompany blood product infusions; the tail of the Y-set consists of a single tubing end that connects directly to the IV cannula in the patient's vein (Fig. 38-13).

Figure 38-12 Blood administration Y-set.

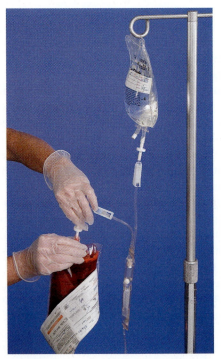

Figure 38-13 Blood administration Y-set primed with NS, showing insertion of the piercing pin into the unit of blood.

IV Tubing Extenders

There are various devices that may be used either to add length to the primary IV tubing or to connect the IV tubing directly to the IV cannula that is inserted into the vein.

- **Extension tubing** is a 6- to 24-inch length of tubing inserted between the patient's IV cannula and the primary IV tubing, for the purpose of extending the length of tubing to provide the patient with more mobility, or to provide additional injection ports where medications can be injected directly into the patient's IV line.
- **Intermittent infusion lock or PRN lock** is a small device that attaches to the IV cannula inserted into the vein and provides an injection port on the end of it through which IV fluids or medications can be administered either continuously or at intervals (Box 38-2). Though technically not an IV tubing "extender," it may have a 1- to 4-inch length of tubing built into it (refer to Fig. 38-10).

Knowledge Connection

What is the difference between a continuous IV infusion and a PRN lock? What does the term *patent mean?* What danger is inherent when using heparin to maintain patency of a PRN lock?

Box 38-2

Heparin Flushes

PRN locks are used to maintain venous access without continuously infusing fluids. To keep the vein *patent,* or open, the lock and IV cannula must be flushed intermittently with 3 to 10 mL NS, dependent upon physician's orders and facility policy, usually once every 8 hours. Though it is now rare to see, you may see a physician's order for heparin to flush a PRN lock. Flush-strength heparin is available in strengths from 10 units/mL to 100 units/mL. It is a very low-dose anticoagulant that was created solely for use in PRN locks. However, there are more concentrated strengths of heparin that are used for anticoagulation therapy. Though flush-strength heparin was heavily used in the past, this is no longer the case. An excessive number of accidental overdoses occurred due to inadvertently flushing PRN locks with the higher concentrations of heparin intended only for anticoagulant use. Some of these overdoses resulted in serious hemorrhages and some in death. Normal saline has been shown to be equally as effective at maintaining vein patency without the risk of overdose, and is now used almost exclusively over flush-strength heparin. However, if you should receive an order for heparin to flush a PRN lock, remember the following safety guideline. *Safety: When flushing a PRN lock with heparin, make certain to use the correct flush strength. Heparin also comes in much higher concentrations for treatment of life-threatening blood clots. It comes in 1,000 units/mL, 5,000 units/mL, 10,000 units/mL, and 20,000 units/mL* (see the Real-World Connection box).

Reduced-strength Heparin Versus Regular-strength Heparin

A 7-month-old infant presented to the hospital's emergency room (ER) with *status epilepticus,* back-to-back seizures that would not stop. Over the course of several hours, the ER staff treated the infant with intermittent doses of IV anticonvulsant medication via an intermittent infusion lock. In between the doses of seizure medication, the nurse was to administer a dose of reduced-strength heparin, 10 units per 1 mL, to maintain the patency of the IV cannula. Later, after the infant had received at least seven doses of the anticoagulant, it was discovered that the nurse had mistakenly been administering full-strength heparin, at a concentration of 5,000 units per 1 mL, rather than the reduced-strength heparin designed for flushing intermittent infusion locks. Even though a dose of vitamin K was given as an antidote, the infant developed the signs of severe pallor, bleeding from the gums, and constant oozing from the intermittent infusion lock site. When the infant began to develop a decreased level of consciousness and vital signs became unstable, the infant was Medi-flighted to a specialty children's hospital for intensive care. The problem? The accidental but massive overdose of anticoagulant had resulted in hemorrhaging within the brain. The infant did survive, but suffered death of sufficient brain cells to result in major neurological deficits, leaving the child in a vegetative state. The infant's mother filed a lawsuit against the first hospital and the nurses who made the mistake. What a horrible tragedy for the infant and the infant's loved ones. But the tragedy does not really end with the lawsuit. Imagine the burden of guilt that the nurses must live with, knowing that something as *basic* as *reading the label* could have prevented this immeasurable loss.

Each manufacturer produces various versions of each of these types of tubing, many to be used only with specific brands or models of IV pumps or infusers. You will need to familiarize yourself with the specific IV equipment and supplies used at the facility where you work.

Drop Factor

A characteristic that differs from one IV tubing to another is the *drop factor,* which represents the number of drops it takes for that specific tubing to equal 1 mL of volume of IV fluid (Fig. 38-14). The drop factor number may be found on the tubing package. If the drops produced by the tubing are large, it requires fewer drops to equal 1 mL of volume than it takes if the drops are smaller. The range of drop factors in IV tubing includes drop factors of 10, 15, 20, and 60, with 10 being the largest drop size and 60 being the smallest (Box 38-3). A drop factor of 10 simply means that it takes 10 of these *largest* drops to equal 1 mL of fluid. On the opposite end of the scale, a drop factor of 60 means that it takes 60 of these tiniest drops to equal 1 mL of fluid (Fig. 38-15).

The size of the fluid drop produced by the tubing is categorized as either a micro-drop or a macro-drop. The tiny

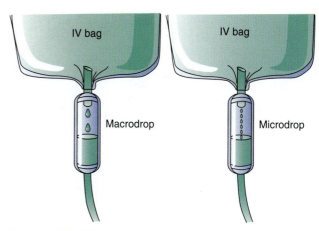

Figure 38-14 Drip chamber and number of drops equaling 1 mL.

Box 38-3

IV Tubing Drop Factors

The drop factor represents the number of drops that an IV tubing delivers to deliver 1 mL of fluid. The drop factor can be found on the tubing box.
- **Drop factor of 10:** 10 drops equals 1 mL
- **Drop factor of 15:** 15 drops equals 1 mL
- **Drop factor of 20:** 20 drops equals 1 mL
- **Drop factor of 60:** 60 drops equals 1 mL

---

drops produced by tubing with a drop factor of 60 are known as *micro-drops*. All the other drop factors produce larger drops and are known as *macro-drops*. The drop factor number is important because it is used in the formula to calculate IV infusion rates that you will be learning later in this chapter.

Knowledge Connection

Explain what is meant by *drop factor*. Where can you locate this information?

Needleless IV Systems and Safety Needles

In an attempt to reduce contaminated needle sticks among health care workers, manufacturers have devised several needleless IV systems that do not require the use of sharp needles to inject medication into the tubing injection ports. The systems have incorporated the technology used in the manufacturing of medication vials that do not require the use of sharps to withdraw their contents. Numerous safety needles have been invented to make administration of intramuscular, subcutaneous, and intradermal injections safer as well.

The Occupational Safety and Health Administration (OSHA) has mandated that hospitals must use either safety needles, safety syringes, or needleless systems to decrease risk of transmission of blood-borne pathogens such as HIV

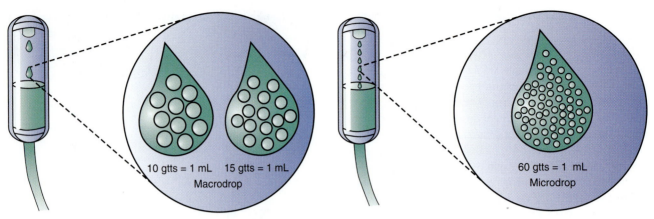

Figure 38-15   A tubing with a drop factor of 10: The drops are larger and it takes 10 of these larger drops to equal 1 mL of fluid. On the opposite end of the scale, a tubing with a drop factor of 60: The drops are quite tiny and it takes 60 of these tiniest drops to equal 1 mL of fluid.

and hepatitis B via contaminated needle sticks. There are many such systems, each a little bit different than the other. Figure 38-16 presents an example of one type of safety syringe and how it works. It is your responsibility to be knowledgeable regarding the system that is used in your facility. Most of the current systems allow you to screw a Luer-Lok–tipped syringe directly to the injection port to inject medication into the IV line. Others require a needleless piercing device, or blunt-tipped adapter, that inserts into the injection ports. Figure 38-17a shows a close-up of a syringe with an attached needleless piercing device.

Intravenous tubing was also adapted to work with the safety needles and needleless systems. The rubber ports had to be designed so that blunt-tipped piercing devices could be inserted without destroying the rubber stopper, which would cause leakage and provide an open entry site for microorganism access. By gaining access to the once-sterile IV tubing, microorganisms had a direct route into the sterile cardiovascular system of the patient, resulting in sepsis and even death. Figure 38-17b shows an injection port with a white ring that indicates it is a needleless port designed to receive blunt-tipped piercing devices. Figure 38-18 shows a variety of needleless devices.

However, it is important to know that, even though these safety needles and needleless systems are in place in most facilities, there are still some older styles of IV tubing and medication vials in use that do not accept these needleless piercing devices. *Safety: Needleless blunt-tip adapters cannot be inserted into vials and injection ports*

Figure 38-17a   A syringe with a needleless piercing device attached.

Figure 38-16   An example of one type of safety syringe before and after activation.

Figure 38-17b   The needleless piercing device inserts into the needleless port designated by the white ring around the rubber port.

Figure 38-18 Various needleless supplies. From left to right: piercing device that secures with a clothespin-like clip; "pigtail" PRN lock; short PRN lock; safety syringe with attached piercing device inserted into a short PRN lock; safety syringe with attached piercing device ready for use; "blunt needle" piercing device; vial converter cap, converting a regular vial to a needleless access vial.

Figure 38-19 An example of an IV pump.

of systems that are not designed to be needleless. To do so carries the potential of punching out a small core from the rubber stopper that falls into the solution and inside the IV tubing. This is known as "coring" and is not a safe practice. Most needleless systems are identified by a white or blue ring painted around the edge of the injection ports.

IV Infusion Pumps and Controllers

Intravenous infusion pumps and controllers provide an immeasurable amount of protection against accidental infusion of too much fluid, as is possible when an IV solution is infused solely by gravity. When infusing by gravity, a 1,000-mL bag of IV solution could conceivably accidentally infuse the complete volume in an hour or less. This would present a very dangerous situation for the patient. Many patients would be unable to tolerate that much fluid instilled into their cardiovascular systems that quickly and could go into circulatory fluid overload and pulmonary edema. Elderly individuals and children are especially prone to fluid overload. You will learn more about this complication later in this chapter.

Each manufacturer produces an infusion pump that looks and works a little differently than other available products, but the premise is the same: They can be programmed to control the total volume of fluid to be infused and the rate of infusion, and to coordinate primary fluid infusion with intermittent infusion of IVPB medications. Pumps provide accurate total volume infused over a particular period of time, such as an 8- or 12-hour shift (Fig. 38-19). They also have alarms to indicate when:

- The IV line is occluded
- Air is present in the line
- The IV bag is empty
- The preset volume of fluid has infused

It is easy to understand how infusion pumps increase the safety of IV therapy for the patient, and save time for you, as well as providing an extra measure of safety for you.

Knowledge Connection
How does use of an IV pump or controller provide a measure of safety for the patient?

IV Start Kit

Many companies package the basic supplies that are used to initiate, or start, an IV access device (Fig. 38-20). These kits are designed exclusively for the health care worker's convenience: It saves you the time of gathering the

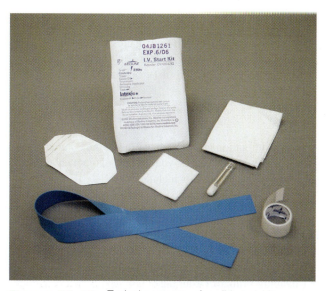

Figure 38-20 Typical contents of an IV start kit.

individual generic supplies that are required for virtually every IV access start. Usually included in these kits are:

- **Tourniquet:** to block venous blood return while selecting a vein and making the initial stick
- **Antiseptic prep pad:** to cleanse the skin site to be punctured
- **Sterile 2×2-inch (5×5-cm) gauze pad:** to dry the puncture site before applying adhesive dressing
- **Sterile 2×3-inch (5×7.6-cm) transparent occlusive, semipermeable adhesive dressing (TOD):** applied over the needle insertion site to reduce contamination by microorganisms
- **Label:** placed on the site dressing with date and initials to indicate when the IV access was started
- **Tape:** to secure the VAD

Asepsis and IV Therapy

As you have previously learned, the body's first line of defense against invasion by microscopic organisms is the skin. *Safety: When this first line of defense is broken by piercing the skin with an IV cannula needle, you must use strict aseptic technique.* Even with use of aseptic technique, the patient remains at risk for infection of the IV site. Infection at the site can progress to infection of the bloodstream, known as *sepsis,* which can be fatal. Even a local infection at the IV site, without progression to the bloodstream, can:

- Increase the patient's discomfort and anxiety; risk of **thrombus,** or blood clot, formation; length of hospital stay, and expense of hospitalization
- Decrease the patient's trust and rapport with health care providers
- Increase the nurse's workload and liability

Therefore, use of asepsis during IV therapy cannot be adequately emphasized.

Handwashing

You must thoroughly wash your hands for at least 15 seconds immediately prior to handling any of the supplies you will be using for initiation of IV access or maintenance of IV therapy.

Gloves

Clean examination gloves are worn for any nursing care of IV therapy that places you at risk of contact with the patient's body fluids. This includes:

- Initiating the IV access
- Changing the occlusive IV site dressing
- Touching a leaking IV site dressing
- Discontinuing an IV line
- Converting an IV infusion to a PRN lock
- Changing primary IV tubing

- Any care that requires you to come in contact with the insertion site or supplies used at the insertion site
- Any other nursing care of IV therapy that places you at risk of contact with patient body fluids

Supplies

Certain parts of IV supplies must be kept sterile at all times (Box 38-4). Once the IV access has been initiated, everything is connected, and fluids are infusing, you should have an enclosed sterile system from the inside of the solution bag through the tubing into the patient's vein. Any intrusion into the inside of this system requires that principles of strict asepsis be followed. This includes introduction of a needle, blunt-tipped adapter, or Luer-Lok syringe tip into either the solution bag or IV tubing at any injection port or connection.

The Infusion Nurse's Society (INS) recommends that you change "continuously infusing" primary and secondary IV tubing at least every 72 hours and any time that contamination of tubing is even suspected. If a facility's rate of IV-related infections increases using the 72-hour schedule, INS recommends changing the continuous infusion tubing every 48 hours. INS also recommends that tubing used for "intermittent infusions," such as secondary tubing used for infusion of IVPB medication, be changed every 24 hours. The increased frequency of opening the sterile system to spike the next IVPB medication bag provides more opportunities for contamination, thus requiring more frequent changing. A bag of IV solution should never be allowed to

---

Box 38-4

IV Supplies That Must Be Kept Sterile

Maintaining sterile technique during IV initiation is paramount. Because there are "specific parts" of each supply item that must be kept sterile, you will need to be able to identify them on sight while you are manipulating the supplies during IV initiation. You may find it helpful to locate the parts listed below on the actual items. If so, obtain (1) an IV needle with cannula, (2) a primary IV tubing, (3) a bag of IV solution, (4) a PRN lock, and (5) a transparent occlusive dressing (TOD). Identify the parts on each item that must be kept sterile.

- Entire length of the IV needle barrel and cannula or butterfly
- Opening to the hub of the IV cannula or butterfly that connects directly to the IV tubing end
- Open end of the IV tubing that connects into the IV cannula or needle hub
- IV tubing spike, or *piercing pin,* that enters the sterile IV solution bag
- IV solution bag insertion port into which the IV tubing spike enters
- IV solution being infused
- Adhesive side of the TOD prior to application over the IV insertion site
- All direct connection points of tubing extensions or adaptors

infuse longer than 24 hours. It is common practice to dispose of remaining solution and hang a new sterile bag of solution every 24 hours.

A tourniquet must be used on only one patient before discarding it. Studies have shown that use of a tourniquet on multiple patients increases nosocomial infections.

Patient's Skin

The skin site to be pierced with the IV cannula or needle must be thoroughly cleansed to reduce skin surface microorganisms using the antiseptic agent specified in facility policy. The four solutions recommended by the INS include:

1. 10% povidone-iodine
2. 2% tincture of iodine
3. 2% aqueous chlorhexidine gluconate
4. 70% isopropyl alcohol

If povidone-iodine is to be used, assess the patient for allergy to iodine or shellfish. If the patient has no allergy, use alcohol to remove skin oils, then proceed with the iodine solution. Vigorously scrub the selected site for at least 20 seconds, beginning in the center and working outward in concentric circles until a 3-inch diameter circle has been cleansed. Avoid retouching the center of the cleansed area with the wipe that has touched the outer edges of the circle and the contaminated skin next to it. Touching the cleansed site with the gloved finger requires recleansing of the site prior to piercing the skin with a needle. Allow the solution to dry. If alcohol is the sole agent used, extend the scrub time to 30 seconds. Avoid using alcohol *after* povidone-iodine because it has been shown to negate the effect of the iodine.

Knowledge Connection
Explain why asepsis is so important during IV initiation and maintenance therapy. Which parts of the IV catheter must be kept sterile? Which parts of the primary or main IV tubing must be kept sterile? For how long should you cleanse the skin site to be punctured?

Calculation of Infusion Rate

Many formulas have been devised to calculate the IV infusion rate. The authors have selected one formula that is simple to understand and works for calculation of both gravity infusion and infusion by pump. Before proceeding with the formula itself, there are a few things you must understand first:

1. You will hear several terms used to describe the rate at which an IV solution is to infuse into the patient. They include *infusion rate, flow rate, drop rate,* and *drip rate.*

2. These terms are not to be confused with the *drop factor.*
3. When infusing an IV solution by *gravity,* the drop factor is printed on the tubing container. It will be stated as a number of "*drops per mL.*" Do not confuse this factor with "*drops per minute,*" which refers to the rate of infusion. The drop factor tells you how many drops that specific tubing must "drip" to equal 1 mL of fluid, or "*drops per mL.*"
4. When using a *pump or controller,* the *drop factor is always 60.* It does not matter which drop factor is printed on the tubing box, because the machine is electronically designed to equal the drop factor of 60, since the pump is set in milliliters per hour (mL/hr) rather than drops per minute (gtts/min).
5. When the IV solution is to infuse via *gravity,* the infusion rate (or flow rate, drop rate, or drip rate) is measured by visually counting the number of *drops per minute.*
6. When the IV solution is to infuse via an IV *pump or controller,* the pump electronically measures the infusion rate in *milliliters per hour.*
7. The abbreviation for *drops* is *gtts.*

Until you have a working knowledge of calculating IV infusion rates, you should memorize the above seven points. This will make using the following formula easier to learn. There are three numbers required for use of this formula:

1. Specified volume of fluid that is to infuse
2. Amount of time, in minutes, in which the specified volume of fluid is to infuse
3. Drop factor of the tubing/pump

The formula to calculate an IV infusion rate is:

$$\frac{\text{Volume} \times \text{drop factor}}{\text{Time}} = \text{rate of infusion}$$

where *Volume* is the volume of fluid to be infused, *Time* is the time (in minutes) in which the specified volume of fluid is to infuse, and the rate of infusion is measured in mL/hr if an IV pump is used or in gtts/min if gravity flow is used.

For this formula to work, you must make certain the *Volume* and *Time* are directly related. For example: if you are calculating the rate for the *Volume* of the entire bag, the *Time* must be the number of minutes, not hours, for the entire bag to infuse. If the entire bag of *1,000 mL* of fluid is to infuse in 2 hours; you would perform the calculation using *120 minutes* for *Time.* If the *1,000 mL* is to infuse in 4 hours, you would use *240 minutes* for *Time.* If the order is to run the *1,000 mL* bag for 8 hours, you would use *320 minutes* for *Time* in the formula.

However, if you are just calculating the rate of infusion for a 50-mL bag of IVPB antibiotic that must infuse within *1 hour,* you would use *50 mL* for *Volume* and *60 minutes* for *Time.* Remember, the *Volume* of fluid to infuse must correlate with the *Time* in which it is to infuse. Skill 38-4 (page 951) covers calculation of the IV infusion rate.

Most IVPB medications will be infused over a period of 15, 30, 45, 60, or 90 minutes. If the physician and pharmacy both fail to provide you with the length of time for infusion of a specific medication, you can find this information in a drug book. It is your responsibility to know the appropriate length of time to infuse medication.

Practice

The only way to be able to correctly calculate IV infusion rates is to practice until you are competent and confident that you fully understand the formula and what each number represents, the actual working steps of the problem, and the application of the process to specific situations. Some sample problems are included in Table 38-3, in the workbook, and on the student CD.

Knowledge Connection

If you are to infuse D5W 500 mL at 30 mL/hr to keep the vein open, at how many drops per minute would you set the gravity flow rate? You must administer the following IVPB antibiotic: ampicillin 500 mg in D5W 50 mL over 20 minutes. At how many drops per minute would you set the gravity flow rate? At how many milliliters per hour would you set an IV pump for this same IVPB?

Initiating Peripheral Venipuncture

Before you initiate peripheral venipuncture, whether it is to infuse fluids or to place an intermittent infusion lock, review the facility's policy for the procedure and review the patient's medical record for several pieces of information.

Medical Record Review

Review the physician's orders for verification of what is to be done. Review the patient's medical record to determine the patient's condition, including his or her medical diagnoses and reason for IV access, as well as the patient's age, mental cognition, and allergies.

Table 38-3 Sample Calculations of IV Infusion Rates

Infusion Order	Calculations for	
	Gravity Infusion (measured in gtts/min)	**Pump Infusion** (measured in mL/hr)
Infuse Unasyn 500 mg in D5W 50 mL IVPB over 15 minutes (Tubing drop factor is 20)	$\dfrac{50\,\text{mL} \times 20}{15\,\text{min}} = 66.6$ or 67 gtts/min	$\dfrac{50\,\text{mL} \times 60}{15\,\text{min}} = 200$ mL/hr
Infuse vancomycin 1 gram in NS 250 mL IVPB over 90 minutes (Tubing drop factor is 10)	$\dfrac{250\,\text{mL} \times 10}{90\,\text{min}} = 27.7$ or 28 gtts/min	$\dfrac{250\,\text{mL} \times 60}{90\,\text{min}} = 166.7$ or 168 mL/hr
Infuse gentamycin 80 mg in D5W 100 mL IVPB over 30 minutes (Tubing drop factor is 15)	$\dfrac{100\,\text{mL} \times 15}{30\,\text{min}} = 50$ gtts/min	$\dfrac{100\,\text{mL} \times 60}{30\,\text{min}} = 200$ mL/hr
Infuse IV LR 1,000 mL over 10 hours (Tubing drop factor is 15)	$\dfrac{1{,}000\,\text{mL} \times 15}{600\,\text{min}} = 25$ gtts/min	$\dfrac{1{,}000\,\text{mL} \times 60}{600\,\text{min}} = 100$ mL/hr
Please note that the above order would be the equivalent of infusing 100 mL in 1 hour. These numbers came from dividing the total volume (1,000 mL) by the number of hours (10) in which it all should infuse (1,000 ÷ 10), to get the number of mL that should infuse in 1 hour (1,000 ÷ 10 = 100 mL/hr). It allows you to work with smaller numbers than calculating the entire 1,000-mL bag.	$\dfrac{100\,\text{mL} \times 15}{60\,\text{min}} = 25$ gtts/min	$\dfrac{100\,\text{mL} \times 60}{60\,\text{min}} = 100$ mL/hr

Physician's Order

Make certain that the physician's order includes the date, time, type of solution, size of solution container, route, and infusion rate. Note whether there is an order for additives such as vitamins or potassium chloride.

Patient's Medical Condition

You need to know not only the patient's current admission diagnosis, but also his or her medical history. Does the patient have congestive heart failure or other cardiac problems? Is there renal disease? Are there chronic respiratory problems? All of these affect the patient's ability to receive different types of fluids and rates of infusion. Is this patient stable or unstable? Is the patient at risk of hemorrhaging or going to surgery? Why does the patient need IV access? All of these things help to determine what gauge of IV intracatheter would be appropriate, what type of fluid is needed, and whether or not the patient can receive faster rates of infusion.

Patient's Age and Mental Cognition

How old is the patient? Is he or she an infant, child, teenager, adult, or older adult? Infants and children do not require the same fluid volumes as a teenager or adult. They are also unable to tolerate a fast rate of infusion. Many older adults are intolerant of faster rates of infusion also. Intravenous infusion of fluids in infants, small children, and elders must be controlled and observed even more frequently than in the average adult for signs and symptoms of circulatory fluid overload. Younger children and confused patients have added risk due to their inability to call for a nurse when needed.

Allergies

Assess whether the patient is allergic to iodine, medications, latex, or tape. Non-latex gloves and tourniquets are available for use with patients with latex allergies. A blood pressure cuff can also be used in place of a tourniquet in patients who are allergic to latex or rubber. Numerous types of tape are available for use when the patient is allergic to a particular type, including paper, silk, plastic, micropore, and old-fashioned adhesive tape. As you read earlier in this chapter, other types of antiseptic solutions are available for site preparation if the patient is allergic to iodine.

Knowledge Connection

What assessment data should you collect prior to initiating an IV access? Why should you review the facility policy for a skill you are about to perform?

Preparing the Equipment

Identify your patient using two methods of identification. Introduce yourself and explain the procedure, answering any questions the patient might have. To assist you in determining which gauge of IV cannula to bring, assess the patient's veins for size and characteristics.

Wash your hands for at least 15 seconds. Obtain the correct volume container of the ordered IV solution. Check the label three times as you would any medication, checking the type of solution and the expiration date. Check the bag for leaks by squeezing the bag and inspecting for pinhole leaks. If there are any leaks in the bag, the solution is considered contaminated and should be discarded. Inspect the solution for clarity, assuring there is no cloudiness or any floating particulates.

Calculate the rate of infusion, in mL/hr for pump infusion and in gtts/min for gravity infusion. Label the solution container, including the patient's name, room number, date, rate of infusion, time infusion is to start, and your initials. If an additive is ordered, fill out a red or other bright-colored medication label as dictated by facility policy and attach it to the solution container. Add the appropriate dose of additive to the solution. Skill 38-5 (page 951) provides more information on adding medications to a primary IV solution.

Obtain an infusion pump or controller if available and an IV pole. Following the instructions accompanying the pump or controller, set the pump button labeled "Primary VTBI" (volume to be infused) for the total volume of primary IV solution that is to be infused; also set the physician-ordered rate of infusion button that is labeled "Primary Rate." The rate will be measured and marked with "mL/Hr" as the unit of measurement. It is helpful to set the VTBI setting at a few milliliters less than the actual total volume in the bag. This will prevent the bag from running dry, which can allow air to enter the drip chamber and proximal end of the IV tubing. For example: if the solution bag holds 1,000 mL, set the pump VTBI setting around 940 or 950 mL. When the pump alarm signals that the VTBI has been infused, you will still have fluid left in the bag. You can then set a new VTBI at 30 or 40 mL, giving you adequate time to obtain the next bag of solution and hang it before the original bag runs dry.

Obtain the required tubing administration set that works with the pump, or one designed for infusion by gravity flow if a pump is not available for use. Inspect the packaging of the sterile IV tubing administration set, ensuring that it is still intact and not expired. Remove the tubing from package and close the roller clamp. Remove the cap from the solution container port. Aseptically insert the piercing pin of the tubing set into the port on the solution container. Read the instructions on the package for priming the tubing set because each set is designed to prime differently, especially those with a cassette feature that inserts into the pump mechanism. Prime the tubing according to instructions, assuring that all air is removed from the tubing set. Replace the sterile cap on the end of the tubing. Do not insert the IV tubing into the IV pump until after cannulation has been verified by free flow of IV fluid in the drip chamber by gravity. You do not want it attached to the pump to force fluid into the vein until you are certain that the site is not going to swell.

Most nurses prefer to bring the two different sizes of IV cannulas or winged butterflies that would work for the patient's medical diagnosis, condition, and reason for IV access as well as the preview of vein size and characteristics. The final selection of cannula size and length will be made after you make further assessment at the bedside. Get a towel or waterproof pad to protect the bed. Gather an IV start kit or the individual supplies that would be contained in the kit.

Knowledge Connection
What preparation does the container or bag of IV solution require? What should you assess before opening packages containing IV tubing administration sets? What data must you enter into an IV pump or controller prior to use?

Selecting a Vein

The most common veins used in peripheral IV therapy include the veins of the forearm. On the forearm, the cephalic, basilic, median cubital, median antebrachial, and accessory cephalic veins are the superficial veins commonly used (Fig. 38-21).

If there are no suitable veins on the forearm, the dorsal side of the hand may be used, but this is not the best choice due to the proximity of nerves and tendons. Cannulation of hand veins can limit the patient's use of the hand, so use of the non-dominant hand is preferred over the dominant hand. If use of the hand veins becomes necessary, the basilic vein, metacarpal veins, and cephalic veins are used (Fig. 38-22). Leg veins are the farthest veins from the heart, and are used only as a last resort, although they are sometimes the only veins accessible in infants or small children. It is not advisable to use the leg or foot veins in elders or anyone with peripheral vascular disease, due to the decreased circulation to the extremities. A facility may have a policy requiring a physician's order before an IV access can be initiated in a lower extremity.

Once a vein has been pierced and cannulated, the vein should not be accessed distally for IV restarts. An IV restarted distal to a previously used site has an increased chance of infiltration. A site proximal to the previous site should be used if another IV cannula must be inserted into the same vein. If the patient is apt to have IV therapy for several days, it is best to select the most distal vein that is suitable.

Knowledge Connection
Locate and name the common forearm veins used for IV therapy on your arm and on another classmate's arm. If an IV restart becomes necessary, what are the limitations for selecting the next vein to cannulate?

Apply the tourniquet proximal to the elbow; inspect and palpate the veins. Make certain that the distal arterial pulse is still palpable after application of tourniquet. You only want to occlude the venous blood flow, not the arterial blood flow. Select a vein that is large enough to accommodate the gauge of IV cannula needed for the patient's condition. You also want to choose a vein that is stable and does not roll when you palpate it. Feel for bumps and observe for vein *bifurcations,* which are where veins separate into two branches. These are both indications of valves in the veins,

Figure 38-21 The superficial veins of the forearm.

Figure 38-22 The superficial veins of dorsal aspect of hand.

whose purpose is to control the direction of blood flow back toward the heart. Inserting the IV needle into a valve may result in damage that can cause blood to pool distally from the damaged valve. Anytime blood pools, there is an increased risk of thrombosis.

A good vein should feel slightly rounded, spongy, resilient or elastic, and bouncy, but not flat. It is always best to initiate an IV access in the patient's nondominant arm if at all possible. This allows the patient free use of the dominant hand. Do not use extremities on the same side as a mastectomy, paralysis, or a dialysis access device. Avoid selecting a vein site that:

- Extends over a flexible joint
- Feels **sclerosed** or hardened
- Is bruised, red, or edematous
- Lies adjacent to an infected area
- Has been recently used for IV therapy or is distal to a recent stick site
- Is too small for the IV cannula
- Has a bump or bifurcation indicating a valve
- Rolls

Once the vein has been selected, remove the tourniquet to allow return of blood flow while you set up your work site. There are several ways to increase the blood flow to the veins if further dilation is needed (Box 38-5). If the vein selected for IV initiation is located over a flexible joint due to lack of other suitable sites, you will want to stabilize the joint after the IV access has been initiated. This is done by placing the hand or arm on top of an arm board and wrapping it securely, but not so tightly as to impair venous return, with an Ace bandage, roller gauze, or Coban, a stretchable roller bandage that is secured when it sticks to itself (Fig. 38-23).

Knowledge Connection
What are the characteristics of a *good* vein for IV therapy? Why should you avoid puncturing a vein where there is a known valve? Which vein sites should be avoided for IV therapy?

Performing Final Preparation of Supplies

After selecting the vein, place a towel underneath the patient's extremity to protect the bed from blood drips. It will save you a linen change. Open and arrange all your supplies on the towel so that each item is within easy reach. You want to avoid reaching or turning to pick up an item while you are holding the cannula, which cannot be bent or crimped. Inspect the cannula and needle bevel for intactness and burrs. Open several alcohol wipes to use to clean the puncture site after cannulation of the vein and prior to applying the dressing. Place the capped sterile end of the IV tubing or PRN lock on the towel so it can be easily reached when it is time to connect it to the cannula hub. Label the IV tubing set according to facility policy so nurses will know when to change the tubing.

Box 38-5
Tips for Dilating Veins

At times the patient on whom you need to start an IV will not have a clearly visible or palpable vein. There are several simple techniques you may use to help stimulate vein dilation. In almost all situations except life-and-death emergencies, the few extra minutes that it may take you to perform one, or even all, of these techniques will serve you well. The majority of the time, being patient and working to stimulate the veins will provide you with a more appealing vein, increase your confidence, and reduce the number of attempts to cannulate the vein. However, the greatest and most important benefit belongs to the patient who will not be forced to endure more needle sticks than absolutely necessary. Try the following techniques:

- Use gravity by allowing the extremity to hang dependent off the side of the bed to a position lower than the heart for several minutes.
- Apply a BP cuff rather than a tourniquet.
- Have the patient squeeze a rolled-up washcloth or rubber ball, clasping and unclasping the fist several times.
- Apply moist, warm packs to the extremity for 10 to 15 minutes.
- *Using an alcohol wipe and friction, rapidly wipe back-and-forth over the vein for several seconds.
- *Using the thumb and middle finger, gently flick the skin over the vein.

Note: Avoid slapping the patient's skin with your hand. It really stings and is uncomfortable.

*These two methods of stimulation cause release of histamine under the skin, which dilates the vein.

Figure 38-23   Hand with IV secured to arm board with Coban.

If you have not already applied clean examination gloves, do so at this point before proceeding. Position your body in linear alignment with the patient's arm. This is done by positioning the patient's arm in front of you so that, when you look straight ahead, you are looking linearly up the arm. In other words, you are lined up with the arm as if you are an extension of the hand. Avoid trying to start an IV access with your body perpendicular to the arm (standing to the side of the arm). Linear alignment allows you optimal visualization of the IV catheter needle and its relationship to the selected vein you are attempting to cannulate. Because you are lined up with the arm and vein, it also allows you to have a more accurate mental image of the exact location of the vein as it extends beyond your point of needle insertion.

Once you have determined the exact site where you will puncture the vein, use a cap taken from a needle or tubing to *mark the vein*. Do this by pressing the open end of the cap against the patient's skin to make an indention or impression directly over the vein where you intend to make the stick. Hold the cap in place for a couple of seconds to leave a circle indention in the patient's skin. Make a second indention over the vein about 1 inch (2.5 cm) proximal to the first one. This provides a visual *marker* to help you know the exact location and path of the vein even when you cannot see the vein but can palpate it. This may help prevent the need to palpate the vein location again after you have already cleansed the site, thus contaminating the intended insertion site.

Prepare the sterile end of the primary IV tubing by making certain the cap over the sterile end has been slightly loosened so that you will be able to easily remove the cap once you have advanced the cannula into the vein. Place the tubing end, with the cap loose but still covering the sterile tip, within easy reach on your work surface, towel, or waterproof pad. This decreases the risk of inadvertently pulling the cannula out of the vein while reaching for the tubing to connect it to the cannula.

Knowledge Connection

Why is positioning of your body in relationship to the patient's arm important? Explain the purpose of arranging all IV initiation supplies on the towel or protective pad work surface directly in front of you prior to attempting vein cannulation.

Cleaning the Site

Next, cleanse the site with the antimicrobial agent indicated by facility policy. Use the method of cleansing described earlier in this chapter under Asepsis and IV Therapy.

Knowledge Connection

Describe the proper technique for cleansing the site chosen for venipuncture, including the length of time to spend scrubbing the site. Is it a problem to confirm the location of the vein by palpating the site with your gloved hand immediately prior to puncturing the skin? Explain your answer.

Performing Venipuncture and Cannulation

Without contaminating the cleansed site, apply the tourniquet 6 inches proximal to the selected site. (Refer to Chapter 34, Skill 34-1, page 818, for application instructions.) Place your nondominant hand distal to the intended puncture site. Use your thumb to pull the skin taut, to stabilize the skin and underlying vein. This should help to prevent the vein from rolling. Make sure your hand pulling the skin taut is an adequate distance from the site to prevent contamination of your needle and cannula when you perform the venipuncture. If the selected site is the distal portion of the forearm, flex the patient's wrist to help pull the skin taut.

Safety: The needle must be inserted in the same direction that the venous blood flows, back toward the heart. Hold the flashback chamber of the needle in your dominant hand with the bevel up. Line the needle up linearly with the vein, as if the vein were an extension of the IV catheter needle. Inform the patient of the ensuing prick. Hold the needle at a 20- to 30-degree angle to perform the venipuncture. A very superficial or fragile vein may necessitate decreasing the angle to 15 degrees, while a deeper vein on an obese patient may require an increase in the needle's angle up to 45 degrees. Pierce the patient's skin and vein using one of following two methods: direct or indirect.

- **Direct method:** a one-step method that consists of puncturing the skin and the vein in one motion or movement of the needle. Useful for entry into rolling veins, fragile veins, and hand veins, and when using smaller gauge needles, such as 22 G (0.7 mm) or 24 G (0.6 mm).
- **Indirect method:** a two-step method; first, the skin is pierced parallel to the vein; the tip of the needle is then angled toward the vein and gently inserted into the vein. Useful for entry into all veins.

Once the bevel of the needle enters the vein, you will see blood enter the flashback chamber, commonly known as a *flash* or *blood return*. Lower the angle of the needle and advance the needle and cannula as one unit just far enough to ensure that the entire bevel of the needle and the end of the over-the-needle cannula are inside the vein and stop. *Safety: Never advance the full length of the needle while still inside the cannula as one unit into the vein.* Use your nondominant thumb and index finger to carefully advance the over-the-needle cannula off the end of the needle into the vein lumen.

If the cannula remains in the vein as you advance it, you should observe a steady backflow of blood. While advancing the cannula off the needle, make certain your dominant hand holding the flashback chamber does not move. If you experience difficulty advancing the cannula all the way, sometimes it helps to "float" it in with IV solution. After advancing the cannula as far as it will go:

- Remove the needle
- Attach the IV tubing
- Open the roller clamp on the IV tubing
- Allow a slow infusion of solution
- Use your nondominant hand to reapply traction to the vein
- Use your dominant hand to attempt further advancement of the cannula into the vein

After you have advanced the full length of the cannula into the vein, use the nondominant hand to gently release the tourniquet. Then place the middle or ring finger of your nondominant hand on the vein proximal to the end of the cannula to block venous flow. Use your thumb and index finger to stabilize the needle hub against the patient's skin, without contaminating the skin puncture or the sterile open end of the hub. Use your dominant hand to activate the needle retraction device or remove the needle manually from the inside of the cannula. Quickly pick up the end of the IV tubing or PRN lock, remove the cap from the sterile end, and insert the end into the needle hub without contaminating the tubing end or needle hub.

Safety: Never use your teeth to remove the cap from the sterile end of the tubing, and avoid trying to remove the cap from the end of the tubing one-handedly. You are bound to contaminate the end of tubing. It is safer to make certain the cap is loosely attached to the tubing just before performing the venipuncture. Then when you pick up the tubing with your dominant hand, you can place the capped end between two of the fingers of your nondominant hand that is occluding the vein and securing the cannula hub. A gentle grasp of the cap by the two fingers will allow you to easily and gently pull the tubing end from the cap with your dominant hand and yet maintain its sterility. This requires good fine motor skills and practice. Initially, until you have become skilled using this or an equivalent technique, you may want to simply have a classmate or instructor present who can assist you by removing the cap from the sterile end of the tubing.

Encountering Difficulty

If your initial venipuncture does not produce a blood return into the flashback chamber indicating that you are in the vein, you will simply continue using the indirect method: The skin has been punctured, but you are not in the vein. Continue to use your dominant hand to hold the needle in place. Before moving the needle again, use the index finger of your nondominant hand to relocate the vein. Feel the skin just proximal to the insertion site. Without contaminating the insertion site, locate the end of the needle and its position in relation to the intended vein. When a needle is not in the vein, it has to be in one of four places: on top of the vein, to the right side of the vein, underneath the vein, or to the left side of the vein. It is important to know the needle's location and proximity to the vein before you make further attempt to enter the vein.

Lower or increase the needle's angle, according to the depth of the vein. Try again to enter the vein. If you are at the side of the vein, you will need to angle the needle *just slightly* toward the vein. If you are under the vein, you will need to *pull the needle back slightly* to reposition it for entry. *Safety: If using an over-the-needle cannula, you must place your dominant hand's index finger on the colored hub of the plastic needle while you gently pull the needle and cannula back as one unit. If you do not hold the cannula hub, the*

inner needle will pull back without the cannula. Once this occurs, you cannot reinsert the needle into the plastic cannula. This could sever the tip of the cannula, creating a migrating embolism requiring emergency surgical removal of the severed cannula tip. After repositioning the needle, gently insert the needle into the vein, avoiding quick movements such as jabbing or stabbing, as they cause pain and can damage nerves and veins.

You will want to limit the number of unsuccessful venipuncture attempts on a patient to no more than two. Then it is best to ask another nurse to try to start the IV access. No one likes to "miss" the vein during venipuncture, but all of us will be unsuccessful at one time or another, even nurses who are highly skilled at venipuncture. So, do not allow initial unsuccessful attempts to discourage you. Continue to take advantage of opportunities to perform venipuncture until you become confident and skilled. Skill 38-6 (page 953) provides more information on initiating peripheral venipuncture.

Knowledge Connection

What degree of angle is commonly used to puncture the vein? If it is a fragile vein lying close to the surface, what degree of angle will serve you better? What area of the IV catheter needle do you hold while inserting it? How will you initially determine you have accessed the vein? Which part of the IV catheter and needle is advanced its full length into the vein lumen?

Determining Proper Cannulation

Once you have connected the IV tubing to the cannula hub, open the roller clamp on the IV tubing and observe for rapid free flow of fluid in the drip chamber of the tubing. Observe the venipuncture site for swelling as the fluid flows in. Site swelling is indicative of displacement of the IV cannula outside the vein. Immediately close the roller clamp and remove the cannula from the vein.

If the fluid free flows rapidly and without site swelling, you know that the cannulation is successful. If the fluid only drips slowly with the roller clamp wide open, there is some type of problem with the cannulation. You may try pulling the cannula back just slightly, not even 1/8 inch. If it is just lying against a valve or the wall of the vein, this will allow it to free-flow. It is also wise to assess that all the clamps on the tubing are open and that there are no crimps in the tubing that might slow the fluid flow. Once you have verified free flow of fluid by gravity with no site swelling, you may proceed to secure the site.

Securing the IV Site

Secure the Luer-Lok by screwing it onto the cannula hub. Avoid screwing it tightly; the Luer-Lok connects securely without excessive tightening. Clean all blood from the connection and skin with alcohol wipes, using care not to bend the cannula where it attaches to its hub. Use the sterile 2×2-inch

(5×5-cm) gauze pad to dry the skin. Peel the backing from and apply the transparent occlusive dressing (TOD) over the site and the hub of the cannula. Do not cover the Luer-Lok connector on the IV tubing (Fig. 38-24). Doing so would necessitate removal of the primary sterile dressing just to change the IV tubing. (If your facility does not use TODs, apply the type of sterile dressing dictated by facility policy.)

After applying the TOD, apply several 3- to 4-inch (7.6- to 10-cm) pieces of tape to secure the Luer-Lok connection and the first 6 to 8 inches (15 to 20 cm) of the IV tubing to the patient's arm. Place a small label on the dressing indicating the date and time of venipuncture, gauge and length of needle, and your initials (Fig. 38-25).

Knowledge Connection

Why is it important to determine proper cannulation of the vein with gravity free flow of IV solution prior to inserting the tubing administration set into the pump? Why is it recommended to cover the puncture site with a sterile TOD?

Starting the IV Pump

Place the IV tubing in the IV pump according to the manufacturer's instructions. Open all tubing set clamps. Check that the volume to infuse and the rate of infusion are both correctly set. Start the pump and assess its proper function.

Figure 38-24 Applying transparent occlusive dressing (TOD) to new IV site.

Figure 38-25 The nurse initials the label of a newly inserted IV site.

Reassess the venipuncture site for swelling or leaking. Make certain the patient is feeling no discomfort at the site before leaving the room.

Setting Gravity Infusion Rate

If the solution is to infuse by gravity, hold your watch with a second hand next to the drip chamber on the IV tubing. Count the number of drops that fall during 1 minute. Does it match your calculations? Use the roller clamp to adjust the flow until you achieve the desired rate (Fig. 38-26).

Here is a time-saving hint: Divide by 4 the total number of drops per minute that you calculated prior to beginning the infusion. That will be the number of drops that should infuse per 15 seconds. Adjust the flow with the roller clamp and re-count the drops until you obtain the desired number of drops per 15 seconds. Once you have regulated the drip rate for the 15 seconds, count the drops for an entire minute to ensure that the rate is correct. By counting the number of drops for 15 seconds, you will save 45 seconds every time you have to regulate the roller clamp. This generally will save you anywhere between 1 and 5 minutes; this may not sound like much time, but over the course of a shift, every 5 minutes you can save is better used somewhere else. Refer to the Calculation of Infusion Rate section earlier in this chapter for further assistance.

Knowledge Connection

What is the formula for calculating the infusion rate? What unit of measurement is used for gravity flow infusion rates? An infusion controlled by a pump?

Monitoring IV Infusions

You should monitor the rate of infusion and the condition of the IV site frequently. The site and surrounding tissue should be assessed for the signs and symptoms of infiltration

Figure 38-26 Counting the number of drops per minute to calculate a gravity flow infusion rate.

(Box 38-6), phlebitis (Box 38-7), and infection. The accepted nursing standard for frequency of IV site assessment is to assess and document it at least every 2 hours in an adult, and every 1 hour in children, the elderly, and those patients who might be prone to circulatory fluid overload. Some experts even recommend assessment of the site every hour in adults. Your facility may have policies that differ from these standards. If the facility policy dictates assessment to be done at *shorter* intervals, you must perform accordingly. However, if the facility policy dictates *longer* intervals, such as every 4 hours, you are ethically and legally held to the more frequent schedules.

Monitor the volume of solution remaining in the primary bag so that you are prepared and have time to obtain the next ordered bag of solution prior to the hanging bag running completely dry. Plan to prepare the next bag of solution when there is still a minimum of 50 to 100 mL of solution remaining. Skill 38-7 (page 957) provides more information on adding a new bag of IV solution to the existing IV line.

Documenting the Venipuncture

Document the venipuncture, including the date and time; gauge, length, and type of needle; site of placement; number of attempts it took; type of fluid and size of fluid container;

Box 38-6

Signs and Symptoms of Infiltration

Assess adult IV sites at least every 2 hours, and more often if indicated, for the following signs and symptoms of infiltration. Assess IV sites every 30 to 60 minutes in infants, children, and older adults.
- Blanching or pallor of skin around site
- Complaint of tightness or discomfort around site
- Edema at site
- Lack of blood return upon lowering IV solution bag or aspirating with needle and syringe
- Site cool to touch
- Sluggish flow or lack of infusion
- Solution leakage at site
- Taut skin around site

Box 38-7

Signs and Symptoms of Phlebitis

Each time you assess the IV site for infiltration, also assess for the following signs and symptoms of phlebitis, or vein inflammation.
- Edema of site
- Erythema at site
- Increased warmth at site compared to surrounding area
- Reports of burning or discomfort at IV site or along vein track
- Sluggish infusion rate
- Vein feels like a hard cord when palpated

---

whether it is flowing by gravity or pump; rate of infusion; site assessment; any difficulties experienced; and how the patient tolerated the procedure. (Refer to the sample documentation at the end of Skill 38-6.)

Knowledge Connection
How frequently should you assess an IV site in a child? In an adult without risk of fluid overload?

People and Places Connection

Performing Venipuncture in Elders
Venipuncture of elderly persons can present different challenges. Their skin is sometimes very thin, fragile, and even somewhat transparent. Their veins are often tiny, fragile, and sclerosed, making it easy to go completely through the vein with the needle. Here are some hints to make venipuncture of elders a little easier:

- **Avoid use of a tourniquet if possible:** Fragile veins often "blow" or rupture, causing a hematoma, when a tourniquet is used. If a tourniquet is needed, it is less uncomfortable and easier on their fragile skin to apply the tourniquet less tightly and over the sleeve of the patient's gown.
- **Use a blood pressure (BP) cuff in place of a tourniquet:** Position it at least 6 inches proximal to the site of intended venipuncture. Pump it only 10 to 20 mm Hg higher than the diastolic pressure.
- **Avoid excessive friction or prolonged tapping as methods to distend the vein:** It is best to use the smallest gauge needle and cannula that is available, usually a 22-G × 1-inch (0.7-mm × 25-mm) length. Use no more than a 15-degree angle of the needle during venipuncture.
- **Be selective when choosing tape to use on fragile skin:** Silk or micropore tape will usually come off without tearing the fragile skin, as plastic and adhesive tape can do. Some nurses prefer paper tape for fragile skin, while others feel that, if any moisture comes in contact with paper tape once applied to the skin, it becomes similar to glue.
- **Be careful when removing tape:** When removing any type of tape from fragile skin, use adhesive remover to loosen the adhesive. Then, after lifting the end of the piece of tape, *use your fingers to gently pull the skin from the tape* as opposed to *peeling the tape from the skin.* This helps to prevent skin tears.

Problem-Solving

If the IV solution stops infusing or the pump alarms *occlusion,* take the following steps:

- Make certain the solution container is not empty or that the pump setting for *volume to be infused* has not been completed.

- Inspect the IV tubing from the solution container all the way to the insertion site in the patient's vein, ensuring that all clamps are open and that the tubing has not been inadvertently pinched by the bed rails or by the patient lying on it.
- Also ensure that there are no air bubbles in the tubing or pump cassette. Assess the site for signs and symptoms of infiltration and phlebitis.

If everything appears to be within normal limits:

- Remove the solution container from the pump and IV pole. Lower the bag below the level of the vein. Observe for a blood return in the cannula hub. This is an indication that the cannula is still in the vein.
- If no blood return is obtained, hang the container back on the IV pole. Use a syringe to connect to the injection port closest to the vein, being careful to cleanse the port with alcohol first. Pinch the tubing proximally to the port while aspirating with the syringe. Observe for a blood return. If no blood is returned, the cannula is no longer in the vein and must be removed. If there is a vacuum when you attempt to aspirate (if the syringe does not allow you to aspirate), there is most likely a blood clot obstructing the end of the cannula. The cannula should be discontinued and the IV restarted. *Safety: Do not use NS to force-flush or push the clot from the end of the cannula.* The clot then becomes an embolism that can migrate to and occlude vessels in major organs, causing necrosis of tissue. You may see other nurses do this, but it is not acceptable and presents a clear danger to your patient.

Discontinuing an IV Infusion

When you have a physician's order to discontinue an IV infusion or PRN lock, or there is a problem that necessitates removal, turn off the IV pump. Close the roller clamp. Apply clean examination gloves and gently remove the tape securing the tubing set to the arm. Use adhesive remover if needed.

While securing the cannula hub with your nondominant hand, lift each of the four TOD edges toward the insertion site. Use caution to avoid crimping or bending the plastic cannula where it attaches to the hub. Once the TOD is completely loosened from the patient's skin, use your nondominant hand to apply pressure with a sterile 2×2-inch (5×5-cm) gauze pad *proximal* to the end of the cannula that is still within the vein. *Safety: Do not apply pressure over the cannula itself, or you can dislodge the cannula from the hub and free it to migrate through the vascular system as an embolism.* Allow your hand applying pressure on the vein to slide toward the puncture site as you carefully remove the cannula from the vein using your dominant hand.

While removing the cannula, maintain a pull that is parallel to the vein. Inspect the cannula to be sure that it is intact and that a small piece has not been broken off the tip. Once the cannula is completely out of the vein, apply firm pressure with the 2×2-inch (5×5-cm) gauze pad directly over the puncture site to prevent bleeding and bruising while

allowing the blood time to clot. Hold pressure for 1 to 2 minutes, depending on the size of cannula and vein. The larger they are, the longer you may need to hold pressure. If the vein is fragile, as in some elderly patients, or if the patient is taking anticoagulant medications, hold pressure for 3 to 5 minutes before lifting the gauze to assess cessation of bleeding. While holding pressure on the site cleanse the surrounding skin with alcohol wipes and allow to air dry. Once bleeding has ceased, apply a bandage or apply a piece of tape to hold a clean 2×2-inch (5×5-cm) gauze pad in place. Instruct the patient to remove the bandage or tape within 24 hours. Skill 38-8 (page 958) provides more information on discontinuing an IV infusion or PRN lock.

Knowledge Connection

Explain the danger of forcing a blood clot from the end of the IV cannula so that the IV solution will drip again. What are the steps you should take in problem-solving a pump warning of *occlusion?* What is the risk of applying manual pressure against the cannula in the vein during removal? How long do you hold pressure on the site after removal of the cannula?

Supervision/Delegation Connection

IV Push and IVPB Medications

Intravenous access initiation and administration of IV push and IVPB medications should not be delegated to CNAs or UAPs. These invasive skills should be performed by either a trained and certified LPN/LVN or RN. It is helpful and provides a certain degree of protection for a nurse to have documented proof that he or she has received formal IV therapy training and testing. While some practical and vocational nursing schools include IV certification in their programs, others do not. Some state Nurse Practice Acts prohibit the practical/vocational nurse from performing IV therapy.

Complications of Peripheral IV Therapy

Due to the invasive nature of IV therapy, it has potential for numerous complications that can have serious or fatal consequences. Possible complications include:

- **Infiltration**: leakage of nonvesicant IV fluid or medication into the tissue surrounding the IV insertion site; **nonvesicant** means that it does not cause blistering and death of tissue
- **Extravasation**: leakage of vesicant IV fluid or medication into the tissue surrounding the IV insertion site; **vesicant** means that it causes blistering, necrosis, and sloughing of tissue
- **Phlebitis:** inflammation of the inner layer, or *intima,* of a vein
- **Thrombophlebitis:** inflammation of a vein in conjunction with the formation of a thrombus

- **Localized infection:** infection at the IV cannula insertion site
- **Septicemia:** life-threatening infection of the bloodstream
- **Severed cannula:** a piece of the IV cannula breaks off inside the vein
- **Air embolism:** obstruction of a blood vessel by an air bubble traveling through the circulatory system
- **Circulatory fluid overload:** excessive fluid volume within the cardiovascular system
- **Speed shock:** shock caused by rapid IV infusion of medication/solution

Infiltration

Infiltration can be caused by displacement of the IV cannula outside of the vein, either at the insertion site or by piercing through the other side of the vein, allowing nonvesicant fluid to leak from the vein into the surrounding tissues. Other causes of infiltration can include puncturing the other side of the vein during venipuncture, excessive movement of the cannula inside the vein, or too-rapid a rate of infusion of IV fluid. Signs and symptoms of infiltration include:

- Edema around or dependent to the site; a good way to detect edema is to compare both arms
- Cool, pale, or taut skin around site
- Absence of or decreased blood return upon lowering the solution bag below the level of the insertion site, or when aspirating with a syringe at an injection port close to the IV site
- IV fluid will not infuse at all or will only infuse at a slow rate, even when the tubing clamp is wide open
- Complaint of discomfort at the IV site or proximal to it
- Blanching around the insertion site or proximal to the end of the IV cannula

Prevention

Assess the IV site for edema, erythema and increased skin warmth, pallor and coolness of skin, leaking of IV solution, drainage, patency of site, and patient reports of discomfort at least every 1 hour in infants, children, older adults, and anyone who might be at risk for fluid volume overload. Keep the IV site well secured to reduce movement of the cannula.

Nursing Care

The IV infusion should be immediately discontinued and restarted as needed. The extremity should be elevated and positioned according to patient comfort. Warm or cool packs may be applied to the site according to facility policy.

Extravasation

Extravasation, the leakage of vesicant medications into the subcutaneous tissues, can have serious consequences. The initial indications of extravasation will be the same as those for infiltration. An alert patient may complain of significant pain at or proximal to the IV site, or the site may exhibit erythema or edema.

The extent of tissue damage will be dependent upon the specific type and concentration of medication, as well as the volume of vesicant fluid that has leaked into the tissues. There may be blistering and death of tissue. The necrotic tissue sloughs and can leave an extensive crater that will have to granulate and heal by second or third intention or be surgically covered with grafts. Extravasation can result in disfigurement, loss of function, and even amputation of the extremity. Box 38-8 provides a list of vesicant medications.

Prevention

When infusing vesicant medications, the dorsal hand should not be used for IV placement, as it is more prone to tendon and nerve damage. Assess the IV site at least every 2 hours for adults, and every 1 hour for infants, children, older adults, and anyone who might be at risk for fluid volume overload. Always assess IV site condition prior to administering IV medications. Be knowledgeable regarding all medications you administer intravenously so that you are aware of which ones are vesicants.

Nursing Care

As soon as extravasation is even suspected, stop the infusion, leave the cannula in place, estimate the volume of extravasated vesicant fluid, and notify the physician immediately.

Box 38-8
Vesicant Medications

When allowed to extravasate into surrounding tissues, a vesicant medication causes blistering. Some of the more commonly used vesicants are listed below by drug classification.

Antibiotics
Amphotericin B
Cefoxitin sodium (Mefoxin)
Erythromycin
Nafcillin
Tetracycline
Vancomycin

Anticonvulsants
Phenytoin
Valium

Antiemetics
Promethazine

Chemotherapy Drugs
Cisplatin
Streptozocin
Vincristine

Electrolytes
Calcium chloride and calcium gluconate
Potassium chloride

Stat response and treatment must be carried out to reduce the amount of damage to tissues. The prescribed antidote is instilled into the tissues after aspirating any residual vesicant solution from the cannula. Elevate the affected extremity and apply either cold or heat packs according to the drug manufacturer's recommendations or facility policy. Document the situation in the patient's medical record. Depending upon the extent of damage, long-term wound care, surgical débridement, skin grafts, cosmetic surgery, or amputation may be required.

Phlebitis and Thrombophlebitis

Inflammation of the intima of the vein without a blood clot is known as *phlebitis,* while inflammation in conjunction with a thrombus is termed *thrombophlebitis;* both cause burning, tenderness, or pain at the IV site. The skin at the site will become erythematous and feel warmer than the unaffected skin surrounding the phlebitis. There may or may not be edema present. The vein may feel hard or cord-like. The infusion rate may become sluggish. The presence of a thrombus adds the additional risk that it will break away from the vein wall and become a moving embolus.

Factors contributing to development of phlebitis include:

- Using a vein that is too small
- Using an IV cannula that is too large
- Failure to change the IV site at least every 72 hours
- Infusion of irritating or caustic medications
- Poorly secured IV site allowing excessive motion of the IV cannula inside the vein
- Contamination of insertion site during IV initiation
- Failure to use strict asepsis during IV therapy
- Failure to treat infiltration quickly

Prevention

When proactive steps are not taken to prevent it, phlebitis becomes a fairly common complication of peripheral IV therapy, though thrombophlebitis does not occur as often. Be proactive and do not let any of the factors on the above list occur.

Nursing Care

There are numerous actions you should take to help prevent phlebitis. As previously noted, it is important to select the correct size of both IV cannula and vein. Maintain strict asepsis during IV initiation and during IV maintenance. Secure the IV cannula hub to the extremity with tape to prevent movement or dislodgment. Also secure to the arm the first 6 to 8 inches (15 to 20 cm) of the IV tubing from where it connects into the IV cannula. Infuse concentrated or irritating drugs only through larger central venous lines whenever possible. Assess the IV site at least every 2 hours for signs and symptoms of infiltration and phlebitis. As soon as any are noted, take immediate action to remedy the problem.

If phlebitis develops, stop the flow of the IV fluid and discontinue the IV cannula. Elevate the affected arm on pillows. Apply warm moist packs to the site for 20 to 30 minutes every 2 hours until signs of phlebitis are gone. If there is purulent drainage from the puncture site, or red streaks going up the arm, or if fever develops indicating infection, the site should be cultured. Antibiotics most likely will be required. If thrombophlebitis develops, administration of an anticoagulant may be necessary.

Knowledge Connection

What signs and symptoms indicate infiltration? Phlebitis? Contrast infiltration to extravasation. Why is it important to know which drugs are vesicants? What nursing intervention should you perform after removal of a cannula due to phlebitis?

Localized Infection

Once a needle pierces the skin, the body's first line of defense against infection is breached. Even though the skin is cleansed and the needle is sterile, there is a great risk of site infection. If microorganisms gain access to the site, infection sets in. Infection is manifested by erythema, edema, discomfort, purulent drainage, and fever.

Prevention

Prevention is key. Strict asepsis is required for all contact with any parts of the infusion system, during IV initiation, and throughout the span of the entire infusion. Included in prevention are:

- Handwashing thoroughly for at least 15 seconds prior to contact with any aspect of the IV setup
- Use of alcohol-based hand cleanser following handwashing according to facility policy
- Visually examining IV solution containers for cloudiness of fluid, leaks, and expiration date
- Using the facility's approved antiseptic pads to thoroughly cleanse the skin prior to needle stick
- Maintaining strict asepsis of the IV needle, cannula, or winged butterfly
- Covering the site with a sterile dressing, preferably a clear adhesive dressing that allows visual observation of the immediate site
- Firmly securing the IV cannula hub and IV tubing
- Assessing and documenting the condition of the IV site at least every 2 hours in adults and every 1 hour in children, elders, and patients prone to circulatory fluid overload
- Changing the IV site dressing if it becomes moist or soiled
- Removing the IV cannula at the first sign of inflammation or contamination
- Never allowing a solution container to hang longer than 24 hours
- Changing the IV site and IV tubing every 48 to 72 hours based on facility policy

Nursing Care

The initial treatment is the same as for phlebitis: discontinue the IV cannula and apply warm packs to the site for 20 to 30 minutes every 2 hours until drainage and erythema have abated. The physician will probably order antibiotics. Monitor the patient for further worsening of his or her condition.

Septicemia

Once a vein becomes inflamed and infected, it is possible for the microorganisms to travel through the bloodstream and cause system-wide infection, known as *septicemia.* Left untreated, septicemia quickly becomes life threatening. More than one-fourth of septicemias due to IV therapy are fatal. Signs and symptoms include:

• High fever
• Chills and shivering
• Diaphoresis
• Nausea, vomiting, and diarrhea
• Tachycardia
• Tachypnea
• Hypotension
• Confusion
• Backache

Prevention

Assess for signs and symptoms of localized infection and discontinue the IV infusion upon detection. Notify the physician for new orders.

Nursing Care

The top priority once you suspect septicemia is to stop the IV flow and notify the physician stat. Discontinue the IV infusion and, according to facility policy or the physician's orders, culture the cannula tip, tubing, and fluid. Restart a new IV infusion in the other extremity using a completely new setup, including cannula, tubing, and fluids. The physician will generally order blood cultures and IV antibiotics to be administered. It will be necessary to monitor the patient and vital signs closely for worsening of the patient's condition.

> ### Knowledge Connection
> What are the signs and symptoms of local infection at the IV site? Of septicemia? What is the difference between the two diagnoses? List at least eight ways you can help prevent these infections.

Severed Cannula

The plastic IV cannula that is left in the vein after removing the steel needle is extremely fragile and bends or crimps very easily. Crimping and flexing of the cannula increases the risk of the cannula separating from the hub, or a piece of the cannula breaking off to become an embolus. An embolus

can result in occlusion of vessels, including those of the heart and lungs, and can be fatal. Signs and symptoms include sudden sharp pain at the IV site, chest pain, cyanosis, tachypnea, tachycardia, and hypotension.

Prevention

Prevention is the best course of action. Take care to avoid bending the cannula during IV initiation and maintenance. Secure the site to minimize movement of the cannula. Avoid applying pressure directly over the cannula while removing an IV cannula from the vein. During IV initiation, use caution to prevent bending the cannula while you are connecting the tubing and securing the site. Avoid insertion of the IV cannula across a flexible joint.

Nursing Care

If a cannula does break away from the hub or a piece of the cannula breaks off inside the vein, immediately apply strong manual pressure on the vein several inches proximal to the insertion site. The goal is to prevent the cannula embolism from traveling from the periphery into the central circulation. Some facilities have policies dictating application of a tourniquet just proximal to the antecubital area. Notify the physician and radiology personnel stat. Start a new IV line in the opposite arm. Measure the remaining cannula length that you removed to determine the length of the severed cannula now acting as an embolism.

Air Embolism

An air embolism can occur if a large volume of air is introduced into the patient's vascular system. The occurrence of air embolism is rare in peripheral IV therapy, but the risk is there. It is more commonly seen with cannulation of central veins. The exact amount of air deemed to be fatal is not known, and a rapid rate of infusion of the air is as important as the amount of air infused. Signs and symptoms of air embolism are cyanosis, dyspnea, chest or shoulder pain, hypotension, tachycardia, and loss of consciousness.

Prevention

The first step in prevention of air embolism is to prime the IV tubing, PRN devices, and extensions before connecting them to the IV cannula. Remove all air from the syringe before injecting medication into the IV line. All tubing connections should have Luer-Loks if possible. If they do not have Luer-Lok connections, make certain the connections are snugly connected. Never allow the solution container to run dry; hang the next container of solution while there is still 30 to 50 mL of fluid remaining in the original container.

Nursing Care

If air should enter the IV line during infusion, stop the infusion, use a needle or blunt-tipped adapter attached to a syringe to pierce the injection port closest to the air in the tubing, and aspirate to remove all the air before restarting the flow of solution. If you suspect an air embolism, call for help to notify the physician and bring the crash cart. Place the patient on his or her left side in the Trendelenburg position. Once the air enters the right atrium of the heart, this position causes the air to rise to the top of the atrium, which reduces the chance of the air entering the pulmonary artery, traveling to the lungs and back to the left side of the heart, and then out into the systemic circulation. Apply supplemental oxygen and monitor vital signs until the physician arrives. Talk factually, firmly, and calmly to the patient to achieve compliance with your requests but to avoid frightening the patient more than necessary.

Circulatory Fluid Overload and Pulmonary Edema

Too much fluid infused into the cardiovascular system can result in fluid overload. Extreme fluid volume overload can result in pulmonary edema, where the excess fluid is forced into the pulmonary tissues. Patients with cardiovascular, renal, or respiratory disease, children, and elders are most susceptible to these complications. Fluid overload causes a rise in BP as the circulatory volume increases the pressure against the walls of the vasculature. Heart rate increases as the heart works harder to pump the increased fluid volume through the cardiovascular system. If the initial signs and symptoms are not detected and the infusion rate slowed, the hypertension, tachycardia, and tachypnea worsen; the patient begins to manifest signs of anxiety and restlessness; and moist breath sounds called *crackles* can be auscultated. The severity increases very quickly, and respirations become labored and gurgling. The patient becomes extremely dyspneic and cyanotic and starts coughing up pink frothy fluid. Box 38-9 presents other signs and symptoms of fluid overload.

Box 38-9

Signs and Symptoms of Circulatory Fluid Overload

It is important to detect circulatory fluid overload as early as possible. The patient may only exhibit one or two signs before the vital signs begin to change and the patient begins to rapidly decline. Each patient will be different. Be alert to the following signs in all patients receiving IV fluids and be ever-vigilant in infants, children, older adults, and any patient with a diagnosis or medical history of diseases such as congestive heart failure.

- Anxiety without identifiable cause
- Cough
- Distention of neck veins
- Facial, hand, or foot edema
- Headache
- Increased blood pressure
- Increased pulse rate
- Crackles in lungs
- Restlessness
- Shortness of breath

Causes of fluid overload include:

- Infusion of an excessive volume of fluid above the needs of the patient
- Too much sodium chloride for the needs of the patient
- An infusion rate that is too fast

An excessive infusion of isotonic fluid can result in overloading the circulatory system even though it does not cause third-space shifting. Infusion of hypertonic fluid, especially one with sodium chloride, when the patient does not need a hypertonic solution will pull excess fluid into the vascular spaces.

Once the overload has progressed to pulmonary edema, the patient's situation becomes critical. Without immediate treatment including, among other things, supplemental oxygen and IV diuretics, this patient will die.

Prevention

It is better to prevent fluid overload than to try to treat it after it occurs. Using an infusion pump is the best way to control the rate of infusion. Always make certain that you are aware of the reason for infusion of the IV fluids as well as the patient's medical history so that you will be able to identify the potential for development of fluid overload and pulmonary edema. Monitor intake and output, auscultate breath sounds, and monitor vital signs for tachycardia, hypertension, and tachypnea. You must monitor the type and osmolality of fluid infusing as well as the infusion rate. Do not be afraid to discuss the type of fluid or infusion rate with the physician if you are concerned that either one does not match the patient's needs. Be respectful and tactful, but by all means, talk to the physician about your concerns. The physician may very well appreciate it when you point out something that he or she may have overlooked. Remember that you are the patient's advocate. The best nurses are the ones who will seek answers and clarification of orders from physicians when they have a concern, doubt, or question regarding a patient's care. Be one.

Nursing Care

At the first sign or symptom of fluid overload, decrease the IV infusion rate and apply supplemental oxygen. Assess the vital signs and auscultate breath sounds after placing the patient in the high Fowler's position. Notify the physician immediately.

Speed Shock

When an IV solution or medication is infused rapidly, causing a harmfully elevated blood level, it can result in a condition known as speed shock. It is characterized by flushed skin, dizziness, headache, chest tightness, hypotension, irregular pulse, syncope or fainting, and cardiac arrest.

Prevention

The best care is prevention by monitoring the rate of infusion of the primary IV solution. Again, if you are concerned about the rapid rate of infusion, talk to the physician. Administer

IVPB and IV push medications slowly and according to the manufacturer's recommendations. Make it a habit to use a drug reference book and look up the safe rate of administration. Use an IV pump when available, especially for medications, or use micro-drip tubing (60 gtts/mL) administration sets if the solution is infused by gravity.

Nursing Care

If signs and symptoms of speed shock occur, stop the medication infusion and notify the physician. Call for assistance and the crash cart. Administer a medication antidote if there is one. Continually assess the patient's response to each intervention. Document the episode thoroughly afterward.

Knowledge Connection
Explain why it is dangerous to reinsert the needle into the cannula once it has been pulled partially out. What should be your first intervention if the cannula is severed while in the patient's vein? List the signs and symptoms of circulatory fluid overload.

Blood and Blood Products

Blood has many functions, but it primarily serves as the transporter of oxygen and nutrients to body cells and transporter of waste substances removed from the cells. There are many variations of blood and blood products that may be transfused to meet various patient needs (Box 38-10).

Not all cultures and organized religions believe in or approve of transfusing blood or blood products. Some actually prohibit their members from receiving blood transfusions, an example of which is Jehovah's Witnesses.

Box 38-10
Examples of Blood Products and Their Uses

Research and technology have made it possible to isolate individual components and factors that compose the blood. It is no longer necessary to transfuse whole blood to every patient who only needs specific components. These are examples of specific blood components and possible situations in which they might be administered.
- **Albumin:** increase plasma volume
- **Cryoprecipitate:** replace coagulation factors I, VII, and XIII
- **Fresh frozen plasma:** replace coagulation factors V and XI, drug reversal of warfarin (Coumadin)
- **Liquid plasma:** replace plasma proteins
- **Packed red blood cells:** acute blood loss, hemoglobin less than 8–10 g/dL, symptomatic anemia
- **Platelets:** prevent/control bleeding related to low platelet count, acute leukemia, thrombocytopenia
- **Whole blood:** rarely used but restores blood volume along with all its components; mostly broken down for use of its individual components

Transfusion

A written physician's order is required for both the transfusion of blood or blood products and the pretransfusion laboratory tests. An informed consent for transfusion of blood or blood products is also required. The patient who is to receive transfusion of blood or blood products must have his or her own blood tested for its specific ABO type and Rh grouping. The blood of both the potential recipient and the blood donor are tested for compatibility and screened for antibodies. Known as *typing and crossmatching tests,* they are necessary to prevent antigen-antibody reactions during transfusion therapy. After the typing, crossmatching, and compatibility tests have been completed and verified by the laboratory or blood bank staff, a specific identification number is assigned to the blood product and is used for verification that it is the correct blood product for the specified patient.

Safety: Blood and blood products are not compatible with any IV solution other than 0.9% sodium chloride (NS). Therefore, no other IV solutions are used in conjunction with blood product infusion. Dextrose can cause **hemolysis**, meaning lysis or destruction of red blood cells. Even medications cannot be mixed with blood products. If infusion of IV medication is scheduled during the transfusion, a separate IV line should be established. The transfusion is initiated by infusing NS, and completion of transfusion is followed by infusion of the same. The NS is also used to dilute packed red blood cells to a thinner consistency so they can be infused. **Packed red blood cells (PRBCs)** are those that have been separated from **plasma**, the liquid portion of the blood.

Transfusion Reactions
Because transfusions have the potential for serious risks to the patient, you are responsible to be knowledgeable regarding safe administration, signs and symptoms of reactions, steps to prevent reactions, and interventions to treat reactions. There are at least a dozen types of transfusion reactions that create significant risks to the patient, but we will only address six primary types of reaction in this chapter:

- Acute hemolytic
- Bacterial
- Allergic
- Febrile
- Circulatory overload
- Anaphylactic reactions

Table 38-4 presents descriptions and treatments of these reactions.

Knowledge Connection
Which IV solution must always be used to begin and end blood product transfusions? Contrast the signs and symptoms of an acute hemolytic reaction to those of an allergic reaction.

Table 38-4   Transfusion Reactions

Reaction Type	Description	Signs & Symptoms	Nursing Interventions
Acute hemolytic	Very serious Related to ABO incompatibility Causes lysis (destruction) of blood cells Can result in shock and death	Chest pain Back pain Bleeding Vein burning ↑ R rate, ↑ P rate, ↓ BP	**Stop transfusion stat.** Call a code. Apply oxygen. Start new IV line. Administer colloidal plasma expanders to ↑ BP. Monitor vital signs.
Febrile	Related to release of proteins by white blood cells during blood storage Transient fever	Nausea/vomiting ↑ Temp Chills Headache Chest pain	Stop transfusion. Start NS. Notify physician. Administer antipyretics as ordered. Monitor vital signs.
Mild allergic	Related to sensitivity to proteins in transfusion	Flushed Urticaria Itching Watery eyes Shortness of breath Mild wheezes	Stop transfusion. Start NS. Notify physician. Administer antihistamines as ordered. Monitor vital signs.
Anaphylaxis (severe allergic)	Very serious Life threatening Previously developed antibodies related to sensitivity to proteins in transfusion Can result in shock and death	Wide-eyed appearance Anxiety Extensive urticaria ↓ BP Severe wheezing Cyanosis	**Stop transfusion stat.** Start NS. Notify physician. Administer antihistamines and corticosteroids as ordered. Start a new IV line. Administer fluids to maintain BP. Call code prn.
Circulatory overload	Related to decreased cardiac output or transfusion rate too rapid, or patient was at risk for fluid excess	Wide-eyed appearance Anxiety Dyspnea Crackles Frothy sputum ↓ SpO$_2$ ↑ BP, ↑ P rate, ↑ R rate	Stop transfusion. Raise head of bed. Apply O$_2$. Notify physician. Administer diuretic as ordered. Monitor vital signs.
Bacterial contamination	Related to earlier contamination of blood product Can result in renal failure and shock	Very high fever Flushed ↓ BP, then compensatory ↑ BP	Stop transfusion. Notify physician. Administer steroids and antibiotics as ordered.

Supplies

Transfusions are generally administered with a special Y-shaped administration set, often referred to as a *Y-set*. Each of the two top branches of the Y-set end in piercing pins, one of which is used to spike the bag of blood product and the other to spike the bag of NS solution. The long tail of the Y-set contains an in-line filter and attaches to the cannula hub at the site of insertion into the patient's vein (refer to Figs. 38-12 and 38-13). Most commonly an 18-G (1.2-mm) or 20-G (0.9-mm) IV cannula is used to administer blood products. Infusing blood through a cannula that is too small is likely to lyse the blood cells.

Nursing Care Pretransfusion

Once blood products are ordered, inquire if the patient has ever received a blood transfusion before. Provide the appropriate level of patient teaching regarding the transfusion process. Discuss signs and symptoms that the patient should report to you if they are experienced during the transfusion, making certain that none of these signs and symptoms are present prior to initiating the transfusion so as not to be misinterpreted as reactions to the transfusion.

Assess the patient's vital signs immediately prior to beginning the blood or blood product transfusion, for use as a baseline against which you can compare vital signs taken during the transfusion. If the patient's temperature is elevated, you should notify the physician before proceeding with initiation of the transfusion. The physician may order an antihistamine such as diphenhydramine hydrochloride to be administered prior to beginning a transfusion. During the transfusion, it is not uncommon for the patient to experience a low-grade fever, but you will still report it to the physician.

Safety Measures

Just prior to initiating a blood product transfusion, most facilities require that two nurses, usually RNs, double-check the physician's order, comparing it to the actual blood product to make certain that the correct blood components have been prepared for transfusion. The nurses are responsible for ensuring that the patient's name and identification number on the blood product container match those on the patient's identification band and those on the patient chart. Each unit of blood product will also have its own specific identification number assigned to it during typing and crossmatching. The nurses must verify that this identification number on the blood product container matches the number on the blood bank form. Once all data have been matched and verified, both nurses are required to sign the blood bank form. *Safety: If any type of discrepancy exists, the transfusion should not be started and the blood product should be returned to the blood bank.*

Preparing Blood Product for Infusion

Wash your hands and apply clean examination gloves for preparation of blood products. Prepare the NS, blood administration set, and blood product container for use prior to going to the patient's room. Follow the manufacturer's instructions on the blood administration Y-set package for spiking NS and blood product containers, maintaining sterility of appropriate parts of the equipment. Label the tubing with the date and time. Prime the entire Y-set with the NS solution, including *back-priming* the branch of tubing that will insert into the blood product container. Skill 38-9 (page 959) provides more information on preparing, initiating, and monitoring infusion of blood and blood products.

Nursing Care During Transfusion

To initiate the transfusion, start the flow of NS first and reassess patency of the IV site. Assess vital signs. Then you can close the clamp to the NS and begin infusion of the blood product at a rate of 2 to 5 mL/min according to facility policy. Once the transfusion has been initiated, you will remain at the patient's bedside to monitor the patient for the first 15 minutes of the transfusion, as this is the most likely time for reactions to occur. Assess the patient's responses and vital signs every 5 minutes during this first 15 minutes. Also, this is a good time to complete documentation that may not have been done yet regarding pretransfusion assessments, patient teaching, and initiation of the transfusion.

If there are no indications of a problem during the first 15 minutes, increase the rate to a rate that will ensure completion of the transfusion within a 2- to 4-hour window. After 4 hours, the unit of blood is at risk for contamination because it is the perfect medium for bacterial growth. The only exception to this rate of infusion is during emergency volume replacement, which may be infused more rapidly. Assess the patient's vital signs every 15 to 30 minutes according to facility policy throughout the remainder of the transfusion, obtaining one last set after the completion of the transfusion.

If there are any signs or symptoms of reaction during the transfusion, immediately stop the infusion of blood and resume the infusion of NS to keep the vein open. Refer to Table 38-4 for specific nursing interventions for different types of reactions.

Nursing Care Post-transfusion

When the blood has completely infused, close that tubing clamp and reopen the one to the NS solution, allowing the NS to flush the line. If there is no need to infuse another unit of blood product or wait for laboratory results, the IV infusion is usually discontinued as soon as the NS has flushed the line. Again, this will be according to facility policy and the physician's orders. The physician will generally order a blood count to be done 12 to 24 hours post-transfusion to determine the effect on the blood cell counts.

Knowledge Connection

What gauge of needles may be used for blood product transfusions? Why is it not adequate for one nurse to verify that identification data assigned to the unit of blood product correspond with data on the chart, patient ID band, and transfusion form?

Skill 38-1 Administering IV Push Medication via PRN Lock or IV Line

Assessment Steps

1. Review the physician's order for IV push medication *to improve accuracy and decrease the risk for error.*

2. Unless you are familiar with the medication, use a drug book to research its therapeutic action, purpose, compatibility with the primary IV solution, drug-drug interactions, dosage, route, side effects, and length of time to infuse. *This reduces the risk of administration of inappropriate solution and allergic reactions and better prepares you to detect problems. It also increases your ability to detect side effects and potential problems, evaluate whether or not the medication does what is intended, and reduces risk of errors.*

3. Review the patient's diagnoses, medical history, and allergies to medications *to ensure that it is safe to administer this medication to the specific patient.*

4. Perform any pertinent physical assessments such as blood pressure, apical pulse, urine output, or auscultation of breath sounds *for comparison after medication administration.* Review pertinent laboratory results. *Some medications should not be given unless specific laboratory results are within designated parameters.*

5. Assess the patient's IV access. Is it a continuous infusion or a PRN lock? Or does it connect to a Luer-Lok syringe or require a needle or blunt-tipped adapter? *This allows you to know what type of adapters you need.*

6. Calculate the volume of medication you will draw up. Recheck your calculations *to decrease risk of error.* There are specific medications that MUST be rechecked by another nurse, such as heparin and insulin.

Planning Steps

1. Gather needed equipment and supplies: syringe, needle or blunt-tipped adapter if required, two NS flushes (prefilled syringe if available), alcohol wipes, correct form and dosage of ordered medication, examination gloves. *Being prepared saves you time and effort, and helps you to appear more confident and competent in the patient's eyes.*

2. Inspect packages for intactness and expiration date *to ensure continued sterility.*

Implementation Steps

Before Going to the Patient's Room

1. *Safety: Wash hands to prevent cross-contamination.*

2. *Safety: To prevent error, compare the medication label to the medication administration record (MAR) three times, checking the patient name, medication name, dosage, route, and time. IV administration is so critical if errors are made. Check the labels an extra time before going to the patient's room. Check allergies.*

3. Cleanse the medication stopper with alcohol *to remove any microorganisms.*

4. Draw up the ordered dosage of medication. *Safety: If the medication is insulin, an anticoagulant, or certain other drugs that may require verification by a second nurse, have another nurse verify the dosage before removing the needle from the medication vial.*

5. *Safety: Recap the sterile needle using the scoop method* you learned in Chapter 37. *You should never carry an uncovered needle down the hallway.*

After Entering the Patient's Room

6. Follow the Initial Implementation Steps located on the inside front cover.

7. *Safety: To prevent error, compare the medication label to the medication administration record (MAR) a third time, checking the patient name, medication name, dosage, route, and time.*

8. Explain to the patient what you are about to do. Provide any necessary patient teaching *to reduce patient anxiety and increase compliance.*

9. *Safety: Wash hands again to prevent cross-contamination.*

10. Assess the patient's IV site for signs of infiltration and phlebitis. *You must not infuse IV solution or medications into a site that shows possible indication of infiltration or phlebitis.*

If Injecting Into the IV Line of a Continuous Infusion of IV Solution

11. Locate the Y-injection port closest to the insertion site in the patient's extremity. Cleanse the port with an alcohol wipe *to remove microorganisms.*

12. Even though a medication may be compatible with the primary IV solution, many facilities have policies in place dictating that all prn or routine IV push medications should be both preceded and followed by an NS flush. To do so, attach the Luer-Lok NS flush syringe to the Y-injection port (or insert a needle or blunt-tipped adapter into the Y-injection port) and aspirate for blood *to confirm catheter placement in the vein* (refer to Fig. 38-2). Inject NS as dictated previously and disconnect the syringe from the Y-injection port.

13. Making certain the medication syringe contains no air, then attach the syringe to the Y-injection port after cleansing the port with an alcohol wipe *to reduce the risk of air embolism.* Slowly inject the medication, evenly distributing the volume over the designated time frame. For example, if you have 3 mL of medication to inject over 3 minutes, inject about 1 mL over the first minute, 1 mL over the second minute, and the last milliliter over the third minute.

    a. To inject the medication, pinch off the primary IV tubing just proximal to the Y-injection port, stopping the flow of IV solution. While pinching off the IV tubing, inject a small portion of the medication, and then release the IV tubing, allowing the IV solution to flow behind the medication.

    b. When it is time to inject another small amount of the medication, again pinch off the primary IV tubing and inject the designated portion of the medication. Release the IV tubing in between injecting the medication.

    c. Repeat this process over the designated period of time until all the medication has been instilled. Follow medication with 2 to 3 mL NS flush according to facility policy. *Safety: Never administer an IV push too quickly. Injecting IV push medication*

Skill 38-1 (continued)

over the recommended time span helps to protect the patient from too great a response in too short a time span and helps to protect against speed shock (refer to Fig. 38-2).
Safety: Continually monitor the patient's skin around the injection site for edema to ensure that the medication is still infusing into the vein and not infiltrating.

Note: *If the medication is incompatible with the primary IV solution, rather than trying to adequately flush the IV line with NS before and after administering the medication, it is best to inject the medication via another access device or directly into a different vein using a needle.*

14. After all medication is injected, remove the syringe or needle from the injection port.

15. Dispose of all contaminated supplies appropriately.

16. Remove and dispose of contaminated gloves. Wash hands *to reduce microorganisms and risk of cross-contamination.*

17. Follow the Ending Implementation Steps located on the inside back cover.

18. Document the administration of the medication in the nurses' notes only if it was a one-time order or a prn order. Otherwise, it is only documented on the MAR. Document any adverse or side effects exhibited as well as the effectiveness of the medication.

If Injecting into a PRN Lock

11. Cleanse the PRN lock injection port with alcohol *to reduce microorganisms.*

12. While maintaining sterility of the syringe tip, dispel air from the Luer-Lok syringe and attach the syringe with 3 to 5 mL NS to the Y-injection port of the PRN lock (or insert a needle or blunt-tipped adapter into the injection port). Open the slide clamp on the PRN lock *to reduce the risk of air embolism and infection.*

13. Aspirate with the syringe *to verify blood return* into the PRN lock. If blood return is noted, flush the PRN lock with part of the NS flush solution. Use the amount of NS dictated by facility policy. It should be a minimum of 2 to 3 mL but may vary up to 10 mL. If there is *no* blood return, do not infuse the IVPB. Establish a new venous access site for the IVPB.

14. After completing the flush, disconnect the NS flush syringe from the PRN lock injection port.

15. Wipe the injection port with an alcohol wipe *to reduce microorganisms.*

16. Making certain there is no air in the medication syringe, connect the Luer-Lok of the syringe holding the medication to the injection port of the PRN lock (or insert the needle or blunt-tipped adapter that is attached to the syringe into the injection port). *This helps to reduce risk of air embolism.*

17. Slowly inject the medication, evenly distributing the volume over the designated time frame *to reduce the risk of adverse reactions and speed shock.*

18. Once the medication is completely infused, disconnect the syringe from the injection port and repeat the NS flush as before, using the remaining NS solution or another prefilled syringe of NS flush, depending on facility policy.

19. Close the slide clamp on the PRN lock and remove the NS syringe or needle from the injection port.

20. Remove contaminated gloves and dispose of all contaminated supplies.

21. Wash hands *to reduce cross-contamination.*

22. Follow the Ending Implementation Steps located on the inside back cover.

23. Document the administration of the medication in the nurses' notes only if it was a one-time order or a prn order. Otherwise, it is only documented on the MAR. Document any adverse or side effects exhibited as well as the effectiveness of the medication.

Evaluation Steps

1. *Safety: Make any assessments that should be made after administration of the medication, such as respiratory or pulse rate, to detect any untoward effects.*

2. Assess for effectiveness of the medication. *This helps to determine if the medication needs to be changed.*

3. Assess the IV site one last time before leaving the patient's room *to ensure that it is not becoming erythematous or edematous.*

4. Evaluate the adequacy and balance of patient's intake and output *to detect possible signs of fluid imbalance.*

Sample Documentation

4-6-11   0415   *Respirations 17 per minute. MS 6 mg diluted in NS 6 mL and administered slowly IV push over 5 minutes for C/O pain at a 6 on a scale of 0 to 10. States pain is down to a 2. Respirations 14 per minute.* ————————————
——————————————— *Nurse's signature and credentials*

Skill 38-2 Administering IV Piggyback Medication

Assessment Steps

1. Review the physician's order for IVPB medication and rate of infusion *to clarify the order and reduce the risk of error.*

2. Unless you are familiar with the specific medication, use a drug book to research its therapeutic action, purpose, compatibility with primary IV solution and IVPB solution, possible drug-drug interactions, dosage, route, side effects, and length of time to infuse. *This reduces the risk of administration of inappropriate solution and allergic reactions, and better prepares you to detect problems. It also increases your ability to detect side effects and potential problems, evaluate whether or not the medication does what is intended, and reduces the risk of errors.*

3. Review the patient's diagnoses, medical history, and allergies to medications *to make certain it is safe to administer the medication.*

4. Assess to determine whether short secondary or IVPB administration tubing is already hanging. If so, was it used for this medication or a different medication? If it was a different medication, are they compatible or do you need to obtain another IVPB tubing to be used solely for administration of this specific medication? What date is the IVPB tubing due to be changed? Will a needle or a needleless piercing device be required to access the Y-injection port, or does it screw on with a Luer-Lok? *Obtaining this information helps you to be properly prepared and have all the supplies that you will need to reduce the number of trips made to the supply room. It will save you time and energy. It also helps to raise the patient's perception of your competency.*

5. Assess the patency of the IV line and assess the IV site for signs and symptoms of infiltration and phlebitis.

IVPB INFUSION INTO PRIMARY IV LINE WITH CONTINUAL INFUSION OF IV SOLUTION

Planning Steps

1. Gather needed equipment and supplies: correct form and dosage of medication, solution (type and volume) in which to instill the medication if the IVPB medication is not premixed, medication label, IVPB secondary tubing administration set, alcohol wipes, examination gloves. *Being prepared increases your efficiency, saves time and footwork, and helps to increase the patient's perception of your competence.*

2. Calculate the recommended rate of infusion according to facility policy, a pharmacist, or a drug book: mL/hr for pump flow and gtts/min for gravity flow. *This reduces the risk of error.*

3. Inspect packages for intactness and expiration dates *to ensure sterility.*

Implementation Steps

Before Going to the Patient's Room

1. *Safety: Wash hands to prevent cross-contamination.*

2. *Safety: Compare the medication label to the medication administration record (MAR) twice, checking the* patient name, medication name, dosage, route, and time, *to prevent error.*

3. Inspect the IVPB tubing administration set package for intactness and expiration date *to ensure continued sterility.*

4. Remove the tubing from the package and close the roller clamp. *Closing the clamp reduces the risk of introducing air bubbles as the solution begins to flow.*

5. Locate the tubing port on the IVPB bag of medication and remove the rubber plug, maintaining the sterility of the port *to reduce the risk of infection.*

6. Remove the cap from the tubing's piercing pin, maintaining the sterility of the pin *to reduce the risk of infection.*

7. Placing your thumb and index finger behind the flange *to reduce the risk of contaminating the sterile piercing pin,* insert the pin into the tubing port on the IVPB medication bag. Use a twisting motion to aid insertion. *Safety: Use caution to prevent the piercing pin from piercing the sides of the port.*

8. If the injection ports on the patient's primary IV tubing are not compatible with the Luer-Lok ends on the IVPB tubing, attach a needle or blunt-tipped adapter to the end of the IVPB tubing before continuing. *Safety: Be careful to maintain sterility of the tubing end as well as both ends of the needle or blunt-tipped adapter.*

9. Squeeze the drip chamber on the IVPB tubing, filling it one-third to one-half full. *This leaves adequate room in the drip chamber to observe the solution dripping.*

10. Remove the cap from the end of the IVPB tubing (or the attached needle or blunt-tipped adapter). Maintain sterility of the Luer-Lok end of IVPB tubing (or the attached needle or blunt-tipped adapter) *to reduce the risk of infection.*

11. Open the roller clamp on the IVPB tubing, allowing only enough solution to run through the tubing to displace all air. *Safety: Avoid allowing excessive amount of solution to flow once all air has been removed from the tubing. The smaller volume in a piggyback, usually only 50 or 100 mL, necessitates that there be no excessive wastage of medication-containing fluid.*

12. Close the roller clamp *to prevent premature dripping of solution* and replace the sterile cap on the end of the IVPB tubing (or needle or blunt-tipped adapter) without contaminating it *to reduce the risk of infection.*

After Entering the Patient's Room

13. Follow the Initial Implementation Steps located on the inside front cover.

14. *Safety: Compare the medication label to the medication administration record (MAR) a third time, checking the patient name, medication name, dosage, route, and time, to prevent error.*

15. Explain to the patient what you are about to do. Provide any necessary patient teaching. *This reduces patient anxiety and increases patient compliance.*

Skill 38-2 (continued)

16. *Safety: Wash hands again to remove microorganisms.*
17. Reassess the patient's IV site for signs of infiltration and phlebitis.
18. Hang the IVPB medication bag on the IV pole. If infusing by pump, hang both bags at the same height. **Note:** *If infusing by gravity rather than IV pump, use the extender wire to hang the primary IV solution bag lower than the IVPB medication bag. This allows the higher IVPB bag to infuse before the primary bag starts to run again.*
19. Locate the highest Y-injection port on the primary tubing. Cleanse the port with an alcohol wipe. **Note:** *Some pump tubing has plastic cassettes that insert into the pumping mechanism of the controller or pump. The highest injection port may be located on the top of these cassettes.*
20. Remove the cap from the end of the IVPB tubing (or needle or blunt-tipped adapter), maintaining sterility of the end *to prevent contamination and reduce the risk of infection.*
21. Cleanse the Y-injection port on the primary IV tubing with alcohol *to remove microorganisms.* Connect the IVPB tubing Luer-Lok adapter or blunt-tipped adaptor to the primary tubing Y-injection port (refer to Fig. 38-4).
22. **If using an IV pump:** Program the settings for the IVPB: the *secondary volume to be infused* and the *secondary rate of infusion.* Open the clamp on the IVPB tubing and start the pump. Once the IVPB medication has entirely infused, the primary IV solution will resume its set rate of infusion.

    If using gravity flow: Open the roller clamp on the IVPB tubing and adjust the rate to the number of gtts/min that you previously calculated. Once the IVPB medication has completely infused, the lowered bag of primary IV solution will resume dripping at its previous rate of infusion.
23. Remove contaminated gloves and dispose of them properly.
24. Wash hands before leaving room *to reduce risk of cross-contamination.*
25. Follow the Ending Implementation Steps located on the inside back cover.
26. Because routine medications are only documented on the MAR, the IVPB infusion itself is not documented in your nurses' notes. However, document the IV site assessment, any problems that develop, and the effectiveness of medication in the nurses' notes.

INFUSING INTO A PRN LOCK WITHOUT A CONTINUOUS IV INFUSION

Planning Steps

1. Gather needed equipment and supplies: smaller volume IVPB bag of IV solution containing the ordered type and dosage of medication; two NS flushes (in prefilled syringes if available); primary IV tubing (rather than the short IVPB tubing) *because it is longer and will reach from the medication bag hanging from the top of the IV pole to the PRN lock on the patient's arm;* alcohol wipes; examination gloves.

2. Calculate the recommended rate of infusion in gtts/min for gravity flow.
3. Inspect packages for intactness and expiration dates *to ensure continued sterility.*

Implementation Steps

Before Going to the Patient's Room
1. *Safety: Wash hands to prevent cross-contamination.*
2. *Safety: Compare the medication label to the MAR twice, checking the patient name, medication name, dosage, route, and time to prevent error.*
3. Inspect the primary tubing administration set package for intactness and expiration date *to ensure continued sterility.*
4. Remove the tubing from the package and close the roller clamp *to prevent solution from premature dripping.*
5. Locate the tubing port on the IVPB bag of medication and remove the rubber plug, maintaining the sterility of the port *to prevent contamination and lower the risk of infection.*
6. Remove the cap from the IV tubing's piercing pin, maintaining sterility of the pin *to avoid contamination.*
7. Placing your thumb and index finger "behind the flange," insert the pin into the tubing port on the IVPB medication bag. *This prevents your fingers from contaminating the sterile piercing pin.* Use a twisting motion to aid insertion. *Safety: Use caution to prevent the piercing pin from piercing the sides of the port.*
8. Squeeze the drip chamber on the tubing, filling it one-third to one-half full, *leaving room to observe the drip rate.*
9. Remove the cap from the end of the IV tubing, maintaining sterility of the Luer-Lok end *to avoid contamination.*
10. Open the roller clamp on the IV tubing, allowing only enough solution to run through the tubing to displace all air. *Safety: Avoid allowing excessive amount of solution to flow once all air has been removed from the tubing. The smaller volume in a piggyback, usually only 50 or 100 mL, necessitates that there be no excessive wastage of medication-containing fluid.*
11. Close the roller clamp and replace the sterile cap on the end of the IV tubing.

After Entering the Patient's Room
12. Follow the Initial Implementation Steps located on the inside front cover.
13. *Safety: Compare the medication label to the MAR a third time, checking the patient name, medication name, dosage, route, and time to prevent error.*
14. Explain to the patient what you are about to do. Provide any necessary patient teaching *to reduce anxiety and increase patient compliance.*
15. *Safety: Wash hands again to prevent cross-contamination.*
16. Reassess the patient's IV site for signs of infiltration and phlebitis.

(skill continues on page 950)

Skill 38-2 (continued)

17. Hang the IVPB medication bag on the IV pole.

18. Apply clean examination gloves if not already wearing them, *to protect you from contact with the patient's body fluids.*

19. Cleanse the injection port on the PRN lock with an alcohol wipe *to remove microorganisms.*

20. Remove the sterile cap from the first NS flush syringe, press down on the plunger *to remove air from the syringe,* and attach the Luer-Lok tip to the injection port on the PRN lock while maintaining sterility.

21. Assess for continued placement of cannula within the vein: open the slide clamp on the PRN lock and pull back on the plunger of the NS syringe to aspirate blood return from the vein into the PRN lock. *A blood return indicates correct placement of the cannula.* Inject the NS slowly over 1 minute. Observe for swelling at the IV site. (If it begins to swell or the cannula is clogged and will not allow you to aspirate blood or flush with the NS, discontinue the PRN lock.)

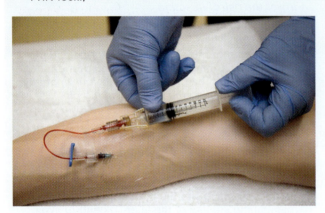

22. After completion of the NS flush, disconnect the syringe from the injection port. Remove the cap from the sterile end of the IV tubing without contaminating the tubing end.

23. Cleanse the injection port with an alcohol wipe and attach the IV tubing's Luer-Lok end to the injection port, maintaining sterile technique. You may remove and dispose of gloves until you are ready to discontinue the IVPB.

24. Open the IV tubing roller clamp and adjust the flow rate to the number of gtts/min you calculated earlier. *This is necessary to infuse the medication in the desired time frame.*

25. Assess the IV site for swelling, redness, coolness or increased warmth of skin, and patient report of discomfort, which are signs and symptoms of infiltration or phlebitis. Monitor the rate and appearance of the site closely throughout the infusion *to ensure continued correct rate and early detection of problems.*

26. Once the IVPB is infused, wash hands and apply clean examination gloves.

27. Close the roller clamp on the tubing and disconnect the tubing from the injection port.

28. Cleanse the injection port with alcohol *to remove microorganisms.*

29. Remove air from the second NS flush syringe and attach the Luer-Lok to the PRN lock injection port. Aspirate for blood return to verify continued placement in vein. Then slowly inject the NS flush over at least 1 minute *to clear blood and medication from the cannula, monitoring the site for swelling. Administering NS faster may cause irritation of the vein and cause the patient discomfort.*

30. Close the slide clamp on the PRN lock *to prevent blood from reentering the lock.* Disconnect the syringe from the injection port and dispose of it.

31. Remove contaminated gloves and dispose of them properly.

32. Wash hands before leaving the room *to reduce risk of cross-contamination.*

33. Follow the Ending Implementation Steps located on the inside back cover.

34. Because routine medications are only documented on the MAR, the IVPB infusion itself is not documented in your nurses' notes. However, document the IV site assessment, any problems that develop, and the effectiveness of medication in the nurses' notes.

Evaluation Steps

1. During IVPB infusion, assess the IV site *to make certain problems have not developed. Safety: At the first sign of infiltration, stop the infusion. If vesicant drugs are being infused, follow the appropriate facility protocol.*

2. Evaluate the effectiveness of the infused medication *to determine whether the medication is doing what was intended.*

3. Evaluate the adequacy and balance of the patient's intake and output *to detect possible signs of fluid imbalance.*

Sample Documentation

2-4-10   1205   Noted 1/2-in. edematous area just proximal to IV cannula during ampicillin IVPB infusion. Able to obtain blood return. C/O of site beginning to burn. IV DC'd. IV restarted in Lt. forearm with 22-G × 1-in. intracath with 1 attempt, no difficulty. IV infusing IVPB at 100 mL/hr. ——————————
——————————— *Nurse's signature and credentials*

Skill 38-3 Converting an IV Infusion to a PRN Lock

Assessment Steps

1. Review the physician's order for conversion to a PRN lock *to reduce the risk of error.*
2. Assess whether the patient has IV tubing that connects directly to the cannula hub or has a PRN lock connecting the tubing to the cannula hub *to determine the type of supplies you need.*
3. Assess the IV site for signs of infiltration or phlebitis.

Planning Steps

1. *Safety: Wash your hands to prevent cross-contamination.*

If Patient Has IV Tubing Connected Directly to the Cannula Hub

2. Gather needed equipment and supplies: PRN lock device, NS flush, needle or blunt-tipped adapter, alcohol wipes, tape.
3. Inspect packages for intactness and expiration dates *to ensure continued sterility.*
4. If the PRN lock device does not allow use of Luer-Lok device, apply a needle or blunt-tipped adapter to the NS flush syringe. Maintain sterility of the tip of the NS flush syringe and the needle or blunt-tipped adapter *to prevent contamination.*
5. Cleanse the injection port end of the new PRN lock device with alcohol *to remove any microorganisms.*
6. Connect the sterile Luer-Lok tip of the syringe to the injection port, or insert the needle or blunt-tipped adapter into the injection port of the PRN lock, while maintaining sterility.
7. Prime the new PRN lock by injecting the NS into the lock until all air has been displaced with NS. *This helps to prevent air embolisms.*

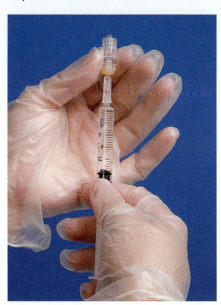

8. Leave the syringe with the remaining NS attached to the PRN device so *it is ready to flush once connected to the cannula hub.*

If Patient Has a PRN Lock Device Connecting the Cannula Hub to the Tubing

2. Gather needed equipment and supplies: NS flush, needle or blunt-tipped adapter if needed, alcohol wipes.
3. Inspect packages for intactness and expiration dates *to ensure continued sterility.*

Implementation Steps

1. Follow the Initial Implementation Steps located on the inside front cover.
2. Explain to the patient what you are about to do. Provide any necessary patient teaching *to reduce patient anxiety and increase compliance.*
3. *Safety: Once in the patient's room, wash hands again to prevent cross-contamination.*
4. Reassess the patient's IV site *to ensure there are no signs of infiltration and phlebitis.*
5. Tear several 3- to 4-inch strips of tape to use for securing the PRN lock.
6. Stop the IV solution flow by turning off the IV pump or closing the tubing clamp if infusing by gravity flow.
7. *To protect you from possible contact with patient body fluid,* apply clean examination gloves.

If Patient Has IV Tubing Connected Directly to the Cannula Hub

8. Gently loosen the tape securing the IV tubing to the extremity and cannula hub, taking care not to lift the cannula hub away from the skin. *Safety: Lifting the hub bends the attached plastic cannula that is inserted into the vein, increasing the risk of a severed cannula. Pull the tape ends toward the cannula to decrease the risk of dislodging or bending the cannula.* Try not to disturb the TOD over the insertion site.
9. Once the tape is removed, place a sterile 2×2-inch (5×5-cm) gauze pad underneath the cannula hub connection *to reduce the risk of contamination.* Disconnect the IV tubing end from the cannula hub, maintaining the sterility of the cannula hub.

(skill continues on page 952)

Skill 38-3 (continued)

10. Remove the end cap from the connecting end of the new PRN lock device without contaminating the connecting end.

11. Insert the end of the PRN lock device into the sterile hub of the cannula in the patient's vein.

12. Screw the Luer-Lok connection device to the cannula hub *to ensure that the PRN lock device will not be accidentally disconnected from the cannula hub.*

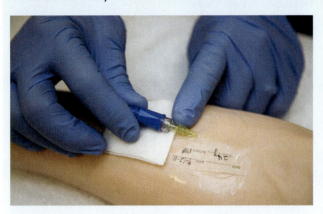

13. Secure the PRN lock device to the extremity with strips of tape *to reduce risk of displacement of the cannula from the vein and reduce irritation of the vein due to movement.*

14. Aspirate with the NS flush syringe and observe for a blood return from the cannula hub. *Blood return indicates the cannula is still in the vein.*

15. Taking at least 1 minute, inject the remaining NS flush solution *to clear blood out of the tip of the cannula to prevent clotting and obstruction of the cannula.*

16. Close the sliding clamp on the PRN lock device.

17. Disconnect the NS flush syringe from the cannula.

18. Remove contaminated gloves and dispose of all contaminated supplies.

19. Wash hands *to prevent cross-contamination.*

20. Follow the Ending Implementation Steps located on the inside back cover.

21. Document the conversion from IV infusion to PRN lock.

If Patient Has a PRN Lock Device Connecting the Tubing to the Cannula Hub

8. Disconnect the IV tubing from the injection port of the PRN lock device.

9. Cleanse the injection port with an alcohol wipe *to remove microorganisms.*

10. Connect the Luer-Lok tip of the NS flush syringe to the PRN lock device injection port or insert a needle or blunt-tipped adapter into the injection port of the PRN lock device.

11. Aspirate by pulling the syringe plunger back while observing for blood return *to ensure placement of the cannula in the vein.* If blood return is observed, flush the PRN lock device and cannula by injecting the NS flush slowly over at least 1 minute.

12. Close the slide clamp on the PRN device *to prevent blood from backing up into the device, where it can clot.*

13. Disconnect the NS syringe.

14. Remove contaminated gloves and dispose of all contaminated supplies.

15. Wash hands *to prevent cross-contamination.*

16. Follow the Ending Implementation Steps located on the inside back cover.

17. Document the conversion from IV infusion to PRN lock.

Evaluation Steps

1. Reassess the site *to ensure that there are no signs of infiltration before leaving the room.*

Sample Documentation

7-18-11   1520   IV converted to PRN saline lock. Site without edema or erythema. No C/O discomfort. ─────────────
──────────────── Nurse's signature and credentials

Skill 38-4 Calculating IV Infusion Rate

Assessment Steps

1. Review the physician's order for size of IV solution bag and rate of infusion *to reduce the risk of error.*
2. Assess whether you will infuse the IV solution by gravity flow or with an IV pump or controller.
3. Assess for correct drop factor. If using gravity flow, check the tubing administration set box for the drop factor. If you are going to use a pump/controller, use 60 as the drop factor. *This information is required to calculate the rate of infusion.*

Planning Steps

1. Plan to use this formula to calculate the infusion rate using the three pieces of data obtained during assessment:

$$\frac{\text{Volume} \times \text{drop factor}}{\text{Time}} = \text{rate of infusion}$$

where *Volume* is the volume of fluid to be infused, *Time* is the time (in minutes) in which the specified volume of fluid is to infuse, and the rate of infusion is measured in mL/hr if an IV pump is used or in gtts/min if gravity flow is used.

2. Obtain the needed supplies: administration set package (for gravity flow), calculator or pen and paper.

Implementation Steps

1. Multiply the volume of fluid you want to infuse times the drop factor.
2. Divide the total by the number of minutes in which you want this volume of fluid to infuse.
   Note: Remember that, if you use the volume of the entire bag, you will have to use the total number of minutes in which you want to infuse the entire bag. If you use a lesser volume, such as the volume that is to infuse per hour, you must use only the number of minutes in 1 hour (60 minutes). If the volume is 50 mL and it must infuse in 20 minutes, then use these same two figures. The volume and time must be related to each other.

Evaluation Steps

1. Evaluate your calculations and result, making certain you calculated the rate in gtts/min if it is to infuse by gravity flow and mL/hour if it is to infuse by pump.

Skill 38-5 Adding Medications to Primary IV Solution

Assessment Steps

1. *Safety: Review the physician's order to verify for type, route, and dosage of medication; type, size, and route of primary IV solution; and rate of infusion. This reduces the risk for error, reduces the risk of administration of inappropriate solution and allergic reactions, and better prepares you to detect problems.*
2. *Safety: Determine medication compatibility with primary IV solution and other drugs the patient is receiving. This prevents incompatibility errors.*
3. *Safety: Assess patient's allergies to make certain it is safe to administer the medication.*
4. Collect data regarding the medication's action, purpose, side effects, dosage, drug-drug interactions, and nursing implications. *This provides you with the required knowledge to evaluate the appropriateness of the medication order and to be prepared to detect problems.*
5. If the patient already has the primary IV solution infusing, assess the IV site *to rule out any signs and symptoms of infiltration and phlebitis.*

Planning Steps

1. Gather needed equipment and supplies: correct type and size of bag of IV solution; correct type, form, and dosage of medication; syringe large enough to draw up medication; 20- or 21-G (0.9- or 0.8-mm) needle; alcohol wipe; orange or other bright-colored medication label. *Being prepared saves you time and unnecessary footwork. Being prepared also helps you to appear more competent and confident, both of which are important to the patient's perception of and trust in you.*

2. Complete the "medication added" label, including the patient's name and room number; name, dosage, and rate of infusion of medication; date and time; and your initials. Apply it to IV bag to which you will instill the medication *to clarify what is infusing and help to reduce medication errors.*

3. Inspect packages for intactness and expiration dates *to prevent use of unsafe supplies.*

Implementation Steps

1. Follow the Initial Implementation Steps located on the inside front cover.
2. *Safety: Check the medication label a minimum of three times to prevent medication error.*
3. *Safety: Use two methods of identifying the patient according to facility policy to reduce the risk of error.*
4. Explain to the patient what you are about to do. Provide any necessary patient teaching *to reduce patient anxiety and increase compliance.*
5. *Safety: Wash hands to prevent cross-contamination.*

(skill continues on page 954)

Skill 38-5 (continued)

6. Using aseptic technique, attach the needle to the syringe. *Safety: The needle hub and the tip of the syringe must stay sterile to reduce the risk of infection.*

7. Cleanse the rubber stopper of the medication vial with an alcohol wipe *to remove any microorganisms.* If the medication requires dilution, add an appropriate volume of the proper diluent and mix well.

8. Using aseptic technique, instill an equal volume of air to displace the number of milliliters of medication you will remove from vial. *Safety: The cleansed rubber stopper on the vial and the needle must be kept sterile to reduce the risk of infection.*

9. Withdraw the correct volume/dosage of additive and remove the needle from the vial.

10. Locate the medication port on the IV solution bag. It normally does *not* have a cap or cover. Cleanse the port with an alcohol wipe *to remove any microorganisms.* **Note:** Do not confuse it with the port for the IV tubing, which has a rubber plug/cover over the end of it.

11. Using aseptic technique, insert the needle through the medication port, using care to avoid puncturing the back side of the IV bag or port with the needle, *which would require a new bag and tubing. Safety: The cleansed port and needle must be kept sterile.*

12. Instill the medication and remove the needle.

13. *Safety: Activate the needle safety mechanism and dispose of it in the sharps container.*

14. Gently invert the IV bag several times *to distribute medication* and hang it back on the IV pole.

15. Reassess the IV infusion rate *to ensure it is still flowing at the ordered rate.*

16. Follow the Ending Implementation Steps located on the inside back cover.

Evaluation Steps

1. Evaluate for even distribution of medication and inspect for precipitation or clouding.

2. After the solution is infusing, again assess the patient's IV site *to rule out any signs and symptoms of infiltration or phlebitis.* Make certain the patient feels no discomfort.

3. Monitor for therapeutic effects, side effects, and adverse reactions *to evaluate the effectiveness of the medication.*

4. Evaluate the adequacy and balance of the patient's intake and output *to detect possible signs of fluid imbalance.*

Sample Documentation

12/31/11 1430 One vial MOI added to hanging IV bag of D5W with approximately 900 mL left in bag. Infusing @ 125 mL/hr. IV site intact, clean, dry, without edema, erythema, or discomfort.
——————————————— *Nurse's signature and credentials*

Skill 38-6 Initiating Peripheral Venipuncture

Assessment Steps

1. Review the physician's order for venipuncture; type and size of bag of IV solution; and rate of infusion. *This provides you with the required knowledge to evaluate the appropriateness of the order and reduce errors.*

2. Review the patient's diagnoses, medical history, risk factors for circulatory fluid overload, reason for IV access, age, mental cognition, and allergies to medications, solution, latex, iodine, and tape. *This reduces the risk of administration of inappropriate solution and allergic reactions and better prepares you to detect problems.*

3. Assess whether the patient has ever had an IV before and determine what patient teaching needs to be done. *Patient teaching reduces patient anxiety and increases patient compliance.*

4. Assess which side is the patient's dominant hand; assess the size and caliber of the veins in the non-dominant extremity *to determine the best site for IV initiation.*

Planning Steps

1. Gather needed equipment and supplies: IV pole; IV pump if available; correct type and size of bag of IV solution; correct primary IV tubing administration set that works with pump; extension tubing if desired; two sizes of IV needle catheter that will be suitable for the patient's needs; IV start kit or the components normally found in one (antiseptic wipe, tourniquet, sterile transparent occlusive dressing [TOD], roll of tape, sterile 2×2-inch [5×5-cm] gauze pad, IV site label); labels for tubing and bag of solution; towel or waterproof pad; clean examination gloves. *Adequate preparation saves you time and footwork and helps you appear more confident and competent.*

2. *Safety: Check the solution label at least three times to avoid medication error.*

3. Calculate the rate of infusion in mL/hr for a pump or gtts/min for gravity, whichever applies. *This reduces the risk of an incorrect administration rate.*

4. Inspect packages for intactness and expiration dates *to ensure sterility and reduce the risk of infection.*

Implementation Steps

Before Going to the Patient's Room

1. *Safety: Wash hands to prevent cross-contamination.*

2. If a pump will be used, program or set the pump for the volume to infuse and rate of infusion.

3. Inspect the outer wrapper of the IV solution bag for intactness and moisture before removing the outer wrapper, *to detect leaking of solution, which would indicate breach in sterility.*

4. Inspect the IV solution bag for name or type of solution and expiration date. Inspect the solution for clarity. Make certain the fluid is clear, not cloudy, and contains no particulates. *This helps to ensure the use of the correct solution and clarify whether it is safe for use.* Squeeze the bag *to observe for pinhole leaks.*

5. Apply a label to the bag of solution, including patient name, room number, date, time, and rate of infusion. *This communicates the appropriate information to each nurse providing care to the patient.*

6. Verify that you have the correct primary IV tubing administration set for the type of pump being used or for gravity infusion. *This increases efficiency and helps to control cost and waste of opening incorrect supplies.*

7. Open the package and remove the tubing administration set. Review the manufacturer's priming instructions if you are not familiar with this set *to save time and increase competency.* Close the roller clamp on the tubing *to prevent premature dripping of solution into the administration set. This helps to reduce the risk of air bubbles while priming the tubing.*

8. Locate the port on the IV bag of solution into which the tubing administration set piercing pin will be inserted. Remove the rubber plug or cover from the port. *Safety: Use caution to maintain sterility of the port.*

9. Remove the protective cap from the piercing pin, or spike, at the end of the tubing administration set. *Safety: Use care to maintain sterility of the piercing pin to reduce the risk of infection.*

10. Insert the piercing pin into the port of the IV bag without contaminating the piercing pin. Be certain to hold the port of the bag straight as you insert the piercing pin, *to prevent piercing the side of the port with the piercing pin. Once the piercing pin pierces the side of the port, it is no longer sterile and a new bag of solution and a new primary IV tubing administration set would be required.*

(skill continues on page 956)

Skill 38-6 (continued)

11. Squeeze the drip chamber on the tubing administration set and fill it approximately one-third to one-half full of solution. *This leaves adequate room in the drip chamber to observe the solution dripping.*

12. Hang the IV bag on an IV pole. Follow any special priming instructions from the manufacturer. Otherwise, remove the cap from the end of the tubing administration set, maintaining sterility of the tubing end. Next, prime the tubing by opening the roller clamp and allowing solution to run through the tubing set *to displace all the air within the solution to reduce the risk of air embolism.* Once all the air has been removed, close the roller clamp and recap the end of the tubing, maintaining sterility of the tubing end and the cap *to reduce the risk of infection.*

13. Complete the label with the date and time started and date the tubing is due to be changed. Attach the label to the tubing. *This communicates when the tubing should be changed to reduce the risk of infection.*

14. Drape the tubing over the top of the pole. *Safety: In order to prevent contamination, do not allow tubing to touch the floor.* If using a pump, do not insert the tubing into the pump mechanism until free flow of solution has ensured proper cannulation of the vein.

After Entering the Patient's Room

15. Follow the Initial Implementation Steps located on the inside front cover.

16. Explain to the patient what you are about to do. Provide any necessary patient teaching *to reduce anxiety and increase patient compliance.*

17. *Safety: Wash hands again to prevent cross-contamination.*

18. Place a towel or moisture-proof pad under the patient's nondominant arm. *This saves you the extra work of changing soiled linens.* Prepare supplies for use and arrange them on the towel or pad so that they are within easy reach *to prevent you from searching for supplies, or turning around or reaching for supplies during initiation. Unnecessary movement before the IV cannula is secured to the patient's arm increases the risk of displacing the cannula from the vein.*

19. Apply a tourniquet and use recommended methods for dilating veins until adequate vein distention is obtained. *This increases successful cannulation of the vein with fewer needle sticks for the patient.*

20. Assess and palpate veins to select a vein. If desired, you may use a needle cap to make an indentation to mark the point of intended venipuncture and another indention to show the path of the vein 1 inch proximal to the first indentation. *This helps to identify the path of the vein, assists you to "line up" the needle with the marks, and helps to reduce the need for palpation of the site once the site has been cleansed.*

21. Remove the tourniquet *to allow venous circulation.*

22. *Safety: Apply clean examination gloves to protect you from blood-borne pathogens.*

Skill 38-6 (continued)

23. Cleanse the site with facility-preferred antiseptic wipe. Start in the center where you intend to perform the venipuncture. Using vigorous friction, cleanse in widening, concentric circles for at least 20 seconds until a 3-inch diameter circle has been cleansed. Allow the site to air dry. *This removes microorganisms and reduces the risk of infection.*

24. Reapply the tourniquet 4 to 6 inches proximal to the venipuncture site without contaminating the cleansed site. The tail of the tourniquet should be tucked from the top side (proximal) rather than from below (distal). This results in both ends of the tourniquet coming out of the top side *so that they do not contaminate the cleansed site.*

25. Carefully remove the cap from the sterile IV needle cannula, maintaining sterility of the entire length of needle and cannula *to reduce the risk of contamination and infection.*

26. Place your nondominant hand *several inches distal* to the intended venipuncture site *to reduce the risk of contaminating the IV cannula with your nondominant hand during initiation.* Use the thumb on your nondominant hand to pull the skin taut *to ease needle insertion through the skin and decrease patient discomfort.*

27. Hold the IV needle in your dominant hand with the bevel up. Use a 30- to 45-degree angle, depending on the location and depth of the vein. If the vein is shallow and appears fragile, decrease the needle angle to 15 degrees. *The bevel-up position eases needle insertion and reduces trauma to the vein, which decreases patient discomfort. Using too much angle will increase the risk of going through the vein.*

28. Inform the patient of the impending prick *to avoid surprising the patient, which can cause the patient to jump or move.* Insert the needle through the skin and into the vein with one motion if possible, *which reduces the discomfort of probing.*

29. Upon obtaining blood return in the flashback chamber, advance the entire IV needle and cannula just far enough into the lumen of the vein to ensure that the end of the cannula is within the vein, usually less than ⅛ inch. *Safety: Do not insert the entire length of both the needle and cannula into the vein, which would increase the risk of the needle going through the vein.*

30. Once the bevel of the needle and the end of the cannula are inside the vein, use aseptic technique to carefully advance the cannula over and off the end of the needle into the vein lumen.

Avoid forcing the cannula, *which can cause displacement of the cannula from the vein and damage to the vein walls.* If resistance is met, gently apply traction to the vein or try to turn the cannula ever so slightly. If the cannula still does not advance with ease, it may be helpful to wait for further advancement of the cannula until you have connected the administration set tubing and slowly initiated flow of the solution. *This sometimes helps to "float" the cannula into the vein.*

31. Once the cannula is fully inserted, use the thumb and index finger of your nondominant hand to secure the cannula hub. *Safety: Do not contaminate the open end of the hub.* Then use the middle or ring finger of your nondominant hand to apply pressure over the vein, beyond the end of the cannula, *to prevent excessive bleeding during connection of the tubing.* While your nondominant hand secures the cannula hub without contaminating it, use your dominant hand to carefully remove the needle from the cannula. Dependent upon the type and style of needle and cannula used, the needle may be removed from the cannula and vein by pressing the retracting button so that the needle retracts into the needle guard, or some other method may be used.

(skill continues on page 958)

Skill 38-6 (continued)

Some needle types require that you actually *pull* the needle from inside the cannula before the safety device will activate. Know your equipment and supplies and how they work prior to attempting IV initiation. Avoid "learning how to use" them at the bedside, *which may increase patient anxiety and decrease the patient's perception of your competence.*

32. Using aseptic technique, quickly remove the cap from the end of the IV tubing. With your nondominant hand, use a finger to apply pressure against the vein proximal to the cannula while securing the cannula hub with your thumb and index finger. With your dominant hand, aseptically insert the tubing end into the cannula hub, securing attachment by gently screwing on the Luer-Lok.

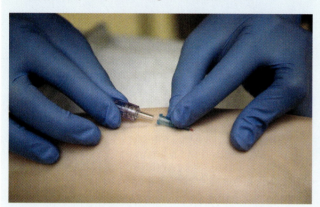

Safety: Avoid using a one-handed method of removing the cap from the tubing. It is virtually impossible to do without contaminating the sterile tubing end.

33. Do not apply a site dressing yet. Continue to hold the connection between the cannula hub and tubing securely against the patient's skin, preventing bending or crimping of the cannula. *To ensure proper cannulation of the vein,* open the roller clamp on the tubing and observe for free flow of solution. As solution is infused, make certain that there is no swelling at the site. Once free flow of solution is confirmed, partially close the roller clamp to prevent rapid infusion of solution while securing the site.

34. To secure the site, peel backing from a sterile TOD and apply, covering the insertion site and the hub of the cannula only. *This helps to secure the cannula and maintain the sterility of the puncture site, and allows tubing to be changed at the hub connection without having to remove the TOD.*

35. Use strips of tape to secure the tubing to the extremity *to reduce the risk of displacement of the cannula and infiltration.* Avoid application of tape strips over the TOD unless absolutely necessary. *This allows tubing to be changed at the hub connection without having to remove the TOD.*

36. Apply a small label with the date, time, cannula gauge, and your initials on the IV site. *This communicates to staff when the IV should be changed to reduce the risk of phlebitis.*

37. Insert the tubing into the pump mechanism, set the volume to be infused (volume of bag) and rate of infusion (mL/hr), open the roller clamp all the way, and start the pump. This step will be different when using different manufacturer's IV pump models, so be certain to read the instructions prior to use.

38. Dispose of used supplies, and discard the needle in the sharps container *to reduce the risk of contaminated needle sticks.*

39. Follow the Ending Implementation Steps located on the inside back cover.

Skill 38-6 (continued)

Evaluation Steps

1. Observe the infusion site *to make certain there is no swelling with infusion of the solution.* Inquire of the patient regarding discomfort. *Swelling and discomfort are both indicative of possible infiltration.*

2. Before leaving the room, reassess that the pump is working, solution is flowing, and the site remains clean, dry, and without edema or erythema.

3. Evaluate the adequacy and balance of the patient's intake and output *to detect possible signs of fluid imbalance.*

Sample Documentation

2/1/11   1915   IV initiated per physician's orders, using aseptic technique, in Rt. forearm with 22-G × 1-in. intracath, one attempt, without difficulty. 1000 mL D5W infusing per pump at 125 mL/hr. Site clean, dry, intact, and without erythema or edema. Voices no discomfort. ————————— Nurse's signature and credentials

Skill 38-7 Adding a New Bag of IV Solution to Existing IV Line

Assessment Steps

1. Review the physician's order for type and volume of IV solution and rate of infusion *to ensure correctness of the order.*

2. Review the patient's diagnoses, medical history, and allergies to medications *to determine the appropriateness of the order.*

3. If the infusion rate is to be different from the rate at which the IV solution is now infusing, calculate the new rate in mL/hr for a pump or gtts/min for gravity flow.

Planning Steps

1. Obtain the ordered type and volume of solution and a new label for the bag. *Being prepared saves time and effort.*

2. Inspect packages for intactness and expiration dates *to ensure continued sterility.*

3. Fill out the label and apply to the bag *for communication of contents to staff members.*

Implementation Steps

1. Follow the Initial Implementation Steps located on the inside front cover.

2. Explain to the patient what you are about to do. Provide any necessary patient teaching *to decrease patient anxiety.*

3. *Safety: Wash hands to prevent cross-contamination.*

4. Assess the patient's IV site for signs of infiltration and phlebitis.

5. Remove the rubber stopper covering the tubing port on the new IV solution bag, maintaining sterility.

6. *If using an IV pump or controller,* press the button to stop the infusion. *If infusing by gravity,* clamp the tubing.

7. Remove the IV solution bag from the IV pole and invert the bag (upside down) *to prevent leakage of solution after removing the piercing pin.*

8. Remove the piercing pin, maintaining its sterility *to lower the risk of infection.*

9. Insert the piercing pin into the tubing port on the new bag of IV solution, using care to maintain sterility of the piercing pin and the inside of the port.

10. Right the bag and hang it on the IV pole.

11. Squeeze the tubing drip chamber to fill the chamber one-third to one-half full. Do not overfill the chamber; leave room *to observe dripping of the solution.* If you accidently overfill, invert the bag and squeeze the drip chamber so that the extra fluid runs back into the bag.

12. *If using an IV pump,* set the volume to be infused and the rate of infusion on the pump. *If infusing by gravity,* count the drops falling in the drop chamber, setting the drop rate to the precalculated rate.

13. Follow the Ending Implementation Steps located on the inside back cover.

14. If the new solution bag was added solely because the previous one had completely infused, document the bag of IV solution only on the medication administration record (MAR). If a new physician's order prompted discontinuation of the infusing bag to hang a different new one, it should be documented in the nurses' notes as well as the MAR.

Evaluation Steps

1. Assess the IV site *to ensure that there is no edema or erythema.*

2. Evaluate the adequacy and balance of the patient's intake and output *to detect possible signs of fluid imbalance.*

Sample Documentation

6-25-11   0235   IV solution D5W discontinued and 1000 mL NS hung & infusing at 80 mL/hr per physician's order. IV site without erythema or edema. ————————————
————————————— Nurse's signature and credentials

Skill 38-8 Discontinuing an IV Infusion or PRN Lock

Assessment Steps

1. Review the physician's order to discontinue the IV infusion or PRN lock *to reduce the risk of error.*

Planning Steps

1. Gather needed supplies: alcohol wipes, sterile 2×2-inch (5×5-cm) gauze pad, bandage, examination gloves. *Being prepared saves you time and effort.*

Implementation Steps

1. Follow the Initial Implementation Steps located on the inside front cover.
2. Check the patient's identification using two methods according to facility policy.
3. Explain to the patient what you are about to do. Provide any necessary patient teaching. *This reduces patient anxiety and increases patient compliance.*
4. *Safety: Wash hands to prevent cross-contamination.*
5. Apply clean examination gloves *to protect you from blood-borne pathogens.*
6. Close the tubing clamp and turn the IV pump off if one is in use.
7. While securing the cannula hub with your gloved nondominant hand, use your gloved dominant hand to remove tape securing the tubing to the extremity, pulling the tape ends toward the IV site *to avoid tearing skin at the puncture site.*
8. Continuing to secure the cannula hub, lift all four edges of the transparent occlusive dressing (TOD) toward the insertion site until the TOD is no longer secured to the patient's skin. *This reduces the risk of crimping or breaking the cannula from the hub and decreases the risk of tearing the skin at the puncture site.*
9. Using your nondominant hand, apply gentle pressure to the vein immediately proximal to the inserted end of the cannula or needle, with a sterile 2×2-inch (5×5-cm) gauze pad, *without* applying pressure over the cannula itself. *Doing this proximally reduces the risk of accidental pressure on the cannula causing it to separate from its hub and become an embolism.* As you use your dominant hand to gently remove the cannula from the vein, keeping the cannula parallel to the skin, slide the gauze pad in your nondominant hand toward the insertion site, so that once the cannula tip is out of the vein, you can increase pressure being applied to the insertion site to prevent formation of a hematoma. *This helps to reduce the risk of hematoma at the site.*

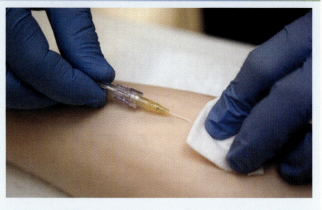

10. Immediately inspect the tip of the cannula upon removal *to ensure that the cannula tip is intact.*
11. Hold pressure on the insertion site while cleansing the surrounding area of any blood using alcohol wipes. Maintain pressure to the site for 1 minute before lifting the gauze pad to inspect for cessation of bleeding. If the patient takes anticoagulants or bleeds easily, hold pressure for 3 to 5 minutes. *This helps to reduce the risk of hematoma formation.*
12. Apply a bandage *to reduce the risk of contamination with microorganisms.*
13. Remove and dispose of the contaminated gloves and cannula in proper biohazard bags.
14. Wash hands *to prevent cross-contamination.*
15. Follow the Ending Implementation Steps located on the inside back cover.

Evaluation Steps

1. Evaluate to determine whether the tip of the cannula is intact as soon as it is withdrawn from the vein *to ensure that the tip did not break off inside the vein, making it an embolism.*
2. Assess the site for bleeding or bruising.
3. Assess and record the total volume infused as noted on the IV pump on the I&O record. Assess intake and output for imbalance.

Sample Documentation

8-27-11   1325   IO discontinued with intact 22-G cannula, according to physician's order. No erythema, edema, or bruising noted at site. Total IO volume infused 635 mL. ————————
——————————————— Nurse's signature and credentials

Skill 38-9 Preparing, Initiating, and Monitoring Infusion of Blood and Blood Products

Assessment Steps

1. Verify that informed consent has been obtained. *The patient's informed consent is required for administration of blood.*

2. Assess the patient's diagnoses and evaluate risk factors for fluid imbalance.

3. Assess the patient's knowledge level regarding transfusion *to determine teaching needs.*

4. Assess the patient's IV site *to ensure there are no signs of infiltration or phlebitis.* If there is *not* an IV access device already in place, initiate IV access using a 20-gauge or larger cannula depending upon facility policy.

Planning Steps

1. Perform any necessary patient teaching and explain signs and symptoms the patient should report during the transfusion. *This helps to reduce patient anxiety and increase patient compliance.*

2. *Safety: Verify with a second nurse that the physician's order matches the blood components about to be infused; that the patient name and ID number on the unit of blood product container matches the one on the patient's ID band and the one on the transfusion record; that the unit of blood product identification number on the unit's label matches the one on the transfusion record; that the ABO blood type and Rh factor of the unit of blood matches that of the patient's; and finally that the blood's expiration date has not passed. Follow facility policy closely for this safety check.*

3. Gather needed equipment and supplies: blood administration Y-set, container of blood product that you have previously verified, container of 0.9% sodium chloride IV solution, alcohol wipes, tape, clean examination gloves. *Preparation saves you time and footwork.*

Implementation Steps

Before Going to the Patient's Room

1. *Safety: Wash hands and apply clean examination gloves to protect you from contact with blood-borne pathogens.*

2. Inspect the blood administration Y-set package for intactness and expiration dates *to ensure continued sterility.* Remove the Y-set from the package.

3. Close the clamps on both of the Y-shaped branches of the blood administration set *to prevent premature dripping of solution.* Label the tubing with date and time.

4. Remove the cap from one of the piercing pins and, *to prevent contamination,* aseptically spike the NS container port. *Safety: Use only 0.9% sodium chloride as companion to blood and blood products, due to incompatibility of all other solutions.*

5. Prime the entire Y-set with the NS solution. *Priming the Y-set removes air from the tubing.*
   a. Begin by back-priming the branch of tubing that will insert into the blood product container. This is done by opening the clamp to the NS and priming the long tail of the tubing that will eventually connect to the patient's IV cannula.
   b. Now close the main roller clamp on the long tail of the tubing and proceed with back-priming the second branch of the Y-set that is going to be inserted into the blood product container. Open the roller clamp on the second branch of the Y-set. This will allow NS to flow from the NS branch through the Y-set into the blood branch. As soon as all air in the blood branch of the Y-set has been replaced with NS, close the roller clamp.
   c. Remove the cap from the piercing pin and aseptically spike the blood product container.
      • If the unit to be transfused is PRBCs, NS will need to be back-primed into the unit of PRBCs to dilute it to a consistency that will infuse through the Y-set and cannula. Open the roller clamp and allow NS to flow into the unit of PRBCs until the desired dilution is attained. Close the roller clamp.
      • After you close the roller clamp, it should remain closed while you initiate the flow of NS. The roller clamp on the blood product side of the Y-set is not to be opened again until you are ready to start the transfusion. *The blood product is not infused until the NS has been initiated.*

After Entering the Patient's Room

6. Follow the Initial Implementation Steps located on the inside front cover.

7. Use two methods of identifying the patient according to facility policy *to reduce the risk of error.*

8. Explain to the patient what you are about to do. Provide any necessary patient teaching. *This reduces patient anxiety and increases patient compliance.*

9. *Safety: Wash hands to prevent cross-contamination.*

10. Aseptically connect the NS-primed Y-set to the IV cannula in the patient's vein.

11. Open only the clamp to the NS and set it to infuse at TKO rate or as dictated by facility policy.

12. Assess the patient's vital signs. Report any abnormal results to the physician *prior to starting the blood transfusion.*

13. If vital signs are normal, close the NS roller clamp and open the blood roller clamp. Start the transfusion at a rate of 2 to 5 mL/min for the first 15 minutes

(skill continues on page 962)

Skill 38-9 (continued)

and according to facility policy. *The initial slower rate of infusion limits the volume of blood infused should the patient have a reaction within the first 15 minutes.*

14. Remain with the patient for the first 15 minutes *to assess for reactions.* Assess vital signs every 5 minutes during this time. Monitor for signs and symptoms of reactions. If any are experienced, stop the transfusion immediately, open the roller clamp to begin infusion of NS, perform appropriate nursing interventions (refer back to Table 38-4), and notify the physician stat. Save the Y-set tubing, the unit of blood, and the bag of NS *for return to the laboratory for testing.* Leave the Y-set attached to the blood bag and NS. Also obtain a urine specimen from the patient and deliver it to the laboratory.

15. If there are no signs or symptoms of reaction, increase the rate of infusion so that the transfusion will complete within a 2- to 4-hour window according to facility policy and patient's ability to tolerate rapid infusion of blood. Do not allow blood to hang longer than 4 hours.

16. Remove and dispose of contaminated gloves. Then wash hands *to reduce microorganisms.*

17. Assess the patient's vital signs every 30 minutes during the remainder of transfusion time, or more often if facility policy dictates.

18. At completion of the blood transfusion, reapply clean gloves and close the blood clamp. Open the NS clamp and flush the line *to ensure that the patient receives any blood product that might remain in the line.*

19. Once the line has been flushed with NS, the IV site is maintained at TKO rate until it is determined that no further blood transfusion will be administered.

20. Some facilities require that the empty blood bag be returned to the laboratory even when there were no problems during transfusion.

21. After you have completed nursing care requiring contact with the blood bag and Y-set, remove and dispose of contaminated gloves.

22. Assess one final set of vital signs.

23. Wash hands *to prevent cross-contamination.*

24. Follow the Ending Implementation Steps located on the inside back cover.

25. Document the transfusion procedure, including all assessment findings, any reactions experienced, vital signs, volume infused, time the transfusion was completed, and patient's condition post-transfusion.

Evaluation Steps

1. Evaluate the patient's tolerance of the transfusion throughout the entire infusion.

Sample Documentation

4-6-11   1730   *Awake & alert. No C/O of pain, nausea, or discomfort. Skin pink, warm, & dry. IV Saline lock with 20-G cannula intact in left forearm, site without erythema or edema. Teaching done RE: blood transfusion procedure. States she has had numerous transfusions in the past and has no questions or concerns. Informed consent signed earlier and in the medical record.* ———
——————————— *Nurse's signature and credentials*

4-6-11   1755   *Physician's order, plasma component, Pt. ID band, Type & Crossmatch results, Unit of plasma type, Rh factor, and ID number, plasma expiration date of 4-7-11, all checked by me and L. Cook, RN. Blood transfusion record completed and signed by Cook and Me.* ——— *Nurse's signature and credentials*
1757   *I concur with the above entry.* ———
——————————— *Nurse Cook's signature and credentials*

4-6-11   1800   *NS infusion initiated via 20-G cannula. BP 116/68, T – 98° F orally, AP – 73 reg & distinct, R – 19 reg & even. 1810 First unit, 250 mL of A + plasma, ID#329776105, began per gravity flow, infusing at 2 mL/min.* ———
——————————— *Nurse's signature and credentials*

4-6-11   1815   *BP – 118/72, T – 98° F, P – 76, R – 21. No C/O voiced.* ——— *Nurse's signature and credentials*
4-6-11   1820   *BP – 122/66, T – 98.2° F, P – 69, R – 22. No C/O voiced.* ——— *Nurse's signature and credentials*
4-6-11   1825   *BP – 118/70, T – 98.2° F, P – 73, R – 20. No C/O voiced. Rate of plasma infusion increased to 125 mL/hr.* ———
——————————— *Nurse's signature and credentials*

4-6-11   1855   *BP – 122/72, T – 98.4° F, P – 78, R – 21. No C/O voiced. IV site intact, no erythema or edema. Still infusing at 125 mL/hr. No S&S of reaction.* ———
——————————— *Nurse's signature and credentials*

4-6-11   1940   *BP – 124/74, T – 98.4° F, P – 74, R – 22. No C/O voiced. IV site intact, no erythema or edema. Still at 125 mL/hr. No S&S of reaction.* ——— *Nurse's signature and credentials*

4-6-11   2015   *Transfusion completed. NS started & infusing TKO. IV site intact, no erythema or edema. BP – 124/70, T – 98.4° F, P – 73, R – 22.* ———
——————————— *Nurse's signature and credentials*

Post Conference

Your experiences today were very valuable in helping you learn about IV therapy. You did have to discontinue your patient's current IV and start a new one. His veins were fragile, and you learned the value of not using a tourniquet the second time you attempted to initiate IV therapy. You were successful that time and were able to re-establish his IV fluids. Your patient began to have some complications of hypotonic solution infusion, which you recognized because you had studied your chapter carefully. You reported them immediately to your instructor, who then notified the charge nurse. The physician decreased the rate of infusion and changed the IV fluid to normal saline to prevent further problems.

KEY POINTS

- Purposes of IV therapy include providing daily body fluid and electrolytes, replacing abnormal loss of fluids and electrolytes, and providing IV administration of medications.

- Medications and IV solutions mixed or administered at the same time must be compatible.

- Movement of excessive volumes of fluid from the vascular space into the interstitial spaces is known as third-space shifting, which lowers BP and causes edema and swelling of individual cells.

- It is important for you to understand the differences between isotonic, hypotonic, and hypertonic fluids and when each is appropriate for use.

- Strict aseptic technique must be utilized during preparation of supplies, initiation of IV access, and maintenance of IV therapy.

- Infusion rate is calculated by multiplying the volume times the drop factor; dividing the total by the time in minutes. Gravity flow is measured by gtts/min. Pump flow is measured in mL/hr.

- The best veins to consider for IV therapy are the cephalic vein, basilic vein, median cubital vein, and accessory cephalic vein.

- Never stick a patient more than twice before seeking the assistance of another nurse.

- Complications of IV therapy include infiltration, extravasation, phlebitis, thrombophlebitis, localized infection, septicemia, severed cannula, air embolism circulatory fluid overload, and speed shock.

- The classic signs and symptoms of infiltration include edema; cool, pale, or taut skin; absence of blood return; sluggish flow or lack of infusion; site discomfort; and blanching of skin.

- The classic signs and symptoms of phlebitis include erythema, edema, increased warmth of skin, sluggish infusion rate, cord-like vein, and burning or discomfort.

- Extravasation requires immediate intervention to reduce the amount of tissue damage.

- Informed consent is required for blood product transfusion.

- Vital signs must be monitored closely along with other signs and symptoms of reactions during blood product transfusion.

- Blood products are compatible ONLY with 0.9% sodium chloride.

- A type and crossmatch test must be performed prior to blood or blood component transfusion.

- Two nurses must check and confirm that the blood component matches the physician's order, the correct blood type and Rh factor, the patient name and ID number, that the blood unit ID number matches those on the transfusion record, and the blood's expiration date. Both must sign the documentation.

REVIEW QUESTIONS

Select the answer that is most appropriate for each of the following questions. Some questions may have more than one correct answer. Check all that apply.

1. The minimum length of time that is safe for administration of IV push medication is:

a. 1 hour.

b. 30 seconds.

c. 5 minutes.

d. the amount of time designated by the medication manufacturer.

e. 1 minute per 1 milligram.

2. The difference(s) between a primary IV administration set and a secondary IVPB administration set include(s) which of the following?

   a. The secondary IVPB administration set is used for administering IV push medication.

   b. The primary IV administration set always has a drop factor of 60.

   c. The primary IV administration set is longer than the secondary IVPB administration set.

   d. The secondary IVPB administration set has a drip chamber for visualizing the drip rate, while the primary administration set does not.

   e. There is no difference except the drop factor.

3. If set up correctly, through which of the following could you directly administer an intermittent infusion of medication?

   a. Secondary IVPB administration set

   b. PRN lock

   c. Primary IV administration set

   d. Y-set blood tubing

4. Which of the following strengths of heparin could you use for flushing a PRN lock?

   a. 1,000 units/mL

   b. 10 units/mL

   c. 5,000 units/mL

   d. 10,000 units/mL

   e. 100 units/mL

5. Which of the following preparations should be performed at the bedside?

   a. Mixing of IV medication

   b. Verification of physician's IV order with MAR

   c. Site selection

   d. Priming primary IV administration set

   e. Calculation of infusion rate for gravity flow

6. If an IV order says to infuse 1,000 mL of fluid at the rate of 125 mL/hr, how many hours will it take to complete the infusion?

   a. 8 hours

   b. 6 hours

   c. 12 hours

   d. 10 hours

   e. 125 hours

7. Hypovolemia refers to a condition resulting from:

   a. dehydration caused by loss of intracellular and extracellular fluids.

   b. water losses that are greater than electrolyte losses.

   c. excessive loss of equal proportions of extracellular fluid and electrolytes.

   d. excessive loss of electrolytes in greater proportions than the loss of fluids.

SHORT ANSWER QUESTIONS

8. List at least five situations or conditions that might place a patient in need of IV access or infusion of IV fluids.

9. What substances can be administered through routine peripheral IV infusion? List at least three.

10. Does it take fewer macro-drops than micro-drops to equal 1 mL of solution? Explain your answer.

CRITICAL THINKING EXERCISES

11. Describe what you should do if your patient rings the call light and says, "My IV is not dripping anymore and the pump alarm is going off."

    For Questions 12-14: Calculate the rate of infusion or length of time it will take to complete the infusion for each of the following scenarios.

12. The physician's order says to infuse 1,000 mL D5W at 125 mL/hr. You must infuse the solution by gravity, because all the IV pumps are in use at this time. The drop factor on the primary administration set is 15 gtts/mL. How many gtts/minute will you set the solution to infuse?

13. You know that the physician has ordered dextrose 5% in 0.45% sodium chloride 1,000 mL to infuse over the next 10 hours. If you use an IV pump, at what rate will you set the pump?

14. The patient asks you how long it will take her bag of IV solution to complete its infusion. The size of the bag is 500 mL. The rate of infusion is 80 mL/hr. What do you tell her?

ADDITIONAL RESOURCES

For additional Resources, Questions, and Activities, please see:

 Student Resource Disk

http://davisplus.fadavis.com

 Student Study Guide

REFERENCES

David K. IV fluids: do you know what's hanging and why? *RN.* 2007;70(10):35-40.

Etzel-Hardman D. Teaching IV therapy to pediatric nurses: specialized training programs alleviate pain for both patients and practitioners. *RN.* 2008;71(11):24-28.

Hadaway L. Emergency infiltration and extravasation. *Am J Nurs.* 2007;107(8):64-72.

Hadaway LC. I.V. rounds: Managing vascular access device occlusions, part I. *Nursing2009.* 2009;39(1):10.

I.V. Essentials: Complications of peripheral IV therapy. *Nurs Made Incredibly Easy.* 2008;6(1):14-18.

LPN Expert Guides: I.V. Therapy. Philadelphia: Lippincott Williams & Wilkins; 2006.

Ludeman K. I.V. essentials: Which vascular access device is right for your patient? *Nurs Made Incredibly Easy.* 2008;6(4):7-11.

Phillips LD. *Manual of IV Therapeutics.* 5th ed. Philadelphia: FA Davis; 2010.

Polovich M, White JM, Kelleher LO, eds. *Chemotherapy and Biotherapy Guidelines and Recommendations for Practice.* 2nd ed. Pittsburgh: Oncology Nursing Society; 2005.

Rhoads J, Meeker BJ. *Davis's Guide to Clinical Nursing Skills.* Philadelphia: FA Davis; 2008.

Rosenthal K. Intravenous fluids: the whys and wherefores. *Nursing2006.* 2006;36(7):26-27.

Scanlon V, Sanders T. *Essentials of Anatomy and Physiology.* 5th ed. Philadelphia: FA Davis; 2007.

Venes D, ed. *Taber's Cyclopedic Medical Dictionary.* 21st ed. Philadelphia: FA Davis; 2009.

Wilkinson JM, Van Leuven K. *Fundamentals of Nursing: Theory, Concepts & Applications.* Philadelphia: FA Davis; 2007.

Williams LS, Hopper PD. *Understanding Medical Surgical Nursing,* 3rd ed. Philadelphia: FA Davis; 2007.

Answers to Review Questions

Chapter 1. The Vista of Nursing

1. b
2. c
3. d
4. b
5. a
6. c
7.
   a. Registered Nurse, Associate Degree
   b. Masters of Science in Nursing
   c. Licensed Practical/Vocational Nurse
   d. Registered Nurse, Baccalaureate Degree
   e. Registered Nurse, Diploma Program
8. Inform the instructor immediately, no matter how difficult or embarrassing it may be for you. Be prepared to follow through by notifying the charge nurse and the physician.
9. While nurses in today's world are responsible for a great deal of technical and scientific knowledge, the personal touch in nursing cannot be negated. Nursing is a blend of both art and science, requiring thinking <u>and</u> caring people to work with all aspects of a patient's needs.

Chapter 2. Health Care Delivery and Economics

1. b, d
2. c
3. a
4. d
5. b
6. a
7. c
8. a, c
9. Make an appointment with the PCP to evaluate the skin condition. If the PCP is unable to treat it, then he or she will give the patient a referral to see a specialist.

10. Responses should include the following points:
    • Various scenarios can occur where people are working and still do not have health insurance
    • The focus of all nurses is on caring for the patient, not on how their bill is paid

Chapter 3. Nursing Ethics and Law

1. a, b, d, e
2. a, b, c, d, e, f
3. a
4. c, e, f
5. Protect the public's health, safety, and welfare from harm related to nursing care
6. It was not done.
7. Negligence
8. Court order
   Marriage
   History of living independently and being self-supporting
   Service in the military
9. You must notify the physician.
10. You are responsible for explaining the importance of remaining under the physician's care. If Mr. Jones still wants to leave, then ask him to sign a Leaving Against Medical Advice (AMA) form.

Chapter 4. The Nursing Process and Decision Making

1. a, b, c, d, e
2. b, d
3. d
4. b
5. Answers will vary, but *dependent* should be an example of an intervention requiring a health care provider's order, such as diet, activity, medications. *Independent* should be a nursing action that does not require an order,

such as intake and output. *Collaborative* should include interventions in which health care professionals work together, such as with a physical or respiratory therapist.
6. Assessment, Diagnosis, Planning, Implementation, Evaluation
7. *Participates in:* Implementation, Evaluation. *Contributes to:* Assessment, Diagnosis, Planning

8. Any two of the following:
   Nausea
   Deficient fluid volume
   Readiness for enhanced fluid balance
   Nutrition: less than body requirements
9. Any two of these:

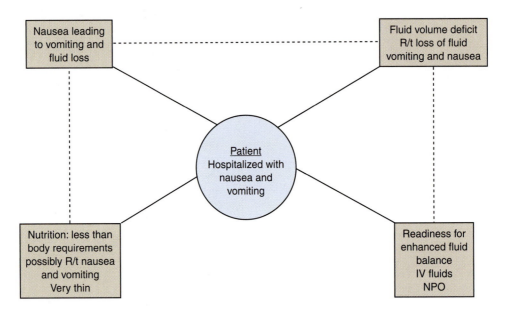

Chapter 5. Documentation

1. c, e
2. b
3. a, c, d, f

4. b, d
5. c, d, e

Table A-1

Section of Source-Oriented Record		Data Found in Record Sections
6. Graphic Data	j	a. nurse's physical assessment data
		b. physician's physical assessment data
7. Admission Record	i	c. respiratory therapy treatment notes
		d. patient's response to initiation of IV infusion
8. Nurse's Notes	a, d, f, j	e. notation of strength training exercise session
		f. voiced patient complaint
9. Advance Directive	g	g. living will
		h. report of chest x-ray results
10. Rehabilitation Therapy	c, e	i. consent for treatment
		j. 0800 vital sign results

11. The answer should be succinct, without unnecessary words such as: the, is, you. The word "patient" should be avoided. Should include date, time, name, credentials. The entry should be organized and sequential. It should be similar to the following example:

8-12-11 1330 IV initiated in Rt. dorsal forearm with 20-G intracath, one attempt. D5W 1000 ml infusing at 80 mL/hr per pump. Site without edema or erythema. Instructed to call for assistance before getting up to prevent injury trying to move IV pole & pump. Verbally acknowledged understanding. Bed left in low position. Brakes locked. 2 rails at head of bed raised. ────────────
─────────────────────────── R. Reherman, RN

12.

Stelling, Lindsey #0621199 Rm. 758 BD 6-11-86 Admit 8-9-12		Mission Regional Hospital
Date	Time	*Nurse's Notes*
8-11-12	*1115*	*P - #3 --*
		I - Tylenol 650 mg given po for T-102.4°F. Cool cloth applied
		to brow & neck.--------------------------------S. May, LPN
	1255	*E - Supine with eyes closed. Snoring softly. Face no longer*
		flushed. Skin warm and damp. Awakened to voice. Denies
		restlessness. States aching is decreasing. T - 100.2°F.
		P - 84 reg & strong. Pillow case & top sheet changed.
		--S. May, LPN

13.

Stelling, Lindsey #0621199 Rm. 758 BD 6-11-86 Admit 8-9-12		Mission Regional Hospital
Date	Time	*Nurse's Notes*
8-11-12	*1115*	*S - C/O aching & restlessness. -----------------------------*
		O - T - 102.4, P - 104 strong & irr. Face & neck flushed.
		Skin hot & dry.---
		A - Fever and discomfort.------------------------------
		P - Monitor temp within 90 min. after PRN Tylenol
		administered. -------------------------------------
		I - Tylenol 650 mg given po for T - 102.4°F orally. Cool cloth
		applied to brow & neck.----------------------S. May, LPN
	1255	*E - Supine with eyes closed. Snoring softly. No longer*
		flushed. Awakened to voice. T - 100.2°F. Skin warm &
		damp. Denies restlessness. States achiness decreasing.
		Top sheet & pillow case changed. ---------------------
		R - None required.------------------------------S. May, LPN

14.

Stelling, Lindsey #0621199 Rm. 758 BD 6-11-86 Admit 8-9-12		Mission Regional Hospital
Date	Time	*Nurse's Notes*
8-11-12	*1115*	*C/O aching & restlessness. Skin flushed, hot & dry. T - 102.4°F*
		oral. P - 104, irr & strong. Tylenol 650 mg given po. Cool cloth
		applied to brow and neck. -------------------S. May, LPN
	1255	*Supine with eyes closed. Snoring softly. No longer flushed.*
		Awakened to voice. T - 100.2°F orally. P - 84 irr & strong.
		Denies - achiness or restlessness. Skin warm & damp. Pillow-
		case & top sheet changed. -------------------S. May, LPN

Chapter 6. Communication and Relationships

1. d

2. a, b, c, d

3. b, d

4. d

5. a, c, d

6. b, d

7. c

8. a, b, c, d

9. Speak slowly and use short sentences when you are talking to Mrs. Jones. Watch her facial expressions and gestures for clues as to what she is trying to communicate. Show respect and caring, always speaking in a normal tone of voice. Ask her to point to what she wants. Give limited choices, such as "Would you like to wear your red robe or your sweater?"

Chapter 7. Promoting Health and Wellness

1. a, b, d
2. b
3. a, b, c, d
4. F
5. F
6. F
7. T
8. F
9. The physiological response would be the same. Your brain engages the sympathetic nervous system, which stimulates the endocrine glands to pump cortisol, adrenaline, and other hormones into the bloodstream, enabling you to hit harder, jump higher, see farther, and think or run faster. These hormones cause the bronchial airways to dilate and the respiratory rate to rise, both helping to increase oxygen intake. The hormones also cause the heart rate to increase, blood vessels in the skin to constrict, and central blood vessels to dilate, in an effort to deliver more oxygen-rich blood to the brain, heart, and muscles needed for the fight or flight response. Glycogen is converted to glucose to provide additional fuel and energy. The pupils of the eyes dilate to allow better vision. The sense of hearing is heightened to detect warning sounds. Salivary glands decrease their secretions and peristalsis slows in the digestive track in order to prevent the need for bowel elimination during this "emergency" or high-stress time. Arm and leg muscles tense in preparation for running or physical fighting. When the threat is removed, the parasympathetic nervous system dominates and reverses these responses.

Chapter 8. Ethnic, Cultural, and Spiritual Aspects of Care

1. c
2. c
3. d
4. a
5. d
6. b
7. b, d, f, h
8. e
9. T
10. T
11. F
12. Demonstrated barriers to health care in this situation include stereotyping, prejudice, and discrimination. To improve the situation, the nurse may use therapeutic communication, remain unbiased, avoid taking the patient's response personally, and provide presence. If the nurse is unable to calm the patient and talk with him, she could explain that she has his pain medication and ask him if he would prefer another nurse to provide his care.
13. Mr. Miller might want his family with him for support in case the diagnosis or prognosis may indicate any disability (feared more than death). Families are close-knit. The decision about surgery most likely would be made by the husband and wife, but possibly by the entire family and maybe even the church or community members. Financial considerations may include the amount of community resources that are available to pay for the surgery, and whether the surgery will provide complete restoration of health or not. They believe in rationing money spent on care toward the end of life and do not want to waste any more of community resources if the surgery isn't going to be curative.

Chapter 9. Growth and Development Throughout the Life Span

1. b
2. d
3. c
4. a
5. a, c, d
6. B
7. S
8. E
9. The child is frustrated by a loss of control over his environment. You could remove the medication from the room and attempt to quiet the child. Speak in a calm, controlled voice and offer comfort with a stuffed animal or blanket. Explain that you have to give the child the medication but that, after you do so, you will play a game or read a book to him. Engage the assistance of the parents if possible.
10. You can give the patient the opportunity to talk about her concerns for her son and her parents. You can help her sort through some options for ways to get help for her parents while she is hospitalized, including other family members, friends, and community groups. You can also help her to see that her stress over her family responsibilities could be contributing to her own illness.

Chapter 10. Loss, Grief, and Dying

1. a, b, c, e, f
2. b
3. d
4. b
5. c
6. b
7. c
8. a, c
9. b, b, b, b, a, a
10. b, c, d, e, f
11. Your answer should have included between three and four of the following concepts:
    - Multiple disease processes
    - Original intent of CPR techniques
    - CPR as a violation of patient's right to die with dignity
    - Patient advocacy
    - Survival rates for the frail and chronically ill
    - Burdens of CPR
    - Chain of events put into motion with CPR
    - Who can make the choice for DNR
    - Assurance of care that will be given (airway maintenance, pain control and other symptom management)
12. Your answer should have included the following concepts:
    - Hunger in the healthy person
    - Comforting aspects of dehydration
    - Burdens of full hydration
    - Increased pain
    - Edema
    - Pulmonary edema
    - Death rattle
    - Increased frequency of urination and defecation
    - Repositioning necessary for bathing associated with incontinence
    - Decreased need for food and fluids

Chapter 11. Complementary and Alternative Medicine

1. b
2. f
3. c
4. a
5. b, c, e, f, i
6. functional change; chronic illness
7. Acupuncture/acupressure
8. A history of blood clots in the legs or lungs, a cancerous tumor that has not been removed, certain heart conditions, and in some types of massage, severe osteoporosis
9. Ask if the herbal blend contains Echinacea since it can increase the effectiveness of warfarin and cause excessive bleeding. Ask what other herbs are in the blend in case there are other herbs that could interact with her prescription medications. Educate her about the interactions of warfarin with Echinacea and feverfew, as well as any other herb-drug interactions that could affect her. Encourage her to keep her physician informed about any herbal supplements she may be taking.

Chapter 12. Patient Teaching

1. d
2. d
3. a, b, c, e, f
4. a
5. a
6. b
7. The patient may be in denial about her own illness and therefore not ready to learn how to use the glucometer. She also may feel that you did not assess her level of knowledge before you began teaching and are not giving her credit for what she knows.
8. "Deficient knowledge related to high blood pressure manifested by a lack of awareness of cardiac complications"
9. It might be helpful to ask the patient to tell you what he has learned about his disease and treatment. As he tells you, you can make notes of any misinformation or misinterpretation of information that you hear. Then you can praise him for what he does know and gently correct any misinformation. You could also ask about the web sites he used and, if need be, steer him toward more reliable sites.

Chapter 13. Safety

1. b
2. c
3. a
4. d
5. a
6. d
7. b
8. Explain that patients may fall or injure themselves if they do not get help promptly. They may try to get up and walk alone when it is unsafe for them to do so.
9. Call your place of work and ask if you are needed either there or at another location as a volunteer.
10. You would first determine if fall precautions were in use. Was this patient identified as a fall risk? If not, why not? If precautions were in use, how did the fall occur? Could it have been prevented? If so, how?

Chapter 14. Medical Asepsis and Infection Control

1. d
2. b

3. c

4. a, d, e, f

5. a

6. You would explain the reason for the use of PPE, and re-assure the patient that he is not considered unclean because of his illness. Show that you respect and value him even though PPE is necessary when entering the room. Offer to spend extra time with the patient, and to bring him diversionary activities such as newspapers, magazines, and puzzle books.

7. Rest is needed for the immune system to repair damage and function at full capacity. Without it, the chance for developing infection increases.

8. Any answer that includes an appropriate illustration and all the links in the chain of infection is acceptable. The links are: infectious agent, reservoir, portal of exit, mode of transmission, portal of entry, and susceptible host.

9. Mask, goggles, gown, and gloves

Chapter 15. Personal Care

1. b

2. d

3. a, d, e, g, h

4. a, c, e

5. a

6. Make a surgical bed for easy stretcher access. Position the bed in reverse Trendelenburg so the patient's head is up but the leg is straight.

7. Make and use a padded tongue blade turned to hold the mouth open during mouth care.

8. Check for perfumed room deodorizer spray; check for staff or visitors wearing perfume, cologne, or aftershave.

9. Explain that differences in culture influence people's bathing preferences, and that not all women shave their legs and armpits. Ask the patient for permission for the CNA to assist with the bath. Determine if she would prefer that a family member be present during the bath. Ask the patient's usual frequency of bathing and explain any necessity for more frequent bathing while in the hospital.

Chapter 16. Moving and Positioning Patients

1. c, e

2. d: 1, c: 2, f: 3, a: 4; e: 5, b: 6

3. a, c, e

4. d

5. a

6. 2: a, c, d, e

7. a, c, f

8. Follow the physician's orders for ambulation, even if the patient feels like walking further. It is important to slowly increase the distance, keeping in mind that the patient has to ambulate back to her room as well as make it to the end of the hall.

9. Lower the patient down your leg to the floor. Call for help. Prepare to perform CPR if no pulse or respirations are present. Check vital signs. Do not leave the patient alone. Obtain a lift to return her to bed after she has regained consciousness.

Chapter 17. Vital Signs

1. b, d, e

2. c, d

3. a, d

4. c

5. d

6. Rate, rhythm, and volume or strength

7. Use a pain scale such as 0 to 10, with 0 being no pain and 10 being the worst pain the patient has experienced. Ask for descriptors such as sharp, stabbing, cramping, continuous, intermittent, dull, and aching. Assess the location of pain and what if anything set it off.

8. Systolic pressure is the measurement of the force exerted by the blood against the walls of arteries during contraction of the heart. This is when the pressure is the highest. Diastolic pressure is the measurement of the pressure exerted by the blood on the artery walls while the heart is not contracting, which is the lower of the two pressures. During diastole the ventricles are at rest.

9. Assess the patient's BP lying supine. Then have the patient arise to a sitting position, wait for 1 minute, then assess BP while sitting. Then have the patient arise to a standing position, wait for 1 minute, then assess BP while standing. Record all three BPs with corresponding positions.

10. Irregular pulse rate, high or low BP, weak or thready pulse, capillary refill longer than 3 seconds in an adult or 5 seconds in an older adult, nonpalpable pulse, pale or cold extremities

Chapter 18. Applying Heat and Cold

1. d

2. a, c, d

3. a

4. b, e, f

5. b, c, d

6. Whether the physician wants it to be dry or moist, temperature setting, length of time to leave on the heat application

7. It widens the vessel lumen diameter so more blood flow will be delivered to the site, providing more oxygen and nutrients to support healing. It also delivers more white blood cells to help fight infection.

8. Assess the patient's age and cognitive level of function, orientation, sedation, sensory impairment, and impairment

of circulation to determine if there are any contraindications. Assess the site where heat is to be applied, noting the appearance, color, presence of edema, temperature of site and surrounding skin, integrity of skin, and any discomfort. This provides a baseline against which you can measure the effects of the application. Continue to reassess skin every 10 to 15 minutes, inquiring of the patient about discomfort. After removing the heat pack, assess the site for objective data such as color, temperature, and edema. Assess the subjective data related to effectiveness of the heat application by inquiring of the patient about any change in discomfort/comfort level at the site.

9. You should tell him that applying heat at this stage of recovery will increase the swelling even more. Explain that ice will help prevent further swelling, but to avoid use of heat until the swelling stops increasing.

Chapter 19. Pain Management, Rest, and Restorative Sleep

1. a, b, e
2. c
3. a
4. d
5. Phantom
6. NSAID
7. Five of the following should be included: ethnic and cultural beliefs, developmental stage, individual values, previous pain experiences, personal support system, emotions, and fatigue.
8. The brain works to repair the minute injuries to the body, mind, and emotions that occur as part of the natural wear and tear of daily living, including such things as cellular repair and synthesis of protein. The brain also works to heal and repair the damages of illness and trauma, and to restore the body to optimum health.
9. NREM Sleep:

Stage I: Relaxation begins during this stage. It is the period of lightest sleep, where one is easily aroused and lasts a few minutes. The metabolism and vital signs begin to slow. If awakened, the patient feels as if he or she has been daydreaming.

Stage II: Relaxation continues; sleep becomes more sound and lasts 10 to 20 minutes. Arousal is still relatively easy as the metabolism continues to slow.

Stage III: Muscles are completely relaxed and the body becomes immobile. This is the beginning of deep sleep, making arousal more difficult. The parasympathetic nervous system slows the vital signs; this stage lasts 15 to 30 minutes.

Stage IV: The deepest level of sleep that rests and restores the body. The patient is very difficult to arouse; this stage lasts 15 to 30 minutes. If the patient is sleep deprived, he or she will spend more time in stage IV. The eyes are still, but the patient may dream during this stage.

REM Sleep: REM sleep occurs at end of each NREM cycle and does not serve to be as restful as NREM. The first cycle occurs about 90 minutes after sleep begins. The patient has rapid eye movement and fluctuating vital signs. Vivid dreams occur and may be remembered. The brain is very active. The duration increases with each cycle, averaging 20 minutes.

10. Modify the room temperature to the patient's preference. Provide blankets and pillows. Turn on a night-light or provide dim lighting. Offer a snack or cup of warm milk. Straighten and remove wrinkles in the patient's gown and bed linens, reposition the patient, and provide support with pillows. Administer a back massage. Sit with the patient and listen to his concerns about his cat. Be an active listener. Validate his feelings. Play soft, relaxing music.

Chapter 20. Admission, Transfer, and Discharge

1. b, d, e, f, g
2. a, b, c, d, e, f
3. b
4. b
5. a, b, f, g
6. b, c, d, f
7. The Joint Commission
8. On the day of admission or shortly thereafter.
9. Name, room number, hospital identification number, age, birthdate, physician's name
10. Knock
11. Telephone the receiving facility to report the impending transmission so the appropriate personnel can receive the fax.
12. Smile and greet the child and the parent in a calm and somewhat quiet voice. Take your time approaching the child. If possible, allow the parent to hold the child. If the child has brought a toy or book from home, comment on the toy or book to draw the child's attention away from you to something pleasant that he or she is familiar. Allow the child to handle your stethoscope and listen to mom's heart before trying to listen to the child.
13. Avoid using terms other than what you can see objectively, such as "white metal ring, with 1 clear stone and 6 green stones." The stones may not be real diamonds and emeralds and the metal may not be gold. The hospital would be liable for replacing them with real gems should the ring be lost. Or the patient could claim that the "real" gems had been replaced with fake ones, again holding the hospital liable.

Chapter 21. Physical Assessment

1. a, c, e, f, g, k
2. b
3. d

4. c

5. b

6. c

7. e

8. Inquire about nausea, vomiting, indigestion, gas or flatus, or anorexia; edentulous or missing teeth; shape of abdomen, whether abdomen is firm or soft, tenderness upon palpation; bowel sounds; time of last BM, color, amount, & consistency of stools; cramping or pain

9. General appearance, position of patient, does patient appear to be comfortable, snoring, ease of breathing, shortness of breath, use of accessory respiratory muscles, affect, skin color, response to verbal stimuli, picking at covers, fidgeting, relaxed, watching TV, unkempt, visiting with guests, talking on phone, mood or emotional tone, smiling, frowning, coughing, movement of extremities, eye contact, wide-eyed, eyes darting about, splinting, moaning, jugular vein distention, speech

10. A sign is objective, and can be observed by the nurse. A symptom is subjective, cannot be observed by the nurse, and can only be reported by the patient or family.

11. Cardiovascular, respiratory, integumentary, nervous, muscular, skeletal, digestive, and genitourinary; also provides some information on the immune system

12. The two systems are directly related to each other. Many assessments of one system will also relate data regarding the other system. Some examples include: Assessment of heart rate can also provide data related to the respiratory system. A faster heart rate will be seen with respiratory distress and a lower SpO_2 level. Assessment of hydration and intravascular fluid level in the cardiovascular system can also provide data related to the respiratory system. If the neck veins are distended, there may be fluid or congestion in the lungs. Full, bounding pulses can also direct you to assess for adventitious sounds in the lungs. If peripheral pulses are strong in all four extremities and capillary refill time is brisk, but cyanosis is present in the feet, it reflects impaired function of the respiratory system rather than the cardiovascular system. Severe congestion in the lungs may be a direct result of impaired cardiac output. An increased respiratory rate will usually result in a faster heart rate.

Chapter 22. Surgical Asepsis

1. a

2. c

3. a, c

4. a, c, f, g

5. b

6. d

7. Report what you saw to the circulating nurse. Even if a physician breaks technique, it is important that it be recognized and corrected for the safety and protection of the patient.

8. The pathogens in the patient's home are those that the patient's body is used to fighting off. Hospitals have many more and stronger pathogens present, so surgical asepsis is a must in a hospital setting. At home, the patient may be able to use clean technique and still prevent infection.

9. Remove street clothes and put on hospital-laundered scrubs

   Don shoe covers, head cover, goggles (if needed), and mask

   Perform a surgical hand scrub

   Don a sterile surgical gown

   Don sterile gloves completely

   Enter operating room by backing through the door

Chapter 23. Nutrition

1. c

2. d

3. a

4. d

5. c, e

6. c

7. b

8. d

9. a

10. b

11. Mr. Baze should avoid processed foods such as pickles, canned vegetables, bologna, canned soups, wieners, and sausages. He should be taught to read food labels and look for foods labeled low sodium or sodium free.

12. Ms. Havner should be advised to go to *www.mypyramid. gov* to complete an online nutritional assessment. MyPyramid can be individualized and is interactive. She can also go to websites that end in .gov, .edu, or .org for science-based information.

Chapter 24. Nutritional Care and Support

1. d

2. c

3. d

4. d

5. b

6. c

7. a, b

8. a = 1st

   d = 2nd

9. Anorexia nervosa and bulimia nervosa. She seems to be obsessed with food, exercise, and her weight. The sore throat is possibly due to excessive vomiting, retching, and excoriation from gastric acid.

10. The care plan should include the priorities of maintaining a patent airway and prevention of aspiration through

positioning, use of a thickening agent, and five or six small feedings spread out over 24 hours to reduce the volume to be administered at any one time. The number of calories with the percentage of carbohydrate, protein, and fat needs should be calculated by a dietitian to determine the type and amount of foods that will best meet her nutritional requirements. It would be important to determine if she handles a pureed diet better than solids. A target goal of fluid intake should also be addressed in the care plan.

11. Probably clear liquids until diarrhea and nausea resolve. Then advance according to the patient's tolerance of each advancement. Higher percentages of calories and protein might be helpful in an attempt to regain some of his weight loss. Interventions should include those of monitoring I&O, frequency of BMs along with description of characteristics of stools, assessment of urine color, reassessment of bowel sounds every 4 hours, and assessment for abdominal distention or cramping.

12. Yes, you should re-instill the aspirate because it has electrolytes in it and is less than half of the previous feeding volume. This indicates that the formula is being adequately absorbed.

Chapter 25. Diagnostic Tests

1. a, d, f
2. c, d, e
3. a, c
4. a
5. a, b, d, e, f
6. b
7. d
8. b
9. Inform the patient that he or she will be asleep during the procedure and feel no discomfort. Assure the patient that the staff will do their best to provide privacy and protect the patient's modesty. After awakening after the examination, the patient will most likely be unable to remember anything about the procedure.
10. To decrease the patient's anxiety and fears and to increase the patient's ability to be compliant with examiner's requests and be more helpful, making the performance of the procedure easier to accomplish.

Chapter 26. Wound Care

1. b, c
2. b
3. b
4. e
5. c
6. c
7. a, c, d, e, g, h

8. a, b, d, e, g
9. a
10. Answers will vary but should include four of the following indicators:
    - Erythema is present around sutures, staples, and edges of wound.
    - Drainage is malodorous.
    - Drainage increases rather than decreses over successive days.
    - Patient has an elevated temperature and heart rate.
    - WBC count is elevated.
    - Patient complains of increasing rather than decreasing pain in days after wound repair.
    - You note open areas between the sutures or staples closing the wound.
11. Answers will vary, but should include one or both of the following:
    - When you begin to remove the staples, the wound edges begin to gap open.
    - Wound is not healed with edges completely approximated, so gaps are apparent before removing the staples.

Chapter 27. Musculoskeletal Care

1. c
2. a, b, c
3. a
4. b
5. d
6. b
7. c
8. It will heal in a squared-off shape and then not fit into the socket of a prosthetic arm later.
9. The muscles are pulled from their normal position, leading to muscle spasms, which are quite painful.
10. How is she walking with the crutches? How is she supporting her weight? How did the fall occur? Correct any misunderstandings about how to use the crutches.

Chapter 28. Respiratory Care

1. a, c, d, f
2. a
3. b
4. a, b, c
5. b
6. c
7. Take on the earlobe or forehead. Do not take time to remove nail polish.
8. Acidosis
9. Call for help. Elevate the head of the bed to facilitate chest expansion. Check the output in the chest tube for increase of more than 100 mL/hr or increase in bleeding, since these symptoms could indicate loss of blood and

hypoxia. Assess lung sounds for bilateral expansion in case of tension pneumothorax and notify physician.

10. You suspect possible crepitus and subcutaneous emphysema. You will palpate the edematous area for the typical feeling of crepitus, like crunching Rice Krispies under the skin. If present, you will notify the physician immediately since this indicates an air leak. If not present, you will assess the neck for signs of infection in the tracheostomy or surrounding tissue.

Chapter 29. Fluids, Electrolytes, and Acid-Base Balance

1. b, e
2. c, d, f
3. c
4. d
5. a
6. d
7. b
8. b
9. a
10. a
11. d
12. c
13. Ask if she has checked his weight. If not, have her do so. If he has gained 2 pounds or more, the patient is probably holding onto fluid because of his heart condition and should be asked to come in for an appointment with the doctor right away.

Chapter 30. Bowel Elimination and Care

1. b
2. a, d, f, g
3. c
4. b, c, d, f
5. b
6. a
7. a, b, d
8. d
9. Answer should include most of the following factors: age, general anesthetic, pain, dentures at home, edentulous diet (decreased fiber), bedrest preventing her normal physical activities, morphine sulfate.
10. It would be helpful to explain the A&P of the colon so that he will understand why this colostomy will not produce formed feces and cannot be trained to move at a certain time each day. He also needs to know about the different types of appliances and products that are available for use. He must be taught how to empty the appliance bag, how to measure the size of the stoma for selection of the correct faceplate and bag, how to apply the

faceplate and bag, skin care for the stoma and peristomal skin to avoid skin breakdown, and foods that may increase production of flatus. He should be referred to the local ostomy support group and introduced to at least one member of the group. He will need emotional support not only from the support group, but also from his closest family members. It is possible that, because his colostomy produces only liquid and mushy stools that cannot be regulated, he may suffer worse problems with self-esteem than if it were a trainable colostomy. Usually the closest family members are included in all the teaching sessions so they can understand how to provide colostomy care as well as how to support the patient emotionally.

Chapter 31. Urinary Elimination and Care

1. b, c, d
2. a: 2, b: 4, c: 3, d: 1, e: 5
3. b
4. a
5. a
6. c
7. a
8. Open the thumb clamp on the irrigation bag and increase the flow to irrigate out any clots that might be blocking the catheter openings. Observe the output and, as the urine becomes light pink again, decrease the irrigation rate.
9. Most UTIs occur because bacteria from bowel movements enters the urethra and moves into the bladder. Your urethra is located very close to the anus, so the bacteria does not have to travel very far. In addition, vaginal secretions are no longer as acidic as they were when you were younger, so they do not fight off invading bacteria as well as they did before.
10. What type of fluid does she drink? How much in a day? Does it contain caffeine? Does she take any medications with diuretic effects?

Chapter 32. Care of Elderly Patients

1. c
2. a
3. b
4. b
5. a
6. d
7. b
8. a, b, e, g, h, i, j
9. You can learn a great deal from the elderly: history, perspective, and wisdom are available if you take the time to listen and to learn. You can also benefit by having long-term relationships with residents, getting to know them on a deeper level than is possible in the acute care

setting. And, you can be the person who helps brighten their days by being a positive caregiver.

10. Your approach would be different for each of these age groups because their concerns may be different. For example, a young-old person may be able to perform most ADLs for himself or herself, while an old-old person may require more assistance. Each person is an individual, however, and age is not the primary factor in determining the amount of assistance a patient requires. No matter the age, you will assist all patients with their needs, whether they are physical, psychosocial, emotional, or spiritual.

11. You need to report your concerns. Find out as much as you can about the person and his or her business of investing money. Encourage your patient to ask for references. Check with the Better Business Bureau for complaints against this person. Discourage the patient from giving personal information to this person until he or she has been completely checked out and is proven not to be running a scam.

Chapter 33. Care of the Surgical Patient

1. c
2. b
3. a, d, e
4. c
5. a
6. Answer should reflect any six of the following:
   - Turning, coughing, and deep breathing exercises
   - Incentive spirometry
   - Early ambulation
   - Type of device to be used to stimulate venous return (antiembolism stockings, leg exercises, sequential compression devices)
   - Approximate time in operating room and recovery
   - Importance of asking for pain medication before the pain becomes severe
   - Importance of informing staff of nausea as soon as it is detected
   - Showing the family where to wait for the physician's report
   - Necessary preoperative preparations, procedures, or required laboratory or other tests:
     - Cessation of smoking 24 hours preoperatively, with option for nicotine patches
     - NPO status
     - Medications to stop before surgery
     - Skin or intestinal preparation
   - IV infusion, type of anesthesia
7. Answer should reflect any three of the following:
   - Leg and ankle exercises:
     - Ankle circles 10 times in each direction
     - Ankle pumps (flexion and extension) 10 times each
     - Flex and extend knees 10 times each

- BRP and ambulation as soon as allowed
- SCDs and TED hose, with physician order

8. Three purposes of administering preoperative medication might include any of the following: relief of preoperative anxiety, fear, apprehension, pain, or discomfort; decreasing production of gastric juices and preventing postoperative nausea and vomiting; preventing aspiration during anesthesia and recovery; increasing ease of anesthesia induction and decreasing amount of anesthesia requirements; providing a degree of postoperative amnesia; preventing risk of allergic reactions and development of blood clots; and decreasing the risk of infection in the surgical incision or in those patients with risk factors for bacterial endocarditis.

9. Primary responsibilities of the circulating nurse in surgery include the following:
   - Being the primary patient advocate, ensuring that the correct procedure is performed, ensuring that the patient's dignity and modesty are protected, consistently standing up for "what is best" for the patient
   - Obtaining supplies
   - Coordinating the surgical team
   - Calling for "time-out" before surgery; sponge and needle count at end of surgery
   - Observing patient condition from arrival in OR until he or she goes to PACU

10. Assessment findings that you might detect in a postoperative patient that could be cause for concern include:
    - Respiratory distress, possibly indicating airway blockage due to laryngeal edema, secretions, or tongue; shallow and irregular respirations or oxygen saturation levels below 95% could also indicate a reaction to anesthesia, pain medications, or a chronic respiratory condition. Could indicate a pulmonary embolus or atelectasis.
    - Elevated heart rate and decreased blood pressure, possibly indicating hemorrhage and shock.
    - Irregular heart rate or bradycardia, possibly indicating cardiac dysfunction, adverse medication or anesthesia reaction, central nervous system depression, or excessive analgesic administration.
    - Increased bleeding from the surgical wound site, possibly indicating external hemorrhage.
    - Rigid abdomen, possibly indicating internal hemorrhage.
    - Elevated temperature, possibly indicating infection; excessively elevated temperature could be indicative of malignant hyperthermia.
    - Subnormal temperature; may be due to extended exposure to cold environmental temperature in OR or anesthesia-induced hypothermia
    - Decreased level of consciousness, possibly indicating an adverse reaction to the anesthetic or increased intracranial pressure.

Chapter 34. Phlebotomy and Blood Specimens

1. b, d
2. b, c
3. d
4. a, d
5. a, e
6. d
7. F
8. F
9. T
10. T
11. F
12. Blood culture
13. Wipe it off.
14. Use correct size needle, between 20 G and 23 G for an adult; gently invert tubes after blood is drawn, do not shake them; if using a needle and syringe for draw, change to an 18-G or 20-G needle to instill blood into specimen tubes, pierce the rubber stopper at an angle, and allow it to run slowly down the sides of the tubes.

Chapter 35. Researching and Preparing Medications

1. d
2. a, c, d, e
3. b
4. c
5. a
6. b
7. a
8. The route by which the medication is to be administered
9. 12 mL
10. You would not leave the medications at the bedside. You are responsible for administering the medications that you prepare. While the medications sit unattended, they could be tampered with or be taken by someone else, such as the patient's roommate. You cannot delegate administering medications that you have prepared to another nurse, an assistant, or a patient's relative. You also need to perform the third safety check as you open and administer the medications.

Chapter 36. Administering Oral, Topical, and Mucosal Medications

1. d
2. c, d
3. a, b, c, d
4. b

5. a, b, c
6. a
7. b
8. c
9. Ask the patient to describe how the medication makes him feel. Explain that some side effects are often felt for the first few weeks of therapy, then subside. Explain the need for lowering his blood pressure and the consequences of sustained hypertension. Respect the patient's informed decision. Inform the prescriber of the patient's refusal and objections to the medicine. Document according to facility policy for a refused medicine; generally you will circle the time the medicine was to have been given and explain this in the nurse's notes.
10. If you administer the medicine through the nasogastric tube and then reconnect it to suction, the medicine will quickly be removed from the stomach. You will need to administer the medication, then keep the tube disconnected from the suction and clamped for 30 minutes. This will allow time for the medication to coat the ulcer prior to restarting the intermittent suction. You can then unclamp the tube and reconnect it to suction so the gastric juices do not remain sitting in the stomach.

Chapter 37. Administering Intradermal, Subcutaneous, and Intramuscular Injections

1. a, e
2. b
3. d
4. b, d
5. a, b, c, e
6. c
7. a
8. b, c, e
9. a, b, e
10. Size and weight of patient, muscle mass, type and volume of medication to be injected, gauge and length of needle
11. Various depths of tissue are injected via different routes: ID, subcutaneous, and IM; do not aspirate for ID or subcutaneous routes; do not massage injection site afterward for ID or subcutaneous routes; prime choice of muscle for IM is gluteal muscles at ventrogluteal site for all ages over 2 years, deltoid only for volume less than 2 mL for adults and 1 mL in small children; Left inner forearm for ID of PPD, abdomen for best absorption of insulin.
12. Neither the NS (multiple-dose vial) nor the Water for Injection (multiple-dose vial) can be used. They both contain a bacteriostatic preservative that is contraindicated in newborns. Only the Water for Injection (single-dose vial) can be used due to the lack of the preservative.

Chapter 38. Peripheral Intravenous Therapy

1. d
2. c
3. a, b, c
4. b, e
5. c
6. a
7. c
8. NPO status, excessive vomiting/diarrhea, inability to swallow, any type of GI tract disease, decreased LOC, NG tube connected to suction, decreased cognition, dehydration from excessive environmental exposure, need for administration of medications via the IV route, or any other situation the student can identify that could interfere with ingestion or cause excessive loss of fluids
9. Any three of these: water, vitamins, electrolytes, glucose or dextrose, medication
10. Yes, it takes fewer drops because they are larger.
11. Answer should reflect a broad coverage of the following areas and not be limited to only assessment of the site or inspection of the IV pump. Assess the IV solution bag: Is it empty and infusion completed? Or does it still contain solution? Assess the IV pump: Look to see what message is flashing on the IV pump. Has the set volume to be infused been reached? Check the IV tubing: Are all the clamps open? Is it crimped or pinched off in the bed rail or underneath the patient? Is there air in the tubing? Assess the IV site for: edema, erythema, temperature difference between site and surrounding area, blanching of skin, pallor, fluid leakage, or complaints of any type of discomfort. Assess for a blood return. Attempt to flush the cannula with NS. Discontinue the cannula if signs and symptoms of infiltration or phlebitis are present.
12. 31 gtts/min
13. 100 mL/hr
14. Approximately 6 hours or 6 hours 15 minutes (either answer is acceptable)

Except as noted below, all photographs are by Kris Piersall.

Unit 1

Chapter 1

Figure 1-1: Neeb KC. *Fundamentals Mental Health Nursing.* 3rd ed. Philadelphia: FA Davis; 2006.

Figure 1-2: Wilkinson JM, Van Leuven K. *Fundamentals of Nursing: Theory, Concepts & Applications.* Vol 1. Philadelphia: FA Davis; 2007.

Chapter 3

Figure 3-1: Courtesy of Kingfisher Regional Hospital, Kingfisher, OK.

Figure 3-2: Courtesy of Kingfisher Regional Hospital, Kingfisher, OK.

Box 3-1: American Nurses Association. *Code of Ethics for Nurses with Interpretive Statements.* © 2001 Nurses-books.org, Silver Spring, MD.

Box 3-2: American Hospital Association. *The Patient Care Partnership: Understanding Expectations, Rights and Responsibilities.* © 2003 American Hospital Association.

Box 3-4: National Association for Practical Nurse Education and Service, Inc. (NAPNES). *Standards of Practice and Educational Competencies of Graduates of Practical/Vocational Nursing Programs.* © 2007 National Association for Practical Nurse Education and Service, Inc.

Chapter 4

Figure 4-1: Doenges M, Moorhouse MF. *Application of Nursing Process and Nursing Diagnosis.* 5th ed. Philadelphia: FA Davis; 2008.

Figure 4-2: Williams LS, Hopper PD. *Understanding Medical-Surgical Nursing.* 3rd ed. Philadelphia: FA Davis; 2007.

Figure 4-3, parts 1,2: Courtesy of Kingfisher Regional Hospital, Kingfisher, OK.

Figure 4-4: Wilkinson JM, Van Leuven K. *Fundamentals of Nursing: Theory, Concepts & Applications.* Vol 1. Philadelphia: FA Davis; 2007. (Adapted from Maslow A. *The Farther Reaches of Human Nature.* New York: Viking Press; 1971; and Maslow A, Lowery R, eds. *Toward a Psychology of Being.* 3rd ed. New York: Wiley & Sons; 1998.)

Figure 4-5: Courtesy of Kingfisher Regional Hospital, Kingfisher, OK.

Figure 4-6: Townsend M. *Psychiatric Mental Health Nursing.* 6th ed. Philadelphia: FA Davis; 2010.

Figure 4-7: Courtesy of Canadian Valley Technology Center, El Reno, OK.

Chapter 5

Figure 5-1: Wilkinson JM, Van Leuven K. *Fundamentals of Nursing: Theory, Concepts & Applications.* Vol 1. Philadelphia: FA Davis; 2007.

Figure 5-2: Courtesy of Kingfisher Regional Hospital, Kingfisher, OK.

Figure 5-4: Courtesy of Kingfisher Regional Hospital, Kingfisher, OK.

Figure 5-5: Wilkinson JM, Van Leuven K. *Fundamentals of Nursing: Theory, Concepts & Applications.* Vol 1. Philadelphia: FA Davis; 2007.

Figure 5-13: Wilkinson JM, Van Leuven K. *Fundamentals of Nursing: Theory, Concepts & Applications.* Vol 1. Philadelphia: FA Davis; 2007.

Figure 5-15: Courtesy of Parkview Hospital Home Health, El Reno, OK.

Figure 5-16: Courtesy of Parkview Hospital Home Health, El Reno, OK.

Unit 2

Chapter 6

Figure 6-1: Wilkinson JM, Van Leuven K. *Fundamentals of Nursing: Theory, Concepts & Applications.* Vol 1. Philadelphia: FA Davis; 2007.

Figure 6-3: Williams LS, Hopper PD. *Understanding Medical-Surgical Nursing.* 3rd ed. Philadelphia: FA Davis; 2007.

Chapter 7

Figure 7-1: Wilkinson JM, Van Leuven K. *Fundamentals of Nursing: Theory, Concepts & Applications.* Vol 1. Philadelphia: FA Davis; 2007.

Figure 7-2: Wilkinson JM, Van Leuven K. *Fundamentals of Nursing: Theory, Concepts & Applications.* Vol 1. Philadelphia: FA Davis; 2007. (Source: Dunn HL. High level wellness for man and society. *Am J Public Health.* 1959;49(6):786-788.)

Chapter 8

Figure 8-1: Williams LS, Hopper PD. *Understanding Medical-Surgical Nursing.* 3rd ed. Philadelphia: FA Davis; 2007.

Figure 8-2: Imagine ID: 72421026 from City Hospital 2 CD on http://www.punchstock.com.

Figure 8-3: Wilkinson JM, Van Leuven K. *Fundamentals of Nursing: Theory, Concepts & Applications.* Vol 1. Philadelphia: FA Davis; 2007.

Chapter 9

Figures 9-1 through 9-4: Dillon PM. *Nursing Health Assessment: A Critical Thinking Case Studies Approach.* 2nd ed. Philadelphia: FA Davis; 2007.

Figure 9-5: Wilkinson JM, Van Leuven K. *Fundamentals of Nursing: Theory, Concepts & Applications.* Vol 1. Philadelphia: FA Davis; 2007.

Figure 9-6: Polan E, Taylor D. *Journey Across the Life Span: Human Development and Health Promotion.* 3rd ed. Philadelphia: FA Davis; 2007.

Chapter 10

Figure 10-1: Oklahoma's Advance Directive for Health Care. Public domain.

Figure 10-2: Public domain.

Figure 10-4: City Hospital 2 CD on http://www.punchstock.com.

Unit 3

Chapter 13

Figure 13-1a,b: Wilkinson JM, Van Leuven K. *Fundamentals of Nursing: Theory, Concepts & Applications.* Vol 2. Philadelphia: FA Davis; 2007.

Figure 13-3: Courtesy of Kingfisher Regional Hospital, Kingfisher, OK.

Unnumbered Figures 13-2 and 13-6 through 13-9: Wilkinson JM, Van Leuven K. *Fundamentals of Nursing: Theory, Concepts & Applications.* Vol 2. Philadelphia: FA Davis; 2007.

Table 13-1: Morse J. *Preventing Patient Falls.* 2 ed. New York: Springer Publishing Company; 2008:54.

Chapter 14

Figure 14-1: Scanlon V, Sanders T. *Essentials of Anatomy and Physiology.* 5th ed. Philadelphia: FA Davis; 2007.

Figure 14-2: Wilkinson JM, Van Leuven K. *Fundamentals of Nursing: Theory, Concepts & Applications.* Vol 1. Philadelphia: FA Davis; 2007.

Unnumbered Figures 14-1 through 14-8a,b: Wilkinson JM, Van Leuven K. *Fundamentals of Nursing: Theory, Concepts & Applications.* Vol 2. Philadelphia: FA Davis; 2007.

Chapter 15

Figure 15-1: Wilkinson JM, Van Leuven K. *Fundamentals of Nursing: Theory, Concepts & Applications.* Vol 2. Philadelphia: FA Davis; 2007.

Figure 15-3: Wilkinson JM, Van Leuven K. *Fundamentals of Nursing: Theory, Concepts & Applications.* Vol 1. Philadelphia: FA Davis; 2007.

Figure 15-4 and 15-5a,b,c: Wilkinson JM, Van Leuven K. *Fundamentals of Nursing: Theory, Concepts & Applications.* Vol 2. Philadelphia: FA Davis; 2007.

Unnumbered Figures 15-8 through 15-13 and 15-16 through 15-30: Wilkinson JM, Van Leuven K. *Fundamentals of Nursing: Theory, Concepts & Applications.* Vol 2. Philadelphia: FA Davis; 2007.

Chapter 16

Figures 16-1, 16-2, 16-5, and 16-6: Wilkinson JM, Van Leuven K. *Fundamentals of Nursing: Theory, Concepts & Applications.* Vol 1. Philadelphia: FA Davis; 2007.

Figures 16-3 and 16-4: Wilkinson JM, Van Leuven K. *Fundamentals of Nursing: Theory, Concepts & Applications.* Vol 2. Philadelphia: FA Davis; 2007.

Unnumbered Figures 16-9 through 16-12, 16-14, 16-21, 16-24, and 16-25: Wilkinson JM, Van Leuven K. *Fundamentals of Nursing: Theory, Concepts & Applications.* Vol 1. Philadelphia: FA Davis; 2007.

Unnumbered Figures 16-15, 16-16, 16-18 through 16-20, 16-22, and 16-23: Wilkinson JM, Van Leuven K. *Fundamentals of Nursing: Theory, Concepts & Applications.* Vol 2. Philadelphia: FA Davis; 2007.

Unnumbered Figures 16-26 through 16-30: © 2009 Hill-Rom Services, Inc. Reprinted with permission—All rights reserved.

Chapter 17

Figures 17-2, 17-3, and 17-6 through 17-8: Wilkinson JM, Van Leuven K. *Fundamentals of Nursing: Theory, Concepts & Applications.* Vol 1. Philadelphia: FA Davis; 2007.

Figures 17-4 and 17-9: Wilkinson JM, Van Leuven K. *Fundamentals of Nursing: Theory, Concepts & Applications.* Vol 2. Philadelphia: FA Davis; 2007.

Figure 17-5: Scanlon V, Sanders T. *Essentials of Anatomy and Physiology.* 5th ed. Philadelphia: FA Davis; 2007.

Figure 17-11: Courtesy of Kingfisher Regional Hospital, Kingfisher, OK.

Unnumbered Figures 17-1 through 17-16, 17-18, and 17-19: Wilkinson JM, Van Leuven K. *Fundamentals of Nursing: Theory, Concepts & Applications.* Vol 2. Philadelphia: FA Davis; 2007.

Unnumbered Figure 17-17: Dillon PM. *Nursing Health Assessment: A Critical Thinking Case Studies Approach.* 2nd ed. Philadelphia: FA Davis; 2007.

Unnumbered Figures 17-20 through 17-22: Dillon PM. *Nursing Health Assessment: A Critical Thinking Case Studies Approach.* 2nd ed. Philadelphia: FA Davis; 2007.

Chapter 18

Figures 18-2 and 18-3: Wilkinson JM, Van Leuven K. *Fundamentals of Nursing: Theory, Concepts & Applications.* Vol 1. Philadelphia: FA Davis; 2007.

Chapter 19

Figure 19-1: Williams LS, Hopper PD. *Understanding Medical-Surgical Nursing.* 3rd ed. Philadelphia: FA Davis; 2007.

Figure 19-3: Wilkinson JM, Van Leuven K. *Fundamentals of Nursing: Theory, Concepts & Applications.* Vol 2. Philadelphia: FA Davis; 2007.

Chapter 20

Figure 20-5: Courtesy of Kingfisher Regional Hospital, Kingfisher, OK.

Chapter 21

Figures 21-2, 21-4, 21-5a,b, and 21-7 through 21-11a: Dillon PM. *Nursing Health Assessment: A Critical Thinking Case Studies Approach.* 2nd ed. Philadelphia: FA Davis; 2007.

Figures 21-3 and 21-17: Wilkinson JM, Van Leuven K. *Fundamentals of Nursing: Theory, Concepts & Applications.* Vol 1. Philadelphia: FA Davis; 2007.

Figure 21-6: Myers E, Hopkins T. *LPN Notes.* 2nd ed. Philadelphia: FA Davis; 2006.

Figures 21-11b through 21-15: Dillon PM. *Nursing Health Assessment: A Critical Thinking Case Studies Approach.* 2nd ed. Philadelphia: FA Davis; 2007.

Figures 21-16 and 21-19: Williams LS, Hopper PD. *Understanding Medical-Surgical Nursing.* 3rd ed. Philadelphia: FA Davis; 2007.

Figure 21-18: Venes D, ed. *Taber's Cyclopedic Medical Dictionary.* 21st ed. Philadelphia: FA Davis; 2009.

Figure 21-20: Courtesy of Kingfisher Regional Hospital, Kingfisher, OK.

Unnumbered Figures 21-1 and 21-3: Dillon PM. *Nursing Health Assessment: A Critical Thinking Case Studies Approach.* 2nd ed. Philadelphia: FA Davis; 2007.

Unnumbered Figures 21-2 and 21-4 through 21-10: Dillon PM. *Nursing Health Assessment: A Critical Thinking Case Studies Approach.* 2nd ed. Philadelphia: FA Davis; 2007.

Table 21-2: Teasdale G, Jennett B. Assessment of coma and impaired consciousness: A practical scale. *Lancet.* 1974;304:81-84, with permission from Elsevier.

Chapter 22

Figure 22-3: Wilkinson JM, Van Leuven K. *Fundamentals of Nursing: Theory, Concepts & Applications.* Vol 2. Philadelphia: FA Davis; 2007.

Figure 22-7: Wilkinson JM, Van Leuven K. *Fundamentals of Nursing: Theory, Concepts & Applications.* Vol 1. Philadelphia: FA Davis; 2007.

Unnumbered Figures 22-3, 22-4, and 22-6: Wilkinson JM, Van Leuven K. *Fundamentals of Nursing: Theory, Concepts & Applications.* Vol 2. Philadelphia: FA Davis; 2007.

Unit 4

Chapter 23

Figure 23-1: Wilkinson JM, Van Leuven K. *Fundamentals of Nursing: Theory, Concepts & Applications.* Vol 1. Philadelphia: FA Davis; 2007.

Figure 23-2: U.S. Department of Agriculture; 2005.

Chapter 24

Figures 24-4, 24-6, and 24-10: Wilkinson JM, Van Leuven K. *Fundamentals of Nursing: Theory, Concepts & Applications.* Vol 1. Philadelphia: FA Davis; 2007.

Figure 24-7: Williams LS, Hopper PD. *Understanding Medical-Surgical Nursing.* 3rd ed. Philadelphia: FA Davis; 2007.

Figure 24-8: Wilkinson JM, Van Leuven K. *Fundamentals of Nursing: Theory, Concepts & Applications.* Vol 2. Philadelphia: FA Davis; 2007.

Figure 24-9: Phillips L. *IV Therapy Notes: Nurse's Clinical Pocket Guide.* Philadelphia: FA Davis; 2005.

Unnumbered Figures 24-1 and 24-3 through 24-7: Wilkinson JM, Van Leuven K. *Fundamentals of Nursing: Theory, Concepts & Applications.* Vol 2. Philadelphia: FA Davis; 2007.

Unnumbered Figure 24-2: Scanlon V, Sanders T. *Essentials of Anatomy and Physiology.* 5th ed. Philadelphia: FA Davis; 2007.

Chapter 25

Figure 25-3: Scanlon V, Sanders T. *Essentials of Anatomy and Physiology.* 5th ed. Philadelphia: FA Davis; 2007.

Unnumbered Figure 25-1: Wilkinson JM, Van Leuven K. *Fundamentals of Nursing: Theory, Concepts & Applications.* Vol 1. Philadelphia: FA Davis; 2007.

Chapter 26

Figure 26-2: Wilkinson JM, Van Leuven K. *Fundamentals of Nursing: Theory, Concepts & Applications.* Vol 1. Philadelphia: FA Davis; 2007.

Figure 26-3a-f: Dillon PM. *Nursing Health Assessment: A Critical Thinking Case Studies Approach.* 2nd ed. Philadelphia: FA Davis; 2007.

Figure 26-4: Wilkinson JM, Van Leuven K. *Fundamentals of Nursing: Theory, Concepts & Applications.* Vol 1. Philadelphia: FA Davis; 2007.

Figure 26-6: Wilkinson JM, Van Leuven K. *Fundamentals of Nursing: Theory, Concepts & Applications.* Vol 1. Philadelphia: FA Davis; 2007.

Figure 26-7: Williams LS, Hopper PD. *Understanding Medical-Surgical Nursing.* 3rd ed. Philadelphia: FA Davis; 2007.

Figures 26-8 through 26-12: Wilkinson JM, Van Leuven K. *Fundamentals of Nursing: Theory, Concepts & Applications.* Vol 1. Philadelphia: FA Davis; 2007.

Unnumbered Figures 26-1 through 26-3: Wilkinson JM, Van Leuven K. *Fundamentals of Nursing: Theory, Concepts & Applications.* Vol 1. Philadelphia: FA Davis; 2007.

Unnumbered Figures 26-5 through 26-7: Wilkinson JM, Van Leuven K. *Fundamentals of Nursing: Theory, Concepts & Applications.* Vol 2. Philadelphia: FA Davis; 2007.

Unnumbered Figures 26-13 through 26-25: Wilkinson JM, Van Leuven K. *Fundamentals of Nursing: Theory, Concepts & Applications.* Vol 1. Philadelphia: FA Davis; 2007.

Chapter 27

Figures 27-1 and 27-2: Williams LS, Hopper PD. *Understanding Medical-Surgical Nursing.* 3rd ed. Philadelphia: FA Davis; 2007.

Figure 27-3: Scanlon V, Sanders T. *Essentials of Anatomy and Physiology.* 5th ed. Philadelphia: FA Davis; 2007.

Figures 27-4 and 27-5: Williams LS, Hopper PD. *Understanding Medical-Surgical Nursing.* 3rd ed. Philadelphia: FA Davis; 2007.

Figures 27-6 and 27-7: Wilkinson JM, Van Leuven K. *Fundamentals of Nursing: Theory, Concepts & Applications.* Vol 1. Philadelphia: FA Davis; 2007.

Unnumbered Figures 27-2 and 27-3: Wilkinson JM, Van Leuven K. *Fundamentals of Nursing: Theory, Concepts & Applications.* Vol 2. Philadelphia: FA Davis; 2007.

Chapter 28

Figure 28-1: Williams LS, Hopper PD. *Understanding Medical-Surgical Nursing.* 3rd ed. Philadelphia: FA Davis; 2007.

Figures 28-2 through 28-4: Wilkinson JM, Van Leuven K. *Fundamentals of Nursing: Theory, Concepts & Applications.* Vol 1. Philadelphia: FA Davis; 2007.

Figures 28-6 and 28-7: Wilkinson JM, Van Leuven K. *Fundamentals of Nursing: Theory, Concepts & Applications.* Vol 1. Philadelphia: FA Davis; 2007.

Figure 28-8: Williams LS, Hopper PD. *Understanding Medical-Surgical Nursing.* 3rd ed. Philadelphia: FA Davis; 2007.

Figure 28-9: Wilkinson JM, Van Leuven K. *Fundamentals of Nursing: Theory, Concepts & Applications.* Vol 2. Philadelphia: FA Davis; 2007.

Unnumbered Figures 28-1 through 28-21: Wilkinson JM, Van Leuven K. *Fundamentals of Nursing: Theory, Concepts & Applications.* Vol 2. Philadelphia: FA Davis; 2007.

Chapter 29

Figures 29-1 and 29-2: Wilkinson JM, Van Leuven K. *Fundamentals of Nursing: Theory, Concepts & Applications.* Vol 1. Philadelphia: FA Davis; 2007.

Figures 29-4 and 29-5: Wilkinson JM, Van Leuven K. *Fundamentals of Nursing: Theory, Concepts & Applications.* Vol 1. Philadelphia: FA Davis; 2007.

Figure 29-6: Scanlon V, Sanders T. *Essentials of Anatomy and Physiology.* 5th ed. Philadelphia: FA Davis; 2007.

Chapter 30

Figures 30-3 through 30-7: Wilkinson JM, Van Leuven K. *Fundamentals of Nursing: Theory, Concepts & Applications.* Vol 2. Philadelphia: FA Davis; 2007.

Unnumbered Figures 30-1 through 30-9: Wilkinson JM, Van Leuven K. *Fundamentals of Nursing: Theory, Concepts & Applications.* Vol 2. Philadelphia: FA Davis; 2007.

Chapter 31

Figure 31-2: Wilkinson JM, Van Leuven K. *Fundamentals of Nursing: Theory, Concepts & Applications.* Vol 1. Philadelphia: FA Davis; 2007.

Figure 31-4: Williams LS, Hopper PD. *Understanding Medical-Surgical Nursing.* 3rd ed. Philadelphia: FA Davis; 2007.

Figures 31-5 through 31-11: Wilkinson JM, Van Leuven K. *Fundamentals of Nursing: Theory, Concepts & Applications.* Vol 1. Philadelphia: FA Davis; 2007.

Figures 31-12 and 31-13: Williams LS, Hopper PD. *Understanding Medical-Surgical Nursing.* 3rd ed. Philadelphia: FA Davis; 2007.

Unnumbered Figures 31-1 and 31-2: Wilkinson JM, Van Leuven K. *Fundamentals of Nursing: Theory, Concepts & Applications.* Vol 2. Philadelphia: FA Davis; 2007.

Unnumbered Figures 31-4 through 31-8: Wilkinson JM, Van Leuven K. *Fundamentals of Nursing: Theory, Concepts & Applications.* Vol 2. Philadelphia: FA Davis; 2007.

Unnumbered Figure 31-10: Wilkinson JM, Van Leuven K. *Fundamentals of Nursing: Theory, Concepts & Applications.* Vol 2. Philadelphia: FA Davis; 2007.

Chapter 32

Figures 32-1 and 32-2: Polan E, Taylor D. *Journey Across the Life Span: Human Development and Health Promotion.* 3rd ed. Philadelphia: FA Davis; 2007.

Figure 32-3: Williams LS, Hopper PD. *Understanding Medical-Surgical Nursing.* 3rd ed. Philadelphia: FA Davis; 2007.

Figure 32-4: Getty Images.

Figures 32-5 and 32-6: PunchStock.

Chapter 33

Figures 33-1 and 33-2: Wilkinson JM, Van Leuven K. *Fundamentals of Nursing: Theory, Concepts & Applications.* Vol 1. Philadelphia: FA Davis; 2007.

Figure 33-3: Courtesy of Kingfisher Regional Hospital, Kingfisher, OK.

Figure 33-4: Williams LS, Hopper PD. *Understanding Medical-Surgical Nursing.* 3rd ed. Philadelphia: FA Davis; 2007.

Figure 33-5: Courtesy of Kingfisher Regional Hospital, Kingfisher, OK.

Figures 33-6 and 33-7: Williams LS, Hopper PD. *Understanding Medical-Surgical Nursing.* 3rd ed. Philadelphia: FA Davis; 2007.

Figures 33-8 and 33-9: Wilkinson JM, Van Leuven K. *Fundamentals of Nursing: Theory, Concepts & Applications.* Vol 1. Philadelphia: FA Davis; 2007.

Figure 33-12: Williams LS, Hopper PD. *Understanding Medical-Surgical Nursing.* 3rd ed. Philadelphia: FA Davis; 2007. (Modified from Barnes TA. *Respiratory Care Principles.* Philadelphia: FA Davis; 1991:425.)

Chapter 34

Figures 34-1 and 34-2: Wilkinson JM, Van Leuven K. *Fundamentals of Nursing: Theory, Concepts & Applications.* Vol 1. Philadelphia: FA Davis; 2007.

Figure 34-4: BD Tube Guide. Courtesy of and © 2008 Becton, Dickinson and Company.

Figure 34-6: Wilkinson JM, Van Leuven K. *Fundamentals of Nursing: Theory, Concepts & Applications.* Vol 1. Philadelphia: FA Davis; 2007.

Figures 34-8 through 34-10: Wilkinson JM, Van Leuven K. *Fundamentals of Nursing: Theory, Concepts & Applications.* Vol 1. Philadelphia: FA Davis; 2007.

Unnumbered Figure 34-6: Wilkinson JM, Van Leuven K. *Fundamentals of Nursing: Theory, Concepts & Applications.* Vol 2. Philadelphia: FA Davis; 2007.

Unnumbered Figures 34-8 and 34-9: Wilkinson JM, Van Leuven K. *Fundamentals of Nursing: Theory, Concepts & Applications.* Vol 2. Philadelphia: FA Davis; 2007.

Chapter 35

Figure 35-2: Wilkinson JM, Van Leuven K. *Fundamentals of Nursing: Theory, Concepts & Applications.* Vol 1. Philadelphia: FA Davis; 2007.

Figure 35-4: Wilkinson JM, Van Leuven K. *Fundamentals of Nursing: Theory, Concepts & Applications.* Vol 1. Philadelphia: FA Davis; 2007.

Unit 5

Chapter 36

Figures 36-1 through 36-5: Wilkinson JM, Van Leuven K. *Fundamentals of Nursing: Theory, Concepts & Applications.* Vol 1. Philadelphia: FA Davis; 2007.

Unnumbered Figures 36-1 through 36-11: Wilkinson JM, Van Leuven K. *Fundamentals of Nursing: Theory, Concepts & Applications.* Vol 2. Philadelphia: FA Davis; 2007.

Chapter 37

Figures 37-1 through 37-8b: Wilkinson JM, Van Leuven K. *Fundamentals of Nursing: Theory, Concepts & Applications.* Vol 2. Philadelphia: FA Davis; 2007.

Figures 37-9 through 37-15a: Wilkinson JM, Van Leuven K. *Fundamentals of Nursing: Theory, Concepts & Applications.* Vol 2. Philadelphia: FA Davis; 2007.

Figures 37-16 through 37-24b: Wilkinson JM, Van Leuven K. *Fundamentals of Nursing: Theory, Concepts & Applications.* Vol 2. Philadelphia: FA Davis; 2007.

Figures 37-26 through 37-29: Wilkinson JM, Van Leuven K. *Fundamentals of Nursing: Theory, Concepts & Applications.* Vol 2. Philadelphia: FA Davis; 2007.

Chapter 38

Figure 38-2: Wilkinson JM, Van Leuven K. *Fundamentals of Nursing: Theory, Concepts & Applications.* Vol 2. Philadelphia: FA Davis; 2007.

Figure 38-4: Wilkinson JM, Van Leuven K. *Fundamentals of Nursing: Theory, Concepts & Applications.* Vol 1. Philadelphia: FA Davis; 2007.

Figure 38-13: Wilkinson JM, Van Leuven K. *Fundamentals of Nursing: Theory, Concepts & Applications.* Vol 2. Philadelphia: FA Davis; 2007.

Figures 38-16 through 38-17b: Wilkinson JM, Van Leuven K. *Fundamentals of Nursing: Theory, Concepts & Applications.* Vol 1. Philadelphia: FA Davis; 2007.

Figure 38-19: Wilkinson JM, Van Leuven K. *Fundamentals of Nursing: Theory, Concepts & Applications.* Vol 2. Philadelphia: FA Davis; 2007.

Figure 38-22: Wilkinson JM, Van Leuven K. *Fundamentals of Nursing: Theory, Concepts & Applications.* Vol 1. Philadelphia: FA Davis; 2007.

Figure 38-24: Wilkinson JM, Van Leuven K. *Fundamentals of Nursing: Theory, Concepts & Applications.* Vol 2. Philadelphia: FA Davis; 2007.

Unnumbered Figure 38-1: Wilkinson JM, Van Leuven K. *Fundamentals of Nursing: Theory, Concepts & Applications.* Vol 2. Philadelphia: FA Davis; 2007.

Unnumbered Figure 38-3: Wilkinson JM, Van Leuven K. *Fundamentals of Nursing: Theory, Concepts & Applications.* Vol 2. Philadelphia: FA Davis; 2007.

Unnumbered Figures 38-6 through 38-10: Wilkinson JM, Van Leuven K. *Fundamentals of Nursing: Theory, Concepts & Applications.* Vol 2. Philadelphia: FA Davis; 2007.

Unnumbered Figures 38-17 and 38-18: Wilkinson JM, Van Leuven K. *Fundamentals of Nursing: Theory, Concepts & Applications.* Vol 2. Philadelphia: FA Davis; 2007.

Unnumbered Figure 38-20: Wilkinson JM, Van Leuven K. *Fundamentals of Nursing: Theory, Concepts & Applications.* Vol 2. Philadelphia: FA Davis; 2007.

Note: Page numbers followed by *f* refer to figures; page numbers followed by *t* refer to tables.

A

Abandonment, 38
Abbreviations, document, 88–91, 89t
Abdomen
    abdominal binders, 573
    abdominal paracentesis, 544f
    bowel and bladder status and, 442
    bowel sounds and, 440–441
    dressings and equipment and, 442
    four abdominal quadrants, 440f
    palpation contraindications, 441
    skin color and, 441
    skin integrity and, 411–422
    skin turgor and, 411
    temperature and moisture and, 441
Abductor pillow, 593t, 596, 596f
Ability to understand, patient, 234
Abnormal breath sounds, 436–437
Abrasions, 558
Absorption
    digestion and, 478
    drug effects on, 506–507
Accommodation response, 431
Accountability, 81
Acculturation, 493
Accurate order transcription, 109
Acetaminophen, 397–398
Acid-base balance
    acidosis and, 667
    alkalosis and, 667
    bicarbonate buffer system and, 666
    brain and, 667
    compensation and, 668
    kidneys role and, 667
    lungs and, 668
    metabolic imbalances, 667
    pH scale and, 665, 665f
    regulation and, 666–667
    respiratory system role and, 666–667
    treatment and nursing care for, 668
Acidosis, 667
Activated partial thromboplastin time (APTT),
    773, 896
Active bowel sounds, 440
Active listening, 118–119
Active range-of-motion exercises, 314
Activity intolerance, 60
Activity level, bowel elimination and, 679, 682
Acupressure, 214
Acupuncture, 214
Acute care hospitals, 18–19
Acute hemolytic actions, transfusions and, 944t
Acute illness, 139
Adaptation and stress, 139–144
Adequate intake (AI), 476
Admission
    admission forms, 53f–54f
    admission kit, 412, 413f
    admitting procedures, 411
    anxiety and, 409–410
    attire and modesty and, 410–411
    authority to treat and, 412

clothing and personal item inventory and, 413
common patient reactions and, 409
cultural considerations and, 411
data analysis and, 414
data collection and, 413–414
decision making and, 411
discharge planning and, 414
fear and, 409
financial concerns and, 410
first impressions and, 408, 408f
identification bands and, 412, 412f
initial physical assessment and, 414
loss of control and, 410
loss of identity and, 411
nursing responsibilities during, 412–414
orientation checklist and, 413
patient and family introduction and, 412
patient rooms and, 411
reactions to, 409–411
separation anxiety and, 409–410
supervision/delegation and, 414
Adolescents
    ambivalence by, 177
    cognitive development and, 177
    experimentation and, 179
    firearms and, 179
    health teaching and, 180
    Internet social networking and, 179
    menarche and, 176
    moral and spiritual development and, 177
    nursing implications and, 180
    nutritional needs and, 491
    physical development and, 176
    psychosocial development and, 176–177
    puberty and, 176
    safety concerns and, 179–180
Adult development, 180–182. *See also* specific
    age grouping
Advanced directives. *See* End-of-life
    documentation
Adventitious breath sounds, 362, 436–437
Advocating for patient, 31–32
Aerobic organisms, 815
Afebrile, 355
Age. *See also* Elderly patients; specific age groups
    age group classifications, 746–747
    ageism and, 747
    blood pressure readings and, 346
    bowel elimination and, 680–681
    infections and, 261
    injection variations and, 901
    medication administration concerns and, 847
    myths about aging, 747
    patient safety and, 234
    positive aspects of, 758
    pulse rate and, 358t
    respiratory rate and, 361t
    wound healing and, 566t
Aggressive behavior style, 119
Air embolism, intravenous therapy and, 941–942
Air-fluidized bed, 318t
Air-lock, injections and, 897

Airborne infection isolation rooms, 265
Airborne transmission of infections, 265, 266t
Alanine aminotransferase, 546
Albumin, 546, 943
Alcock catheter, 720–721
Alcohol abuse, 137
Alcohol-based hand gels, 263
Aldosterone, 650
Alginate dressings, 573t
Alkaline phosphatase, 546
Alkalosis, 667
Allergic reactions
    medications and, 830
    peripheral venipuncture and, 931
    transfusions and, 944t
Allopathic medicine, 211
Aloe vera, 215
Altered urinary functions. *See also* Urinary
    catheters
    urinary catheters and, 719–725
    urinary diversions, 725, 725f
    urinary tract infections, 725–730, 729t–730t
Alternative bowel elimination
    appliance application and, 691–692, 691f
    colostomy irrigation and, 690, 690f, 692,
        705–706
    colostomy with descending colon, 692–697,
        695t–697t
    ileostomy, 690
    nursing care and, 691–692
    ostomy appliances and, 703–704
    skin care and, 692
Alternative therapy. *See* Complementary and
    alternative therapy
Alzheimer's disease, 748–753
Ambivalence, 177
Ambulation, 235, 326–327, 338–339
Ambulation devices
    canes, 598, 599f
    crutches, 598, 599t
    walkers, 599–600, 599f
Ambulatory care clinics, 21
Ambulatory surgery, 20
American Heart Association (AHA) diet, 478
American Hospital Association's patient care
    partnership, 31–32
American Nurses Association (ANA) Code of
    Ethics, 30, 189
Ampules, 888, 889f, 903
Amputation, 592, 597–598
Anabolism, 480
Anaerobic organisms, 567, 815
Analgesics, 838t
Anaphylaxis, 501, 544, 831, 944t
Ancillary staff, 18t
Anesthesia
    anesthesia provider, 781–783
    conscious sedation, 784–785
    epidural anesthesia, 785–786
    general anesthesia, 784
    local anesthesia, 786
    peripheral nerve block, 786

Anesthesia (*continued*)
  postanesthesia assessment and care, 788–790
  regional anesthesia, 785
  spinal anesthesia, 785, 785f
Anesthesiologist, 783
Aneurysms, 548
Anger in communication, 120–121
Angioedema, 432, 432f
Animal-assisted therapy, 216
Anisocoria, 431
Anorexia nervosa, 440, 491, 505
Anoxia, 168
Antacids, 835t
Anterior auscultation sites, 438f
Antianginals, 833t
Antianxiety medications, 838t
Antiarrhythmics, 833t
Antibacterial soaps, 285
Antibiotics, 257, 837t
Anticholinergics, 835t
Anticoagulants, 833t
Anticonvulsants, 838t
Antidepressants, 838t
Antidiabetics, 836t
Antidiuretic hormone, 650
Antiembolism hose, 315, 778, 778f, 799–800
Antiemetics, 506, 836t
Antifungals, 837t
Antigen-avoidance diet, 504
Antihistamines, 839t
Antihyperlipidemics, 834t
Antihypertensives, 834t
Antiinflammatories, 837t
Antioxidants, 216, 484
Antipyretic medications, 356
Antitussives, 839t
Antiviral medications, 257, 838t
Anuria, 711
Anxiety
  admission process and, 409–410
  blood pressure readings and, 346
  immobility and, 319–320
  respiratory rate and, 361t
  restorative sleep and, 401
Aphasia, 128, 433, 748
Apical pulse, 356–357, 356f, 369–370, 439–440
Apnea, 200, 361, 434t
Appearance and behavior, 9–10
Appendicitis, 379
Appropriate level of care, 16–22
Approximation, wound infection and, 794
Aquathermia pads, 380, 380f, 386
Arcus senilis, 431, 431f
Arm boards, 322t, 323
Aromatherapy, 216
Arrhythmias, 773
Arterial blood gases, 616–617, 618t, 669
Arteriography, 548
Artificial eyes, 289–290
Ascites, 425, 485, 649
Asepsis. *See also* Sterile technique; Sterilization
  airborne transmission and, 265, 266t
  CDC guidelines and, 264–266
  clean environment and equipment, 262
  direct and indirect contact transmission and,
    265–266, 266t
  droplet transmission and, 265, 266t
  hand hygiene and, 262–263, 271–272
  injections and, 884–885, 885f
  personal protective equipment and, 272–273
  psychological aspects of, 266–267
  responsibilities for, 262
  standard precautions and, 264–265, 264t
  supervision of, 266
  transmission-based precautions, 265–266

Asepsis and IV therapy
  gloves and, 928
  handwashing and, 928
  skin sites and, 929
  supplies and, 928–929
Aspartate aminotransferase, 546
Aspiration prevention techniques, 517
Aspiration procedures, 551–552
Aspirin
  children with viruses and, 356
  pain management and, 398
Assault and battery, 36
Assertive behavior style, 119
Assessment, 51–55, 53f–54f
  blood pressure readings and, 348
  body temperature and, 353–355, 353t–354t
  flow sheet or checklist form, 446f
  interviewing, 51–55
  physical assessment, 55
  subjective and objective findings, 61
Assisted care, 283
Assisted living facilities, 18, 20
Assisted or help bath, 284
Assisted suicide, 188–189
Assisting patient to dangle, 337–338
Associate degree nurse, 6
Atelectasis, 315, 547, 614, 776, 793
Atherosclerosis, 429
Atrial natriuretic factor, 650
Attachment, infant, 173
Attire, patient, 410–411
Attitude and communication, 118
Auditory distraction, 397
Auditory learning, 222
Auscultation
  abnormal and adventitious breath sounds,
    436–437
  anterior auscultation sites, 438f
  apical pulse and, 357
  auscultatory gap, 349
  breath sounds and, 435–437, 451
  heart sounds and, 438–439, 439f, 452
  landmarks, 434–435, 434f–435f
  lateral auscultation sites, 438f
  physical assessment and, 426
  posterior auscultation sites, 438f
Authority to treat, 412
Autoclaving, 456
Avoidant behavior, 119, 143t
Axillary temperature measurements, 354

B

Babinski's reflex, newborns, 172, 172f
Bacilli, 256
Back massages, 286, 286f, 298
Bacteria, 256–257, 257f
Bacterial contamination, transfusions and, 944t
Bad cholesterol, 481
Barium enema, 542t
Basal metabolic rate, 350
Basophil levels, 544
Bathing
  administering complete bed bath, 294–296
  antibacterial soaps and, 285
  assistance and, 283
  bath blankets, 284
  bed baths, 294–296
  benefits of, 281
  circulation and, 281
  comfort and relaxation and, 281
  cultural issues and, 282–283
  delegation and, 283
  nurse-patient relationship and, 281–282

  nursing responsibilities and, 285
  patient abilities and, 283
  patient preferences and, 282–285
  safety and, 285
  self-esteem and, 281
  sensation and, 281
  skin assessment and, 281
  timing and, 282
  types of, 284–285
Bathroom privileges, 683
Bedmaking
  bed positions and, 293, 293t–294t
  closed beds and, 292
  mitered corners and, 293
  nursing responsibilities and, 292–293
  occupied beds and, 292, 306–307
  open beds and, 292
  surgical beds and, 292
  unoccupied beds and, 292, 304–305
Bedpans, 712, 712f, 731–732
Beds, specialty, 318t–319t
Bedside commode, 683
Bedsores. *See* Pressure ulcers
Belching, 426
Benign prostatic hypertrophy, 721
Bicarbonate, 656t, 666
Bier block, 786
Bilious wound drainage, 570
Bilirubin levels, 545–546
Binge eating, 505
Biofeedback, 216
Biological hazards, 245
Bioterrorism, 242
Biot's respirations, 362t, 434t
Black hairy tongue, 432, 432f
Bladder function. *See also* Urinary elimination
  abdomen and, 442
  altered, 717–719
  bladder training and, 718–719
  functional incontinence and, 718
  nocturia and, 717–718
  overflow incontinence and, 718
  residual urine and, 717, 717f
  stress incontinence and, 718
  urge incontinence and, 718
  urinary incontinence and, 718–719
  urinary retention and, 717
Bladder irrigation, 739
Bladder training, 718–719
Blanket rolls, 322t, 323
Blebs, 891, 892f
Blood. *See also* Phlebotomy; Transfusion
  administration Y-set, 923, 924f
  blood clots, 314, 777
  blood count normal values, 544t
  blood culture specimens, 815, 821
  blood glucose tests, 545
  cell production, 541
  chemistry tests, 545–546
  products, 943–945
  specimen labels, 813–814
  volume, pulse rate and, 358t
Blood pressure
  in adults over 18 years, 347t
  assessment sites, 348, 364–366
  auscultatory gap and, 349
  automatic vital sign machines and, 347
  cardiac output and, 345
  circulatory qualities and, 345
  components of, 346
  diastolic pressure and, 346
  equipment and, 346–348
  factors affecting, 346
  hypertension and, 349
  hypotension and, 349–350

initial assessment and, 429
Korotkoff's sounds and, 348–349
measurement and, 349
pulse pressure and, 346
sphygmomanometers and, 346–347, 347f
stethoscopes and, 347–348, 348f
stroke volume and, 345
systolic pressure and, 346
Blood urea nitrogen (BUN), 545–546, 719
Bloodshot eyes, 431
Blunt percussion, 426
Body composition, 650
Body fluids. *See also* Fluid volume disturbances;
Water
abnormal movement of, 649
body composition and, 650
bowel elimination and, 679, 683
diffusion and, 648, 648f
distribution and movement of, 646–649
excess and, 653–654
filtration and, 648
fluid wave test, 426
hormonal regulation and, 650
intravenous therapy and, 914–915
loss and gain per 24 hours, 652t
normal fluid losses and, 650–651
osmosis and, 647–648, 647f
postoperative balance and, 792
pulse rates and, 359t
regulation of, 650–651
requirements for, 445
volume deficits and, 653
water functions, 649–650
water intake, 650
water movement from gastrointestinal tract,
648–649
withholding and diagnostic testing, 540
Body language, 116
Body mass index (BMI), 485–487, 486t
Body mechanics, nursing staff safety and,
243–244, 250
Body system deficits, aging and, 749t–752t
Body systems, physical assessment and, 427,
427t–428t
Body temperature
assessment of, 367–369
assessment routes and, 353–355, 353t–354t
axillary temperature readings, 354
elevated temperature, 355–356
factors affecting, 352
fahrenheit-celsius conversion formula, 351
fever signs and symptoms, 355
heat therapy and, 379
hypothermia and, 356
infections and, 261
initial assessment and, 429
measurement scales and, 350
normal temperature by selected routes, 355,
355t
nursing care and fever, 355–356
oral temperature readings, 354
pulse rate and, 359t
ranges of, 351f
rectal probes and, 354
skin probes and, 354
temporal artery temperature, 355
thermogenesis and, 350
thermometer types and, 352–353, 352f
thermoregulation and, 351–352
tympanic thermometers and, 354
water and maintenance of, 649
Bolus feedings, 514–515
Bone marrow, 542t, 551–552
Borborygmus, 440, 682
Borrelia burgdorferi, 258

Bowel elimination. *See also* Alternative bowel
elimination; Constipation; Diarrhea
abnormal characteristics and, 677–678, 678t
adequate fluid and fiber intake and, 683
alternative bowel elimination, 689–692
constipation and, 678–681
diarrhea and, 679–681
dietary considerations and, 684
digital removal of impaction, 688–689
distention and, 677
elimination needs and, 445
enemas and, 685–688, 698–699
fecal impaction and, 681, 702
fecal incontinence and, 681, 689
feces characteristics and, 677–678
frequency of, 677
gastrointestinal tract and, 676–677
guaiac testing, 701
impaction and, 678
increased activity and, 682
medications and, 684–688
normal characteristics and, 677, 678t
nursing interventions and, 682
objective assessment and, 682
ostomy appliances and, 703–704
perineal care and, 688
peristalsis and, 676
positioning and, 683
preventing recurrent constipation, 684
privacy and, 683
promotion of, 681–684
stool specimens and, 688, 700
subjective assessment and, 681–682
timing of, 677
Bowel sounds, 426, 440–441, 677
Brachial pulse, 357, 370
Braden scale for predicting pressure sore risk,
562f
Bradycardia, 358
Bradypnea, 360, 434t
Brain, acid-base balance and, 667
Brain protection, water and, 649
Breastfeeding, 480
Breath sounds, auscultation of, 435–437
Breathing mechanics, 612–613
Bronchodilators, 839t
Bronzing, skin, 441
Bruising, pressure ulcers and, 561
Bruit, 426
Bruxism, 402t
Buccal route, medication, 852
Buddhism, 142t
Bulimia nervosa, 491, 505–506
Business office notification, discharge and, 417
Butterfly needles, 922–923
Butterfly or winged infusion sets, 812, 813f

C

Cachexia, 506
Caffeine, blood pressure readings and, 346
Calcium
deficiency and excess and, 662
functions and sources of, 485t
imbalances and, 659t
levels of, 546
nursing care and, 662–663
ranges of, 657t
Calorie-restricted diet, 503
Cancers, 140, 598, 599f
Candida albicans, 259, 432
Cannulation, 920–922
determining proper, 935
performing, 934–935
severed cannula, 941

Capillary refill time, 360, 443
Caplets, medication, 852–853
Capsaicin, 215
Capsules, medication, 853
Carbamazepine (Tegretol), 855
Carbohydrates
complex carbohydrates, 482–483
deficiency of, 487
dietary fiber and, 483
digestion and, 483
simple carbohydrates, 482
Cardiac glycosides, 834t
Cardiac ischemia, 550
Cardiac output, 345, 356
Cardiac patients, heat therapy and, 379
Cardiac rehabilitation, 21
Cardiopulmonary resuscitation (CPR), 241
Cardiovascular system
assessment of, 427t
cardiovascular medications, 833t–835t
elderly patients and, 750t, 753
immobility effects on, 314–315
postoperative care and, 789
presurgical review and, 773
pulse rate and, 359t
Care continuity, documentation and, 80–81
Care plans
computerized plans, 64
critical pathway and, 69, 69f
interventions and evaluations, 74t–75t
multidisciplinary care plans, 64–69, 65f–68f
standardized care plans, 64
student care plans, 70–76, 71f–73f
Career advancement, 7, 7t
Carotid body, 360
Carotid pulse, 357, 370
Carts, medication, 844
Case management, 23
Casts, 593t, 594–595
Catabolism, 480
Cataracts, 753
Catheters. *See* Urinary catheters
Celiac disease, 487
Cellulitis, 380
Centers for Disease Control and Prevention
(CDC), 36, 262
Central nervous system, presurgical review and, 773
Central obesity, 492
Central venous catheters, 519, 519f
Cephalocaudal pattern of growth, 168
Cerebrovascular accidents
blood clots and, 314
neurological functioning and, 748
nursing care with a PEG tube, 520–527,
524t–527t
Certified registered nurse anesthetist (CRNA), 783
Cerumen, 427
Chain of infection, 257–260, 260f
Chair monitors, 236, 237f
Chamomile, 215
Charitable organizations, 25
Charting methods, 96–103
charting by exception, 100
computerized charting, 102–103, 103f
focus charting, 99
narrative charting, 100–101
PIE charting, 98, 99f
SOAPIER charting, 96–98, 98f
Cheilitis, 432
Cheilosis, 432
Chemical changes, bowel elimination and, 680
Chemical cold packs, 384
Chemical disinfection, 456
Chemical exposure, infections and, 261
Chemical hazards, 244–245

Chest assessment
  apical pulse and, 439–440
  auscultation landmarks, 434–435, 434f–435f
  auscultation of breath sounds, 435–437
  auscultation of heart sounds, 438–439
  dressings and equipment and, 442
  impaired oxygenation and, 615–616
  respiratory patterns and, 434t
  stethoscope placement and, 437
  view with landmarks and ribs numbered, 437f
Chest tubes
  chamber one and, 625–626
  chamber three and, 626
  chamber two and, 626
  draining system, 625–626
  maintaining, 640–641
  nursing interventions and, 616–627
  placement of, 625
Chest x-rays, 547, 617t
Chewable tablets, 853
Cheyne-Stokes respirations, 200, 362t, 434t
Child Protective Services, 36
Children
  administering medications and, 857
  admission reactions and, 409, 409f
  avoiding salicylate use and, 356
  catheters and, 726
  delegating care of, 180
  heat therapy and, 382
  injections and, 901
  medication administration and, 847
  pain and, 394
  personal care considerations and, 283
  teaching of, 226
Chiropractic medicine, 212–213, 212f
Chlamydia, 256
Chloride
  deficiency and excess, 660
  functions and regulation, 656t
  imbalances and, 658t
  levels of, 546
  nursing care and, 660–661
Choking, infants and toddlers and, 178
Cholesterol, 481
Chronic illness
  characteristics of, 139
  infections and, 261
  lung disease, 613
  metabolic conditions, 560
  wound healing and, 566t
Chronic obstructive pulmonary disease (COPD),
    426, 627–629, 629t–630t
Chronic pain, 393, 396
Chvostek's sign, 663f
Chyme, 676
Circadian rhythms, 346, 358t
Circular cyanosis, 199
Circulating nurse, 461, 783
Circulation, bathing and, 281
Circulatory changes, dying process and, 200
Circulatory overload, 942, 944t
Clean-catch midstream urine specimens,
    732–733
Clean-contaminated wounds, 558–559
Clean wounds, 558
Cleaning wounds, 571–572
Cleansing enemas, 685–686
Clear liquid diets, 502–503
Client-centered care, 23
Clinitron II Air Fluidized Therapy System, 318t
Clinitron Rite Hite Air Fluidized Therapy
    System, 319t
Closed beds, 292
Clostridia bacteria, 567
Clostridium difficile, 258, 263

Clostridium perfringens, 258
Closure, wound, 569–570
Closure and dying, 196
Clothing, inventory of, 413
Clubbing, fingertip, 443, 443f
Clutter, hospital room, 292
Code Blue, 241–242
Code teams, 241–242
Cognitive development
  adolescents and, 177
  characteristics of, 169
  infants and, 173
  middle adults and, 181
  older adults and, 182
  preschoolers and, 175
  school-age child and, 176
  toddlers and, 174
  young adults and, 181
Cold therapy
  chemical cold packs, 384
  cold compresses, 384
  edema and, 383
  effects of, 383t
  fever reduction and, 384
  hemostasis and, 383
  indications and, 383–384
  methods of, 384
  muscle spasms and, 384
  numbing sensation and, 383
  nursing care during, 384–385
  pain management and, 396
  pain relief and, 383
  pallor and, 385
  refillable ice bags, collars, gloves and, 384
  refreezable commercial cold packs, 384
  tepid baths and, 384
  vasoconstriction and, 383
Colectomy, postoperative care and, 795–799,
    797t–799t
Collaboration in care planning, 51
Collaborative interventions, 62
Colon perforation, enemas and, 688
Colonized wound, 559
Colonoscopy, 549
Colostomy, 690
Colostomy irrigation, 692, 705–706
Colostomy with descending colon, 692–697,
    695t–697t
Comatose patient, 430
Combination air-fluidized and low air-loss bed,
    319t
Comfort, dying process and, 202
Commercial heat packs, 380
Comminuted fracture, 592
Communicable diseases, 265–267
Communication. *See also* Special communication
    needs
  abilities and safety, 235
  active listening and, 118–119
  anger and hostility in, 120–121
  attitude and, 118
  body language and, 116
  body position and, 117
  congruence and, 117
  crisis communication, 120–121
  cultural aspects and, 118
  culturally savvy communication, 412
  developmental stages and, 130
  emotion and, 118
  factors affecting, 117–118
  health care team and, 121–123
  humor and, 121
  language and, 117–118
  learning new styles of, 119
  nervous system role in, 129

  nonverbal communication, 116–117
  older adults and, 130
  personal space and, 117
  physical assessment and, 424
  process of, 116
  shift-to-shift reporting, 123–125
  special communication needs, 127–130
  styles of, 119
  therapeutic communication, 119–120
  types of, 116–117
  verbal communication, 116–117
  written communication, 125–126
Comorbidity, 188
Compensation, 142t
Competency, 39
Complement cascade, 261
Complementary and alternative medicine
  acupuncture and acupressure, 214
  alternative *vs.* complementary therapy,
    210–211
  chiropractic medicine, 212–213
  Eastern medicine, 211
  herbal supplements, 214–215
  lifestyle changes that reverse disease, 215
  massage therapy, 213
  mind-body connections and, 211
  nursing care and, 216
  Western medicine and, 211
  yoga, 214–215
Complete bed bath, 284
Complete blood cell count (CBC), 541, 774
Complete metabolic panel, 545–546
Complex carbohydrates, 482–483
Comprehensive health assessment, 422
Compression devices, 801
Compression neuropathy, 317
Computed tomography (CT), 548
Computerized cabinets, medication, 843–844,
    844t
Computerized care plans, 64
Computerized charting, 102–103, 103f
Concept maps, 76–77, 76f
Condition Blue, 241–242
Condom catheter, 720, 722, 740
Confidentiality of documentation, 82–83
Conflict resolution, 121
Confusion, 749t
Congestive heart failure, 433
Congruent communication, 117
Connotative meaning, 118
Conscious sedation, 784–785
Consciousness level, 429–431
Consensual reflex, 431
Constipation. *See also* Bowel elimination
  activity level changes and, 679
  aging process and, 680–681
  dietary and fluid intake and, 679
  laxative abuse and, 680
  medication side effects and, 679
  older adults and, 492
  pregnancy and, 680
  preventing recurrent, 684
  stress levels and emotional problems and,
    680
  structural changes and, 680
  surgery side effects and, 679–680
Contact lenses, 289
Contaminated wounds, 559
Contamination, 457
Continent ostomy, 690
Continuing education, 39–40
Continuous bladder irrigation, 721–722, 722f
Continuous infusion feedings, 516
Continuous IV infusion, 915
Continuous lateral-rotation bed, 319t

Continuous passive motion machines, 597, 605–606
Contractures, 312, 443
Controlled-release tablets, 853
Controlled substances, 398
Contusions, 558
Conversion reaction, 143t
Coping skills, 137
Corrective surgery, 770
Cosmetic surgery, 770
Costovertebral angle, 426
Coudé catheter, 720
Coughs
    cough etiquette, 264t
    immobility and, 316
    impaired oxygenation and, 615
    physical assessment and, 433
Crackles, 362, 436
Cradle cap, 288
Creams, 858
Creatinine, 546, 710, 773
Crepitus, 616
Crisis communication, 120–121
Critical pathways, 69, 69f
Crohn's disease, 487, 678
Crutches, 598, 599t
Cryoprecipitate, 943
Cultural considerations, 132–138. *See also*
    Health care barriers
    admission process and, 411
    barriers to health care and, 139–141
    bathing and, 282–283
    communication and, 118
    cultural awareness, 131
    cultural competence, 131
    cultural diversity defined, 131
    cultural sensitivity, 131
    culturally savvy communication, 412
    death and dying and, 138–139, 189, 197t–198t
    delivering culturally sensitive care, 130
    ethnic cultural beliefs, 133t–137t
    folk healing, 133t
    illness beliefs and, 132t–133t
    naturalistically or holistically based beliefs, 132t
    needs assessment and, 445
    nutrition and, 492–493
    pain and, 394
    personal space and touch preferences, 117
    physical assessment and, 425
    religiously based beliefs, 133t
    scientifically based beliefs, 132t
    transcultural nursing defined, 131
Cultures, wound, 572, 582
Curative care, 189–190
Cutaneous pain, 394
Cyanosis, 432, 443, 615
Cyanotic skin, 441
Cystic fibrosis, 427

D

Dangle assistance, 337–338
DAR notes, 99, 99f–100f
Data collection, admission process and, 413–414
Data needing documentation, 96, 97t–98t
Deaf patients, 127–128
Death. *See* End-of-life care
Debridement, 567
Decision making, critical thinking skills and, 48–49
Decision making, patient, 411
Decubitus ulcers. *See* Pressure ulcers

Deep breathing, 316, 776
Deep somatic pain, 394
Deep tissue injury, 560
Deep tissue massage, 213
Deep venous thrombosis, 314, 380, 777
Defecation. *See* Bowel elimination
Defecation reflex, 677
Defense mechanisms, 141, 142t–143t
Dehiscence, 568
Dehydration, 652
Delayed assistance and safety, 235
Delirium, 748, 749t
Deltoid injection site, 900, 900f
Dementia, 748, 749t
Denial, 142t
Denotative meaning, 118
Dental caries, 432–433
Denture care, 287, 287f, 300–301
Dependency phase of illness, 139
Dependent interventions, 62
Depression, 319–320, 749t
Depth of respiration, 361
DESC method, 119
Detoxification, 19, 890
Development. *See* Growth and development
Diabetes
    diabetic diet, 503
    laboratory and diagnostic testing and, 504
    patient teaching and, 505
    wound healing and, 566t
Diagnosis in nursing process
    determining diagnoses, 57–60
    environmental problems and needs, 59
    physiological problems and needs, 57
    prioritizing diagnoses, 56
    psychosocial problems and needs, 58–59
    selecting nursing diagnoses, 56–57
    simplified divisions of, 57–59
    writing diagnosis, 60
Diagnosis-related groups (DRGs), 24
Diagnostic testing
    aspiration procedures, 551–552
    barium enema, 542t
    bone marrow aspiration, 542t
    graphic recording tests, 549–551
    intravenous pyelograms, 542t
    laboratory tests, 541–547
    lumbar puncture, 543t
    nursing's role in, 540–541
    oral glucose tolerance test, 543t
    paracentesis, 543t
    performing 12-lead electrocardiogram, 552–553
    preparing patient for, 541
    radiology and imaging tests, 547–549
    withholding food and fluids and, 540
Dialysis, 711
Diaphoresis, 351
Diarrhea. *See also* Bowel elimination
    activity level changes and, 679
    aging and, 680–681
    chemical changes and, 680
    dietary and fluid intake and, 679
    food allergies and, 680
    laboratory and diagnostic tests and, 681
    medication side effects and, 679
    surgery side effects and, 679–680
Diastolic pressure, blood pressure readings and, 346
Dietary approaches to stop hypertension (DASH) eating plan, 477–478
Dietary Guidelines for Americans, 477
Dietary intake, bowel elimination and, 679
Dietary reference intakes (DRIs), 476
Diets modified by consistency, 502–503

Diffusion, 648, 648f
Digestion, 478–480
    carbohydrates and, 483
    fats and, 482
    proteins and, 481
Digestive tract, 509f, 650
Digital removal of impaction, 688–689
Dilutional hyponatremia, 657
Diplococci, 256
Diploma programs, 6
Direct contact transmission of infections, 265–266, 266t
Disaster response, 242
Discharge
    business office notification and, 417
    criteria and, 61
    discharge instructions and, 415
    discharge teaching, 415
    final nursing responsibilities and, 417
    gathering belongings and valuables, 417
    initial planning of, 414
    instruction form and, 415, 416f
    leaving against medical advice, 415
    physician's order and, 415
    planning for, 414–415
    reconciling medications and, 415
    terminal cleaning and, 417
    typical process, 414
Discrimination, 140–141
Disinfectant cleaning agents, 262
Displacement, 143t
Dissociation, 142t
Distal pulse, 359
Distention, 677
Distraction, pain management and, 397
Diuretics, 711, 835t
Diverticulitis, 680
Do-not-resuscitate (DNR) orders, 185f, 193–194
    characteristics of, 33
    documenting, 194
    ethics and, 189
    following, 194
    history of, 194
Documentation. *See also* Medical records
    accountability and, 81
    accuracy of, 83
    care plans, 87
    charting methods, 96–103
    confidentiality of, 82–83
    continuity of care and, 80–81
    data to document, 96, 97t–98t
    forms of, 83
    guidelines for, 87–93
    home health care, 104, 106f–107f
    incident reports, 85–86
    Kardex, 83, 85, 86f
    long-term care and, 103–104
    medical record ownership and, 82
    medication and, 862–865
    not charted, not done, 82
    patient chart or medical record, 87
    patient teaching and, 226
    permanent record of care and, 81
    postoperative, 792
    problem-oriented records, 95
    providing legal record and, 82
    purposes of, 80–82
    report forms, 83–85, 84f
    source-oriented records, 93–95, 94t–95t
Documentation guidelines
    accuracy and, 89–92
    approved abbreviations and, 88–91, 89t
    being succinct, 88, 88t
    blank lines and, 92
    continued notes and, 92, 93f

Documentation guidelines (*continued*)
  follow chronological order, 87–88
  include date and time, 87
  keep medical records intact, 92–93
  punctuation and, 88
  sign each entry, 87
  subjective *vs.* objective entries, 92t
  timeliness and, 88
  use black or blue ink, 87
  write neatly and legibly, 87
Documentation mistakes
  documenting on wrong chart or MAR, 105–108
  failure to accurately document physician's orders, 108
  failure to document assessment findings, 104
  failure to document medications administered, 104
  failure to document pertinent health history, 104–105
Dorsalis pedis pulse, 358, 371
Dorsogluteal injection site, 900–901, 901f
Double-barreled colostomy, 690
Double-lumen catheters, 719–721
Downward communication, 123
Drainage, 570–571
Draining sinus tracts, 563
Draping, surgical patient and, 787
Drawing up, medications, 886–888
Drop factor, 925, 925f
Droplet transmission of infections, 265, 266t
Drowning, infants and toddlers and, 178
Drugs. *See* Medications
Dry heat application, 385
Dry-powder inhalers, 861
Dunn's theory of high-level wellness, 135, 135f
Durable power of attorney, 190–193
Dying process. *See also* End-of-life care
  circulatory changes and, 200
  comforting and, 201
  dehydration and malnutrition and, 201–202
  dyspnea and, 203
  elderly patients and, 756–757
  elimination and, 202
  emotional and spiritual distress, 202
  end-stage disease signs and symptoms, 198
  eyes and, 200
  fluid intake and, 201–202
  gas exchange and, 202
  just being there and, 204
  listening and, 200, 201f
  mental changes and, 199
  mucous membrane moisture and, 202
  narcotics use and, 202
  nursing care and, 200–204
  observation and provision of comfort, 202
  pain and nausea and, 202–203
  pain management and, 203
  physical activity and, 200
  physical changes and, 199–200
  positioning and, 202
  psychological and emotional changes, 199
  respiratory changes and, 200
  skin changes and, 199
  symptom management and, 203
  teaching and, 201
  typical calendar of, 199
  vital signs and, 199
Dysphasia, 433, 748
Dyspnea, 203, 361, 615
Dysuria, 713

E
E-cylinder, 620f
Ear care, 289–291

Ear medications, 859, 869
Ear wax, 427
Eastern and alternative health care, 211
Eating assistance, 500
Eating disorders, 505–506
Ecchymotic skin, 441
Echinacea, 215
Economics-related health care barriers, 139
Edema, 379, 383, 443–444, 444f, 559
Education-related health care barriers, 139
Effleurage, pain management and, 396
Eggcrate mattress, 318t
Egocentricity, toddler, 174
Elastic bandages, 593t, 606–607
Elbow protectors, 563f
Elderly patients
  administering medications and, 857
  ageism, 747
  aging myths, 747
  Alzheimer's disease and, 748–753
  assessment and, 75, 755, 762
  body system deficits and, 749t–752t
  cardiovascular functioning and, 753
  chronic illness and, 183
  cognitive development and, 182
  communication with, 130
  confusion and, 183, 748
  dietary recommendations and, 477
  documentation and, 762
  elder abuse, 757
  elite old, 747
  endocrine and genitourinary functioning and, 754
  financial concerns and, 757–758
  fluid intake and, 652
  gastrointestinal functioning and, 754
  health teaching and, 183
  heat therapy and, 382
  injections and, 901
  integumentary functioning and, 755
  long-term care and, 758–762
  loss, grief, and dying and, 756–757
  medication administration and, 847
  medication metabolization and elimination, 754
  middle-old group, 746–747
  modesty concerns and, 411
  moral and spiritual development and, 182
  musculoskeletal functioning and, 755
  neurological functioning and, 748–753
  nursing care for, 763–766, 765t–766t
  nutritional needs and, 492
  old-old group, 747
  orientation changes and, 749t
  pain and, 394
  performing venipuncture and, 937
  personal care considerations and, 283
  physical development and, 181, 182t
  polypharmacy and, 762–763
  positive aspects of aging, 758
  pressure ulcers and, 560
  preventing falls and, 183
  psychosocial development and, 182
  psychosocial problems and, 756–758
  reproductive functioning and, 755
  respiratory functioning and, 753–754
  safety concerns and, 183
  scams and crimes and, 757
  sensory function and, 753
  teaching and, 226
  vital sign assessment and, 762
  wound care and, 574
  young-old group, 746
Elective surgery, 770
Electrocardiograms (EKG), 549–550, 550f, 552–553, 774

Electroencephalography (EEG), 551
Electrolytes, 658t–659t
  bicarbonate imbalances and, 664
  calcium imbalances and, 662–663
  chloride imbalances and, 660–661
  magnesium imbalances and, 663–664
  nutritional sources and, 655t–657t
  phosphorus imbalances, 664
  potassium imbalances and, 661–662
  ranges, functions, regulation and, 655t–657t
  sodium imbalances and, 655–660
  testing levels and, 545
Electronic MAR documentation, 863
Elevated body temperature, 355–356
Elimination. *See* Bowel elimination
Emaciation, 505, 560
Emancipated minors, 41
Emergency response. *See* Safety
Emergency surgery, 771
Emotions
  blood pressure readings and, 346
  bowel elimination and, 680
  communication and, 118
  dying process and, 199
  intimacy and young adults, 180
  pain and, 395
  pulse rate and, 358t
Empathy, 32, 126
End-of-life care. *See also* Dying process
  cultural and religious differences and, 197t–198t
  dying process and, 198–200
  facing loss, 194
  family role reversal and, 194
  fearful patients and, 188
  five stages of grief, 194–198
  hospice care, 189–190
  living until they die, 190
  medications and, 188–189
  palliative care and, 189–190
  postmortem care and, 204–205
  reconciliation and closure and, 196
  respect for human dignity and, 188
End-of-life documentation
  advance directives, 42, 191f–193f
  do-not-resuscitate orders, 193–194, 195f
  durable power of attorney, 190–193
  living will, 190
End-stage disease signs and symptoms, 198
Endocrine medications, 836t–837t
Endocrine system
  elderly patients and, 751t, 754
  presurgical review and, 773
Endorphins, 393
Endoscopic examinations, 548–549
Endotracheal airways, 624
Endotracheal suctioning, 637–638
Endotracheal tube, 624, 786, 786f
Enemas
  administration of, 698–699
  cleansing enemas, 685–686
  colon perforation and, 688
  complications of, 687–688
  contraindications to, 687
  delegating administration of, 688
  hypertonic solutions and, 686
  medicating enemas, 687
  normal saline enemas, 686
  oil retention enemas, 686–687
  return flow enemas, 687
  soapsuds enemas, 686
  tap water enemas, 686
  types and solution volumes and, 686t
  vagal response and, 687
Energy conservation, impaired oxygenation and, 619–620

Entamoeba histolytica, 259
Enteral nutrition
  bolus feedings, 514–515
  checking feeding tube placement and, 416
  checking residual gastric volume and,
    516–517
  continuous infusion feedings, 516
  enteral feeding methods, 514–517
  feeding tubes and, 513, 514f
  formula types, 515t
  home healthcare and, 520
  intermittent tube feedings, 514, 516f
  jejunostomy tubes and, 513
  nursing care and, 517
  percutaneous endoscopic gastrostomy tubes,
    513, 513f
  tube feeding formulas, 513–514
Enteral tube uses, 508–509
Enteral tubes, medication administration and,
  855–857
Enteric-coated tablets, 853
Enterobius (pinworm), 259
Environment
  body temperature and, 352
  environmental quality, 138
  equipment considerations and, 292
  growth and development and, 168–169
  hospital room clutter, 292
  learning environment, 222
  noise and, 291
  odors and, 291–292
  respiratory rate and, 361t
  restorative sleep and, 401–402
  water needs and, 480
Envision E700 Low Air Loss Therapy System,
  318t
Enzyme testing, 545
Eosinophil levels, 544
Epidural anesthesia, 785–786
Epispadias, 723
Erectile dysfunction, 755
Erikson, Erik, 169, 170t
Erikson's stages of psychosocial development,
  169, 170t
Eructation (belching), 426
Erythema, 431, 559, 561
Erythematous skin color, 441
Eschar, 561
Escherichia coli, 258, 567
Esophagogastroduodenoscopy (EGD), 548–549
Essential amino acids, 480
Essential hypertension, 349
Estimated average requirement (EAR), 476
Estimated glomerular filtration rate, 773
Ethics
  advocating for patient, 31–32
  committees, 33
  ethical dilemmas, 30–31
  laws and, 33–38
  reporting unethical behavior, 32
Ethnicity. *See* Cultural considerations
Eupnea, 360, 433, 434t
Euthanasia, 188–189
Evacuated tube system, 809–810, 810f
Evisceration, 568
Exacerbations, illness, 139
Exception charting, 100
Excoriation, 281
Excretion, drugs effect on, 507–508
Excursion, chest, 433
Exercise. *See also* Physical activity
  blood pressure readings and, 346
  body temperature and, 352
  infections and, 261
  pulse rate and, 358t

respiratory rate and, 361t
  water needs and, 480
Exertional dyspnea, 615
Exhalation, 613
Exhaustion phase and stress, 140
Expected outcomes, 61
Expectorants, 839t
Experimentation, adolescents, 179
Expiration, 360
Exploratory surgery, 770
Expressive aphasia, 128
Extended-release tablets, 853
Extension tubing, 924–925
External fixators, 593, 593f
External respiration, 360, 613
Extracellular fluids, 646
Extravasation, intravenous therapy and,
  939–940
Extremity assessment
  lower extremities, 443–444
  upper extremities, 442–443
Extremity restraint, 240t
Extubation, 788
Eye care
  artificial eyes and, 289–290
  assessment and, 431
  contact lenses and, 289
  eye and ear irrigations, 859, 870–871
  eye protection, 264t, 273, 274
  eye response, 430t
  medications and, 858–859, 869
Eyes, dying process and, 200

F
Face shields, 264t
Face tents, 622t
FACES Pain Rating Scale, 393, 393f
Facility report form, 84f
Fahrenheit-celcius conversion formula, 351
Fall prevention
  fall assessment rating scales, 235, 236t
  infants and toddlers and, 178
  monitors and, 236
  nursing care plan for, 245–246, 246t–247t
  restraint alternatives and, 235–240
  soft devices and, 236
  strategies and, 237
False imprisonment, 36
Fat-restricted diet, 504
Fatigue, 211, 396
Fats
  cholesterol and, 481
  digestion and, 482
  high-density lipoproteins, 482
  lipid profile and, 482, 482t
  low-density lipoproteins, 481–482
  monounsaturated fats, 482
  polyunsaturated fats, 482
  saturated fats, 481
  trans fats, 481
Fauna, 256
Fear
  admission process and, 409
  immobility and, 319–320
  respiratory rate and, 361t
Febrile reactions, transfusions and, 944t
Fecal impaction, 681, 702
Fecal incontinence, 680, 681, 689
Feces characteristics, 677–678
Feeble pulse, 359
Feedback, communication process and, 116, 123
Feeding, patient assistance with, 527–528
Feeding pumps, 534–535
Femoral pulse, 358, 371

Fever
  nursing care and, 355–356
  postsurgical, 793
  reduction, 384
  signs and symptoms of, 355
Fiber, dietary, 483, 504, 683
Fight-or-flight response, 140
Filter needles, 888
Filtration, 648
Financial concerns
  elderly patients and, 757–758
  hospital admission and, 410
Finger stick blood sugar (FSBS), 816–817, 816f,
  822
Fingertip clubbing, 443, 443f
Fire drills, 240–241
Fire extinguishers, 241
Fire response, 240–241
Fire types, 241
Firearms, adolescents and, 179
First aid certification, 241
First-pass metabolism, 890
First surgical assistant, 783
Fist percussion, 426
Fistulas, 563, 563f
Fitzpatrick's rhythm method, 135
Five stages of grief, 194–198, 196t
Five to six small, frequent feedings, 504
Flatus (gas), 426
Flora, 256
Fluid volume disturbances. *See also* Body
  fluids
  assessment and diagnostic findings, 652
  fluid volume deficits, 651–653
  fluid volume excess, 653–654
  intake in elders, 652
  nursing care plan for, 669–671, 670t–671t
  treatment and nursing care, 653
Fluoroquinolones, 856
Flushed skin, 441
Focus charting, 99
Focused assessment, 422
Foley catheter, 719–721
Folk healing, 133
Fontanels, 173
Food. *See also* Nutritional care and support
  allergies, 501, 680
  body temperature and, 352
  drug effects and, 506
  intolerances, 501–502
  label example, 477f
  list by consistency, 503t
  withholding and diagnostic testing, 540
Food-drug interactions
  drug effects on absorption, 506–507
  drug effects on excretion, 507–508
  drug effects on food intake, 506
  drug effects on metabolism, 507
  selected interactions, 507t
Foot boards, 314, 314f, 323, 323t
Foot care, 227–s
Footdrop, 293, 314
Footdrop boots, 314
Fowler's stages of spiritual development,
  170–171, 171t
Fracture pan, 712, 712f
Fractures, 592
Free radicals, 216
Fresh frozen plasma, 943
Full liquid diet, 503
Full Trendelenburg position, 350
Functional incontinence, 718
Fungi, 257
Furniture, hospital, 291
Furosemide, 655

G

Gangrene, 567, 592
Garlic, 215
Gaseous disinfection, 456
Gastric decompression, 509–513
Gastric volume, enteral nutrition and, 516–517
Gastroenteritis, 680
Gastrointestinal system
  anatomy and physiology, 508
  assessment and, 428t
  elderly patients and, 750t–751t, 754
  gastrointestinal medications, 835t–836t
  immobility effects on, 316–317
  infections and, 260–261
  postoperative care and, 789
  presurgical review and, 773
  water movement from, 648–649
Gate control theory, 392–393
Gauge, needle, 883–884
Gauze dressings, 573t
Gels, 858
General adaptation syndrome, 140
General appearance, initial assessment and, 428–429
Genitourinary system, 428t, 751t, 754
Geography-related health care barriers, 139
Geri-chairs, 760
Giardia lamblia, 259
Ginger, 215
Gingko, 215
Ginseng, 215
Glands, 282
Glasgow Coma Scale, 430, 430t
Glaucoma, 753
Global aphasia, 128
Glomerular filtration rate, 547, 547t, 773
Glossitis, 432
Gloves, sterile, 263–265, 264t, 273–274, 463–466, 467–469, 814, 928
Glucose levels, 546
Glycemic control, 504
Glycosylated hemoglobin, 504
Good Samaritan Law, 38
Gowns, sterile, 264t, 272–274, 467–469
Granulation tissue, 564
Grapefruit juice, medication interactions and, 832
Graphic recording tests, 549–551
Gravity infusion rate, 936, 936f
Grief stages, 194–198
Grieving, 756–757
Grooming needs, 445
Growling stomach, 682
Growth and development
  adolescence, 176–177
  biological and hereditary factors and, 168
  cephalocaudal pattern and, 168
  development theories and, 169–171
  environmental factors and, 168–169
  factors influencing, 168–169
  infant development, 172–173
  preschoolers and, 175
  principles and, 168, 169t
  proximodistal pattern and, 168
  school-age child and, 175–176
  social factors and, 169
  toddlers and, 173–174
Guaiac testing, 678, 681, 701
Guided imagery, 397–398
Guidelines, medication preparations and, 845–846
Guilt and anger, 121
Gurgling bowel sounds, 440

H

Hair, anatomy and physiology and, 282
Hair care
  lesions and, 287
  lice and nits and, 288
  seborrhea and, 288
  shampooing hair, 288, 288f
  styling hair, 288
  tinea capitus and, 287
Hairline fracture, 592
Halitosis, 426, 432
Hallucinations, 748
Hand hygiene, 262–263, 264t. *See also* Gloves
  hand gels, 272
  handwashing, 928
  patient teaching and, 263
  performing, 263
  scrubbing and, 460–461, 466–467
  steps in, 271–272
  WHO guidelines, 263
Hand rolls, 323, 323t
Handle With Care campaign, 323
Handouts, teaching, 225
Hard of hearing patients, 127–128
Hard palate perforation, 432, 432f
Head and neck assessment
  consciousness level and, 429–431
  dressings and equipment and, 433
  eyes and, 431
  lips and, 432
  neck and, 433
  oral mucous membranes and, 431–432
  pupils and, 431
  speech and, 433
  teeth and, 432–433
Heal protectors, 563f
Healing touch, 216
Health care
  access to, 138
  associated infections, 260, 315
  barriers to, 139–141
  Dunn's theory of high-level wellness, 135
  economic considerations and, 139
  educational considerations and, 139
  Fitzpatrick's rhythm model, 135
  geographical considerations and, 139
  health grid, 135, 135f
  health literacy, 127
  Healthy People 2010, 135–138
  language challenges and, 139–140
  prejudice and discrimination and, 140–141
  promoting wellness and, 135–138
  public health insurance and, 24
  stereotyping and, 140
  wellness-illness continuum, 134–135, 134f
Health Care Financing Administration (HCFA), 104
Health care teams
  communication with, 121–123
  downward communication, 123
  members of, 16, 17t
  telephone and verbal physician orders, 122, 123f
  upward communication, 121–122
  writing physician's orders, 122–123
Health education
  adolescents and, 180
  infants and toddlers and, 178
  middle adults and, 183
  older adults and, 183
  preschoolers and school-age children and, 179
  young adults and, 183
Health Insurance Portability and Accountability Act (HIPAA), 35, 82
Health maintenance organizations (HMO), 25

Health Occupations Students of America (HOSA), 10
Healthy People 2010
  environmental quality and, 138
  focus areas of, 136
  health care access and, 138
  immunizations and, 138
  injury and violence and, 137
  mental health and, 137
  overweight or obesity and, 136
  physical activity and, 136
  responsible sexual behavior and, 137
  substance abuse and, 137
  tobacco use and, 136–137
Hearing aids, 290–291, 290f
Heart attacks, 314
Heart sounds
  auscultation and, 438–439, 439f
  electrocardiogram example of, 439f
  left base heart sound, 438
  left lateral sternal border heart sound, 438
  right base heart sound, 438
Heat therapy
  aquathermia pads and, 380, 380f, 386
  body temperature and, 379
  cold packs and, 387
  commercial heat packs and, 380
  contraindications for, 379
  dry or moist heat application, 385
  edema and, 379
  effects of, 383t
  healing process and, 379
  heating pads and, 380, 382
  hot compresses and, 381
  hot water bottles and, 380
  hyperthermia blankets and, 380
  indications for, 379
  methods of, 379–381
  muscle spasms and, 379
  nursing care during, 382
  pain management and, 379, 396
  rebound phenomenon and, 380
  safety and, 382
  seniors and children and, 382
  sitz baths and, 381, 381f, 386–387
  vasodilation and increased permeability and, 378, 378f
  warm soaks and, 381
  whirlpool baths and, 381–382
Height measurement, 447
Heimlich maneuver, 241
Helminths (parasitic worms), 257
Hematocrit, 346
Hematological system, 541–545, 774
Hematomas, 814
Hematuria, 711
Hemoconcentration, 814
Hemolysis, 810
Hemorrhages, 346, 569
Hemorrhagic stroke, 748
Hemostasis, 383, 563
Hemothorax, 625
Hemovac, 570, 570f
Heparin
  heparin flushes, 924
  reduced-strength *vs.* regular-strength, 925
  subcutaneous injection and, 893t, 896
Hepatomegaly, 485
Herbal supplements, 214–215. *See* Complementary and alternative therapy
Herpes simplex virus, 259
High-calorie, high-protein diet, 504
High-density lipoproteins, 482
Hip joint, 596, 596f

HMO regulations, 25
Holding area, presurgical, 781, 783f
Holistic care, 132t, 143–145, 210
Holter monitors, 551
Home health care
 documentation and, 104, 106f–107f
 medication administration and, 857
 oxygen use and, 241
 parenteral nutrition and, 520
 patient teaching and, 226
 service types and, 21–22
 sterile technique and, 461
 urinary catheters and, 726
 wound care and, 574
Homeostasis, 141
Hormonal regulation, 650
Hormones, pulse rate and, 358t
Hospice care, 22, 189–190
Hospital-acquired urinary tract infection, 723
Hospital admission kits, 412, 413f
Hospital outpatient departments, 20, 771
Hospitals, Language, and Culture: A Snapshot of the Nation, 130
Hostility, patient, 120–121
Hot compresses, 381
Hot water bottles, 380
Human chorionic gonadotropin (hCG) test, 774
Humor in communication, 121
Hydration
 blood pressure readings and, 346
 wound healing and, 566t
Hydrocolloid dressings, 573t, 585–586
Hydrofiber dressings, 573t
Hydronephrosis, 717
Hydrostatic pressure, 648
Hyperbaric chamber, 568
Hypercalcemia, 203, 659t, 662–663
Hyperchloremia, 658t, 660–661
Hyperglycemia, 894, 895t
Hyperkalemia, 659t, 661–662
Hypermagnesemia, 659t, 663–664
Hypernatremia, 657, 658t
Hyperphosphatemia, 659t, 664
Hypertension
 blood pressure readings and, 346, 347t
 risk factors for, 349
 treatment of, 349
Hyperthermia, 355, 786
Hyperthermia blankets, 380
Hypertonic solutions, 686, 918–920, 920t, 921f
Hypervolemia, 653–654
Hypoactive bowel sounds, 440
Hypocalcemia, 659t, 662–663
Hypochloremia, 658t, 660–661
Hypoglycemia, 894, 895t
Hypokalemia, 658t, 661–662
Hypomagnesemia, 659t, 663–664
Hyponatremia, 657, 658t
Hypophosphatemia, 659t, 664
Hypospadias, 723
Hypostatic pneumonia, 315
Hypotension, 349–350
Hypothermia, 356, 379, 789
Hypothermia blankets, 380
Hypotonic solution, 918, 919t, 921f
Hypovolemia, 429, 651–652, 915
Hypoxemia, 315, 360, 361, 566t, 614–615
Hypoxia, 359t, 614–615

I

Identification bands, 412, 412f
Ileostomy, 690
Ilizarov frame, 594

Illness
 acute, 139
 chronic, 139
 cultural beliefs and, 132t–133t
 phases of, 139
 remissions and, 139
 risk factors and, 139, 140t
 types of, 138–139
Illusions, 748
Immobility
 ambulation assistance and, 326–327
 appropriate positions and devices and, 320–322
 cardiovascular system and, 314–315
 common positions and their purposes, 321t–322t
 complications of, 313t
 devices for lifting and moving patients, 323–326
 gastrointestinal system and, 316–317
 impaired mobility and safety, 235
 integumentary system and, 317
 manual transfers and, 326
 musculoskeletal system and, 312–314
 neurological system and, 317–319
 patient positioning and, 320–322, 321t–322t
 physiological effects of, 312–319
 positioning devices and, 320–323, 322t–323t
 pressure ulcers and, 560
 psychological effects of, 319–320
 respiratory system and, 315–316
 support surfaces and specialty beds, 318t–319t
 turning, deep breathing, and coughing, 316
 urinary complications and, 317
Immobilizers, 593t
Immune system medications, 837t–838t
Immunizations, mandated, 138
Impaction, 678, 688–689
Impaired circulation, pressure ulcers and, 560
Impaired oxygenation
 arterial blood gases and, 616–617, 618t
 causes of, 614
 chest assessment and, 615–616
 cough and, 615
 diagnostic tests and, 616–617, 617t
 energy conservation and, 619–620
 hypoxemia and, 614–615
 hypoxia and, 614–615
 incentive spirometry, 617–618
 mucous membranes and, 615
 nebulizer treatments and, 618
 nursing interventions and, 617–618
 oxygen delivery and, 619
 patient care and, 614–617
 respiratory assessment and, 615–617
 respiratory effort and, 615
 skin color and, 615
 supplemental oxygen and, 618–619
 turn, cough, and deep breath, 617
Impaired swallowing, 524t–525t
Implementation in nursing process
 individualized interventions, 62–63
 initial intervention steps, 63
 intervention types, 61–62
Incentive spirometry, 316, 316f, 617–618, 632–633, 776–777
Incident reports, 42, 85–86
Incontinence, pressure ulcers and, 560
Independent interventions, 62
Independent living facilities, 18
Indian Health Service (IHS), 24
Indicator tape, sterilization and, 456, 457f
Indirect contact transmission of infections, 265–266, 266t
Indirect patient care, 61–62

Individual emergency response, 241–242
Individual values, pain and, 394–395
Individualized interventions, 62–63
Indwelling catheters, 719–721, 721f, 742
Infants
 administering medications and, 857
 attachment and, 173
 cognitive development and, 173
 delegating care of, 180
 fontanels and, 173
 health concerns and, 177–178
 health teaching and, 178
 injections and, 901
 moral development and, 173
 nursing implications for, 178
 pain and, 394
 physical development and, 172–173
 preventing choking and, 178
 preventing drowning and, 178
 preventing falls and, 178
 psychosocial development and, 173
 reflex development and, 172, 172f
 safety concerns and, 178
 weight and length measurement and, 448–449
Infections. *See also* Medical asepsis
 bacterial infections, 256–257
 causes of, 256–257
 factors that decrease defenses, 261
 fungal infections, 257
 healthcare associated, 260
 helminths, 257
 infected wounds, 559
 infection chain, 257–260, 260f
 infectious drainage, 427
 inflammatory process and, 261
 localized infections, 260, 940–941
 medical asepsis and, 262–266
 microbes and, 257, 258t–259t
 nursing care plan for, 267–269, 269t–271t
 pathogen types and, 256–257
 prevention of, 261–266
 primary defenses against, 260–261
 primary infections, 260
 protozoal infections, 257
 secondary defenses against, 261
 secondary infections, 260
 standard precautions and, 262
 systemic infections, 260
 tertiary defenses against, 261
 transmission-based precautions and, 262
 types of, 260
 viral infections, 257
Infiltration, intravenous therapy and, 937, 940
Influenza, 259
Information validation, 48
Informed consent, 41, 779–781, 780f, 781f
Infusion pumps and controllers, 927, 927f
Infusion rate calculation, 929–930, 930t
Inhalation, 613
Inhaled medications, administering, 873–874
Initial head-to-toe shift assessment, 422–423
 abdomen and, 440–442
 assessment flow sheet or checklist form, 446f
 blood pressure and, 429
 chest and abdomen and, 433–442
 documentation and, 445–447, 447f
 extremities and, 442–444
 general appearance and, 428–429
 head and neck and, 429–433
 needs and comfort and, 444–445
 neurological examination and, 429
 performance of, 449–450
 pulse and, 429
 respirations and, 429
 SpO$_2$ levels and, 429

Initial head-to-toe shift assessment *(continued)*
  temperature and, 429
  vital signs and, 429
Injections
  administering insulin subcutaneously, 904–905
  administration routes and, 890–891
  advantages of, 880
  age considerations and, 901
  decreasing discomfort and, 901
  delegation and, 881
  disadvantages of, 880
  getting ready and, 884
  handling syringes and needles, 884–886
  intradermal injections, 891, 891f, 903–904
  intramuscular injections, 896–901, 906–907
  maintaining asepsis and, 884–885, 885f
  mixing medications and, 888–890
  needles and, 883–884, 883f
  preventing needlestick injuries, 885–886, 885f
  reconstituting and withdrawing medication
    from vial, 902
  reconstitution and drawing up and, 886–890
  subcutaneous injections, 892–896
  supplies and equipment, 881–884
  syringes, 881–883
  tissue anatomy and, 890
  tuberculin skin testing and, 892
  withdrawing medication from ampule, 903
  Z-track injections, 907–908
Injury and violence, 137
Insensible fluid loss, 650
Insomnia, 402t
Inspection, physical, 424, 424f
Inspiration, 360
Insulin
  hyperglycemia and, 894, 895t
  hypoglycemia and, 894, 895t
  lipoatrophy and, 896
  preferred injection site and, 894
  self-administration of, 894
  sliding scale and, 894, 894t
  subcutaneous injection and, 893–896, 893t
  syringe used, 882, 883f
Intake and output, recording, 528–529
Integrative health care, 210
Integumentary system
  assessment and, 428t
  elderly patients and, 751t, 755
  immobility effects on, 317
Intellectual distraction, 397
Intermittent bolus enteral feedings, 533–534
Intermittent catheter irrigation, 724
Intermittent infusion lock, 924–925
Intermittent tube feedings, 514, 516f
Internal respiration, 360, 613
International normalized ratio (INR), 773
Internet
  medication resources and, 833
  patient teaching resources and, 226–227
  social networking, adolescents and, 179
Interpreter use
  arranging for interpreter, 223
  breaking language barrier and, 140
  learning and, 222
Interstitial spaces, 378
Intervention types, 61–62
Interviews. *See* Patient interviews
Intestinal malabsorption disorders, 487
Intracellular fluid (ICF), 646
Intracranial pressure
  blood pressure and, 346
  early signs of, 921
  pulse rate and, 359t
  respiratory rate and, 361t
Intractable pain, 393

Intradermal injections, 891, 891f, 903–904
Intramuscular injections, 896–901
  administering, 906–907
  air-lock and, 897
  deltoid injection site, 900, 900f
  dorsogluteal injection site, 900–901, 901f
  maximum volume and, 896
  needle length and, 896–897
  preventing complications and, 897–898
  rectus femoris injection site, 900
  repetitive injections, 897
  vastus lateralis injection site, 900, 900f
  ventrogluteal injection site, 898–900, 899f
  Z-track method, 897–898, 898f
Intraoperative interventions, 786–788
Intravascular space, 646
Intravenous equipment
  infusion pumps and controllers, 927, 927f
  needle cannula, 920–922, 922t, 923f
  start kits, 927–928, 927f
  tubing, 923–927
  winged butterfly, 922–923
Intravenous therapy. *See also* Peripheral venipuncture
  adding medications to primary solution,
    953–954
  adding new bag of solution to existing line, 959
  administering push medications, 915–917,
    915f, 946–947
  air embolisms and, 941–942
  asepsis and, 928–929
  bag sizes/volumes, 915, 915f
  blood and blood products and, 943–945,
    961–962
  circulatory fluid overload and, 942
  common solutions and their uses, 919t–920t
  compatibility *vs.* incompatibility, 917
  complications and, 938–943
  continuous infusion and, 915
  converting infusion to PRN lock, 951–952
  discontinuing an infusion or PRN lock, 960
  extravasation and, 939–940
  fluid and electrolyte losses and, 914–915
  hypertonic solution and, 918–920
  hypotonic solution and, 918
  infiltration and, 937, 939
  infusion rate calculation, 929–930, 930t, 953
  initiating peripheral venipuncture, 955–959
  intravenous push and, 915–917, 915f
  intravenous pyelograms, 542t
  isotonic solution, 917–918, 918f
  localized infection and, 940–941
  medication infusion, 915–917
  needle cannula and, 920–922, 922t, 923f
  peripheral venipuncture, 930–938
  phlebitis and, 940
  piggybacking medications and, 916–917,
    916f, 948–950
  pulmonary edema and, 942
  purposes of, 914–917
  safe administration of, 917
  septicemia and, 941
  severed cannula and, 941
  solutions, 917–920
  speed shock and, 942–943
  thrombophlebitis and, 940
  transfusions and, 943–945
Intravenous tubing
  characteristics of, 923
  drop factor and, 925, 925f
  extenders and, 924–925
  needleless systems and, 925–926, 926f, 927f
  safety needles and, 925–926, 926f
  styles of, 923
Intubation, 786, 786f

Ionizing radiation, 456
Iron, 485t
Irregular pulse, 359
Irrigation, wound, 580–581
Ischemia, 559
Ischemic stroke, 748
Isoenzyme testing, 545
Isolation, 143t
Isotonic solution, 917–918, 918f, 919t

J

Jackson-Pratt drain, 570, 570f
Jaundice, 431, 441, 545, 561
Jejunostomy tubes, 513–517
Job instruction, 123
Job rationale, 123
Joint injuries, heat therapy and, 379
Joint lubrication, water and, 650
Joint replacement, 592, 595–597

K

Kardex, 83, 85, 86f
Kegel exercises, 728
Keloids, 564
Ketonuria, 546
Kidney function assessment, 719. *See also*
  Bladder function; Urinary elimination
Kidneys, acid-base balance and, 667
Kinesthetic learning, 222
Kock pouch, 690
Kohlberg's stages of moral development, 171
Korotkoff sounds, 348–349
Kübler-Ross, Elisabeth, 194–198, 196t
Kussmaul's respirations, 362t, 434t
Kwashiorkor, 485
Kyphosis, 433

L

Laboratory staff, 17t
Laboratory tests
  blood chemistry tests, 545–546
  complete blood count normal values, 544t
  glomerular filtration rate, 547, 547t
  hematology, 541–545
  preoperative, 774–775
  urine tests, 546–547
Lacerations, 558
Lactose intolerance, 502, 679
Lancets, handling of, 461
Language and communication, 117–118
Language and learning, 222
Language-related health care barriers, 139–140
Lap guards, 236, 237f
Laparoscopic cholecystectomy, 776
Laparoscopic surgery, 20
Lateral auscultation sites, 438f
Laws. *See also* Legal documents
  areas of potential liability, 38
  civil laws, 36–38
  common legal terminology, 33t–34t
  statutory laws, 34–36
Laxatives and stool softeners, 680, 836t
Least restrictive environment, 238
Leaving against medical advice, 37f, 415
Left base heart sound, 438
Left lateral sternal border heart sound, 438
Left shift, 544
Leg exercises, 777
Leg monitors, 236, 237f
Legal documents
  advance directives, 42
  incident reports, 42
  informed consent, 41

patient charts, 40–41
records, 82
Legal regulation of medications, 829–830
Legal terminology, 33t–34t
Length, needle, 884
Lesions, hair care and, 287
Lethargy, 430
Leukocytosis, 541
Leukopenia, 541
Level of consciousness, 429–431
Levin's tube, 509
Liability insurance, 39
Lice, 287
Licensed practical or vocational nurse
   (LPN/LVN), 6
Licensure, 36
Lifelong learning, 7
Lifestyle
   changes that reverse disease, 215
   restorative sleep and, 401
   wound healing and, 566t
Lifting and moving patients
   lifts, 325–326
   logrolling a patient, 324
   moving patients in bed, 323–324
   obese patients, 327
   sit-to-stand lifts, 325, 325f
   slide boards, 324–325, 325f
   slide sheets, 324, 324f
   transfer belts, 324
   transferring patients, 324–326
   turning a patient, 324
Lipid profile, 482, 482f
Lipoatrophy, 896
Lips, assessment of, 432
Liquid medications, 853–854, 854f
Liquid oxygen unit, 620f
Liquid plasma, 943
Listening, dying process and, 200, 201f
Lithium, 508
Liver spots, 441
Living will, 190
Local anesthesia, 786
Localized infections, 260, 940–941
Location of pain, 393
Logrolling a patient, 324
Long-term care
   activity and entertainment and, 761
   catheters and, 726
   data set for resident assessment and care
      screening, 103
   documentation and, 103–104
   elimination and toileting and, 761
   immobility and, 761
   medical documentation and, 863–864
   medication administration and, 104, 761, 857
   nutrition and hydration and, 760–761
   patient or resident classification, 758–759
   patient populations in, 184
   personal attire and, 759
   personal care and, 283, 759–760
   promoting mobility in, 600
   resident rooms, 759
   resident's needs and, 759–761
   sterile technique and, 461
   weekly assessment data, 103–104
Loop stoma, 690
Lordosis, 433
Loss, elderly patients and, 756–757
Loss of control, admission process and, 410
Loss of identity, patient, 411
Lotions, 858
Low air-loss bed, 318t
Low-density lipoproteins, 481–482
Lower extremity assessment, 443–444

Lower extremity circulation stimulation, 777
Lubb-Dupp heart sound, 439
Luer-Lok tips, 881, 916f
Lumbar puncture, 543t, 544f, 551–552
Lungs. *See also* Chest assessment; pulmonary
   entries
   acid-base imbalance compensation and, 668
   anatomy and physiology of, 435
   lung lobes, 436f
Lymphedema, wound healing and, 566t
Lymphocyte levels, 261, 545
Lymphostasis, 807

M

Maceration, 281
Macro-drops, 925
Macronutrients, 476
Macular degeneration, 753
Magnesium
   deficiency and excess, 659t, 663–664
   functions and sources of, 484t
   nursing care and, 664
   ranges and regulation of, 656t
Magnetic resonance imaging (MRI), 547
Malignant hyperthermia, 786
Malnutrition, 773
Malpractice, 36
Mandatory reporting laws, 36
Mannitol, 648
Manual transfers, 326
Masks, 273, 275
Maslow, Abraham, 56
Maslow's hierarchy of human needs, 56
Mass casualty event, 242
Massage therapy, 213, 213f, 396
Material safety data sheet, 244–245
Mattress overlays, 318t
Mattresses, specialty, 318t
Meal planning assistance, 500
Measurement systems, medication, 842, 842t
Mechanical lifts, 325, 326f
Mechanical soft diet, 503
Mechanical ventilation, 129
Meconium, 677
Medicaid, 24
Medical administration records (AMRs).
   See also Documentation
   characteristics of, 87
   confidentiality and, 82–83
   faxing of, 83
   legal issues and, 40–41
   ownership of, 82
Medical centers, 18–19
Medical necessity, 16
Medical offices, surgical procedures at, 771
Medicare, 16, 24
Medicating enemas, 687
Medication administration
   coordinating with blood specimens, 862
   documentation and, 862–865
   ear medications, 869–870
   enteral tubes and, 855–857, 866–867
   eye and ear irrigation, 870–871
   eye medications, 869–870
   home health care and, 857
   infants and children and, 857
   long-term care and, 857
   mucosal route and, 858–861
   nursing responsibilities and, 861–862
   older adults and, 857
   oral medications, 852–855, 865–866
   organizers and, 857
   punch-card systems and, 857
   rectal suppositories and, 872–873

topical and transdermal medications, 858, 868
vaginal medications, 871–872
Medication administration records (MARs)
   administering medications and, 840, 841f
   electronic documentation and, 863
   long-term care and, 104, 863–864
   paper documentation and, 862–863, 863f
   preventing errors and, 864–865
   special situation documentation, 862–863
   withheld or refused medications, 864
Medications, 833t–839t. *See also* Food-drug interactions; Medication administration; Mixing
   medications
   absorption and, 506–507
   adding to primary IV solution, 953–954
   administration routes and, 829
   adverse effects and, 830
   age-related concerns and, 847
   allergic reactions and, 830
   ampules and, 888, 889f
   anaphylaxis and, 831
   application delegation and, 845
   blood pressure readings and, 346
   body temperature and, 352
   bowel elimination and, 679
   brand names of, 828
   calculations and, 842–843
   categories of, 829
   chemical names of, 828
   computerized cabinets and, 843–844, 844t
   desired effect and, 830
   drug abuse and, 137
   drug dose calculations and, 841–843
   drug interactions and, 831–832
   drug overdoses and, 361t
   errors and, 846, 864–865
   excretion and, 507–508
   food intake and, 506
   generic prescriptions, 828–829
   Internet resources and, 833
   intravenous infusion and, 915–917
   legal regulation of, 829–830
   locked bins in patient rooms, 844
   measurement systems and, 842, 842t
   medication carts, 844
   medication order abbreviations, 841
   medications not administered, 864
   metabolism and, 507
   mixing of, 888–890
   names of, 828–829
   nutritional considerations and, 499
   obtaining, 843–844
   over-the-counter medications, 829
   patient rights and, 845
   polypharmacy and, 762–763
   preoperative medications, 779
   preparation guidelines and, 845–846
   prescription medications and, 829
   professional drug abuse and, 829
   reading medication orders, 840–841, 840f
   reconciling for discharge, 415
   reconstitution and drawing up, 886–888
   researching medications, 832–833
   respiratory rate and, 361t
   rights involving, 844–845
   safety checks and, 845
   scheduled (controlled) drugs, 830
   side effects and, 830
   specific ordered frequencies, 840
   toxicity and, 831
   vials and, 887–888, 887f, 888f
   wound healing and, 566t
Meditation, 216, 358t, 361t
Megakaryocytes, 541
Melena, 678

Menarche, 176
Mental changes, dying process and, 199
Mental health, goals to improve, 137
Meperidine, 398
Meridians, 214
Metabolic acidosis, 361t, 668
Metabolic alkalosis, 361t, 667–668
Metabolic imbalances, 667–668
Metered-dose inhalers, 860–861, 860f
Methicillin-resistant *Staphylococcus aureus,* 567
Micro-drops, 925
Microbes, common illnesses caused by, 257, 258t–259t
Micronutrients, 476
Microorganisms, 256
Middle adults
    development and, 181
    health teaching and, 183
    nursing implications and, 183
    safety concerns and, 183
Mind-body connections, 211
Minerals, 484, 484t–485t, 487
Minimum Data Set for Resident Assessment and Care Screening (MDS), 103
Misunderstandings, 141
Mitered corners, bedmaking and, 293
Mitt restraint, 240t
Mixed incontinence, 718
Mixing medications, 888–890
    compatability/incompatability and, 889
    prefilled syringes and, 890
    ready to mix, 889–890
Modesty, patient, 410–411
Modified-release tablets, 853
Modified Trendelenburg position, 350
Monitors and fall prevention, 236
Monocyte levels, 544
Monounsaturated fats, 482
Montgomery straps, 573, 574t
Moon facies, 507
Moral development, 169–170
    adolescents and, 177
    infants and, 173
    middle adults and, 181
    older adults and, 182
    preschoolers and, 175
    school-age children and, 176
    toddlers and, 174
    young adults and, 181
Morse fall scale, 236t
Motor response, 430t
Mottling of skin, 200, 281
Moving patient up in bed, 332–333
Mucosal administration
    dry-powder inhalers, 861
    ear medications and, 859
    eye and ear irrigations, 859
    eye medications and, 858–859
    metered-dose inhalers, 860–861, 860f
    nasal medications, 859
    rectal medications, 860
    respiratory medications, 860–861
    vaginal medications, 859–860
Mucous membranes, 260, 431–432, 615
Multidisciplinary care plans, 64–69, 65f–68f
Multiple wounds, healing and, 566t
Murmurs, heart, 426, 439–440
Muscle atrophy, 312
Muscle spasms, 379, 384
Musculoskeletal care. *See also* Ambulation devices
    amputation and, 597–598
    applying elastic bandages, 606–607
    assessment and, 428t
    common musculoskeletal conditions, 592–593

continuous passive motion machine set-up, 605–606
    elderly patients and, 751t, 755
    immobilization and, 312–314, 593–594, 593t
    joint replacement and, 595–597
    neurovascular checks, 605
    patients in traction, 59f, 595
    patients with casts, 594–595
    presurgical review and, 773
    testing for musculoskeletal conditions, 593
    total hip replacement and, 595–596, 597f
    total knee replacement and, 597–598
Music therapy, 216
Mycobacterium tuberculosis, 258
Myocardial infarction, 314, 753
Myocardial ischemia, 549
MyPyramid food management system, 478, 479f

N

Nail care, 282, 287, 302–303
Nailbeds, 443
Naloxone (Narcan), 398
Narcolepsy, 402t
Narcotics, 854–855
Narrative charting, 100–101
Nasal cannula, 621t
Nasal medications, 859
Nasogastric tubes, 508–509, 510f. *See also* Gastric decompression
    insertion of, 530–531
    removal of, 532–533
Nasointestinal tubes, 508–509
Nasopharyngeal airway, 623
Nasopharyngeal suctioning, 635–637
National Council Licensure Examination (NCLEX), 6, 36
National Federation of Licensed Practical Nurses (NFLPN), 10, 49
National patient safety goals, 234
National Student Nurse Association (NSNA), 10
Naturalistically based illness beliefs, 132t
Nausea, 203, 794
Nebulizer treatments, 618, 633–634
Neck assessment, 433
Necrotic tissue, 559
Needles
    filter needles, 888
    gauge of, 883–884
    handling of, 461, 461f, 884–886
    length of, 884
    needle-and-syringe method, 810–812, 813f
    needleless intravenous systems, 925–926, 926f, 927f
    needlestick injuries, 884–885, 885f
    one-handed "scoop" method and, 885–886, 886f
    parts of, 883–884
    phlebotomy and, 809–810, 810f, 812f
    recapping and, 885–886, 886f
    safety needles, 925–926, 926f
    standard precautions for, 264t
Negative pressure rooms, 265
Negative pressure wound therapy, 573t
Negligence, 32
Nervous system medications, 838t–839t
Neurogenic bladder, 721
Neurological functioning, aging and, 748–753
Neurological system
    elderly patients and, 749t
    examination and, 427t, 429–430, 450–451
    immobility effects and, 317–319
Neuropathic pain, 394
Neurovascular checks, 605
Neutrophil levels, 544

Nicotine, blood pressure readings and, 346
Night terrors, 402t
Nitrogen balance, 480
Nits (head lice), 287
No lifting programs, 323
Nocturia, 717–718
Nocturnal coughs, 433
Non-opioid analgesics, 397–398
Non-rapid eye movement sleep (NREM), 400, 400t
Non-rebreathing masks, 622t
Nonessential amino acids, 481
Nonintact skin, infections and, 261
Nonpharmaceutical management, pain and, 396–397
Nonproductive cough, 433
Nonskid footwear, 327
Nonsteroidal anti-inflammatory drugs (NSAIDs), 398
Nonverbal communication, 116–117, 127
Normal saline enemas, 686
North American Diagnosis Association-International (NANDA-I) diagnoses, 56–57
Nosocomial infections, 260
Not charted, not done, 82
NPO (nothing per os), 502
Numbing sensation, cold therapy and, 383
Nurse Practice Act, 7, 34–36
Nursing
    adequate rest and appropriate focus, 244
    associate degree nurse, 6
    baccalaureate degree nurse, 6–7
    being caring and, 8, 9f
    being honest and, 8
    being organized and, 9
    being responsible and, 8
    biological hazards and, 245
    body mechanics and, 243–244, 250
    chemical hazards and, 244–245
    developing rapport and, 126
    diploma programs and, 6
    drug use and, 244
    education levels and, 6–7, 6t
    empathy and, 126
    establishing trust and, 126
    hazard types and, 243
    nurse characteristics, 8–9
    nurse-patient relationship, 126–127
    patient-centered communication and, 126
    patient interviews and, 126–127
    radiation hazards and, 244
    specialization and, 7
    staff safety and, 243–245
    theorists regarding, 11, 11t
Nursing Outcomes Classification (NOC), 61
Nursing process
    assessment and, 51–55
    evaluation and, 63
    implementation and, 61–63
    interconnected steps of, 50f
    from non-nursing perspective, 50
    planning and, 60–61
    RNs and LPN/LVNs and, 49–51
    steps in, 49
Nutrition Labeling and Education Act, 476
Nutritional care and support
    adolescents and, 491
    adulthood and, 491–492
    American Heart Association diet, 478
    anorexia nervosa and, 505
    assessment and, 498–499
    bulimia nervosa and, 505–506
    carbohydrate requirements and, 482–483
    clear liquid diets, 502–503
    cultural influences and, 492–493

DASH eating plan, 477–478, 478t
diabetes and, 504–505
Dietary Guidelines for Americans, 477
diets modified by consistency, 502–503
diets modified by disease, 503–504
digestion and, 478–480
eating assistance and, 500
eating disorders and, 505–506
enteral nutrition and, 513–517
enteral tubes and, 508–509
fat requirements and, 481–482
FDA guidelines and food labels, 476–477
feeding assistance and, 527–528
feeding pumps and, 534–535
food allergies and, 501
food-drug interactions and, 506–508
food intolerances and, 501–502
food list by consistency, 503t
full liquid diets and, 503
gastric decompression and, 509–513
infections and, 261
intermittent bolus enteral feedings and,
    533–534
managing tube feeding formulas, 518
meal planning and, 500
mealtime preparation, 499
mechanical soft diets and, 503
medication use and, 499
metabolism and, 476
minerals and, 484, 484t–485t
monitoring intake and output, 500–501
MyPyramid food management system, 478,
    479f
nasogastric and nasointestinal tubes, 508–509,
    510f
nasogastric tube insertion, 530–531
nasogastric tube removal, 532–533
NPO (nothing per os), 502
nursing responsibilities and, 504
nutrient interactions and, 476
odors and, 499
older adults and, 492
overweight and obesity and, 485–487
parenteral nutrition and, 518–520
patient comfort and, 499
patient positioning and, 499
pregnancy and, 490
protein deficiencies and, 485
protein requirements and, 480–481
pureed diet and, 503
recording intake and output and, 520–529
regular diet and, 502
school-aged children and, 491
special nutritional needs and, 501–502
specific population groups and, 477
standard container volumes and, 501
therapeutic diets and, 502–504
toddlers and preschool children and, 490–491
tube feeding complications and, 517–518
USDA food guide and, 477, 478t
vitamins and, 483–484
water requirements and, 480
wound healing and, 566t

O

Obesity
    blood pressure readings and, 346
    body mass index and, 485–487
    moving patients and, 327
    older adults and, 492
    promoting wellness and, 136
Objective data, obtaining, 51–52
Occult blood tests, 678, 681
Occupied beds, 292

Ocular prosthesis, 289–290
Odors, 291–292, 426–427
Oil retention enemas, 686–687
Ointments, 858
Oklahoma advance directives for health care,
    191f–193f
Older adults. *See* Elderly patients
Olfaction, 426–427
Oliguria, 711
Omnibus Budget Reconciliation Act (OBRA),
    103
Open beds, 292
Open-ended questions, 127
Operating room, sterile technique and,
    460–461
Opiate/opioid analgesics (narcotics), pain and,
    398
Oral care
    conscious patient and, 286–287, 299–300
    denture care, 287, 287f
    safety and, 286
    special mouth care, 28
    unconscious patient and, 286, 298–299
Oral glucose tolerance test, 543t
Oral medications
    administering, 865–866
    capsules and, 853
    enteric-coated tablets and, 853
    liquid medications and, 853–854, 854f
    narcotic medications and, 854–855
    sustained-release tablets and, 853
    tablets and caplets and, 852–853
Oral mucous membranes, 431–432
Oral temperature measurements, 354
Orientation changes, elderly patients and,
    749t
Orientation checklist, 413
Oropharyngeal airway, 623
Oropharyngeal suctioning, 635–637
Orthopnea, 361, 433
Orthopneic position, 615
Orthostatic hypotension, 315, 350, 366–367
Orthotopic bladder substitution, 725
Osmosis, 647–648, 647f
Osmotic diuresis, 648
Osteoarthritis, 592
Osteogenic pain, 394
Osteoporosis, 312, 662
Ostomy appliances, 691–692, 691f
Outcome and Assessment Information Set
    (OASIS), 104, 105f
Outpatient care, 20
Outpatient mental health services, 20
Outpatient surgery, 777
Ova and parasite test, 681
Over-the-counter medications, 829
Over-the-needle cannulas, 922, 923f
Overactive bladder, 718
Overflow incontinence, 718
Overhead ceiling lift devices, 326
Oxygen
    circulatory needs and, 445
    concentrator, 621t
    delivery devices and, 619, 621t–623t
    e-cylinder, 620f, 621t
    flowmeter, 619f
    home use and, 241
    liquid oxygen unit, 620f, 621t
    oxygen tanks, 621t
    safety and, 245
    saturation and, 362, 373, 616
    source types, 621t
    supplemental, 618–619
Oxygenation, 612–613, 616. *See also* Impaired
    oxygenation

P

Packed red blood cells, 943
Pain
    acknowledgment and acceptance and, 396
    acupressure and acupuncture and, 396
    acute or chronic pain, 363, 396
    adjuvant analgesics and, 399
    characteristics of, 363, 396
    classifications of, 393–395
    cold therapy and, 383
    cutaneous pain, 394
    deep somatic pain, 394
    developmental stage and, 394
    distraction and, 397
    documenting, 363–364, 364f
    dying patient and, 188–189
    dying process and, 202–203
    emotions and, 395
    endorphins and, 393
    ethnic and cultural beliefs and, 394
    factors affecting, 394–395
    fatigue and, 395
    gate control theory and, 392–393
    guided imagery and, 397–398
    heat therapy and, 379
    holistic view of, 392
    hot and cold packs and, 396
    individual values and, 394–395
    initial assessment and, 429
    intractable pain, 393
    level or extent of, 395–396
    management and treatment of, 395–399
    massage and effleurage and, 396
    nature and physiology of, 392–393
    neuropathic pain, 393–394
    nociceptive pain, 393–394
    non-opioid analgesics and, 397–398
    nonpharmaceutical management and, 396–397
    nonpharmacological interventions for, 202
    nonsteroidal anti-inflammatory drugs and, 398
    opiate/opioid analgesics and, 398
    pain scales and, 363, 393
    patient-controlled analgesia and, 398–399,
        399f
    patient's desires and, 396
    personal support system and, 395
    phantom limb pain, 394
    pharmaceutical management and, 397–399
    postoperative, 778–779, 790, 792
    previous pain experiences and, 394–395
    progressive relaxation and, 397
    radiating pain, 393
    referred pain, 393, 393f
    relaxation and, 396–397
    respiratory rate and, 361t
    responses to, 395
    rest and restorative sleep and, 399–402
    safety concerns and, 235
    signs and symptoms of, 395t
    site or location and, 363, 396
    transcutaneous electrical nerve stimulation,
        396, 396f, 403
    visceral pain, 394
Pale skin, 441
Palliative care, 189–190
Palliative surgery, 770
Pallor, 385, 561
Palpation
    abdominal contraindications, 441
    chest assessment and, 615–616
    physical assessment and, 425
Paracentesis, 543t, 551–552
Parenteral nutrition
    conditions requiring, 518
    home healthcare and, 520

Parenteral nutrition (continued)
  monitoring nutritional status and, 520
  partial parenteral nutrition, 518–519
  total parenteral nutrition, 519–520, 519f
Paresthesia, 441
Partial bath, 284
Partial parenteral nutrition, 518–519
Partial rebreathing masks, 622t
PASS acronym, 241
Passive behavior style, 119
Passive range-of-motion exercises, 327–330
Pathogens, 256–257
Pathological fracture, 662
Patient care partnership, 31–32
Patient-centered communication, 126
Patient chart. See Medical records
Patient-controlled analgesia (PCA), 398–399, 399f
Patient desires, pain management and, 396
Patient history, presurgical assessment and, 772
Patient interviews
  communication during, 126–127
  directive interview, 127
  format of, 126–127
  nonverbal communication during, 127
  nursing process and, 51–55
  open-ended questions and, 127
  physical assessment and, 423–424
Patient positioning, surgery and, 787
Patient rights, medications and, 845
Patient rooms
  management of, 291
  sharing of, 411
Patient teaching. See also Teaching plans
  comfort and, 222
  documentation and, 226
  environment and, 222
  factors affecting learning, 222
  focus of, 224
  health promotion and, 223
  home care considerations, 226
  Internet resources and, 226–227
  interpreters and, 222–223
  language and, 222
  learning styles and, 222
  purposes of, 223–224
  readiness and, 222
  reinforced, 223
  repetition and, 223
  senses and, 222
  teachable moments and, 223–224, 224t
  teaching children, 226
  teaching elderly patients, 226
  teaching handouts and, 225
  teaching plans and, 224–226
  wellness strategies and, 223
Patient transfer
  to another facility, 417–418
  from bed to stretcher, chair, or wheelchair, 335–336
  within the facility, 417
  lifts and, 325
  manual transfers, 326
  mechanical lift and, 336–337
  sit-to-stand lifts and, 325
  slide boards and, 324–325
  slide sheets and, 324
  transfer belts and, 324
  transfer summary form, 417
Peak flow tests, 617t
Peel-apart packs, 457, 457f
Penetrating wounds, 558
Penrose drain, 571
Peppermint, 215
Percussion, physical assessment and, 425–426, 426f

Percutaneous endoscopic gastrostomy (PEG) tubes, 513, 513f, 520–524, 524t–527t
Percutaneous injuries, needles and, 884–885, 885f
Perfusion, 359
Perineal care, 296–297, 688
Peripheral nerve blocks, 786
Peripheral pulse assessment, 370–371
Peripheral pulse scale, 442
Peripheral pulse sites, 357–358, 357f. 359t
Peripheral venipuncture. See also Intravenous therapy; Venipuncture
  allergies and, 931
  determining proper cannulation, 935
  dilating veins and, 933
  discontinuing IV infusion, 938
  documenting venipuncture, 937
  elderly patients and, 937
  encountering difficulty and, 935
  equipment preparation and, 931–932
  final preparation of supplies and, 933–934
  infiltration signs and symptoms and, 937
  initiating, 955–959
  medical record review and, 930–931
  mental cognition and, 931
  monitoring IV infusions, 936–937
  patient's age and, 931
  performing venipuncture and cannulation, 934–935
  phlebitis signs and symptoms and, 937
  physician's order and, 931
  problem-solving and, 937–938
  securing IV site, 935–936
  setting gravity infusion rate and, 936, 936f
  site cleansing and, 934
  starting IV pump and, 936
  vein selection and, 932–933, 932f
Peristalsis, 316, 440, 676
PERLA documentation, 431
Permeability, heat therapy and, 378, 378f
Pernicious anemia, 432, 432f
Personal care
  back massages and, 286, 286f, 298
  bathing, 281–282
  bedmaking, 292–294
  children and, 283
  complete bed bath, 294–296
  conscious patient and, 299–300
  denture care, 300–301
  elderly and, 283
  environment and, 291–292
  eye and ear care, 289–291
  furniture, 291
  hair care, 287–288
  making an occupied bed, 306–307
  making an unoccupied bed, 304–305
  nail care, 287, 302–303
  oral care, 286–287
  patient room, 291
  perineal care, 296–297
  piercings and, 288–289, 289t
  routinely scheduled care, 280
  shampooing hair with patient in bed, 303–304
  shaving patient, 287, 301–302
  special settings and, 283
  types of care, 283
  unconscious patient and, 298–299
Personal items, 413
Personal protective equipment, 264t, 272–275
Personal space, 117
Personal support system, pain and, 395
Pet therapy, 216
Petechiae, 814
pH scale, 665, 665f, 711
Phagocytes, 261

Phagocytosis, 379, 564
Phantom limb pain, 394
Pharyngeal airways, 623
Phenytoin (Dilantin), 855
Phlebitis, 379, 937, 940
Phlebotomy. See also Venipuncture sites
  blood culture specimen collection, 821
  butterfly needles and, 923
  butterfly or winged infusion sets, 812, 813f
  complications of, 815–816
  delegation and, 817
  drawing blood culture specimens, 815
  equipment and supplies, 809–814
  evacuated tube system and, 809–810, 810f
  gloves and, 814
  needle-and-syringe method, 810–812, 813f
  needles and, 809–810, 810f, 812f
  patient preparation and, 506
  performing venipuncture and, 814–815
  plastic tube holders and, 810, 810f
  puncture for finger stick blood sugar, 822
  purpose of, 806
  site cleansing and, 809
  skin punctures and, 816– 817, 816f, 919f
  specimen labels and, 813–814
  tourniquets and, 808, 813–814, 818
  tubes with color-coded tops, 812–813, 813t
  vein and artery anatomy/physiology, 807
  venipuncture and, 819–820
  venipuncture site selection, 807–809, 807f
Phosphorus, 485t, 657t, 659t, 664
Physical activity. See also Exercise
  blood pressure readings and, 346
  body temperature and, 352
  dying process and, 200
  respiratory rate and, 361t
Physical assessment
  abnormal findings and, 423
  auscultation and, 426
  body systems and, 427, 427t–428t
  comprehensive health assessment, 422
  cultural beliefs and, 425
  focused assessment, 422
  initial head-to-toe shift assessment, 422–423
  inspection and, 424, 424f
  interviewing and, 423–424
  levels of, 422–423
  olfaction and, 426–427
  palpation and, 425
  percussion and, 425–426, 426f
  presurgical, 774
  purpose of, 422
  rapport and communication and, 424
  signs and symptoms and, 423
  techniques for, 423–427
  therapeutic communication and, 424
  timing of, 423
  weight and height and, 424–425
Physical development
  adolescence and, 176
  infants and, 172–173
  middle adults and, 181
  older adults and, 181, 182t
  preschoolers and, 175
  school-age child and, 175
  toddlers and, 173–174
  young adults and, 180
Physical mobility, impaired, 526t–527t
Physical therapists, 592
Physicians, communication with, 122
Physician's Desk Reference, 832–833
Physician's discharge order, 415
Phytonutrients, 216
Piaget, Jean, 169–170

Piaget's four stages of cognitive development, 169–170
PIE charting, 98, 99f
Piercings care, 288–289, 289t
Pillow, as positional device, 322t
Piped-in oxygen, 621t
Pitting edema, 443–444, 444f
Planning in nursing process, 60–61
Plantar flexion, 293, 317
Plasmodium, 259
Plastic tube holders, 810, 810f
Platelets, 943
Play therapy, 216
Playground safety, preschoolers and school-age children, 179
Pleura, 613
Pleural effusion, 616
Pleural friction rub, 436
Pneumonia, 627–629, 629t–630t
Pneumothorax, 616
Pocket-brains, 83, 85f
Point of maximum impulse (PMI), 356–357, 438
Point-of-service (POS) plan, 25
Polydipsia, 653
Polypharmacy, 762–763. *See also* Medications
Polyunsaturated fats, 482
Polyuria, 711
Polyvinyl dressings, 573t
Popliteal pulse, 358, 371
Portal circulation, 649
Positioning, bowel elimination and, 683
Positioning devices, 320–323, 322t–323t
Positioning patients, 320–322, 321t–322t, 331–332
Post-cerebrovascular accident with a PEG tube
    assessment and, 521–522
      evaluation and, 524
      impaired physical mobility and, 526t–527t
      impaired swallowing and, 524t–525t
      implementation and, 524
      nursing diagnoses and, 522
      planning and, 523
Postanesthesia assessment and care, 788–790
Postanesthesia care unit (PACU), 773
Posterior auscultation sites, 438f
Posterior tibialis pulse, 358, 371
Postmortem care, 204–205
Postoperative care
    cardiovascular problems and, 789
    colectomy and, 795–799, 797t–799t
    continued assessments and, 792
    discharge and, 790
    documentation and, 792
    equipment and supplies needed, 791
    first priority and, 791
    fluid and electrolyte balance and, 792
    fluids and related equipment and, 791–792
    gastrointestinal problems and, 789
    hypothermia and, 789
    initial assessment and, 790–792
    pain and discomfort and, 778–779, 790, 792
    postanesthesia assessment and care, 788–790
    postoperative orders and, 792–793
    respiratory problems and, 788
    room preparation and, 790
    safety interventions and, 792
    second priority and, 791
    surgical site and, 791
    vital sign frequency and, 792
Postsurgical complications
    atelectasis, 793
    fever, 793
    nausea and vomiting, 794
    pulmonary embolism, 793, 794f
    urinary retention, 794
    wound infection, 794

Postural hypotension, 315, 350
Potassium
    deficiency and excess and, 661
    functions and sources of, 484t
    imbalances and, 658t–659t
    levels of, 546
    regulation and, 656t
    treatment and nursing care and, 661–662
Potassium chloride, 661
Povidone-iodine, 929
Prealbumin, 520
Precedents, legal, 34
Precipitate, 917
Preferred provider organization (PPO), 25
Prefilled syringes, 882–883, 883f, 890, 916f
Pregnancy
    blood pressure and, 346
    bowel elimination and, 680
    dietary recommendations and, 477
    nutritional needs and, 490
    water needs and, 480
    weight gain and diet, 491
Prejudice, 140–141
Preoperative care
    checklist and, 781, 782f
    laboratory tests and, 774–775
    medications and, 779
    patient history and, 772
Presbyopia, 183
Preschoolers
    development and, 175
    health teaching and, 179
    nursing implications for, 179
    nutritional needs and, 490–491
    playground safety and, 178–179
    safety concerns and, 178–179
    stranger danger and, 178
    water safety and, 179
Prescription medications. *See* Medications
Pressure ulcers
    Braden scale and, 562f
    common sites for, 559, 559f
    deep tissue injury, 560
    depth of, 561
    immobility effects and, 317
    prevention of, 561–563
    risk factors for, 560
    shearing force and, 559
    stage I, 560
    stage II, 560–561, 575–576, 577t–578t
    stage III, 561
    stage IV, 561
    unstageable, 561
Previous pain experiences, 394–395
Primary care nursing, 23
Primary care physicians, 25
Primary hypertension, 349
Primary infections, 260
Primary intravenous administration sets, 923
Privacy, bowel elimination and, 683
Private health insurance, 24–25
PRN lock devices, 915–917, 922f, 924–925
Problem-oriented records, 95
Prodromal phase of illness, 139
Productive cough, 433
Professional liability insurance, 39
Professional organizations, 10–11
Professionalism
    accountability and, 38–40
    appearance and, 9–10
    behavior and, 9–10
    role boundaries and, 39
Progressive relaxation, 397
Projection, 143t
Prostaglandins, 393

Protective devices. *See* Restraints
Proteins
    anabolism and, 480
    deficiencies, 485
    digestion and, 481
    essential amino acids, 480
    nitrogen balance and, 480
    nonessential amino acids, 481
    primary bodily function of, 481
    protein-restricted diets, 504
Proteinuria, 546
Proteus infection, 427
Prothrombin time, 773, 896
Proton pump inhibitors, 856
Protozoa, 257
Proxemics, 117
Proximal pulse, 359
Proximodistal pattern of growth, 168
Pseudomonas infection, 427
Psychological effects
    dying process and, 199
    immobility and, 319–320
Psychosocial development
    adolescents and, 176–177
    infants and, 173
    middle adults and, 181
    older adults and, 182
    preschoolers and, 175
    school-age child and, 175–176
    toddlers and, 174
    young adults and, 180
Psychosocial needs, 445
Ptosis, 431
Puberty, 176
Pulmonary edema, 615, 942
Pulmonary embolisms, 314, 315, 777, 793, 794f
Pulmonary function tests, 617t
Pulmonary rehabilitation, 21
Pulse
    apical pulse, 356–357, 356f
    assessment of, 358–360, 369–372, 429
    blood pressure readings and, 346
    factors affecting rate of, 358t–359t
    peripheral pulse scale and, 442
    peripheral pulse sites, 357–358, 357f, 359t
    pulse deficit, 357, 439
Punch-card systems, medication, 857
Puncture wounds, 558
Pupil assessment, 431
Pupil size, 431f
Pureed diet, 503
Purging, 505
Purulent drainage, 559, 570
Pyloric sphincter, 676
Pyrexia, 355

R

Race, blood pressure readings and, 346
RACE acronym, 241
Radial pulse, 357, 369–371
Radiating pain, 393
Radiation exposure, 566t
Radiation hazards, 244
Radiography, 547
Radiology staff, 18t
Radionucleotides, 541
Radiopaque substances, 541
Rales, 362, 436
Range-of-motion exercises, 314
Rapid eye movement sleep (REM), 400, 400t
Rapport, 126, 424
Rationalization, 142t
Reaction formation, 142t
Readiness, learning, 222

Rebound phenomenon, 380
Rebound tenderness, 425
Receptive aphasia, 128
Recommended dietary allowance (RDA), 476
Reconciliation and closure, 196
Reconstitution, medications, 886–888
Recovery phase of illness, 139
Rectal medications, 860
Rectal suppositories, 872–873
Rectal thermometers, 354
Rectus femoris injection site, 900
Red, beefy tongue, 432, 432f
Red blood cell (RBC) counts, 541, 545, 774
Referrals, 25
Referred pain, 393, 393f
Refillable ice bags, 384
Reflex development, infants, 172, 172f
Reflexology, 213
Refreezable commercial cold packs, 384
Refused medications, documentation and, 864
Regional anesthesia, 785
Registered nurse first assistant (RNFA), 783
Regression, 142t, 179
Regular diet, 502
Regular syringe, 881–882
Rehabilitation facility, 19
Reinforced learning, 223
Relaxation
    pain management and, 396–397
    restorative sleep and, 402
    therapy and imagery, 216
Religious beliefs
    death and dying and, 197t–198t
    illness beliefs, 133t
    tenets and, 141–143, 142t–143t
Remissions, illness, 139
Renal caliculi, 715
Renal diet, 504
Renal system, presurgical review and, 773
Renin-angiotensin-aldosterone system, 651f
Repetition, learning and, 223
Report forms, 83–85, 84f
Reporting unethical behavior, 32
Repression, 142t
Reproduction system deficits, elderly patients
    and, 751t, 755
Research, medication, 832–833
Residential care, 18
Residual urine, 717, 717f
Resistance phase and stress, 140
Resorption, 662
Respiration
    abnormal respiratory patterns, 362t
    adventitious sounds, 362
    assessment of, 360–362, 372–373, 428t
    Biot's respirations, 362t
    Cheyne-Stokes respirations, 362t
    depth of, 361
    dying process and, 200
    elderly patients and, 753
    expiration and, 360
    factors affecting, 361t
    initial assessment and, 429
    inspiration and, 360
    Kussmaul's respiration, 362t
    postoperative care and, 788
    rales or crackles, 362
    rate per minute and, 360–361
    regulation, 613
    related characteristics and, 362
    respiratory effort, 361, 615
    respiratory hygiene, 264t
    respiratory imbalances, 667
    respiratory medications, 839t, 860–861
    respiratory patterns, 361, 434t

rhonchi, 362
    stertorous breathing, 362
    stridor, 362
    wheezes, 362
Respirators, 273, 275
Respiratory acidosis, 667
Respiratory alkalosis, 667
Respiratory care
    breathing mechanics, 612–613
    chest tubes and, 625–627, 640–641
    chronic lung disease and, 613
    chronic obstructive pulmonary disease and,
        627–629, 629t–630t
    endotracheal airways and, 624
    endotracheal suctioning and, 624, 637–638
    impaired oxygenation and, 613–614
    incentive spirometry and, 632–633
    internal and external respiration, 613
    nasopharyngeal suctioning and, 635–637
    nebulizer treatment and, 633–634
    normal oxygenation and, 612–613
    nursing interventions and, 623–625
    oropharyngeal suctioning and, 635–637
    pharyngeal airways and, 623
    pneumonia and, 627–629, 629t–630t
    respiration regulation, 613
    sputum specimens and, 630–631
    suctioning with pharyngeal airways in place,
        623–624
    supplemental oxygen and, 634–635
    throat culture specimens and, 632
    tracheostomy and, 624–625, 625t, 637–640
Respiratory medications, 839t, 860–861
Respiratory system
    acid-base balance and, 666–667
    diseases, respiratory rate and, 361t
    elderly patients and, 750t
    immobility effects, 315–316
    presurgical review and, 773
Respite, family caregivers and, 190
Rest
    adequate, 244
    blood pressure readings and, 346
    infections and, 261
    pain management and, 399–402
    pulse rate and, 358t
    respiratory rate and, 361t
    rest and activity needs, 445
Restitution, 143t
Restless legs syndrome, 402t
Restorative sleep
    amount required, 400–401
    characteristics of, 399–400
    comfort and, 402
    environmental factors and, 401
    illness and health problems and, 401
    interventions and, 401–402
    lifestyle and, 401
    pain relief and, 402
    relaxation and, 402
    sleep cycle and, 400, 400t
    sleep medications and, 402
    stress and anxiety and, 401
Restraints
    alternatives and, 235–236
    application of, 238, 248–249
    avoiding use of, 237
    delegation and, 238
    flowsheet for, 239f
    guidelines regarding, 238
    least restrictive environment and, 238
    legal issues and, 36
    physician's order for, 238
    threatening patients with, 237
    types of, 239t–240t

Retractions, 434
Return flow enemas, 687
Reye's syndrome, 356
Rhonchi, 362, 436
Rhythm and pattern, respiration and, 361
RICE treatment for sprains, 592
Rickettsia rickettsi, 258
Rickettsial infections, 256
Right base heart sound, 438
Right shift, lymphocytes and, 545
Risk factors, for illness, 139, 140t
Role boundaries, 39
Role modeling, 123
Role reversals, 194
Room preparation, postoperative, 790
Rooting reflex, newborns, 172, 172f
Routinely scheduled care, 280

S

Safety. *See also* Nursing staff safety
    adolescents and, 179–180
    age and ability to understand and, 234
    bed/chair or leg monitors and, 247–248
    cardiopulmonary resuscitation and, 241
    communication abilities and, 235
    decision-making chart and, 244f
    delayed assistance and, 235
    disaster response and, 242
    fire extinguishers and, 241
    fire response and, 240–241
    Heimlich maneuver and, 241
    hospital equipment and, 235
    impaired mobility and, 235
    individual emergency response and, 241–242
    infants and toddlers and, 178
    interventions, postoperative, 792
    medication checks and, 845
    middle adults and, 183
    national patient safety goals, 234
    needs regarding, 445
    nursing staff and, 243–245
    older adults and, 183
    oxygen home use and, 241
    pain and discomfort and, 235
    preschoolers and school-age children and,
        178–179
    preventing falls and, 235–240
    unsafe environments and, 234–235
    young adults and, 181, 183
Safety needles, 925–926, 926f
Salem sump tube, 509
Saline lock, 916
Salivary amylase, 478
Salvage surgery, 771
Same-day surgery, 20
Sanguineous drainage, 570
Satiety, 483
Saturated fats, 481
Saw palmetto, 215
Scalp-vein needle, 922–923
Scheduled (controlled) drugs, 830
School-age children
    cognitive development and, 176
    health teaching and, 179
    moral and spiritual development and, 176
    nursing implications for, 179
    nutritional needs and, 491
    physical development and, 175
    playground safety and, 178–179
    psychosocial development and, 175–176
    regression and, 179
    safety concerns and, 178–179
    stranger danger and, 178
    water safety and, 179

School nurses, 184
Scientifically based illness beliefs, 132t
Scleral cover shell, 289
Scoliosis, 434
Scrub nurse, 461, 783
Seborrhea, 287
Secondary data, 52
Secondary hypertension, 349
Secondary infections, 260
Secondary medication tubing administration set, 923
Sedation, conscious, 784–785
Sedative and hypnotic medications, 839t
Sediment, urinary, 711
Seeking help phase of illness, 139
Self-care, 283
Self-esteem, 281
Self-pay, 25–26
Self-worth, immobility and, 319–320
Senior citizens. *See* Elderly patients
Sensory functioning, elderly patients and, 749t–750t, 753
Separation anxiety, admission process and, 409–410
Septicemia, 260, 815, 941
Sequential compression devices, 315, 778, 778f, 801
Seropurulent wound drainage, 570
Serosanguineous drainage, 570
Serous wound drainage, 570
Serum creatinine testing, 545
Severed cannulas, 941
Sexual behavior, 137
Sexual drive, elderly patients and, 755
Sexual harassment, 36–37
Shampooing hair, 288, 288f, 303–304
Shared meaning, 116
Shaving, 287, 301–302
Shearing, 317
Shiatsu, 213
Shift reports, 123–125, 124t–125t
Shivering, 350, 355
Short-term goals, 61
Showering, 284
Simple carbohydrates, 482
Simple face mask, oxygen delivery and, 621t
Single-lumen catheter, 720–721
Sit-to-stand lifts, 325, 325f
Sitz baths, 381, 381f, 386–387
Skeletal traction, 595
Skin
    bathing and, 281
    breakdown and, 317
    color, 441
    dying process and, 199
    impaired oxygenation and, 615
    infections and, 260
    integrity and, 411–422
    ostomy appliances and, 692
    punctures and, 816–817, 816f, 919f
    readings, body temperature and, 354
    traction, 595
Sleep. *See also* Restorative sleep
    pulse rate and, 358t
    requirements for, 400–401
    respiratory rate and, 361t
    sleep apnea, 402t
    sleep cycle, 400, 400t
    sleep disorders, 401, 402t
    sleep medications, 402
Sleepwalking, 402t
Slide boards, 324–325, 325f
Slide sheets, 324, 324f
Sliding scale, insulin injection and, 894, 894t
Slip-tip syringe, 881

Smoking, respiratory rate and, 361t
Smoking cessation, 136–137
SOAPIER charting, 96–98, 98f
Soapsuds enemas, 686
Sodium, 655–660, 655t
    deficiency and excess of, 657–658, 658t
    functions and sources of, 484t
    levels of, 546
    sodium-restricted diets, 503–504
    treatment and nursing care and, 658–660
Soft spots, infant, 173
Soft tissue pain, 394
Solar lentigines (liver spots), 441
Somnambulism, 402t
Sordes, 432
Source-oriented records, 93–95, 94t–95t
Soy, 215
Special communication needs
    aphasia, 128
    deaf or hard of hearing patients, 127–128
    patients on mechanical ventilation, 129
    speech and language impairments, 128
    unresponsive patients, 129–130
Special mouth care, 286
Special situation documentation, 862–863
Specialized health insurance plans, 25–26
Specialized mattresses, 318t
Specialty beds, 318t–319t
Specific gravity, 711
Speech assessment, 433
Speech impaired patients, 128
Speed shock, intravenous therapy and, 942–943
Sphincter control, toddlers, 174, 174f
Sphygmomanometer, 346–347, 347f
Spinal anesthesia, 785
Spinal cord protection, 649
Spirilla, 256
Spiritual care, 143–144
Spiritual development
    adolescents and, 177
    middle adults and, 181
    older adults and, 182
    preschoolers and, 175
    school-age child and, 176
    toddlers and, 174
    young adults and, 181
Spiritual distress, 144–145
Spirometry, 316, 316f, 776–777
Splints, 593t
SpO$_2$ levels, 429
Sprains, 592
Sputum specimens, 615–616, 630–631
St. John's wort, 215, 832
Stage I pressure ulcers, 560
Stage II pressure ulcers, 560–561, 575–576, 577t–578t
Stage III pressure ulcers, 561
Stage IV pressure ulcers, 561
Stand-alone surgery center, 771
Standardized care plans, 64
Standards of care, 39
Staphylococci, 256
Staphylococcus aureus, 258
Staples, removing, 578–579
Start kits, intravenous, 927–928, 927f
Startle reflex, newborns, 172, 172f
Stasis ulcers, 563
Stat nursing, wound care and, 568–569
Statutory laws, 34–36
Steatorrhea, 677–678
Sterile dressings, 582–585
Sterile liquids, pouring, 461–462
Sterile packs, opening, 457f, 458–460, 459f

Sterile technique
    adding items to sterile field, 459
    circulating nurse and, 461
    circumstances requiring, 460
    donning sterile gloves–closed method, 467–469
    donning sterile gloves–open method, 463–466
    donning sterile gown, 467–469
    entering operating room and, 460
    handling needles, syringes, and lancets, 461, 461f
    home setting and, 461
    long-term care setting and, 461
    nursing judgments and, 460
    opening sterile packs, 458–462
    opening sterile supplies, 458
    pouring sterile liquids, 461–462
    scrub nurse and, 461
    setting up sterile field, 458–459, 461–462
    surgical hand scrub, 466–467
    technique principles, 457–458
    working with a sterile field, 460
Sterilization
    delegation and, 458
    indications of, 456–457, 457f
    patient care activities and, 457
    patient's bedside and, 457
    sterile conscience, 458
    sterile settings, 457
    types of, 456
Sternotomy, 285
Steroids, 837t
Stertorous breathing, 362
Stethoscopes, 347–348, 348f, 437
Stirrups, 323t
Stoma, 689, 691f
Stools
    foul smelling, 427
    occult blood testing and, 688
    specimens, 688, 700
Straight catheters, 720–721, 737–738
Stranger danger, preschoolers and school-age children, 179
Step throat, 616
Streptococcus group A, 258
Streptococcus group B, 258
Stress
    adaptation and, 139–144
    alarm phase and, 140
    blood pressure readings and, 346
    body temperature and, 352
    bowel elimination and, 680
    coping mechanisms and, 140–141
    coping strategies and, 141
    defense mechanisms and, 141, 142t–143t
    exhaustion phase and, 140
    fight-or-flight response and, 140
    general adaptation syndrome and, 140
    homeostasis and, 141
    illness and, 141
    infections and, 261
    patient teaching and, 144
    pulse rate and, 358t
    recognizing symptoms of, 141
    resistance phase and, 140
    respiratory rate and, 361t
    restorative sleep and, 401
    stress incontinence, 718
    symptoms of, 144
Stretchers, safety tips for, 326
Stridor, 362, 436–437
Stroke
    blood clots and, 314
    blood pressure and, 345
    stroke volume, 356

Structural changes, bowel elimination and, 680
Student care plans, 70–76, 71f–73f
Subcutaneous injections
    administering, 892
    heparin and, 893t, 896
    insulin and, 893–896, 893t
    maximum volume and, 892–893
    sites of, 892, 892f
Subjective data, obtaining, 51
Sublimation, 143t
Sublingual route, medication, 852
Substance abuse, 137
Substance P, 393
Sucking reflex, newborns, 172, 172f
Suction catheter, 623–624
Suctioning with pharyngeal airway in place,
    623–624
Sundowning, 402t
Supplemental oxygen, 618–619, 634–635
Supplements, increased bleeding and, 898
Support surfaces, 318t–319t
Suprapubic catheter, 720, 721f
Surgery. See also Anesthesia; Postoperative care;
    Postsurgical complications; Preoperative care;
    Sterile technique; Sterilization
    anesthesia provider and, 781–783
    antiembolism hose and, 778, 778f, 799–800
    bowel elimination and, 679–680
    circulating nurse and, 783
    degrees of urgency and, 770–771
    final intraoperative interventions and, 788
    first surgical assistant and, 783
    hand scrubbing and, 460–461, 466–467, 787
    holding area and, 781, 783f
    incentive spirometry and, 776–777
    informed consent and, 779–781, 780f, 781f
    inpatient surgery, 771
    intraoperative interventions and, 786–788
    intubation and, 786, 786f
    leg exercises and, 777
    lower extremity circulation stimulation and,
        777
    needle, sponge, and instrument counts,
        787–788
    outpatient surgery, 771
    patient draping and, 787
    patient positioning and, 787
    physical examination and, 774
    postoperative pain and discomfort control,
        778–779
    presurgical assessment, 772–774
    purposes of, 770
    scrub nurse and, 783
    sequential compression devices and, 778,
        778f, 801
    standard preoperative laboratory tests, 774
    suite preparation and, 784
    surgical bed, 292
    surgical incisions, 563, 564f, 565
    surgical procedure and, 787
    surgical scrub and, 787
    surgical shave and, 787
    surgical suite preparation, 784
    surgical team members, 781–783
    systems review and, 772–774
    tissue specimens and, 787
    turn, cough, and deep breathing exercises and,
        776
Sustained-release tablets, 853
Suture/staple care, 570
Sutures, removing, 578–579
Swallowing, impaired, 524t–525t
Swedish massage therapy, 213
Symptomatic phase of illness, 139
Syncope (fainting), 350, 806

Synergy Air Elite mattress, 318t
Syringes, 881–883, 881f
    barrel of, 881
    handling of, 461, 461f, 884–886
    insulin syringe, 882, 883f
    Luer-Lok tip, 881
    parts of, 881, 882f
    plunger of, 881
    prefilled syringes, 882–883, 883f
    regular syringe, 881–882
    slip-tip, 881
    tips of, 881
    tuberculin syringe, 882, 883f
Systemic infections, 260
Systolic pressure, 346
Systolic sound, heart, 439

T
T-piece, 623t
Tablets, medication, 852–853
Tachycardia, 358
Tachypnea, 360, 434t
Tactile distraction, 397
Taenia infection, 259
Tap water enemas, 686
Teaching plans, 224–226. See also Patient teaching
    assessment and, 225
    evaluation and, 226
    implementation and, 225–226
    nursing diagnosis and, 225
    planning and, 225
Team nursing, 22–23
Teenage pregnancy, 491
Teeth assessment, 432–433
Telemetry monitoring, 550–551
Telephone physician orders, 122, 123f
Temper tantrums, 174
Temperature. See Body temperature
Temporal artery temperature, 355
Temporal pulse, 357, 370
Tension pneumothorax, 616
Tepid baths, 384
Terminal cleaning, 417
Tetany, 661
Texas catheter, 720
Therapeutic baths, 284
Therapeutic communications, 119–120, 424
Therapeutic diets, 502–504
Therapeutic touch, 216
Therapy staff, 17t
Thermogenesis, 350
Thermometers, 352–353, 352f
Thermoregulation, 351–352
Third-spacing of fluids, 649
Thready pulse, 359
Three-way catheters, 720–722
Throat culture specimens, 616, 632
Thromboembolic disorder, 778
Thrombophlebitis, 940
Thrombosis, 548
Thrombus, 777, 928
Thyroid replacement hormones, 837t
Tidal volume, respiration and, 361
Time of day, body temperature and, 352
Timed urinary collection, 713
Tinea capitis, 287
Tissue anatomy, 890
Tissue fluid, 649
Tissue specimens, surgery and, 787
Tobacco use, 136–137
Toddlers
    cognitive development and, 174
    health concerns for, 177–178
    health teaching and, 178

    injections and, 901
    moral and spiritual development and, 174
    nursing implications for, 178
    nutritional needs and, 490–491
    physical development and, 173–174
    preventing choking and, 178
    preventing drowning and, 178
    preventing falls and, 178
    psychosocial development and, 174
    safety concerns and, 178
Tolerable upper intake level (UL), 476
Topical medications, 857–858, 868
Tort law, 36
Total bilirubin levels, 545–546
Total care, 283
Total hip replacement, 595–596, 597f
Total knee replacement, 597–598, 600–602,
    602t–604t
Total parenteral nutrition, 519–520, 519f
Total protein levels, 545–546
Total serum calcium level, 662
TotalCare SpO2RT bed, 319t
Tourniquets, 808, 813–814, 818
Towel baths, 284–285, 285f
Toxicity, drug, 831
Trace mineral imbalances, 487
Tracheostomy, 624–625, 625t, 639–640
Tracheostomy collar, 623t
Tracheostomy suctioning, 637–638
Traction, 59f, 593t, 595
Trans fats, 481
Transcultural nursing. See Culture and ethnicity
Transcutaneous electrical nerve stimulation
    (TENS), 396, 396f, 403
Transdermal medications, 858, 868
Transfer. See Patient transfer
Transfusions
    hemolysis and, 943
    nursing care during, 945
    nursing care preparation, 944–945
    post-transfusion care, 945
    preparing, initiating, and monitoring, 961–962
    preparing blood product and, 945
    reactions to, 943, 944t
    safety measures and, 945
    supplies and, 944
Transient ischemic attacks, 748
Transmission-based precautions, 265–266
Transparent dressings, 585–586, 936f
Transurethral resection of the prostate (TURP), 721
Trapeze bar, 323
Triple-lumen catheter, 720–722
Triple-lumen central venous catheter injection
    ports, 519, 519f
Trochanter roll, 314, 323, 323t
Tropical sprue, 487
Trousseau's sign, 663f
Trust establishment, 126
Tub bath, 284
Tube feeding complications, 517–518
Tube feeding formulas, 513–514, 518
Tuberculin skin testing, 617t, 892
Tuberculin syringe, 882, 883f
Tubes with color-coded tops, 812–813, 813t
Tubing, intravenous. See Intravenous tubing
Turgor, skin, 411
Turn, cough, and deep breathing exercises, 776
Turning, patient, 316, 324, 333–335
Twilight sleep, 784–785
Tympanic thermometers, 354

U
Ulcerations, 432
Ultrasonography, 548

Unconscious patient, 129, 286, 298–299
Unethical behavior, reporting, 32
Uninsured patients, 138
Unoccupied beds, 292
Unprofessional conduct, 10
Unresponsive patients, 129–130
Unstageable pressure ulcers, 561
Unusual occurrence reports, 42, 43f–44f
Upper extremity assessment, 442–443
Upward communication, 121–122
Urea, 710
Urge incontinence, 718
Urgent surgery, 770–771
Uric acid, 710
Urinals, 712, 712f, 731
Urinalysis, 546–547, 713, 714t–715t, 774
Urinary catheters
    bladder irrigation and, 739
    catheter care, 725
    catheter size, 722
    condom catheter, 720, 722, 740
    continuous bladder irrigation and, 721–722, 722f
    Coudé catheter, 720
    discontinuing catheters, 725
    draining urine from bladder, 724
    home health care and, 726
    indwelling catheters, 719–721, 721f, 742
    insertion of, 722–724, 723f, 733–738
    intermittent catheter irrigation, 724
    long-term care and, 726
    obtaining urine specimen and, 736–737
    pediatric considerations and, 726
    straight catheters, 720–721, 737–738
    suprapubic catheters, 720, 721f
    three-way catheters, 720–722
    troubleshooting low output, 724
    types of, 719–722
Urinary complications, immobility and, 317
Urinary diversions, 725, 725f
Urinary drainage system irrigation, 741
Urinary elimination. *See also* Altered urinary
    function; Bladder function
    altered urinary function, 719–726
    anatomy and physiology and, 711–712
    anuria and, 711
    assistance with, 712, 712f
    bedpans and, 731–732
    clean-catch midstream urine specimens,
        732–733
    color and clarity and, 710–711
    intake and output measurement, 715–717
    irrigating closed urinary drainage system, 741
    normal voiding patterns, 712
    odor and, 711
    oliguria and, 711
    pH and, 711
    physical assessment and, 713
    polyuria and, 711
    reagent testing and, 713–715, 716f
    specific gravity and, 711
    specimen collection and, 713–715
    straining urine and, 715, 716f
    timed urinary collection and, 713
    urinals and, 731
    urinalysis and, 713, 714t–715t
    urine characteristics and, 710–712
Urinary incontinence, 718–719
Urinary retention, 717, 794
Urinary sepsis, 712
Urinary tract infections, 711, 723, 725–730,
    729t–730t
Urine dipsticks, 716, 716f
Urine strainers, 715, 716f
Urine testing, 713–715
USDA food guide, 477, 478t

V
Vacutainer tube guide, 811f
Vagal response, enemas and, 687
Vaginal medications, 859–860, 871–872
Valerian, 215
Validation, information, 48
Valuables, gathering for discharge, 417
Values, 31
Variance reports, 42
Vasoconstriction, 352
Vasodilation, 285, 351, 378, 378f, 835t
Vastus lateralis injection site, 900, 900f
Vectors, 256
Vein dilation tips, 933
Venipuncture. *See also* Peripheral venipuncture;
    Phlebotomy
    equipment, 809–814
    finding vein and, 808
    finding vein with eyes closed, 808
    locating and assessing difficult veins, 808–809
    performing, 814–815, 819–820
    site selection, 807–809, 807f
    sites to avoid, 807–808
    vein selection and, 932–933, 932f
Venography, 548
Venous access devices (VADs), 915
Venous return, 281
Venous stasis, 314
Venous thrombosis, 314
Ventilation, 360
Ventrogluteal injection site, 898–900, 899f
Venturi masks, 622t
Verbal communication, 116–117
Verbal orders, 122–123
Verbal response, 430t
Vesicant medications, 939
Vessel lumen, 378
Vest restraint, 239t
Vials, withdrawing medications from, 887–888.
    See also Injections
Violence, 137
Viruses, 257
Visceral pain, 394
Visual distraction, 397
Visual learning, 222
Vital signs
    assessment of, 762
    blood pressure, 345–350
    body temperature, 350–356
    delegation and, 344–345
    designated times and, 345
    dying process and, 199
    initial assessment and, 429
    oxygen saturation, 362
    pain assessment, 363–364
    postoperative, 792
    pulse, 356–360
    respiration, 360–362
Vitamins
    deficiencies and, 487, 488t–489t
    medication interactions and, 832
    nutrition and, 483–484
    vitamin C megadosing, 487
Vomiting, postoperative, 794

W
Waist restraints, 240t
Walkers, 599–600, 599f
Warfarin (Coumadin), 507, 855–856
Warm soaks, 381
Water
    brain and spinal cord protection and, 649
    electrolyte, minerals, vitamin, and waste
        transport, 649

functions of, 649–650
intake of, 650
joint and digestive tract lubrication and, 650
maintaining temperature and, 649
movement from gastrointestinal tract,
    648–649
total body weight and, 646
water balance, 480
Water safety, preschoolers and school-age
    children, 179
Weekly assessment data, long-term care and,
    103–104
Weight and height measurement, 424–425, 448
Weight gain, 485–487
Wellness. *See* Health and wellness
Wellness-illness continuum, 134–135, 134f
Wellness strategies, patient teaching and, 223
West Nile virus, 259
Western medicine, 211
Wet-to-damp dressings, 572, 582–585
Wet-to-dry dressings, 572
Wheezing, 362, 436
Whirlpool baths, 381–382
White blood cell (WBC) counts, 541, 544, 774
WHO Guidelines for Hand Hygiene in Health
    Care, 263
Whole blood, 943
Wilson's disease, 487
Winged butterfly, 922–923
Withheld medications, documentation and, 864
Wong-Baker FACES Pain Rating Scale, 393,
    393f
Wound care
    applying hydrocolloid dressings, 585–586
    applying transparent dressings, 585–586
    changing sterile dressings, 582–585
    changing wet-to-damp dressings, 582–585
    cleaning wounds, 571–572
    closure and, 564, 565f, 569–570
    complications and, 565–569
    documentation of, 574
    drainage device care and, 579–580
    drainage observation and, 571
    draining sinus tracts, 563
    drains and drainage, 570–571
    dressings and, 572–574
    elderly patients and, 574
    evisceration, 568–569
    factors affecting, 566t–567t
    healing process and, 563–564
    hemorrhage and, 569
    home health care and, 574
    infection and, 567–568
    inflammatory process and, 564–565
    inflammatory stage, 563–564
    irrigating a wound, 580–581
    maturation phase, 564
    obtaining wound cultures, 572, 582
    patient teaching and, 568
    pressure ulcers, 559–563
    reconstruction phase, 564
    removing sutures and staples, 578–579
    stasis ulcers, 563
    surgical incisions, 563, 564f, 565
    suture/staple care, 570
    unlicensed assistive personnel and, 574
    wound contamination, 558–559
    wound dehiscence, 568–569
    wound measurement, 571
    wound types, 558, 559f
Wound dressings
    abdominal binders and, 573
    hydrocolloid dressings, 585–586
    Montgomery straps and, 573, 574f
    nursing responsibilities and, 574

Wound dressings *(continued)*
  securing, 572–573
  sterile dressings, 582–585
  tape dressings, 574
  transparent dressings, 585–586
  types and purposes of, 573t
  wet-to-damp dressings, 572, 582–585
  wet-to-dry dressings, 572
Wound infection, postoperative, 794
Wound tension, 567t
Writing physician's orders, 122–123
Written communication, 125–126

Y
Yankauer suction catheter, 624, 624f
Yoga, 214–215
Young adults
  cognitive development and, 181
  emotional intimacy and, 180
  health teaching and, 183
  moral and spiritual development and, 181
  nursing implications and, 183

physical development and, 180
psychosocial development and, 180
safety concerns and, 183

Z
Z-track injections, 897–898, 898f, 907–908
Zinc, 485t